Anaesthetic physiology and pharmacology

Edited by

William McCaughey MD, FRCA, FFARCSI
Consultant Anaesthetist, Craigavon Area Hospital, Co. Armagh; Lecturer, Department of Anaesthetics,
The Queen's University of Belfast, Belfast, Northern Ireland

Richard S. J. Clarke BSc, MD, PhD, FRCA, FFARCSI
Emeritus Professor of Anaesthetics, The Queen's University of Belfast,
Belfast, Northern Ireland

J. P. Howard Fee MD, PhD, FFARCS
Professor of Anaesthetics, The Queen's University of Belfast, Belfast; Consultant Anaesthetist,
Royal Victoria Hospital and Musgrave Park Hospital, Belfast, Northern Ireland

William F. M. Wallace BSc, MD, FRCP, FRCA
Professor of Applied Physiology, Department of Physiology, The Queen's University of Belfast,
Belfast; Consultant Physiologist, Belfast City Hospital, Belfast, Northern Ireland

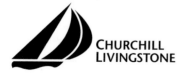

CHURCHILL
LIVINGSTONE

NEW YORK EDINBURGH HONG KONG MADRID MELBOURNE SAN FRANCISCO TOKYO 1997

CHURCHILL LIVINGSTONE
Medical Division of Pearson Professional Limited

Distributed in the United States of America by Churchill
Livingstone Inc., 650 Avenue of the Americas, New York,
N.Y. 10011, and by associated companies, branches and
representatives throughout the world.

First published 1997

ISBN 0-443-05203-4

British Library Cataloguing in Publication Data
A catalogue record for this book is available from the British
Library.

Library of Congress Cataloging in Publication Data
A catalog record for this book is available from the Library
of Congress.

Medical knowledge is constantly changing. As new
information becomes available, changes in treatment,
procedures, equipment and the use of drugs become
necessary. The editors/authors/contributors and the
publishers have, as far as possible, taken care to ensure that
the information given in this text is accurate and up to date.
However, readers are strongly advised to confirm that the
information, especially with regard to drug usage, complies
with latest legislation and standards of practice.

The
publisher's
policy is to use
**paper manufactured
from sustainable forests**

Produced by Longman Asia Ltd, Hong Kong
SP/01

Contributors

J. P. Alexander FRCPI, FFARCS
Consultant Anaesthetist, Belfast City Hospital,
Belfast, Northern Ireland

J. D. Allen MD
Reader, Department of Physiology, The
Queen's University of Belfast, Belfast,
Northern Ireland

A. B. Atkinson MD
Regional Centre for Endocrinology and Diabetes,
Royal Victoria Hospital, Belfast, Northern
Ireland

J. G. Bovill MD PhD, FFARCSI
Professor of Anaesthesia, Department of
Anaesthesiology, University Hospital PO Box
9600, 2300 RC Leiden, The Netherlands

R. S. J. Clarke BSc, MD, PhD, FRCA, FFARCSI
Emeritus Professor of Anaesthetics, The
Queen's University of Belfast, Belfast,
Northern Ireland

Valerie M. Cox PhD
Research School of Medicine, University of
Leeds, Leeds, England

H. J. L. Craig MD, FRCA, FFARCSI
Consultant Anaethetist, Royal Victoria
Hospital, Belfast, Northern Ireland,

N. Damani MSc, MB BS, MRCPath
Consultant Microbiologist, Craigavon Area
Hospital, Co Armagh, Northern Ireland

C. D. Doherty MD, FRCP, FRCPI
Consultant Nephrologist, Regional Nephrology
Unit, Belfast City Hospital, Belfast, Northern
Ireland

R. Dwyer MD, FFARCSI
Consultant Anaesthetist, Beaumont Hospital,
Dublin, Ireland

J. P. H. Fee MD, PhD, FFARCS
Professor of Anaesthetics, The Queen's
University of Belfast, Belfast; Consultant
Anaesthetist, Royal Victoria Hospital and
Musgrave Park Hospital, Belfast, Northern
Ireland

Tess M. Gallagher MD, FFARCSI, MRCPI
Consultant Anaesthetist, Royal Belfast Hospital
for Sick Children, Belfast, Northern Ireland

D. F. Goldspink PhD, DSc
Professor of Cell Biology, Research School of
Medicine, University of Leeds, Leeds, England

R. Hainsworth MD, PhD, DSc
Professor of Applied Physiology, Academic
Unit of Cardiovascular Studies, University of
Leeds, Leeds, England

J. P. Howe MD, FFARCSI
Consultant Anaesthetist, Belfast City Hospital,
Belfast, Nothern Ireland

J. P. Jamison BSc, MD, MRCPI
Consultant in General Medicine, Department
of Physiology, The Queen's University of
Belfast, Belfast, Northern Ireland

J. R. Johnston MD, FFARCSI
Consultant in Intensive Care Medicine,
Regional Intensive Care Unit, Royal Victoria
Hospital, Belfast, Northern Ireland

J. G. Kelly PhD
Chief Executive, Irish Board of Medicines,
Earlsfort Centre, Dublin, Ireland

G. G. Lavery MD, FFARCSI
Consultant in Anaesthesia and Intensive Care
Medicine, Robert C. Gray Regional Intensive
Care Unit, Regional Intensive Care, Royal
Hospitals Trust, Belfast, Northern Ireland

W. B. Loan MD, FFARCSI
Consultant Anaesthetist, Belfast City Hospital,
Belfast, Northern Ireland

K. G. Lowry MMedSc, FFARCSI
Consultant in Anaesthesia and Intensive Care
Medicine, Regional Intensive Care Unit, Royal
Victoria Hospital, Belfast, Northern Ireland

C. McAllister MB, MRCPI, FFARCSI
Consultant Anaesthetist, Craigavon Area
Hospital, Co. Armagh, Northern Ireland

Dympna McAuley MD, FFARCSI
Consultant Anaesthetist, Ulster Hospital,
Dundonald, Belfast, Northern Ireland

S. J. McBride BSc, MRCP
Registrar in Chemical Pathology, Royal
Victoria Hospital, Belfast, Northern Ireland

W. T. McBride BSc, MD, FRCA, FFARCSI
Consultant Anaesthetist, Department of
Anaesthetics, Royal Victoria Hospital, Belfast,
Northern Ireland

G. McCarthy MD, FRCA
Consultant Anaesthetist, Belfast City Hospital,
Belfast, Northern Ireland

W. McCaughey MD, FRCA, FFARCSI
Consultant Anaesthetist, Craigavon Area
Hospital, Co. Armagh; Lecturer, Department of
Anaesthetics, The Queen's University of
Belfast, Belfast, Northern Ireland

N. McClure MD, MRCOG
Senior Lecturer, Department of Obstetrics and
Gynaecology, The Queen's University of
Belfast; Consultant Obstetrician and
Gynaecologist, The Royal Maternity Hospital,
Belfast, Northern Ireland

J. G. McGeown BSc, MB, PhD
Senior Lecturer in Physiology, Department of
Physiology, Medical Biology Building,
Belfast, Northern Ireland

A. C. McKay MD, FFARCSI
Consultant Anaesthetist, Belfast City Hospital,
Belfast, Northern Ireland

C. McLoughlin MD, FFARCSI
Consultant Anaesthetist, Belfast City Hospital,
Belfast, Northern Ireland

T. J. McMurray MD, FRCA, FFARCSI
Consultant Anaesthetist, Royal Victoria
Hospital, Belfast, Northern Ireland

P. McNamee MD
Consultant Nephrologist, Department of
Nephrology, Belfast City Hospital, Belfast,
Northern Ireland

R. K. Mirakhur MD PhD, FRCA, FFARCSI
Senior Lecturer in Anaesthetics, Department of
Anaesthetics, The Queen's University of
Belfast, Belfast; Consultant Anaesthetist,
Royal Victoria and Belfast City Hospital Trusts,
Belfast, Northern Ireland

J. M. Murray MD, FFARCSI
Consultant Anaesthetist, Ulster Hospital,
Dundonald, Belfast, Northern Ireland

S. D. Nelson BA, MB, FRCPI, FRCPath
Consultant Haematologist, Craigavon Area
Hospital, Portadown, Co. Armagh, Northern
Ireland

C. C. Patterson BSc, MSc, PhD
Senior Lecturer in Medical Statistics, The
Queen's University of Belfast, Belfast,
Northern Ireland

D. L. Paxton MD, FFARCS
Consultant Anaesthetist, Craigavon Area
Hospital, Portadown, Co. Armagh, Northern
Ireland

Barbara J. Pleuvry BPharm, MSc, PhD, MRPS
Senior Lecturer in Anaesthetics and
Pharmacology, Department of Physiological
Sciences, University of Manchester,
Manchester, UK

I. C. Roddie MD, FRCPI
Emeritus Professor of Physiology, The Queen's
University of Belfast, Belfast, Northern Ireland

W. Thompson BSc, MD, FRCOG
Department of Obstetrics and Gynaecology,
The Queen's University of Belfast, Belfast,
Northern Ireland

W. F. M. Wallace BSc, MD, FRCP, FRCA
Professor of Applied Physiology, Department
of Physiology, The Queen's University of
Belfast, Belfast; Consultant Physiologist, Belfast
City Hospital, Belfast, Northern Ireland

Contents

Preface

The practice of anaesthesia has been described as consisting essentially of applied physiology and applied pharmacology. Our aim is to present concisely concepts and knowledge derived from these disciplines as a basis for anaesthetic practice and postgraduate anaesthetic examinations.

This book is a logical development of the earlier publication *Clinical Anaesthetic Pharmacology*, which covered mainly the pharmacological basis of anaesthetic practice. We have here sought to integrate physiology, pharmacology and anaesthesia and have provided a more detailed physiological and theoretical background to the actions of drugs than is available in other comparable books. We hope that this integrated approach will appeal to the reader and that it will result in a more thorough understanding of the subject.

As a consequence, there is more emphasis on those aspects of human physiology which are of relevance in the ill or critically ill throughout the perioperative period. The nervous, cardiovascular and respiratory systems receive particular attention, and we have aimed to balance the needs of both the practising anaesthetist and the examination candidate. Particular emphasis is given to the pattern of responses to the stresses of disease, trauma and surgery, and of the underlying mechanisms. In addition, because increasing numbers of patients are being treated at an advanced age, the effects of ageing are highlighted.

Rational use of drugs likewise requires knowledge of the principles underlying their actions. Drugs have long been used empirically, the rationale for their use being observation of the results of their administration. A major advance occurring mainly in the past two decades has

been the application of pharmacokinetic principles; especially important in anaesthesia where the time-course of the onset and termination of effect of drugs must be so closely controlled. Although pharmacokinetic data may be scarce for some older drugs, continuing research and improved detection methods mean that the kinetics of most newly introduced drugs are well studied. An emphasis is placed throughout the book on the pharmacokinetics of the drugs described.

Less complete in many cases is knowledge of the mechanisms underlying the actions of drugs — general anaesthesia itself is a case in point. Recent developments in molecular biology affect all branches of medicine, and in pharmacology they are in particular leading to greater understanding of the mode of action of drugs at cellular level. This is at the expense of increased complexity, as receptor subtypes multiply, and any textbook account must be a simplification to be understandable, while giving as up-to-date an account as possible. Again, in the field of intensive care, improvements in understanding mediators of the response to infection offer the possibility of better treatment, and this is reflected in the relevant chapters.

Finally it is our intention that this book, while primarily providing the theoretical background to anaesthetic practice, will also have a role as a practical guide. Thus, the physiological sections address a number of clinical problems; such as nutrition of the critically ill, and perioperative management of diabetes mellitus and other endocrine disorders, and sections on individual drugs include details of their clinical use. We hope that this work, having evolved from a textbook of pharmacology with a significant physiological background into the present integrated *Anaesthetic Physiology and Pharmacology*, will make it easier for the reader to understand the logical background to their everyday practice in the operating theatre, ward and intensive therapy unit.

Sadly the senior editor of *Clinical Anaesthetic Pharmacology*, John Wharry Dundee, died shortly after publication and we pay tribute to his widespread and benevolent influence in the field of Anaesthesia over many decades.

W. McCaughey
R. S. J. Clarke
J. P. H. Fee
W. F.M. Wallace

Belfast
1997

Basics

SECTION CONTENTS

1

Chemistry related to anaesthetic practice

J. G. Kelly

The importance of a knowledge of chemical principles in anaesthetics is not difficult to justify. The nature of anaesthetic agents (both physical and chemical), their stability and compatibility with other agents and with equipment, their modes of action, various structure/activity relationships and the existence of isomeric forms provide clear but not exhaustive examples. In addition, knowledge of various aspects of physical chemistry related, for example, to volatile agents, to diffusion and equilibria and to electrolyte physiology is clearly important.

It is the intention of this chapter to remind the reader of basic aspects of chemical structure and properties related to drugs used in anaesthetics and to highlight relevant aspects of physical chemistry.

With the exception of nitrous oxide, all clinically used anaesthetic agents are organic in nature. Most drugs used as anaesthetics or in combination with anaesthetic agents are synthetic. Some older drugs of relatively complex structure are derived from plant materials, for example morphine and atropine. These complex, nitrogen-containing bases (alkaloids) have no commercially realistic synthesis. Sometimes a substance devised from a plant may be modified chemically (semisynthetic), for example the acetylation of morphine to produce diamorphine (heroin).

Chemical structures of anaesthetic agents range from the simplest types of organic molecules to compounds of considerable complexity, and physically they range from gases and volatile

1

liquids to compounds of fairly high melting point.

CHEMICAL BONDING

There are two major types of chemical bonds, ionic and covalent. Ionic bonding takes place between ionised atoms or groups of atoms. These ions carry an electrical charge. If the charge is positive then the ion is a cation; if negative, the ion is an anion. An ionic bond is formed by the transfer of one or more electrons from one atom to the other and is due to the electrostatic attraction between the oppositely charged ions. This type of bond is found in inorganic compounds such as sodium chloride or other metal salts. When an ionic compound dissolves in water the ions separate (dissociate) owing to the interaction between the ions and water. Covalent bonds are the typical bonds in organic molecules. These are formed by the sharing of a pair of electrons between two atoms. They differ from ionic bonds in that they do not significantly dissociate in water. Electrons will not necessarily be shared equally between the bonding atoms however, and the share will depend on the electronegativities of these atoms. Electronegativity is a measure of the attraction of the nucleus of an atom for its bonding electrons; for example, oxygen and nitrogen are more electronegative than carbon and hydrogen. This means that in such molecules there will be a relative displacement of negative charge towards the more electronegative element, with formation of a *dipole*. For the same reason, water is a polar molecule and will tend to dissolve organic molecules with a polar character. In organic molecules containing hydrogen bonded to a more electronegative atom, the hydrogen ion of that group can also be attracted to an electronegative atom in another molecule. This hydrogen bonding is responsible for the interactive forces between molecules and explains the higher boiling points in polar, hydrogen bonded molecules, such as ethanol, compared with, for example, ether.

Hydrogen bonding has important biological functions. The shape of proteins is due to hydrogen bonding. In DNA, specific hydrogen bonding between complementary base pairs gives rise to the double-helix configuration. Such interactions are responsible for drug–receptor interactions.

STRUCTURAL ORGANIC CHEMISTRY
Saturated hydrocarbons

These are compounds which contain only carbon and hydrogen. In their most straightforward form they are structures in which the four possible bonds formed by a carbon atom are taken either by one of the bonds of another carbon atom or by the single bond of a hydrogen atom. The simplest structure is of course CH_4, methane. The formula of alkanes is C_nH_{2n+2} and it can readily be seen that the result is a homologous series in which each member differs from the last by the addition of CH_2. The structural possibilities will clearly also become much more varied as the number of carbon atoms increases. Ethane, CH_3CH_3, the second member of the series, and propane, $CH_3CH_2CH_3$, the third member, are also clearly defined. The next member, with four carbon atoms, can also be a linear chain (*n*-butane) or a 3-member (propyl) chain with the central carbon having a methyl substituent $CH_3CH(CH_3)CH_3$, 2-methyl propane. It can readily be appreciated then that the complexity and the number of isomeric forms of alkanes, and indeed of any carbon–carbon structure, will rise considerably with increasing numbers of carbon atoms. Cyclic hydrocarbons beginning with cyclopropane, C_3H_6, also form a homologous series, with the general formula C_nH_{2n}, and can also form fused multiring structures. The muscle relaxants pancuronium and vecuronium are good examples of the latter in which the structural core is formed of three 6-membered (cyclohexyl) rings and one 5-membered (cyclopentyl) ring fused to give a steroid structure. The saturated hydrocarbons tend to be quite stable structures. The distribution of electrons between the carbon atoms of C–C bonds is equal and the distribution between the elements of the C–H bond is relatively equal, so that both of these bonds are considered non-polar. As a result there are relatively small inter-molecular attractive forces and, correspondingly, their melting and boiling points are lower than for polar compounds for which an unequal share of electrons between two dissimilar atoms results in greater intermolecular interaction. For that reason also, alkanes are not soluble in water. Chemically they are relatively inert but are rapidly oxidised when ignited in air. Thus cyclo-propane is readily combustible. So far, saturated hydrocarbons have been considered in which carbon atoms have the maximum four substi-tuents; however, carbon can form double and even triple bonds. Where these are formed with other carbon atoms, they form the class of unsaturated hydrocarbons.

Unsaturated hydrocarbons

Hydrocarbons containing a carbon-carbon double bond, C=C, are alkenes and those with a carbon-carbon triple bond, C≡C, are alkynes. Of these, alkenes are by far the most important in the present context. A hydrocarbon may have two, three or many double bonds (dienes, trienes, polyenes) and of course can also form cyclic structures — for example, cyclohexene, which is cyclohexane with one C=C double bond. The nomenclature can become complicated in the case of branched structures but follows the general scheme for alkanes with an indication of the posi-tion of the double or triple bond and replacement of the -*ane* suffix by -*ene* or -*yne* as appropriate. These structures are chemically more reactive than alkanes and characteristically agents add to the double bonds (addition reactions) to produce saturated derivatives. Alkenes, however, are not particularly polar and will not dissolve in water; lower members are gases and they progress to solids as the molecules grow. Alkenes form the basis for the manufacture of some synthetic polymers.

Aromatic hydrocarbons

An important special case arises when the 6-membered cyclohexane ring contains three C=C double bonds. The resulting structure, benzene

(C_6H_6), does not have the expected features of alkenes but forms a structure in which the carbon–carbon bonds are not true single or double bonds, but electron sharing among all of the carbon atoms produces features of six identical hybrid bonds. The result is a molecule more stable than the corresponding theoretical cyclo-hexatriene and this is the foundation of aromatic chemistry. The so-called 'resonance' or 'hybrid' structure of benzene means that it does not undergo the addition reactions described above for conventional unsaturated bonds but under-goes reactions involving substitution of a hydrogen atom component of the benzene ring. Substituted benzene molecules are named by the position of the substituents, with occasional use of an older convention for disubstituted benzenes. Here the name of the substituent is added to the parent name but its position is defined as next to (*ortho*), two places away (*meta*) or three places away, i.e. at the opposite end of the ring (*para*). Thus 1,4-diethylbenzene and *para*-diethylbenzene are equivalent. Aromatic rings can form fused structures; for example, two fused benzene rings form naphthalene and three fused rings can form anthracene or phenathrene, depending on the configuration. Fusion to rings of other sizes can maintain the aromatic nature of the structure if certain rules are obeyed.

Substituted hydrocarbons and heterocyclic substances

Everything in the preceding sections has de-scribed the chemistry of hydrocarbon structures. The ability to form saturated or unsaturated chains (linear or branching), rings (single or multiple) or ring–chain combinations results in a considerable diversity of molecules. However, the ability of carbon to bind to a range of other atoms introduces the huge diversity responsible for the structure and function of all life. In many cases this introduces reactive sites in a molecule. These functional groups will often dictate the chemical and physical properties of the molecule. Some of the most common classes are shown below (R is any carbon–hydrogen structure) together with the name of the class of substances:

R—OH	alcohol
R—O—R	ether
R—CHO	aldehyde
R—CO—R	ketone
R—COOH	carboxylic acid
R—COO—R	ester
R—NH$_2$	amine
R—CONH$_2$	amide
R—Cl	organohalogen (can be F, Cl, Br or I).

Clearly, a description of the structures and properties of the resulting possible classes of chemicals is beyond the capacity of this chapter and only a selective introduction is possible. These functional groups may themselves form homologous series as the attached carbon chain grows. They can be introduced into hydrocarbon rings to produce heterocyclic rings or can be added to aromatic rings via the substitution reactions mentioned earlier. Primary, secondary and tertiary structures can be formed where, for example, the carbon closest to a group such as an alcohol or an amine can be bound to one, two or three adjacent carbon atoms, respectively.

Alcohols

These contain the hydroxyl (—OH) groups. They can be primary, secondary or tertiary, as described above. The hydroxyl group is polar, and in smaller molecular weight alcohols this promotes miscibility with water. As the carbon chain lengthens, the non-polar component increases so that, for example, octanol, C$_8$H$_{12}$OH, is practically insoluble. The hydroxyl groups cause intermolecular interactions, resulting in relatively high boiling points. Primary alcohols are oxidised to aldehydes or acids. Secondary alcohols are oxidised to ketones. Hydroxybenzene is more frequently known as phenol. The central depressant actions of alcohols are well known, as is the social use of ethanol. Ethanol, isopropanol and phenol have disinfectant and antiseptic uses. Thiols, containing the —SH group (the sulphydryl groups), are related substances.

Ethers

Alcohols can be considered as derivatives of water in which one hydrogen is substituted by an organic group. When both hydrogens are substituted, we get an ether:

H—O—H	water
R—O—H	alcohol
R—O—R	ether.

Ethers have boiling points almost the same as those of alkanes of comparable total length and lower than those of corresponding alcohols because of lower intermolecular attractions. Their water solubility is similar to that of corresponding alcohols. Ethers are combustible in the presence of air, oxygen or nitrous oxide. Free radical oxidation in the presence of oxygen yields hydroperoxides, which will explode if heated. Addition of a non-volatile antioxidant will avoid this. Introduction of an oxygen atom into a cyclic hydrocarbon ring will produce a cyclic ether. Three-membered ring ethers (two carbons, one oxygen) are epoxides. Various volatile inhalational anaesthetic agents are ethers. These include diethyl ether and various halogen substituted ethers. Various structurally complex agents used in anaesthetic practice contain cyclic ether groups, including some opioid analgesics and scopolamine.

Organohalides

These include alkyl halides, where the halogen molecule is bonded by a single bond to a carbon, vinyl halides in which the halogen is bound to a carbon, which is bound to another with a double bond, or aryl halides, bound to one of the carbons of an aromatic ring. They are of interest in anaesthetics and include chloroform, halothane and trichloroethylene. This group will include the halogenated ethers mentioned above. The halogens in volatile anaesthetics are fluorine, chlorine or bromine. This group also includes the refrigerant chlorofluorocarbons (CFCs), the various halogenated dry cleaning solvents, the aromatic, polyhalogenated insecticides, such as dicophane (DDT), and the 'non-stick' polymer polydifluoromethane (Teflon).

Carboxylic acids and their derivatives

The carboxylic acids contain a carbonyl group, —C=O, and also the hydroxyl group —OH bound to a single carbon, often written as —COOH. They are very polar and lower members are miscible with water. Larger members have progressively less water solubility. Strong intermolecular attractions result in higher boiling and melting points for these substances. Small carboxylic acids are well known — formic acid (HCOOH) and acetic acid (CH₃COOH). Long chain carboxylic acids comprise the fatty acids (e.g. stearic acid, $CH_3(CH_2)_{16}COOH$), so called because of their origins as esters in fats and oils. Fatty acids from animal sources tend to be solid and saturated. Those from plants tend to be oils and are polyunsaturated. Prostaglandins are C_{20} carboxylic acids containing a substituted cyclopentane ring and with various degrees of unsaturation.

Derivatives of carboxylic acids resulting from replacement of the hydroxyl groups by, for example, —NH₂, give amides (RCONH₂), or by an alcohol give an ester (RCOOR).

Aldehydes and ketones

These also possess the carbonyl or —C=O group. In an aldehyde this is bonded to a carbon and a hydrogen (RCHO), with the exception of the simplest member of the group, formaldehyde, where the carbonyl group is bonded to two hydrogen atoms, HCHO. In a ketone the carbonyl group is bonded to two hydrocarbon or substituted hydrocarbon residues, RCOR. Physically they are polar and lower members are miscible with water. Oxidation of aldehydes produces primary alcohols and that of ketones produces secondary alcohols. While some (notably formaldehyde) are extremely pungent, others have pleasant odours or flavours. Paraldehyde is a polymer of acetaldehyde.

Amines

Amines are derivatives of ammonia in which one or more hydrogen atoms are replaced by a carbon atom. They can be primary, secondary or tertiary, in a similar fashion to alcohols. Amines are of great importance in biological systems. Most substances of pharmacological interest contain nitrogen. *Alkaloid* is a general name given to nitrogen-containing naturally occurring substances — for example, morphine, atropine, nicotine, cocaine, tubocurarine or ergotamine. The amine group is a very common feature of drugs and neurotransmitters. Noradrenaline, dopamine and histamine are primary amines. Adrenaline is a secondary amine. Many drugs acting at adrenergic and cholinergic receptors are amines. Many local anaesthetics are tertiary amines. Quaternary ammonium compounds are a special case in which a nitrogen atom bonds to four carbon atoms. The resulting amine has a positive charge and can form quaternary ammonium salts. Acetylcholine is a quaternary ammonium compound. Many other substances having actions at autonomic ganglia, at the post-ganglionic parasympathetic receptors and at the neuromuscular junction are quaternary ammonium compounds, including neostigmine, suxamethonium and tubocurarine.

Amino acids, peptides and proteins

All amino acids contain a basic amino group and a carboxylic acid group. The nature of the side-chains is responsible for their variations in structure and these side-chains differ quite considerably in both structure and properties such as polarity. Amino acids are the monomeric components of peptides and proteins of the 20 amino acids prominently found in proteins, all but two are primary amino acids (proline and hydroxyproline are pentacyclic secondary amino acids). These are α amino acids, that is the amino group is contained on the carbon atom which is α (next to) the carbon in the —COOH group. In peptides and proteins amino acids are joined by peptide bonds, R—CONH—R, in which the carboxyl group of one molecule joins to the amine group of the neighbouring molecule to form an amide linkage. A peptide formed from two amino acids is a dipeptide, from three is a tripeptide, and so on. Proteins are simply large peptides. The distinction is rather arbitrary, with proteins having more than about 50 amino acids. Proteins can be structural and insoluble, such as those found in connective tissue, bone and hair, or functional, often soluble, such as enzymes, or conjugated to a non-protein group, as in haemoglobin or in lipoproteins.

THE SHAPE OF MOLECULES: STEREOCHEMISTRY AND ISOMERISM

Although chemical structures are often portrayed in two-dimensional forms on paper, it is important to realise that they exist in three dimensions, that atoms and molecules will take up specific orientations in respect to each other and that particular orientations may be favoured for reasons of stability and in the interests of producing a minimum energy conformation. In proteins and other macromolecules there are different levels of structure. In the case of a protein there is a primary structure, which is the sequence of amino acids. Molecular interactions will cause these amino acid chains to take up a shape, often a helix. This is the secondary structure. For larger molecules the secondary structure can itself adopt a folded structure, the tertiary structure. Larger scale interactions between protein subunits dictate the quaternary structure. The secondary, tertiary and quaternary interactions give a protein its shape and are essential for proper function of an enzyme, the recognition sites in receptors or the functioning of multiple unit systems such as haemoglobin or ion channels in cell membranes. This complex architecture is disturbed, sometimes irreversibly, by placing the molecule in an inappropriate environment in which the intermolecular interactions are disturbed.

Simpler molecules can also adopt different forms. Isomerism is the term applied to the existence of compounds with the same molecular formula but which are different either in the order in which their atomic and molecular components are joined together or in the possible existence of differently preferred conformations. Compounds with the same molecular formula but with atoms arranged differently are structural isomers. At the simplest level the compound of molecular formula $C_4H_{10}O$ could be diethyl ether, $CH_3CH_2OCH_2CH_3$, or could be one of several alcohols, $CH_3CH_2CH_2CH_2OH$ (butan-1-ol), $CH_3CH_2CH(OH)CH_3$ (butan-2-ol) or $(CH_3)_3COH$ (the tertiary alcohol, 2-methyl-2-propanol or *tert*-butyl alcohol). The greater the number of carbon atoms the greater the number of structural isomers — for example, three isomeric structures can be drawn for pentane and 75 for decane ($C_{10}H_{22}$).

More subtle forms of isomerism exist relating to the way in which substituents on a carbon atom are arranged in space. Such isomers are known as stereoisomers and the study of these properties is known as stereochemistry. There are various types of stereoisomer.

The substituents located on adjacent C–C single bonds have a certain freedom to rotate about that bond. Such isomers are called conformational isomers. There are two extremes: in one conformation the substituents on each adjacent carbon orient in opposite directions (staggered form); in the other, orientation of bonds on adjacent carbons is the same (eclipsed form). While a molecule can exist in either arrangement, or indeed in intermediate arrangements, it will spend most of its time in the more stable, staggered conformation, especially if the substituent groups are bulky, so that there is greater intermolecular repulsion.

If adjacent carbons cannot rotate, as in alkenes or in cyclic structures, then substituent groups can be oriented so that they are on the same side of the double bond or on the same side of the ring, that is in the *cis* position relative to each other, or they can be on opposite sides of the bond or of the ring, that is in the *trans* configuration. This is known as *cis-trans* isomerism.

From the biological point of view, optical isomerism is of importance. This form of stereoisomerism is associated with so-called asymmetric or chiral-bonded carbons. When carbon is bonded to four hydrogen atoms (methane), the bonds point towards the four corners of a tetrahedron with carbon in the centre and the angle between each bond 109.5°. Substitution of one hydrogen always leads to the same compound.

Substitution of two hydrogens also always leads to the same compound. By that is meant that no matter which hydrogens are replaced, simple reorientation of the molecule always produces compounds which are superimposable. However, the situation changes when three hydrogen atoms are replaced by three different substituents — that is, each 'arm' of the tetrahedron has a different substituent. The substituent groups can be placed in two different ways so that the resulting two isomers are not superimposable, whichever way the molecules are placed; however, they are mirror images of each other. This is a general finding and the carbon atom in question is a chiral centre (from the Greek *kheir* = hand). These molecules are called enantiomers. Such a subtle difference results in only very small differences in physical properties, and indeed it is not possible to separate enantiomers on the basis of differing physical properties. However, when a beam of polarised light is passed through a solution of each of the isomers, they rotate the plane of the light by the same amount but in different directions. A compound rotating light to the right is known as the (+) or *d* (dextrorotatory) isomer and an enantiomer rotating light to the left is known as the (–) or *l* (for laevorotatory) isomer. Conventional chemical synthesis usually results in production of each enantiomer with equal probability. The result is a so-called racemic mixture, which is not optically active because it contains equal proportions of the enantiomers. However, in biologically synthesised molecules, in which a substrate is contained in a fixed orientation by an enzyme based system, the product is often an enantiomer. Biological synthetic procedures usually produce the *l* enantiomer, and in pharmacology, where a substance is optically active, the pharmacological activity is almost always chiefly possessed by the *l* isomer. Thus *l*-isoprenaline has effects on β adrenoceptors that are orders of magnitude greater than those of *d*-isoprenaline. The prefixes *d* and *l* or (+) or (–) do not give information about the orientation of the substituents in a chiral carbon. This is conventionally done by arranging the substituents in an order of priority using a systematic scale. The molecule is orientated so that the lowest priority group points back towards the observer. The order (clockwise or anticlockwise of the remaining three substituents, highest to lowest) is then defined. If the direction is clockwise, the configuration is *R* (rectus); if anticlockwise, the configuration is *S* (sinister). This convention draws no conclusion about the optical properties of the compound, which need separate determination and correlation with the absolute configuration. A molecule may have more than one chiral centre.

PROPERTIES OF GASES AND VAPOURS

A few inhalational general anaesthetics are gases (e.g. nitrous oxide and cyclopropane). Most however, are vapours (ethers, halogenated hydrocarbons). Gases represent one of the three states of matter (together with liquids and solids). A vapour is formed by molecules escaping from a liquid and, in a closed system, forming an equilibrium with the liquid.

Gases

Gases are characteristic in that many of their properties are not related to their chemical nature and may be defined by well known gas laws. The interaction between molecules in the gas phase is very much lower than that for liquids, and gases form a state of freely moving atoms or molecules, which are entirely miscible. Gases are subject to relatively large volume changes associated with changes in temperature and pressure and this can be described by a series of simple relationships.

Boyle's law states that at constant temperature the volume (V) of a fixed mass of gas varies inversely as its pressure (P), i.e.

$$PV = \text{constant.}$$

Charles' Law states that at constant pressure the volume (V) of a fixed mass of gas varies as its absolute temperature (T), i.e.

$$\frac{V}{T} = \text{constant.}$$

These relationships can be combined to produce the general gas equation

$$PV = nRT.$$

where n represents the number of moles of gas present and R is a constant, the gas constant. The above relationships apply to a so-called ideal gas and hold well enough at lower pressures and higher temperatures. Real gases tend to deviate from this behaviour because gas molecules themselves occupy volume and molecules demonstrate attractive forces.

The pressure exerted by a gas on the walls of a container may be considered as the force of the molecules of gas striking the container walls. In the case of a mixture of gases, the total pressure will be the sum of the contribution of the various components. Each gas exerts the same pressure as if it alone occupied the whole of the available volume and this pressure is the partial pressure of the gas. This is Dalton's law of partial pressures. In this case, the general gas equation may be rewritten as

$$PV = (n_1 + n_2 + \ldots n_n)RT,$$

where $n_1, n_2 \ldots n_n$ are the number of moles of the various gases in the mixture.

An important and interesting property of gases relevant to this is defined by Avogadro's law, which states that equal volumes of gases under the same conditions of temperature and pressure all contain equal numbers of molecules. Specifically, a mole (molecular weight in grams) of a gas under standard conditions (101 kPa, 0°C) will contain a fixed number of molecules (Avogadro's number, 6.022×10^{23}) and occupy a volume of 22.4 litres, the gram molecular volume.

Vapours

When a liquid is placed in a closed container, molecules within the liquid moving with sufficient velocity are able to escape and become vapour. These molecules, if they collide with the liquid surface, will again become liquid. At equilibrium, the escape rate will equal the capture rate and the vapour will be saturated. The pressure over the liquid at this time is the vapour pressure.

The saturated vapour pressure of a liquid depends on the kinetic energy of the molecules in the vapour and hence on the temperature. The vapour pressure in fact rises exponentially with temperature. When the kinetic energy is high enough, so that the vapour pressure equals atmospheric pressure, bubbles form in the liquid and the liquid boils. The saturated vapour pressure is independent of the volume of the liquid remaining. Hence one cannot predict the amount of liquid in a cylinder of liquefied gas (e.g. nitrous oxide or carbon dioxide) by measuring the pressure because as long as any liquid remains the pressure will be that of the saturated vapour. The amount remaining has to be determined by weighing.

BEHAVIOUR OF MOLECULES IN SOLUTION

Solutions and solubility

Formation of a solution requires an interaction between the molecules of the solute and the molecules of the solvent. As a general rule, a solute dissolves most readily in a solvent of comparable polarity. Non-polar solvents, such as benzene, hexane or carbon tetrachloride, will dissolve non-polar compounds, such as greases or oils. Polar solvents, such as water, methanol or ethanol, will dissolve polar and ionic substances, such as sodium chloride or the salts of many drugs. Thus pentobarbitone and theophylline, for example, are only slightly soluble in water, whereas sodium pentobarbitone or the EDTA complex of theophylline (aminophylline) are water soluble. Molecules with detergent or surface active properties, for example $CH_3(CH_2)_{16}COO^-Na^+$ (sodium stearate) or long hydrocarbon chains with quaternary ammonium residues at the end, can interact with both polar and non-polar components and enhance interaction of otherwise incompatible phases. When two immiscible solvents are in contact there is an interface between them. If a solute is added it will partition between each of the two immiscible solvent phases according to its solubility in each.

The ratio of the concentration of the solute in each solvent is its partition coefficient. The octanol:water partition coefficient is an important property of drugs and a high coefficient will be reflected in an increased lipid solubility and interaction with cell membranes. General anaesthetic potency is reflected in the octanol:water partition coefficient for a given series of agents.

Osmotic pressure and the Donnan effect

A common feature of biological systems is that of solutions kept apart by selective membranes. Semipermeable membranes allow the passage of some molecules but not of others. For example, dialysis membranes allow passage of smaller molecules but will not allow passage of molecules of molecular weight greater than a particular cut-off weight. Thus a more concentrated solution of the macromolecule may be produced on one side of the membrane and there is a tendency for solvent molecules to move in this direction until there is isotonicity. This process is osmosis and the pressure required to prevent this is the osmotic pressure. An erythrocyte placed in a hypotonic aqueous environment will have a relatively increased concentration of solute molecules, osmosis will cause external water molecules to flow into the cell and the resulting osmotic pressure will cause the cell to swell and rupture. Where components of such systems are ions and there is, for example, a system that allows transport of solvent molecules and small ions but does not allow transport of large ions, such as proteins, then there will be an asymmetric distribution of ions, leading to a transmembrane potential. This phenomenon is the Donnan effect and the transmembrane potential is known as the Donnan potential. In a simple case, an aqueous sodium chloride solution is present on both sides of a semipermeable membrane, and a negatively charged macromolecule is present on only one side. As a result, sodium ions will accumulate on the macromolecule side and chloride ions on the opposite side, resulting in a transmembrane potential. If the macromolecules are polyelectrolytes, then the Donnan effect will itself contribute to the osmotic pressure.

Ionisation, acids and bases

In aqueous solutions of ionic molecules there is a tendency for the latter to dissociate. This is due to the strong attractions between the charged ions and water molecules resulting in the ions becoming surrounded by water molecules. This is clearly seen for strong electrolytes such as sodium chloride or for strong acids (e.g. HCl) or strong bases (e.g. NaOH). Many organic materials are weakly ionised, and indeed water itself is weakly ionised. This results in a more complicated system in which an equilibrium is set up between the ionised and unionised components. Water can dissociate to form two ions, the hydronium ion H_3O^+ and the hydroxyl ion OH^-. An equilibrium is set up, represented by the following reaction:

$$2H_2O \leftrightarrow H_3O^+ + OH^-.$$

At equilibrium there will be no net change in the concentrations of the components, so that there will be constant proportions of these components, written as

$$K = \frac{[H_3O^+][OH^-]}{[H_2O]^2},$$

where the square brackets denote concentrations in moles per litre (M) and K is the equilibrium constant for water. Clearly since water is only slightly ionised and the concentration of H_2O is very high, then the concentration of H_2O is practically unaffected by the concentration of the ions (1×20^{-7} mol l^{-1} each at 25°C). Therefore the equation may be rewritten as

$$K_w = [H_3O^+][OH^-],$$

where K_w is the ionic product of water.

pH is the negative log (to the base 10) of the hydronium (H_3O^+) ion activity, so that

$$pH = -\log_{10}[H_3O^+]$$

and, since at 25°C this is 1×10^{-7}, then the pH of water at 25°C is $-\log_{10}(1 \times 10^{-7}) = 7.0$.

The commonly employed definition of acids and bases in organic systems is based on the Bronsted–Lowry concept of acids as donors of hydrogen ions (protons) and bases as proton acceptors. In the case of a strong acid, such as the mineral acids, or a strong base, dissociation will be virtually complete and the pH will be essentially a direct function of the concentration of the acid or base; for example, the pH of a 0.1 mol l^{-1} aqueous solution of hydrochloric acid will be 1. Organic acids and bases are relatively weak and dissociation will be incomplete; for example, in the case of an acid there will be an equilibrium represented by the equation

$$HA \leftrightarrow H^+ + A^-$$

and an equilibrium constant calculated as

$$K_a = \frac{[H^+][A^-]}{[HA]}.$$

K_a is the dissociation constant at a given temperature. Similarly to the calculation for pH, the negative log of the dissociation constant is defined as the pK_a. Thus the pH of such systems will be a function of the concentration of the proton donor (acid) and proton acceptor (base) and can be written as

$$pH = pK_a + \frac{[base]}{[acid]}.$$

This is the Henderson–Hasselbalch equation and is fundamental to quantitative calculations of acid–base equilibria in biological systems. It is worth noting that, for any such species, if pH is adjusted to the value of the pK_a then the molecule is 50% ionised. It is also worth noting that drug molecules and macromolecules may have more than one ionisable site and may have more than one value of pK_a.

2

Cell physiology

J. G. McGeown
W. McCaughey
W. F. M. Wallace

This chapter reviews cellular features of relevance to the understanding of physiology as applied to anaesthesia, and will focus particularly on the principles controlling signalling at the cellular level. This is of considerable importance because all messenger molecules, whether they be naturally occurring transmitters or synthetic drugs given for therapeutic purposes, must ultimately act through these signalling pathways to modify cell function. Consideration of these physiological issues cannot be divorced from an understanding of relevant structure, however, and so we will begin with an overview of some important cellular components.

CELL STRUCTURE

The cells of a multicellular organism, such as the human body, are specialised in a multitude of ways, but all are based on a common basic structure. An outer plasma membrane separates the contents of the cell from the external environment. Within the confines of this membrane there are a variety of specialised organelles surrounded by the intracellular fluid or cytoplasm. In most cells there is also a nucleus bounded by a nuclear membrane. The nucleus contains, among other things, the reproductive mechanisms of the cell.

Structure in relation to function

Advances in knowledge of cell function are facilitated by parallel advances in knowledge of structure. In understanding cell, and indeed organ, function it is most helpful to correlate constantly the two aspects of structure and function. Structure gives a hint of function and assumed function must always be consistent with structure. For example, the absence of a nucleus in a red blood cell correlates with the cell's inability to reproduce, while abundant mitochondria in a cell suggest a high level of oxidative metabolism for the production of energy. In the kidneys, the cells of the proximal convoluted tubule have microvilli and many mitochondria; this rightly suggests that they have a powerful absorptive capacity and use much energy in the process. The relatively abundant cytoplasm and organelles of the cells of the thick ascending limb of the loop of Henle suggest that they have a more active role in altering lumen contents than have cells of the thin limb, which have little cytoplasm and are believed to behave more passively, rather like the capillaries whose structure they resemble. It is also worth noting that the cells of the proximal convoluted tubule bear quite a strong resemblance to the enterocytes in the intestinal villi and this correlates with some parallel functions in active absorption of electrolytes and nutrients.

Cell size

In thinking of cellular physiology it is helpful to remember the scale of cells. Very large cells, such as the ovum, the pyramidal cells of the cerebral cortex and the anterior horn cells of the spinal cord, measure about 100 μm — or one-tenth of a millimetre in diameter — a size just visible to the naked eye. Most cells are smaller and the red blood cell, at 7–8 μm in diameter, is a useful reference scale when looking at histological sections. Because of this minute size, and because the interior of the cell is subdivided by many subcellular organelles, the properties of structures and fluids with which we are familiar do not necessarily apply in the cell. Conventional diagrams and even electronmicrographs give only a hint of what cells are like and how they function. It is also useful to remember that the tiny distances involved in and between cells allow chemicals to

diffuse and react in a remarkably short time. For example, synaptic transmission includes entry of calcium ions to the presynaptic terminal, vesicular movement and fusion with the cell membrane, exocytosis and diffusion of the transmitter, reaction of transmitter with receptor, channel opening and diffusion of sodium ions. Nevertheless, the entire synaptic delay is only about 1 millisecond.

Cell membrane

The membrane that encompasses cells, the cell membrane or plasma membrane, both separates its contents from the rest of the body and provides a highly sophisticated system for the interaction of the cell with other cells and, in particular, for the control and regulation of cell function. The membrane is believed to have a fluid lipid nature, with specific minute structures, mainly protein in nature, floating in it (Fig. 2.1). These provide the structural basis for functions such as accepting external chemical signals (at receptors), allowing ionic flow across the membrane (through channels) and actively extruding or exchanging specific ions (by energy-consuming pumps).

Membrane lipids

The basic framework of all membranes is a double layer (bilayer) of lipid molecules, usually phospholipids, which have a hydrophilic 'head' composed of a phosphate linked to a residue (choline, ethanolamine, serine or inositol), and a hydrophobic 'tail' which is a fatty acid chain. These molecules have the remarkable property that, in a watery environment, they spontaneously line themselves up into a bilayer. Because of the essentially lipid nature of the membrane, lipid soluble substances, such as steroid hormones and fat soluble drugs, cross it freely, while water soluble particles, such as ions, do not. For this reason, the cell can maintain high concentration gradients of ions across its plasma membrane, as is the case with sodium, potassium and chloride. In addition, most hormones and

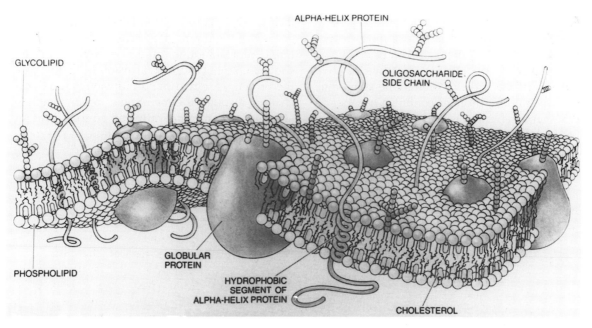

Figure 2.1   Plasma membrane. (Reproduced with permission from Bretscher MS 1985 The molecules of the cell membrane. Scientific American 253: 86–90.)

many drugs, which are water-soluble chemicals, tend to act on external receptor sites on the plasma membrane.

Membrane proteins

The (mainly protein) structures floating in the lipid of the cell membrane are present in large numbers, making up more than half of the mass of the membrane. Some are exposed on one surface only, but many span the membrane (Fig. 2.1). These proteins serve a number of functions. Some are structural and are attached to the protein framework of the cell itself, the cytoskeleton. Others act as carriers that transport ions or other substances across the membrane. This may facilitate the passive movement of substances down an electrochemical gradient (facilitated diffusion) or involve the active transport of some substrate against a diffusion gradient (active transport). Proteins involved in active transport include both adenosine triphosphate (ATP) degrading ion pumps (e.g. the Na^+, K^+-ATPase) and ion exchange systems, which use the passive movement of one species to drive

the active transport of another (e.g. Na^+, Ca^{2+} exchange). These are examples of primary and secondary active transport systems, respectively. Other membrane proteins include ion channels, membrane receptors for chemical messengers, such as neurotransmitters, hormones or drugs, and enzymes. It is also the surface proteins which determine the antigen status of a cell and thus how other cells will recognise it. This may decide whether such cells will be rejected immunologically after tissue transplantation and it is these antigens which are identified in the process of tissue typing. The most common application of this principle is in blood grouping, in which surface antigens glycoproteins (carbohydrate chains linked to protein) known as agglutinogens lead to red cell agglutination, when masses of cells are linked together by the multivalent, antigen specific antibodies (agglutinins).

Protein structure and folding. Proteins are constructed of long chains of amino acid residues whose sequence determines the primary structure of the protein molecule. This chain folds into different shapes, such as the α helix and the β sheets, which make up the secondary structure of the protein. Finally, the various helical and sheet-like elements are folded into a more or less globular shape, the detailed morphology of which constitutes the tertiary structure, or conformation, of the protein. Membrane-spanning, or transmembrane, proteins contain a number of helical segments, and these are arranged parallel to each other and are the portion that actually spans the membrane. Figure 2.2 shows a digrammatic representation of the α subunit of the sodium channel as a typical example. In this case, the protein is folded in such a way as to form a channel through the membrane, an ion channel, as shown diagrammatically in Figure 2.3. Protein

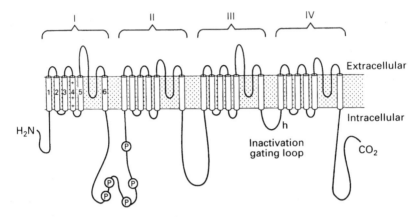

Figure 2.2 Proposed transmembrane folding of the primary structures of the Na^+ channel. (Reproduced with permission from Catterall W A 1991 Structure and function of voltage-gated sodium and calcium channels. Current Opinion in Neurobiology 1: 5–13.)

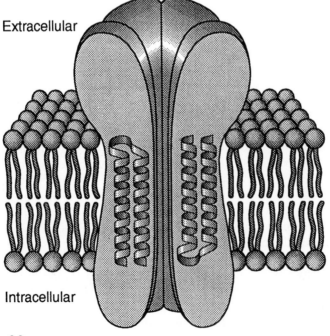

Figure 2.3

folding is determined by attraction and repulsion between charges on different parts of the chain. Thus, if a messenger molecule, whether endogenous or a drug, has a structure that allows it to bind to a region of a surface protein molecule, it may, by its interaction with the charges on the protein, cause this to change its tertiary shape. This can be used by the cell to activate a sequence of events that allows the extracellular signal to modify cell function in a controlled way, often through the formation of an intracellular, or second messenger. These events are said to constitute the relevant signal transduction pathway in the cell.

The protein make-up of the membrane can change rapidly; for example, each cardiac muscle cell has many β adrenoceptors but the numbers of these vary from time to time depending on external stimuli. Thus when catecholamine levels rise, the number of β adrenoceptors decreases (downregulation), and when the level of catecholamines falls, the receptors increase in number (upregulation). This is accomplished by internalisation and externalisation of the receptors (see below).

Endocytosis and exocytosis

About 2% of the surface of the cell membrane is undergoing a process of endocytosis at any one time. In this, a portion of the membrane forms a pit, then invaginates, and finally pinches off to form a closed vesicle. This process is used to remove active receptors from the surface — internalisation — and also as a transport mechanism to take certain substances into the cell; for example, iron is absorbed as ferric ions (Fe^{3+}) bound to transferrin, which binds to receptors on the membrane. The iron–transferrin–receptor complex enters the cell by endocytosis of a patch of membrane; the iron is released and transferred to an intracellular lysosome, and the empty vesicle then fuses again with the plasma membrane. Exocytosis is the opposite process, responsible for secretion of cell products, such as transmitter substances, hormones and exocrine secretions, as well as the externalisation of membrane receptors.

Cytoplasm

The cytoplasm or cytosol is the intracellular fluid in which the organelles, such as the nucleus and mitochondria, are contained. It allows free movement of molecules, including oxygen and carbon dioxide, from and to the cell membrane. However, it is not a formless mass of jelly — it is highly structured, being criss-crossed by the filaments of the cytoskeleton, a network of fibres and microtubules composed of protein — mainly actin. This has functions in maintaining cell shape and locomotion, and in movement of vesicles within the cell as well as the assembly of the plasma membrane.

The ionic composition of cytoplasm is very different from that of extracellular fluid — it is high in potassium and low in sodium and chloride. Non-diffusible anions, mainly proteins and phosphates, provide most of the negative charge to balance the potassium ions. These differences between intracellular and extracellular fluid provide the basis for the transmembrane voltage gradients, which exist in most cells and which are a central feature of excitable tissues, such as nerve and muscle. The concentration gradients favour ion and hence current flow when the appropriate channels open, and this can lead to rapid changes in membrane potential, e.g. during an action potential. Just as extracellular fluid is the external environment of body cells, so the cytoplasm is the external environment of cellular organelles. Its temperature and composition must be optimal if chemical reactions in the organelles are to proceed normally. Hydrogen ions are one such critical component, and pH, usually slightly lower than in extracellular fluid, is maintained by an extensive intracellular buffering capacity and by proton and bicarbonate pumps in the cell membrane.

Nucleus

This organelle, bounded by its own nuclear membrane (another phospholipid bilayer), is the major site controlling the structure and function of the cell, and also, where appropriate, cell replication. The relevant information is contained in the chromosomes, each of which consists essentially of an enormous molecule of deoxyribonucleic acid (DNA). The structure of DNA molecules is well adapted to the storage of information on the sequence of amino-acids required to synthesise necessary cell proteins. The DNA sequence within each chromosome is currently being documented in the human genome project. All cell nuclei contain all the information used by all the different cell types in the body and therefore much of this information is normally suppressed in a given cell. This information may, however, be used by abnormal cells so that, for example, lung tumours may produce vasopressin or adrenocorticotrophic hormone.

Gene structure, function and nomenclature

The 'unit' of stored hereditary information is the gene: a gene is a region of DNA that codes for a particular polypeptide or protein. DNA itself consists of a series of nucleotides, each made up of a pentose sugar residue, deoxyribose, attached to phosphate groups on the outside and a nitrogenous base on the inside. The nucleotides are connected into a long strand through phosphate linkages and two strands are held in the familiar double-helix arrangement by hydrogen bonds between the bases. Each amino acid in the gene product is designated by a base triplet, i.e. a sequence of three nitrogenous bases selected from adenine, guanine, cytosine and thymine. Each base can only associate with one of the other bases, i.e. adenine only pairs with thymine and cytosine with guanine. This provides the basis for DNA replication, in which the normal double strand becomes unzipped, leaving the bases on each single strand unpaired. Since each base will only pair with one other, these single strands act as the templates for two new double strands, each identical to the original. Similarly, this base complementarity rule ensures that the messenger ribonucleic acid (mRNA) formed during transcription mirrors the original code, albeit with the base uracil replacing thymine. In this way the nucleotide sequence of mRNA consists of a series of codons, each complementary to the base triplets on the original gene (Fig. 2.4).

The conversion of mRNA into the required polypeptide (translation) occurs outside the nucleus in association with ribosomes (which also contain ribonucleic acid, rRNA). These facilitate the association of the base triplets on the mRNA with complementary base sequences (anticodons) on transfer RNA (tRNA) molecules in the cytoplasm. A tRNA molecule carrying a given anticodon will also bind to a specific amino acid, so that, as tRNA molecules line up along the mRNA, the amino acids are also lined up in the appropriate order and can then form permanent peptide links.

The DNA sequence for a single gene includes regions that do not actually code for any peptide product. These introns act as spacers dividing up the gene into a number of separate peptide coding regions, or exons. Both introns and exons are transcribed into mRNA initially but subsequent modification leads to removal of the introns and splicing of the exons end to end to produce an uninterrupted sequence which codes for the product protein. The mRNA also carries stop codons transcribed from the original DNA: when these sequences are reached during translation the ribosome releases a completed polypeptide.

Any abnormality in the nucleotide sequence of the gene, a mutation, will ultimately lead to an abnormal sequence of amino acids in the polypeptide product and may have serious structural and functional consequences. Detailed mapping of individual human genes could have important implications in identifying individuals with susceptibility for specific diseases or whose metabolism might predispose them to certain adverse drug reactions. This will require not just the identification of genes in the genome but an understanding of the function of their peptide products within the cell. A gene's location may be described in terms of the number of the chromosome on which it is found (1–22 for the autosomes, X or Y for the sex chromosomes), whether it lies on the short arm (p) or long arm (q) of that chromosome, and its position along the length of the arm (related to a series of bands that show up on histological staining). Thus the location of the gene that causes cystic fibrosis is described as

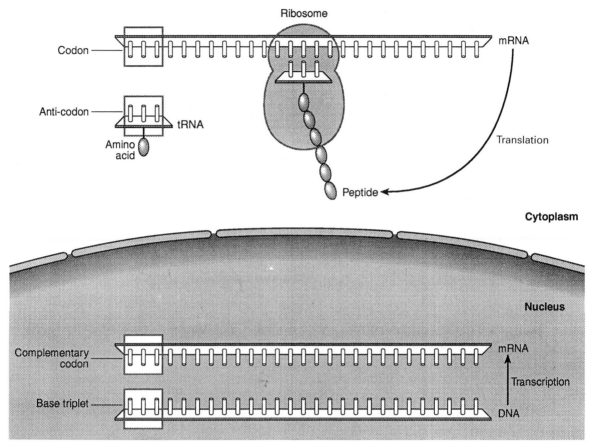

Figure 2.4   Summary of the main events in gene expression.

7q31, i.e. it lies in the first band of the third region along the long arm of chromosome 7.

The nomenclature applied to genes is complex and confusing, not least because of the widespread use of abbreviations that have become detached from their original meanings. For this reason gene names should be taken as arbitrary codes to which functions will be ascribed as further information is gathered. These names often reflect normal or abnormal cell functions related to a given gene, e.g. a mutant gene in the fruitfly *Drosophila*, which is associated with rapid shaking of the insect's legs when anaesthetised with ether, has been dubbed the *shaker* gene. This is now known to code for an abnormal potassium channel. Other ion channel related genes in *Drosophila* have names such as *ether-a-go-go* (*eag*) and *seizure* (*sei*). Genes may also be named for the proteins they produce, with abbreviations in italics indicating the gene. Thus, one may refer to the gene producing a chloride channel, known as the cystic fibrosis transmembrane conductance regulator (CFTR), as the *cftr* gene. Abnormalities in this gene are responsible for cystic fibrosis.

Oncogenes and proto-oncogenes

Other genes of considerable pathological significance include the oncogenes, which promote uncontrolled cell multiplication leading to tumour formation. A wide range of such genes has been implicated in the pathogenesis of various forms of human tumours. A thread common to many haematological and solid tumours, however, seems to be mutations in a family of genes known as *ras* genes. These code for ras proteins (members of the G protein superfamily, see below) involved in normal growth factor signal transduction pathways, and the tumorigenic mutation favours persistent activation of the ras proteins. It may be that this ultimately leads to stimulation of uncontrolled cell replication.

Oncogenes are mutations of the closely related proto-oncogenes, which are normal genes involved in controlling growth. These are also known as immediate early genes, as they are capable of being induced within minutes, unlike the late response genes, whose mRNA can only be transcribed after the synthesis of other, regulatory proteins. Proto-oncogenes form part of the signal transduction cascade controlling nuclear function and have been called 'third messengers'. The proto-oncogenes *c-fos* and *c-jun* have also been shown to be involved in pain pathways. *c-fos* activation appears to be an important link in the transmission of painful stimuli in the spinal cord, and may be important in the development of more lasting changes in response to pain, such as hyperalgesia and chronic pain syndromes (see Ch. 16).

Mitochondria

Mitochondria carry out the oxygen dependent, energy producing reactions in the cell. They are contained within their own outer membrane and have an internal membrane folded to produce partitions, or cristae, which are the sites for a series of enzymes that progressively oxidise substrates and convert the resultant energy into the high energy phosphate bonds of ATP, a process known as oxidative phosphorylation. ATP is then available as an energy source and its hydrolysis to adenosine diphosphate (ADP) and phosphate powers energy dependent processes in both animal and plant cells. The mitochondria are also the main source of carbon dioxide and heat in the cell. Not surprisingly, the oxygen partial pressure in the mitochondria approaches zero, thereby providing the gradient for oxygen diffusion into them. Thyroid hormones increase the cell content of certain mitochondrial enzymes and this contributes to the hormonally induced increase in cellular metabolism, energy and heat production.

These organelles provide an interesting example of correlation between structure and function at a cellular scale. Being the site of oxidative phosphorylation they are abundant in cells that operate at a high level of aerobic metabolism. Thus, they are more common in slow oxidative skeletal muscle fibres than in fast glycolytic fibres and are abundant in the cells of the renal proximal convoluted tubule — cells requiring considerable energy to drive their ionic pumps.

Endoplasmic reticulum and other structures

The endoplasmic reticulum is a network of membranous channels within the cytoplasm of the cell. In some areas the defining membranes carry ribosomes on their outer surface and this rough endoplasmic reticulum is associated with protein synthesis, while smooth (ribosome-free) endoplasmic reticulum is a site for various other metabolic processes. In secretory cells, membranes continuous with the endoplasmic reticulum may be arranged into flattened stacks of cisternae and vesicles known as the Golgi apparatus. This is analogous to the transmitter vesicles in nerve terminals, as in both cases cell products are stored while they await exocytosis. A further important specialisation of the endoplasmic reticulum involves storage of calcium ions, which may be released to trigger cellular activity and taken up again to maintain the low basal level of cytoplasmic calcium. Skeletal muscle, with its highly organised sarcoplasmic reticulum, provides a good example of this type of activity, but many other contractile and secretory cells appear to function in a similar way.

Cells contain many other organelles, the dominant features of which vary according to the tissue of origin and functional specialisations required. Actin and myosin, for example, are prominent molecules in contractile cells, particularly skeletal and cardiac muscle cells where the contractile and regulatory molecules are highly organised in the form of evenly spaced thick and thin myofilaments. This produces the familiar striated pattern in these cell types.

CELL SIGNALLING

The exchange of information between cells displays a vast diversity in detail but is largely dependent on two types of signalling: electrical and chemical. The following sections provide a brief overview of these processes, with a particular emphasis on how cells can generate and respond to these signals.

Membrane potential, ion channels and membrane pumps

A fundamental property of most cells is a trans-membrane electrical gradient, which varies from tissue to tissue over the range of about –9 mV to –100 mV but is often 70–80 mV in amplitude, with the inside of the cell negative. This resting membrane potential is generated by ionic gradients across the membrane and is largely dependent on K^+ because this is the ion to which the cell membrane is most permeable under resting conditions. The high concentration of K^+ inside the cell favours its outward diffusion through K^+ leak channels, leaving a net negative charge on the inside because the large intracellular anions cannot escape from the cell. The Na^+ concentration gradient favours ion movement in the opposite direction but has much less influence on the resting membrane potential because the membrane permeability to Na^+ is normally low. During the action potential in nerves or striated muscle, however, the Na^+ permeability rises dramatically owing to the opening of voltage sensitive Na^+ channels and this allows a large Na^+ current to flow into the cell. This depolarises the cell, producing a positive potential peak at about +20 mV. The inward Na^+ current soon declines again, however, as a result of voltage dependent closure, or inactivation, of the Na^+ channels, and there is a simultaneous increase in the outward K^+ current due to voltage dependent opening of K^+ channels. This repolarises the cell back to its resting potential.

Ion channels

The movement of lipid insoluble ions across the cell membrane is largely dependent on the existence of ion channels, transmembrane proteins which are envisaged as providing aqueous pores that cross the full thickness of the membrane bilayer (Fig. 2.1). Some are open continuously, but many are only opened or gated in response to a specific stimulus. They can either be voltage gated, i.e. they open in response to an electrical impulse, or ligand gated, i.e. they open when a specific molecule binds to their receptor site(s). Some are very specific in their permeability, with a given channel type being selective for one ion, while other, non-selective channels allow several different ions to permeate through them.

At any given time an individual channel may be in an open or closed state and it is only when it is open that ions can move through the channel. The direction of ion movement is determined by the electrical and concentration gradients across the membrane, and the net force driving ions in or out of the cell is referred to as the electro-chemical gradient for that ion. The actual size of the resulting current also depends, however, on the number of open ion channels available to conduct the current. For example, when the membrane of a nerve is depolarised, sodium channels open and the membrane resistance to the flow of current carried by these ions decreases (sodium conductance increases). The resulting passive diffusion of sodium ions into the cell produces the inward sodium current, which further depolarises the cell, producing the rising phase of the action potential as described above. This voltage dependent increase in the number of open channels is referred to as activation. Sodium channels then close again under the continued influence of membrane depolarisation, and this inactivation is followed by opening of potassium channels. The resultant efflux of potassium ions produces an outward current that repolarises the membrane.

Experimental recordings from individual channels show that these spontaneously oscillate between the open, or conducting, and closed, or non-conducting, states. A large increase in the probability of channel opening may be triggered by voltage changes or by the action of a chemical messenger, or ligand. Voltage gated channels account for action potential conduction in excitable tissues, while ligand gated channels may be activated by neurotransmitters, e.g. when acetylcholine binds to the receptors at the neuromuscular junction. It can be appreciated from this that ion channels play an important role in controlling cell function and in cell–cell communication, which often involves modulation of ion channels by messenger molecules. In addition, it is now clear that Ca^{2+} plays a vital intracellular signalling role in most cell types (see below), so it is not surprising that manipulation of Ca^{2+} channels has important functional consequences, making them a significant drug target.

Membrane pumps

The electrical events described above require that the normal concentration gradients for Na^+ and K^+ be maintained across the cell membrane, despite continuous diffusion of each ion down its gradient. This is achieved by an energy consuming sodium–potassium pump, the enzyme Na^+,K^+-ATPase, which degrades ATP to pump K^+ into the cell in exchange for Na^+, which is pumped out. The pump directly contributes a small amount to the recorded membrane potential (<5 mV in nerves) because the number of sodium ions extruded exceeds the number of potassium ions pumped in ($3Na^+$ out: $2K^+$ in), resulting in a small outward or polarising current. Such a pump is said to be electrogenic. It should be emphasised, however, that the main role of the Na^+,K^+ pump is to maintain the appropriate ionic gradients, and it is these which generate most of the observed potential.

Many other ion pumps have been identified, including the gastric proton pump, which can maintain a millionfold gradient (six log units) between the inside (pH 7.2) and outside (pH 1–2 in gastric secretions). A variety of calcium pumps and exchangers maintain very low intracellular concentrations of free Ca^{2+}, while renal tubular pumps reabsorb most of the filtered electrolytes and vary urinary acidity according to body needs. Overall, membrane pumps contribute significantly to the basal metabolic rate.

Messengers, receptors and signal transduction

Messenger molecules influence cell function by binding to cell receptors. These may be located within the cell but in the majority of cases the messenger remains extracellular, interacting with membrane bound surface receptors. This often leads to the production of intracellular, or second, messengers. In many cases second messenger pathways ultimately activate protein kinases (enzymes that phosphorylate proteins) or phosphatases (enzymes that dephosphorylate proteins) and it seems to be the change in the level of phosphorylation that alters the performance of the target protein. Despite these rather complex interactions, however, responses may be very rapid owing to the close approximation of the relevant substrates within the cell.

Surface receptors

An extracellular messenger binds to membrane bound proteins which incorporate receptor sites in their structure. These sites are situated on the external part of the protein, often residing in glycosylated sugar residues. Binding sites demonstrate a messenger specificity that is dependent on their structure and shape and it is this need for conformational complementarity that determines the tissue selectivity of a given messenger or agonist. Only cells expressing appropriate receptors can be stimulated by a given molecule. Binding is normally mediated by hydrogen bond formation and is reversible; rarely, covalent bonds form, greatly reducing the reversibility of the binding reaction. The interaction with the messenger molecule (the ligand) causes a change in the tertiary shape or conformation of the receptor, and it is this which triggers the transduction pathway leading to a change in cell function (Fig. 2.5). This may involve the opening of an ion channel, the activation of a second class of protein on the intracellular side of the membrane (G proteins) leading to second messenger production,

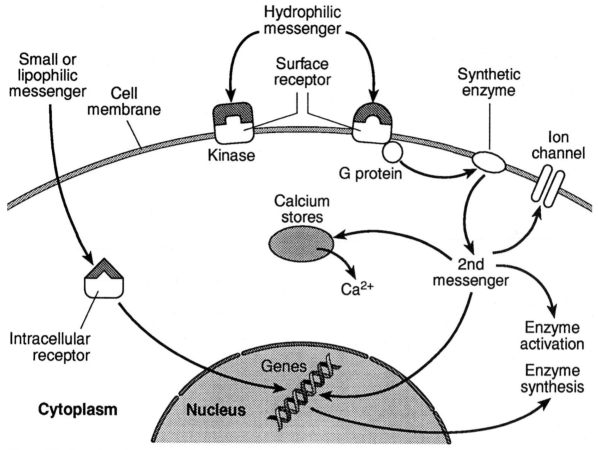

Figure 2.5 Some important pathways in signal transduction.

or the activation of a receptor linked enzyme known as a tyrosine kinase. Some of these pathways will be considered in more detail below.

G proteins

Many receptors belong to a superfamily of closely related transmembrane proteins, including adrenoceptors, opioid receptors, etc. Linkage between these receptors and other intracellular molecules in the transduction pathway depends on a receptor associated protein known as a guanosine-nucleotide binding protein, or, simply, a G protein. This consists of three distinct chains or subunits, α, β and γ (Fig. 2.6). In the resting state (Fig. 2.6A), the G protein, bound to a molecule of guanosine diphosphate (GDP), is situated on the inner side of the membrane. Activation of the receptor (Fig. 2.6B) causes the G protein to exchange GDP for GTP (guanosine triphosphate), and the α subunit dissociates from the βγ complex (Fig. 2.6C). It is these activated G-protein components that interact with nearby effector molecules in the membrane, thus modifying their function. For example, the G protein may activate or inhibit an enzyme that catalyses the production of an important intracellular messenger (see Second messengers, below). Alternatively, it may act on an ion channel, opening or closing it, and so influence membrane potential. Whatever its action, the G protein cycle is completed as the α subunit converts its bound GTP to GDP and reassociates with the other two subunits (Fig. 2.6A).

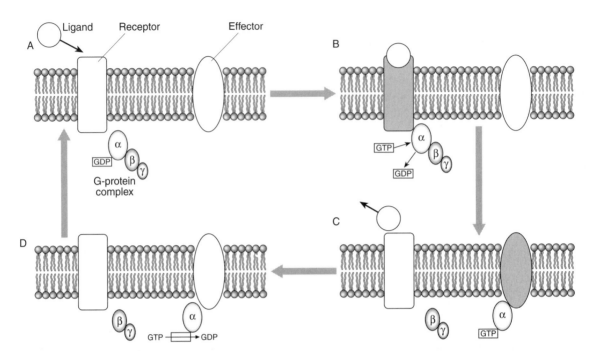

Figure 2.6   Main steps in the activation of a receptor coupled G protein (A). Ligand binding to the receptor leads to displacement of GDP from the α subunit by GTP (B) and dissociation of the α and βγ subunits (C). These dissociated elements activate other effector molecules (C). The cycle of events is completed when the α subunit degrades GTP to GDP (D) and the G protein complex reforms (A).

There are approximately 1000 different G proteins with different names and actions. Thus, G_s stimulates cyclic adenosine monophosphate (cAMP) production, whereas G_i inhibits it. Some G proteins are involved in sensory systems, e.g. in the photoreceptors of the retina. Still other G proteins include the ras proteins, which form part of the signal transduction pathways for a variety of growth factors. Some variant on the cycle of G protein activation and inactivation described above seems to apply in each case, however.

Second messengers and their release/ production

Calcium. This is the most important ion involved in intracellular communication; it triggers responses as diverse as contraction in muscle and secretion of chemical transmitters from neurones and endocrine cells. The cell maintains an intracellular Ca^{2+} concentration which is 10 000 times lower than the extracellular level. Calcium may enter from outside through one of the several types of calcium channel in the plasma membrane — for example, voltage sensitive calcium channels, which are activated by depolarisation. This explains the rationale of using calcium channel blocking agents to reduce intracellular calcium levels in cardiac and vascular muscle, thereby reducing myocardial contractility and vascular tone. Alternatively, calcium may be released from internal stores, e.g. from the endoplasmic reticulum (sarcoplasmic reticulum in muscle). These intracellular stores release their contents by opening channels in the membranes which surround them, thus allowing the calcium they contain to diffuse into the cytoplasm where it has its effects. Two important intracellular calcium channels have been identified so far, one sensitive to ryanodine and the other to inositol 1,4,5-trisphosphate. The ryanodine receptor/ channel is sensitive to the plant alkaloid ryanodine, which can activate or inhibit the opening of this channel in a dose dependent fashion. It is this ryanodine channel which allows the calcium in the sarcoplasmic reticulum of skeletal muscle to be released in response to plasma membrane depolarisation, thus activating muscle contraction. An abnormality in the ryanodine receptor, due in some cases to an inherited mutation in chromosome 19, leads to susceptibility to malignant hyperthermia (see Chs 19 and 51).

Calcium signalling is dependent on interactions with a number of calcium binding proteins, such as calmodulin (found in nearly all tissues) or troponin (found in striated muscle). Through these, calcium can initiate other reactions in the relevant pathways, e.g. by activating calcium calmodulin dependent kinases or phosphatases.

Adenylyl and guanylyl cyclase. These are large membrane-spanning proteins with an intracellular portion acting as an enzyme, which are activated by the action of stimulatory G_s proteins and inhibited by inhibitory G_i proteins in response to activation of different receptors. Adenylyl cyclase catalyses the conversion of ATP to cAMP, while guanylyl cyclase performs the same function in the formation of cyclic guanosine monophosphate (cGMP) from GTP. These cyclic nucleotides act as second messengers, which activate specific protein kinases (PKA and PKG, respectively), leading to the phosphorylation of other enzymes and functionally important proteins.

The cardiac β adrenoceptor is a typical example of a cAMP dependent signalling pathway. The cascade of events starts when noradrenaline (the first messenger) binds to the extracellular aspect of the receptor protein, leading to its activation. This activates a G_s protein which stimulates adenylyl cyclase, and this catalyses the production of cAMP. This initiates a cascade of enzymatic processes leading, for example, to increased cardiac contractility.

Phosphodiesterases degrade the cyclic nucleotides, e.g. catalysing the conversion of cAMP to adenosine monophosphate (AMP). Thus, drugs that inhibit the action of phosphodiesterase may be used to elevate cAMP levels, and these may be tissue selective, e.g. methylxanthines are used as bronchodilators, enoximone as a cardiac inotrope.

Phospholipase C. The lipids of the cell membrane are not simply inert structural components but act as important substrates for second messenger production. Phosphatidylinositol is a minor lipid existing mainly in the inner leaflet of the bilayer. Receptors are coupled by G proteins to an enzyme, phospholipase C, on the inner surface of the membrane. This cleaves the phosphorylated form of the lipid, phosphatidylinositol, to produce inositol 1,4,5-triphosphate (IP_3) and diacylglycerol (DG or DAG), both of which have important second messenger actions. IP_3 releases calcium from internal stores, thus raising the cytoplasmic concentration of free Ca^{2+}. In many cells this calcium then binds to calmodulin, leading to a wide variety of functional responses, e.g. contraction in smooth muscle. (It should be noted that this IP_3-sensitive calcium store is believed to be pharmacologically distinct from the ryanodine-sensitive store mentioned above.)

The actions of DAG, produced as a coproduct with IP_3, depend not on Ca^{2+} release but rather on its ability to activate protein kinase C (PKC), another membrane bound enzyme. This in turn phosphorylates the relevant target proteins, many of which are ion channels.

Phospholipase A_2. Another important second messenger system consists of the metabolites of the fatty acid arachidonic acid. This is released from membrane lipids by the action of the enzyme phospholipase A_2, another G-protein regulated enzyme, and is rapidly metabolised to produce a wide range of short lived but biologically potent intermediates, including the prostaglandins and thromboxanes. These messengers can act intracellularly but as they are very lipid soluble they can also cross the cell membrane to act as extracellular messengers affecting other cells.

Tyrosine kinases. Some receptors function as tyrosine kinases when activated by their agonists. The intracellular active site is an integral part of the receptor molecule and no G-protein linkage is required. This type of receptor leads to phosphorylation of tyrosine residues on target proteins and is important in the transduction pathways of a number of peptide growth factors. Mutations leading to permanent activation of such receptors may be one cause of uncontrolled growth in cancer cells.

Nuclear and cytoplasmic receptors

Some receptors are actually located within the cell itself and these are activated by lipid soluble messengers which can diffuse through the cell membrane (Fig. 2.5). Steroid and thyroid hor-

mones are good examples of messengers that act on intracellular receptors. This often leads to an increase in the rate of DNA transcription to mRNA within the nucleus, ultimately promoting an increase in the cell content of the proteins coded for by specific genes. The resulting changes in cell function may require some time to develop fully, however, and responses to intracellular receptors are generally slower in onset (hours to days) than those mediated by surface receptors (seconds to minutes).

FURTHER READING

Alper J S 1996 Genetic complexity in single gene diseases. British Medical Journal 312: 196–197
Bannister L H 1995 Cells and tissues. In: Williams P L, Bannister L H, Berry M M et al (eds) Gray's anatomy, 38th edn, pp 17–63. Churchill Livingstone, New York
Clapham D E 1996 The G-protein nanomachine. Nature 379: 297–299

Connolly D L, Shanahan C M, Weissberg P L 1996 Water channels in health and disease. Lancet 347: 210–212
Somlyo A P, Somlyo A V 1994 Signal transduction and regulation in smooth muscle. Nature 372: 231–236
Sperelakis N 1995 Defining ischaemia — when cells start screaming for help. British Medical Journal 311: 890–891

3

Pharmacodynamic aspects of drug action

W. McCaughey

A major goal in clinical pharmacology is to understand how the administration of a drug in a particular way may lead to a particular therapeutic action. The study of this has led to the separation of two aspects of drug action — pharmacokinetics and pharmacodynamics.

Study of the absorption, distribution, metabolism and elimination of a drug can often predict remarkably well how the drug concentration at the site of action will vary. This will help predict the time course and magnitude of the drug effect, but will tell nothing of the type of effect that will occur. The study of the underlying mechanisms of action of the drug and how the presence of the drug at its site of action is related to its therapeutic effect is known as pharmacodynamics. In brief, pharmacokinetics is the effect of the patient on the drug, while pharmacodynamics is the effect of the drug on the patient.

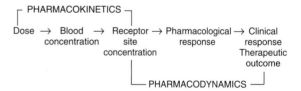

To understand the effects of drugs on the body it is necessary to have a good understanding of the structure of cell and other membranes, receptors and the pathways that the body normally uses for communication between organs and cells. These have been described briefly in Chapter 2.

DRUG ACTION AT RECEPTORS

Receptor sites are designed for intercellular communication, and are acted on by endogenous substances. They become drug receptors when an exogenous substance, a drug, that also has an affinity for the site is found.

The glycoproteins which form receptors are able to fold their tertiary shape into at least two different states. This is a dynamic equilibrium but generally, in the absence of a ligand (endogenous messenger or drug), the receptor protein will spend all or most of its time in the inactive configuration. If the drug binds to the receptor and has a higher affinity for the active than the inactive configuration of the receptor (which is another way of saying that it activates the receptor), then the equilibrium moves toward the active state, and this is the first step in initiating an intracellular response in the effector tissue. This drug action is described as *agonist* activity. Pure agonist drugs have high affinity for the active state of the receptor and thus have high intrinsic activity or efficacy.

The ability of a drug to mimic the action of an endogenous ligand implies a similarity in structure between the drug and its natural counterpart, at least in the region that interacts with the receptor site, but the rest of the molecule may be very different. A good example is the contrasting chemistry of the enkephalins, which are peptides, and morphine, an unrelated plant alkaloid. Here the benzene ring A of morphine and a benzene ring in the tyrosine group of enkephalin are in exactly the same orientation, so that their molecules can fit the same protein template.

When the drug or endogenous transmitter binds to a pharmacologically active receptor site, it changes the receptor and this initiates a sequence of events leading to the drug's characteristic action. This is not an 'all or none' effect. Usually binding is reversible, and so an equilibrium is set up. This can be represented as:

$$\text{drug} + \text{receptor} \underset{k_2}{\overset{k_1}{\longleftrightarrow}} \text{drug–receptor complex} \rightarrow \text{effect},$$

where k_1 and k_2 are rate constants for the association and dissociation of drug and receptor. In this simple model, drug effect is proportional to the fraction of receptor occupied, and maximal effect will occur when all receptors are occupied.

Dose–response curves

When the dose of drug is plotted against the effect obtained, as shown in Figure 3.1A, this gives a dose–response curve. This is approximately a rectangular hyperbola. If, however, the plot is of *log* dose against effect, this gives the familiar sigmoidal curve shown in Figure 3.1B. This not only allows a greater range of doses to be represented but, because there is a straight line relationship between log dose and response over a substantial part of this curve, it is easier to compare the actions of different drugs by its use.

Affinity

Affinity is a measure of the ability of the drug to bind to the receptor site and form a stable complex. Affinity is often represented by an IC_{50} value, which is the concentration producing 50% inhibition of the binding of a highly selective ligand. There is a high correlation between the IC_{50} of a drug and its potency. The relative affinity of the drug for the receptors may be defined as the concentration required to produce half the maximal effect; however, this simplification may be invalid if other factors, e.g. second messengers, are involved and are the limiting factor in the degree of drug effect.

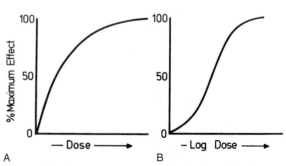

Figure 3.1   Dose–response curves for a drug plotted on (A) linear and (B) semilogarithmic scales.

Efficacy or intrinsic activity

The efficacy, or maximal efficacy, of a drug is simply the maximum effect that it is capable of producing, and it is represented by the plateau of the dose–response curve (although in some cases it may be limited by other factors, such as the ability to deliver a sufficient drug concentration to the receptor sites). The use of these terms is restricted to drugs with agonist actions.

Potency

The potency of a drug is an expression of the position of the dose–response curve along the dose axis. Thus two drugs (for example morphine and fentanyl) might have similar efficacy, but the potency of one — expressed as milligrams per kilogram required to produce a given effect — might be many times greater than that of the other. A difference in potency of two drugs is of itself not important, unless the actual mass of drug to be given is so large that it causes problems in administration.

It is often useful to compare two drugs by their relative potency — the ratio of equieffective doses. This apparently simple concept will work well for similar drugs with parallel dose–response curves, but if this is not so, as in some of the cases described below, then the relative potencies of the two drugs will be different at different dose levels.

Agonist and partial agonist activity

If a drug binds to the receptor but has only slightly greater affinity for the active than the inactive state of the receptor, then even in high concentration it will not cause all the receptor sites to be activated, and thus the maximal effect of the drug will be less. Such a drug may be referred to as a partial agonist, in contrast to the drug whose affinity is strongly in favour of the active receptor and which is referred to simply as an agonist. It may also be said that the partial agonist has a lower intrinsic activity or efficacy than the agonist drug.

With some β-adrenergic blocking drugs a different terminology is often used: they are described as having 'intrinsic sympathomimetic activity', but this is simply another way of describing partial agonist activity.

Antagonists

A drug that has no preference for the active or inactive conformation of the receptor protein, or one that encourages the inactive state, will act as an antagonist by competing with an agonist for receptor sites. This type of antagonism is known as competitive antagonism. Antagonism may also be non-competitive, where the antagonist inactivates the receptor so that an agonist cannot combine with it to cause activation. Non-competitive antagonism may be reversible or irreversible. A partial agonist, by binding to receptors but failing to produce a maximal response, can act as a competitive antagonist to a full agonist, and for this reason such drugs are also referred to as agonist-antagonists. The opioid agonist-antagonists are discussed in Chapter 17.

Dose–response curves are useful in determining some of the characteristics of a drug. Two drugs of similar efficacy but differing in potency will have parallel curves, as in Figure 3.2A, where drug (b) is of lower potency. A common example would be morphine and fentanyl, each capable of producing the same degree of analgesia but at very different milligram doses. The same displacement of the dose–response curve to the right would be seen in the presence of a competitive antagonist. In this case, the potency of the drug (a) is reduced, so that it follows curve

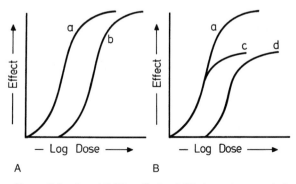

A   B

Figure 3.2 A and B: The effects of differing potency and of partial agonist activity on dose response (see text for explanation).

(b), but it is still able to achieve its maximal effect if given in sufficient concentration.

A different situation occurs (Fig. 3.2B) if the drug is unable to obtain the maximum effect from the system. This might occur if a non-competitive antagonist had removed some of the receptor potential from the system (for example by binding with them), or if the drug is by nature a partial agonist. In this case, as compared with the normal response to a full agonist (curve a), the maximal response is reduced (curve c). Thus the potency of the drug, at least over the lower part of the dose range, is relatively unchanged, but the maximal efficacy is reduced. A useful quantifiable parameter in studying drug–receptor interaction, particularly when several receptors may be involved, as with the opioids, is the pA_2. This is the negative logarithm of the concentration of drug necessary to produce a particular level of response. If a series of agonists acts on the same receptor, then, although a different concentration of each may be required to produce the same effect, the pA_2 will be the same. Studies examining the antagonism by naloxone of the analgesia produced by a wide variety of μ-agonist opioids, including morphine and β-endorphin, give uniform pA_2 values of approximately 7. In contrast, the pA_2 value with (D-Ala2, D-Leu5 enkephalin), a δ-receptor agonist, is approximately 6, that is it takes 10 times more naloxone to antagonise DADL than morphine. This suggests that these two classes of agents act on different receptor populations for which naloxone has differing affinities.

OTHER FACTORS IN DRUG RESPONSE

Drugs do not all act, as has been implied in this simplified description of drug action, by a single action occurring at a single receptor site. More than one receptor type or subtype may be involved, and many other factors come into play, so that actual dose–response curves may differ widely from those shown above. The opioids again provide a good example of drugs that produce similar and also different effects at different receptors (see Ch. 17).

Some drugs act by mechanisms not involving receptor sites, for example by competing for transport systems, or by purely physical effects, like osmotic diuretics.

The clinical usefulness of the drug may be influenced by some other features of its action.

Selectivity

Selectivity, the ability of the drug to produce its desired effect with a minimum of other undesired or side-effects, is important in this context.

Therapeutic index

Therapeutic index is a measure of the safety of the drug in normal use. It is the ratio of the dose of the drug which produces the desired effect to the dose which produces an important toxic effect. If the slope of the dose–response curve is steep, then increasing the dose will more easily raise the effect to levels where toxic effects can arise, so that the drug must be treated more carefully.

VARIATION IN RESPONSE
Normal distribution

Individual patients vary in their response to a drug, and the same patient may exhibit a different response on different occasions. This can be seen either as different responses to the same dose, or as different doses being required to produce the same response. In either case the variation between individuals can almost always be seen to follow the usual normal distribution or gaussian curve of variation (Fig. 3.3A) when, for example, the number of individuals having each degree of response is plotted. This simply represents the random differences between people, as would be found with height, weight, etc.

ED_{50} and LD_{50}

When different doses of a drug are given, and a certain end-point sought, a dose can be found

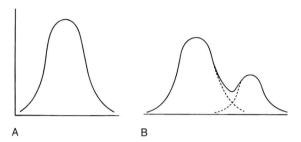

Figure 3.3 A: Continuous or gaussian distribution. B: Discontinuous or bimodal distribution.

when half the individuals produce the effect sought. The dose at which 50% of individuals show a specified effect is the median effective dose, or ED_{50}. The dose to produce an effect in a different percentage of individuals could also be estimated. In animal testing of drugs the dose to produce a toxic effect is also used — if the endpoint is death, this is the median lethal dose or LD_{50}. The therapeutic index can then be defined as the ratio of these:

$$\text{therapeutic index} = \frac{LD_{50}}{ED_{50}}.$$

In some situations another toxic effect might be used to define toxicity — for example, in testing a respiratory stimulant, the ratio of the dose to produce a therapeutic stimulation and that to produce convulsions. The therapeutic index of a drug is important in determining its safety in use and is a useful comparison between drugs.

Pharmacogenetics

Some of the variation between individuals is genetically determined. This may be pharmacodynamic in origin — a variation in responsiveness to the drugs, leading to the normal gaussian distribution curve described above (Fig. 3.3A). More of the important variations are pharmacokinetic — there is an altered handling of the drug by the body. When the distribution of drug responses is measured in some of these cases it can be seen that there exist two (or more) distinct populations, which behave differently in response to the drug, and which also have

a normal variation within each population (Fig. 3.3B).

Such different populations are likely to be due to genetic polymorphism, and the different populations are maintained from one generation to the next by inheritance of different genes. One of the most common causes of pharmacokinetic differences between subpopulations is difference in expression of cytochrome p450 enzymes in the liver, leading to different patterns of metabolism of drugs in different individuals. This is explored in more detail in Chapter 4. A classical example in anaesthetic practice is the rare occurrence of an abnormally prolonged response to suxamethonium, resulting in abnormally prolonged paralysis and apnoea. Here there are at least four different genetically determined variants of the cholinesterase enzyme (see Ch. 20), which break down suxamethonium at different rates.

These are examples of altered pharmacokinetic handling of drugs, but there are many examples of altered response at molecular level in the type of response — pharmacodynamic differences. The most dramatic in anaesthesia is the rare syndrome of malignant hyperpyrexia (see Ch. 50) in which an abnormality in one gene (in chromosome 19 in some cases) codes for an abnormality in the calcium channel in the sarcolemma. In susceptible individuals certain drugs, including suxamethonium and volatile anaesthetic agents, may trigger a massive and potentially fatal hyperpyrexic response.

Other clinically relevant examples of genetically determined conditions in which there is an altered response to drug therapy include the porphyrias and some of the conditions due to haemoglobin variants.

Factors modifying the degree of response to drugs

While there is inherently a variability in the response of patients to drugs, some factors can be identified and, when they are taken into account, the dosage of a drug can be better tailored to the patient's needs. Not all are relevant to anaesthetic practice but some are described in the following section.

Psychological factors

These include the willingness and ability of the patient to take the prescribed drug, and of the nurse or doctor to prescribe the drug appropriately and accurately. Medication errors are in practice extremely common.

The placebo response is also important in many cases, the response to the drug being modified by the patient's mental attitude, so that a response may be obtained from an inert substance, or an exaggerated — or reduced — response obtained from an active drug. For this reason many clinical trials to test the efficacy of a drug must use a protocol that assesses or eliminates the placebo response. A variant of this type of response is seen in the fact that it has been shown that a preoperative visit to a patient by the anaesthetist has an equal anxiolytic effect to that produced by administration of a barbiturate.

Age

The young, particularly the neonate, may differ profoundly from the adult in handling of and response to drugs. In the elderly, too, there are differences, partly due to changes in physiological variables and partly due to an increased incidence of disease. These are discussed in later chapters.

Body weight and volume of distribution

These pharmacokinetic factors are discussed elsewhere.

Body rhythms

The influence of circadian or other rhythms on drug treatment has not been well studied but may be important — for example, the anticoagulant effect of a constant dose of heparin may vary by as much as half between night and morning, and other drugs might theoretically vary in their effect and toxicity, depending on the time of administration.

Physiological and pathological variables

There are marked variations in the response to drug therapy caused either by physiological variations in respiration, cardiac output, blood flow and distribution of blood flow, renal function, etc., or by changes in these and similar variables caused by acute or chronic disease. Some of these are described in other chapters.

Tolerance, addiction and sensitivity

The response to a drug does not always remain the same. In some cases a greater response is achieved initially rather than later — the body becomes tolerant to the effects of the drug. This may take several days to months to develop, or may occur very rapidly in minutes or seconds. In the latter case it is known as acute tolerance or tachyphylaxis. This occurs with several drugs, including local anaesthetics. Conversely, situations exist in which the response is exaggerated — there is a state of sensitivity or supersensitivity to the drug (the term hypersensitivity is used only to describe conditions of an allergic nature).

Tolerance that develops very rapidly to a drug, so that there is decreasing response to repeat doses given within a short time, is known as tachyphylaxis. The mechanism of this is different with different drugs. Another phenomenon that develops in an extremely short time, and presumably is due to a change at cellular level, is the acute tolerance seen with barbiturate anaesthetics. Patients who receive thiopentone regain consciousness while the blood concentration of thiopentone is still higher than that at which they lost consciousness.

Altered sensitivity to a drug may occur by one or several mechanisms:

- Continued administration may lead to a change in its absorption or to an increase in its rate of elimination, or there may be a change in its passage to its site of action; these are all pharmacokinetic mechanisms.
- Homeostatic mechanisms may compensate for its action: patients taking thyroid hormone may become tolerant to its effects because of feedback involving pituitary and thyroid glands.
- Antibodies may develop, as in some cases of insulin resistance.
- With indirectly acting sympathomimetic amines such as ephedrine, tachyphylaxis

occurs because stores of noradrenaline become depleted.

Some cases may be mixed: tolerance to chronic use of barbiturates or alcohol is partly due to increased drug metabolism, but tolerant individuals will show less response to the drug even when brain levels are identical to those in non-tolerant individuals. There may be cross-tolerance between drugs of similar pharmacological classes.

• In many cases there has been a change or changes as cellular level. Many different mechanisms may be involved in different cases, and knowledge of these is scanty.

Tolerance to β-adrenergic receptors may initially involve uncoupling of β adrenoceptors from the stimulatory guanine nucleotide binding protein G_s, and at the same time reduction in the number of active β receptors as these are internalised or sequestrated, so that adenylate cyclase activity is reduced. With prolonged exposure to β agonists, the total number of receptors is reduced. Chronic alcohol exposure may lead to uncoupling of G_s protein in several receptors, and also perhaps to changes in cell membrane lipids.

Tolerance, dependence and addiction to opioid drugs occurs, related to their action on receptors normally occupied by enkephalins. This too may involve changes in the coupling of G proteins. Occupation of the receptor by an opioid may also activate a feedback mechanism to reduce the amount of enkephalin, either by reducing the quantity released (for which there is some evidence) or by increasing the rate of its breakdown — there is a considerable increase in the enzyme that degrades enkephalin. Thus, with lack of endogenous enkephalin at the receptor site, more opioid is needed to replace it — tolerance has occurred. In addition, when opioid is withdrawn, the lack of inhibitory effect, which activation of the enkephalin receptor causes, is seen as a withdrawal syndrome. This may be due to increased activity of certain noradrenergic neurones in the locus ceruleus region of the brain (see also Ch. 17). The activity of these can be reduced, and the withdrawal syndrome suppressed, by low doses of the α_2 agonist clonidine.

Increased sensitivity to a drug or natural transmitter substance may also be due to an increase in the number of receptor molecules. Following denervation of a muscle, it can be shown that the muscle end-plate region expands to cover virtually the whole of the muscle fibre, leading to increased sensitivity (and also to the danger of excessive release of extracellular potassium when suxamethonium is administered). An increase in the number of receptor sites can also be found as a result of drug therapy. Long term treatment with β-adrenergic blocking drugs may cause an increase in the number of adrenergic receptor sites, and abrupt cessation of these drugs in patients can sometimes lead to cardiac arrhythmias or myocardial infarction.

• There may be interplay between different receptors and nervous pathways; for example, glutamate antagonists have been shown to prevent morphine withdrawal in mice and guinea pigs, suggesting that the activation of excitatory amino acid receptors, mainly the NMDA (*N*-methyl-D-aspartate) receptors, plays a role in the expression of opiate abstinence (Tanganelli et al 1991). Nitric oxide may also be involved in development of tolerance to morphine and to ethanol, as this can be prevented by blockade of nitric oxide synthase (Khanna et al 1993, Kolesnikov et al 1993).

REFERENCES

Khanna J M, Morato G S, Shah G, Chau A, Kalant H 1993 Inhibition of nitric oxide synthesis impairs rapid tolerance to ethanol. Brain Research Bulletin 32: 43–47
Kolesnikov Y A, Pick C G, Ciszewska G, Pasternak G W 1993 Blockade of tolerance to morphine but not to kappa opioids by a nitric oxide synthase inhibitor. Proceedings of the National Academy of Sciences of the United States of America 90: 5162–5166
Tanganelli S, Antonelli T, Morari M, Bianchi C, Beani L 1991 Glutamate antagonists prevent morphine withdrawal in mice and guinea pigs. Neuroscience Letters 122: 270–272

4

Pharmacokinetics

W. McCaughey

BASIC CONCEPTS

A drug causes an effect by acting on some body process — often by interfering with an existing neurotransmitter or hormonal pathway or some intracellular process, and often, but not always by acting on a receptor. These pharmacodynamic concepts were discussed in Chapters 2 and 3. Pharmacodynamic factors determine what the effect of a certain concentration of drug at its site of action will be. Pharmacokinetics is concerned with how the drug gets to its site of action, what influences its concentration there and how this will change with time.

Equilibria and transport across membranes

The various compartments of the body are separated by different kinds of membrane. Many substances cross by simple passive diffusion or filtration or by osmosis. These do not require energy, and obey simple laws of physics. Others cross by specialised processes: active transport, facilitated diffusion, exchange diffusion.

Lipid solubility and ionisation

The main factors influencing the rate at which a drug crosses a membrane are the *permeability* of the membrane to the drug molecules, and the *concentration gradient* between one side and the other.

  Body fluids are aqueous solutions so, in order to be distributed around the body, a drug must be soluble in water. The cell membrane is, however, composed mainly of phospholipid and most membranes therefore behave as though they were mostly made of lipid, and the ability of a drug to cross is mainly dependent on its solubility in lipid — although water and some small molecules that are water soluble (hydrophilic) can cross reasonably easily, if their molecular weight is below about 100.

Lipid solubility is a property that may be quantified as a partition coefficient λ (lambda) by measuring how a drug in solution will divide itself between a water phase and an oily phase, which has been chosen to simulate the lipids of body membranes. In the early work by Overton and Meyer, olive oil was used, but now other substances such as butanol, octanol or heptane are more commonly chosen. These different substances may each be more appropriate to model different body membranes.

Many drugs are weak electrolytes — acids or bases, which can exist in an ionised or an un-ionised form, the degree of ionisation depending on the pH of their surroundings. Usually only the unionised form of the drug is sufficiently lipid soluble to diffuse through biological membranes — lipophilicity falls by a factor of about 10 000 when ionisation occurs — and the ionised drug can cross only if it is of sufficiently low molecular size to penetrate the aqueous channels in the membrane.

The ionised and unionised forms of the drug are in equilibrium. From the Henderson–Hasselbalch equation (see Ch. 1), it can be seen that when the pH is close to the pK_a of the drug (the pH at which the drug is 50% ionised), then small changes in pH will result in large changes in the degree of ionisation of the drug, and in its behaviour. Strong acids have low pK_a values and strong bases high values, so that both are highly ionised at the range of pH found in the body. However the degree of ionisation of weak acids and weak bases with pK_a values close to body pH (6.5–8.5) will be markedly affected by pH changes. Increased acidity, i.e. a decrease in pH, will cause a weak acid to become less ionised and therefore more highly lipid soluble — thus phenobarbitone, for example, will be readily absorbed from the acidic surroundings of the gastric juice. The reverse situation will occur with weakly basic drugs, such as local anaesthetics, in which acidification will increase ionisation and decrease lipid solubility (see Ch. 7, p. 92 and Table 7.2).

Membrane transport mechanisms

Passive mechanisms

Drugs cross membranes by a number of means. Passive mechanisms do not require the expenditure of energy, and diffusion is driven by a concentration, osmotic or electrochemical gradient. The rate of movement depends on a number of factors: the concentration difference between the two sides of the membrane, lipid solubility and state of ionisation of the drug (as described above), molecular weight, and in addition the surface area available for diffusion, the thickness of the membrane, and the temperature. A few small molecules diffuse through aqueous pores in the membrane, but this is important only for those of mol. wt. 100–200 or less; nevertheless it explains why the lipid-insoluble morphine molecule actually diffuses relatively well from the epidural space to cerebrospinal fluid (CSF). For most drugs lipid solubility is more important.

Specialised transport mechanisms

Carrier mediated active transport is the means by which many amino acids, sugars, etc. are transported across cell membranes. This is an energy consuming process in which the drug or other substance is carried across the membrane while associated with a carrier molecule. It is able to act against the concentration gradient.

Facilitated diffusion is similar, in that movement is increased or facilitated by a carrier molecule, but differs in that it does not consume energy and cannot cause movement against the concentration gradient. Both these mechanisms are specific for a particular type of chemical structure and can be saturated. Thus one substance which is a substrate for such a pathway can interfere with movement of another by competition with it. The classical example is competition for excretion by the organic anion pathway in the kidney by penicillin and probenecid.

Pinocytosis is the process in which a portion of cell membrane invaginates and pinches off to form a vesicle containing the molecule to be transported. This is used to transport large molecules such as proteins and glycoproteins.

Special membranes: blood–brain barrier

The blood–brain barrier separates two of the major compartments of the central nervous system (the brain and the CSF) from the third compartment (the blood). It exists to regulate the access of substances in the blood to the nervous system. The barrier is located at the endothelial layer of brain capillaries. In most tissues, endothelial cells are separated by gaps of 10 nm (100 Å) or more, forming fenestrations or a 'small pore system' through which molecules in aqueous solution can exchange. Within the central nervous system, the plasma membranes of endothelial cells partially fuse to form 'tight junctions', with the result that they act almost like a continuous layer of cells. At barrier sites, substances that can most easily cross are those which are highly lipid soluble, so that they are able to pass directly through the layer of cells. The blood–brain barrier is highly impermeable to ions and macromolecules like proteins, although they can still cross at a very slow rate, probably through the tight junctions.

The blood–brain barrier is situated at the interface between the blood and the other compartments: at the choroid plexus and the blood vessels of the brain and subarachnoid spaces, and also at the arachnoid membrane. Peripheral nerves have a barrier at the blood vessels of the endoneurium and at the perineurium, which surrounds nerve bundles. The eye, being derived directly from nervous tissue, also has a barrier. The blood–brain barrier is not complete, and there are special sites where normal fenestrated capillaries exist. These sites are required for and involved in transfer of hormones between blood and nervous tissues. Sites include the chemoceptor trigger zone. Peripherally, olfactory receptor cells, terminal endings of peripheral nerves, and sensory ganglia also have no barrier.

CSF is produced at the choroid plexus. Here the choroidal epithelial cells are joined by tight junctions, and passive exchange of water and solutes between blood and CSF is restricted. Sodium is actively transported into the CSF, accompanied by Cl^- and HCO_3^-, and water follows passively down the osmotic gradient. Many other substances cross the choroid plexus by processes such as facilitated diffusion and active transport. These include mono- and divalent ions, glucose, amino acids and various organic acids and bases, some of which are drugs. The purpose of this activity is to maintain an environment around neurones and glia that is homeostatic and distinct from plasma.

The CSF may be considered together with the brain, as there is no barrier to diffusion between these two compartments, so that drugs that do not have ready access to the brain may sometimes be given by injection into the CSF.

The blood–brain barrier, as well as some other aspects of brain development, such as myelination, seems to be incomplete at birth, and the penetration of drugs in the neonate may differ from that in adults.

Drug transfer across the blood–brain barrier

The major feature of the blood–brain barrier is that, as described above, it behaves mainly like a continuous lipid membrane. Many of the drugs used in anaesthetic practice are weak acids or bases, and are largely unionised at body pH, so that they readily penetrate the blood–brain barrier. Substances that are highly ionised, such as strong acids or bases, or quaternary ammonium compounds, would not be expected to be able to cross in any detectable quantity. In fact ions also have a finite though small lipid solubility, and may be able to cross in amounts that are pharmacologically significant.

The permeability of the blood–brain barrier may be increased if the tight junctions between cells are opened up. This may be caused by inflammation, as in meningitis or encephalitis, or in other pathological situations, such as hypertensive encephalopathy, cerebral ischaemia or head injury. It may also be caused by osmotically active substances — for example, contrast media used in cerebral angiography or concentrated glucose solutions. If this occurs, then drugs or other substances may enter the brain more readily. The dangers of this are obvious but it may also be useful in allowing better access of antibiotics in treatment of meningitis, or antimitotic drugs in tumour therapy.

MATHEMATICAL CONCEPTS IN PHARMACOKINETICS

First order kinetics

The law of mass action states that the rate at which a chemical reaction proceeds is proportional to the active masses of the reacting substances. This is simply because the rate of reaction is proportional to the rate at which the molecules involved collide with each other and thus have an opportunity to react. This law leads to several principles fundamental to drug disposition. In chemical reactions, generally if two compounds X and Y are reacting, the rate of reaction is proportional to [X] * [Y]. This is a second order reaction. However, in situations such as diffusion across a membrane, the two things that are reacting are a limited amount of substance X and a very large number of molecules of the membrane. This second number is so much in excess of the other that it can be regarded as constant. Thus rate is proportional to [X]. The same applies most of the time to a drug reacting with an enzyme system that is metabolising it — the reactive sites in enzyme molecules are more than able to react with any molecule of drug which passes, and rate of reaction is proportional to [X]. This is first order kinetics.

If rate of reaction is proportional to concentration of X, then rate = k_x [X], where k_x is a constant known as the rate constant or velocity constant of the reaction. A constant proportion of the remaining substance X disappears in any given time, independent of the initial concentration.

The equation describing this process is an exponential — concentration of drug falls exponentially, and so the concentration at any time (') can be calculated using the equation:

$$C = C_0e^{-kt},$$

where C_0 is the initial concentration, k is the rate constant, and e = 2.718.

The time constant τ (tau) is equal to $1/k$, and is the time at which concentration falls to $1/e$ or 36.8% of its initial value (Fig. 4.1). It is also the time that it would have taken for the concentration to drop to zero if the rate of decay had continued at its initial rate. This is a difficult concept (and not immediately useful), and so it is customary to quote a half-life ($t_{1/2}$) for the process — the time required for the amount to fall to half its initial value. One half-life is equal to 0.698τ.

A graph of concentration of X against time is an exponential curve (Fig. 4.2), but log concentration is proportional to time, and so if plotted on semilogarithmic paper, the curve is transformed into a straight line. A reaction of this type is known as a first order reaction, or as a process following first order kinetics.

This concept applies not only to reactions in which substances react chemically, but also to processes such as diffusion between compartments of the body. Again the rate can be described in terms of a rate constant. Often movement is bidirectional, and in this case a different rate constant may apply to movement in each direction.

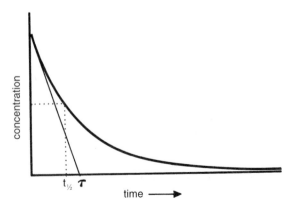

Figure 4.1 Exponential decay.

$$\xleftarrow{\ k_1\ }$$
$$\overrightarrow{k_2}$$

Actually the rate of fall of the concentration will not be exactly exponential, as there are two opposing movements going on, and the result is the sum of these.

Enzyme kinetics: zero order and Michaelis–Menten kinetics

The situation is different if we are dealing with an enzyme system or with, for example, a transport system where there is not a great excess of capacity to deal with the drug — the process is saturable. Then a situation can occur in which a constant amount of substance is changed per unit time, independent of the concentration of the substance present. These are known as zero order reactions, or reactions following zero order kinetics. A zero order reaction will give a straight line plot on a linear concentration–time plot (Fig. 4.2).

To see why processes in the body should be zero and first order, it is useful to look superficially at the kinetics of reactions involving enzymes acting on a substrate. From a mathematical treatment known as the Michaelis–Menten equation, it can be shown that a graph of velocity of reaction versus substrate concentration is a rectangular hyperbole (Fig. 4.3). The velocity of reaction, v at concentration C is given by:

$$v = C \times v_{max} / (C + K_m),$$

where K_m is a constant, the Michaelis constant.

In the majority of cases, the substrate concentration is relatively low, so that the lower, straight part of the graph is used, and in the presence of an excess of enzyme the concentration of substrate is the controlling factor, and first order kinetics prevail. Occasionally the enzyme system is easily saturated, for example in metabolism of alcohol, and thus the reaction is occurring at its maximum rate, and a zero order reaction results.

It is obvious that there will also be some drugs that, at clinically used doses, will fall into an intermediate position. These are said to have dose dependent kinetics. Phenytoin is an example of such a drug, but this phenomenon is relatively unusual at therapeutic concentrations.

Often reactions proceed by several steps, and in these cases the step that proceeds most slowly is known as the rate limiting step. If the rate limiting stage is not the first, there may be a build-up of intermediate substances, which can be an important factor in drug toxicity.

A different type of dose dependent variability in drug response can be due to the effect of a drug on, for example, cardiac output.

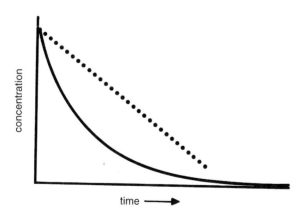

Figure 4.2   Zero order (····) and first order (—) kinetics.

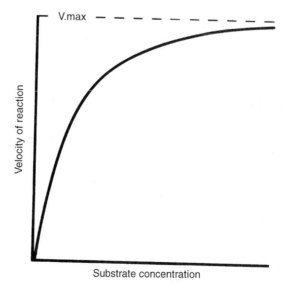

Figure 4.3   Kinetics of enzyme reactions.

Pharmacokinetic models

Volume of distribution (V_D)

When a drug is injected into the body, the plasma concentration found should, in the simplest case, be the dose given divided by the volume through which it distributes itself — or V_D = dose/concentration; however, because drugs do not all cross membranes equally easily, some may distribute into a volume less than the whole body. On the other hand, some may give a low plasma concentration, having apparently distributed into a volume larger than that of the whole body. This is possible because some tissues may be able to take up large amounts of drug — for example, into fat if the partition coefficient for fat is high, or by binding to tissue proteins. Because of these factors, the V_D is described as the *apparent volume of distribution*, but although it is an artificial concept, it is useful in allowing correct prediction of the relationship between total drug content of the body and plasma concentration of the drug.

The volume of distribution of many drugs is reduced in the elderly, partly because of reduced binding of the drug to proteins. Some disease states may also be important — for example, decreased cardiac output from heart failure or haemorrhage, by reducing perfusion of tissues, may lead to a reduced volume of distribution and thus an increased plasma level of the drug.

Because drugs and other substances do not distribute equally rapidly to all compartments of the body, it is possible to have more than one measurement of the volume of distribution, depending on whether it is measured early, when the drug is largely in the hypothetical 'central' compartment (V_{D_1}), or later, when it has equilibrated further, or when it is assumed to have reached a steady state ($V_{D_{ss}}$), and more sophisticated models of drug kinetics may require even further definitions.

Multiple compartment models

Attempts to apply mathematical analysis to the processes of absorption, distribution and elimination of drugs has led to the practice of re-garding the body as made up of one, two or three or more compartments, depending on the drug studied and the sophistication of the mathematics applied, and thus constructing mathematical models of the rate of transfer of drug from one to the other, which can be matched with actual measured values. Although the 'central' compartment is composed largely of the plasma and richly perfused tissues, and the 'peripheral' or tissue compartment of the less well perfused tissues, the compartments do not represent accurately any anatomical or physiological reality. In practice it has turned out that too-complex models have been less successful than simpler ones, because the quality of information available as to the exact constants involved in various intercompartmental movements is insufficient. The behaviour of many drugs is fairly closely described by two- or three-compartment models.

If a drug is given rapidly into the bloodstream, i.e. into the central compartment of the body, its initial plasma concentration will approximate to the dose distributed within the central compartment, i.e.:

$$C = \text{dose}/V_D.$$

The concentration will then begin to fall as the drug leaves the central compartment, both by elimination from the body and by distribution to the peripheral compartment.

The rate of elimination of the drug from the body, by metabolism or excretion, will be (at least at the beginning) proportional to the concentration in the central compartment. However, initially most of the transfer of drug out of the central compartment is to equilibrate with the peripheral compartment. The rate of this transfer is proportional to the difference between drug concentrations in central (C_1) and peripheral (C_2) compartments (Fig. 4.4). As distribution and elimination continue, C_2 will increase to equal C_1 and then, as elimination continues to lower C_1, C_2 will exceed it, and the drug is thereafter moving from peripheral to central compartments and thence to elimination. The result of these interrelated processes is that an initial rapid distribution phase is succeeded by a slower elimination phase.

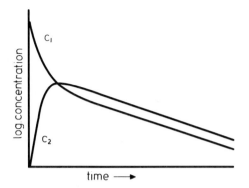

Figure 4.4 Log concentrations in both compartments of a two-compartment open model after an intravenous dose.

The curve of plasma (central compartment) concentration after such a bolus intravenous injection is the algebraic sum of two exponential curves (commonly described as a biexponential curve), and can be expressed as:

$$C = A\,e^{-\alpha t} + B\,e^{-\beta t},$$

where α and β are the rate constants for the two exponential components, and half-lives can be calculated for each of the components. These are described as distribution or α phase, with a half-time $t_{\frac{1}{2}}\alpha$, and elimination or β phase, with a half-time $t_{\frac{1}{2}}\beta$.

On a graph of log concentration versus time, these phases can be separated (Fig. 4.5). As in the later phases, elimination is the dominant process and is a first order process, the later part of the

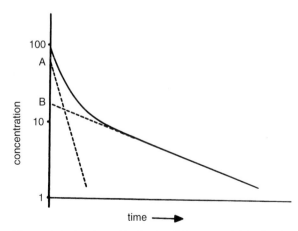

Figure 4.5 Semilogarithmic plot of biexponential decline in plasma concentration.

graph is approximately a straight line. By extrapolating this line back to intercept the y axis, and subtracting it from the original combined plot, a second straight line can be derived, which represents the component due to drug distribution. The intercepts A and B of these lines are the constants that appear in the equation for the curve.

In studies of drug pharmacokinetics, an attempt is made to find the mathematical model that best parallels the actual measurements made. A two-compartment model may give a reasonable fit, or it may be necessary to use a more complicated model. Any such descriptions, as fitting two- or three-compartment models for example, must be approximate, for reasons already stated.

If a model with more than two compartments is used, then other terms may be introduced. In a three-compartment model, it is usual to use π as the constant for the first, most rapid phase of distribution, followed by a slower α phase and by a β elimination phase. Thus:

$$C = P e^{-\pi t} + A e^{-\alpha t} + B e^{-\beta t}$$

However, terminology is not entirely constant: the two early phases may also be termed α_1 and α_2 and the idea of a late 'γ' phase following α and β has been used in describing, for example, the very slow terminal elimination of a drug such as gentamicin, which is only slowly released from tissue binding sites.

An old multiple compartment model, which is familiar to anaesthetists, is the division of the body tissues in terms of tissue perfusion into a vessel-rich group (VRG), a muscle group (MG) and a fat or vessel-poor group (VPG). This was used in particular in describing the disposition of intravenous induction agents.

Clearance

With first order kinetics, the rate of elimination of a drug is constantly changing as the concentration falls. Measurement of plasma half-life is one way to express the elimination kinetics of the drug; another concept that is used widely is clearance.

If the rate of elimination is proportional to concentration, this is the same as saying that at any point in time, rate of elimination = concentration × a constant, or, rate of elimination/concentration = constant. It we call this constant 'clearance', then clearance = rate of elimination/concentration, and looking at the units, this will be measured as volume per unit time (for example, millilitres per minute) and it is thus defined as the volume of plasma cleared totally of the drug or other substance in unit time.

The total clearance of the drug from plasma may be due to contributions by different organs, e.g. total clearance = hepatic clearance + renal clearance. For an individual organ, or compartment, the clearance (Cl) (volume of plasma cleared in unit time) is flow × fraction of drug removed in unit time; i.e. $Cl = Q \times (C_a - C_v)/C_a$, where Q is the flow and C_a and C_v are the concentrations entering and leaving the compartment. The fraction $(C_a - C_v)/C_a$ is the *extraction ratio*.

Extraction ratio

In general, drugs are not completely cleared from the plasma in one passage through the eliminating organ. The proportion that is removed is the extraction ratio, which is the ratio of clearance to total blood flow through the organ. For example, if an opioid drug eliminated by the liver has a clearance of 1200 ml min^{-1}, and the total hepatic blood flow is 1500 ml min^{-1}, then the extraction ratio for this drug will be 80%. It could be predicted from such figures that this drug would be relatively ineffective by the oral route because of the high rate of first pass metabolism.

Area under the curve

The drug concentration–time curve may be used as a measure of the total amount of drug in the body.

If the equation for clearance, *rate of elimination = clearance × concentration* is modified for a small interval of time, dt [multiply across by time (dt)], then it becomes:

mass eliminated = clearance × concentration × dt

Concentration × dt is the corresponding small area under the curve (AUC) for the time interval dt. The total amount eventually eliminated will be the sum of all these small increments, and so will be the total AUC × clearance. For an intravenous dose, this will be equal to the total dose administered, and so dose = Cl × AUC.

The AUC may be used in several ways; for example, in determining the contribution of renal and other routes to the total clearance of a drug, the total clearance may be calculated from the dose administered and the area under the plasma concentration–time curve, while the renal clearance is estimated from the total amount eliminated in the urine and the urinary excretion rate.

If a drug is given other than directly intravenously, then the total amount administered may not enter the circulation in an active form. After oral administration, not only may absorption be incomplete but metabolism of the drug to a different form may occur in the gut wall or liver before the drug reaches the systemic circulation. AUC for the plasma concentration–time curve following oral administration may be used to estimate the amount of the drug absorbed, and compared with the dose administered (or with the AUC after an intravenous dose), to estimate the oral bioavailability of the drug as a percentage.

Single and multiple dosing: infusion kinetics

Anaesthetic practice is unusual in that a majority of drugs are given as a single dose and by the intravenous route. Where repeated doses are given, then the principles just described can be used to calculate the effect of later doses of drug. Usually the aim is to maintain the plasma level of the drug at a certain therapeutic level or within a therapeutic range.

Using the simplest, one-compartment model, if a drug is given intravenously then the plasma concentration $C = dose/V_D$. After administration, the concentration declines exponentially, and so if a second equal dose is given before elimination is complete, a higher peak plasma drug concentration will be reached (Fig. 4.6). This

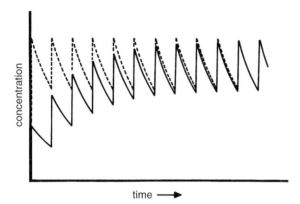

Figure 4.6 One-compartment model of drug accumulation with multiple dosing: —, no loading dose; - - - - -, correct loading dose given.

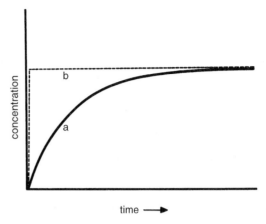

Figure 4.7 One-compartment model of (a) infusion and (b) loading dose and infusion.

will occur with each succeeding dose, but eventually a steady state will be reached as the tendency to accumulate is balanced by the increased rate of elimination at higher plasma concentrations. The rate at which the steady state is reached will depend on the elimination half-life of the drug: 50% of steady state is reached in one half-life, and 97% in five half-lives. There will of course be a fluctuation between peak and trough values with each dose, even when the steady state has been reached, and this will be more marked if the dosage interval is relatively long in comparison to the half-life of the drug, and vice versa. The steady state reached will depend on the dose and interval between doses, as well as the half-life and volume of distribution of the drug.

In order to avoid the delay between starting treatment and achieving therapeutic drug concentrations, a loading dose may be given, followed by appropriate maintenance doses of the drug.

Intravenous infusions

The fluctuation of plasma levels between peak and trough values may be minimised by giving smaller doses of drug at more frequent intervals, and the logical conclusion of this process is to use a constant intravenous infusion. During a steady-state infusion, the plasma concentration will rise exponentially toward a steady-state value. This curve (Fig. 4.7a) is often referred to as a 'wash-in' curve, as opposed to the more familiar 'wash out' curve. Again the steady state will be achieved in approximately five half-lives, while it could be achieved immediately by giving a loading dose equal to the desired steady-state concentration $\times V_D$ and maintained by a constant infusion at a rate equal to the rate of elimination (Fig. 4.7b).

In practice of course, the one-compartment model described falls far short of describing what actually occurs, as redistribution must be taken into account as well as elimination, and this is to one or more peripheral compartments. In the real-life situation, the rate of infusion for maintenance is still as described, but the idea of a loading dose must be modified because of the time taken for diffusion into various compartments. Figure 4.8 shows the pattern of change in plasma concentration with different approaches to this problem. From this diagram, it would seem that 'e', a combination of bolus + loading infusion + exponentially decreasing maintenance infusion, would achieve the ideal, but in practice the difficulty in obtaining the numerical values needed and interindividual variation make this difficult to achieve. The various regimens that are used for total intravenous anaesthesia with propofol are approximations to this principle.

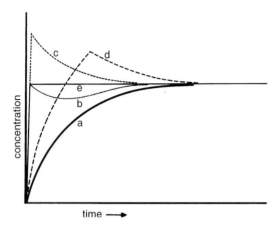

Figure 4.8   Theoretical changes in plasma concentration of drug with various intravenous infusion techniques: (a) maintenance infusion alone; (b) loading dose ($C \times V_{D_{initial}}$) + maintenance infusion; (c) loading dose ($C \times V_{D_{ss}}$) + maintenance infusion; (d) loading infusion + maintenance infusion; (e) loading dose + exponentially reducing loading infusion + maintenance infusion.

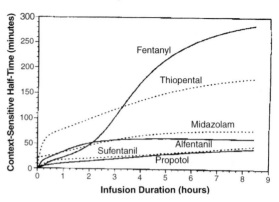

Figure 4.9   Context-sensitive half-times as a function of infusion duration for computer simulations of pharmacokinetic models. (Reproduced with permission from Hughes, Glass, Jacobs 1992 Anesthesiology 76: 334–341.)

Context-sensitive half-time

The rate of recovery from the effect might reasonably be assumed to be related to its elimination half-life ($t_{1/2}\beta$). This is largely the case for recovery from a single dose, but following repeated dosing or infusions the situation is often very different, and more complex. Pharmacokinetic data are usually quoted for single bolus doses of a drug. When an infusion is given, drug continues to diffuse into the slow or peripheral compartment during the infusion. When infusion stops, the rate at which plasma concentration falls will depend not only on the rate of removal of drug by metabolism and excretion, but also on the rate at which it diffuses back from the peripheral compartment. This in turn depends on the rate constant for diffusion between central and peripheral compartments, the size of the peripheral compartment, and the time which it has had to fill. The time for concentration to fall to half that at the end of infusion has been described as the context-sensitive half-time.

Figure 4.9 shows a computer simulation of how the recovery time from infusion of some drugs (as represented by the context-sensitive half-time) increases with duration of infusion. It can be seen from this that there is not a simple relationship between the commonly quoted half-life, derived from studies of single doses, and the context-sensitive half-life after infusion or repeat dosing.

Elimination by other processes

A small number of drugs are inactivated by processes that may not require intercompartment transfer. Examples are the chemical breakdown of atracurium by Hofmann elimination, and the breakdown of this and other drugs by esterases. An increasing number of newer drugs, e.g. remifentanil, are being designed to be eliminated in this way. The pharmacokinetics of these drugs will obviously be very different, and recovery times much less subject to cumulation.

Routes of absorption

Oral

This is the most common route for medication, and drugs are absorbed from the gastric mucosa or from lower parts of the alimentary tract. Drugs need to be in aqueous solution, and a number of factors in the chemical nature and pharmaceutical preparation of the drug are important. These include pharmaceutical factors — the rate of disintegration of tablets, and rate of dissolution after disintegration; and physicochemical factors — the aqueous and lipid solubility of the drug, and the factors influencing these, i.e. pK_a and the pH of the environment. The rate of emptying of the stomach is important in determining rate of absorption, and this may be influenced by disease, other drugs (delayed by opioids, speeded by prokinetics) or the presence of food.

Drugs may be enteric coated, either to protect the stomach from the action of the drug (aspirin and non-steroidal anti-inflammatory drugs (NSAIDs)) or to protect the drug from being inactivated by stomach acid (omeprazole, etc.). Sustained release preparations (e.g. morphine MST tablets) dissolve slowly and in a controlled fashion for prolonged effect; these should not be prescribed generically as different formulations will not be equivalent.

Orally administered drugs are subject to first pass metabolism in gut wall and liver. This reduces bioavailability, although a few preparations (e.g. pivampicillin) take advantage of the process by being prodrugs, which become active after metabolism.

Transmucosal

Sublingual, transnasal. Lipid soluble drugs are rapidly absorbed through mucosal surfaces. The buccal or sublingual routes are well known: buprenorphine achieves a bioavailability by the sublingual route 50% of that after intramuscular injection. First pass hepatic metabolism is avoided, although some of the drug is likely to be swallowed and thus metabolised in this way.

Nasal sprays are less commonly used but transnasal sufentanil and butorphanol have recently been investigated, with some success.

Rectal. As with sublingual administration, rectal drug therapy may avoid first pass metabolism, depending on the exact site of absorption. Absorption is more erratic than when given orally, and some drugs are less well absorbed, but others, including morphine, may be better absorbed. Local irritation is a recognised problem with some drugs, including NSAIDs. Explanation to the patient is mandatory.

Parenteral, intramuscular, subcutaneous

Absorption by these routes is variable, depending on factors to do with drug chemistry and formulation, as well as the characteristics of the tissue into which the drug is injected. It will be absorbed most rapidly if in aqueous solution, more slowly if the solution is viscous, of low pH, or if it is not water soluble so that precipitation occurs. The solvent used is very important in determining rate of absorption, and depot preparations are used where the solvent is oily, or where the drug is adsorbed to a crystalline vehicle (e.g. protamine zinc insulin).

Absorption can vary widely depending on the vascularity of the tissue used: muscle is different from subcutaneous tissue, and different muscle sites differ — absorption is more rapid from deltoid than from gluteal muscle. Movement also increases absorption from intramuscular sites by increasing local blood flow.

Intratracheal

This route may be used during resuscitation, for drugs such as adrenaline, if venous access is not possible; however, absorption is unreliable and much larger doses are required than when the drugs are given intravenously.

Transdermal

This is in theory an attractive route, as it is pain free and avoids first pass metabolism. It is used widely and successfully for hormone replacement therapy. In treatment of acute as opposed to chronic states, the kinetics of absorption by this route become less attractive. Drug has to diffuse through the stratum corneum and into the dermis before encountering blood vessels for absorption. This requires the establishment of a concentration gradient of drug through a significant depth of skin before blood levels rise, and there is thus a delay in onset. On removal of the patch, there is still a reservoir of drug that continues to absorb. In the case of fentanyl, plasma concentration rises to reach a plateau only after about 18 hours, and after removal the elimination half-life from plasma is also of the same order. There has also been great inter-individual variation between patients studied in plasma levels achieved. These factors mean that currently available preparations would not be safe as the sole or main analgesic for treatment of acute pain. However, transdermal fentanyl is approved for cancer pain in opioid tolerant patients. Transdermal hyoscine is marketed for motion sickness.

Iontophoretic transdermal administration, where diffusion is increased, or controlled, by a small electric current, is being investigated and may provide an answer to some of the problems of the transdermal route.

Transport: protein binding

During transport of the drug in the circulation, some drugs are simply dissolved in serum water, but many are partly associated with plasma proteins. Binding to albumin is, for most drugs, by far the most important of these, and often accounts for almost the entire drug binding in plasma, but drugs also bind to α_1-acid glycoprotein, haemoglobin, lipoproteins and certain other globulins. Albumin binds mainly *acidic* drugs, while α_1-acid glycoprotein binds mainly *basic* drugs and some acidic drugs, and some lipophilic drugs bind more to lipoproteins. Tubocurarine binds mainly to γ globulin. These proteins can also bind endogenous substances.

This method of transport has important effects on the fate of drugs in the body. Only the free, unbound drug can diffuse through the capillary walls and reach the sites of drug action, or sites of biotransformation and excretion (although this is a simplification which I will come back to); however, the drug–albumin binding is easily reversible, and thus the complex forms a reservoir of drug, smooths out peaks and troughs in the intensity of drug action, and in *most* cases delays excretion and prolongs the action of the drug. Drugs also bind to proteins in the tissues and this may constitute a large reservoir of drug and delay its final elimination.

The extent of binding of drug to albumin varies widely, from very low values to 98–99% binding

in the case of warfarin or diazepam. The drug binds to specific sites on the albumin molecule, and for different drugs there may be one or several sites.

Binding sites

On the albumin molecule, six or more sites bind drugs and endogenous compounds. Drugs bind mainly to two independent sites, known as site I and site II, and to a small extent to a third, site III. Site I, which is less specific, binds several structurally diverse drugs such as warfarin, phenylbutazone, etc. It may be described as the warfarin site, and the ability to displace warfarin is used as a measure of a drug's binding to site I. In the same way, diazepam has been used as a marker for site II. Apart from the benzodiazepines, the drugs that bind to site II are mainly carboxylic acids such as NSAID analgesics. There may also be non-specific sites.

In the fetus, α_1-fetoprotein plays the same transport role as albumin in the adult; however, although it has the same site I as albumin, it seems to lack sites II and III, which could lead to lower binding and greater toxicity of drugs that bind to these sites in the adult.

α_1-Acid glycoprotein, the main transport protein for many basic drugs, such as psychotropic drugs and β blockers, occurs in three genetic variants, leading to differences in binding and activity of these drugs.

Drug binding

The type of bond formed varies but will be covalent only where irreversible bonds form. The more usual reversible bond obeys the law of mass action, and thus an equation can be written:

$$\text{unbound drug} + \text{albumin} \underset{k_2}{\overset{k_1}{\longleftrightarrow}} \text{(drug–albumin complex)},$$

where k_1 and k_2 are the rate constants for the forward and reverse actions. This equation can be written as:

$$\frac{[\text{bound drug}]}{[\text{unbound drug}] \times [\text{albumin}]} = \frac{k_1}{k_2}$$

and the affinity of the drug for albumin expressed as an affinity constant, which is the ratio of bound drug concentration to the product of albumin and unbound drug concentrations. This constant, $K_a = k_1/k_2$. More commonly used is a dissociation constant, K_d:

$$K_d = 1/K_a = k_2/k_1.$$

Thus a drug with a high affinity for albumin has a low value of dissociation constant. As there may be more than one binding site on each molecule, and each may have a different dissociation constant, the concentration of the drug left unbound will depend on the total drug concentration, the albumin concentration, the number of binding sites and the dissociation constant(s).

A high degree of binding of the drug to albumin will have several important effects. These could be anticipated from the facts that only free drug diffuses into and is in equilibrium with the water of the extracellular fluid and other body compartments, and that the drug–albumin binding is easily reversible. Firstly, the plasma concentration of the drug as commonly measured is an estimate of the total amount of the drug, bound and unbound, and will often be much higher than the concentration of drug dissolved in body fluids and available to produce a therapeutic effect. The level of free drug in body fluids can be measured using a physical separation technique, such as ultrafiltration of plasma, or by measuring levels in a relatively protein-free body fluid, such as saliva, and such values should correlate better with biological effects than do plasma total drug levels. When a bolus injection of the drug is given, much of this will bind to albumin, so that the tendency to produce an instantaneously high blood level and pharmacological effect is smoothed out. However, occasionally, if a very rapid intravenous injection is given, which does not have time to mix with the whole blood volume, then the binding capacity of albumin molecules in the limited volume of blood with which the drug mixes initially may be exceeded, and a higher level of free drug and pharmacological effect will result.

Secondly, there may be an influence on the metabolism and excretion of the drug. The organs that eliminate drugs can only act on the drug which they can get at, which is the free drug. In the glomeruli, ultrafiltration occurs, and only free drug passes into the tubules. As there is no concentrating effect there is no tendency for the bound drug to dissociate, and thus only the free drug is exposed to excretion processes, while that part that is bound to albumin is protected from excretion, so a high degree of protein binding will reduce excretion of the drug by the kidney. However, if a drug is actively excreted, as in the liver or the kidney tubules, this process reduces the concentration of free drug in plasma, bound drug dissociates immediately to replace this and is excreted — so albumin binding has little effect on the rate of elimination of the drug. Therefore drugs which are excreted by passive filtration through the glomeruli, and which are highly albumin bound, will have long half-lives, as much as a year for some iodinated contrast media. When excretion is by active tubular secretion, as in the case of penicillins, then even if the drug is highly albumin bound, rapid excretion may occur, and in fact the rate of excretion may be increased by albumin binding, as this acts in effect as a transport mechanism carrying more drug to the site of excretion. Albumin binding will also hinder removal of drug from the circulation by haemodialysis or peritoneal dialysis.

Competition for binding sites

When more than one drug is given to the patient, the drugs may compete for protein binding sites, and this can result in the displacement of one or other drug from its binding sites and lead to an increase in the concentration of free drug, and an increase in the pharmacological effect of the drug. This interference of one drug with the binding of another may be due to competitive inhibition, in which the drugs simply compete for binding to the same site on the albumin molecule, or to non-competitive inhibition, in which the binding of the drug to albumin results in a change in the tertiary conformation of the albumin, and thus alters the number or affinity of the sites accessible to the second drug.

Endogenous compounds such as bilirubin or

fatty acids also bind to serum proteins, and may be displaced by drugs competing for the same sites. In the newborn with jaundice this may lead to development of kernicterus, while administration of heparin by raising free fatty acid levels causes an increase in free diazepam fraction by several fold. Similar interaction may take place with drugs, like diazepam or tricyclic antidepressants, that are extensively bound to *tissue* proteins, but the clinical importance of this is unknown.

Drug competition for binding sites is most likely to occur to a significant degree if both drugs are highly albumin bound, and if high concentrations of the drug are reached either by rapid administration of a large dose, or by repeated administration. The potentiation of the effect of one drug by another by this process is likely to be transient, as an increase in the concentration of the free drug results in an increase in its rate of elimination, and a new state of equilibrium is soon reached. The converse will occur when the competing drug is stopped (Fig. 4.10). However although the effect is short lived, if the drug has a narrow range of therapeutic concentrations or if the therapeutic and toxic doses are close, it may be clinically important. This compensating safety factor may not apply to drugs with high extraction ratios, where protein binding is helping to accelerate elimination, and adverse reactions will be more likely in these cases.

When drug concentrations are high, the binding sites on proteins may become saturated, so the concentration of free drug will be relatively higher, and this may be another reason for non-linear kinetics. (But, whereas saturation of enzymes leads to a situation where the clearance of the drug is reduced at higher drug concentrations, saturation of protein binding sites will cause it to increase — provided the metabolising enzymes are not also saturated.) For example, phenylbutazone in low doses has a plasma half-life of 3 days, whereas at high doses which saturate binding proteins, this falls to 3 hours.

Biotransformation: sites of metabolism

Drugs are modified by the actions of enzyme systems within the body. Most drug metabolism occurs in hepatic microsomes but biotransformation also occurs elsewhere in the body, including the plasma, gastrointestinal tract, lungs and non-microsomal systems in the liver.

The main useful purpose of biotransformation is to rid the body of the drug. Highly polar substances may easily be excreted by the kidney, and are often excreted unchanged, at least in part. Those which are non-polar and highly lipid soluble are rapidly reabsorbed from the kidney tubules after filtration by the glomeruli, and thus not easily excreted. Biotransformation to more polar and less lipid soluble metabolites will make excretion easier. Metabolic degradation will also often change the drug to an inactive form before it is excreted, and lead to a termination of its action — suxamethonium is metabolised rapidly by plasma pseudocholinesterase — but metabolic change may have different

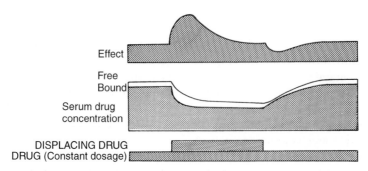

Figure 4.10 Changes in concentration and effect of a drug caused by a second drug which competes for binding sites.

effects. In some cases an active drug is metabolised to a still active metabolite (diazepam to desmethyldiazepam) or an inactive 'prodrug' to an active metabolite (codeine to morphine), which is responsible for its therapeutic effect. A metabolite may also be responsible for the toxic effects of a drug — for example, the hepatotoxicity of paracetamol overdosage.

These metabolic processes have evolved both to deal with substances produced by the body, often degraded by specific enzymes, and to deal with toxic chemicals introduced into the body, which in evolutionary terms were mainly from plants in the diet but now include drugs.

It is also possible for a drug to be degraded by purely chemical reactions, for example Hofmann elimination in the case of atracurium.

Enzymatic processes involved in drug elimination are described as phase I and phase II. Phase I, or non-synthetic reactions, involve inactivation of the drug by oxidation, reduction, hydrolysis, dealkylation or similar modifications of the administered molecule in which a polar group is added. A majority of these are carried out in the liver by a versatile group of enzymes known as mixed function oxidases, a system in which one of the most important components is cytochrome P-450.

Cytochrome P-450

The cytochromes P-450 consist of a large number of genetically related enzymes. The name is derived from the fact that light of wavelength 450 nm is absorbed. In mammals, 12 families of P-450 are described at present, of which four are mainly concerned with metabolism of foreign substances, xenobiotics, including drugs, and the others mainly with endogenous substances, in particular steroids and bile acids. At least 30 different individual P-450 enzymes occur in humans.

The cytochromes P-450 are named systematically as CYP, followed by a numeral indicating family, a letter indicating subfamily, and a numeral for individual form — for example, P-450 3A4 or CYP3A4. Classification is based on the closeness of their amino acid sequences. The CYP2 and CYP3 families are the most important in drug metabolism — CYP3A4 forms up to 60% of all P-450 in some livers. It is responsible for metabolism of a large number of drugs, including opioids and nifedipine, the latter being used as a marker to measure the activity of CYP3A4.

There is a large interindividual variation in the levels of expression of the enzymes, which is a major factor in leading to differences in individual patient's responses to drugs — for example, the considerable variation in elimination clearance of alfentanil has been related to CYP3A4 activity. The best studied cause of important variability in drug metabolism, which affects many cardiovascular, psychotropic and other drugs, is the existence of poor and good metabolisers, due to polymorphism of debrisoquine 4-hydroxylase (CYP2D6). There is a correlation between blood levels of antidepressants and measured CYP2D6 activity. Volatile anaesthetic drugs are metabolised mainly by CYP2E1, which also oxidises alcohol. This enzyme is also genetically polymorphic.

In addition to the cytochromes P-450, a number of other enzymes carry out phase I processes. These include alcohol and aldehyde dehydrogenases, glutathione-s-transferase, sulphotransferases, xanthine oxidase, etc. These also show considerable polymorphism and thus variation in activity.

Phase II, or synthetic, reactions are also known as conjugation reactions. These involve coupling of endogenous compounds with the drug, or with the products of phase I reactions. The endogenous substance is usually a carbohydrate or amino acid, or a derivative of these, or acetic acid or inorganic sulphate. The common conjugation reactions are therefore glucuronidation, other glycosylations, sulphation, acetylation, conjugation with amino acids or with glutathione, and methylation. Phase II metabolism occurs in the liver but the gut is almost as rich in conjugating enzymes (though not in phase I enzymes), and so drugs that are metabolised largely along these pathways — for example, morphine — are subject to extensive first pass metabolism.

A drug is often metabolised simultaneously along several pathways; for example, glucuronidation of morphine at the 6 position gives rise to the active metabolite morphine-6-glucuronide, while conjugations at the 3 position account for about 60% of morphine elimination, and the products are inactive. *N*-demethylation, a phase I reaction, gives normorphine, which is then conjugated to a glucuronide. As well as these, other pathways, such as methylation to codeine, exist, and also 10% of morphine is excreted unchanged. The relative importance of different pathways changes under different circumstances; for example, halothane metabolism is normally mainly oxidative but under hypoxic conditions an alternative reductive pathway becomes more important and, in this case, reactive intermediates may be formed, which have been suggested as a cause of hepatic damage. Reactive intermediates formed in this way by phase I reactions are usually made harmless by inactivation of their reactive groups in a phase II or synthetic reaction. Because the phase II reactions may depend on an available supply in the liver of, for example, glutathione, it is possible for the capacity of this pathway to be overwhelmed if a large amount of the toxic intermediate compound is made. This might occur with paracetamol (acetaminophen *USP*) in overdose, and liver damage can then occur as irreversible binding to macromolecules in the liver cells occurs. In the case of paracetamol, this may to some extent be prevented by administering to the patient a glutathione precursor such as acetylcysteine.

Modification of metabolism

There are genetically determined differences in drug metabolism which may result in up to a sixfold difference in the rates of metabolism in different individuals. Much of this difference can be accounted for by the normal gaussian distribution of any property between individuals. However, in a number of instances this variability is due to variant alleles resulting from mutations in genes encoding these enzymes, as mentioned above. An example is metabolism of

drugs by acetylation: patients may belong to one of two populations, 'fast' or 'slow' acetylators, and the dose regimen of a drug eliminated by this pathway — for example, isoniazid — must be greatly modified depending on its rate of metabolism. A similar example is genetic polymorphism in suxamethonium.

Genetic polymorphism is important — for example, in CAST (Cardiac Arrhythmia Suppression Trial), serious problems occurred with encainide and flecainide because of polymorphic metabolism by CYP2D6.

The rate at which an enzyme system carries out its activity is largely dependent on the amount of substrate present; however, certain substances are able to stimulate enzyme activity without a change in the amount of enzyme present — enzyme stimulation or enzyme activation. More importantly, it is also possible to increase the amount of enzyme in the system.

Enzymes are proteins, which, like other proteins, are assembled from amino acids according to instructions transferred by messenger RNA from a structural gene. Exposure to environmental substances or drugs can increase the level of expression of the gene, and thus the amount of the enzyme present — this is *enzyme induction*.

There are at least five types of enzyme induction, named after model inducers (Brockmoller & Roots 1994): polycyclic aromatic hydrocarbon type (CYP1A), phenobarbital type (CYP2 and CYP3A), steroid or pregnenolone 16α-carbonitrile type (CYP3A), alcohol (CYP2E1), and clofibrate or peroxisome proliferator type (CYP4). Within each of these, there is a wide range of potencies for different inducers.

Induction of enzymes by a drug not only leads to an increase in its own metabolic degradation, but often also that of other drugs. This is one of the most important mechanisms of drug interaction. The mixed function oxidases of the liver microsomes are involved in the biotransformation of many different drugs. Barbiturate drugs are among those that are particularly effective in causing induction of oxidation enzymes. Thus, for example, if a patient maintained in a steady state of anticoagulation by warfarin then starts barbiturate treatment, an increase in warfarin metabolism will ensue, and with a fall in plasma warfarin levels there will be a decrease in anticoagulation effect. If a metabolite is toxic, then induction of metabolism may result in increased toxicity — for example, the nephrotoxic potential of methoxyflurane may be potentiated.

Inhibition of metabolism may also occur. It may be due to inhibition of enzymes, or more commonly to competition between drugs for the same metabolic pathway. With most drugs, which are eliminated by processes obeying first order kinetics, competition rarely causes significant inhibition of metabolism, but competition is more important in those eliminated by zero order kinetics, where the enzyme system is easily saturated.

Inhibition may also be due to temporary or permanent inactivation of enzymes. The most important example in anaesthetic practice is inhibition of cholinesterase. Similarly, inactivation of hepatic enzymes can occur.

The breakdown of drugs that depend on hepatic metabolism may be greatly influenced by changes in liver blood flow. In general, a reduction in hepatic blood flow will lead to a reduction in metabolism of the drug, but this may not always be so.

The detailed knowledge of hepatic metabolism is rapidly increasing and leading to changes in how we think about drug biotransformation. One paper has stated it thus:

Study of liver function is moving away from a physiological approach assessing liver clearance toward a biochemical and molecular biological approach. Major improvements in understanding of drug disposition in humans have resulted . . . analysis of metabolites has grown in importance in comparison to clearance, as metabolite analysis is more suitable for analysis of enzyme function . . . In clinical research, non-specific deterioration of liver function by disease, drug-specific liver function impairment by enzyme inhibition, enzyme induction and pharmacogenetics should all be taken into account. (Brockmoller and Root 1994)

First pass metabolism

First-pass metabolism occurs to a significant extent after absorption of many drugs from the gastrointestinal tract. Since the drug is absorbed into the splanchnic circulation, it must pass through the liver before it can reach the systemic circulation and its target. It may therefore be metabolised both in the liver and, usually to a lesser extent, by enzymes in the gut wall.

Drugs that are mainly eliminated by phase II metabolism (e.g. oestrogens and progestogens, morphine, etc.) undergo significant first pass gut metabolism. This is because the gut is rich in conjugating enzymes. The role of the lung in first pass metabolism is not clear, although it is quite avid in binding basic drugs such as lignocaine (lidocaine *USP*), propranolol, etc.

If a significant proportion is metabolised by the liver (i.e. the hepatic clearance of the drug is relatively high), then the amount reaching the systemic circulation will be greatly reduced. Thus the drug, even if it is absorbed well, will be relatively ineffective when given orally, as with, for example, morphine. Where the drug is used by the oral route, the dose administered will be much larger than when given parenterally. When the rate of metabolism of the drug by the liver is high, hepatic blood flow may be the limiting factor. Thus any situation in which hepatic blood flow is reduced will result in a reduction in hepatic clearance of the drug.

If the drug is metabolised according to zero order kinetics, it will be a low extraction drug, and an increase in hepatic blood flow will allow more of the drug to pass through the liver unaffected; in this case increased hepatic blood flow can result in an increase in drug action, in contrast to the general rule described above.

Although the fetus is able to metabolise xenobiotics, even in the early stages of gestation, newborn babies still have immature metabolic processes; however, their capacity to carry out phase I processes such as oxidation is relatively well developed, although the situation is different in many other animal species. Phase II processes of conjugation are not carried out well in the human newborn and therefore there is a reduced capacity to deal with drugs that are detoxified by these processes.

Drug elimination

Drugs are eliminated by a variety of routes:

renal and hepatobiliary are the most important in the majority of drugs, although pulmonary excretion is the main route for volatile and gaseous anaesthetics. There are a number of minor routes: sweat, faeces, breast milk, etc.

Renal excretion

In the proximal renal tubule many organic acids, bases and metabolites are excreted by active tubular secretion. The carrier systems can be bidirectional so that some drugs are both secreted and reabsorbed. In the proximal and distal tubules, non-ionised forms of weak acids and bases undergo passive reabsorption, and the concentration gradient is determined by reabsorption of water, sodium and other inorganic ions. Passive reabsorption of some substances is pH dependent. Alteration of urine pH can result in significant change in drug elimination if pH dependent passive reabsorption can be influenced. Thus alkalinisation of urine can produce a 4–6-fold increase in excretion of a relatively strong acid such as acetylsalicylic acid ($pK_a = 3.5$) and of phenobarbitone ($pK_a = 7.2$) when urinary pH is changed from 6.4 to 8.0. Excretion of bases ($pK_a > 7.5$) such as amphetamine and quinine is enhanced by acidification of urine, but has no practical application.

REFERENCES AND FURTHER READING

Berner B, John V A 1994 Pharmacokinetic characterisation of transdermal delivery system. Clinical Pharmacokinetics 26: 121–123

Brockmoller J, Roots I 1994 Assessment of liver metabolic function. Clinical implications. Clinical Pharmacokinetics 27: 216–248

Hervé F, Urien S, Albengres E, Duche J C, Tillement J P 1994 Drug binding in plasma. A summary of recent trends in the study of drug and hormone binding (review). Clinical Pharmacokinetics 26: 44–58

Hughes M A, Glass P S, Jacobs J R 1992 Context-sensitive half-time in multicompartment pharmacokinetic models for intravenous anesthetic drugs. Anesthesiology 76: 334–341

Krauer B, Dayer P 1991 Fetal drug metabolism and its possible clinical implications. Clinical Pharmacokinetics 21: 70–80

Motwani J G, Lipworth B J 1991 Clinical pharmacokinetics of drug administered buccally and sublingually. Clinical Pharmacokinetics 21: 83–94

Tam Y K 1993 Individual variation in first-pass metabolism. Clinical Pharmacokinetics 25: 300–328

van Hoogdalem E, de Boer A G, Breimer D D 1991 Pharmacokinetics of rectal drug administration, part I. General considerations and clinical applications of centrally acting drugs. Clinical Pharmacokinetics 21: 11–26

5

Clinical trials and statistical methods

C. C. Patterson

1. PRINCIPLES OF CLINICAL TRIALS

1.1 Phases of drug development

New drugs must undergo assessment for efficacy and safety before receiving a product licence. During drug development toxicological and pharmacodynamic studies will have been conducted using animal models. The first administration of a drug to humans will typically take the form of a *phase I* trial in which the aims will be to elucidate a drug's mode of action and to determine non-toxic methods of administration and dosage schedules. Such trials may be performed either with patients or with healthy volunteers. *Phase II* trials are a first attempt to assess whether or not a drug is efficacious. These trials do not always involve randomisation and may be conducted in an open fashion (i.e. the clinician knows the treatment the patient is receiving). Many drugs are rejected as unpromising at this stage. In *phase III* trials the effectiveness of a drug will be compared with the effectiveness of an existing treatment or a placebo treatment. Such trials are usually randomised. However, even large phase III trials cannot hope to detect rare side-effects and accordingly *postmarketing surveillance* studies are carried out on new drugs. In the United Kingdom the *yellow card* system encourages doctors to report suspected adverse drug reactions.

1.2 Design considerations

A key aspect of the trial design is the decision

about which treatment (or treatments) the patient will receive. In *controlled* trials, in addition to a group of patients receiving a new treatment, there will be another group who receive an existing treatment or a placebo (dummy) treatment. The outcome for this latter group provides a standard for comparison. Very rarely is an *historical control group* (i.e. a control group comprising patients from a previous time period) satisfactory.

In *parallel group* designs each patient receives only one of the treatments under study. Comparison between treatments must be made on a between-patient basis. In *cross-over* designs the patient receives more than one treatment, and such designs specify the order in which treatments are received. Comparisons between treatments are made on a within-patient basis, with patients acting as their own controls. The design of a typical two-period cross-over trial is illustrated in Figure 5.1. Patients are allocated to two treatment groups which receive treatments in a different order (i.e. AB/BA). Assessments are performed at the end of each treatment period, although in some trials baseline measurements may also be taken at the start of each treatment period. Usually a *washout period* is required between treatment periods to avoid contamination or *carry-over* effects. Also a *run in period* may

be necessary to minimise practice or order effects. This design is typically used for the comparison of treatments which provide short term relief from a chronic condition or for the study of the short term effects of fast acting drugs. This is because it is desirable for the patient's condition to be similar at the start of each treatment period. A *Latin square* design may be used for a cross-over trial of more than two treatments. For example, if three treatments (A, B and C) are being compared, the design allocates each treatment the same number of times in each treatment period. Patients are allocated at random to one of the three groups.

	Treatment period		
	1	2	3
Group 1	A	B	C
Group 2	C	A	B
Group 3	B	C	A

Often in trials of anaesthesia a patient can receive an anaesthetic agent only once, and therefore only a parallel group design is possible. However, in a phase II pharmacodynamic study a volunteer might receive a series of treatments at weekly intervals in accordance with a Latin square design.

Randomisation is the allocation of treatments to

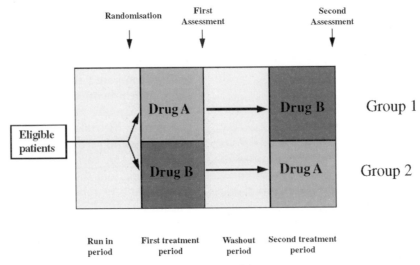

Figure 5.1 Format of the two-period cross-over trial.

patients using some random process, such as the toss of a coin. In practice, specially prepared tables of random numbers are available in statistical textbooks, or a computer may be used to generate the allocations. The purpose of randomisation is to ensure that the groups of patients receiving treatments are comparable. The comparison of treatments will be fair (unbiased) and the statistical analysis will be valid only if randomisation has taken place. The allocation is implemented using a *randomisation list*. If there is scope for manipulation, then the allocations on the list should be hidden in *sealed envelopes*; only after the name of an eligible patient has been written on the outside of the envelope should the seal be broken to reveal which treatment the patient has been allocated. Refinements of the randomisation process include *restricted randomisation*, in which treatment groups are restricted to be of equal size, and *stratified randomisation*, in which subgroups of patients defined by some important prognostic variable are equally distributed between treatment groups. In the following example, random permutations of two As and two Bs have been used to restrict the randomisation and so achieve balance after every fourth allocation. The randomisation has also been stratified by the American Society of Anesthesiologists grade of the patient so that this balance is achieved within each stratum.

Stratum 1 ASA grade 1 or 2															
Block	1	1	1	1	2	2	2	2	3	3	3	3	4	4	4	4
Patient	1	2	3	4	5	6	7	8	9	10	11	12	13	14	15	16
Treatment	A	B	B	A	B	B	A	A	A	B	A	B	B	A	B	A

Stratum 2 ASA grade 3 or 4															
Block	1	1	1	1	2	2	2	2	3	3	3	3	4	4	4	4
Patient	1	2	3	4	5	6	7	8	9	10	11	12	13	14	15	16
Treatment	B	A	B	A	A	B	A	B	A	B	B	A	A	B	A	B

In many trials, assessment of the patient's condition is made in the absence of knowledge of the treatment the patient has received. This avoids bias on the part of the assessor or patient, which might occur if the treatment were known. If either the assessor or the patient does not know which treatment the patient received the trial is called *single blind*; if neither knows the trial is *double blind*. To maintain blindness it may be necessary to include a *placebo* treatment. This is a pharmacologically inert preparation included in the trial to eliminate effects attributable to suggestion. The trial is then said to be *placebo controlled*. The placebo elicits a non-specific response which would be obtained with any treatment. The placebo should mimic the active treatment as closely as possible in presentation (i.e. size, shape, colour, method of administration). If a drug administered by injection is to be compared with a drug given in tablet form a *double placebo* may be used, patients receiving either the active tablet and a placebo injection or an active injection and a placebo tablet.

Finally, estimation of the *trial size*, the number of patients required, is an indispensable step in the design stage, but consideration will be deferred to section 4.1 after some necessary statistical terms have been introduced. A *multi-centre* study may be necessary if the trial size is so large as to preclude the study being performed in a single centre. In contrast to the fixed-size trial, a trial employing a *sequential* design permits results to be analysed repeatedly as they accumulate, and the trial to be stopped as soon as a significant result is obtained (section 6.1). This approach minimises potential ethical problems that can otherwise arise towards the end of a trial when some patients may be given a treatment that is becoming more and more obviously inferior.

1.3 The trial protocol

The *trial protocol* is an essential document which should provide a detailed description of the trial. It ensures that everyone involved is properly informed about the trial, and it will form an important part of the submission to the research ethics committee. Included in the protocol should be the following:

- title of trial
- names, job titles, addresses and contact numbers of trial organisers
- statement of aims and the rationale for performing the trial

- brief review of relevant literature
- trial design
- specific hypotheses to be tested, distinguishing between primary and secondary trial end-points
- detailed description of drugs, regimens and method of administration, and any necessary instructions about packaging, labelling and storage
- patient recruitment procedures, including entry criteria (e.g. age, gender, verification of diagnosis, severity of condition) or exclusion criteria (e.g. previous/concurrent treatments or diseases, contraindication to any trial treatment)
- statistical justification for trial size
- method of randomisation and its implementation
- patient information sheet and consent form
- assessment procedures
- patient record sheet together with any instructions for its completion
- criteria for withdrawal
- mechanism for discovering a patient's treatment in a blinded trial in the event of an emergency
- arrangements for data handling, quality control checks
- plan for the statistical analysis, including any proposed interim analyses
- arrangements for any ethical review of interim analysis and for early termination
- publication and authorship policy.

2. ETHICAL CONSIDERATIONS

2.1 Protection of the patient

It is not uncommon for the ethics of randomisation to be questioned. In response, it may be argued that, when compared with the possible alternatives, properly conducted randomised trials are ethical because they result in improved medical knowledge, which benefits both patients and society at large. Poorly conducted trials or trials the results of which are never published are, however, unethical because they may place patients at unnecessary risk without any gain in knowledge.

Certain safeguards are necessary for the protection of the patient if a trial is to be considered ethical. All research involving human subjects should be approved by a *research ethics committee*, which will include both doctors and lay people. The primary role of such a committee is to check that patients' interests are being looked after. The purpose of any proposed trial must be worthwhile and any extra risks to which patients are exposed as a consequence of the trial must be minimal and must be justifiable in relation to the purpose of the trial. Some groups of patients (e.g. women of childbearing age) may need to be excluded if the risks associated with participation are too great. It has been suggested that anaesthesia may normally be prolonged for 20 or 30 minutes to facilitate a clinical trial, provided that there are no signs of danger to the patient. A useful yardstick for deciding if a proposed trial is ethical is whether or not one would be happy for a close relative or friend to participate. Proper arrangements should be in place to ensure that any patient who suffers harm as a result of participation in a trial is adequately compensated.

2.2 What is informed consent?

Patients must be invited to participate in a trial voluntarily, and only after providing *informed consent*. This requires that the following steps have been taken:

- An adequate explanation of the purpose of the trial has been given using language and terminology appropriate for the patient.
- The patient is made aware that the trial is a research project.
- The extent and duration of the patient's involvement is made clear.
- It must be explained that the treatment given to the patient may be decided on the basis of chance, and in some trials that this means the patient may receive a placebo (dummy) treatment.
- Any likely risks or discomfort to the patient arising from participation are fully explained.
- Patients are made aware of their right to refuse to participate or to withdraw at any time

without giving a reason, and without prejudice to their continued medical care.

- The name of an investigator is made available should the patient need clarification or further information about the trial.
- The patient should be advised that all information obtained during the trial will be treated confidentially, although in certain trials information may need to be disclosed to regulatory authorities for inspection purposes.

A *patient information sheet* should be provided for the patient to retain.

Generally, written consent should be obtained in preference to verbal consent; if the latter is used it should be witnessed by a third party. In the case of patients who cannot give informed consent, e.g. children, those with mental illness or patients who are unconscious, the informed consent of a parent or guardian must be sought, but the wishes of the patient (whether expressed verbally or by their actions) should always be respected.

Remuneration must not be used as an inducement for patient recruitment, although payments to cover travelling expenses or loss of earnings are permissible.

3. BASIC STATISTICAL CONCEPTS

3.1 The need for statistical analysis

In common with other research in medicine and the biological sciences, differences between treatments which the investigator wishes to identify in a clinical trial are usually masked by variation (inter- and intrapatient variation, measurement error, etc.). Consequently there is a need for the results of a trial to be assessed objectively using valid techniques. Unfortunately reviews of the statistical methodology in published trials show that many are poorly designed and that the selection of inappropriate techniques or incorrect interpretation of analyses are commonplace (Altman & Gore, 1982). This section describes some of the fundamental statistical concepts necessary for the design and analysis of trials. Some other statistical issues that arise at the planning stage are considered in section 4. Section 5

deals with some of the simpler, more commonly used methods of statistical analysis, the majority of which are described in detail in introductory statistical textbooks (Armitage & Berry 1987, Bland 1987, Campbell and Machin 1993, Hill 1977).

3.2 Scales of measurement

Any qualitative or quantitative assessment may be assigned to one of three scales of measurement — nominal, ordinal or interval:

1. The lowest scale of measurement is the *nominal* scale. This is the scale of measurement for categorical variables. Any assignment of numbers to the categories of such a variable is arbitrary. Examples are assessing intubating conditions (satisfactory or unsatisfactory) and occurrence of nausea (present or absent).

2. In the *ordinal* scale of measurement, the assignment of numbers to categories is again arbitrary, but does impose an ordering or ranking on the categories. Examples are a patient's anxiety level (none, slight, moderate or severe) or the level of sedation (responds to speech, responds to painful stimulus or unresponsive).

3. An *interval* scale variable requires an underlying unit of measurement, so that sums and differences may be validly calculated. Examples are systolic blood pressure (mmHg) and oxygen saturation level (%). Some researchers would regard an assessment of pain on a 100 mm visual analogue scale as an interval scale measurement. Others argue that the relationship between the actual level of pain and the visual analogue scale score is complex, and that a 10 mm difference at one end of the pain scale is not the same as a 10 mm difference at the other; consequently visual analogue scale scores are often regarded as ordinal scale measurements.

The scale of measurement is an important consideration in selecting the appropriate technique for statistical analysis.

3.3 Measures of location and dispersion

In summarising the distribution of some quantitative variable there are two aspects that are typically of interest. An indication of where the distribution is centred is given by a *measure of location*, while a *measure of dispersion* indicates the amount of scatter or spread in the distribution.

For an interval scale variable, x, measured in a group of n patients the usual measure of location is the *(arithmetic) mean* obtained by summing the values $x_1, x_2, \ldots, x_n$ and dividing by n

$$\bar{x} = \frac{1}{n} \sum_{i=1}^{n} x_i$$

Another possible measure of location that can also be employed for an ordinal scale variable is the *median*, the middle value (if n is odd) or the average of the two middle values (if n is even) obtained when the n values are arranged in ascending order. A family of other measures of location may be similarly defined; for example, there are three *quartiles* dividing the group into four equal parts, nine *deciles* dividing the group into 10 equal parts and 99 *percentiles* dividing the group into 100 equal parts. For nominal scale data the *mode*, the most commonly occurring value, is the only suitable measure of location.

For an interval scale variable the basic measure of dispersion is the *variance*, s^2, given by

$$s^2 = \frac{1}{n-1} \sum_{i=1}^{n} (x_i - \bar{x})^2$$

Apart from the use of $n-1$ as opposed to n in the denominator, the variance is simply the average of squared deviations from the mean. Usually the square root of the variance is taken to give the *standard deviation*, s, because it provides a measure in the original units of the variable. Alternative measures of dispersion are the *range*, defined as the difference between the maximum and minimum values, and the *interquartile range*, defined as the difference between the third and first quartiles. The *coefficient of variation* is the standard deviation expressed as a percentage of the mean and provides a measure of dispersion that is independent of the units of measurement. It is useful for comparing relative dispersions — for example, comparing the variability of heart rates in children and adults, while taking into account the higher heart rates in children. It also permits a comparison of dispersion between variables that are measured in different units.

Certain interval scale variables (e.g. height) will follow the bell-shaped *normal* (or *gaussian*) distribution. The properties of this distribution show that 90% of values will fall within 1.64 standard deviations of the mean, 95% within 1.96 standard deviations and 99% within 2.58 standard deviations. If such a variable is measured in a large representative sample of the healthy population, these properties of the normal distribution provide a method for defining *reference ranges*. For example, a 95% reference range will be given by

$$\bar{x} \pm 1.96\,s$$

For variables that do not follow the normal distribution, reference ranges must be defined using percentiles. Such reference ranges are to be found in routine biochemistry reports.

3.4 Statistical inference

In general, statistical techniques require the assumption that a group under study may be considered to be a *random sample* from the population about which inferences are to be made. A random sample is one selected in such a way that every member of the population has the same chance of being included in the sample. In practice, there could be considerable practical difficulties in mounting a clinical study of a random sample from the population of, for example, all patients undergoing general anaesthesia in a particular health authority in some specified year; frequently, for convenience, a consecutive series of patients attending a single hospital will be studied. However, the potential for biased conclusions resulting from not using random samples must be carefully assessed. The investigator must therefore be cautious not to extrapolate findings beyond the population from which the sample was drawn. Statistical methods only take account of *sampling error* (i.e. variation arising from the process of random sampling); they cannot quantify the extent of biases attributable to non-random sampling. In the context of the clinical trial, the need to apply entry and exclusion criteria during patient recruitment limits the generalisability of trial findings to a *target population* comprising of patients who meet these eligibility criteria. The purpose of the randomisation is to ensure that each treatment group in the trial may be considered as a random sample from this target population. Consequently any significant differences in outcome between the treatment groups may reasonably be attributed to the treatments given during the trial.

When calculated in a sample, a measure of location or dispersion is often referred to as a *statistic*. A statistic is generally regarded as providing an *estimate* of the corresponding measure in the population, which is called a *parameter*. A simple example is the use of the sample mean (a statistic) to estimate the population mean (a parameter). Typically the value of a parameter is not known, and furthermore any given estimate will differ somewhat from the parameter value because of sampling error. Statistical theory can at least help to determine how repeatable this *estimation* process is. It requires consideration of the rather abstract notion of the *sampling distribution*. This is simply the distribution obtained by calculating the statistic in every single possible random sample from the population. The standard deviation of this distribution is called the *standard error* (SE) of the statistic, and provides the basic measure of how much the statistic will vary from one sample to the next. In practice, formulae are available that enable an estimate of the standard error to be obtained from only one sample. For example, the standard error of the mean may be obtained as

$$SE\,(\bar{x}) = s\,/\,\sqrt{n}$$

In many situations (especially when the sample size is large) the sampling distribution of a statistic will follow the normal distribution, the mathematical properties of which are well known. This makes it possible to derive formulae that involve the standard error and which may be used to conduct tests of hypothesis and to calculate confidence intervals.

A proper understanding of *hypothesis tests* or *significance tests* is vital for the successful application of statistical methods in clinical trials. Any significance test is a formalised decision making procedure. Formally a test begins with the supposition that a *null hypothesis* is true. In a clinical trial comparing two treatments, this will typically specify that the treatments are, in reality, equally effective. In a more general situation, the null hypothesis might state that two samples are drawn from populations with the same mean, or alternatively that any difference between two sample means may reasonably be ascribed to sampling error. An *alternative hypothesis* is also necessary, which is often simply a negation of the null hypothesis. In a clinical trial it will typically specify that the treatments are, in reality, not equally effective. The test of significance is a method for deciding between the following two courses of action:

1. Reject the null hypothesis in favour of the alternative, and conclude that the treatments in reality differ in their effectiveness.
2. Do not reject the null hypothesis, and conclude that there is insufficient evidence to state that in reality the treatments differ.

Under the assumption that the null hypothesis is true, the probability, P, of encountering (in hypothetical repetitions of the trial) as large a difference in treatment outcomes as that actually observed in the trial is obtained. Modern computer software will usually supply the value of P directly. If P is small, then a difference between treatment outcomes of the magnitude which has been observed will only occur very rarely by chance. Sampling error is therefore an unlikely explanation for the observed difference in outcomes, and consequently the null hypothesis is rejected (action 1). However, if P is large then the observed difference may very reasonably be ascribed to chance, and there is no evidence to reject the null hypothesis (action 2). Values of P which are considered small depend on the *significance level* (α) chosen for the test. A test at the conventional 5% significance level will result in rejection of the null hypothesis if $P<0.05$.

Unfortunately errors do occur in this decision making process. A *type I error* occurs if the null hypothesis is rejected when it is true. So two treatments are considered to differ in their effectiveness when, in reality, they are equivalent. By choosing the 5% level of significance, the investigator as a consequence accepts a 1 in 20 chance of rejecting the null hypothesis when it is true. On the other hand, a *type II error* occurs if the null hypothesis is not rejected when it should have been because the alternative is true. In such a situation it is concluded that two treatments do not differ in their effectiveness when, in reality, they do.

True situation	Result of test	
	Reject null hypothesis	Do not reject null hypothesis
Null hypothesis true	Type I error (α)	—
Alternative hypothesis true	—	Type II error (β)

The risk of a type II error (β) can be calculated for an alternative hypothesis which specifies a particular difference between treatments. The probability of not committing a type II error is called the *power* of the test and is $(1-\beta)$. This concept of power is important in ensuring that a trial is of adequate size (section 4.1).

Although much emphasis in the medical literature has been placed on significance tests, additional knowledge may be gained from the calculation of *confidence limits*. Taking a simple example, the confidence limit for a population parameter is usually derived from an estimate of the parameter and its standard error. So 95% confidence limits for the population mean may be obtained from a large sample using the formula

$$\bar{x} \pm 1.96 \text{ SE } (\bar{x})$$

The range between the confidence limits is called *confidence interval*. If one were to repeatedly take samples from the population, then 95% of the samples would provide confidence intervals that include the population (or true) mean. This concept may be extended, and in clinical trials confidence intervals for differences in means, differences in medians, differences in proportions and relative risks may usefully be calculated (Gardner and Altman, 1989). In comparison with significance tests, such intervals provide more information about the likely magnitude of the true differences between treatments. Additionally such confidence intervals usually allow a test of significance of the difference between treatments to be conducted implicitly.

Irrespective of whether confidence intervals or hypothesis tests are employed, an important consideration in the statistical analysis is how to handle results from *drop-outs* (patients who quit the trial), *withdrawals* (patients who must have treatment stopped because of some side-effect or adverse reaction) and *protocol deviants* (patients whose treatment does not follow that which was specified in the trial protocol). When possible, observations should continue to be made on such patients, as this allows greatest flexibility in the analysis. The recommended approach is usually that the analysis be conducted with the treatment groups as they were randomised. This is the *intention to treat principle*, which, in effect, gives a comparison of treatment policies as opposed to the treatments that were actually received. Such an analysis usually reflects clinical practice most closely. However, occasionally it may be of some scientific interest to compare treatments in an analysis restricted to those patients who completed the trial without deviation from the protocol, although there is a risk of bias because the depleted patient groups may no longer have comparable characteristics.

4. STATISTICAL CONSIDERATIONS AT THE PLANNING STAGE

4.1 Estimating trial size

The importance of ensuring a trial is of adequate size cannot be overemphasised. If a trial is too small its findings may be inconclusive or even misleading, while too large a trial is wasteful of resources and may expose patients needlessly to inferior treatments. Although some indication about the adequacy of trial size may be obtained at the analysis stage through consideration of the width of confidence intervals for the difference in treatments, this is not a satisfactory substitute for a proper assessment of trial size at the planning stage.

The primary aim of most trials is the comparison of two groups, although methods for assessing trial size can be extended to the comparison of three or more groups. Simple techniques are available both for outcome variables that are interval scale, and so typically summarised for a group of patients using the mean, and for outcomes that are binary or nominal scale (e.g. success or failure) and so typically summarised using a proportion. In the former case, information is required about the magnitude of inter-patient variability in a between-patient trial or intrapatient variability in a within-patient trial. In the latter case a rough estimate of the magnitude of the proportion is necessary. Such information may be obtained either from a pilot study or from previous work in the same field. Also required is an assessment of the *clinically worthwhile difference*. This is the smallest difference in outcome between treatments which, if it existed in reality, would be considered likely to have some clinical impact. This difference supplies a specific value for the alternative hypothesis in a test of significance. The number of patients required for a trial to have a high chance (i.e. 80% or 90% power) to detect this difference as statistically significant (e.g. at the 5% significance level) may be estimated by formula (Armitage & Berry 1987), using tables (Machin & Campbell 1987) or with nomograms (Altman & Gore 1982).

4.2 Minimising measurement error

An important part of the planning for a trial is the training and appraisal of those who will assess the patients during the trial. Clearly this needs to take place before the trial begins, although some form of quality assurance is also valuable as the trial proceeds.

Measurement error in the assessment of an outcome may be considered as consisting of a systematic component (*inaccuracy* or *bias*) and a random component (*imprecision* or *unreliability*). The observer may introduce systematic error into a measurement through knowledge of which treatment a patient has received. Such bias is best avoided by arranging, where possible, for assessments to be conducted in a blinded fashion. Sometimes this requires measurements to be performed by an observer who is not part of the clinical team providing care for the patient. Other possible sources of bias arise from faulty measurement technique or from the use of incorrectly calibrated instruments. In multicentre studies particular care must be taken to achieve comparability of assessment. The remainder of this section describes statistical methods which may be useful for analysing interobserver and intraobserver error.

For an interval scale outcome variable, there is potential to reduce the magnitude of the random component of error by increasing the number of measurements. For example, a better assessment of forced expiratory volume may be obtained from an average (or maximum) of three readings than from a single reading. If a series of measurements can be repeated by the same observer in similar circumstances then a simple method is available for obtaining the standard deviation or the coefficient of variation for measurement error (Bland 1987). The use of the correlation coefficient for this purpose is not recommended. Assuming measurement error is normally distributed, it is also possible to derive a measure called the *repeatability*, which indicates the magnitude of the difference between a pair of measurements which will only rarely be encountered. Note, however, that if the measurements are repeated by a different observer or using a different method, then *interobserver bias* or *method comparison* is likely to be of primary interest and different approaches to statistical analysis are appropriate (Bland 1987).

Subjective clinical gradings (for example, a patient's intubating condition or sedation level) typically give rise to nominal or ordinal scale data. Such measurements can be assessed for reliability and interobserver error using the κ statistic, (Siegel & Castellan 1988). This statistic provides a measure of agreement that takes into account the amount of agreement which might have been anticipated purely by chance. A value of 1 indicates perfect agreement, while a value of 0 indicates no more agreement than would be expected by chance. Although ranges of κ representing fair, moderate and almost perfect agreement have been suggested, the values obtained are probably best judged in the context of previous work.

5. SIMPLE STATISTICAL METHODS

5.1 Preliminary analysis

It is important that the trial sample is adequately characterised in terms of demographic and clinical characteristics. The first step in the statistical analysis is therefore pictorial presentation and the calculation of appropriate summary statistics. *Histograms* will indicate if an interval scale variable has a frequency distribution which is symmetric. For such a variable the usual measure of location is the mean, while the usual measure of dispersion is the standard deviation, but for a heavily skewed variable the median and range or interquartile range are more appropriate. Nominal scale data or ordinal scale data in the form of ordered categories are usually summarised with percentages.

Additionally, it is vital to demonstrate that the randomisation has produced study groups that are comparable. It is therefore necessary to supply suitable descriptive statistics for each treatment group. By convention, statistical tests of significance are usually performed to compare the baseline characteristics of the groups (section 5.2), although if the randomisation has been properly performed some statisticians regard such tests as superfluous. In practice if there are important imbalances between groups on baseline variables which are related to outcome, then the comparison of treatments may be *confounded*. Statistical techniques to adjust for such imbalances are mentioned briefly in section 5.3.

5.2 Comparisons between groups

The selection of an appropriate statistical technique for comparing groups depends on the study design, on the scale of measurement of the variable in question, and on whether or not certain assumptions are satisfied. Table 5.1 provides a guide to selection of tests of hypothesis. Descriptions of the methods can be found in standard statistical texts.

The techniques shown in the first line of Table 5.1 are called *parametric methods*. These methods typically require certain parametric assumptions. For example, in addition to the need for the variable to be interval scale, the independent samples *t* test and one-way analysis of variance require that, within each treatment group:

Table 5.1   A guide to selecting the appropriate statistical test for comparisons of treatment groups in a clinical trial

Scale of measurement	Two Groups		R Groups (R>2)	
	Independent	Paired	Independent	Matched
Interval scale (parametric assumptions satisfied)	Independent samples *t* test*	Paired samples *t* test*	One-way analysis of variance	Randomised block analysis of variance
Ordinal scale **Interval scale** (parametric assumptions not satisfied)	Mann–Whitney *U* test *or* Wilcoxon rank sum test	Wilcoxon signed rank test	Kruskal–Wallis analysis of variance	Friedman two-way analysis of variance
Nominal scale 2 categories	χ^2 test for 2 × 2 table *or* Fisher's exact probability test	McNemar's test	χ^2 test for R × 2 table	Cochran's *Q* test
C categories (C > 2)	χ^2 test for 2 × C table	—	χ^2 test for R × C table	—

*Or equivalent large-sample *z* test.

1. the variable should follow the normal distribution.
2. the variable should have approximately the same standard deviation.

Although statistical methods can help in the assessment of whether or not a variable follows the normal distribution, the techniques are not as useful as they might appear. Tests of hypothesis are insensitive unless sample sizes are large, and in this situation the normality requirement is often less critical. Graphical methods for assessing normality are also available, but these require subjective interpretation. A *transformation* may be applied to give transformed results that more closely satisfy the necessary assumptions. Often the *logarithmic* transformation is used to rectify positive skew, and it also permits a convenient interpretation in terms of multiplicative effects.

If the assumptions necessary for the parametric methods do not hold, then the *non-parametric methods*, shown in the second line of Table 5.1, may still be employed even though these methods are primarily intended for the analysis of ordinal scale variables. When used for interval scale data, the methods are slightly less efficient (i.e. there is a small sacrifice in power in using a non-parametric method on occasions when a parametric method could validly have been employed). Also, methods for calculating confidence intervals for means are much simpler and more widely available than are the corresponding methods for medians (Gardner & Altman 1989). Parametric methods are therefore recommended when the necessary assumptions can be justified. Nevertheless non-parametric methods must often be used, especially when sample sizes are small, as in such situations it is difficult to assess the validity of the parametric assumptions.

For nominal scale variables, the tests shown in the final line of Table 5.1 may be used. Most of these tests are *contingency table methods*. The calculation of confidence intervals for proportions is also relevant in such instances (Gardner & Altman 1989). A comprehensive yet readable account of both contingency table methods and non-parametric methods is available (Siegel & Castellan 1988).

Analyses involving more than two treatment groups may be complicated by the difficulty of interpreting a multitude of statistical tests. If the aim of an analysis is to test only a small number of hypotheses about pairs of groups that were specified in advance and stated in the trial protocol, then multiple testing is less of an issue. However, for the investigator who is testing hypotheses other than these (e.g. hypotheses formulated after looking at the results), a conservative approach is necessary to limit the risk of type I errors. This issue often arises when a significant result has been obtained in a one-way analysis of variance and the investigator wishes to state which groups differ from which other groups. Special *multiple comparison procedures* have been devised to address this problem (Armitage and Berry 1987). Each procedure permits comparisons to be performed, while offering certain safeguards against type I error. Associated methods are available for non-parametric techniques (Siegel & Castellan 1988) but they are seldom used.

5.3 Methods for the study of association

This section deals primarily with regression and correlation analyses, both of which are used to study associations between interval scale variables. Although these are key statistical techniques, their use in the analysis of clinical trials is limited. However, the techniques can be helpful in identifying baseline variables which are associated with an interval scale outcome variable, and which may therefore *confound* the comparison between treatment groups. Also, extensions of regression methodology may be used to adjust treatment comparisons for any such confounding variables which should happen to show differences in distribution between the groups. *Correlation analysis* is appropriate only if the relationship between two variables is linear, so a vital preliminary step is to plot a scatter diagram. The *correlation coefficient*, r, provides a measure, on a scale from −1 (perfect negative relationship) through 0 (no association) to +1 (perfect positive relationship), of the degree of linear relationship.

One might, for example, expect to obtain quite a strong positive correlation coefficient of, say, 0.7 between the weights and heights of a sample of men or women. Most computer packages provide a test of whether or not the correlation coefficient differs significantly from zero, and methods are also available for calculating 95% confidence limits.

Often *regression analysis* is more informative than correlation analysis, providing a better description of the relationship and permitting the making of predictions. *Simple* or *linear regression* specifies that the following relationship exists between a *dependent* (response or outcome) variable, y, and an *independent* (explanatory or predictor) variable, x.

$$y = a + bx$$

where a is the intercept (on the y axis) and b is the slope, the average increase in the y variable associated with unit increase in the x variable. An example might be the relationship between systolic blood pressure (in mmHg) and age (in years). A positive slope would be anticipated and would provide an estimate of the average increase in systolic blood pressure per year increase in age. Simple regression may be extended by adding further x variables to give a *multiple regression* analysis.

$$y = a + b_1x_1 + b_2x_2 + \ldots + b_mx_m$$

The slope b_j ($j = 1, \ldots, m$) is now interpreted as the average increase in the y variable associated with unit increase in the x_j variable with all other x variables held constant (or adjusting for all other x variables).

Multiple regression provides the basis for a technique called *analysis of covariance* in which a comparison between treatment groups on an interval scale response variable can be adjusted for chance imbalances in an interval scale *confounding variable* (or *covariate*). The technique can be extended to accommodate nominal scale confounding variables. For a trial whose outcome variable is nominal scale and binary (e.g. success/failure), an analogous technique called *multiple logistic regression* analysis may be employed.

Non-parametric methods are available for the study of associations between ordinal scale variables (e.g. *Spearman's rank correlation coefficient*), but they are not as flexible and useful as regression analysis.

Tests for association between qualitative (nominal scale) variables may be obtained using the contingency table methods in Table 5.1. Measures of association are also available (Siegel & Castellan 1988).

6. MORE SPECIALISED STATISTICAL METHODS

6.1 Sequential analysis

In most clinical trials the number of patients to be included is estimated in advance (section 4.1), and statistical analysis is performed once at the end of the trial. Occasionally for ethical reasons *interim analyses* are performed so that a trial may be terminated early if there is clear evidence of a difference between treatments. A single analysis at the conventional 5% significance level restricts the risk of type I error to 0.05 (or 1 in 20). However, if several interim analyses are performed on accumulating data, each at the 5% significance level, then the risk of type I error for the entire analysis will considerably exceed 5%. If such interim analyses are to be performed they must be conducted according to established protocols for *group sequential* analysis which restrict the risk of type I error to some specified level.

An alternative strategy is to employ *sequential analysis* methods, which permit an analysis to be performed after each patient completes the trial. Accumulating results are plotted on a chart and the trial stops when a boundary on the chart is crossed. Figure 5.2 shows an example of a sequential trial of two cough suppressants, pholcodine and diamorphine, given in a cross-over design (Armitage 1975). For each patient the outcome was a preference for one or other treatment. The excess preferences for pholcodine were plotted against the total number of preferences, patients with no preference being omitted from the analysis. The boundaries of the design were chosen to give 95% power to detect a differ-

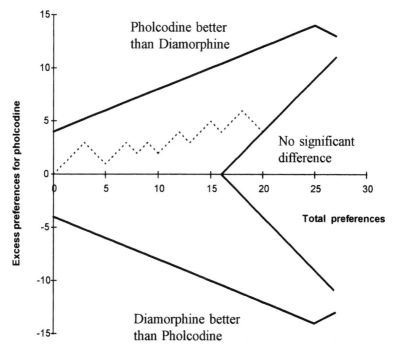

Figure 5.2   Sequential analysis of patient preferences for pholcodine and diamorphine cough suppressants showing the plot crossing the no significant difference boundary. The plot moves 'north east' after a preference for pholcodine and 'south east' after a preference for diamorphine. (Reproduced with permission from Snell ES, Armitage P 1957 Clinical comparison of diamorphine and pholcodine as cough suppressants. Lancet 6974: 860–682. © The Lancet Ltd.)

ence in preferences as extreme as 85% in favour of one treatment, and 15% in favour of the other as statistically significant at the 5% level. After 20 patients had contributed to the analysis the central boundary was crossed and consequently it was concluded there was no evidence of a difference in the effectiveness of the two treatments. Sequential designs are particularly suitable for comparisons of two treatments involving a single binary outcome (e.g. success or failure) which may be ascertained shortly after the patient enters the trial.

6.2 Repeated measures designs

Many trials in anaesthetics require serial readings of a response variable to be taken on each subject at prespecified times over an observation period. For example, in a trial comparing opioid analgesic premedicants, measurements of blood pressure may be recorded at 5 minute intervals to check for hypotension, while visual analogue

scale scores might be used to assess pain levels postoperatively at hourly intervals. Such data are called *repeated measures*, and are characterised by the tendency for measurements made at adjacent times to be highly correlated. Separate statistical analyses performed at each time point are not satisfactory because of the difficulty of interpreting multiple tests and because the analyses are not independent. Although special forms of analysis of variance for repeated measures are possible, certain important assumptions rarely hold. A multivariate analysis of variance approach requires fewer assumptions, but the technique is complex and findings are difficult to interpret. Furthermore these methods often do not address hypotheses of most clinical interest.

The recommended approach for the analysis of such data (Matthews et al 1990) is to define a suitable *summary measure* for the responses from each subject. The choice of measure will depend on the study. Often, as in the trial of premedicants, the minimum or maximum response may be satisfactory. For response variables that rise to a peak/fall to a nadir and return to baseline thereafter, other suitable measures could be the time to the peak/nadir or the area under the curve approximated using the trapezium rule. In other situations a rate of change with time may be obtained from the slope in a simple regression analysis using each subject's results as the dependent variable and time as the independent variable. Rates of absorption or excretion may be summarised using estimates of the time constant for a fitted exponential washin or washout function. Once values for the summary measure have been derived they are analysed using straightforward statistical methods, such as those in Table 5.1.

The summary measure method typically addresses issues of clinical interest more directly. It also has the advantage that it can usually cope with occasional items of missing data. It is recommended that the conventional plot of group means versus time is, when feasible, replaced by plots of the profiles of individual patients (Matthews et al 1990).

6.3 Analysis of cross-over trials

Although cross-over trials are extensively used in studying the pharmacological properties of drugs, they are less often used in clinical anaesthetic studies. However, they have been employed in the intensive care setting to assess treatments given to patients whose conditions are relatively stable. Two-period cross-over designs of the type illustrated in Figure 5.1 can be analysed using the paired samples techniques described in section 5.2, but more refined methods of analysis are available which make adjustment for period effects and which test for carry-over (Hills & Armitage 1979). However, the latter test often lacks statistical power and is therefore not recommended as a means for justifying the choice of length of washout period. The presence of carry-over invalidates the use of a two-period cross-over approach. The design of the trial must therefore ensure that the washout period is long enough to rule out the possibility

of carry-over. Otherwise a parallel-groups design should be used.

6.4 Estimation of ED_{50}

In some dose-finding studies, it is not possible to determine the exact dose required to produce some desired response in any given patient. All that can be observed is whether or not some chosen dose generates the response. An example is whether or not an induction dose of midazolam produces a response such as the loss of eyelash reflex. By repeating the process for a group of patients the proportion responding at any given dose may be observed. The aim is often to estimate the *median effective dose* (ED_{50}), the dose required to produce a response in 50% of patients. Typically the data for such a study take

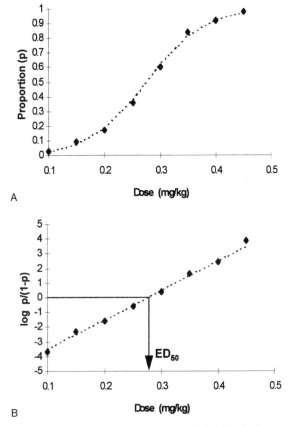

Figure 5.3 Proportion of patients with loss of eyelash reflex before (A) and after (B) application of the logistic transformation plotted against midazolam dose, showing estimation of the median effective dose (ED_{50}).

the form of the proportion of patients responding (p) at a number of equally-spaced doses chosen to straddle the expected ED_{50} result. A plot of the proportion responding against dose (or the logarithm of dose) produces a sigmoid curve, as illustrated in part A of Figure 5.3.

If the *logistic* transformation is applied to the proportions plotted on the vertical axis the effect will be to linearise the plot, as shown in part B of Figure 5.3, making it more suitable for regression analysis. However, simple regression analysis is not adequate because points must be given different weights during the fitting process. Suitable statistical software is available to estimate the ED_{50} and provide confidence limits. Alternatively the *probit* transformation may be used if the distribution of dose threshold in the population is thought to be normal; typically ED_{50} estimates differ very little from those obtained with the logistic transformation.

REFERENCES

Altman D G, Gore S M 1982 Statistics in practice. British Medical Association, London

Armitage P 1975 Sequential medical trials, 2nd edn. Blackwell Scientific, Oxford

Armitage P, Berry G 1987 Statistical methods in medical research, 2nd edn. Blackwell Scientific, Oxford

Bland J M 1987 An introduction to medical statistics. Oxford University Press, Oxford

Campbell M J, Machin D 1993 Medical statistics — a commonsense approach, 2nd edn. Wiley, Chichester

Gardner M J, Altman D G (eds) 1989 Statistics with confidence. British Medical Journal, London

Hill A B 1977 A short textbook of medical statistics. Hodder & Stoughton, London

Hills M, Armitage P 1979 The two-period cross-over trial. British Journal of Clinical Pharmacology 8: 7–20

Machin D, Campbell M J 1987 Statistical tables for the design of clinical trials. Blackwell Scientific, Oxford

Matthews J N S, Altman D G, Campbell M J, Royston P 1990 Analysis of serial measurements in medical research. British Medical Journal 300: 230–235

Siegel S, Castellan N J 1988 Nonparametric statistics for the behavioral sciences, 2nd edn. McGraw-Hill, New York

Nervous system

SECTION CONTENTS

6

The axon and synapse

A. C. McKay

THE NEURONE, AXON AND SYNAPSE

The nerve cell, or neurone, is the basic functional unit of the nervous system. Figure 6.1 is a representation of the most common type of neurone, as found, for example, in the cerebral motor cortex. It consists of three parts: a nucleated cell body (soma), a number of branching dendrites, which are projections of the soma, and a single axon. The axon may branch many times, each branch terminating on the dendrites or soma of

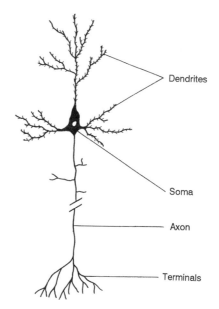

Dendrites

Soma

Axon

Terminals

Figure 6.1 Structure of a large neurone in the brain. (Modified with permission from Guyton AC 1991 Textbook of medical physiology, 8th edn. WB Saunders, Philadelphia.)

another cell. The terminal axons of other neurones — numbering as few as one or as many as 200 000 — form excitatory and inhibitory synapses on the neuronal membrane of the dendrites and the soma itself. These parts of the cell function as an input zone, through which information enters the neurone in the form of changes in membrane potential. The region at the origin of the long axonal process, termed the axon hillock or initial segment, has a lower threshold of excitability than the rest of the cell membrane and acts as an integrator of the various depolarising and hyper-polarising changes in membrane potential occurring in the neurone as a whole at a given moment. A sufficient depolarisation at the initial segment triggers an action potential, which is propagated both back over the soma and dendrites and distally along the axon.

There are many variants of this model. There are, for example, axoaxonal and dendrodendritic synapses. However, this generalised description does serve to distinguish the two modes of information transfer in the nervous system: synaptic transmission and axonal conduction. At a typical neuronal postsynaptic membrane, binding of the appropriate neurotransmitter causes a local change in ionic conductance and thus a change in membrane potential, which can summate with other similar changes. This membrane potential change is not propagated, so that its effects decrease with distance from the synapse and also with time. Axonal conduction, on the other hand, is by means of action potentials, which are large all-or-none depolarisations, caused by large, transitory, self-limiting ionic conductance changes, that may be propagated unchanged over long distances. The graded, non-propagating properties of neural postsynaptic potentials are similar to muscle end-plate potentials and the generator potentials of sensory receptors, while action potentials are the basis of contraction in skeletal, cardiac and some types of smooth muscle.

AXONAL TRANSMISSION
Resting membrane potential

The interior of an excitable cell membrane is electronegative with respect to the exterior, to an extent varying from about -30 mV in smooth muscle to -65 mV in the neuronal soma and -90 mV in large nerve and skeletal muscle fibres. The origin of the potential lies mainly in the distribution of ions inside and outside the cell and the differential permeability of the membrane to these ions. Large organic anions are confined to the interior of the cell. The distribution of monovalent cations, with sodium (Na^+) predominating in the extracellular fluid and potassium (K^+) in the cytoplasm, is due ultimately to the action of the ion pump Na^+,K^+-ATPase, which uses the energy of the terminal phosphate ester bond of adenosine triphosphate (ATP) to transport Na^+ out of and K^+ into the cell. In the resting state the membrane is more permeable to K^+ than to Na^+ by a factor of about 100, and the resting membrane potential is much closer to the electronegative equilibrium potential, which balances the tendency of K^+ to leak out of the cell, than the electropositive potential, which would balance the tendency of Na^+ to leak in. Na^+,K^+-ATPase, by pumping three Na^+ ions out of the cell for every two K^+ pumped in, also contributes to the electronegativity of the interior of the cell. The value of the resting membrane potential is the result of the summation of these factors. A change in the resting potential towards a less negative value is termed a depolarisation, and a change in the opposite direction a hyperpolarisation.

Chloride ion (Cl^-) contributes only slightly to the resting potential, even though there is a Cl^- concentration gradient from outside to inside the cell, because at a potential of -90 mV the distribution of this ion is close to electrochemical equilibrium.

Action potential

The mechanism of the nerve action potential depends on the presence in the excitable membrane of voltage gated Na^+ and K^+ ion channels. These channels, which are closed in the resting state, allow changes in the permeability of the membrane to these ions to occur, with consequent changes in the membrane potential. The Na^+ channel has an activation mechanism at the outer end of the channel and an inactivation mechanism at the inner end. The sequence of changes in the membrane potential that occur during an action potential is shown in Figure 6.2. If the membrane becomes depolarised to a threshold value, usually about –55 mV in a nerve fibre, a conformational change is induced in the voltage gated Na^+ channels so that they open. Since there is a large electrical and chemical gradient from outside to inside the membrane for Na^+ ions, these begin to flow inwards through the channels. This in turn further depolarises the membrane, opening more Na^+ channels and further increasing the flow of ions, giving rise to an explosive rise in membrane Na^+ conductance, which increases by a factor of up to 5000. During this time the membrane potential moves towards zero and usually, depending on the type of nerve fibre, overshoots, so that the interior of the fibre becomes positive with respect to the exterior by about 35–50 mV. This depolarisation is short lived. The initial electrochemical gradient

driving Na^+ ions into the cell declines, and in addition the channel inactivates after a short time. By this means the rapid influx of Na^+ ions is terminated, and the duration of the action potential spike is limited to about 1 ms. The channel remains closed until the membrane potential returns almost completely to the resting level. Voltage gated K^+ channels are less numerous in the axonal membrane than Na^+ channels, and the importance of their role in the action potential varies in different nerve fibres. As already noted, membrane permeability to K^+ in the resting state is much higher than that to Na^+ due to K^+ leak channels, so that even without voltage gated K^+ channels a certain amount of K^+ redistribution in response to depolarisation can occur. Typically, the depolarising current causes a slow opening of the K^+ channel so that K^+ conductance rises to a maximum by about 1.5 ms, by which time the Na^+ channels are already closed. The effect of opening the K^+ channels is to cause K^+ ions to flow out of the cell down their electrochemical

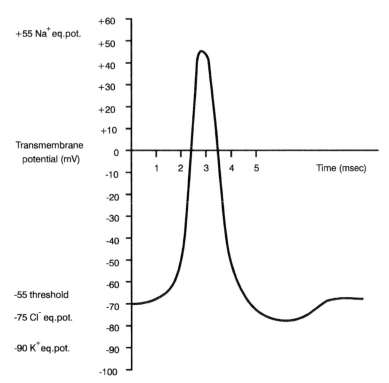

Figure 6.2 Nerve action potential, showing the relationship of the changes in membrane potential to the equilibrium potentials of the important ions.

gradient, increasing the electronegativity of the interior. After the Na^+ channels have closed, this unopposed K^+ current initially facilitates the return of the potential to the resting value and then, because the K^+ channels remain open for several further milliseconds, causes a transitory hyperpolarisation of the membrane.

Despite the large changes that occur in the membrane potential during this process, the number of ions that actually cross the membrane is extremely small compared to the overall numbers in the extracellular fluid and cytoplasm in the immediate vicinity. No measurable change in ionic concentrations occurs until many thousands or even millions of action potentials have taken place, and in the short term the ability of the nerve fibre to produce action potentials does not depend on the functioning of Na^+,K^+-ATPase.

Refractory period

Inactivation of the Na^+ channels means that the membrane is absolutely refractory to the effect of a further depolarising current, no matter how large. For a somewhat longer time following this absolute refractory period, a greater than normal depolarisation is required to initiate an action potential. This is termed the relative refractory period and is due to the after-hyperpolarisation resulting from the increased K^+ permeability during this phase.

Initiation and propagation of the action potential

An action potential is triggered by local depolarisation of the membrane to a threshold value. Experimentally, this depolarisation can be brought about by applying an electric stimulus.

In the axon, propagation of the action potential occurs by the creation of local electrotonic circuits. The structure of the membrane, with two layers of ions separated by an insulating lipid bilayer, gives it the properties of an electrical capacitor. The sharp increase in Na^+ permeability at the onset of the action potential causes discharge of the capacitor, with an inward flow of charge and local reversal of the membrane potential. The local circuit is completed by the flow of charge through resistances, both across the membrane and longitudinally in the cytoplasm. The flow of current across the membrane adjacent to the site of the action potential depolarises it and triggers an action potential there, thus enabling the action potential to be propagated over the whole length of the axon. Although local currents flow in both directions from the centre of excitation, the section which has just been depolarised is normally refractory to restimulation, so that, although the axon is capable of transmitting in either direction, under normal circumstances the action potential is propagated in one direction only.

Experimentally, the ability of a local current to initiate an action potential depends not only on the size of the current but also on its duration, as it is the total quantity of charge which is the determining factor. A weaker current needs to be applied for longer to allow depolarisation to reach threshold, and currents weaker than a certain value, termed the rheobase, will not trigger a response no matter for how long they are applied.

Conduction velocity in axons: myelination

The current flow in the local circuit, caused by the discharge of the membrane capacitance through the adjacent membrane resistance, decays exponentially over time. The larger the capacitance and the resistance, the greater will be the time required for this exponential decay, and thus the slower will be the electrotonic conduction of action potentials. The relationship of these properties to the size of the axon is such that, as the diameter of the fibre increases, there is an increase in membrane capacitance but a proportionately greater decrease in overall resistance. Therefore, the larger the fibre, the greater the conduction velocity; a fibre with twice the diameter of another will conduct faster than it by a factor of approximately 1.4 (square root of 2).

Conduction velocity is increased by a factor of about 100 when the larger nerve fibres are myelinated, as in many vertebrate central and peripheral axons. Myelin sheaths are composed of oligodendrocytes in the central and Schwann cells in the peripheral nervous systems. During development, the Schwann cell envelopes the axon and rotates around it, wrapping it in many layers of lipid membrane (Fig. 6.3). Every 1–3 mm along the axon are the gaps — the nodes of Ranvier — between the individual Schwann cells, each node 2–3 μm in length. The effects of myelination on the electrical properties of the axon are greatly to decrease the capacitance and increase the membrane resistance, while the resistance to longitudinal current flow is not affected. As well as increasing the velocity of local current flow, the increased membrane resistance improves the efficiency of the fibre as an electric cable, so that a local current declines less with distance along the axon. Since the membrane resistance of the myelinated sections is too high to allow sufficient ion flow for action potentials to be generated, these occur only at the nodes of Ranvier, which become much more densely populated with Na^+ channels than elsewhere. Action potentials thus jump from node to node in the process termed *saltatory conduction*, which allows larger mammalian peripheral nerves to transmit at velocities in the region of 100 m s^{-1}, compared to about 1–2 m s^{-1} in an

unmyelinated fibre. Saltatory conduction is also much more energy efficient than that in unmyelinated fibres because the transfer of ions across the membrane, and therefore the number that have eventually to be actively transported to maintain resting Na^+ and K^+ concentrations, is greatly reduced.

Factors affecting membrane excitability

The duration of the absolute refractory period dictates the upper limit of firing frequency for an axon, which may be as high as several hundreds of action potentials per second in a large mammalian nerve fibre.

The rate of rise of the depolarising current also has an important bearing on excitability. If this is lower than a critical rate, allowing some of the Na^+ channels to close, and K^+ channels to open, before the explosive opening of Na^+ channels, the membrane accommodates to the current and an action potential is not triggered. If a subthreshold depolarising current is short lasting, so that the opening of Na^+ channels is dominant, the threshold for depolarisation for an immediately following stimulus is reduced and excitability increased. A prolonged subthreshold depolarising current, on the other hand, raises the threshold of excitability to a following brief stimulus as the later events opposing excitation come into play. Thus the abruptness of the depolarisation is a crucial factor in deciding whether or not the membrane fires, and the system is afforded some protection against random potential changes. If a constant depolarising current is sufficiently large, however, accommodation is abolished and the membrane fires repetitively, at a rate that depends on the refractory period of the fibre.

The threshold depolarisation required to fire the membrane, and the propensity to fire repetitively, are affected by the extracellular calcium ion (Ca^{2+}) concentration. If extracellular $[Ca^{2+}]$ is lower than normal, the threshold is reduced and excitability increased. It is believed that normally Ca^{2+} binds to sites at the extracellular end of the Na^+ ion channel in a way that decreases the

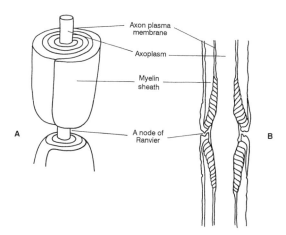

Figure 6.3   A: Schwann cell enveloping an axon to form a myelin sheath. B: Cross section through a myelinated axon near a node of Ranvier. (Reproduced with permission from Berne RM, Levy MN 1988 Physiology, 3rd edn. CV Mosby, St Louis, Missouri.)

likelihood of voltage induced activation. A fall in extracellular $[Ca^{2+}]$, caused for example by respiratory alkalosis, will lead to repetitive firing, which manifests itself clinically as *tetany*. Sensory fibres are similarly stimulated (paraesthesiae), as are central fibres (increased risk of convulsions). The same effect results from competitive displacement of Ca^{2+} in hypermagnesaemia. Conversely, hypercalcaemia increases the threshold for depolarisation, and its clinical effects include hypotonia and reflex depression.

In the earlier stages of hypoxia in excitable membranes, effects similar to those of hypocalcaemia are observed: the firing threshold for action potentials is reduced, leading on to repetitive firing, before eventually excitability falls. The mechanism is probably derangement of the oxygen dependent Na^+,K^+-ATPase pump, allowing accumulation of Na^+ ions in the cell and hence partial depolarisation of the membrane. Local anaesthetic drugs act on nerve fibres by blocking the Na^+ channel.

Nerve action potentials are thus a solution to the problem of how to convey signals over long distances quickly to a specific destination. The transmission of an action potential has been aptly compared to the movement of a spark along a trail of gunpowder. The amplification of the signal, required to overcome the inefficiency of the axon as a cable conductor, is provided by the properties of the axon itself. Since, however, action potentials are all-or-nothing phenomena, the only way in which information about, for example, a change in the strength of a stimulus can be conveyed by a single fibre is by a change in the frequency of firing. In most parts of the nervous system increasing strength of stimulation is signalled both by increased frequency of firing of individual fibres and by recruitment of increasing numbers of fibres with progressively higher thresholds.

Mixed peripheral nerves: compound action potential, classification, response to damage

In the periphery, nerve fibres run in mixed nerves containing fibres of various diameters and conduction velocities, some myelinated and some not, all wrapped in the fibrous perineural sheath. When such a nerve is stimulated at one point and a recording made from another, a *compound action potential* is obtained (Fig. 6.4). It is a complex series of waves comprised of the algebraically summed action potentials of fibres of differing conduction velocity, related to diameter, myelination and distance between nodes of Ranvier. Several classifications of peripheral nerve fibres have been made on the basis of the compound action potential, of which perhaps the most comprehensive is that of Erlanger and Gasser, who divided them into three groups, the first of which is further subdivided as shown in Table 6.1. The relative size and conduction velocity of the different fibre types is well adapted to their function, as the fibres subserving proprioception and movement, functions requiring the fastest possible responses, are in fact the fastest conducting.

Effects of local anaesthetic drugs and local hypoxia

The different fibre types are differentially sensitive to various forms of disturbance. The fact that sensitivity to the blocking action of local anaesthetics is highest in the smallest fibres is made use of clinically, for example in the 'walking epidural', in which the aim is to block the smaller fibres which carry pain signals, while leaving the larger motor and proprioceptive fibres intact.

On the other hand it is the largest myelinated fibres that are most sensitive to the effects of hypoxia or pressure, the small, unmyelinated C fibres being relatively protected.

Response to injury

Unlike central axons, those in the peripheral nerves can regenerate after injury, provided the cell body is intact. After section of a nerve, the axon distal to the injury undergoes degeneration but remains surrounded by its Schwann cell sheath. Proximal to the injury, there is chromatolysis of the cell nucleus, and the sectioned end of the fibre begins to grow at a rate of about

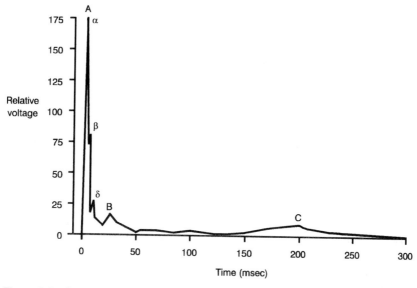

Figure 6.4 Compound action potential recorded from a mixed peripheral nerve, showing the latency and amplitudes of the recordings from the different classes of nerve fibre.

Table 6.1 Classification of nerve fibre types

Fibre type	Function	Diameter (μm)	Conduction velocity (m s^{-1})
A			
α	Proprioception, somatic motor	12–20	70–120
β	Touch, pressure	5–12	30–70
γ	Motor to muscle spindles	3–15	15–30
δ	Pain, cold, touch	2–5	12–30
B	Preganglionic autonomic	< 3	3–15
C			
Dorsal root	Pain, temperature, some mechanoreceptors, reflex responses	0.4–1.2	0.5–2
Sympathetic	Postganglionic	0.3–1.3	0.7–2.3

1 mm day^{-1} into the connective tissue sheath distal to the cut. However, the growing axon of a particular cell is unlikely to connect with the same channel that the nerve occupied before the injury, so that motor neurones may become connected to sensory receptors and sensory fibres to neuromuscular end-plates. In practice this can be minimised by careful surgical apposition of the severed fascicles. Eventually there is often compensation for residual deficit by hypertrophy of muscles whose nerve supply has been successfully restored. In crush injuries to nerves, where the anatomical alignments are preserved, complete recovery of function may occur. However, the conduction velocity in regenerating nerves is lower than normal, taking perhaps 6 months to be restored to half the preinjury value.

SYNAPTIC TRANSMISSION

General principles

The synapse is the junction point between one neurone and the next, or between a neurone and a muscle fibre. In the great majority of cases transmission is chemical, involving the transfer of a neurotransmitter substance from one cell to the other.

The sequence of events in synaptic transmission begins with the release of neurotransmitter from the presynaptic nerve terminal and its rapid diffusion across the very narrow synaptic gap. At the postsynaptic cell membrane, transmitters bind to their specific receptor proteins to initiate electrical changes. Neurotransmitters fall broadly into two groups according to their structure and the kind of effects they produce on the post-synaptic cell. In one group are acetylcholine and a number of comparatively low molecular weight amines and amino acids, synthesised within the presynaptic axonal terminal, which act mainly by altering membrane ionic permeabilities and hence altering the membrane potential of the postsynaptic cell. They are the mediators of the rapid responses that are characteristic of the mammalian nervous system. In the other, and much larger, group are the neuropeptides, larger molecules that are synthesised in the cell body of the presynaptic neurone and transported down the axon to its terminal. Their actions are much more prolonged than those of the small-molecule transmitters and include such effects as long term changes in neuronal excitability and in receptor numbers as well as altered intracellular metabolic activity. Although a presynaptic terminal may release one or more neuropeptide transmitters as well as a small-molecule transmitter, it is a general rule that not more than one small-molecule transmitter is released by the terminals of a given neurone. In circumstances where stimulation of a nerve leads to excitation at some synapses and inhibition at others, for example in the tendon stretch reflex, it is found that an inhibitory interneurone is interposed in the pathway.

In this chapter we are primarily concerned with rapid synaptic processes mediated by the small-molecule transmitters.

Release of transmitter at the presynaptic nerve terminal

The termination of a nerve fibre at the synaptic junction with the postsynaptic neurone is characteristically widened to form a terminal bouton or synaptic knob (Fig. 6.5). Within the cytoplasm of the synaptic knob are vesicles that contain quanta of transmitter, so termed because they are released all at once as the vesicle ruptures. Also contained in the cytoplasm are many mitochondria, which are involved in the active process of transmitter synthesis.

The most intensely studied and best understood example of neurotransmitter release is that in the neuromuscular junction, which is described later in the chapter, but the mechanism is believed to be essentially similar at all fast transmitting synapses in the central nervous system (CNS). In the resting state small amounts of transmitter are released through random fusion of vesicles with the presynaptic membrane. The arrival of an action potential at the presynaptic terminal, however, triggers the release of many quanta of transmitter, by a mechanism that involves the opening of voltage gated Ca^{2+} channels in the presynaptic membrane, and the consequent inward flow of Ca^{2+} ion. This increase in intracellular Ca^{2+} concentration brings about fusion of several hundred transmitter-containing vesicles with release sites on the presynaptic cell membrane, and their subsequent rupture, with the release of the transmitter into the synaptic cleft. Inhibition of voltage gated Ca^{2+} channel opening may be a significant part of the basis of general anaesthesia.

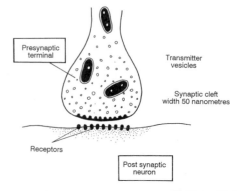

Figure 6.5 Structure of a synaptic junction in the CNS. (Reproduced with permission from Guyton AC 1991 Textbook of medical physiology, 8th edn. WB Saunders, Philadelphia.)

Fate of released transmitter

The width of the synaptic cleft separating the pre- and postsynaptic membranes is of the order of 50 nm and contains a reticular matrix. Molecules of transmitter diffuse rapidly across this space and bind to receptor proteins. Binding, however, is transitory, and molecules are removed from their sites of action within milliseconds of their arrival, not only by diffusion away from the site but also by destruction by specific enzymes that are present in the matrix of the synaptic cleft, such as cholinesterase in the case of cholinergic synapses, and, in other cases such as that of noradrenaline, by reuptake into the presynaptic terminal for reuse.

Action at the postsynaptic receptor

The receptors in the postsynaptic neuronal membrane are predominantly complex proteins, consisting of a transmitter binding component on the outer surface of the membrane and an ion channel which passes through the membrane to the interior. The nicotinic acetylcholine receptor, shown below in Figure 6.9, is one type whose structure has been worked out in detail. Binding of the appropriate transmitter activates the receptor by producing the conformational change which opens the ion channel. The effect of activation depends ultimately upon the type of channel rather than the transmitter.

Excitatory synapses

The most common type of excitatory synaptic receptor is the transmitter ligand gated channel which, when open, allows the free passage of sodium ions. Permeability to all cations is increased, but Na^+ is overwhelmingly the cation most affected by the increased conductance, so that there is a rapid influx of Na^+ from the extracellular fluid. As shown in Figure 6.6, this influx of positive ions causes a local, transient change in the intracellular potential to a less negative value, i.e. a partial depolarisation, termed an excitatory postsynaptic potential (EPSP). A single EPSP, resulting from discharge of a single presynaptic

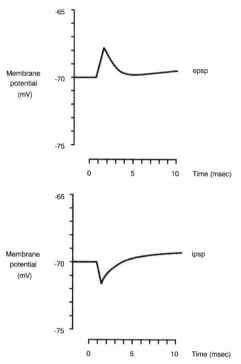

Figure 6.6 Excitatory (above) and inhibitory (below) postsynaptic potentials.

nerve ending, depolarises the membrane by about 0.5–1.0 mV and lasts about 1–2 ms, after which the Na^+ channel once more becomes inactive. The membrane potential then returns to normal over about 15–20 ms as the local potential change is dissipated by current flow in the neuronal soma and K^+ and Cl^- ions flow across the membrane. The effect of a single EPSP, therefore, is usually to produce only a transient, local, partial depolarisation of the postsynaptic cell membrane.

The EPSP and the nerve action potential are thus both initiated by an increase in Na^+ permeability, but while in the action potential the increase is self-regenerating because of the positive feedback effect of Na^+ inflow on the voltage gated Na^+ channel, the ligand gated channel does not have this property and its open time is limited by the short interaction of the transmitter and receptor. A further important property of the EPSP is that, unlike the action potential, it is not followed by a refractory period. This allows consecutive EPSPs to summate (see below) until a sufficiently large depolarisation, usually in the region of 20 mV, is reached to fire the neurone.

Postsynaptic inhibition

At inhibitory synapses transmitter is released from the presynaptic nerve ending by the same mechanism as at excitatory synapses, but its binding to the receptor causes opening of an associated K^+ or Cl^- ion channel. Usually the effect of the increased membrane permeability to either of these ions will be to cause an efflux of K^+ or an influx of Cl^- through the membrane. In either case a transient, local *hyperpolarisation* of the membrane, termed an inhibitory post-synaptic potential (IPSP) is produced, comparable in size and duration to an EPSP but opposite in sign (Fig. 6.6). Thus the membrane is rendered less excitable and the effect of an EPSP occurring at the same time on another part of the membrane will be opposed.

Response of the postsynaptic neurone

Spatial and temporal summation

A neurone in the CNS may well have many thousands of excitatory and inhibitory synapses impinging on its soma and dendrites. In such a neurone a single EPSP will not result in firing, but its excitability is subject to very fine control by *summation* of EPSPs and IPSPs. The neuronal soma has a high electrical conductance, so that the effect of an EPSP, producing a depolarisation of about 1 mV, which gradually declines over 10–15 ms, will spread throughout its extent. Other excitatory synapses acting elsewhere on the surface at the same time will also produce depolarisations, while inhibitory inputs will produce hyperpolarisations, so that at a given moment the effect on the membrane potential of the neurone as a whole corresponds to the algebraic sum of these positive and negative influences from different parts of the membrane. This effect is termed spatial summation. A comparable effect, known as temporal summation, occurs through repeated stimulation of the same

receptor. For example, since the opening of a Na^+ channel for 1–2 ms results in an EPSP lasting up to 15 ms, a second opening of the same channel within this time will cause a further depolarisation of the soma superimposed on the first. In this way repeated stimulation of a single excitatory synapse can cause firing of the postsynaptic neurone.

Excitability and firing of the postsynaptic neurone

If the balance of the above effects is excitatory the neurone may be held in a state of facilitation, so that a further small excitation causes firing. It is the state of the membrane potential at the initial segment, at the origin of the neuronal axon, that determines whether or not the neurone will fire an action potential. This is primarily because this part of the membrane contains a much higher concentration of voltage gated Na^+ channels than either the soma or the dendrites. A depolarisation of about 20 mV at the initial segment will trigger an action potential which, as well as travelling distally along the axon, spreads back over the soma. In the soma, the spike of the action potential is followed by a period of hyper-polarisation, and hence reduced excitability, which is largely due to opening of voltage gated K^+ channels by the action potential. This hyper-polarisation gradually diminishes over about 50 ms, so that over this time the excitatory state of the neurone increases and the degree of depolarisation required to cause it to fire a second time decreases. If the neurone is subjected to a constant bombardment of excitatory stimulation, as happens in some parts of the CNS, it will fire repeatedly, and the rate of firing will depend on three factors: the level of stimulation from the balance of excitatory and inhibitory synapses; the speed of the membrane potential's recovery from the hyperpolarisation following the last action potential; and the background level of the resting potential at the initial segment. This last factor is influenced by the activity of the slowly acting neuropeptide transmitters which also affect the neurone. The mechanism of control of long term excitability is primarily through the activity of slow K$^+$ channels, which have been shown to be affected by some general anaesthetics.

Presynaptic inhibition

In many parts of the CNS there are neurones whose axons terminate, not on the membrane of a postsynaptic cell, but on the axon of another neurone, just proximal to the termination of this second axon as it forms an excitatory synapse on a postsynaptic neurone. This is the anatomical basis of presynaptic inhibition. The mechanism appears to be that the transmitter released by the presynaptic inhibitory neurone partially depolarises the membrane of the terminal excitatory fibre, thereby reducing the peak amplitude of the excitatory action potential and consequently the number of vesicles of excitatory transmitter released at the synapse. Of the two types of inhibition (Fig. 6.7), presynaptic is the more precise mechanism of control, in that it regulates some excitatory inputs to the postsynaptic neurone without altering the latter's own excitability; postsynaptic inhibition, on the other hand, has a non-specific depressant effect on all excitatory inputs.

Advantages of synapses

In contrast to the limited capacity of the action potential for coding information, the integration of nerve impulses which occurs at synapses provides enormous scope for fine adjustment of signals, which may be blocked, amplified and modified in many ways. One of the most important properties of chemical synapses is that they act as valves, allowing transmission in one direction only, while the existence of inhibitory synapses, allowing transmission of negative as well as positive signals, adds a further dimension. Signals may *converge* from a number of different sources on to one neurone, which may require input from two or more of these sources before it will fire. Firing of the neurone will then show 'coincidence' in the firing of the presynaptic neurones.

Divergence, by branching of axons so that one presynaptic neurone can excite several in the next relay, allows signals to be amplified, and branches can also inhibit surrounding neurones. This *surround inhibition* operates at several relays in sensory transmission; stimulation of a point on the skin, for example, excites peripheral afferents, which both excite the second order neurones corresponding to the centre of stimulation and, via inhibitory interneurones, inhibit those corresponding to its periphery, with the overall effect of improving localisation of the initial stimulus.

Recurrent inhibition is a negative feedback mechanism found in association with the motor neurones of the spinal cord anterior horn. Collateral branches arise from the first node of Ranvier of the axons of these cells to synapse with an inhibitory interneurone, known as a Renshaw cell. The Renshaw cell axon branches and synapses with several motor neurones. A single discharge of a motor neurone produces a long chain of impulses from the appropriate Renshaw cell, each impulse causing an IPSP in the motor neurone which originally fired and in its neighbours. The effect is to act as a brake on the firing of motor neurones and limit the duration of muscle contraction.

Most centrally acting drugs act at synapses. In some cases, notably the opioids, there is direct agonist or antagonistic competition with the endogenous transmitter for sites on the receptor, while in other cases, such as the benzodiazepines, the drug binds on a different part of

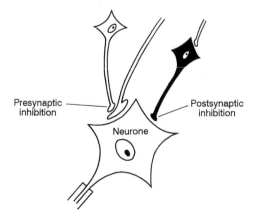

Figure 6.7 Presynaptic and postsynaptic inhibition. (Reproduced with permission from Ganong WF 1989 Review of medical physiology, 14th edn. Appleton & Lange, East Norwalk, Connecticut.)

the receptor from the transmitter. Actions of the latter kind on the γ-aminobutyric acid (GABA) receptor probably play a major role in the mechanism of general anaesthesia, although, because the activity of synaptic networks as described above is so delicately tuned, a minor anaesthetic induced disruption at any point would be expected to have far reaching consequences. The number of quanta of transmitter released at the presynaptic membrane is also reduced by some anaesthetics, possibly by means of an effect on the voltage gated Ca^{2+} channels.

INTEGRATED AXON–SYNAPSE UNIT IN THE CNS

Spinal cord dorsal horn

A neurone in one of the laminae of the dorsal horn of the grey matter of the spinal cord, whose axon projects centrally in, for example, the lateral spinothalamic tract, exemplifies how the balance of inputs from many sources may provide fine control of the volume and quality of onward transmission of sensory information from the periphery. Fibres carrying pain signals from the periphery are of two types: the faster myelinated Aδ and the slower unmyelinated C fibres. These fibres have their cell bodies in the dorsal root ganglia. C fibres, which make up 80% of pain afferents, terminate in the substantia gelatinosa of the dorsal horn, an area containing closely packed neurones and short interneuronal axons. The former include second order neurones of the pain pathways, which project centrally to the thalamus and reticular formation. Many nerve terminals synapse on these neurones and influence the onward transmission of the pain signals. The primary pain fibres, as well as synapsing directly on second order neurones, influence them indirectly through excitatory and inhibitory interneurones. Large diameter Aβ fibres, which carry touch and vibration sensation from the periphery, give off collateral branches to excite interneurones, which in turn inhibit second order neurones of the pain pathways through a presynaptic action on the terminals of primary pain afferents. This antinociceptive action of other afferents explains the well known beneficial

effect of rubbing a painful part, and is the theoretical basis for the analgesic use of transcutaneous nerve stimulation. Descending fibres from higher parts of the CNS also synapse on the interneurones, thus enabling pain signals to be influenced by the state of the whole CNS.

It is thus clear that many influences converge on the first synaptic relay in the pain pathway. The balance between these excitatory and inhibitory inputs determines whether or not pain signals are transmitted towards the brain.

Neuromuscular junction

The mammalian skeletal neuromuscular junction is a special example of an excitatory synapse, which has been intensely studied.

A motor unit comprises a lower motor neurone in the anterior horn of the spinal cord, its long axon, which divides into many terminal branches, and the associated skeletal muscle fibres, one for each branch of the axon. The motor neurone receives excitatory and inhibitory synaptic inputs from higher brain levels, muscle and tendon afferents, nociceptive and other skin afferents, Renshaw cells and others. Its Aα myelinated axon, which leaves the spinal cord via the ventral root and becomes part of a mixed peripheral nerve, is among the largest and fastest conducting in the body, with a diameter of up to 20 μm and a conduction velocity of 50–120 m s^{-1}. An axon supplying a large muscle may have up to 1000 branches.

Structure of the neuromuscular junction

At its terminal each branch of the motor nerve loses its myelin sheath and further divides to end in a depression, the junctional cleft, approximately in the centre of the surface membrane of the muscle fibre (Fig. 6.8). Within the nerve terminal the transmitter, acetylcholine (ACh), is synthesised from choline and acetylcoenzyme A under the control of the enzyme choline O-acetyltransferase. About 80% of the ACh in the nerve terminal becomes incorporated into synaptic vesicles, which, having been synthesised in the cell body and transported to the terminals, accu-

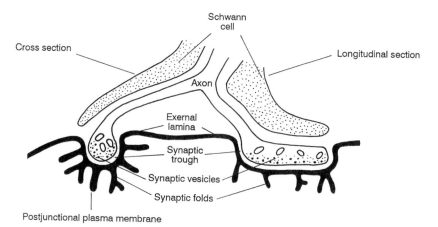

Figure 6.8 Ultrastructure of the skeletal neuromuscular junction. (Reproduced with permission from Berne RM, Levy MN 1988 Physiology, 3rd edn. CV Mosby, St Louis, Missouri.)

mulate in the centre of the nerve ending, from whence they move to sites of release, known as active zones, on the presynaptic membrane.

The junctional gap, about 50 nm wide, which separates the prejunctional (presynaptic) membrane from the muscle fibre membrane, is filled with a collagen-like matrix. As shown in Figure 6.8, the muscle (postjunctional) membrane immediately underlying the nerve ending is deeply folded, forming depressions known as secondary clefts. ACh receptors are concentrated on the folds between these clefts, i.e. closest to the nerve ending, and the active zones on the prejunctional membrane are positioned opposite the receptors. There is indirect evidence that there are also ACh receptors on the prejunctional ending itself.

ACh release at the neuromuscular junction

Two types of spontaneous release of ACh from the prejunctional membrane are recognised. The larger of these in terms of quantity of transmitter is the leakage of ACh dissolved in the cytoplasm, rather than contained in vesicles; the other is due to vesicles randomly discharging their contained quanta of ACh into the synaptic gap. These quanta, containing some 8000 ACh molecules, diffuse across the gap and occupy ACh receptors, causing opening of ion channels and characteristic small depolarisations of the muscle mem-

brane, which can be recorded within the fibre as *miniature end-plate potentials* (MEPPs). These normally occur with a frequency of about 1 Hz, but become more frequent if the resting potential of the presynaptic membrane is reduced, for example by increasing the extracellular K^+ concentration, or if the extracellular Ca^{2+} concentration is high.

The arrival at the presynaptic terminal of an action potential triggers the release of about 300 quanta of ACh, which diffuse across the junctional gap to produce a depolarisation of the postsynaptic membrane, termed an excitatory postsynaptic potential (EPP), which is normally of more than sufficient size to cause contraction of the muscle fibre. Voltage gated Na^+ channels are not present on the presynaptic ending itself, and depolarisation of the ending is thought to occur by electrotonic spread distally from the most distal Na^+ channels. This depolarisation opens membrane Ca^{2+} channels, causing an inrush of Ca^{2+} which brings about the release of ACh from the vesicles by a process that is not understood but may involve the calcium binding protein calmodulin. This calcium dependent release of ACh is antagonised by magnesium ion. At the same time membrane K^+ channels also open, permitting an outflow of these ions along their electrochemical gradient and restoration of the membrane potential to the resting level.

There is now indirect evidence that prejunctional ACh receptors, on the surface of the presynaptic membrane, have a role in the regulation of ACh release by enhancing the availability of ACh-filled vesicles at release sites. The mechanism of this process is not known, but it is thought to provide fine control of ACh availability, linking it to the frequency of nerve stimulation.

There is also evidence of a negative feedback control of ACh release through the action of adenosine and adenosine phosphates, which are also released from the nerve ending. Adenosine reduces the number of ACh quanta in the MEPP and EPP.

ACh action at the postjunctional membrane

Released ACh molecules cross the junctional gap and bind to a type of nicotinic ACh receptors, which, as noted above, are concentrated on the folds between the secondary clefts in the surface of the muscle membrane. The ACh receptor (Fig. 6.9) is made up of five helical protein subunits, each of which crosses the membrane five times in such a way as to form a channel with a hydrophilic core, allowing the passage of cations and water molecules. Two of the subunits, designated the α subunits, are identical and each contains one recognition site that binds reversibly to one molecule of ACh, and occupation of both sites brings about the conformational change in the receptor that opens the ion channel. This in turn causes a flow of cations along their electrochemical gradients, in which the inward flow of Na^+ predominates, resulting in a short lived inward current that depolarises the membrane. The discharge of one quantum of ACh from the prejunctional membrane causes the opening of about 2000 ion channels, while, as noted above, some 300 quanta are released in response to a nerve impulse. These depolarisations summate in a manner analogous to the temporal summation of EPSPs in a postsynaptic neurone, described above, and when a critical depolarisation of about 40 mV is reached an action potential is triggered in the muscle fibre. The processes by which this action potential

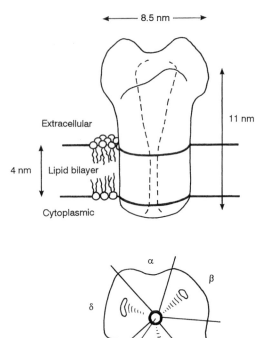

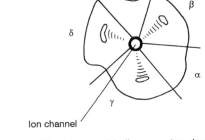

Figure 6.9 Nicotinic acetylcholine receptor, showing the membrane, ion channel and receptor subunits. (Reproduced with permission from Ganong WF 1989 Review of medical physiology, 14th edn. Appleton & Lange, East Norwalk, Connecticut.)

leads to muscle contraction are described in Chapter 19.

Using sophisticated electrophysiological techniques, such as patch clamping, to study the behaviour of individual channels, it has been shown that in frog skeletal muscle stimulated by ACh, mean channel open time is about 1 ms, and that this time is reduced if the membrane is partially depolarised. This appears to correspond to the duration of attachment of an ACh molecule to the receptor. It is thought that each ACh molecule binds to one receptor only and detaches from it when the channel closes. Experimentally, it can be shown that receptors become desensitised to the effects of ACh which is continuously applied and recover slowly when it is removed. This desensitisation, which is enhanced by increased Ca^{2+} and by some volatile anaesthetic agents, and opposed by increased Na^+ concentrations, may be a key to the blocking action of the depolarising agents decamethonium and suxamethonium.

The non-depolarising muscle relaxants, on the other hand, form bonds with the ACh receptor but are unable to induce the conformational change to open the channel. They thus block transmission by preventing ACh molecules from gaining access to the receptor.

Fate of ACh at the neuromuscular junction

Various molecular forms of the enzyme acetyl-cholinesterase are present in the neuromuscular junctional gap, especially in the region close to the receptors. An ACh molecule making contact with the catalytic subunit of the enzyme is hydrolysed to choline and acetic acid very rapidly — in about $100\,\mu s$ — so that under normal circumstances there is no accumulation of ACh in the gap, even during very high frequency stimulation. The choline and acetic acid are taken up by the nerve ending to be recycled into ACh.

In the presence of an anticholinesterase drug such as neostigmine, however, accumulation of ACh does occur, enabling individual molecules to bind on multiple occasions to receptor sites.

FURTHER READING

Agnew W S 1984 Voltage-regulated sodium channel molecules. Annual Review of Physiology 45: 517

Eccles J C 1968 The physiology of nerve cells. Johns Hopkins Press, Baltimore

Erlanger J, Gasser H S 1937 Electrical signs of nervous activity. University of Pennsylvania Press, Philadelphia

Hodgkin A L 1963 The conduction of the nervous impulse. C C Thomas, Springfield, IL

Keynes R D 1979 Ion channels in nerve-cell membranes. Scientific American 240: 126

Peper K, Bradley R J, Dreyer F 1982 The acetylcholine receptor at the neuromuscular junction. Physiological Reviews 62: 1271–1340

Simpson J A, Fitch W 1988 Applied neurophysiology with particular reference to anaesthesia. Wright, London

7

Local anaesthetics

J. P. Howe

Local anaesthetics are substances that reversibly depress impulse transmission in nerves. They are a closely related group of relatively simple aromatic compounds known as amino esters and amino amides. Although there are numerous local anaesthetic agents, only a few of them are clinically relevant to anaesthetists. These are, in chronological order of introduction, the esters — cocaine, benzocaine, procaine, amethocaine, chloroprocaine; and the amides — cinchocaine, lignocaine, mepivacaine, prilocaine, bupivacaine, etidocaine and ropivacaine (Fig. 7.1). The ester drugs are no longer used in regional anaesthetic practice in the UK but amethocaine and chloroprocaine are still used for subarachnoid and epidural anaesthesia, respectively, in the USA. Of the amide drugs only lignocaine, prilocaine and bupivacaine are available for anaesthetic use in the UK. Ropivacaine is due for release shortly. The remaining amides have been abandoned in favour of these agents. A diverse group of substances other than local anaesthetics can inhibit conduction, to varying degrees, in nerves and other excitable tissues. These include anticonvulsants, class 1 antiarrhythmics, antihistamines, β-adrenoceptor antagonists, opioids (especially pethidine) and a number of marine biotoxins.

CHEMICAL STRUCTURE

Local anaesthetics are a homogenous group of drugs of similar size and structure and fit the general description of poorly water soluble, weakly basic, aromatic amines. The molecule is

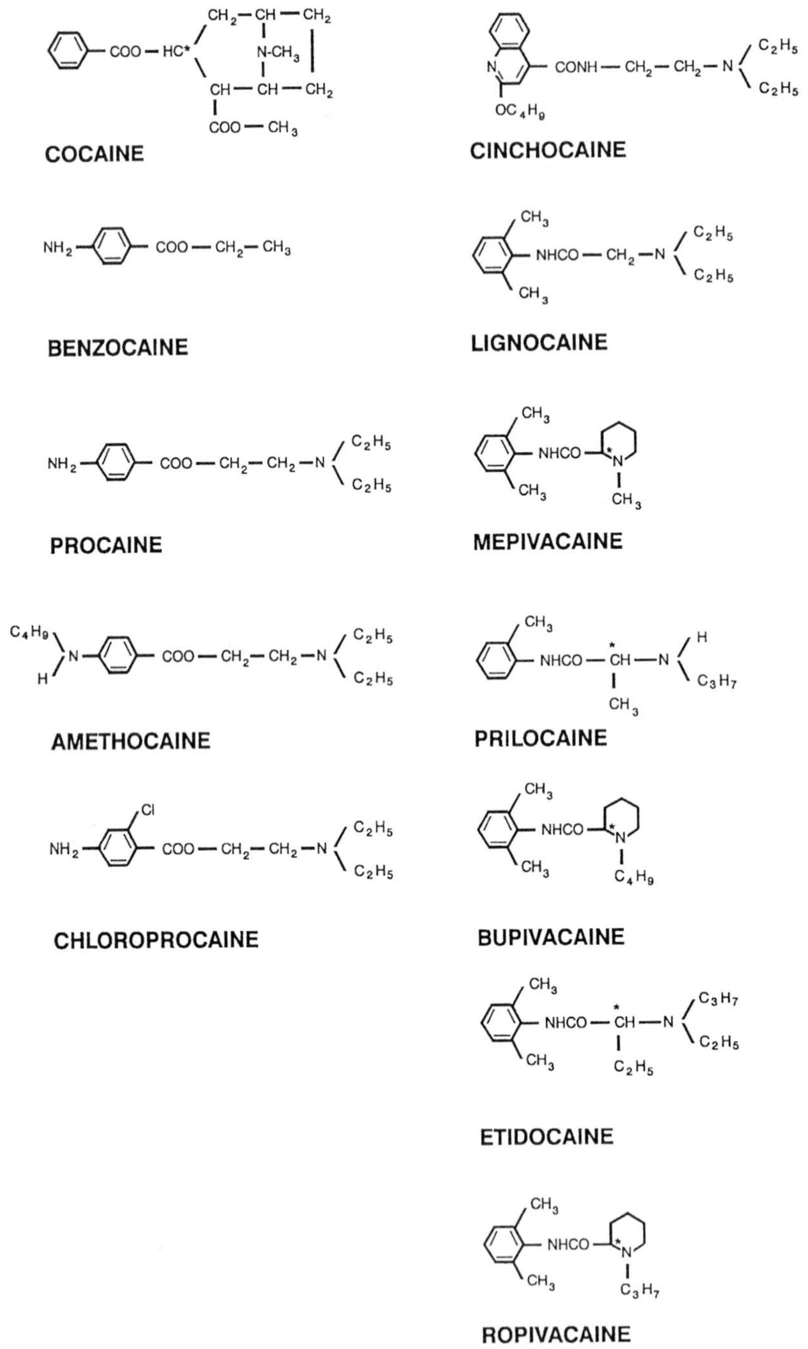

Figure 7.1 Chemical formulae of amino esters and amino amides. * denotes asymmetrical carbon atom.

composed of an aromatic 'head' and an amino 'tail' joined by an intermediate linkage (Fig. 7.2). Each of the three components confers different

properties on the molecule and it is these properties in turn which account for the clinical profile of each agent. All the clinically relevant local

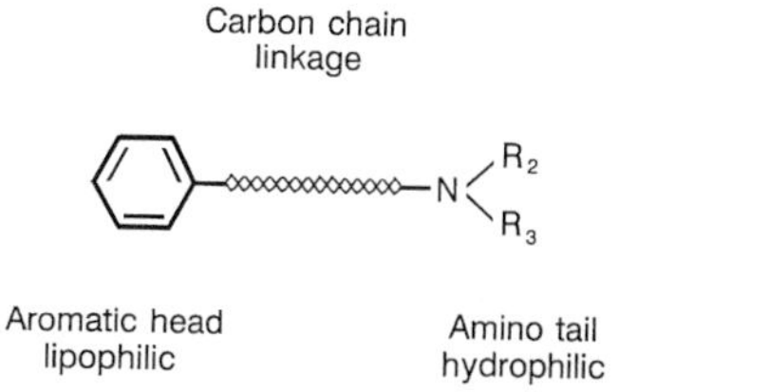

Carbon chain
linkage

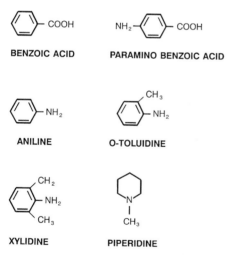

Aromatic head
lipophilic

Amino tail
hydrophilic

Figure 7.2 The three components of a local anaesthetic molecule.

anaesthetics are synthetic with the exception of cocaine.

Aromatic 'head'

The fundamental building block is a cyclical benzene ring, which is responsible for the physical 'bulk' of the molecule and also its lipid soluble properties. Cocaine is derived from benzoic acid and the remaining esters are derived from *p*-aminobenzoic acid. The amides are derived from aniline, methylation of which yields *o*-toluidine, the precursor of prilocaine (Fig. 7.3). Further methyl substitution gives xylidine, the precursor of all the remaining amide drugs except cinchocaine, which is a quinoline derivative.

BENZOIC ACID   — COOH

PARAMINO BENZOIC ACID   NH$_2$ — — COOH

ANILINE   — NH$_2$

O-TOLUIDINE   CH$_3$ — NH$_2$

XYLIDINE   CH$_2$ — NH$_2$ — CH$_3$

PIPERIDINE   N — CH$_3$

Figure 7.3 Structural elements of local anaesthetics.

Intermediate linkage

This is a carboxy chain of 6–8 nm in length made up of 1–3 carbon atoms. Chemically the

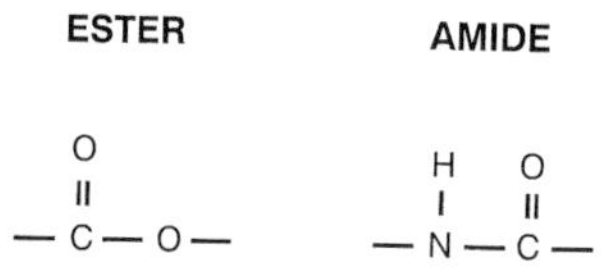

ESTER

$$-\overset{\overset{\displaystyle O}{\|}}{C}-O-$$

AMIDE

$$-\overset{\overset{\displaystyle H}{|}}{N}-\overset{\overset{\displaystyle O}{\|}}{C}-$$

Figure 7.4 Ester and amide linkages.

linkage is either an ester (—COO—) or an amide (—NHCO—) moiety (Fig. 7.4). The ester link is synthesised from an aromatic acid and an amino alcohol and the amide link is synthesised from an aromatic amine and an amino acid. This subdivision forms the basis of the classification of local anaesthetics because of the central role of the linkage in the synthesis and subsequent metabolism of the molecule. Esters are unstable compounds that undergo rapid ester hydrolysis in plasma, while amides are very stable compounds that require extensive hepatic biotransformation. Increasing the complexity of the linkage is associated with enhanced toxicity.

Terminal amine

This moiety is a tertiary amine, with the exceptions of prilocaine, which is a secondary amine, and benzocaine, which lacks a terminal amine. Amino compounds are weak bases (proton acceptors) that are partially water soluble. The unionised and the ionised forms coexist in dynamic equilibrium in solution as tertiary amine and quaternary ammonium compounds respectively (Fig. 7.5). The water solubility of the molecule is enhanced by the presence of the amino group but is restricted by the aromatic component. The nitrogen atom of the amino group of mepivacaine, bupivacaine and ropivacaine is contained within a cyclical piperidine ring (Fig. 7.3).

Structure and function

Local anaesthetics are aliphatic, i.e. they combine the properties of lipid and water solubility. The former is essential to the passage of drug across phospholipid cell membranes and the latter is essential to the ionisation of the drug, which is necessary for sodium channel inactivation. The active species extraneurally is the unionised form but the active species intraneurally is the ionised

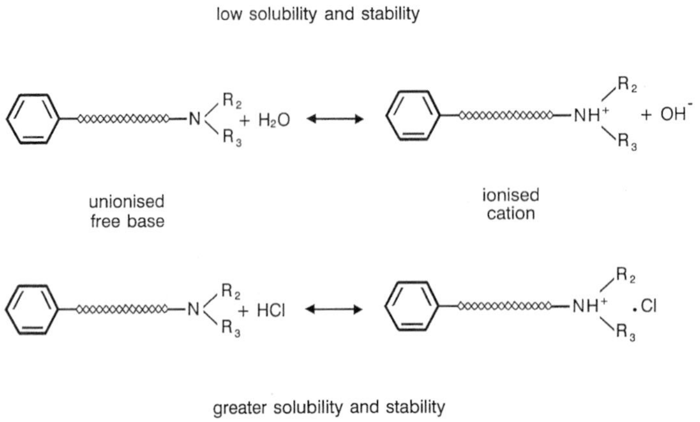

low solubility and stability

unionised
free base

ionised
cation

greater solubility and stability

Figure 7.5 Ionisation of local anaesthetic drug in solution. Combining the weak base with a strong acid increases its solubility.

form. Unionised, lipid soluble base will not produce impulse blockade when applied to the internal surface of the axon, and water soluble cation will not produce impulse blockade when applied to the exterior.

There are marked structural similarities among the drugs. The esters, procaine, amethocaine and chloroprocaine, are closely related compounds. Lignocaine, prilocaine and etidocaine are also structurally similar, as are mepivacaine, bupivacaine and ropivacaine (Fig. 7.1).

PHYSIOCHEMICAL PROPERTIES

The physical and chemical properties of local anaesthetics (Table 7.1) are important determinants of clinical effects. Lipid solubility, ionisation and protein binding are the most important but other factors such as spatial configuration and molecular size also play a role. The clinical profile of each drug is the sum of its physiochemical properties, no one of them being of overriding importance.

Table 7.1 Physical and chemical properties of local anaesthetics

Agent	Dissociation constant (pK_a)	Molecular weight	Protein binding (%)	Relative lipid solubility	Relative potency	Toxicity
Esters						
Cocaine	8.8	303	91	—	—	High
Benzocaine	3.5	165	—	—	—	Low
Procaine	8.9	236	6	<0.1	0.5	Low
Amethocaine	8.5	264	76	5	4	High
Chloroprocaine	9.1	271	—	0.2	?	Low
Amides						
Cinchocaine	8.5	343	—	—	—	High
Lignocaine	7.9	234	64	1	1	Med
Mepivacaine	7.6	246	78	0.5	1	Med
Prilocaine	7.9	220	55	0.6	1	Low
Bupivacaine	8.1	288	95	8	4	Med
Etidocaine	7.9	276	95	19	3	Med
Ropivacaine	8.1	274	95	3	3	Med

Lipid solubility

This is an index of a drug's affinity for lipid-rich tissues and therefore of its capacity to penetrate the axonal lipid bilayer, the neurilemma. It is quantified as the partition coefficient or ratio of distribution of a drug between a lipid and a non-lipid phase at equilibrium. The greater the partition coefficient, the greater the lipid solubility. The degree of lipid solubility is independent of ester or amide classification and is usually inversely proportional to water solubility. Only amethocaine, bupivacaine, etidocaine and ropivacaine are regarded as highly lipid soluble. High lipid solubility is associated with a slow onset or latency and prolonged duration of action. Both of these characteristics reflect the drug's affinity for non-specific perineural lipid sites, which act as a reservoir for drug storage. Conversely agents with low lipid solubility, such as procaine, have a rapid onset and a short duration of action. Modification of the procaine molecule by chlorination to yield 2-chloroprocaine increases its lipid solubility, and further substitution in the *para* position to yield amethocaine dramatically increases lipid solubility. Butyl substitution of mepivacaine yields bupivacaine, an agent with much greater lipid solubility. Etidocaine is the most lipid soluble of all the local anaesthetics and, while it has a long duration of action, it has a fast onset time. This is probably due to its relatively low pK_a (see below).

Aqueous solubility

Local anaesthetic base is poorly water soluble and is difficult to prepare in an effective and stable solution. Combining the weak base (B) with a strong acid (HCl) to form the hydrochloride salt increases aqueous solubility and stability, allowing more drug to reach the neural target (Fig. 7.5). It also renders the solution acidic with a pH in the range 3–5. When the resultant solution is injected into the tissues, which are alkaline, local buffering by bicarbonate yields the free unionised base (B), which is then available for neuronal penetration:

$$BH^+.Cl^- + HCO_3^- \Leftrightarrow B + H_2O + CO_2 + Cl^-.$$

pK_a

In the extracellular fluid a dynamic equilibrium is established between the unionised tertiary amine base and the ionised quaternary ammonium cation (Fig. 7.5). The relative proportion of the two forms is determined by the pK_a of the local anaesthetic, i.e. the pH at which half the drug is unionised free base and the other half is cation. The pK_a ultimately determines the amount of unionised drug that is available for diffusion across the neural membrane and subsequently the amount of ionised drug that is available for sodium channel binding. Applying the Henderson–Hasselbach equation:

$$\log([base]/[cation]) = pH(\text{of tissues}) - pK_a$$

where [ ] denotes concentration. In other words the *ratio* of base to cation is determined by the difference between the pH of the tissues and the pK_a of the drug. For lignocaine:

$$\log([base]/[cation]) = 7.4 - 7.9 = -0.5.$$

and converting the log gives a base to cation ratio of 0.33. Therefore only about 25% of lignocaine is unionised base at plasma pH and the other 75% is ionised. From this it is apparent that a high concentration of unionised base, and therefore rapid membrane penetration, is favoured by a low pK_a. Mepivacaine has the lowest pK_a of the amides, with a value of 7.6, and is 38% unionised at plasma pH (Table 7.2). Were a drug to have a pK_a of 7.4 it would of course be 50% unionised, and at a pK_a of 6.4 it would be 90% unionised.

After the unionised drug has crossed the neurilemma into the aqueous environment of the axoplasm the equilibrium between base and cation is re-established. Here a high concentration of cation is desirable and is favoured by a

Table 7.2 Dissociation of local anaesthetic agents: effect of pH and pK_a on the *unionised* portion expressed as a percentage of total drug

Tissue pH	Drug pK_a					
	9.1	8.8	8.5	8.1	7.9	7.6
7.6	3	5	11	24	34	50
7.4	2	3	7	17	24	38
7.2	1	2	5	11	17	29

high pK_a. Chloroprocaine, for example, has a pK_a of 9.1 and, while it is less than 5% unionised outside the axon, it is over 95% ionised inside the axon.

Stereoisomerism

The amide drugs prilocaine, etidocaine, mepivacaine, bupivacaine and ropivacaine contain an asymmetric carbon atom in the intermediate chain and exhibit spatial asymmetry or optical stereoisomerism (Fig. 7.1). During preparation equal amounts of the S and R varieties or enantiomers are formed, yielding a racemic mixture. The two enantiomers differ in their intrinsic potency, vasoactivity, biotransformation and toxic potential. Laboratory evidence indicates for example that the R(+) enantiomer of bupivacaine is about 30% more cardiotoxic than the S(−) enantiomer. Ropivacaine is the first local anaesthetic to be synthesised in a single enantiomeric form, namely S(−). This agent is an analogue of bupivacaine, with which it is nearly equipotent but much less cardiotoxic.

Protein binding

The major impact of protein binding on local anaesthetics is on drug kinetics after absorption into the bloodstream. This will be dealt with later. Binding of local anaesthetic to tissue proteins at perineural sites also occurs. High tissue binding delays systemic absorption and prolongs the concentration gradient of diffusable drug between the perineural tissues and the neural target. Drugs with low protein binding have a rapid onset and short duration of action and those with high protein binding have a slow onset and long duration. Only bupivacaine, etidocaine and ropivacaine are considered highly protein bound, 95% or more, and these are also the most highly lipid soluble drugs. High affinity for tissue and plasma proteins is probably associated with high affinity for the sodium channel binding protein.

MODE OF ACTION

The transmembrane resting potential of the axon is maintained at 70 to 90 mV, the interior being negative with respect to the exterior, by the selective impermeability of the nerve membrane to sodium ions. Nerve impulse transmission is due to self-propagating depolarisation, which results from a rapid increase in membrane conductance resulting in massive sodium influx into the cell and reversal of the electrical gradient. The nerve membrane contains complex proteins that function as ion channels for sodium. These are inactive under resting conditions and prevent sodium ion entry into the neurone but actively facilitate sodium ion influx during depolarisation. This mechanism is *voltage sensitive*. If a localised depolarisation fails to achieve the nerve threshold potential of approximately 55 to 65 mV, the sodium channel remains inactive and ion influx is prevented. At values greater than the threshold potential the channel is activated, allowing accelerated sodium ion influx and depolarisation. Local anaesthetic agents bind to and inactivate the sodium channel. By preventing sodium ion influx they prevent depolarisation. They have no effect on the value of the resting membrane potential or the threshold potential but produce a dose related fall in the velocity and magnitude of the action potential.

Sites of action

The local anaesthetic molecule has three possible routes of access to the sodium channel: the external opening of the channel, the internal opening of the channel, and from within the nerve membrane itself (Fig. 7.6). The substances best known for their ability to block the channel at its external opening are the marine biotoxins tetrodotoxin and sagitoxin. These are highly polar compounds that form tight bonds with the channel protein and dissociate slowly from the resultant complex, causing an irreversible block. An intramembrane site of action is the basis of the so-called membrane expansion theory of local anaesthetic action. This postulates a physiochemical alteration of the phospholipid matrix of the axonal membrane by the local anaesthetic molecule, leading to some, as yet unidentified, change in the sodium channel. Benzocaine is the clearest example because it exists only in the

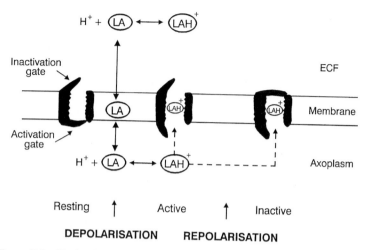

Figure 7.6 Mechanism of sodium channel inactivation by local anaesthetic. LA (local anaesthetic base) LAH (ionised local anaesthetic) ECF (extra cellular fluid).

unionised state and is ineffective if delivered directly into the axoplasm of the neurone. All the remaining clinically relevant local anaesthetics demonstrate only minor degrees of membrane expansion activity. By far the most important site of action of local anaesthetics is the axoplasmic opening of the sodium channel, where the ionised species induces an electrochemical change which prevents the inward passage of sodium ions. Most agents produce their effects by a combination of membrane expansion and ion channel inactivation, the latter being much more important. It has been estimated that for lignocaine over 90% of the block is due to ion channel inactivation.

Sodium channel gating

The massive influx of sodium ions during depolarisation is brought about by a configurational change in the sodium channel protein that is usefully explained in terms of a sequential gating mechanism (Fig. 7.6). Under resting conditions the activation gate of the channel is closed, inhibiting the inward passage of sodium ions. The arrival of a threshold potential opens the activation gate, thereby switching the channel from the resting to the active state and allowing sodium influx and depolarisation. The influx of sodium ions continues until the inactivation

gate closes, at which point depolarisation ceases and repolarisation begins. The channel has now switched from the active to the inactive state. Because the switch from resting to active to inactive is triggered by the arrival of a threshold potential, the gating mechanism is said to be 'voltage sensitive'.

Local anaesthetics function as non-depolarising sodium channel blockers. By binding to the sodium channel they prevent the configurational change which facilitates the inward passage of sodium ions. The exact mechanism probably involves a specific binding area within the channel protein and the bond is most likely electrostatic in origin, given that the local anaesthetic must be in its cationic form and that proteins contain anionic fragments. According to the modulated receptor hypothesis, local anaesthetics preferentially bind to the channel in the active and inactive states when access is relatively uninhibited (Fig. 7.6). Binding and dissociation are characterised as 'fast in, fast out' for all the local anaesthetics.

Other ions

There is also an ion channel for potassium, which is gated in the same voltage sensitive manner as the sodium channel. It can be inactivated by large doses of local anaesthetics but this is unnecessary for normal local anaesthetic activity. Under experimental conditions calcium interacts with local anaesthetics, perhaps by altering the surface charge on the nerve membrane. Elevation of extraneural calcium concentration decreases local anaesthetic potency and vice versa.

Frequency dependent block

Repetitive artificial depolarisation of a nerve results in the sodium channels being in the open state more frequently, recruits more of them and maintains them in the open state for longer. When a nerve is artificially stimulated during the application of a local anaesthetic the onset of block is hastened and the degree of block is enhanced compared with an unstimulated nerve. Drug uptake by the sodium channel is facilitated because the channel is maintained in the open state by stimulation. This is known as frequency dependent block, sometimes called use dependent block or phasic block. Only local anaesthetic cation can produce frequency dependent block; unionised base is ineffective.

Minimum blocking concentration (C_m)

This is the minimum concentration of a local anaesthetic that will prevent impulse conduction in vitro in a specified nerve within a specified time. It is analogous to minimum alveolar concentration for the inhaled anaesthetics and is of value when comparing the potencies of individual agents. For example, the in vitro concentration of prilocaine required to inhibit conduction in frog sciatic nerve is greater than the required concentration of lignocaine, which is greater than the required concentration of bupivacaine. Bupivacaine has the lowest C_m value in this setting and is therefore the most potent drug. Another nerve type will yield three different C_m values for these three agents, usually with the same rank order. The C_m has a specific value for each combination of drug and fibre type. A typical C_m for lignocaine and a medium-sized motor nerve is 0.1%, its low value being due to the fact that the drug is applied directly to the nerve in vitro. This concentration is ineffective in clinical anaesthesia where much higher con-

centrations are needed to overcome the various tissue barriers and the dispersion, dilution and absorption of the drug.

Differential block

Clinical observation indicates that nerves differ in their sensitivity to local anaesthetics. For lignocaine the rank order of block onset is vasodilatation (B fibres), loss of pain and temperature (C and Aδ fibres), muscle spindle reflex (Aγ), motor and pressure (Aβ) and large motor and proprioception (Aα). This phenomenon is known as differential block and is based on the assumption that some nerves are intrinsically more difficult to block than others. However, the apparent differences in sensitivity of the various fibre types can be accounted for by differences in local anaesthetic access posed by neural diffusion barriers. The most important of these are the Schwann cell, which is almost impenetrable to local anaesthetic drugs, and the myelin sheath, which is devoid of sodium channels. The local anaesthetic target site is an area of high sodium channel density located at the nodes of Ranvier of the myelin sheath. Large A fibres have a long myelin sheath segment between each node and it is known that the establishment of an effective block requires the inactivation of two or even three consecutive nodes to prevent saltatory conduction 'jumping' a blocked segment of only one node. Therefore a large nerve fibre with a large internodal distance will require more drug to produce an effective block than a small fibre with a short internodal distance or a fibre without any myelin sheath. Recent in vitro evidence indicates that desheathed nerves have similar C_m values during steady-state conditions, irrespective of fibre type. This supports the view that differential block is largely due to the diffusion barriers mentioned above.

PHARMACOKINETICS: LOCAL DISPOSITION AND SYSTEMIC ABSORPTION

The sequence of kinetic processes affecting local anaesthetics differs from that of other drugs used by the anaesthetist. Intravenous drugs undergo instantaneous absorption into the bloodstream, followed by the distribution of a high drug concentration to many organs of the body, only one of which is the target site. Local anaesthetics, on the other hand, are deposited at or near the target site and only after systemic absorption into the bloodstream are they distributed to other organs in relatively low concentrations. While absorption and distribution are essential to the efficacy of intravenous drugs, the same processes will reduce the efficacy of local anaesthetics by decreasing their perineural concentration and hastening their elimination. Drug absorption, distribution and elimination are dynamic processes that begin before the onset of conduction block and continue after its cessation.

Local disposition

The first process to impact on the kinetics of local anaesthetics is local disposition, i.e. drug dispersal at the injection site. The main components are bulk flow and diffusion.

Bulk flow

Bulk flow is the physical mass movement of drug at the site of administration. Its contribution to the spread of analgesia depends on the administration site and is difficult to assess. During tissue infiltration drug movement by bulk flow is limited by the physical constraints of the surrounding tissues. In the subarachnoid space hydrodynamic factors are important and in the interpleural space gravity is important. Provided the total dose of local anaesthetic is adequate for the purpose, neither the volume nor the concentration of the injectate is a reliable predictor of spread of analgesia. Increasing the concentration of the local anaesthetic solution can shorten the onset time but does not appreciably influence the extent of the block. Likewise, speed of injection does not influence local disposition to any great extent. Age has been shown to limit the spread of local anaesthetic in the epidural space. Hyaluronidase is a mucolytic enzyme that has been used to assist the tissue spread of local anaesthetics but in general has not established

itself because the commonly used drugs have good penetrating powers. Increasing use of regional anaesthesia for ophthalmic surgery, where extensive tissue penetration is important, has led to a resurgence of interest.

Diffusion

Once the immediate effect of bulk flow has ceased, further spread of anaesthetic solution away from the injection site is by diffusion and is largely governed by the ability of the drug to cross cell membranes. Diffusivity is a function of the molecular weight and lipid solubility of a drug, the effective concentration gradient and the properties of the cell wall. In general, local anaesthetics have a sufficiently low molecular weight and sufficiently high lipid solubility to ensure that the rate of diffusion is relatively uninhibited. The *net transfer* of drug across a membrane on the other hand is influenced by factors other than diffusivity. The rate at which bupivacaine can diffuse across cell membranes is extremely high, yet the absolute amount transferring into neural tissue is limited by extensive tissue binding and by tissue perfusion.

Physical barriers. The most important physical impediments to free drug diffusion are the tissue barriers of the Schwann cell, the myelin sheath and the perilemma. Equivalent blocks produced by the epidural and subarachnoid routes require substantially different doses of local anaesthetic, one of the reasons being the relative lack of covering of the nerves in the cerebrospinal fluid. The physical architecture of a mixed peripheral nerve means that access to the outer mantle fibres will be easier than access to the inner core fibres. It is for this reason that the onset of proximal analgesia precedes the onset of distal analgesia in brachial plexus block.

Drug properties. The importance of high lipid solubility and low molecular weight to rapid diffusion have already been mentioned. Perineural tissue binding of local anaesthetics limits their net transfer across the neural membrane. Extensive tissue binding is also associated with a depot effect, which prolongs the effective diffusion gradient between tissue and neurone, resulting in a slow onset and a long duration of action. Bupivacaine, etidocaine and ropivacaine fall into this category. The importance of drug pK_a has also been mentioned. A low pK_a facilitates diffusion by increasing the base to cation ratio.

Ambient pH. This is also an important determinant of base to cation ratio and is normally fixed at about 7.4 for extracellular fluid. It can change in a number of ways. Local sepsis, for example, can markedly reduce tissue pH. At an ambient pH of 6.8 the unionised fraction of lignocaine is reduced from its normal value of 25% to approximately 10%, with severe loss of efficacy. Repeated administration of acidified local anaesthetic solutions with a pH in the range 4–6 into areas of limited buffering capacity, such as the subarachnoid and epidural spaces, causes a progressive fall in tissue pH, resulting in loss of efficacy that is manifest as tachyphylaxis. Sodium metabisulphite is an acidic antioxidant used as a preservative in some local anaesthetic solutions and can also contribute to tissue acidosis. The inherently unstable ester drugs are stabilised in solution by maintaining the pH at a low value, as low as 3, and the injection of large volumes of these solutions carries a substantial acid load which may exceed the local buffering capacity. All of these will reduce the amount of unionised drug available for neural diffusion (Table 7.2). Intracellular acidosis also increases the fraction of ionised drug retained within the cell. This phenomenon is the basis of ion trapping.

Carbonation of local anaesthetic solutions has been used to reduce latency and increase efficacy. This involves the addition of carbon dioxide, instead of hydrochloric acid, to the local anaesthetic solution under two atmospheres pressure. When the solution is injected into the tissues the evolved carbon dioxide acidifies the axoplasm and increases the amount of cation available for sodium channel blockade. The potential reduction in diffusable base owing to acidification of the extracellular fluid is offset by the increased concentration of intraneuronal cation. The technique has not produced any discernible clinical gain.

Alkalinisation of a local anaesthetic solution with sodium bicarbonate immediately before injection will raise the pH from its normal value of 4–5 to more than 7. This will increase the amount of unionised drug, the main clinical benefit being a reduction in onset time. The clinical benefits have not been impressive and precipitation of the mixture in the syringe can occur.

Systemic absorption

This is the process by which local anaesthetic is removed from the tissues into the circulation. It is the link between local disposition and systemic disposition. The two main factors involved are the tissue concentration of freely diffusable drug and tissue blood flow. Blood concentration data indicate that absorption kinetics usually follow a biphasic pattern. Initial absorption is rapid owing to the high concentration gradient between tissue and circulation, and this is followed by a slower phase as tissue binding and neural uptake slow the rate of further absorption.

Site of injection

The uptake of readily diffusable local anaesthetic into the circulation is rapid and largely determined by tissue perfusion. The more vascular the injection site, the more rapid the uptake. Blood concentration of local anaesthetic after a single bolus injection is highest with interpleural and intercostal blocks, followed by the caudal, epidural and brachial plexus routes. The most widely studied technique is epidural administration, where bupivacaine, for example, appears in the blood within minutes of injection. A typical biphasic picture gives a peak plasma concentration at about 1 hour, followed by a terminal half-life of about 2.5 hours.

Drug properties

As expected, high lipid solubility and high protein binding promote local sequestration of drug, which delays absorption. This is associated with a prolonged time to peak plasma concentration and slow elimination. Increasing the concentration of the local anaesthetic solution will have minimal effects on absorption and plasma concentration except in poorly vascular areas. With most routes of administration there is a consistent relationship between total dose and plasma concentration. Prolonged epidural administration, on the other hand, can cause a progressive rise in plasma concentration, which is due to cumulation rather than increased absorption.

The vascular activity of a local anaesthetic can influence its own absorption. The most notable example is cocaine, a potent vasoconstrictor by virtue of its inhibition of catecholamine reuptake. The vasoconstrictor activity of cocaine limits the absorption of what is the most toxic of all local anaesthetics. The only other agent causing clinically relevant vasoconstriction is ropivacaine. The lower toxicity of $S(-)$ ropivacaine compared to $R(+)$ ropivacaine is due in part to lower systemic absorption secondary to vasoconstriction. In clinical doses all the remaining agents are vasodilatory to a greater or lesser extent, the most potent being procaine and chloroprocaine, followed by lignocaine, bupivacaine and prilocaine. When injected intra-arterially these five are all marked vasodilators. Drugs with poor local binding, such as lignocaine, are most susceptible to enhanced absorption secondary to vasodilatation. Other circulatory considerations that can influence systemic absorption are the vasodilatory effects of sympathetic blockade and the direct cardiovascular effects of absorbed drug.

Additives

The effect of a vasoconstrictor on the absorption of a local anaesthetic depends on the agent, the dose and the site of administration. Generally there is a reduction in the peak plasma concentration (C_{max}) with or without a delay in the time to C_{max}. Clinical benefits include a reduced risk of systemic toxicity and an extended duration of block. In highly vascular areas, such as the intercostal space, the addition of 1: 200 000 adrenaline to the anaesthetic solution will reduce the peak blood concentration by up to 50%. Vasoconstric-

tors are most effective at limiting the absorption of drugs of short to medium duration of action with low tissue binding. Vasoconstrictors can also improve the quality of a block.

Adrenaline remains the vasoconstrictor of choice in a concentration of 5 µg ml^{-1} (1:200 000), to a maximum dose of 200 µg. Larger doses do not confer any advantages and carry the risk of cardiac arrhythmias. Phenylephrine, noradrenaline and octapressin have been used from time to time but with no particular advantage. Clonidine has been tried recently but is ineffective.

Patient factors

There is minimal influence on absorption due to patient factors. Advancing age causes some reduction in absorption after epidural administration as a result of anatomical changes in the intervertebral spaces. Weight and pregnancy have no effect. Generalised conditions such as renal and cardiac disease may have a small and variable effect due to altered haemodynamics.

PHARMACOKINETICS: SYSTEMIC DISPOSITION

Distribution

Local anaesthetics appear in the blood within minutes of administration, the profile of the plasma concentration versus time curve being influenced largely by the characteristics of the individual agent, the dose, the site of injection and the presence or absence of vasoconstrictors. After systemic absorption local anaesthetics are widely distributed throughout the body, where organ blood flow and tissue affinity are important considerations in drug uptake. The plasma concentration at any given time depends on the rate at which drug is absorbed from the injection site into the bloodstream, distributed into and out of the various tissues and cleared from the plasma. Because of the difficulty in examining distribution kinetics following many local anaesthetic blocks when plasma concentrations are often negligible, kinetic profiles are derived from concentration/time data after intravenous injection. For example, plasma lignocaine concentration declines in a typical biexponential fashion, with a distribution half-life of a few minutes followed by an elimination half-life of about 100 minutes (Table 7.3). The vessel-rich organs equilibrate rapidly with arterial blood, within minutes, in a manner similar to induction agents.

Plasma protein binding

This has an important influence on drug distribution because only the unbound, free drug is available for transfer out of the plasma and into the tissues. The extent of protein binding differs among agents (Table 7.1) and this will affect the rate of transfer of drug out of the plasma. Binding to α_1-acid glycoprotein (AAG), a high affinity, low volume system, is more important than binding to albumin, a low affinity, high volume system. AAG is an acute phase protein which is affected by a multiplicity of conditions, such as pregnancy, malignancy and surgery. A rise in AAG concentration will reduce the amount of free drug in the plasma. Low AAG concentrations, present in the neonate for example, will have the opposite effect. Since the AAG system is saturable a sudden rise in total drug plasma concentration will cause a proportionately greater rise in the unbound fraction, with the risk of organ toxicity. Where a concentration gradient of unbound drug exists between plasma and tissue, for example across the placenta, the dissociation of the drug from its protein binding site and its transfer out of the plasma are instantaneous processes.

Tissue uptake

The lung is the first organ to be exposed to local anaesthetics and has an especially high tissue affinity for prilocaine. High first pass pulmonary extraction is an important protective mechanism for reducing the amount of free drug delivered to the systemic arterial circulation, particularly the vulnerable coronary and carotid vessels. There is some evidence that pulmonary extraction is greatest when plasma concentration rises rapidly and that sequestration of local anaesthetic may be due to ion trapping caused by the relatively low pH of 6.5 of lung tissue fluid. In the case of

prilocaine there is probably pulmonary detoxification in addition to sequestration because the clearance of prilocaine from the plasma exceeds total hepatic blood flow. Tissue uptake from the arterial circulation by the remaining vessel-rich organs is rapid owing to good perfusion and moderate to high tissue affinity, resulting in a rapid decline in arterial drug concentration. It is known that over 70% of a dose of lignocaine is removed from the systemic circulation of the rat by the vessel-rich organs within 1 minute of intravenous injection. The spleen and the lung have the highest tissue:plasma partition coefficients, followed by kidney, fat, brain and heart. Prolonged intravenous or epidural infusion of local anaesthetic will eventually cause the plasma concentration to rise as tissue storage becomes saturated.

Volume of distribution

The apparent volume of distribution at steady state V_{ss} is an indication of the extent of the spread of local anaesthetic throughout he body. The V_{ss} of the amide drugs are in the moderate range at about $1 \, \mathrm{l \, kg^{-1}}$, except for prilocaine which is about twice as high (Table 7.3). There is little information available on the ester agents. Extensive protein binding can be associated with a low V_{ss} value but is greatly outweighed in the case of local anaesthetics by high lipid solubility and intracellular ion trapping. When the unbound fraction only is used to calculate the volume of distribution, $V_{u_{ss}}$, the value for lignocaine rises to $4 \, \mathrm{l \, kg^{-1}}$, and that for bupivacaine to $15 \, \mathrm{l \, kg^{-1}}$ (Table 7.3). The large increase for bupivacaine suggests that the unbound fraction is small.

Metabolism and elimination

Ester and amide drugs differ in the method, site and rate of metabolism. Neither type undergoes neuronal metabolism, and renal excretion of unchanged drug is minimal. The metabolism and elimination of local anaesthetics bear little relationship to their clinical effects. Amethocaine, for example, has a duration of action of several hours because of extensive tissue binding but has

Table 7.3 Pharmacokinetic values for local anaesthetic drugs

	Lignocaine	Prilocaine	Bupivacaine	Ropivacaine
$t_{1/2}$ (h)	1.6	1.6	2.7	1.9
V_{ss} (l)	91	191	73	59
$V_{u_{ss}}$ (l)	253	320	1028	742
Cl (l min^{-1})	0.95	2.37	0.58	0.73
E_H	0.65	—	0.38	0.49

$t_{1/2}$, half-life; V_{ss}, volume of distribution at steady state; $V_{u_{ss}}$, volume of distribution (unbound fraction) at steady state; Cl, clearance; E_H, hepatic extraction ratio.

a plasma half-life of only a few minutes. Bupivacaine can be detected in plasma for a prolonged period after many blocks because of continuing absorption from the injection site.

Esters

These are hydrolysed by plasma cholinesterases and by esterases in erythrocytes and the liver. In vitro procaine, chloroprocaine and amethocaine are rapidly hydrolysed by plasma cholinesterases, with a half-life of the order of a few minutes. Their presence in human plasma during regional blockade is almost undetectable. A great advantage of rapid ester hydrolysis is the protection it affords against systemic toxicity due to inadvertent intravascular injection. The main metabolic by-products of the procaine derivatives are p-aminobenzoic acid and diethylaminoethanol. Cocaine is metabolised by liver rather than plasma esterases and has a much longer half-life than procaine and chloroprocaine. The main metabolites are ecgonine derivatives which may be active. There is little information available on the clearance of ester drugs.

Amides

These drugs undergo extensive hepatic biotransformation to more polar products and are then excreted in the urine. The important metabolic pathways are N-dealkylation, aromatic hydroxylation and amide hydrolysis and involve mixed function oxidases, cytochrome P-450, and amidases. The main metabolite of lignocaine is monoethylglycinexylidide (MEGX); that of bupivacaine and ropivacaine is pipecoloxylidide. Both these metabolites are pharmacologically active and MEGX in particular is associated with central nervous system (CNS) side-effects. Prilocaine is metabolised to o-toluidine and then to hydroxytoluidine. Amides have moderate to high hepatic extraction and their clearance is dependent on liver blood flow (Table 7.3). The estimated clearance of prilocaine exceeds total hepatic blood flow, suggesting an additional non-hepatic site of metabolism, probably the lung. The elimination half-lives of the amides vary between 1.6 and 2.7 hours and are prolonged in liver disease. Clearance is reduced in heart failure and liver disease. Renal disease tends to cause accumulation of polar metabolites but has minimal effects on the parent drugs. The addition of adrenaline to bupivacaine for epidural use can increase its clearance by altering cardiovascular haemodynamics.

Repeat epidural bolus administration of local anaesthetic in the postoperative period can lead to systemic accumulation and increasing plasma concentration. This is more marked with short acting drugs like lignocaine, which need to be given frequently. Even though total drug concentration may increase to toxic levels the unbound fraction is frequently unchanged, possibly due to an increase in AAG binding capacity in the postoperative period. The use of combined opioid and local anaesthetic mixtures has resulted in a substantial reduction in local anaesthetic requirements and greatly lessened the risk of cumulation.

ADVERSE EFFECTS

These are due to systemic toxicity, drug interactions, hypersensitivity and agent specific effects. Serious adverse reactions are nearly always due to toxicity caused by absolute or relative overdose.

Systemic toxicity

Local anaesthetic toxicity is a function of plasma free drug concentration and is influenced by the drug, the dose and the injection site. Transient symptoms of mild CNS toxicity can occur during properly performed regional anaesthetic procedures when the maximum recommended drug dose is administered. There is a progressive and predictable onset of symptoms that are rarely life threatening. The most common cause of serious toxicity is not overdose but inadvertent intravascular injection. Here the rate of rise of the plasma concentration is as important as the peak value. The brain and the heart are the organs most at risk during acute toxicity and symptoms correlate best with the arterial rather than the venous drug concentration. The predictable progression of symptoms which is a feature of lignocaine toxicity may be absent when toxicity is due to bupivacaine. There is no sound evidence for basing maximum dose on body weight.

CNS toxicity

The spectrum of CNS toxicity extends from mild and non-threatening to cardiorespiratory collapse and death. Even though the signs of CNS toxicity are excitatory, local anaesthetics are neuronal depressants. It is thought that depression reduces inhibitory activity initially. Benzodiazepine pretreatment and general anaesthesia delay the onset of CNS related toxic symptoms by enhancing inhibitory influences in the CNS.

The early symptoms of toxicity are numbness of the tongue and circumoral region, lightheadedness and tinnitus and are encountered most frequently in patients on intravenous antiarrhythmic therapy. They appear at plasma lignocaine concentrations of about $5 \, \mu g \, ml^{-1}$, the normal therapeutic range for antiarrhythmic activity being $2–4 \, \mu g \, ml^{-1}$. The early signs of toxicity with prilocaine occur at roughly similar plasma concentrations to lignocaine, and bupivacaine toxicity appears at plasma concentrations approximately half those of lignocaine. Further progression of toxic manifestations beyond mild CNS symptoms is an indication of impending seriousness. Drowsiness, visual disturbances and muscular twitching occur at lignocaine concentrations of $5–10 \, \mu g \, ml^{-1}$. Above $10 \, \mu g \, ml^{-1}$ convulsions, coma and respiratory arrest are likely. Serious CNS toxicity is indicative of imminent and potentially more lethal cardiac toxicity, direct cardiovascular depression occurring at plasma lignocaine concentrations greater than $20 \, \mu g \, ml^{-1}$. In some circumstances — for example, when drug plasma concentration rises very rapidly — the premonitory signs may be shortened or absent and cardiac toxicity can be the presenting feature. The usual time course of progression of symptoms can also be severely shortened when local anaesthetic is injected directly intra-arterially or intradurally in the region of the head and neck.

Cardiovascular system toxicity

Local anaesthetics directly depress myocardial conduction and myocardial contractility in a dose dependent manner. They bind to and inactivate myocardial sodium channels, reducing the velocity of the cardiac action potential and prolonging the QRS interval. Therapeutic antiarrhythmic activity predominates at low plasma concentrations such as those encountered during intravenous lignocaine therapy. When plasma concentration rises towards toxic levels more and more sodium channels become inactivated until there is a generalised reduction in automaticity accompanied by negative inotropy. Again, the rate of rise of plasma drug concentration is important. The progressive rise during antiarrhythmic therapy is better tolerated than the sudden rise of inadvertent intravascular injection.

Selective cardiotoxicity. The heart is more resistant to the toxic effects of local anaesthetics than the brain. The ratio of plasma drug concentration required to produce cardiovascular collapse (CC) relative to CNS toxicity, the CC:CNS ratio, is different for each agent. Lignocaine has a ratio of 7:1 and has a wider safety margin than bupivacaine, which has a ratio of 4:1.

Differences in toxic potential are due to different myocardial sodium channel binding affinities, which are in turn due to the physiochemical properties of the drugs. Binding is said to be state dependent. Lignocaine binds to the channel in the open and inactivated states, while bupivacaine is believed to bind in the inactivated state only. Dissociation or unbinding is greatest in the closed and resting states for both agents but is approximately 10 times slower for bupivacaine than for lignocaine. Lignocaine binding therefore can be characterised as 'fast in, fast out' and bupivacaine as 'fast in, slow out'. Prolonged binding of bupivacaine to the sodium channel is believed to be the basis of so-called selective cardiotoxicity. Prolonged binding is also believed to be the reason for the difficulty in resuscitation, from resistant ventricular fibrillation. Bretylium may be of value in the management of life threatening arrhythmias and resuscitation should be prolonged.

The sodium channel binding kinetics of the enantiomers of racemic bupivacaine, and probably other agents, are stereospecific. The binding affinity of $S(-)$ bupivacaine is less than $R(+)$ bupivacaine, hence the reduced cardiotoxicity of the former. The low cardiotoxicity of ropivacaine is of similar origin.

CNS mediated cardiotoxicity. There may also be indirect effects of local anaesthetics on the heart mediated by the CNS. Neurogenically mediated cardiotoxicity has been reproduced in the experimental animal by perfusing the cerebral ventricles with dilute bupivacaine. The early onset of life threatening ventricular arrhythmias is a prominent feature. The dose of bupivacaine required to produce this effect is much less than that needed to produce direct cardiotoxicity. Moreover the onset of bupivacaine cardiotoxicity of CNS origin can occur before the onset of other CNS symptoms such as convulsions.

Hypoxia, acidosis and pregnancy. Hypoxia, hypercarbia and acidosis will exacerbate local anaesthetic toxicity. The ensuing intracellular acidosis promotes trapping of local anaesthetic cation. Pregnancy may exacerbate the cardiotoxic effects of bupivacaine, but not lignocaine, by a combination of reduced drug binding by plasma proteins and progesterone sensitisation of the myocardium, so-called gestational cardiotoxicity.

Drug interactions

These are plentiful. Concurrent administration of lignocaine decreases the requirements of nitrous oxide and halothane in an additive fashion, i.e. reduces halothane minimum alveolar concentration (MAC). Anaesthesia with nitrous oxide and halothane also decreases the clearance of lignocaine due to reduced liver blood flow and enzyme inhibition. Propranolol reduces the clearance of lignocaine and bupivacaine by a similar mechanism. Verapamil displaces lignocaine from AAG binding sites, thereby raising unbound drug concentration. Pretreatment of non-parturients with cimetidine, but not ranitidine, decreases the clearance of lignocaine by reducing liver blood flow and by enzyme inhibition. Enzyme induction with barbiturates and phenytoin increases the clearance of lignocaine. Intravenous infusions of lignocaine and bupivacaine can increase liver blood flow, thereby hastening their own clearance. High concentrations of lignocaine depress the twitch response at the neuromuscular junction and can prolong the action of non-depolarising muscle relaxants. Adrenaline can increase the clearance of local anaesthetics by altering cardiovascular system dynamics.

Allergy

Many so-called allergic reactions to these drugs are reactions to their additives and preservatives and not to the local anaesthetics. Methylparaben, a preservative, and sodium metabisulphite, an antioxidant, are the most common offenders. True allergy to the amide drugs is extremely rare. Reactions to ester drugs are more common and are due to a *para*-aminobenzoic acid metabolite in a manner somewhat similar to sulphonamide reactions.

Drug specific

These are uncommon. Prilocaine induced methaemoglobinaemia is due to accumulation of a metabolite, 6-hydroxytoluidine, and is dose related, not allergic, in origin. Cocaine is alone in causing dependence, the result of its cerebral stimulating and euphoric effects. Neurological damage in the form of cauda equina syndrome has been reported after the combined use of lignocaine and microspinal catheters. It is probably due to neuritis caused by poor dispersion at the catheter tip of highly concentrated hyperbaric 5% lignocaine. Neurological damage has also been associated with the accidental administration of large doses of chloroprocaine intrathecally and is due to its preservative sodium metabisulphite. Myotoxicity is common to all the local anaesthetics after intramuscular injection and is maximal with cocaine.

PLACENTAL TRANSFER

Most drugs cross the placenta by simple diffusion. The *rate* of transfer depends on placental blood flow, the presence of an adequate concentration gradient and certain characteristics of the drug, the most important being lipid solubility and molecular weight. Amide local anaesthetics have a sufficiently low molecular weight and sufficiently high lipid solubility to ensure that transfer is almost entirely flow dependent. These drugs effectively equilibrate across the placenta in a single circulation. Since only unbound drug is available for transplacental diffusion the *amount* transferred will be governed by the extent of protein binding in the mother and fetus. Protein binding of local anaesthetic to AAG is greater in the mother than in the fetus because of low fetal AAG concentration at term. At similar total drug plasma concentrations the percentage of bound drug is greater in the mother than in the fetus and the percentage of unbound drug is greater in the fetus than in the mother. Consequently distribution of local anaesthetic across the placenta will favour the maternal circulation. An agent which is highly protein bound has a relatively lower fetal to maternal (F:M) ratio of plasma concentrations than an agent with poor protein binding. High protein binding therefore reduces the risk of toxicity in the fetus. The pH of fetal plasma is typically 0.1 lower than maternal plasma and can be substantially lower during fetal distress. Lower pH favours greater ionisation of drug in fetal plasma than in maternal plasma and promotes ion trapping in the fetus. Worsening fetal acidosis therefore produces a rise in F:M total drug ratio.

Equilibration of free local anaesthetic base between maternal and fetal circulations after a single bolus injection is almost immediate. This is followed by a decrease in plasma concentration in mother and fetus and a rise in fetal tissue concentration, until all three equilibrate at about 1 hour. When administration is by continuous low dose epidural infusion, equilibration of free drug between mother and fetus takes several hours. The F:M ratio of plasma concentrations of total drug at equilibrium is 0.3 for bupivacaine and ropivacaine, 0.6 for lignocaine and 1.0 for prilocaine. The low value for bupivacaine and ropivacaine reflect their extensive protein binding in the mother rather than tissue uptake from fetal plasma. At equilibrium the F:M ratio of free drug approaches unity for all the local anaesthetics.

Because of its short duration of action, and therefore the need for repeat dosing, continuous epidural infusion of lignocaine is associated with systemic cumulation and can cause toxicity in the mother and 'floppy baby' syndrome in the neonate. Prilocaine has the same problem and in addition carries the unacceptable risk to the fetus of methaemoglobinaemia. Bupivacaine is the agent of choice for analgesia in labour because of its long duration of action and has the added benefit of causing minimal neurobehavioural upset in the newborn. Ropivacaine can be expected to have a similar profile to bupivacaine, with the advantage of lower cardiac toxicity. The disposition of amide local anaesthetics in the neonate is broadly similar to the adult but clearance is much slower. Elimination half-life of all the amide drugs is prolonged in the neonate, exceeding 20 hours for bupivacaine. Hepatic metabolism yields similar breakdown products to the adult. Chloroprocaine is the only ester drug used for obstetric epidural anaesthesia, for which it is used infrequently. It has the advantage of limited fetal exposure to the drug owing to rapid ester hydrolysis in maternal plasma.

INDIVIDUAL AGENTS

Lignocaine

This is the most widely used agent and is the gold standard by which the others are judged. It has a quick onset and a medium duration of action and has medium potency and medium toxicity. It is available as the injectable hydrochloride salt in solutions of 0.5–2.0%. Topical preparations are available in concentrations of 2% and 4% in viscous, gel and metered aerosol forms. It is employed for infiltration analgesia, peripheral nerve block, intravenous regional anaesthesia, spinal and epidural anaesthesia as well as for topical application. Duration of anaesthesia after infiltration is of the order of 1 hour, increasing to 2 hours in the presence of adrenaline. The maximum safe dose by single injection is 300 mg, increasing to 500 mg with the addition of adrenaline. Since toxic symptoms depend on plasma concentration, it is possible to use a larger dose in areas of low vascularity. Normal therapeutic doses do not directly affect cardiac output, blood pressure or total systemic vascular resistance. Sustained low plasma concentrations, such as those encountered during intravenous antiarrhythmic therapy, can produce tachycardia and an increase in arterial blood pressure, believed to be due to central sympathetic stimulation. Lignocaine is a class Ib antiarrhythmic drug and is used to treat ventricular arrhythmias (see Ch. 24). It has also been used in the management of neonatal convulsions, chronic pain syndromes in adults and as a parenteral analgesic. This versatile drug has also been shown to possess anti-inflammatory, antithrombotic and antimicrobial activity.

Prilocaine

This agent has a quick onset of action and is equipotent with but somewhat longer acting than lignocaine. The main advantage over lignocaine is a reduced risk of toxicity due to more rapid clearance from the circulation. There is a good case for making it the drug of choice for routine use because the safe maximum dose is only likely to be exceeded when very large doses are employed. Injectable preparations are available in 0.5–2.0% solution, with and without felypressin as a vasoconstrictor. The addition of the vasoconstrictor approximately doubles its duration of action. Its main uses are infiltration analgesia and intravenous regional anaesthesia, where its low toxicity makes it the drug of choice. It is not recommended for epidural use in obstetrics because of the need for repeat dosing. The safe maximum dose is 400 mg, increasing to 600 mg with a vasoconstrictor. Doses in excess of 600 mg cause methaemoglobinaemia, which can be reversed with methylene blue 1 mg kg^{-1} intravenously. There are no overt direct cardiovascular effects attributable to prilocaine. Unlike lignocaine it is a poor local vasodilator. A topical preparation is available in combination with lignocaine (EMLA 5%). This eutectic mixture of local anaesthetic is a combination of equal amounts of crystalline 2.5% prilocaine and 2.5% lignocaine. The mixture has a lower melting point than the individual drugs and becomes an oil at room temperature, which is then emulsified in water to yield EMLA cream. Most of the drug combination is in the unionised readily diffusable form. Application 30–60 minutes before venepuncture is essential to allow transdermal delivery of EMLA. Application for 120 minutes allows partial skin grafting.

Bupivacaine

This agent has a slow onset and a long duration of action, typically about 3 hours. Bupivacaine hydrochloride solution is available as 0.25%, 0.5% and 0.75% and its main uses are infiltration anaesthesia, peripheral nerve block, epidural and subarachnoid anaesthesia. The incidence of motor block increases progressively with increasing concentration. Bupivacaine is not recommended for intravenous regional anaesthesia and the 0.75% preparation is not recommended for epidural use in obstetrics because the safe maximum total dose is easily exceeded. The safe single dose for general use is 150 mg and the maximum daily dose is 400 mg. The addition of adrenaline has only a marginal effect on these recommendations. High potency and prolonged duration of action make bupivacaine a suitable agent for repeat administration as the risk of cumulation is greatly reduced. Incremental, as distinct from bolus, epidural dosing for operative procedures further reduces the risk of toxic plasma concentrations. The use of dilute infusions of epidural bupivacaine combined with opioids such as fentanyl and alfentanil has proved a satisfactory method of providing prolonged analgesia without cumulation or toxicity.

Ropivacaine

This is the propyl homologue of bupivacaine, with which it is nearly equipotent. The onset time is shorter than bupivacaine and the duration of action is similar. Its main advantages are a reduction in motor block and a lesser risk of cardiotoxicity than bupivacaine. Infiltration analgesia, peripheral nerve block and epidural anaesthesia are its main uses. It is prepared as the hydrochloride salt and is available in solutions of 0.5–2.0%. The safe dose is 150–200 mg. Clinical doses of ropivacaine do not appear to have any overt cardiovascular effects. Ropivacaine causes localised vasoconstriction and may be of use where a dry operative field is of benefit.

Esters

Cocaine is limited to topical use only, because of its high toxicity and the potential for dependence. Cardiovascular stimulation produces hypertension, vasoconstriction, mydriasis and tachyarrhythmias. Stimulation of the CNS produces restlessness and euphoria. Cocaine is made up as 4% and 10% solutions for surface anaesthesia. The combination of anaesthesia and vasoconstriction make it suitable for minor

nasal procedures and awake nasotracheal intubation. Maximum dose is 100 mg. The addition of adrenaline is not recommended.

Procaine has low toxicity, rapid onset and short to medium duration of action. It has been used for every form of regional anaesthesia and was for many years the gold standard local anaesthetic drug. Prominent features are vasodilator and antiarrhythmic activity. It is no longer employed routinely.

Chloroprocaine has a rapid onset, short duration of action and low toxicity. It is not available in the UK but is still used extensively in the USA, particularly for day procedures, as a 0.5–3.0% solution for infiltration, peripheral nerve block and epidural block. It is not recommended for subarachnoid use. Maximum dose is 800 mg, increasing to 1000 mg with adrenaline. A prominent safety feature is the very short plasma half-life of less than 1 minute.

Amethocaine is the most potent and longest acting of the esters. It is much more toxic than procaine and chloroprocaine and is only available as surface and topical preparations in the UK. In the USA it is still used for subarachnoid block (tetracaine *USP*), where low dosage poses no threat of toxicity.

Sameridine

This is a new type of drug that is currently undergoing investigation as a spinal anaesthetic. It is not a conventional local anaesthetic agent but is a piperidine derivative similar in structure to pethidine. It possesses partial μ opioid agonist and local anaesthetic properties. Sameridine is equipotent with bupivacaine for operative surgery and provides prolonged postoperative analgesia.

FURTHER READING

Local anaesthetics 1993 In: Reynolds J E F (ed) Martindale the extra pharmacopoeia, 30th edn, pp 995–1018. Pharmaceutical Press, London
McCaughey W 1992 Adverse effects of local anaesthetics. Drug Safety 7(3): 178–189
Reiz S, Nath S 1986 Cardiotoxicity of local anaesthetic

agents. British Journal of Anaesthesia 58: 736–743
Tucker G T 1986 Pharmacokinetics of local anaesthetics. British Journal of Anaesthesia 58: 717–731
Wildsmith J A W, Armitage E N (eds) 1993 Principles and practice of regional anaesthesia, 2nd edn. Churchill Livingstone, Edinburgh

8

Physiology of the central nervous system

A. C. McKay

The human brain contains around 100 000 000 000 neurones, and the number of synaptic connections of which it is theoretically capable exceeds most estimates of the number of atoms in the universe. The unique properties of the central nevous system (CNS) as a whole depend on the extremely complex manner in which the simultaneous and sequential activities of the millions of neurones, axons and synapses interrelate. Sensory function, neuropharmacology and the autonomic nervous system are described in separate chapters of this book. This chapter will briefly review the sensory, motor and integrative functions of the CNS as well as aspects of CNS physiology particularly relevant to anaesthesia and intensive care.

Anatomically, the CNS consists of the brain and spinal cord. Anatomical subdivision of the brain is primarily based on gross appearances and, through comparative studies, on the evolutionary history of the various components. Five parts may be distinguished: the forebrain (prosencephalon), midbrain (mesencephalon), medulla oblongata, pons and cerebellum (Fig. 8.1). The forebrain consists of the telencephalon (cerebral cortex and basal ganglia) and the diencephalon (thalamus and hypothalamus). The midbrain, pons and medulla together make up the brainstem and connect the forebrain with the spinal cord, which extends caudally in the vertebral canal. Peripheral nerve fibres connect the CNS to all parts of the body via the brainstem and cord, while posterior to the brainstem, and connected to it by its peduncles, is the cerebellum.

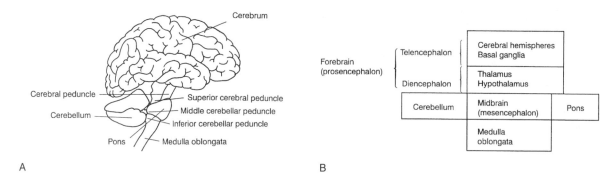

Figure 8.1 A: Outline of the brain. B: Constituents of the CNS. (Modified with permission from Holmes O 1990 Human neurophysiology. Unwin Hyman, London.)

The CNS has evolved from a primitive input–output system that enabled the organism to respond to changes in its environment; hence it consists primarily of sensory and motor components. With increasing complexity a third function, integration, was added, whereby sensory information from both the internal and external environments is processed by the CNS and compared with stored information to determine the appropriate response. In the human, most of the activity of the brain is integrative, including consciousness, memory, conceptual thought and emotion.

Elements of sensory, motor and integrative function are located in all the anatomical divisions of the CNS. As one ascends from the level of the cord towards the cerebral cortex, however, the integrative functions become markedly more complex, with greater flexibility and fineness of control over lower structures.

SENSORY SYSTEMS

Two pathways carry sensory fibres centrally in the spinal cord: the dorsal column-lemniscal and the anterolateral systems.

Dorsal column lemniscal system

Sensory information that needs to be transmitted rapidly and with a high degree of temporal and spatial accuracy is carried in the dorsal column lemniscal system. Its large diameter, myelinated fibres transmit at velocities of 30–110 m s^{-1}, and subserve the sensory modalities of fine touch,

vibration sense and pressure, and position sense of skin, muscle and joints (proprioception), i.e. sensory input which may require a rapid and/or accurate response from the organism.

Peripheral fibres carrying these modalities, the cell bodies of which lie in the dorsal root ganglia, enter the spinal cord through the dorsal roots. Here they divide: one major branch ascending in the dorsal column of the same side, while others synapse with neurones in different parts of the cord grey matter. Many of these are involved in fast spinal cord reflexes, while others ascend to rejoin the dorsal column pathway or to end in the cerebellum.

The fibres that form the dorsal column ascend uninterrupted to the medulla, where they synapse in the cuneate and gracile nuclei. Fibres from the second order neurones of these nuclei here cross to the other side and, forming the medial lemnisci, ascend to terminate in the ventrobasal nuclei of the thalamus. From here third order fibres project to the somatic sensory areas in the postcentral gyrus of the cerebral cortex.

Throughout this system there is accurate spatial representation of the body; in the dorsal columns the lower part of the body is represented medially and fibres from progressively higher levels are added to the lateral aspect of the tracts, while in the somatic sensory area of the cortex the projection of the opposite half of the body is spread from the head laterally and inferiorly, upwards to the lower body medially. In the somatic sensory cortex the different sensory modalities subserved by the dorsal column-lemniscal system are represented by discrete vertical columns of cortical neurones, which extend through all six cortical layers. Signals enter each column at layer IV and from there spread both towards the surface and deeper cortical layers, where there are multiple connections with other cortical regions as well as non-specific input from lower brain centres.

Anterolateral system

The sensory modalities that are carried by the anterolateral system are those for which speed of transmission, sharp localisation and fine intensity discrimination are comparatively unimportant, namely crude touch and pressure, temperature sense and both fast and slow pain. The peripheral fibres that form the input to this system are much smaller and more slowly conducting than those of the dorsal column-lemniscal system, many of them being unmyelinated. They enter the cord via the dorsal roots to synapse mainly in the dorsal horn. Many synapses give rise to interneurones that subserve spinal reflexes, for example the withdrawal (flexor) response to a painful stimulus. Other second order fibres cross in the anterior commissure of the cord to ascend in the opposite anterior and lateral spinothalamic and spinoreticular tracts. Some of these fibres, especially those carrying touch and possibly temperature sensation, terminate in the ventrobasal nuclei of the thalamus, from which third order fibres project, along with those carrying signals originating in the dorsal column system, to the somatosensory cortex. Other fibres, however, notably pain fibres, synapse in the brainstem reticular nuclei, from which fibres pass to the intralaminar thalamic nuclei. These two systems form the basis of the somatic sensory system, whereby sensations are conveyed by direct pathways containing only two synaptic relays from the periphery to the sensory cortex. It is important to note, however, that in the spinal cord, and at each synaptic relay up to the cortex itself, sensory signals can be greatly modified, both by local factors and inputs from other parts of the CNS.

MOTOR SYSTEMS

The spinal cord anterior horn cells (lower motor neurone) and the homologous cranial nerve motor nuclei are the final common pathway of the motor system controlling skeletal muscle activity. During normal movement they are influenced by nerve fibres from many supraspinal areas. Movement is planned and initiated in the cortex and modified by the cerebellum, basal ganglia and brainstem vestibular system, as well as in the cord itself.

Motor and integrative functions of the spinal cord

Motor functions that are mediated solely by the spinal cord are termed spinal reflexes. Spinal reflexes are appropriate and coordinated, but stereotyped, responses to various patterns of sensory input to the cord. They are integrated in the cord grey matter. Interneurones are distributed throughout the grey matter, while the large and much less numerous motor neurones are confined to the anterior horns. Spinal reflexes may be divided into the postural or proprioceptive, which are concerned with muscle and joint position and movement, and protective, which minimise the effects of potential damage to the tissues. Although they are mediated entirely at spinal level, they are under continual tonic control from supraspinal structures.

Postural reflexes

Control of muscle tone and movement at the level of the spinal cord, as well as by higher centres, depends primarily on the muscle spindle. This structure (Fig. 8.2) consists of a fusiform sheath lying within the substance of a skeletal muscle, aligned in parallel with the muscle fibres and attached to them at each end. Within the sheath are intrafusal muscle fibres running longitudinally, with a central, non-contractile region and terminal contractile regions. The receptor can be stimulated either by contraction of the intrafusal fibres or by lengthening of the main (extrafusal) fibres.

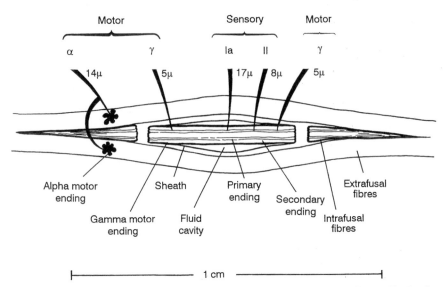

Figure 8.2 Muscle spindle. (Reproduced with permission from Guyton A C 1991 Textbook of medical physiology, 8th edn. WB Saunders, Philadelphia.)

About two-thirds of the motor neurones in the spinal cord anterior horn are the large Aα type, which innervate the extrafusal skeletal muscle fibres. The remainder, the smaller Aγ motor neurones, innervate the contractile ends of the intrafusal fibres of muscle spindles. The stretch receptors are innervated by large, fast-transmitting afferent fibres. These enter the spinal cord by the dorsal root and divide, one branch passing centrally in the dorsal column-lemniscal pathway while other branches terminate either on interneurones or directly on an α motor neurone. Histologically, muscle spindle stretch receptors are of two types, termed primary and secondary, the one responding characteristically only to changes in the degree of stretch by firing transient (phasic) bursts of impulses, and the other firing more steadily and in proportion to the degree of constant (tonic) stretch. In the *knee jerk* response to a tap on the patellar tendon, sudden stretching of the primary receptors in muscle spindles lying in the quadriceps muscle produces a burst of firing of spindle afferent fibres. These synapse directly with α motor neurones supplying the muscle, which briefly contracts, thus tending to oppose the stretch. The briskness of the response depends on the degree

of facilitation of the motor neurones by higher centres. *Clonus*, which is an oscillatory contraction and relaxation of a muscle usually only found when there is considerable facilitation from the brain, is also a form of the stretch reflex. After surgery involving possible stretch of the spinal cord, the demonstration of ankle clonus may be used as an indication, in the lightly anaesthetised patient, that the spinal pathways are undamaged.

In normal voluntary movement there is simultaneous activation of both α and γ efferents. The major role of the muscle spindle apparatus when, for example, lifting a load, is thought to be to provide constant feedback control of the degree of contraction of extrafusal fibres. Activation of the γ efferents stretches the receptors and produces an afferent discharge, which in turn increases α efferent activity via the monosynaptic stretch reflex until the resulting shortening of the extrafusal fibres removes the stretch on the receptor. Thus the degree of muscle shortening is matched to the load efficiently and without necessarily involving higher centres.

The Golgi tendon organ, which is found at the junction of a tendon with its muscle fibres, is a detector of muscle tension rather than length. Signals from it are transmitted in large, rapidly conducting fibres, branches of which synapse on inhibitory interneurones in the grey matter of the cord. These in turn synapse on anterior motor neurones. When the Golgi organ is stimulated by increased muscle tension, muscle contraction is reflexly inhibited, tending to release the tension.

Protective reflexes

Withdrawal reflexes, which have the effect of protecting parts of the body from potential harm, can also be mediated at the purely spinal cord level. These reflexes are most commonly elicited by painful stimuli, but stimulation of other sensory nerve endings can also be effective. Typically, a painful stimulus applied to a limb causes contraction of the limb flexor muscles, with simultaneous reciprocal inhibition of the extensor muscles. This type of reflex is not monosynaptic but involves activation, by stimulation of the faster pain afferents, of interneuronal circuits in the cord grey matter, which both excite the motor neurones controlling the flexor muscles and inhibit the extensors. The pattern of withdrawal depends upon which sensory nerve is stimulated, so that the appropriate movement is produced.

Elicitation of a flexor reflex in a limb may be accompanied by extension of the opposite limb after a 200–500 ms delay. This crossed extensor reflex is the result of activation of multisynaptic interneuronal circuits which cross to the opposite side of the spinal cord to excite and inhibit the appropriate motor neurones.

In injury or disease, stimulation of pain nerve endings can produce tonic contraction of muscles around the area affected. This reflex, which has the effect of protecting the part from further injury, is also mediated at spinal cord level. Examples include the muscle spasm that occurs around a fractured bone and the abdominal guarding that is seen in local or general peritoneal irritation.

Spinal transection

Since neuronal tissue in the CNS does not regenerate, transection of the spinal cord causes permanent loss of communication between the parts of the nervous system above and below the lesion. Immediately after transection there is a profound depression of all cord function below the lesion. This condition, known as *spinal shock*, is due to the abrupt removal of descending tonic facilitatory influences, and is characterised by flaccid paralysis, absent reflexes (including knee jerk, micturition and defecation) and complete anaesthesia, while the permanent absence of higher control of autonomic function below the lesion causes cutaneous vasodilatation and absence of sweating. This leads to hypotension (especially postural), to an extent that depends on the level of the lesion, and impaired temperature regulation. Loss of reflexes leads to urinary retention with overflow, and constipation.

Spinal shock is followed after some days by the beginning of recovery of reflex activity in the cord. The bladder voiding reflex returns, although it is not under supraspinal control. Motor reflexes also reappear, beginning with flexor withdrawal and stretch reflexes, and eventually reflexes become exaggerated, causing spastic paralysis. Although these patients remain completely without sensation below the lesion, autonomic hyperreflexia, with hypertension in response to visceral stimulation, is often a problem during surgery.

Supraspinal control of motor function

Supraspinal control of movement is a highly complex process involving close integration of the activities of the cortex, basal ganglia, cerebellum and vestibular nuclei. Broadly, while the cortex is in overall control, the cerebellum coordinates rapid movements, and the basal ganglia slower, patterned movements and background postural control. These two structures do not initiate activity but act to refine and modify movements initiated elsewhere. The vestibular nuclei of the midbrain are also concerned with posture, mainly with respect to gravity, and are important in the control of eye movements. In some respects the basal ganglia, vestibular and related nuclei can be grouped as an extrapyramidal system responsible for involuntary components of movements initiated in the cortex.

Motor cortex

The primary motor area of the cerebral cortex occupies the convolution of the frontal lobes anterior to the central sulcus, which separates it from the sensory cortex. In it the muscle groups of the body are topographically represented, with the muscles of the feet represented medially and those of swallowing, mastication and speech laterally and inferiorly. The areas are proportional to the precision of movements; thus those controlling the muscles of the hand and of speech occupy more than half of the primary motor cortex, while much less space is devoted to the muscles of the trunk and lower limb.

Anterior to the primary motor cortex is the premotor area. While stimulation of the primary area leads to contractions of individual contralateral muscles or groups of muscles, stimulation of the premotor area produces patterns of movement. It includes the speech area of Broca, as well as areas controlling eye movements and hand skills. The speech area is in the left hemisphere in right-handed and in many left-handed people. The premotor cortex appears to exert a higher level of control over the primary area, with which it connects both directly and via the basal ganglia.

The cells of the primary motor cortex are arranged in vertical columns, which extend through its six layers, each column controlling a single muscle or group of synergistic muscles. Layer V contains the giant pyramidal cells, known as Betz cells, which are unique to the motor cortex, and whose axons project into the spinal cord in the corticospinal tract. Cells in the other layers have multiple connections with other columns and with various parts of the brain.

The corticospinal tract (pyramidal tract), which also contains fibres from the premotor area and the somatosensory cortex, is the main output from the motor cortex. It passes through the posterior limb of the internal capsule and the midbrain into the brainstem where, in the medulla, most of its fibres cross to the other side to continue as the lateral corticospinal tract in the spinal cord, the uncrossed fibres forming the ventral corticospinal tract. Most of the fibres terminate on interneurones in the cord grey matter, although some, especially in the region of the cervical enlargement, where the hands and fingers are represented, synapse directly with anterior motor neurones. Many of the fibres that have arisen in the somatosensory cortex terminate on sensory neurones in the dorsal horn, thereby providing feedback modulation of sensory input.

The motor cortex also projects, mainly by collaterals from the corticospinal tract, to many other parts of the brain, including particularly the basal ganglia, the red nucleus, the brainstem reticular formation and vestibular nuclei, and the cerebellum.

The major input to the motor cortex is from the adjacent somatosensory area, which itself constantly receives feedback on the effects of motor activity from the muscle spindles, joint proprioceptors and skin tactile receptors. Fibres also reach the motor cortex from the auditory and visual cortices, other regions of the cortex, and, via the thalamus, from the basal ganglia, cerebellum and reticular formation. These multiple connections reflect the high degree of complex integration which is involved in motor activity. Although the motor cortex exerts overall control over voluntary movement, this is mainly achieved through control of patterns of activity in lower parts of the CNS. In some cases, however, notably in fine movement of the hands and fingers, it can exert direct control.

The corticospinal tract, with the associated rubrospinal tract from the red nucleus, form a system of motor control with an emphasis on movements of the lateral parts of the body musculature, particularly the distal parts of the limbs. The more medial muscles are more the concern of the brainstem motor nuclei.

Brainstem vestibular nuclei

The reticular and vestibular nuclei of the brainstem are the main controllers of the axial and girdle muscles. Their major role is in the maintenance of posture and equilibrium with respect to gravity. While they normally act under the influence of the higher structures controlling motor activity, they are also the site of integration of complex autonomous postural and other reflexes.

The pontine and medullary reticular nuclei give rise to reticulospinal tracts which are mutually antagonistic. The pontine nuclei receive excitatory connections from the vestibular and deep cerebellar nuclei, and transmit excitatory signals in the pontine reticulospinal tract to the medial anterior motor neurones that supply the muscles of the spinal column and the limb extensor muscles, which provide support against gravity. In contrast, the medullary reticulospinal tract, which is under excitatory control from the motor cortex and basal ganglia, is inhibitory to these muscles. The balance between these two systems, and its manipulation by inputs from other sources, allows the normally tonic activity of the antigravity muscles to be selectively relaxed, so that they can perform other functions. Section of the brainstem between the pons and midbrain leads to decerebrate rigidity and spasticity affecting the antigravity muscles, caused primarily by the removal of excitatory input to the inhibitory medullary nuclei with unopposed activity of the pontine nuclei.

The vestibular nuclei also lie in the brainstem. As well as influencing the pontine reticular nuclei, they directly excite the antigravity muscles via the vestibulospinal tracts. Their main role is to provide the appropriate balance of excitation to these muscles in response to signals from the vestibular apparatus.

The vestibular apparatus of the inner ear, lying within the labyrinth of the petrous temporal bone, is the sensory receptor for the sense of balance. It contains two distinct parts. The utricle and saccule detect the orientation of the head with respect to gravity or any other linear acceleration, while the semicircular canals detect angular rotation of the head.

Signals from the vestibular apparatus pass first to the vestibular nuclei, which have extensive connections with the cerebellum. Signals also project to the cord in the vestibulospinal and reticulospinal tracts, enabling reflex excitation and inhibition, especially of the axial muscles, in response to changes in orientation. An essential component of these reflexes is the direct input that the vestibular and reticular nuclei receive from the neck proprioreceptors, so that the orientation of the head with respect to the trunk is also known. Signals also pass in the medial longitudinal fasciculus to the oculomotor nuclei, serving to stabilise the direction of gaze during rapid movements of the head. The presence or absence of these reflexes is important in the clinical assessment of brainstem function.

Basal ganglia

The term 'basal ganglia' refers to a group of structures with a more or less unitary function that lie in the brain substance, deep to the cortex and mainly lateral to the thalamus. The most prominent component is the corpus striatum, made up of the lentiform and caudate nuclei. The lentiform may be divided into the globus pallidus medially and the putamen laterally, while the caudate is an elongated, C-shaped structure running back in an arc from the lentiform to the amygdaloid nucleus. The subthalamic nuclei and the substantia nigra of the midbrain are also parts of the basal ganglia.

The basal ganglia are intimately connected with the activities of the cortex. They have little direct input from the periphery but send signals to the cord via the red nucleus of the midbrain and the reticular system. Circuits run from the cortex, especially the motor and sensory areas, through various parts of the basal ganglia, and return via the ventroanterior and ventrolateral thalamus to the cortex. The basal ganglia do not themselves initiate motor activity but are ancillary to the motor cortex and corticospinal system. Nevertheless they are essential for normal motor function. The types of movement with which they are most concerned are those that apply complex, subconscious learned skills, such as writing, slowly lifting a cup of liquid, using scissors, cycling or digging. These activities require correct sequencing and timing and constant modification by feedback, as well as associated postural adjustments of the whole body. In cases of severe damage to the basal ganglia, paralysis does not occur but the ability to control complex patterns of motor activity is lost and actions such as writing become crude, stiff and uncoordinated.

Specific lesions of parts of the basal ganglia are associated with characteristic clinical syndromes, of which involuntary movements are a prominent feature. The most common condition is Parkinson's disease, which results primarily from destruction of dopamine-secreting inhibitory neurones in the substantia nigra which project to the caudate, putamen and ventrolateral thalamus. It is characterised by tremor, muscle rigidity and difficulty in initiating movement (akinesia). The exact mechanism by which these symptoms are produced is not clear, although it is likely that tremor and rigidity are due to overactivity of cholinergic pathways, from which the balancing inhibitory dopaminergic input has been lost. Treatment with L-dopa, combined with anticholinergic drugs, is effective in many cases, while increasing numbers of these patients are being treated by ablation of the ventrolateral thalamic nuclei.

Loss of γ-aminobutyric acid (GABA)-secreting neurones in the caudate nucleus, as in the hereditary condition Huntington's chorea, causes increasingly severe involuntary flicking movements. Lesions of the globus pallidus are associated with writhing movements (athetosis).

Cerebellum

The cerebellum is connected to the rest of the CNS through the cerebellar peduncles, the three bundles of fibres that join the brainstem at the level of the pons. Each cerebellar hemisphere is made up of a cortical cellular layer covering the medulla, which consists of white matter and also contains the three paired deep cerebellar nuclei, the dentate, interpositus and fastigial. The two cerebellar hemispheres are joined in the midline by the vermis.

Localisation of function is less marked in the cerebellum than in the cerebral cortex, but three parts may be distinguished, based largely on their connections with other parts of the brain.

Lying posteriorly is the flocculonodular lobe, or vestibulocerebellum, which functions as part of the vestibular mechanism for the control of balance and posture.

The spinocerebellum in the medial cortex receives proprioceptive information from the periphery via the spinocerebellar tracts, and also feedback from the anterior horn cells, so that it is continually updated, not only on the pattern of muscle contraction and the position and orientation of the body at a given moment but also on the total effect of all the various influences acting on the excitability of the motor neurones at that time. The fact that the fibres of the spinocerebellar tract are the fastest conducting in the CNS emphasises the important role of this mechanism. The lateral parts of the cerebellar hemispheres (pontocerebellum) have connections predominantly with the cerebral cortex, via the pontine nuclei and thalamus. This region has a more complex, coordinating role in the planning and execution of movements. Thus the cerebellum exerts control over muscle activity at all levels: spinal cord, brainstem and cerebral cortex. In contrast to the basal ganglia and vestibular system, the cerebellum is primarily concerned with rapid movements of the distal parts of the limbs rather than with posture.

The basic unit of cerebellar function is a neuronal circuit running between the cerebellar cortex and a corresponding deep nuclear region, and centred on a Purkinje cell. These large, GABAergic cerebellar cortical cells continuously inhibit the deep nuclear cells. The two types of cerebellar afferents, the climbing and mossy fibres, are excitatory to both the deep nuclei and the Purkinje cells. The arrangement of the circuit ensures that the arrival of an afferent signal first excites, and then a few milliseconds later inhibits, a group of deep nuclear cells. Efferent signals then go from the deep nuclei to the appropriate other parts of the CNS. It is thought that this circuitry provides the mechanism that enables the cerebellum not only to compute precisely the strength, timing and sequence of reflex and voluntary movements but also to plan, along with the cerebral cortex, the timing and sequence of the next movement that will be required. The cerebellum is particularly concerned with movements that are too rapid to allow feedback control via proprioceptive reflex arcs and thus must be preprogrammed in their entirety, such as rapidly turning a screwdriver or playing a piano. A major part of its role is in the damping of movements and prevention of overshoot. Many of the signs of cerebellar disease may be traced to the absence of this ability and the attempts of the cerebral cortex to compensate for it, notably intention tremor and past pointing. A patient who has had a significant amount of the cerebellum removed is unable subconsciously to predict how far a movement will go and cannot locate the part being moved during rapid motion. This results in uncoordinated movement (ataxia) or speech (dysarthria).

CEREBRAL CORTEX, LEARNING AND MEMORY

The cortex functions in close association with the thalamus, with which all areas have many afferent and efferent connections. Specific thalamic nuclei project to specific cortical regions and, in addition to maintaining a general level of excitation, the thalamus is essential for cortical function.

The six-layered structure seen in the motor and sensory areas is found throughout the cerebral cortex. In all areas two types of neurone can be distinguished: pyramidal cells and stellate cells.

Pyramidal cells, the output cells of the cortex, are found mainly in layers II–III and V–VI. Each has an apical dendrite stretching up towards and ramifying in the cortical surface, while other dendrites surround the soma. Its axon, projecting down into the white matter, has many collateral branches. Stellate cells are more numerous and have short axons. 99% of cortical neurones send axons only to other parts of the cortex.

Other specialised parts of the cortex, apart from the somatosensory and motor areas, include the primary visual and visual interpretive areas of the occipital lobes and the corresponding auditory areas in the temporal lobes.

Parts of the cortex that do not have specific sensory or motor functions are known as association areas, and the comparatively very large proportion of the brain that is occupied by these strikingly distinguishes the human brain from those of other species. Their roles can be broadly inferred from their neural connections and from the effects of lesions. The prefrontal association area, anterior to the motor areas, is the site of intellectual activity and complex planning. The function of the parieto-occipitotemporal association area, which is closely associated with all the sensory areas, is the elaboration of all information to do with the spatial coordinates of the body and its surroundings (stereognosis). It contains Wernicke's area in the posterior superior temporal lobe, where the somatic, visual and auditory interpretive areas all meet. This area, which is fully developed only in the dominant hemisphere, is concerned with the interpretation of sensory information as language, and is essential for intellectual function in man. Broca's area, in the lateral prefrontal and premotor area, has a comparable role in the motor elaboration of speech.

Conscious thought is believed to consist, in neural terms, of sequential patterns of simultaneous activity in many different parts of the brain. Learning is the process by which new neural traces are created by previous synaptic activity, which can then be activated as memory. The synaptic mechanisms by which memories are laid down are not known, but may involve presynaptic facilitation and increased accumulation of Ca^{2+} ion and transmitters at the nerve ending. Short term memory may become long term when permanent structural changes occur, such as an increase in the area of the transmitter vesicle release site. This process of consolidation is particularly susceptible to disruption by drugs, notably benzodiazepines and anticholinergics, which produce anterograde amnesia. Retrograde amnesia, the loss of previously stored material, does not appear to be a feature of the action of drugs, but is found in organic brain disease, notably head injury.

Only a small fraction of the sensory information reaching the CNS is stored as memory. Habituation occurs to repetitive and irrelevant stimuli. Although memories are stored in the cortex, it is input from the limbic system that determines at a subconscious level whether or not information is stored.

LIMBIC SYSTEM

The term 'limbic system' refers to the neuronal circuitry that controls emotional behaviour and motivational drives. It comprises the part of the cerebral cortex lying on the medial aspect of the hemisphere, around the third ventricle, and several interconnected subcortical structures, including the hypothalamus, non-specific thalamic nuclei, hippocampus and amygdaloid nucleus. It is primarily concerned with affect, the perception of sensory information as pleasant or unpleasant, and the regulation of behaviour in response to this perception. Thus, in animals, stimulation of a part of the limbic system produces a behavioural response, such as fear or rage. The role of the hypothalamus in the limbic system is closely related to its function of controlling the autonomic nervous system and other vegetative functions, such as thirst and appetite, so that activity in the limbic system is accompanied by an autonomic change, leading, for example, to a change in heart rate.

Disordered function of the limbic system may be implicated in the development of schizophrenia and other forms of psychosis. It is known that phenothiazine tranquillisers inhibit limbic function in animals.

STATES OF BRAIN ACTIVITY

Consciousness and the reticular formation

Consciousness is expressed through the cerebral cortex but cannot exist without tonic excitatory input from the reticular formation, the diffuse group of nuclei which extend near the midline from the medial thalamus to the caudal medulla. An area of the pontine and midbrain reticular formation is specifically excitatory to the cerebral cortex, via the thalamus. It is activated by sensory input of all kinds from the periphery, especially pain signals, via collaterals from the main sensory pathways in the cord, and it in turn produces general activation of the cortex. The excitatory area also receives excitatory input from the cortex itself, so that a positive feedback mechanism operates, whereby excitation of the

cortex leads to further excitation. The level of cerebral arousal is also controlled by neuro-hormone-secreting systems in the brainstem, which release facilitatory and inhibitory substances directly into the brain substance, producing comparatively long lasting effects. The facilitatory systems include the noradrenergic system of the locus ceruleus at the junction of the pons and midbrain, and the cholinergic area of the excitatory reticular formation. The substantia nigra of the upper midbrain releases dopamine, which is inhibitory to the caudate nucleus and putamen, and the raphe nuclei of the lower pons and medulla secrete serotonin, which is inhibitory to the thalamus and cortex.

The electroencephalogram

The electroencephalogram (EEG) is the electrical activity recorded from electrodes placed over the scalp. Characteristic waveforms (Fig. 8.3) are associated with different states of CNS arousal and depression, both physiological and pathological.

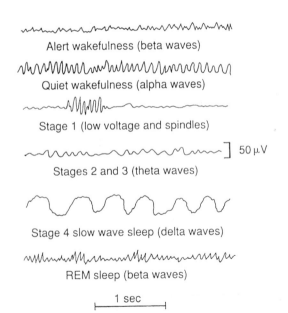

Alert wakefulness (beta waves)

Quiet wakefulness (alpha waves)

Stage 1 (low voltage and spindles)

$] 50\,\mu V$

Stages 2 and 3 (theta waves)

Stage 4 slow wave sleep (delta waves)

REM sleep (beta waves)

1 sec

Figure 8.3 Progressive changes in the EEG during different stages of wakefulness and sleep. (Reproduced with permission from Guyton A C 1991 Textbook of medical physiology, 8th edn. WB Saunders, Philadelphia.)

The α rhythm, which has a frequency of about 8–12 Hz and an amplitude of about 50 μV, occurs most intensely in the occipital region but can be recorded from other areas. It is typically found in awake, relaxed adults with the eyes closed.

Arousal from this state to one of mental activity changes the EEG pattern to a higher frequency, lower voltage, desynchronised waveform, designated the β rhythm. The θ rhythm, with a frequency of 4–7 Hz, is found in normal children and may be seen in adults during emotional disturbance, while δ rhythms, with frequencies of less than 3.5 Hz, are seen in infancy, deep slow wave sleep, and deep anaesthesia, as well as in some organic brain disorders causing coma.

The EEG waves are not action potentials, but represent the summation of very many slow dendritic potentials in the outer (layers I and II) regions of the cortex. However, the rhythms originate in lower parts of the brain. The α rhythm, for example, is due to inhibition, by thalamocortical fibres, of a higher frequency drive originating in the midbrain reticular formation. In desynchronisation the faster rhythm dominates. In general, EEG frequency tends to increase over a broad spectrum of brain states from hypoactivity to hyperactivity.

Sleep

The reticular neurohormonal systems, which exert control over the general state of brain activity, may have a role in cyclical transitions, notably the sleep–wake cycle. It is well established that there are two distinct kinds of sleep, slow wave and rapid eye movement (REM). Slow wave sleep, so called because of its associated EEG pattern, occupies about 75% of sleeping time in a young adult. It is the sleep which immediately follows wakefulness, and is generally regarded as restful and dreamless, although it may be that dreaming occurs but is not remembered. During slow wave sleep there is decreased sympathetic activity, with 10–30% reductions in blood pressure, respiratory rate and metabolic rate. It is now regarded as an active inhibitory process, and its onset and maintenance may be

associated with activity of the serotoninergic system of the pontine and medullary raphe nuclei.

REM sleep normally occurs in bursts lasting about 15 minutes, each separated by about 90 minutes of slow wave sleep. Its characteristics include many features similar to those of wakefulness. The brain is highly active and has a high metabolic rate, and the heart rate and respiration are irregular. However, paradoxically, the subject is harder to rouse than during slow wave sleep, and muscle tone is greatly depressed, with some irregular activity, including the characteristic rapid eye movements. The function of REM sleep is not understood, but processing of recently acquired information is suggested by the content of dreams associated with it. Its occurrence may be related to the noradrenergic output of the locus ceruleus.

It is well known that prolonged wakefulness causes subjective tiredness and deterioration in performance. With further sleep deprivation, however, irritability may turn to psychotic behaviour.

In the EEG four stages of slow wave sleep may be distinguished. In stage 1, as α rhythm disappears, low amplitude 2–7 Hz waves start to appear. In stage 2 these are dominant but are interrupted by sleep spindles, which are short lasting bursts of 12–14 Hz, α-like activity. In stages 3 and 4 the EEG frequency becomes gradually slower until it shows the 2–4 Hz δ rhythm. REM sleep, by contrast, is characterised by a desynchronised waveform similar to that of the awake state.

The importance of REM sleep is suggested by its increase during sleep following sleep deprivation. Both it and slow wave sleep decrease with age. Increased wakening is a cause of concern in the elderly but hypnotic drugs may often further disrupt normal sleep patterns.

Depression of brain activity

In organic brain disease causing depressed function, or in depression due to drugs, there is a progressive loss of higher integrative functions. Initial loss of concentration and volition progresses through disorientation in time and space to confusion and delirium. In stupor there is response to stimulation but no awareness, and the next stage is coma with motor response only to maximal stimulation. Worsening coma is then accompanied by progressive loss of brainstem reflexes in a rostral–caudal sequence. In the Glasgow Coma Scale the degree of depression is graded according to the amount of stimulation required to elicit a response (Table 8.1).

These changes are accompanied by qualitatively similar progressive EEG changes. As consciousness decreases, there is a gradual slowing of frequency until δ rhythm dominates. As coma deepens, isoelectric episodes appear, until gradually the appearance known as burst-suppression activity is seen, with bursts of δ activity against an isoelectric background. With very deep coma and incipient medullary failure, the EEG becomes flat, although recovery can still occur with appropriate life support.

A similar pattern of depression of brain activity is seen in many disturbances of normal physiology, including hypoxia, hypercarbia, hypoglycaemia, acid–base disturbances and disturbed osmolality.

Table 8.1 Glasgow Coma Scale

Motor response		Score
Eye opening		
Spontaneous	E	4
To speech		3
To standardised pain		2
None		1
Best motor response		
Obeying command	M	6
Localising		5
Withdrawal response to standardised pain		4
Abnormal flexion to standardised pain		3
Extension response to standardised pain		2
None		1
Best verbal response		
Oriented in time and space	V	5
Confused conversation		4
Inappropriate speech		3
Incomprehensible (not recognisable words)		2
None		1

Epilepsy

In a subject predisposed to *grand mal epilepsy* an attack may be triggered when the basal level of excitability of the CNS increases to a critical level. Precipitating causes include emotional stimuli, strong sensory stimuli such as flashing lights, and the causes of cerebral depression just described.

In a grand mal attack excessive synchronous neuronal discharges occur in all areas of the brain and spinal cord, causing abrupt unconsciousness and tonic convulsions of all body musculature, possibly accompanied by voiding of urine and faeces and interruption of normal respiration, which may be severe enough to cause cyanosis. Later in the seizure the muscle contractions change to the spasmodic tonic–clonic type, followed by hypotonia as the attack ends and is succeeded by the postictal period of stupor. Grand mal attacks are usually self-limiting, possibly because of activation of inhibitory circuits. Continuous seizures, or attacks occurring so frequently that recovery between them does not occur, constitute status epilepticus, a medical emergency.

During the attack the EEG shows a high voltage, synchronous spiking discharge covering the entire cortex (compare the ECG in ventricular fibrillation), and it can be shown that this also occurs in the thalamus and brainstem reticular formation. The abnormal discharge in grand mal is believed to originate in these lower brain areas, which then activate the cortex.

Petit mal epilepsy is characterised by short periods of unconsciousness, lasting for a few seconds or longer, which usually terminate abruptly without causing further symptoms. The EEG shows a typical spike and dome pattern which covers the entire cortex, indicating that this form of epilepsy also originates in the deeper centres of the brain.

Focal epilepsy, on the other hand, results from a congenital or acquired localised abnormality in some part of the cortex or lower brain. Seizure activity originating in such an area spreads outwards at a variable rate, recruiting other areas. If this involves the motor cortex, a characteristic pattern of progressive involvement of different muscle groups may be seen. Another variant is *psychomotor epilepsy*, during which abnormal emotional behaviour may be observed. The abnormal focus in this type is usually in the limbic area. In focal epilepsy the EEG can often be used to localise the focus.

With minor epilepsy, EEG changes may be revealed by deliberate hyperventilation which depresses brain function by inducing respiratory alkalosis and cerebral vasoconstriction.

CRITICAL REQUIREMENTS OF BRAIN FUNCTION

Although the brain represents only 2% of body mass, its needs account for 15% of the resting metabolic rate. Most of this high energy usage goes to maintain the action of the membrane ion pumps, especially Na^+,K^+-ATPase, which are essential for normal neural function.

As already mentioned, normal brain function depends on normality of a variety of parameters, including glucose availability, oxygen, carbon dioxide and hydrogen ion levels. The brain's vulnerability to hypoxia is increased by the inability of neurones to use anaerobic metabolism to any significant extent. It cannot therefore accrue an oxygen debt and so depends on constant oxygen replenishment from its capillary blood supply. Abrupt failure of the supply leads to loss of consciousness in 5–10 seconds.

The brain's inability to use anaerobic metabolism is related to the very low levels of glycogen available in neurones for conversion to glucose. Under normal circumstances almost all of its energy derives from glucose supplied minute by minute from the capillary blood. Enough glycogen is present to meet glucose requirements only for about 2 minutes. Nevertheless, during global cerebral ischaemia the degree of anaerobic metabolism is sufficient to produce a potentially harmful build-up of lactic acid and hydrogen ion, which remain trapped in the brain due to the relative impermeability of the blood–brain barrier to charged particles. The resulting fall in cerebral pH produces poor conditions for many intracellular enzyme reactions, and may

be a major contributory factor to postischaemic cerebral oedema.

Thus, from the points of view of both oxygen and glucose, the health of neural tissue is critically dependent on the adequacy of the cerebral blood supply. Cerebral blood flow in the adult averages 50–55 ml per 100 g of brain tissue per minute. It has been found that at flows of less than 16–18 ml $100 g^{-1} min^{-1}$ the EEG becomes isoelectric and evoked potentials cannot be elicited, while ionic pump failure occurs at flows below 10 ml $100 g^{-1} min^{-1}$. An area of brain whose blood supply is in the narrow range between these two flow rates, such as might be found surrounding an area of cerebral infarction, is termed an ischaemic penumbra. It is functionally silent, but may be capable of recovery under favourable circumstances, such as the opening of collateral circulation or the resolution of oedema.

Global cerebral ischaemia is most commonly caused by cardiorespiratory arrest and may also occur in less severe forms of circulatory failure. In this situation, the cortex is the first part of the body to suffer irreversible damage. The degree of cerebral damage depends on the duration of the ischaemia, and occurs initially in the arterial border zones at the edges of the supply areas of the major cerebral arteries. Continued global ischaemia leads to permanent loss of cortical function. The EEG becomes isoelectric within about 25 seconds. Levels of high energy compounds fall rapidly while lactate, adenosine monophosphate (AMP) and adenosine diphosphate (ADP) accumulate within 2–3 minutes, followed by ionic pump failure 5–7 minutes after the initial event.

In situations where there is hypoxia without initial ischaemia, the time interval before irreversible damage occurs is slightly longer because blood containing some oxygen is still being delivered to the brain. In a patient under anaesthesia in whom the supply of oxygen is interrupted, this time interval depends on the size of the oxygen reserves in the alveoli and in the blood, and hence on the concentration of oxygen the patient has been breathing previously. The degree of damage to the brain from hypoxia can vary from subtle personality changes, especially in elderly patients, through permanent loss of cortical function, to death from brainstem injury.

In the brain, in contrast to most other tissues, insulin is not required for the transport of glucose into the cells. This affords the neurones some protection in diabetes mellitus; however, the brain is rendered particularly vulnerable to the effects of insulin overdosage, when the preferential movement of glucose into the insulin sensitive cells of other tissues can result in excessively low blood, and hence brain, glucose levels, leading to deranged mental function and eventually coma.

The brain is also particularly vulnerable to the effects of excessively high body temperatures. The degree of damage depends on the temperature and duration of exposure, but body temperatures of around 40°C and above, such as might occur in malignant hyperpyrexia as well as in excessively hot environments, are damaging to neural tissue and require urgent treatment. Hypothermia also depresses cerebral function, leading eventually to coma and death, although it can also protect the brain from the effects of hypoxia by causing a reduction of its metabolic rate. The protective value of hypothermia can be used to advantage in the operating theatre, and also accounts for cases of survival after prolonged immersion in freezing water.

The pattern of damage to the brain is similar whether the insult is ischaemic, hypoxic or metabolic. In a patient in whom cortical function has been lost but the brainstem remains intact, vegetative functions can continue normally. Breathing, heart action and swallowing reflexes are preserved, and with appropriate care survival for years is possible (persistent vegetative state).

In contrast, when brainstem function is lost, functions such as spontaneous breathing and swallowing are absent and survival is only possible with artificial ventilation and other life support measures. Complete brainstem death is followed by cardiac arrest after a few days. The reasons for this are unclear but may be related to increased sympathetic activity. Brainstem damage or death may occur as part of a global insult to the brain, but may also result from mechanical distortion of the brain in head injury.

The development of the means to keep these patients alive for some time in the intensive care unit, despite there being no hope of any recovery of function, together with the increasing use of organ transplants, has raised many ethical dilemmas and has led to the need to have agreed guidelines on the criteria of brainstem death.

In a patient in an apnoeic coma, due to a disorder that can by stated agreement cause brain death, the possibility of any reversible contributing effects from depressant or muscle relaxant drugs, or endocrine, metabolic or electrolyte abnormalities or hypothermia must be excluded before testing. The diagnosis of brain death then depends on there being negative responses to the following tests.

Tests for brain death

1. Absence of grimacing, or other motor responses involving the cranial nerves, to painful stimuli such as supraorbital pressure and others.
2. Fixed pupil diameter with no light response. This reflex depends on the integrity of the brainstem Edinger–Westphal nucleus.
3. Absent lash and corneal reflexes, which are mediated via the facial nerve.
4. Absent oculocephalic reflex, i.e, no movement of the eyes in response to brisk rotation of the head.
5. Absent vestibulo-ocular reflex. The integrity of the external auditory canal and tympanic membrane are checked with an auroscope before slowly injecting 20 ml ice-cold water (caloric test). No movement of the eyes should occur.
6. Absent gag reflex to pharyngeal or bronchial stimulation. This reflex depends on the integrity of the vagal and glossopharyngeal nuclei.
7. Absence of any attempt at spontaneous breathing in response to hypercapnia (hypoxia being avoided by preoxygenation).

These tests should be carried out independently by two suitably qualified observers, usually with an interval of about 2–3 hours.

PHYSICAL ASPECTS OF THE CNS

The brain develops in the embryo as the neural tube, from which the cerebral hemispheres grow as outward expansions. The central cavity of the tube, containing cerebrospinal fluid (CSF), develops into the four ventricles and their interconnections and the central canal of the spinal cord.

The brain and spinal cord are enveloped by the three meningeal membranes: the pia, arachnoid and dura mater. The pia is closely applied to the surface of the brain, while the subarachnoid space, between it and the arachnoid, is filled with CSF and communicates with the ventricular system through the median and lateral apertures of the fourth ventricle. The narrow subdural space lies between the dura and the arachnoid. The dura itself is a thick membrane that lines the inner surfaces of the skull and vertebral canal and extends into the cranial cavity to form sheets separating different parts of the brain. The largest of these is the tentorium cerebelli, which separates the occipital lobe from the cerebellum.

Cerebrospinal fluid

CSF is actively secreted from blood in the choroid plexuses, which invaginate the roof of the fourth ventricle, and also from capillaries within the brain. It circulates through the ventricular system and returns to the blood via the arachnoid villi, which project into the venous sinuses of the skull.

In the adult the CSF volume is about 150 ml. It is formed at a rate of about 500 ml day^{-1} by a process involving mainly active transport of sodium ions. Electrical and osmotic forces ensure that chloride ion and water accompany sodium. Glucose enters the CSF by facilitated diffusion, and there is some active transport of potassium and bicarbonate ion out of the CSF. The electrolyte composition of CSF differs from that of plasma, having less potassium and more chloride and calcium ion. It contains about 30% less glucose than plasma, and is virtually free of protein.

The in vitro weight of the adult brain is about 1.4 kg, and it lacks the mechanical rigidity to support its own weight. The specific gravity of CSF, however, is very slightly less than that of the brain, enabling it to provide a medium in which the brain can float and so maintain its structural integrity. It also protects the brain from the distorting and damaging effects of blows or sudden movements.

Since the rate of formation of CSF at the choroid plexuses is largely constant, CSF pressure, which averages 13 cmH$_2$O in the horizontal position, is regulated by the rate of passive reabsorption by the arachnoid villi, which depends on the pressure gradient between the CSF and the venous blood. An abnormal rise in pressure, from whatever cause, is potentially damaging in itself and through the distortion of brain tissue that may be produced. For example, a space-occupying lesion below the tentorium cerebelli can cause the hindbrain to be forced downwards into the spinal canal. This condition, known as coning, may rapidly cause irreparable brainstem damage if not quickly relieved.

Blood–brain barrier

The composition of the extracellular fluid of the brain is essentially the same as that of CSF. Cerebral capillaries contain tight junctions between cells, and are much less permeable to most substances than those of other tissues. Water, oxygen, carbon dioxide and glucose cross this barrier with ease, but passage of other substances is slow, especially those that are of large molecular size, water rather than lipid soluble, or charged. The blood–brain barrier has the major function of maintaining the constancy of the environment surrounding the brain cells and is profoundly important in determining the activity and potency of drugs in the brain. The barrier is incomplete in infancy. In several areas around the brainstem, known collectively as the circumventricular organs, it is deficient. These areas have functions which necessitate direct communication with the circulation, either to secrete hormones into the blood as in the posterior pituitary, or to detect chemical changes in the blood.

FURTHER READING

Astrup J 1982 Energy-requiring cell functions in ischemic brain. Journal of Neurosurgery 56: 482–497

Bindman L 1981 The neurophysiology of the cerebral cortex. University of Texas Press, Austin

Boyd I A 1985 Muscle spindles and stretch reflexes. In: Swash M, Kennard C (eds) Scientific foundations of clinical neurology. Churchill Livingstone, Edinburgh

Brooks V B 1986 The neural basis of motor control. Oxford University Press, Oxford

Conference of Medical Royal Colleges and their Faculties in the UK 1976 Diagnosis of brain death. British Medical Journal 2: 1187–1188

Creed R S, Denny-Brown D, Eccles J C et al 1972 Reflex activity of the spinal cord. Oxford University Press, Oxford

DeLong M R, Georgopoulos A P 1979 Physiology of the basal ganglia — a brief overview. Advances in Neurology 23: 137–153

Eccles J C 1973 The cerebellum as a computer: patterns in space and time. Journal of Physiology 229: 1–32

Hicks R G, Torda T A 1979 The vestibulo-ocular (caloric) reflex in the diagnosis of cerebral death. Anaesthesia and Intensive Care 7: 169–173

Hossman K A, Kleihues P 1973 Reversibility of ischemic brain damage. Archives of Neurology 29: 375–384

Pallis C 1982 Diagnosis of brain death I and II. British Medical Journal 285: 1558–1560, 1641–1644

Plum F, Siesjo B K 1975 Recent advances in CSF physiology. Anesthesiology 42: 708–730

Rapoport S I 1976 Blood–brain barrier in physiology and medicine. Raven Press, New York

Symon L 1985 Flow thresholds in brain ischaemia and the effects of drugs. British Journal of Anaesthesia 57: 34–43

Teasdale G, Jennett B 1974 Assessment of coma and impaired consciousness: a practical scale. Lancet ii: 81–83

9

Pharmacology of the central nervous system

B. J. Pleuvry

The brain is a unique and irreplaceable organ which harbours the essence of the individual. In view of this it is ironic that man has been tampering with its function by the use of drugs long before this was thought to be a therapeutically useful manoeuvre. Even today, most of the non-prescribed drugs taken by man have actions on the central nervous system (CNS). These drugs include readily available substances, such as ethanol, glue solvents, nicotine and caffeine, as well as those derived from more dubious sources, such as cannabis, opioid analgesics and hallucinogens. While observations of the effects of drugs with CNS activity have been reported for centuries, it is only in the twentieth century that any evidence has been accumulated as to how they may produce their effects.

The brain consists of about 100 billion neurones, each of which may receive thousands of synaptic connections. Transmission at each synapse will involve the release of one or more chemical mediators or *neurotransmitters*, which, combined with pre- or postsynaptic receptor sites, will initiate a signal transduction mechanism resulting in a change in the activity of the neurone. Any drug that has significant pharmacological activity within the CNS must directly or indirectly modify this neurotransmission. Even the classic, structurally non-specific drugs, such as the anaesthetic agents, are now known to have quite selective effects upon neurotransmitter systems, especially those utilising amino acids. There are several well defined neurotransmitter systems (see below) and a vast array of candidate molecules whose exact status is unsure and which have been termed *neuromodulators* in order to hide the uncertainty over their role. The term should more correctly refer to substances that enhance or reduce the actions of an identified neurotransmitter but are not necessarily released into a synapse close to the target neurone. However, the realisation that neuronally active molecules can coexist and be released from a single neurone has blurred the distinctions between modulators and transmitters.

The discovery of neuropeptides and the ready availability of antibodies against them has led to the identification of these substances in a wide divergence of sites throughout the CNS and periphery. Primary sites are those in which a given neuropeptide is consistently present across vertebrate species in a given tissue. However, there are many secondary sites where the distribution of a peptide varies dramatically across vertebrate species. Several studies of neuropeptide function in areas that show great variation in expression have shown equivocal or even negative results with respect to physiological function. In contrast, in areas where the physiological function of a given neuropeptide is well understood, it is restricted to those primary sites, which are invariant between the species. It has been argued that these secondary sites represent superfluous neurotransmitter systems. This hypothesis suggests that the aberrant expression of a single neuropeptide gene could lead to that neurone being classified as being functional for that peptide system. In contrast, non-peptide neurotransmitter neurones would not be similarly misclassified, as the neurone requires uptake mechanisms and special degradation enzymes as well as the synthetic enzyme for a particular transmitter, e.g. γ-aminobutyric acid (GABA). This reinforces the importance of assessing functional relevance as well as anatomical location in all aspects of neuroscience.

A further consideration is that cloning of neurotransmitter receptors has indicated that not all variants exist in all species. The development of drugs acting at receptors that are not present in humans will be largely ignored for the purposes of this chapter. In this overview of CNS pharma-

cology, only the interactions and potential interactions of drugs with known functional neurotransmitter or neuromodulator systems present in man will be discussed.

DRUG INTERACTION WITH NEUROTRANSMITTER SYSTEMS

Acetylcholine

Although acetylcholine was one of the earliest neurotransmitters to be isolated, the lack, until recently, of sensitive methods for the determination of acetylcholine-containing cells, tracts and terminals has left this field some distance behind many of the other transmitters discussed below.

Acetylcholine has both excitatory and inhibitory actions within the CNS. It was first described as a CNS transmitter at the synapse between the α motor neurone and the inhibitory Renshaw cell in the spinal cord. At this site acetylcholine activates a nicotinic receptor that can be blocked by classical neuromuscular blocking agents. In general, however, nicotinic receptors are much less common in the CNS than muscarinic receptors and most behavioural effects of acetylcholine are mediated via the latter. Although five subtypes of muscarinic receptor have been cloned (M_1–M_5), most is known about them in the periphery where the relatively selective M_1-receptor antagonist, pirenzepine, is used to treat benign gastric and duodenal ulceration, but pirenzepine does not cross the blood–brain barrier, and this fact, together with the absence of selective muscarinic agonists, has hindered progress on the defining central role for these receptors.

Physostigmine, an anticholinesterase agent that does cross the blood–brain barrier, causes electroencephalographic (EEG) arousal and has been used to treat overdoses of drugs that cause an anticholinergic syndrome (e.g. tricyclic antidepressants) and of a variety of depressant drugs, including diazepam and morphine, which do not have apparent atropine-like activity. The link between EEG arousal and behavioural activity is confused, as physostigmine itself causes lethargy and anxiety in man. In contrast, the non-selective muscarinic antagonist, atropine, which reduces arousal, may cause excitation. There is considerable evidence that cholinergic transmission is associated with learning and memory. In animals cholinergic agonists increase the ability to learn, and hyoscine has amnesic properties in man as well as lower animals. All this has led to the implication of cholinergic dysfunction in Alzheimer's disease, which is characterized by memory loss. Although there is evidence of loss of acetylcholine-containing neurones in the disease, treatment with cholinomimetics has not been particularly useful and it is clear that many other neurotransmitter dysfunctions occur during the course of Alzheimer's disease.

Amino acid neurotransmitters

Amino acids are the major neurotransmitters within the CNS, although separating their neurotransmitter role from that of their role in intermediary metabolism means that there has been a long hiatus between evidence being presented in the 1950s of apparent neurotransmitter activity and the acceptance of this position in the 1970s and 1980s. The amino acids can be separated into two general classes: excitatory amino acids (glutamic, aspartic, cysteic and homocysteic acids), which cause depolarisation of neurones, and inhibitory amino acids (GABA, glycine, taurine and β-alanine), which hyperpolarise neurones. From a pharmacological point of view, the first two in each of these groups are the most interesting.

Excitatory amino acids (glutamic and aspartic acids)

Most of the early evidence for excitatory amino acid function came from experiments in invertebrates. In mammalian brain the picture was clouded by the fact that glutamate, for example, was involved in detoxification of ammonia and the synthesis of peptides such as glutathione, as well as being a precursor of the inhibitory amino acid GABA. Although no new drugs have been introduced as a result of excitatory amino acid research, it has given us an insight into the

possible mechanisms of action of the dissociative anaesthetics, phencyclidine and ketamine, and many drugs are under development which interact with the system.

The discovery of analogues of glutamic acid, which showed a greater selectivity for some glutamate induced depolarisations, led to the identification of subclasses of excitatory amino acid receptors (Table 9.1). The first three of these were all ligand gated ion channels (or receptor operated channels, ROCs) and have been named for their selective agonists, N-methyl-D aspartate (NMDA), quisqualic acid (AMPA) and kainic acid (KA). NMDA receptors have been the best characterised and the associated channels are blocked by Mg^{2+} and phencyclidine-like drugs. They are usually associated with repetitive activity generated by stimulation of other non-NMDA receptors. Thus they are involved in synaptic plasticity and may be involved in neurogenic or wind-up pain. Particular interest in this receptor has come from the observation that excessive activation of the receptor can result

Table 9.1 Excitatory amino acids: glutamate and aspartate

Receptors	Selective drugs	
	Agonists	Antagonists
NMDA(ROC)	NMDA	D-AP5, etc. (receptor) PCP, ketamine, dizocilipine (channel)
AMPA(ROC)	AMPA	NBQX
KA (ROC)	Kainate	NBQX
L-AP4	L-AP4	None
Metabotropic	Quisqualate	L-AP3

Comment
Agonists are neurotoxins and may be involved in pain transmission and memory. NMDA antagonists are anticonvulsant and may be used in the treatment of ischaemic brain damage; they may prevent tolerance to drugs like opioids.
N.B. Channel blockers — psychotomimetic.
The pharmacology of non-NMDA receptors is sparse.
ROC, receptor operated ion channel; just two non-ROC receptors are shown but at least five more have been cloned.
NMDA, N-methyl-D-aspartate; AMPA, D,L-α-amino-3-hydroxy-5-methyl-4-isoxalone propionic acid; L-AP3, L-amino-3-phosphonopropanoate; L-AP4, L-amino-4-phosphonobutanoate; D-AP5, D-amino-5-phosphonopentanoate; NBQX, 6-nitro-7-sulphamobenzo(f)quinoxaline-2,3-dione.

in cell death and that excitatory amino acids are released during hypoxic conditions such as stroke. Antagonists at the NMDA receptor and receptor channel blockers may be useful for the treatment of stroke and epilepsy, where some derangement of excitatory amino acid transmission has been proposed. Unfortunately all agents so far examined also produce the type of psychotomimetic activity which resulted in the anaesthetic agent, phencyclidine, being withdrawn from medical use and left to pop culture as 'angel dust'. Ketamine, which also exhibits anticonvulsant activity, remains in clinical use, although hallucinatory side-effects are still a problem when it is used as an anaesthetic. It may be that drugs acting on other binding sites associated with the NMDA channel, particularly the glycine modulatory site, could have a better therapeutic profile. Although the AMPA and KA receptors have distinct locations, they appear to subserve similar functions which involve the fast component of the excitatory postsynaptic potential in, for example, the spinal cord, where a role as the primary pain transmitter has been proposed.

In addition to the receptor operated channels described above, excitatory amino acids also act on G protein-linked metabotropic receptors, of which seven have been cloned at the last count. The physiological role of these is unclear but some may be presynaptic and inhibit glutamate release. The therapeutic potential of selective agonists at such a site could be significant.

γ-Aminobutyric acid

GABA is mainly found within the CNS, where it is now believed to be the major inhibitory transmitter. GABA inhibitory neurones can be differentiated from glutamate excitatory neurones by the presence of glutamic acid decarboxylase (GAD), which is a unidirectional enzyme converting glutamate to GABA. An essential cofactor for the action of GAD is pyridoxal phosphate (vitamin B_6), and pyridoxine deficiency is associated with seizures that are rapidly responsive to the vitamin. In view of this observation it is not surprising that enhancement of GABA activity has been a target of anticonvulsant research,

and neuropathological studies do suggest GABA deficiency in at least some cases of epilepsy. Progabide, a GABA prodrug, is commercially available but initial studies suggest that its usefulness is unlikely to be widespread. In general, direct GABA mimetics have not proved therapeutically useful for epilepsy because of the variability of patients' responses to them. Sodium valproate, which inhibits at least two enzymes responsible for GABA metabolism, has a wider spectrum of activity and is one of the few drugs useful for the treatment of absences, grand mal and partial seizures. Vigabatrin has a more selective effect upon a single enzyme, GABA transaminase, and has been introduced as 'add on' therapy for the treatment of epilepsy. As will be seen later, other drugs with anticonvulsant properties modulate GABA activity at the receptor level.

There are two main classes of GABA receptors, $GABA_A$ and $GABA_B$ (Table 9.2). The former is a ligand gated chloride channel, while the latter is G protein linked. Baclofen is the only drug currently in clinical use that acts as an agonist at $GABA_B$ receptors. It is used to treat spasticity associated with multiple sclerosis or spinal injury. Weak antagonists at this receptor, such as 2-OH-baclofen, has been described but have no clinical use. Nevertheless, there is considerable interest in drugs acting at the $GABA_B$ receptor. In the experimental animal $GABA_B$ agonists have

Table 9.2 Inhibitory amino acids: γ-aminobutyric acid (GABA) and glycine

Receptors	Selective drugs	
	Agonists	Antagonists
$GABA_A$ (ROC)	Muscimol	Bicuculline
$GABA_B$	Baclofen	Phaclofen
Glycine	—	Strychnine
Glycine binding on NMDA receptor complex (ROC)	—	7-Chloroknurenate

Comment
Only baclofen has a clinical use (centrally acting muscle relaxant). However drugs enhancing $GABA_A$ transmission (anaesthetics, benzodiazepines, valproate, etc.) are used as anxiolytics, anticonvulsants and anaesthetics.
N.B. Inverse agonists reduce GABA transmission — anxiety, panic and convulsions.
ROC, receptor operated ion channel.

unequivocal analgesic activity, the locus of which appears to be the spinal cord. However, in man, baclofen does not appear to have analgesic activity, although it has been used successfully to treat trigeminal neuralgia. In addition, $GABA_B$ antagonists are potential anticonvulsants.

Interest in $GABA_A$ receptor pharmacology has waned in recent years and research activity has declined. However, the receptor is important to anaesthetists, as a considerable number of anaesthetic and related drugs act on it. These include many general anaesthetics, such as the barbiturates and propofol, as well as the benzodiazepine anxiolytics. All these drugs have been shown to enhance GABA neurotransmission. The benzodiazepines bind to their own receptor, which is located on a subunit of the chloride channel distinct from that of GABA itself. The GABA gated chloride ion channel is a pentamer usually consisting of two α subunits, two β subunits and one γ subunit, although other subunits have been identified. GABA binding requires the presence of the β subunit, but benzodiazepine binding requires both the α and γ subunit. There are many variants to the structure of these subunits, particularly the α subunit, which alter their binding characteristics. This accounts for the subtypes of benzodiazepine (BZ) receptors (1, 2 and 3) (Table 9.3) described in the literature. Some drugs

Table 9.3 Endogenous benzodiazepine-like compounds: diazepam binding inhibitor (DBI), endozepines, carbolines, benzodiazepines

Receptors	Selective drugs	
	Agonists	Antagonists
BZ$_1$ (omega or BDZ*)	Zolpidem Alpidem Triazolopyridazines Clonazepam	Flumazenil
BZ$_2$ BZ$_3$	Clonazepam Alpidem	Flumazenil PK11195

Comment
There are no clear functional correlates of binding to these receptor types. BZ$_3$ is found peripherally and centrally. In the periphery it may be associated with mitochondrial activity. Not all these receptors are associated with the GABA$_A$ receptor.
*Alternative names used in the literature.
PK 11195, 1-(2-chlorophenyl)-*N*-methyl (1-methylpropyl)-3 isoquinolinecarboxamine.

have selectivity for a particular benzodiazepine receptor — for example, zolpidem, a hypnotic which does not have a diazepine ring structure, is selective for BZ$_1$ receptors. However, at present there is no clear functional correlation with receptor selectivity.

Barbiturates and other general anaesthetics are less selective in their actions on the chloride channel and their binding sites are less well characterised. There are differences in the characteristics of the enhancement of GABA transmission by the barbiturates and the benzodiazepines. The former increase the 'chloride channel open time' in response to GABA, while the latter increase the frequency of channel opening. It is obvious that increasing doses of benzodiazepines must have a ceiling effect, at which point the chloride channel opens so fast that it 'flickers' and becomes ineffective. This may account for the higher therapeutic index seen with the benzodiazepines when compared with the barbiturates. There are selective antagonists for the two receptors most clearly defined on the $GABA_A$ gated chloride channel, bicuculline for the $GABA_A$ receptor itself and flumazenil for the benzodiazepine receptor.

The search for the endogenous ligand for the benzodiazepine receptor has yielded a novel and fascinating sideline to receptor pharmacology. Pharmacologically, an agonist is defined as a ligand that binds to a receptor and produces an effect, while an antagonist may bind to the same receptor, denying access to the agonist, but does not produce an effect itself. The first potential endogenous ligand for the benzodiazepine receptor was a β-carboline derivative. However, when this compound binds to the receptor it reduces the effect of GABA transmission and causes anxiety, panic and convulsions. This is diametrically the opposite pharmacology to the benzodiazepines and was antagonised by flumazenil. Compounds of this type are called inverse agonists and are being increasingly described at other receptor types (*see* Further Reading).

It is likely that the endogenous ligand for the benzodiazepine receptor is co-located with GABA, but its true identity has been elusive. As mentioned earlier, β-carboline derivatives have been isolated, but so have peptides such as diazepam binding inhibitor (DBI) and the enzodepines. All of these have inverse agonist properties. However, there is also evidence of benzodiazepine-like structures within the CNS and, in patients with encephalopathy secondary to liver failure, the coma, but not the liver failure, may be partially reversed by flumazenil.

Glycine

Very little progress has been made towards the elucidation of the role of glycine as a neurotransmitter. It is released from the spinal cord, particularly at the Renshaw cell synapse with the α motor neurone, thus preventing repetitive firing of the motor neurone. This effect is antagonised by the convulsant strychnine. There is also a glycine receptor, which is not strychnine sensitive, on the NMDA receptor discussed above. At this site it appears to facilitate glutamate's action and is thus equivalent to the endogenous ligands for the benzodiazepine receptor associated with the $GABA_A$ chloride channel.

Biogenic amines

Biogenic amine-containing neurones make up only a small fraction of those present in the CNS and are confined to distinct nuclei rather than the more diffuse distribution seen with other neurotransmitter systems. Most cells containing noradrenaline are located in the locus coeruleus, while dopamine-containing cells are clustered for the most part in the substantia nigra. 5-Hydroxytryptamine-containing cells are grouped in the raphe nuclei. From these regions fibres spread out to almost all areas of the brain.

In some of these pathways well defined synaptic structures and one-to-one transmission are found; however, in other areas a more diffuse system prevails, in which the transmitter is released some distance from the target cells and needs to reach a critical concentration to cause activation. In these circumstances drug therapy which increases the concentration of the amine in the general area of the target cells can very effectively reverse the effects of reduced activity of

the system, even if there is destruction of cells in the specific nuclei. Thus a given chemical entity may perform a neurotransmitter, a neuromodulator and a hormonal role. This will be illustrated in more detail with the individual amines.

Dopamine

The importance of dopamine as a neurotransmitter, quite separate from its role as a precursor of noradrenaline, became apparent after the observation in the mid-1960s that Parkinson's disease, characterised by tremor rigidity and disturbances of movement, was associated with a massive depletion of dopamine from the striatum. Subsequently it was shown that selective dopamine receptor antagonists induced an extrapyramidal disturbance similar to parkinsonism and that the induction of a Parkinson-like syndrome by a contaminant of synthetic heroin, 1-methyl-5-phenyl-1,2,3,6-tetrahydropyridine (MPTP), was associated with a destruction of nigrostriatal dopaminergic neurones. These observations led to the introduction of the prodrug, levodopa, to ameliorate the signs and symptoms of Parkinson's disease. Levodopa can be converted to dopamine either by the remaining dopaminergic neurones, where it can be stored and released in the normal way, or it can be decarboxylated to dopamine by other cells, thereby raising the concentration of dopamine bathing the striatal neurones. The fact that dopamine agonists other than dopamine, such as bromocriptine, lisuride and pergolide, can reduce the symptoms of the disease suggests that the occupancy of dopamine receptors is more important for the control of movement than the sequence pattern of neuronal firing. Nevertheless, although providing a lower incidence of side-effects, alternatives to levodopa are often less effective and patients may be managed on combinations of dopamine agonists.

Levodopa therapy may be associated with the induction of psychosis and chronic abuse of amphetamine, which releases dopamine and other amines, and is characterised by psychosis which is difficult to distinguish from schizophrenia. Since all effective treatments for schizophrenia are antagonists at dopamine receptors, it is not surprising that excessive dopamine activity has been suggested as a cause of schizophrenic symptoms. However, there is no evidence of consistent changes in dopamine neurotransmission in patients with schizophrenia. In addition, dopamine agonists are rather weak inducers of psychosis and the time course of dopamine receptor blockade is much faster (hours) than the time course of amelioration of schizophrenic symptoms, which can run into several weeks.

At the receptor level the prognosis for future developments may be better. Dopamine receptors have been broadly classified into D_1 receptors, which increase adenylyl cyclase activity, and D_2 receptors, which have either no effect on, or decrease, adenylyl cyclase activity. Most useful drug activity, at least in the CNS, involves agonism or antagonism at D_2 receptors, although it is now clear that D_1 receptors modulate D_2 receptor activity. The brains of schizophrenic patients appear to have larger numbers of D_2 receptors compared with non-schizophrenic controls. Although some of this may result from prior drug therapy, there is also a distinct but less substantial increase in these receptors in patients who have not been prescribed antipsychotic drugs.

Some progress in the possible reduction of the adverse effects of antipsychotic therapy has come from the molecular biologists and the cloning of the complementary deoxyribose nucleic acid (cDNA) and/or genes for several other G protein-linked dopamine receptors. These include D_1 and D_5, which both have the characteristics of D_1 receptors, and D_2, D_3 and D_4, which all have the characteristics of D_2 receptors (Table 9.4). Interest comes from the fact that the distribution of D_3 and D_4 receptors differs from D_2, in that they are poorly represented in the striatal regions which give rise to the parkinsonian side-effects of antipsychotic therapy. Clozapine, an antipsychotic that produces fewer extrapyramidal side-effects than most, has some selectivity for the D_4 receptor.

Noradrenaline

The noradrenergic system is less widespread

Table 9.4 Dopamine

Receptors	Selective drugs	
	Agonists	Antagonists
D_1	SKF 38393	Sch 23390
D_2	Quinpirole	Sulpiride
D_3	7-OH-DPAT	–
D_4	Dopamine	Clozapine
D_5	Dopamine	Sch 23390

Comment
Dopamine receptors were divided into two groups: D_1 and D_2. D_1 receptors (new D_1 and D_5) increase cAMP activity. D_2 receptors (new D_2, D_3, D_4) decrease or have no effect on cAMP. Most useful drugs interact with old D2 group. Clozapine has no effect on prolactin release and causes less extrapyramidal disturbances.
SKF 38393, 2,3,4,5-tetrahydro-7,8-dihydroxy-1-phenyl-1H-3 benzazepine HCl; Sch 23390, 7-chloro-2,3,4,5-tetrahydro-3-methyl-5-phenyl-1H-3-benzazepine-7-ol; 7-OH-DPAT, 7 hydroxy-dipropylaminotetralin.

than the dopaminergic system and no disease states are clearly associated with noradrenaline lack or excess. During the 1980s and early 1990s, genes encoding nine distinct adrenoceptors were cloned: α_{1A}, α_{1B}, α_{1C}, α_{2A}, α_{2B}, α_{2C}, β_1, β_2 and β_3. However, at present, little is known about the physiological function of the subdivisions of α_1 and α_2 receptors in the periphery, let alone the CNS. Thus they can be ignored until selective agonists and antagonists are shown to have a therapeutic role. Noradrenaline generally has inhibitory actions in the CNS mediated via β receptors, although there are well documented excitatory responses mediated by either α or β adrenoceptors. Most of our suppositions concerning the role of noradrenaline in the CNS come from observations of drugs that we know interact with the noradrenergic system. Agonists at α_2 adrenoceptors (e.g. clonidine) have hypotensive, sedative and analgesic actions. It is the last two actions that have particularly interested anaesthetists, as these drugs reduce anaesthetic requirements and can be used epidurally for postoperative pain relief.

In 1965 the monoamine theory of depression was proposed. The theory suggested that depression results from deficient noradrenergic and/or tryptaminergic transmission in the CNS and was based on the observation that antidepressant drugs could facilitate monoamine transmission and that depletion of these transmitters by reserpine resulted in depression. However, facilitation of transmission by inhibition of monoamine uptake (tricyclic antidepressants) or monoamine oxidase inhibition occurs rapidly, while antidepressant activity is delayed. In addition, biochemical studies have not supported any alteration in noradrenergic function in depressed patients. Nevertheless, manipulation of monoamine neurotransmission remains the most successful approach to depression, although the mechanism of success is likely to be due to chronic effects, such as decreased responsiveness of β receptors or increased responsiveness of α_1 receptors.

Adrenaline

The presence of phenylethanolamine-*N*-methyl transferase, which converts noradrenaline to adrenaline in the brain, points to adrenaline being a neurotransmitter. In general, the neurones are intermingled with both noradrenaline and adrenaline fibres innervating the hypothalamus and the dorsal motor nucleus of the vagus nerve. This suggests that adrenaline is involved in blood pressure control and neuroendocrine mechanisms, but the understanding of the CNS adrenaline system is very limited at present.

5-Hydroxytryptamine

In the 1950s 5-hydroxytryptamine (5-HT) (or serotonin) was first located within the CNS and subsequently has been associated with many functions, such as sleep, thermoregulation, pain, sex, learning and memory, aggression, feeding, motor activity and biological rhythms. In addition, it has been associated with the pathological processes of various psychiatric disorders, of which anxiety and depression, particularly of the suicidal type, are the most studied. A proportion of depressed patients show a reduction of 5-hydroxyindoleacetic acid (5-HIAA) in the cerebrospinal fluid, but this persists into recovery, suggesting that it is not a marker of the depressed state. A more consistent depression of 5-HIAA is seen in patients who have attempted to commit suicide. Many antidepressant drugs can poten-

tiate 5-HT as well as noradrenaline (see above) and administration of the 5-HT precursor tryptophan can have beneficial effects in some patients. Selective serotonin reuptake inhibitors, such as fluoxetine (Prozac), are showing increasing favour as they tend to have fewer side-effects than the tricyclic and monoamine oxidase inhibitor (MAOI) antidepressants. While much adverse publicity for fluoxetine was initiated in the USA by a report of suicidal and aggressive behaviour, 'prescription event monitoring' in the UK has failed to confirm these reports, even among patients who had seen the critical television programme. However, selective noradrenaline reuptake inhibitors (maprotiline) are also useful antidepressants and some atypical drugs, such as iprindole and mianserin, do not appear to prevent reuptake of either amine and do not inhibit monoamine oxidase. Thus the basis of the action of any antidepressant drug is still open to debate.

Like adrenoceptors, the advent of molecular biology has spawned a plethora of 5-HT receptors (Table 9.5) whose classification is reorganised at regular intervals as more information emerges. For example the 5-HT$_{1C}$ receptor is

Table 9.5 Hydroxytryptamine

Receptors	Selective drugs	
	Agonists	Antagonists
5-HT$_{1A}$	Buspirone (anxiolytic)	—
5-HT$_{1B}$		
5-HT$_{1D}$	Sumatriptan (antimigraine)	Ritanserin, pizotifen
5-HT$_{2(A \& B)}$	—	Ketanserin (also ritanserin, pizotifen) (vasodilator)
5-HT$_{2C}$	—	Mesulergine
5-HT$_3$ (ROC)	—	Ondansetron (antiemetic)
Also 5-HT$_4$ and 5-HT$_5$	—	

Comment
In addition to the clinical uses shown in the table, drugs interacting with 5-HT sytems have anxiolytic activity (uptake inhibitors and ondansetron as well as buspirone); effects on nociception (ondansetron reduces inflammatory hyperalgesia and ritanserin antagonises the analgesic activity of 5-HT in the spinal cord) and antimigraine activity (ondansetron and pizotifen have been shown to be useful). ROC, receptor operated ion channel.

now reclassified as a 5-HT$_{2C}$ as its predominant effector is on the phosphinositide system, which is common to 5-HT$_2$ receptors, while 5-HT$_1$ receptors predominantly decrease adenylyl cyclase activity. Amongst the wide range of more or less selective agonists and antagonists at these receptors, a few with clear clinical application will be highlighted.

Anxiolytic actions of 5-HT$_{1A}$-receptor agonists such as buspirone have been reported in man and the drug is marketed for this indication. Unlike the benzodiazepines, they do not cause sedation, amnesia or ataxia but there is a delay of several days before any effect is seen. It is interesting to note that buspirone increases the number of benzodiazepine receptors, suggesting an interaction between the two systems. Not all 5-HT$_{1A}$ receptors are identical and there is some evidence that buspirone may act as an agonist at presynaptic 5-HT$_{1A}$ autoreceptors and a partial agonist, or even an antagonist, at postsynaptic 5-HT$_{1A}$ receptors. Some success in treating depression with 5-HT$_{1A}$ agonists has been reported, but again the mechanism of this action is unclear.

5-HT$_{1B}$ receptors are not found in humans and 5-HT$_{1C}$ receptors have been reclassified to 5-HT$_{2C}$. That leaves 5-HT$_{1D}$ receptors, where agonists such as sumatriptan are extremely effective in the acute treatment of migraine and have few side-effects in most patients. Sumatriptan does not penetrate the blood–brain barrier but causes a 5-HT$_1$-like receptor induced constriction of the arteriovenous anastomosis. Dilatation of these vessels is believed to be part of the pathophysiology of migraine. In some vascular beds 5-HT$_{1D}$ receptors are identical with 5-HT$_1$-like receptors (5-HT$_1$-like being defined as having the characteristics of 5-HT$_1$ receptors but not those of 5-HT$_{1A}$, 5-HT$_{1B}$ or 5-HT$_{1C}$), but this is not universally so.

Receptors of the 5-HT$_2$ type were identified early and are the traditional D receptors described by Gaddum and Picarelli in 1957. The classical 5-HT antagonists, cyproheptadine, methysergide and pizotifen, all have high affinity although no great selectivity for this group of receptors. Ketanserin is a selective antagonist at the 5-HT$_{2A}$ receptor and although it has been

tried in a number of disease states it has been marketed only to treat hypertension and intermittent claudication. Ritanserin, an antagonist which does not discriminate between the 5-HT$_2$ subtypes, has been marketed for the treatment of schizophrenia, suggesting a tryptaminergic role in this condition. However, these drugs do interact with other non-tryptaminergic neurotransmitter systems, which may be relevant to the disease process that they treat.

The final group of drugs to be highlighted under the heading of useful modulators of tryptaminergic function are the 5-HT$_3$ antagonists, such as ondansetron. These drugs are useful antiemetics when used in conjunction with cytotoxic drug administration for the treatment of cancers and for postoperative nausea and vomiting. The action of ondansetron probably includes both a peripheral component in the gastrointestinal tract and a central component at the level of the area postrema (chemosensitive trigger zone). 5-HT$_3$ receptors may also be involved in the spinal transmission of nociceptive impulses, as antagonists produce significant analgesia in inflammatory pain.

Histamine

There is compelling evidence that histamine exists in neurones in the CNS as well as in mast cells. All three receptors, H$_1$, H$_2$ and H$_3$ are present and their respective selective antagonists, mepyramine, ranitidine and thioperamide are available. It must be admitted that histamine's functions in the brain are poorly understood. At an electrophysiological level its excitatory actions are usually associated with H$_1$ receptors, whereas inhibitory actions are associated with the H$_2$ type. A role in arousal has been suggested from the observation that H$_1$-receptor antagonists are all sedative. These antagonists also suppress motion sickness, but this is believed by most researchers to be due to atropinic, rather than antihistaminic, activity.

Neuropeptides

Many peptides that were first isolated as

hormones, such as vasopressin and angiotensin, are now known to have a transmitter function in the CNS.

Unlike more traditional neurotransmitters, in which precursors are taken up into the neurone and the transmitter synthesised (e.g. acetylcholine and noradrenaline), the peptide precursors are produced directly by the genetic apparatus. During transport to the nerve terminal, or within it, the propeptide is cleaved to active peptides, which can then be released. The post-translational cleavage of the propeptide may vary from neurone to neurone, depending upon the enzymes present. The whole process is relatively slow and suggests that peptides are associated physiologically with long term changes rather than acute changes. These are more difficult to detect in the experimental situation. Whereas active reuptake of transmitter is common in other neurotransmitter systems, peptides are inactivated only by enzymic breakdown. This may allow enzyme inhibition to be used as a tool for understanding the physiology of neuropeptide mechanisms. Neuropeptides are often found to coexist with other neurotransmitters, such as serotonin, noradrenaline, GABA and other peptides. The details of how the peptides modulate the activity of other cotransmitters awaits elucidation. Peptides usually act on G protein or tyrosine kinase-linked receptors; in general, there are few antagonists, with the notable exception of the opioid peptide receptors, where naloxone is an antagonist. However, research is developing rapidly in this area and the previous statement may be out of date by the time this chapter is published. Peptides themselves do not make good drugs because they are poorly absorbed orally (they are either broken down or not absorbed at all), they are expensive to manufacture, generally they have short half-lives because of rapid metabolism (endorphins are an exception) and they do not cross the blood–brain barrier. Although there are dozens of neuropeptides, some of which are listed in Table 9.6, just two groups, for which there is the greatest current or future potential for drugs useful to the anaesthetist, have been selected.

Table 9.6 Neuropeptides

Neuropeptide	Receptors	CNS role
Angiotensin	AT_1	Promotes drinking, increases blood pressure
Calcitonin and calcitonin gene related peptide	CGRP	Analgesia, satiety, growth hormone release
Cholecystokinin	CCK_A/CCK_B	Functional antagonist of opioid receptor activation, also analgesia and satiety
Opioid peptides	μ, δ, κ	Analgesia
Tachykinins	NK_1, NK_2, NK_3	'Wind-up' pain

Opioid peptides

There are three families of opioid peptides, each family being derived from its own precursor, for which separate genes have been isolated. These are the natural ligands for the opioid receptors at which analgesic drugs such as morphine act as agonists. It is unusual that a non-peptide drug should mimic a peptide, although there is some evidence that the natural ligand of the benzodiazepine receptor may also be a peptide. Opioid drugs and the G protein-linked opioid receptors with which they interact are more fully described in Chapter 17.

Hughes and co-workers were the first to characterise any of the opioid peptides. These were pentapeptides with the structures Tyr-Gly-Gly Phe-Met (methionine enkephalin (Met-enkephalin)) and Tyr-Gly-Gly Phe-Leu (leucine enkephalin (Leu-enkephalin)), which were rapidly broken down by peptidase enzymes. Inhibitors of these enzymes, such as thiophan and kelatorphan, have been shown to have analgesic activity. As neither of these compounds can cross the blood–brain barrier, their clinical potential is uncertain. A new mixed peptidase enzyme inhibitor (RB 101), which does cross the blood–brain barrier, has been developed. Animal tests suggest that it lacks morphine's tolerance and dependence liability but produces effective analgesia. The enkephalins, particularly Leu-enkephalin, have selectivity for the δ subtype of opioid receptor, which has a role in the production of analgesia, but not as much as the μ receptor, for which none of the endogenous opioid peptides show any great selectivity.

The enkephalin precursor, proenkephalin, was demonstrated to have these two peptides in a fixed ratio of six Met-enkephalin sequences to one Leu-enkephalin, although some of the Met-enkephalin sequences may incorporate several more amino acids to produce larger opioids including a heptapeptide, an octapeptide and peptide E (25 amino acids). Proenkephalin-containing cells are extensively distributed throughout the brain and spinal cord as well as more peripheral sites, such as the adrenal medulla, autonomic nervous system and gastrointestinal tract.

Pro-opiomelanocortin (POMC) is the common precursor of the opioid β-endorphin as well as the non-opioid hormones adrenocorticotrophic hormone (ACTH) and α and β melanocyte stimulating hormones (α-MSH and β-MSH). Although the Met-enkephalin sequence is found at the amino terminal of β-endorphin, Met-enkephalin is not derived from POMC. The term endorphin is reserved for those opioid peptides which are derivatives of POMC and the name may be followed by a number to denote the number of amino acids in the sequence, e.g. β-endorphin (1–31). Although the pituitary gland is the major site of POMC biosynthesis, it is also found in specific areas of the brain, such as the hypothalamus, and in diverse sites, including the pancreas, gastric antrum and placenta. However, different forms of β-endorphin may be formed in different brain areas; β-endorphin (1–31) represents the largest constituent in the hypothalamus, while β-endorphin (1–26) and (1–27) are more abundant in the amygdala and mesencephalon. Endorphins are released during stress and may mediate the analgesia often associated with this state.

Prodynorphin, which was known as proenkephalin B, contains Leu-enkephalin sequences but no Met-enkephalin sequences. The opioid peptides derived from this precursor include the dynorphins, α- and β-neoendorphin and leumorphin, which all contain the Leu-enkephalin sequence at the amine terminus. Prodynorphin, like proenkephalin, is synthesised throughout the CNS in a wide variety of neuronal systems. The distribution of dynorphin and enkephalins are often contiguous and they participate through separate receptors in related CNS functions. The dynorphins show some selectivity for the κ subtype of opioid receptor. The role of this receptor in the production of analgesia has probably been the subject of most debate. On balance it is probably true to say that κ agonists can mediate analgesia, but this may depend upon both the site of application and ongoing activity of other opioid and non-opioid transmitter systems. Like the enkephalins, the prodynorphin family are also found in peripheral tissues.

Opioid peptides are involved in many physiological functions as well as analgesia and the reader is referred to the further reading section for a review of some of these functions.

Tachykinins

There are three peptides in this family: substance P, neurokinin A and neurokinin B, acting on NK_1, NK_2 and NK_3 receptors, respectively. They usually produce excitatory responses in neurones, secretory cells and smooth muscle. Traditionally, substance P has been thought of as the primary pain transmitter, but there is no unequivocal evidence that this is the case. Both peptide and non-peptide antagonists are becoming available and it has been shown that NK_1 antagonists are not particularly effective against acute C fibre activity, although NK_2 antagonists are effective to some extent. Tachykinins are coreleased with the excitatory amino acids during chronic C and A fibre activity and may contribute to the wind-up pain described earlier. In addition NK_1 antagonists may have a role in preventing the local effects of substance P in inflammation.

Prostaglandins

Unlike most neurotransmitters, prostaglandins (PGs) are widely and evenly distributed within the CNS. They are formed rapidly on demand, rather than preformed and stored, and are rapidly broken down. All these characteristics make them ideal candidates for a local modulator role in the CNS. The prostanoids mediate their effects through a variety of receptors. The accepted nomenclature is that each receptor is labelled P (for prostanoid) preceded by another letter to denote the active prostaglandin, i.e. $PGF_{2\alpha}$ would act at FP receptors.

Pharmacological interest in the prostaglandins was assured in 1974 by the discovery that non-steroidal anti-inflammatory drugs, such as aspirin, were potent inhibitors of cyclo-oxygenase. This enzyme is responsible for the conversion of arachidonic acid to the cyclic endoperoxides, which in turn are converted to the various prostaglandins. Initially it was believed that the anti-inflammatory action of these drugs was due to a peripheral action of aspirin, while antipyretic activity was due to central cyclo-oxygenase inhibition. The analgesic activity was also ascribed to prostaglandin synthesis inhibition because paracetamol, which is analgesic but not anti-inflammatory at therapeutic doses, appeared to inhibit cyclo-oxygenase in the CNS but not in the periphery. Subsequent work has cast some doubt, or produced voluminous debate, on many of these conclusions. Although all anti-inflammatory agents, including the steroids, prevent the formation of prostaglandins, the correlation between the two properties is not particularly convincing. In addition, inflammatory processes can be influenced by events within the CNS. Fever is associated with a rise in prostaglandin E in the hypothalamus, but the definitive proof of its involvement with fever awaits the development of prostanoid receptor antagonists that will penetrate into the brain. The analgesic activity of paracetamol and aspirin in non-inflammatory pain may be the result of inhibition of cyclo-oxygenase in the spinal cord, where prostaglandins have been shown to be released by persistent C fibre activation. These may act directly or indirectly to influence several other neurotransmitter systems believed to be involved in pain pathways. Nevertheless, there is evidence that some exert analgesic activity by other mechanisms — for example, diclofenac analgesia directly or indirectly involves an opioid component. Finally, the central specificity for paracetamol's inhibitory action on cyclo-oxygenase is also debatable, and tissue rather than CNS speci-

ficity appears to be a more likely explanation of the results observed.

The discovery of an inducible isoform of the cyclo-oxygenase enzyme COX-2 opens up the possibility of selective inhibitors of the two enzymes, COX-1 and COX-2. Some drugs, such as salicylic acid, may have selectivity for COX-2, but preliminary studies with paracetamol suggest that it has no such enzyme selectivity and that its tissue selectivity may be due to the presence of cofactors.

The answers to questions about the relevance of prostaglandin synthesis inhibition to drug activity will only be resolved by the development of water soluble selective prostanoid receptor antagonists.

CONCLUSION

Some drugs defy our attempts to classify them under a particular mechanistic heading. Lithium, unlike the antidepressants discussed previously under the heading of noradrenaline or 5-hydroxytryptamine, controls the manic phase of manic-depressive (bipolar) illness and is effective in unipolar depression. Given prophylactically it prevents the mood swings seen in bipolar depression. Acutely, lithium increases turnover of noradrenaline and 5-HT in the brain and inhibits evoked release of noradrenaline. This evidence could be used in support of the monoamine theory of depression if it is reasoned that the manic phase must be due to excessive activation of monoamines. However, these actions of lithium do not persist during chronic administration, in contrast to the therapeutic effect. Lithium can mimic the actions of other monovalent cations, notably sodium entry into the voltage sensitive channels, that are responsible for the action potential. Since it is only slowly pumped out by Na^+,K^+-ATPase, it tends to accumulate in cells and cannot maintain membrane potentials. This will affect many transmitter systems. In addition, intracellular lithium blocks the phosphatidylinositol pathway which is important as a second messenger for many receptor mediated effects. While this could account for lithium's selective action in the brain, which has a high density of sodium channels through which lithium may enter, the widespread nature of this effect does not help to define the biochemical basis of depression or mania.

In a similar manner, many CNS active drugs are now known to act by the release of nitric oxide, including the opioid analgesics and the benzodiazepine anxiolytics. In the future it may be possible to target drugs to the different steps in the synthetic and signal transduction pathways for this gaseous mediator. However, its ubiquitous involvement in apparently opposing roles, i.e. both long term potentiation and long term depression, prompts one to be cautious in speculating any therapeutic breakthrough.

FURTHER READING

Bowers C W 1994 Superfluous neurotransmitters. Trends in Neurological Sciences 17: 315–320

Bowery N G 1993 GABA$_B$ receptor pharmacology. Annual Review of Pharmacology and Toxicology 33: 109–147

Goodchild C S 1993 GABA receptors and benzodiazepines. British Journal of Anaesthesia 71: 127–133

Hayashi Y, Maze M 1993 Alpha$_2$ adrenoceptor agonists and anaesthesia. British Journal of Anaesthesia 71: 108–118

Lipton S A 1993 Prospects for clinically tolerated NMDA antagonists: open channel blockers and alternative redox states of nitric oxide. Trends in Neurosciences 16: 527–532

McCormack K 1994 Non-steroidal anti-inflammatory drugs and spinal nociceptive processing. Pain 59: 9–43

Maggi C A, Patacchini R, Rovero P, Giachetti A 1993 Tachykinin receptors and tachykinin receptor anatagonists. Journal of Autonomic Pharmacology 13: 23–93

Milligan G, Bond R A, Lee M 1995 Inverse agonism: pharmacological curiosity or potential therapeutic strategy. Trends in Pharmacological Sciences 16: 10–13

Mohler H 1992 GABAergic synaptic transmission regulation by drugs. Arzneimittel-Forschung 42: 211–214.

Pleuvry B J 1993 The endogenous opioid system. Anaesthetic Pharmacology Reviews 2: 114–121.

Sibley D R, Monsma F J 1992 Molecular biology of dopamine receptors. Trends in Pharmacological Sciences 13: 61–69

Zifa E, Fillion G 1992 5-Hydroxytryptamine receptors. Pharmacological Reviews 44: 401–458

10

The brain and anaesthesia

A. C. McKay

MECHANISMS OF ANAESTHESIA

At the clinical level, anaesthesia is a drug induced, reversible disruption of central nervous system (CNS) function. If a comprehensive theory of anaesthesia existed, it would explain how this disruption occurs in terms of functional changes in particular brain structures and pathways, which would be shown to be the result of altered axonal conduction or synaptic transmission in individual neurones, and these in turn would be traced to the interaction between the anaesthetic molecule and neuronal components. This kind of complete explanation is not, however, possible at present. The neurological basis of subjective awareness, the absence of which is the most striking single feature of anaesthesia, is not understood, although it is possible to find neurological correlates for related, objective properties of the CNS, such as response to various forms of stimuli. The effects of anaesthetics on these may be studied, as may their actions on neurotransmission at the level of the single neurone or synapse, but it is not yet possible to make a causal connection between such cellular level effects and effects on systems whose function depends on the integrated activity of billions of neurones and synapses. In the past there has been a similar gulf of scale between anaesthetic actions at the cellular and molecular levels, but in recent years advances in the identification and classification of individual ion channels and neurotransmitter receptor ion channel complexes have enabled the actions of anaesthetics on these structures to be studied directly and the results integrated with neurophysiological findings.

A further difficulty in the study of anaesthetic mechanisms is that anaesthetics have many actions, including not only those known to clinicians as side-effects but also other actions at the molecular and cellular level that are unrelated to the 'main' action of producing anaesthesia. While these are usually readily identifiable in the intact organism, they have been the basis of many false trails in work on isolated brain slices and cellular preparations.

Fortunately, however, all types of study are linked by the common thread that relates them to the observed macroscopic phenomenon of anaesthesia. If an experimental effect of an anaesthetic is to qualify as relevant to the anaesthetic state, it must occur in the concentration range that produces anaesthesia. It must be produced rapidly on exposure to the agent, be sustainable in a steady state over a prolonged period, and be readily reversible by removal of the agent. As a general rule, different agents should show the same rank order of potency for the effect as for anaesthesia.

At least until quite recently, most investigators in this field have assumed that there was a single mechanism of anaesthesia, common to all agents, and that differences among agents, whether in their CNS or other effects, were due to 'side-effects' unrelated to their anaesthetic activity. The origin of this assumption is to be found in the historical development of theories of anaesthesia.

Development of theories of anaesthesia

A number of readily observable features of anaesthetics as a group suggest that they are unusual among pharmacologically active substances. Although as molecules they are comparatively simple, they show considerable variation in size and structure with, for example, a 10-fold difference in size between xenon and the halogenated hydrocarbons and ethers. To the clinician the number of available anaesthetics is comparatively small, but for the experimental pharmacologist it is much larger, including homologous series such as alkanes, alcohols and ethers as well as inert gases. The potency of anaesthetics as a group is low in comparison with other drugs, so that the concentrations necessary to produce an effect are some 10–100 times greater than those of, for example, opioids. Thus, anaesthesia is an effect produced by high concentrations of a large, chemically heterogeneous group of substances, and it was this observation that led the earliest investigators to conclude that their mode of action was non-specific and dependent on physical rather than chemical factors.

Lipid solubility

The discovery at the turn of the twentieth century of the remarkable correlation between anaesthetic potency and olive oil/water partition coefficient lent support to this view, as it implied that solubility in fat was of primary importance in the mechanism of anaesthesia. It led to the first physical theory of anaesthesia, proposed by Overton and Meyer, which stated that anaesthesia was due to the action of the agent on an olive oil-like, i.e. lipid, site in the CNS. The onset of anaesthesia would occur when the molar concentration of the agent reached a critical level, which would be the same for all agents, regardless of their size, shape or chemical nature. Later work confirmed that this correlation holds over a very wide range of anaesthetic potency (Fig. 10.1).

Pressure reversal of anaesthesia and the critical volume hypothesis

The discovery during the 1940s that anaesthesia can be antagonised or reversed by the application of high pressures of up to 200 atmospheres gave, in combination with the lipid solubility correlation, a possible molecular mechanism of anaesthesia. If absorption of anaesthetic molecules caused the site of action — presumably the neuronal membrane — to expand, the pressure reversal phenomenon would be explained, in that pressure would tend to antagonise the expansion and restore the volume of the site towards its former size. This concept was formalised as the critical volume hypothesis. A corollary of it is that all agents share, as well as

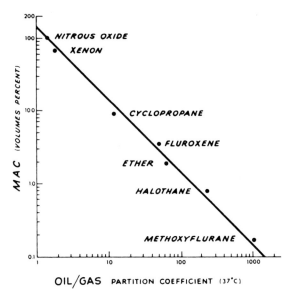

Figure 10.1   Relationship between minimal alveolar concentration and oil:gas partition coefficient for several inhalational anaesthetics.

pressure effects, a common mechanism of action at a common site.

Mammalian cell membranes consist of a lipid bilayer in which are embedded proteins of many types, which, especially in neuronal membranes, include neurotransmitter receptors and ion channels. These continually undergo changes in their conformation in the course of their normal function, switching from active to inactive or open to closed states. The structural integrity of these large membrane-intrinsic proteins depends greatly on the state of the surrounding lipid, so that absorption of anaesthetic molecules by the lipid, disrupting its structure and causing membrane expansion, might easily interfere with the ability of the proteins to function normally.

That membranes do expand when exposed to anaesthetics has been confirmed by experiments using in vitro preparations and model membranes, and the ability of different agents to do this correlates with their known anaesthetic potencies. Various physical mechanisms for the expansion have been proposed — for example, an anaesthetic-induced increase in the fluidity of the bilayer. However, in recent years it has become increasingly apparent that there are serious prob-

lems with theoretical mechanisms of anaesthesia based entirely on membrane expansion.

Firstly, the extent of the expansion caused by appropriate concentrations of anaesthetics has generally been found to be of the order of 0.2–0.6%, and since this small degree of expansion is comparable to that which would be produced by a temperature increase of 1°C, it hardly seems possible that it alone could result in anaesthesia.

A second factor that is difficult to reconcile with the critical volume hypothesis is the occurrence of stereoselectivity among anaesthetics. Agents which can exist in two or more optical isomeric forms are normally used clinically as racemic mixtures; however, potency studies of pure isomers have shown that the laevo isomer is usually approximately twice as potent as the dextro isomer. This stereoselectivity has been demonstrated with barbiturates, ketamine, halothane and isoflurane, and isoflurane is known to have stereoselective effects on ion channels but not on lipid bilayers. These findings strongly suggest that the agent–site interaction is more complex than bulk absorption by a lipid bilayer.

Thirdly, studies of anaesthetic potency have produced some findings that are inconsistent with the predictions of the critical volume hypothesis. The relationship between potency and pressure is non-linear for several intravenous and inhalational anaesthetics, and also the potencies of some mixtures of agents are not additive, showing either synergism or antagonism.

Finally, there is the so-called cut-off effect. In tadpoles, for example, the smaller molecules of the alcohol series are anaesthetics, but dodecanol and larger members of the series are not. This phenomenon, which also occurs with other series, is not due to altered lipid solubility, and obviously implies that the site of anaesthetic action of these substances is limited by size.

These and similar observations have led many to the conclusion that theories involving a simple interaction with membrane lipid greatly underestimate the complexity of anaesthetic action, and coincidentally to the realisation that the unitary theory of anaesthesia would have to be substantially modified. In recent years, most investigative work on molecular mechanisms of anaesthesia has been concentrated on the effects of anaesthetics on membrane proteins rather than lipids.

Actions of anaesthetics on specific neuronal proteins

Both axonal conduction and synaptic transmission depend on the functioning of transmembrane ion channels. In classical axonal conduction these are mainly voltage gated sodium and potassium channels, but the ion channels involved in synaptic transmission are mainly ligand gated and include types that transport calcium and chloride as well as sodium and potassium ions. Ligand gated ion channels occur in association with specific neurotransmitter receptors, while other ligand receptors exert their effects through intracellular second messenger systems. The detailed structures of many of these subcellular components have been elaborated using molecular biological techniques. Most studies of their interactions with anaesthetics involve either recordings of single channel ionic currents, from which the effects on channel function are inferred, or ligand–receptor binding assay. The effects of anaesthetics in these models are frequently consistent with either direct action on the protein itself, on the surrounding lipid, or a combination of actions at both of these.

Sodium and potassium channels

In Na^+ channels incorporated into artificial lipid bilayers, pentobarbitone and propofol reduce fractional channel open time and increase the variability of voltage-dependent activation behaviour. For a number of non-volatile anaesthetic agents there is a correlation between potency for this effect and lipid solubility, but the effect itself is generally found at anaesthetic concentrations that are too high to be relevant to anaesthesia in the intact organism.

There are many varieties of K^+ channel, both voltage and ligand gated, some of which are known to be affected by anaesthetic agents, again mainly at supra-anaesthetic doses. There is evidence from work at the synaptic level that

slow K^+ channels, which control the resting membrane potential of neurones, are influenced by anaesthetics (see below).

Voltage gated Na^+ and K^+ channels do not therefore appear to be major targets of anaesthetic action, which is consistent with the general observation that synaptic transmission is more readily blocked by anaesthetics than axonal conduction; however, it is not impossible that small effects on these ion channels might contribute significantly to the overall picture.

Calcium channels

There are four main subdivisions of voltage gated calcium ion channels, of which one, the N channel, occurs predominantly in neurones. The structures of these channels have been extensively studied by molecular biological techniques and share many of the features of sodium channels. It is of course well known that anaesthetics, as well as other drugs, affect Ca^{2+} channels in sites outside the CNS, notably the myocardium. There is less information on the direct effects, as opposed to those inferred from neurophysiological studies, of anaesthetics on neuronal calcium channels. In rat sensory neurones, halothane and isoflurane block both small and large voltage-activated calcium currents.

Ligand gated ion channels

The structures of the nicotinic acetylcholine (ACh), γ-aminobutyric acid A (GABA$_A$) and glycine receptors are largely known. They are members of a superfamily of receptors which have many common features despite being functionally distinct, and are composed of several membrane-spanning glycoprotein units that form a functional channel with an agonist recognition site.

Nicotinic acetylcholine receptor channels

The nicotinic ACh receptor is believed to have two resting states: normal and desensitised. Binding of two ACh molecules in the normal state switches the receptor to the open channel state, allowing ions to flow. Using ionic current measurements, a number of anaesthetics have been shown to increase the proportion of the receptors in the desensitised state, possibly through a combination of blockage of the ion channel by the anaesthetic molecule and an effect on the lipid surrounding the receptor. Patch clamp experiments on single channels have shown that general anaesthetics change the pattern of channel opening so that openings are more frequent, briefer and appear to be grouped into bursts. In isolated neuronal nicotinic ACh receptor channels the two isomers of isoflurane, at concentrations well within the clinical range, reduce the ACh-induced chloride current to different extents, which correspond to their relative potencies in whole animals. Thus it is clear that ACh receptor channels are sensitive to anaesthetic agents, and the stereoselectivity of the response would favour an effect on the receptor channel itself rather than on the surrounding lipid.

Glycine receptors

Glycine is the major postsynaptic inhibitory transmitter in the brainstem and spinal cord. Its receptor is, like the $GABA_A$ receptor, a chloride ion channel. Some studies have suggested that glycine-mediated Cl^- currents are potentiated by some anaesthetic agents. It is significant that pressure reversal of anaesthesia has been reported to occur only in species in which there is glycinergic transmission; if true, this would suggest that pressure reversal is a specific rather than a general phenomenon. High barometric pressure causes hyperexcitability and convulsions in unanaesthetised animals, therefore one can envisage that pressure may act to prevent a conformational change necessary for activation of the glycine receptor by imposing a volume restriction, and that this effect would be opposed by anaesthetic-induced enhancement of glycinergic transmission.

$GABA_A$ receptors

GABA is the major inhibitory transmitter of the mammalian brain rostral to the brainstem,

about a third of all synapses in the CNS being GABAergic, and virtually every neurone in the mammalian brain is responsive to GABA. Two types of GABA receptor have been identified. $GABA_A$ receptor activation causes an increase in chloride ion permeability by opening of receptor–chloride channels, an action which is blocked by the competitive GABA antagonist bicuculline, while the $GABA_B$ type, activation of which causes opening of K^+ channels, is not blocked by this agent. Activation of the $GABA_A$ receptor–chloride channel complex is responsible for the fast inhibitory postsynaptic potential in the human brain. 15 or more glycoprotein subunits of the $GABA_A$ receptor have been identified, five of which assemble to form an individual receptor channel, giving scope for many subtypes. THIP, a GABA analogue which, unlike GABA itself, crosses the blood–brain barrier, causes sedation and dizziness in humans, and analgesia, sedation and loss of righting reflex in animals.

The interactions of barbiturates with $GABA_A$ receptors have been widely studied, initially using in vivo behavioural models. Loss of righting reflex induced by pentobarbitone is prolonged by THIP and another $GABA_A$ agonist, muscimol, and is reduced by bicuculline. In vitro, barbiturates increase binding of GABA to the receptor, both by increasing the number of available binding sites and slowing dissociation of the ligand from the receptor, and they also modulate allosterically (i.e. by inducing conformational changes) the binding of other ligands, notably benzodiazepines, whose binding is increased. Thus these two groups of drugs appear to act at two distinct binding sites on the receptor. The potencies of barbiturates for this effect correlate well with their potencies as anaesthetics. Studies of chloride ion flux have shown that pentobarbitone itself increases uptake of $^{36}Cl^-$ as well as potentiating uptake induced by muscimol. Pentobarbitone is ten times as potent in this effect as phenobarbitone, suggesting that the effect is related to the anaesthetic, rather than anticonvulsant, action of barbiturates. Single cell studies have shown that normal $GABA_A$ channel opening occurs in bursts of single openings in response to GABA; barbiturates increase both mean channel open time and number of openings per burst.

Like barbiturates, steroid anaesthetics modulate the $GABA_A$ receptor complex, but this action occurs at yet a different site on the complex from those of the barbiturates and benzodiazepines. Alphaxalone also appears to increase Cl^- conductance in the absence of GABA, as well as potentiating the increase produced by GABA by prolonging its decay time.

There is evidence from binding studies that propofol and etomidate also act upon the $GABA_A$ channel complex. Propofol inhibits binding of the convulsant $GABA_A$ blocker TBPS and potentiates muscimol-induced stimulation of Cl^- uptake, while both agents enhance [³H]GABA uptake in rat cerebral cortex. Etomidate has been shown to enhance [³H]diazepam binding in rat forebrain but not cerebellum, indicating selectivity for a particular subgroup of $GABA_A$ receptors.

The volatile anaesthetics, diethyl ether, halothane, methoxyflurane and enflurane, have all been shown to increase ³⁶Cl^- uptake into rat cerebral cortical synaptosomes, an effect which is blocked by the $GABA_A$ receptor blocker picrotoxin. However, this action and others occur at anaesthetic concentrations considerably greater than 1 MAC (minimum alveolar concentration). It has been shown that halothane enhances muscimol stimulated ³⁶Cl^- efflux in cortical slices, and that this effect depends on the presence of extracellular calcium. Studies using radiolabelled GABA suggest that volatile agents can inhibit metabolic breakdown of the transmitter. Single channel electrophysiological analysis has shown that halothane, enflurane and isoflurane, at 2 MAC concentrations, enhance $GABA_A$-mediated currents by increasing channel open probability and mean open time.

There is thus very considerable evidence, from a number of different types of investigation, in favour of the view that all categories of anaesthetic act to enhance $GABA_A$-ergic inhibition, predominantly by increasing the affinity of GABA for the receptor and/or augmenting the GABA-mediated Cl^- conductance. The existence of different molecular sites for different agents and types of agent on the channel–receptor complex, occupation of which leads in each case to the same functional effect (Fig. 10.2), may offer a solution to the problem of how such a group of widely dissimilar substances as anaesthetics produce a generally uniform result. In the past this structural dissimilarity had been a powerful argument in favour of theories of anaesthesia, like the critical volume hypothesis, that postulate a non-specific action of anaesthetics on membrane lipid. The $GABA_A$ receptor with its associated ion channel, however, is not only of fundamental importance to CNS function but is structurally sufficiently complex to provide suitable 'receptor' sites for a wide variety of different anaesthetics. Even some of the effects of anaesthetics on other membrane proteins may conceivably produce their eventual results through modification of the GABA receptor, which is modulated by many other neurotransmitter systems acting on the same neuronal membrane. The importance of the $GABA_A$ system is illustrated by studies in which its contribution was selectively eliminated with specific antagonists, which had the effect of reducing

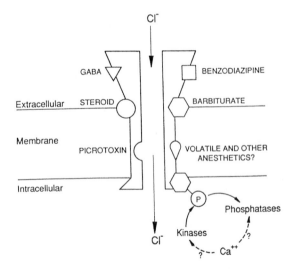

Figure 10.2 $GABA_A$ receptor–Cl^- channel complex showing different sites at which GABA, different groups of anaesthetics, and the channel blocker picrotoxin might act. (Reproduced with permission of Lippincott–Raven, Philadelphia, from Tanelian D L et al 1993 Anesthesiology 78: 757–776.)

the depressant effect of halothane on neuronal excitability in hippocampal slices by 70%.

Furthermore, the GABA$_A$ receptor hypothesis can account not only for the similarities among different agents but also for the differences in their actions. A problem with the critical volume hypothesis is that it does not easily account for these differences. If, however, the predominant mechanism of anaesthesia is GABAergic, the existence of many subtypes of GABA$_A$ receptor complex, which might have subtly different binding sites for different agents, could explain the clinical and experimental variations that are observed among different agents. The actions of anaesthetics on this receptor will no doubt be the subject of much future research, in particular into the relationships between anaesthetic potency and potency for the various in vitro effects on the GABA channel complex. While the GABA receptor is undoubtedly a key site of anaesthetic action, it does not appear likely to be the only site, which is perhaps not surprising when one considers the variety of other channel and receptor proteins, some of them very similar in structure to the GABA receptor, that exist in the CNS.

Other receptors

As glutamate is believed to be the principal excitatory neurotransmitter in the vertebrate CNS, the glutamate-activated ion channel would seem to be a likely site of anaesthetic action. These receptors have been classified into three different types on the basis of their sensitivities to neurotoxin agonists: these are N-methyl-D-aspartate (NMDA), kainate (KA) and quisqualate (AMPA). Phencyclidine and ketamine act as non-competitive antagonists at the NMDA receptor and increase the potency of a range of anaesthetics in intact animals. In *in vitro* preparations, ethanol and diethyl ether, but not barbiturates, inhibit NMDA induced currents; in contrast, pentobarbitone inhibits KA and AMPA induced currents.

All the receptors discussed so far have associated ion channels and are involved in fast transmission. Other transmitter/receptor systems that activate intracellular second messenger systems and mediate slow synaptic modulation include adrenergic, muscarinic cholinergic, dopaminergic, substance P and serotonin receptors. Very little is known about the direct effects of anaesthetics on most of these structures.

The selective α_2-adrenergic agonists clonidine and dexmedetomidine produce sedation and analgesia and increase the potency of several anaesthetic agents in whole animal studies. Halothane reduces noradrenaline turnover in the locus ceruleus, and it is known that agents such as reserpine, which reduce central noradrenergic activity, increase the potency of volatile agents, while monoamine oxidase inhibitors have the opposite effect. It thus appears likely that the central noradrenergic system will be found to play a role in anaesthetic action.

Actions of anaesthetics on synaptic transmission

Whatever the detailed nature and relative importance of these actions of anaesthetics on membranes, ion channels and receptors turns out to be, the overall result at a higher level of function must be interference with the conduction and transmission of neural signals. In view of the complexity of these effects, the response to a specific agent cannot be deduced from first principles. The overall evidence is that general, unlike local, anaesthetics act through interference with chemical transmission across the synaptic gap between axonal endings and postsynaptic neurones, rather than with axonal conduction of action potentials. Thus ether, pentobarbitone and chloroform block axonal conduction only at concentrations much higher than those required to block transmission through mammalian sympathetic ganglia. There is now abundant direct evidence of anaesthetic action on postsynaptic receptors, together with the comparative insensitivity of ion channels to their effects, and it is known that the selectivity of an agent for synaptic block correlates with its lipid solubility, so that there can now be little doubt that the predominant effect of anaesthetics is synaptic. However, there remains a possible role for subtle effects of anaesthetics on conduction, falling short of blockade, which could contribute to their overall effects on neural networks.

Broadly, there are three mechanisms by which anaesthetics could in principle affect synaptic transmission: alteration of the quantity of neurotransmitter released, alteration of the response at the postsynaptic membrane; and alteration of the overall excitability of the postsynaptic neurone.

Anaesthetic effects on presynaptic events

Studies of the effects of thiopentone and pentobarbitone on the excitatory postsynaptic potentials (EPSPs) evoked in cat spinal motor neurones by stimulation of single afferent fibres have shown that, although EPSP amplitude is unchanged by the barbiturates, the calculated mean number of quanta of transmitter released by one afferent impulse is reduced, i.e. synaptic transmission is impaired by a presynaptic effect, while the postsynaptic response to a given quantity of transmitter is unchanged. Volatile agents also depress transmitter release. This depression has been shown in a variety of experimental preparations to affect release not only of the excitatory transmitters glutamate and aspartate but the inhibitory transmitter GABA as well, an action that clearly opposes the enhancing action of anaesthetics on the $GABA_A$ receptor.

In isolated adrenal chromaffin cells, a wide range of volatile and non-volatile clinical anaesthetics, in clinically relevant concentrations, inhibit voltage gated Ca^{2+} channels and reduce Ca^{2+} influx. Halothane and ketamine are the only general anaesthetics that do not show this effect at clinical concentrations. The mechanism of this action of anaesthetics on transmitter/hormone secretion is thus consistent with the findings described above in direct work on Ca^{2+} channels.

Actions on postsynaptic events

The effects of anaesthetics on postsynaptic neurones are comparatively simple to measure, as transmitter may be applied directly, thus excluding any presynaptic influences. Using this method, many anaesthetics have been tested with a wide variety of transmitters and cell types, with the general conclusion that the response to applied excitatory agonists like ACh, glutamate and aspartate is depressed in the presence of anaesthetics. The subtypes of the glutamate receptor appear to be differentially sensitive to anaesthetics; the NMDA type is preferentially depressed by ketamine, phencyclidine, ethanol and ether, while barbiturates are more effective on the KA and AMPA types. There is also evidence of anaesthetic induced depression of muscarinic cholinergic receptors in the CNS.

Anaesthetic effects on inhibitory postsynaptic transmission are more variable. Barbiturates generally enhance postsynaptic inhibition and have also been shown to enhance presynaptic inhibition. Halothane and other agents appear to depress inhibition in some studies, but this finding may be due to depression of excitation of inhibitory interneurones. In keeping with the effects of agents on the $GABA_A$ channel receptor complex, most agents enhance postsynaptic inhibition at most sites, despite the fact that less transmitter is usually released by the presynaptic nerve ending.

Clearly then, anaesthetics have both pre- and postsynaptic effects, but which of these predominates may vary in different sites and different circumstances, for example with the precise type of Ca^{2+} channel and the type of synapse. At a synapse where the amount of transmitter released fully saturates the postsynaptic receptors, any anaesthetic induced change in receptor function would have an immediate effect, while a reduction in transmitter release would have to be sufficient to eliminate the excess transmitter before an effect would be seen. On the other hand, at a synapse where there is an excess of receptors an immediate response would be seen with either a pre- or postsynaptic change.

Actions on the excitability of the postsynaptic neurone and neuronal discharge patterns

A third way in which anaesthetics might affect synaptic transmission is by altering the excitability of the postsynaptic neurone and hence its probability of firing. This could be achieved through modification of either the resting membrane potential or the firing threshold potential; an increase in the difference between these would tend to reduce excitability.

A related factor is the possibility of effects on temporal and spatial patterns of neuronal activity, which would not be detected by the investigations of synaptic effects of anaesthetics outlined above. The effect of the arrival of an action potential at a synapse depends not only on the functional state of the synapse itself, and on the simultaneous overall effect of the thousands of other excitatory and inhibitory synapses that impinge on the same postsynaptic neurone, but also on the recent past of the synapse and the immediately surrounding membrane. Since these factors in turn depend upon the activity of the thousands of neurones from which the postsynaptic cell receives input, it is apparent that the effect of any given synaptic event, and of an anaesthetic agent, depends ultimately upon the activity of the entire CNS. Figure 10.3 illustrates in a simplified way how even small anaesthetic effects alter the subtle balance of spatial and temporal influences. For example, a very slight delay in the arrival of an inhibitory impulse could result in the cell firing when it would not otherwise have done so. The passage of a nerve impulse causes temporary but sometimes quite long lasting changes in axonal membrane excitability and conduction velocity, and the phenomena of fatigue, facilitation and post-tetanic potentiation operate in the CNS, as at the neuromuscular junction.

There is *in vitro* evidence that several volatile agents hyperpolarise pyramidal neurones, reducing their intrinsic excitability. However, the response of these cells to strong depolarising currents (i.e. applied pulses of 600–800 ms duration), which normally produces a burst of 7–8 action potentials followed by a quiescent period due to accommodation, is altered by halothane so that a much longer train of action potentials is produced; in other words, there is partial block of accommodation. These effects are believed to be due to a direct action on one or more of the K^+ channels controlling neuronal excitability.

Summary of the molecular and neuronal mechanisms of action of anaesthetics

The weight of evidence now strongly favours the view that anaesthetics act at protein sites on neuronal membranes rather than by causing bulk perturbations in lipid membranes. Binding assay and single channel ion current studies have clearly shown that anaesthetic agents, in concentrations comparable to those clinically relevant, can modify the functions of ion channels and neurotransmitter receptors. While these observations could perhaps be accounted for by an action on the surrounding lipid, other evidence such as stereoselectivity, and the finding that anaesthetic properties tend to be confined to the smaller molecules of a homologous chemical series (cut-off effect), strongly favours action at a protein site of a specific size, such as a subunit of a protein molecule. The anaesthetic agent may alter the local conformation of the site by an allosteric modification, as barbiturates have been shown to do on the $GABA_A$ receptor–chloride channel complex.

At the synaptic level, two main types of action may be discerned, with the possibility of others. Anaesthetics depress the secretion of neurotransmitter from presynaptic nerve endings in at least some neuronal sites by acting on voltage gated Ca^{2+} channels to reduce the influx of Ca^{2+}. Secondly, anaesthetics act on postsynaptic receptors, both to depress excitatory and enhance inhibitory transmission, the latter most notably at the $GABA_A$ receptor. They may also act via changes in K^+ permeability in the neuronal or axonal membrane to produce more subtle effects on excitability or conduction velocity which, given the extreme complexity and sensitivity of neural networks, may have profound effects.

Thus we have largely abandoned the unitary theory, and are left with the finding that, while general anaesthesia is a single phenomenon, it appears to be produced by a variety of diverse substances whose actions differ from each other at the molecular, cellular and whole animal levels. The human CNS is so complex that it is said to have more potential connections than the

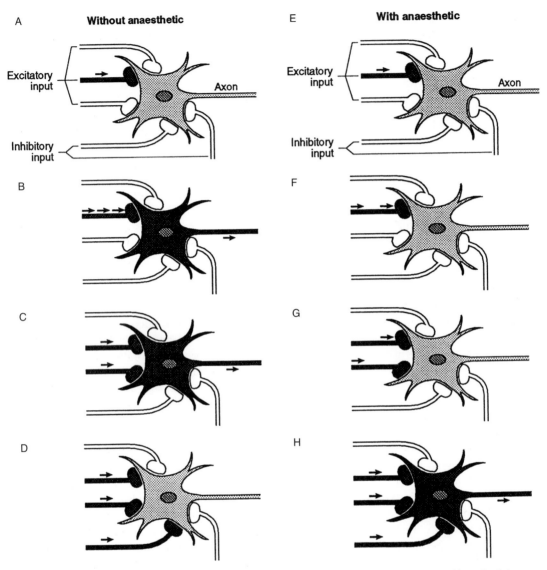

Figure 10.3 Spatial and temporal integration of excitation and inhibition in a model synapse and its potential modification by anaesthetics. Resting fibres are drawn white, grey indicates a non-propagating excitation, black a propagating excitation. The number of arrows indicates the frequency of incoming signals, and their relative shift a temporal shift in signals. Most neurones, even when exposed to an anaesthetic, will not fire in response to a single input (A, E), unless there is temporal (B) or spatial (C) summation, not offset by simultaneous inhibition (D). Anaesthetics could modify the firing rate (F), or cause a temporal shift (G) in incoming signals, or a temporal shift in inhibitory signals (H) might remove inhibition. (Reproduced with permission from Urban B W 1993 British Journal of Anaesthesia 71: 25–38.)

number of atoms in the universe; intuitively one would expect there to be many possible ways of perturbing its function to produce anaesthesia. The extent to which this is so cannot be deduced from investigations at the molecular or synaptic level, but can be approached more closely through investigations of anaesthetic effects on the neuronal pathways and subsystems of the CNS.

Actions of anaesthetics on central neuronal pathways

Because of the lack of knowledge of the detailed location or mechanism of awareness and other subjective phenomena, investigation of the effects of anaesthetics at the level of the integrated CNS has concentrated on the systems that subserve the objective signs of anaesthesia, such as loss of reflex response to sensory stimulation, i.e. the major sensory pathways.

Spinal cord

The first central relay for afferent information, the spinal cord dorsal horn, has an important role in modulating afferent input. A number of anaesthetic agents of various types have been shown to produce dose dependent depression of spontaneous and evoked activity in dorsal horn cells. The cells most affected are generally those in lamina V, which are involved in integration of noxious stimuli, but this appears to be unrelated to any differential analgesic properties of the agents.

At present there is controversy over the role of the spinal cord in modulating the response to stimuli; some animal studies have shown that the ability of volatile agents to prevent movement in response to noxious stimulation is unaffected by precollicular decerebration or spinal cord transection, implying that suppression of reflex movement by these anaesthetics occurs entirely at cord level. Work in other species, however, suggests that descending influences from the brain have a role in the determination of potency. Nevertheless, it is clear that action in the spinal cord is part of the overall picture of anaesthesia.

Reticular formation, thalamus and cerebral cortex

The relationship of the brainstem reticular formation to cortical arousal, and early observations that it could be depressed by anaesthetics, led to hopes that this multisynaptic system would prove to be the key to the action of anaesthetics in the brain. However, results of studies of anaesthetic effects on long latency cortical evoked responses, thought to reflect reticular activity, were inconsistent.

There is a complex interrelationship between the fast dorsal column–thalamocortical sensory pathway and the thalamic reticular nuclei. Using repeated stimulation of the periphery and summated recording techniques, a characteristic somatosensory evoked response consisting of initial and secondary positive and negative waves is recorded from the somatosensory cortex. A large group of anaesthetics, including the barbiturates and all the clinically used gaseous and volatile agents, produced similar, dose dependent increases in the latency and decreases in the amplitude of the initial components of the response. The effect is antagonised by high ambient pressure.

This pathway contains two synaptic relays, at the dorsal column nuclei and the ventrobasal thalamus. Recordings at these sites show that, while the responses of cells in the dorsal column nuclei are very resistant to anaesthetic induced depression, cells in the ventrobasal thalamus showed consistent, dose dependent increases in latency of discharge and decreased probability of response to peripheral stimuli.

Recordings of the responses of somatosensory cortical cells from the different cortical layers show two bands of cells which respond with short latencies, at depths corresponding to the boundaries of layers IV and V and layers V and VI, with a middle band with longer latency responses corresponding to layer V. Anaesthesia produced an increased latency of response and a general decrease in responsiveness in all of these cells. However, while the effects on the cells of the two short latency bands, layers IV/V and V/VI, could be shown in direct stimulation studies to be entirely due to the effects on the input from the ventrobasal thalamus, the cells in layer V showed a greater decrease in response, which was attributable to susceptibility of the cells themselves. Thus, two sites in the pathway are susceptible to anaesthetics: the ventrobasal thalamus and cortical layer V. In the thalamic reticular nucleus, which is adjacent to the ventrobasal nuclei, there are groups of neurones that show spontaneous activity. They form two groups, one of which shows an increase, the other a decrease, in excitability in response to noxious stimuli. All of the group of agents mentioned above produce dose dependent reductions in the discharge frequency of the former group and the opposite in the latter group. Furthermore, these two groups of thalamic reticular nuclear cells receive input from two other groups of neurones in cortical layers V and part of III which have excitatory and inhibitory functions. It is also found that, if the cortex is removed, the reduction of onward transmission at the ventrobasal thalamic relay does not occur; thus it would appear that the primary site of anaesthetic action is on the cells in cortical layers III and V which modulate the thalamic relay cells via corticothalamic and corticoreticular thalamic pathways, causing a preponderance of inhibition over excitation. The resulting reduction in information reaching the cortex could then lead to further corticothalamic inhibition, so that a self-reinforcing circuit is created (Fig. 10.4), leading to partial cortical deafferentation and anaesthesia.

Two groups of agents do not show these effects on somatosensory evoked potentials, one group containing etomidate, propofol and two benzodiazepines, the other the α_2-adrenergic agonists clonidine and medetomidine. Of these, the first group showed similar effects on latency but an increased amplitude of the initial cortical wave, associated with increased response probability of ventrobasal cells; also the cells in all the cortical layers were themselves variously affected by members of this group. The α_2-agonists increased the discharge latency of the ventrobasal cells in such a way that the thalamocortical volley became asynchronous.

Conclusion: anaesthetics and central neuronal pathways

Consciousness depends in a very complex way on the continual activation of the cerebral cortex by subcortical structures. The cortex itself has an input into this process, contributing to its own activation. The effects of anaesthetics on these complex processes are unlikely to be simple, but nevertheless a general pattern begins to emerge of a gradual deafferentation of the cortex, through effects not only on subcortical synaptic relays but on the cortex itself. Feedback inhibition from the sensory cortex to the thalamic relay provides a mechanism capable of explaining many of the objective features of general anaesthesia, while work on auditory evoked potentials shows that the action of anaesthetics on this pathway is similar. However, it is clear that the spinal cord is also a site of anaesthetic action. The serial electroencephalographic changes associated with anaesthesia (see below) are broadly comparable with those of other causes of depression of cerebral function. The view that general anaesthesia is a form of cerebral depression is also supported by the observation that it is associated with a reduction in cerebral metabolic rate. At one time the possibility was considered that this reduction in metabolism might be the primary action of anaesthetics; however, it is now recognised that it is an effect, rather than a cause, of anaesthesia.

CLINICAL EVALUATION OF DEPTH OF ANAESTHESIA

The ability to gauge the depth of anaesthesia clinically is a skill that all anaesthetists develop. It was first quantified by Guedel in 1937, with his well known classification of the continuum of the effects of increasing concentrations of diethyl ether into stages and planes, based on clinical signs. At that time the main concern was that the anaesthetist, using diethyl ether as the sole agent in a spontaneously breathing patient, would be able to avoid overdosage and to adjust the depth of anaesthesia according to surgical requirements.

In more recent years, improved techniques and monitoring, together with the practice of using drugs of several different types during most procedures, have made anaesthesia safer but have made the assessment of anaesthetic depth more difficult, particularly when intravenous infusions rather than volatile agents are used for maintenance. The major concern now is not the danger of excessive depth of anaesthesia so much as the possibility of undetected awareness. An

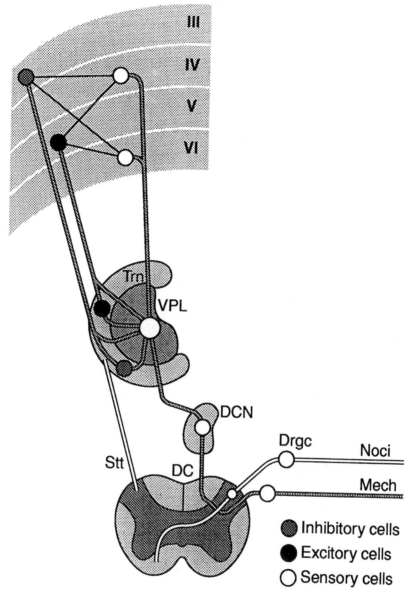

Figure 10.4   The sensory and corticothalamic pathways affected by anaesthetics (see text). III, IV, V, VI, Cortical layers; DCN, dorsal column nuclei; Drgc, dorsal root ganglion cells; Mech, mechanoreceptor input; Noci, nociceptive input; Stt, spinothalamic and spinoreticular tracts; Trn, thalamic reticular nucleus; VPL, ventrobasal thalamus. (Reproduced with permission from Angel A 1993 British Journal of Anaesthesia 71: 148–163.)

increase in the number of reports of awareness under anaesthesia, with accompanying litigation and media attention, has led to the search for a reliable method of detecting awareness in the paralysed subject.

Isolated forearm technique and autonomic responses

In the spontaneously breathing patient it is usually obvious when anaesthesia is inadequate, although there have been reports of patients who were aware yet did not move or otherwise indicate the fact. With these rare exceptions, the problem of potential awareness is confined to cases that involve the use of neuromuscular blockade, which effectively masks the signs by which light anaesthesia or awareness might be detected. The incidence of awareness has been variably reported: in one large series 0.2% of patients having anaesthesia for all types of surgery had recall of intraoperative events. The incidence is higher in situations where light anaesthesia is commonly used, such as obstetric and cardiac surgery.

The isolated forearm technique (IFT) was introduced by Tunstall in the 1970s, and further developed by Russell, as a method of detecting awareness in patients under neuromuscular blockade. The technique consists of the inflation of a tourniquet around one arm during, and for a time after, the administration of a muscle relaxant so that neuromuscular function remains intact in that arm. The patient's response to commands to move the arm may then be tested during surgery. While the IFT has not come into routine or widespread use, it has yielded important information on the relationship between anaesthesia and states of consciousness; in a series of patients anaesthetised with a nitrous oxide–oxygen relaxant technique, over half responded purposefully to commands during surgery, and while none of these had subsequent explicit recall of these events, about half of those who responded showed some degree of recall on more specific questioning and prompting. These and other findings imply that awareness under anaesthesia is not an all-or-none phenomenon. Jones has suggested that a series of states are passed through as anaesthetic concentration increases: (1) conscious awareness with recall, (2) conscious awareness with amnesia, (3) subconscious awareness with amnesia, and (4) no awareness. The last of these may correspond only to very deep levels of anaesthesia, with the implication that in the majority of patients some degree of processing of sensory information continues. This conclusion is supported by psychological studies which suggest that, while information presented during anaesthesia is rarely explicitly recalled, it is possible using appropriate techniques to demonstrate that there may be preservation of implicit memory (defined as memory without conscious recall of the circumstances in which the remembered material was learned). This memory then remains in the patient's subconscious, with unknown and possibly harmful consequences.

The IFT has also been helpful in clarifying the relationship between depth of anaesthesia and autonomic signs. Neuromuscular blocking agents do not of course abolish autonomic reflexes, and the latter have often been used clinically to gauge depth of anaesthesia when these drugs are used. A scoring system based on autonomic signs (the PRST score) has been developed by Evans, based on blood *p*ressure, pulse *r*ate, *s*weating and *t*ear formation. However, the evidence from comparison with the IFT and other studies is that the absence of autonomic responses, such as tachycardia and hypertension, are not reliable indicators that the patient is not aware.

A more promising approach, which is still in the early stages of investigation, may be the analysis of respiratory sinus arrhythmia (RSA), i.e. variation of the heart rate during the ventilatory cycle. RSA is a reflection of brainstem-mediated parasympathetic tone. It has been shown to decrease during anaesthesia and heavy sedation, and this change correlates with changes in mean EEG frequency. Both changes may reflect a common action of anaesthesia in the brain, but measurement of RSA offers a much greater possibility of being capable of adaptation for routine use in the operating theatre.

Monitoring of lower oesophageal contractility, which is known to be positively related to stress, has been assessed as a method of measuring anaesthetic depth and may be of some predictive value with certain anaesthetic techniques and in head injury, but in general, as with other autonomic signs, it is not a reliable indicator of awareness under anaesthesia.

Electromyographic recording of the upper facial muscles has also been evaluated, and although unlikely to be suitable for routine use may be as effective a predictor of awareness as the IFT.

Electrical activity of the brain and depth of anaesthesia

The electroencephalogram

The electroencephalogram (EEG, see Ch. 8) is recorded from conventionally placed scalp electrodes. As anaesthesia deepens progressive EEG changes are seen. There is variation among different agents, but in general, with increasing dose, continuous activity gives way to a pattern showing periods of suppression which gradually increase in duration from less than 1 s to 3 s or more. These periods are separated by bursts of activity of amplitude 100–300 μV, gradually declining as suppressions lengthen to around 50 μV and less, until in the final stage the recording is isoelectric. These changes represent progressive loss of reactivity of the cortex, thalamus and reticular formation. Attempts have been made over several decades to adapt the full EEG for use as a monitor both of depth of anaesthesia and of the integrity of cerebral function in the unconscious patient, and a number of recording devices have been developed. Computerisation of EEG data has led to the emergence of a great many ways of analysing and displaying the information, one of the most widely studied of which is the Fast Fourier Transform of data into power spectra of consecutive time cycles. These may be displayed as the compressed spectral array, which shows the relative distribution of different frequencies over a period of time. The spectral edge, or frequency below which a chosen percentage of activity occurs, falls during anaesthesia. This and other EEG derivatives are useful research tools but so far have had a limited place in clinical anaesthesia.

Evoked responses

The progressive, dose dependent effects of anaesthetics on the transmission of sensory signals via the fast sensory pathways and dorsal thalamus to the cortex have, as described above, been used to study the mechanism of anaesthetic action on the brain. Clinically, evoked responses have been investigated as a means of monitoring anaesthetic depth, the most widely studied modality being the auditory evoked response (AER). Separation of the AER wave from the background EEG activity requires synchronisation of responses to large numbers of signals (auditory clicks) with recording sweeps to average out to zero the background noise, allowing a characteristic 'average' waveform to be identified. In the awake subject, early cortical positive and negative waves, designated Pa and Nb and corresponding to the arrival of the signal at the auditory cortex, are seen at latencies of about 20 and 40 ms. All anaesthetic agents cause a progressive increase in the latency and decrease in the amplitude of these waves, while the presence of noxious stimulation tends to have the opposite effect. It appears that small increases in latency may be associated with suppression of the higher stages of awareness in Jones' classification, but it is not known what degree of alteration of the AER is associated with the guaranteed absence of any degree of awareness. A more reliable indicator may turn out to be the P300, a potential which occurs as a response to a rare stimulus interrupting regular stimuli. This response disappears in the anaesthetised subject. Its absence has been shown to correlate with the absence of recall. However, the more subtle kinds of information processing, as in the third of Jones' states of awareness, probably require longer time periods and are probably not detectable by studies of the evoked response. Evoked responses have also been used to monitor the integrity of the sensory pathways in the anaesthetised patient — for example, the use of the somatosensory response to stimulation of the lower limbs in spinal surgery. Changes in evoked responses are also seen in cerebral hypoxia and hypothermia.

However, as with derivatives of the EEG, the measurement of evoked responses in anaesthesia is so far predominantly performed in a research context. Interpretation of the signals requires account to be taken not only of the various drugs that may be present but also of the degree of noxious stimulation and of cardiovascular and respiratory parameters. Such problems which will have to be solved if they are to have a place in routine clinical practice.

FURTHER READING

Aantaa R, Scheinin M 1993 Alpha$_2$-adrenergic agents in anaesthesia. Acta Anesthesiologica Scandinavica 37: 433–448

Angel A 1993 Central neuronal pathways and the process of anaesthesia. British Jounal of Anaesthesia 71: 148–163

Angel A, LeBeau F 1992 A comparison of the effects of propofol with other anaesthetic agents on the centripetal transmission of sensory information. General Pharmacology 23: 945–963

Charlesworth P, Pocock G, Richards C D 1992 The action of anaesthetics on stimulus-secretion coupling and synaptic activity. General Pharmacology 23: 977–984

Couture L J, Greenwald B, Edmonds H L 1990 Detection of responsiveness during anaesthesia. In: Bonke B, Fitch W, Millar K (eds) Memory and awareness in anaesthesia. Swets & Zeitlinger, Amsterdam

Daniels S, Smith E B 1993 Effects of general anaesthetics on ligand-gated ion channels. British Journal of Anaesthesia 71: 59–64

Evans J M 1987 Clinical signs and autonomic responses. In: Rosen M, Lunn J N (eds) Conscious awareness and pain in general anaesthesia. Butterworth, London

Franks N P, Lieb W R 1994 Molecular and cellular mechanisms of general anaesthesia. Nature 367: 607–614

Frenkel C, Duch D S, Urban B W 1993 Effects of i.v. anaesthetics on human brain sodium channels. British Journal of Anaesthesia 71: 15–24

Guedel A E 1937 Inhalational anaesthesia: a fundamental guide. Macmillan, New York

Isaac P A, Rosen M 1990 Lower oesophageal contractility and detection of awareness during general anaesthesia. British Journal of Anaesthesia 65: 319–324

Jessop J, Jones J G 1992 Evaluation of the actions of anaesthetics in the human brain. General Pharmacology 23: 927–935

Jones J G 1994 Memory of intraoperative events. British Medical Journal 309: 967–968

Pearce R A, Stringer J L, Lothman E W 1989 Effects of volatile anaesthetics on synaptic transmission in the rat hippocampus. Anesthesiology 71: 591–598

Pilkington S N, Hett D A, Pierce J M T, Smith D C 1995 Auditory evoked responses and near infrared spectroscopy during cardiac arrest. British Journal of Anaesthesia 74: 717–719

Plourde G, Picton T W 1991 Long latency auditory potentials during general anaesthesia: N1 and P2 components. Anesthesia and Analgesia 72: 342–350

Pomfrett C J D, Barrie J R, Healy T E J 1993 Respiratory sinus arrhythmia: an index of light anaesthesia. British Journal of Anaesthesia 71: 212–217

Russell I F 1989 Conscious awareness during general anaesthesia: relevance of autonomic signs and isolated arm movements as guides to depth of anaesthesia. Baillière's Clinical Anaesthesiology 3: 511–532

Tanelian D L, Kosek P, Mody I, MacIver B 1993 The role of the GABA-A receptor/chloride channel complex in anesthesia. Anesthesiology 78: 757–776

Wann K T, Southan A P 1992 The action of anaesthetics and high pressure on neuronal discharge patterns. General Pharmacology 23: 993–1004

11

Volatile anaesthetic drugs

J. M. Murray
J. P. H. Fee

The growth of science in the early and middle years of the nineteenth century saw both the synthesis of new chemicals and the rediscovery of forgotten ones. A few of these were intoxicants, notably nitrous oxide and ether, and these were abused as such, their potential as a means of alleviating pain being overlooked or underestimated. Ether and chloroform were the first of two series of lipid soluble, volatile ethers and hydrocarbons which are still being evaluated 150 years after their first use as anaesthetic agents.

PHARMACOKINETICS

Absorption, distribution and elimination

The vast majority of drugs are given orally or by injection and general pharmacology texts tend to ignore drug uptake by the pulmonary route. Like drugs given intravenously or sublingually, inhaled drugs are generally not subject to first pass metabolism. Quite uniquely, this route of administration presents the drug to the heart first, so that it, initially, is exposed to higher concentrations than other tissues.

Modern anaesthetic practice demands that all potent volatile agents be administered through a temperature compensated calibrated vaporiser. In this way volatile anaesthetics in oxygen-containing mixtures can be delivered at a predetermined inspiratory concentration. The safe administration of volatile agents requires a good understanding of their pharmacokinetics. These drugs exert their anaesthetic effect in a way which is not fully understood but the depth of anaesthesia is directly proportional to the tension (or partial pressure) of the agent in the brain or in arterial blood. The speed of induction and recovery are similarly related to the rate at which arterial or brain tensions increase and decrease.

The tension or partial pressure of volatile anaesthetic agents is, in common with other blood gas measurements, such as oxygen tension, measured in units of pressure, i.e. fractions of an atmosphere, or more commonly kilopascals (kPa) or millimetres of mercury (mmHg). The concentration of agent measured variously in units of volume or weight per unit volume, e.g. ml l^{-1}, mg l^{-1}, mmol l^{-1} , or in the gaseous phase as percentage volume, will be different in different compartments and tissues when these are in equilibrium at the same tension. The relationship depends on the differing solubility of the gas or vapour in various tissues with differing composition of lipid and aqueous compartments and is usually expressed in terms of the partition coefficient between different phases, e.g. blood:gas, tissue:gas, and partition coefficients for individual tissues can also be measured. These are discussed in more detail below.

As with drugs given by other routes, the process of uptake and absorption of an inhalational agent is occurring simultaneously with its transport and distribution to the tissues, and later recovery is associated with redistribution, metabolism and excretion. The process must be seen as a cascade where movement from one compartment to another is dependent on the tension gradient between them, and where this gradient depends not only on the rate of delivery to the compartment but also on the rate at which the agent is transferred from it.

The tension of anaesthetic vapour in the brain and in arterial blood is dependent on:

1. alveolar ventilation
2. concentration (or tension) of the agent in the inspired gas mixture
3. transfer of vapour from alveoli to blood in the lungs
4. transfer of vapour from arterial blood to body tissues.

Alveolar ventilation

Each breath transfers some anaesthetic vapour to the lungs. If alveolar ventilation is high the alveolar and arterial tensions increase relatively quickly. On the other hand, an increase in physiological dead space due to pulmonary embolism, emphysema or other ventilation/perfusion inequalities will result in an increased shunt and reduce the amount of volatile agent absorbed. Respiratory depression due to drugs may similarly reduce alveolar ventilation and delay the increase in alveolar and arterial vapour tensions.

Inspired tension

The tension of a vapour in the anaesthetic mixture is directly proportional to its concentration. In clinical practice the inspired tension changes but high inspired percentage concentrations are used during induction to ensure that alveolar and then arterial tensions increase quickly. As anaesthesia deepens, the inspired percentage concentration can be reduced to a maintenance value.

During the inhalation of a constant percentage concentration of anaesthetic vapour, the tension in arterial blood is related to that of the inspired mixture, as shown in Figure 11.1. In the case

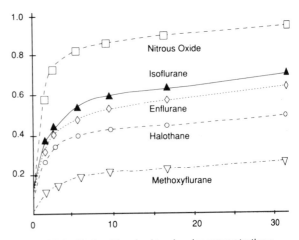

Figure 11.1 Ratio of inspired to alveolar concentrations (F_A:F_I) of some inhalational agents. (Reproduced with permission of Anaquest from Eger E I II 1982 Isoflurane, a compendium and reference. Anaquest.)

of nitrous oxide the arterial tension reaches 90% of the inspired tension in about 20 minutes, compared with about 60% for isoflurane and 45% for halothane. The differences are determined by the solubility of the agents in blood.

Alveolar–blood transfer

As with the majority of drugs, movement of an inhalational anaesthetic agent across body membranes is along a concentration gradient.

The transfer of a volatile agent from the alveoli to blood is dependent on four factors:

1. the condition of the respiratory membrane
2. the solubility of the agent
3. cardiac output
4. the tension of vapour in the alveoli and in blood.

Respiratory membrane

The respiratory membrane is completely permeable to the passage of anaesthetic vapours and gases. The amount transferred across it will depend on the cross-sectional area and thickness of the membrane. Certain pulmonary diseases may impair the transfer of vapour; emphysema will reduce the cross-sectional area of respiratory membrane available. Thus induction of, and recovery from, anaesthesia will be delayed. Other causes of ventilation/perfusion inequality will similarly alter the rate at which vapour passes into the circulation. An increase in the thickness of the respiratory membrane, such as might occur in pulmonary fibrosis, will also tend to delay the transfer of vapour.

Solubility

The true solubility of a particular agent in blood is expressed as its partition coefficient, representing the ratio of anaesthetic concentration in blood to anaesthetic concentration in a gas phase when the two are in equilibrium (Table 11.1). When an agent has a low blood:gas partition coefficient, then the concentration in the blood needed to achieve any given tension will be low, and so the mass of drug that needs to be trans-

ferred into the blood is also low. This also means that the agent is removed from the alveoli at a slower rate and so the alveolar–blood gradient in partial pressure is maintained. Thus, blood and alveolar concentrations approach equilibrium rapidly and induction is rapid (Fig. 11.1). In practice, other factors may compromise this advantage. For instance, the pungency of isoflurane, an agent that is fairly insoluble, may provoke coughing or breath-holding, particularly when administered in high concentrations. The rapidity of induction may, in the end, be no greater, or may even be less, than that achievable with halothane, despite the latter's higher blood:gas partition coefficient. The solubility of anaesthetic vapours is much greater in fat than in blood or vessel-rich tissues such as the brain (Table 11.1). Thus the anaesthetic tension of an agent in fat approaches equilibrium with that of the alveoli only after many hours. In most clinical situations the tension of volatile agents in fat does not reach equilibrium with alveolar tensions.

Cardiac output

A reduction in cardiac output, such as may occur in shocked states, will cause a more rapid increase in the pulmonary arterial concentration of a volatile agent and permit inspired and arterial tensions to equalise sooner. Thus the speed of induction will be increased. Since many volatile agents cause a drop in cardiac output, these drugs may themselves facilitate their own uptake. Similarly, most intravenous induction agents reduce cardiac output, further aiding gaseous uptake and induction.

The tissues with the highest blood flow — brain, kidney, heart (vessel-rich group) — will have a rapid increase in their anaesthetic tension compared with low flow tissues such as fat and bone. Thus the brain anaesthetic tension approaches the inspired tension quickly, resulting in rapid induction of anaesthesia.

Tension in blood

Anaesthetic vapours are taken up by the blood in the lungs and are delivered to all body tissues.

Tissue uptake reduces blood anaesthetic tension, and only when the tissues become saturated does the tension of mixed venous blood approach that of the inhaled anaesthetic vapour. Thus the mass of volatile agent taken into the circulation decreases with time (Fig. 11.2).

Blood–tissue transfer

The uptake of volatile anaesthetic agents into tissues is dependent on the blood:tissue partition coefficient (Table 11.1), tissue blood flow per unit volume, and the inspired concentration. The most important factor is tissue blood flow, and those tissues with high unit flows will take up volatile agents relatively quickly. Mapleson (1963) has devised a system whereby tissues are grouped according to their flow per unit volume and solubility coefficients. This simplifies the problem of how to assess the combined effect of all body tissues on the tension of volatile agent in mixed venous blood. The brain, heart and kidney comprise the vessel-rich group (VRG) with high perfusion per unit volume, and the tensions in these tissues rapidly achieve equilibrium with that of arterial blood.

In contrast, adipose tissue requires a longer time to equilibrate on account of the high fat:blood partition coefficients of the volatile agents and relatively poor blood flow. Muscle and skin also differ from the VRG in having a much lower rate of perfusion per unit volume; consequently equilibration is prolonged. This group occupies an intermediate position in terms of anaesthetic uptake. In general the tissues of the VRG may approach equilibrium with arterial blood during the course of routine clinical anaesthesia, in contrast to both the muscle and fat groups (Fig. 11.2).

Similarly, the rate of elimination is based on tissue perfusion and solubility. The anaesthetic tension in tissues of the VRG decreases much more quickly than that of the muscle group. The fat group is the slowest to release volatile agent on account of its high solubility.

Minimum alveolar concentration (MAC)

MAC is the minimum alveolar concentration of anaesthetic (at 1 atmosphere ambient pressure) that produces immobility in 50% of those patients or animals exposed to a noxious stimulus (Eger 1974). It is a measure of anaesthetic potency and serves as a means of comparing different gaseous and volatile agents. Since it is measured after steady-state conditions have been achieved, MAC is not the sole determinant of the concentration of inspired anaesthetic required for surgical anaesthesia. This latter value is also related to the duration of anaesthesia, the uptake and distribution characteristics of the anaesthetic concerned and the degree of surgical stimulation. In general, to achieve a steady alveolar concentration, high inspired concentrations are required at the commencement of the anaesthetic, with a gradual reduction as tissue tensions come into equilibrium with those of blood.

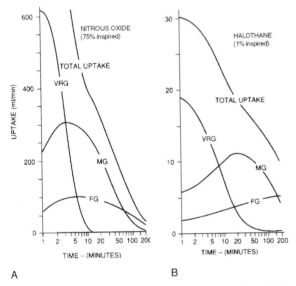

Figure 11.2 Total uptake is the sum of uptake by individual body tissues. The uppermost curve for each anaesthetic is the sum of the three curves beneath it (with a slight time lag). The curves for nitrous oxide and halothane are identical in shape to those for all anaesthetics. Uptake progressively decreases with duration of anaesthesia and with saturation of the tissue depots. The order of saturation is always vessel-rich group (VRG) first, then muscle group (MG) and fat group (FG) last. As noted in the illustration, the inspired concentration is constant at 75% nitrous oxide or 1% halothane. (Reproduced with permission from Eger 1974.)

MAC is determined by maintaining a constant end-tidal (or alveolar) concentration for at least 15 minutes to ensure equilibration between the alveoli, arterial blood and the central nervous system (CNS). It is reasonably assumed that at that point the anaesthetic tensions in the alveoli and at the site of action in the brain and spinal cord are the same, although the concentration in these and in other tissues may differ.

To make the determination in man, the alveolar concentration is adjusted to one of several pre-determined values both above and below the concentration estimated to allow a response to a standard noxious stimulus. Several subjects are anaesthetised at each concentration and the percentage moving is recorded. A dose–response curve can then be constructed from which the concentration (MAC) which prevents movement in 50% of the subjects can be calculated.

MAC is relatively constant within species; even more surprisingly, there is little variability between species: MAC for halothane in man, cat and goldfish is 0.75, 0.82 and 0.76, respectively. MAC appears to be unaffected by duration of anaesthesia, gender, acid–base status and induced hypertension. Induced hypotension, hypothermia, hypoxia and anaemia will reduce halothane MAC, although in the case of the last two this only occurs in the presence of a marked diminution of oxygen delivery. MAC values for a particular anaesthetic agent are highest in neonates and lowest in the elderly, although the explanation for this is uncertain. It is perhaps not surprising that opioids, benzodiazepines and other gaseous or volatile anaesthetics all reduce MAC, but of increasing interest is the role of the α_2-adrenergic receptor in anaesthesia. In animal studies a number of α_2-adrenergic agonists have been shown to reduce MAC.

The clinical usefulness of MAC might seem doubtful in view of the fact that, by definition, 50% of patients move in response to skin incision. Various other measures have been developed from the concept of MAC, notably the median anaesthetic dose required to prevent movement in 50% of patients, AD_{50}, and in 95% of patients, AD_{95}. A typical dose–response curve is shown in Figure 11.3. The AD_{50} corresponds to MAC and is

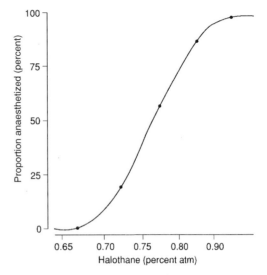

Figure 11.3   Dose–response curve for halothane.

on the steepest part of the curve, thereby allowing accurate measurement of the dosage value. The fact that at this dosage half the patients move makes it a value of limited usefulness to the practising anaesthetist. The AD_{95}, on the other hand, is on a flatter part of the curve and the precision with which this dose can be expressed is somewhat limited. Unfortunately, an AD_{100}, representing the minimum concentration applicable to all patients, cannot be determined from the dose–response curve because of the asymptotic behaviour of the curve at both ends. In general the AD_{95} values are 5–40% greater than MAC.

Another limitation of the concept of MAC, AD_{50} and AD_{95} is that these terms are applicable only to the non-paralysed patient. One of the advantages of blocking neuromuscular function is to enable much lower inspired concentrations of volatile agents to be used. In order to prevent awareness with this technique, the alveolar concentration must be maintained somewhere between MAC and a value at which the patient would be awake — 'MAC awake'. This is an anaesthetic concentration midway between the value when patients can open their eyes on command and the value just preventing this response in 50% of patients during recovery. 'MAC awake' values are in general about 50% of the MAC values.

In the paralysed patient, therefore, a lower concentration than MAC may safely be used to prevent awareness, particularly when anaesthesia is supplemented with nitrous oxide, opioids or other CNS depressants.

Physical characteristics of inhalational anaesthetics

The structural formulae and physical characteristics of the inhaled anaesthetics are given in Table 11.1. These drugs have diverse structures and do not act by forming covalent-ionic bonds with the site of action. It is presumed that the type of bonding involved is due to van der Waals forces produced by the electrostatic attraction between opposite dipoles. Dipoles are electrical charges formed by the unequal distribution of electrons between the atoms of the molecule. These forces allow anaesthetics to bind reversibly to various cell components, including the internal sites of proteins.

HYDROCARBONS

Halothane

```
      F   Cl
      |   |
  F—C—C—H
      |   |
      F   Br
```

HALOTHANE

Halothane is a halogenated fluorocarbon that was introduced into clinical practice in 1956. It rapidly achieved widespread popularity due to its potency, non-flammability and ease of use. As the first non-flammable fluorinated hydrocarbon it provided one of the great landmarks in the development of anaesthesia, and the fact that the drug is still in regular use today bears testament to its safety and versatility. Until recently, it was the standard against which all new inhaled agents were judged, a role which has now passed to isoflurane.

Physical and chemical properties

Halothane (Fluothane) is a halogenated hydrocarbon with the chemical name 1-bromo-1-chloro-2,2,2-trifluoroethane and empirical formula $CHClBrCF_3$. In 1932 Booth and Bixby tested two fluorinated paraffins on mice, and were the first to suggest that this type of compound (Arcton) might have anaesthetic properties. Although their experiment was unsuccessful, research and synthesis of other fluorinated compounds continued after World War II. The objective was to find a molecule that, in addition to its anaesthetic properties, would be non-flammable and chemically inert. Fluorocarbons are inert chemically because of the strong bond between carbon and fluorine; in particular the CF_3 group of halothane was considered highly stable and likely to be of very low toxicity.

Halothane is a heavy colourless liquid with a non-pungent odour. It contains 0.01% thymol to preserve its stability. It has a molecular weight of 197.4 and a boiling point of 50.2°C at 760 mmHg. When exposed to light for several days it will decompose to various halide acids such as HCl, HBr, free chlorine and bromine radicals and phosgene. The presence of thymol helps to prevent the liberation of free bromine. The

Table 11.1 Physical characteristics of inhalational anaesthetics

Formula	Agent	Blood:gas solubility	Oil:gas solubility	Boiling point (°C)	SVP (mmHg)	MAC (O₂ 100%)	MAC (N₂O 70%)
N_2O	Nitrous oxide	0.47	1.4	−89	3900	105	—
$CHClBrCF_3$	Halothane	2.4	220	50.2	243	0.75	0.29
$CHClFCF_2OCF_2H$	Enflurane	1.9	98	56.5	180	1.68	0.57
$CF_3CHClOCF_2H$	Isoflurane	1.4	97	48.5	250	1.15	0.50
$H_2FCOCH(CF_3)_2$	Sevoflurane	0.6	53	58.5	160	2.1	0.6 (64%)
$CF_3CHFOCF_2H$	Desflurane	0.42	18.7	22.8	660	6.1	2.83 (60%)

SVP, saturated vapour pressure.

vapour pressure of halothane is 241 mmHg at 20°C and it is therefore suitable for vaporisation in a 'bubble-through' or a temperature and flow controlled vaporiser.

The MAC of halothane is 1.08% in infants, reducing to 0.64% over 80 years of age. Nitrous oxide (70%) in the breathing mixture can reduce MAC by as much as 60%. Anaesthesia can easily be induced using inspired concentrations of 2–4%, and maintained with inspired concentrations of 0.5–2.5%. Spontaneous breathing will generally increase the inspired concentration; controlled ventilation and opioids will have the opposite effect.

In the absence of water vapour halothane will not attack most metals; however, if water vapour is present it will attack aluminium, brass and lead. Copper is not affected. Halothane is readily soluble in rubber (coefficient 121.1) and less so in polyethylene (coefficient 26.3). This degree of rubber solubility means that the uptake of halothane by rubber can reach significant levels if a low flow or circle absorption technique is used.

Soda lime used to absorb carbon dioxide in low flow or closed system anaesthesia contains 3–5% sodium hydroxide and potassium hydroxide. Therefore, some halogenated alkyls, such as halothane, undergo alkaline hydrolysis in the presence of soda lime. In addition, halothane is also degraded into a small amount of difluorochlorobromoethylene and trifluorochloroethane; however, only small amounts are produced and the concentrations that result are 1/100 of those that cause injury in animals.

Cardiovascular system

Halothane depresses myocardial contractility and reduces stroke volume and cardiac output despite an increase in venous pressure. It causes a decrease in heart rate and arterial blood pressure but the total systemic peripheral resistance is only slightly affected. Myocardial depression is directly related to the depth of halothane anaesthesia. Halothane in increasing concentrations may gradually block the effects of noradrenaline at the effector sites in the heart. On this basis the effect of halothane on the heart would be

to reduce the secretion and activity of noradrenaline at the sympathetic nerve endings in the myocardium and at the same time to sensitise the parasympathetic nerve endings, leading to bradycardia. There is experimental evidence from dogs to show that halothane can inhibit and, in adequate concentration, completely block stellate ganglion transmission. Halothane anaesthesia causes a persistent vasodilatation of the skin and muscle vessels, in addition to a decrease in both the arterial blood pressure and vascular resistance. Halothane does not have a direct action on the vessel wall per se but acts rather by blocking the action of noradrenaline.

Dysrhythmias occurring during halothane anaesthesia bear a direct relationship to hypercapnia from respiratory depression. Adrenaline can safely be used in the presence of halothane, provided the total dose and concentration used are within acceptable limits and the patient is neither hypercapnic nor hypoxic.

Respiratory system

Halothane is non-irritant to the respiratory tract and can be used to produce rapid, smooth induction of anaesthesia. It does not stimulate salivary or bronchial secretions. At higher concentrations it obtunds pharyngeal and laryngeal reflexes and facilitates tracheal intubation. Halothane has a marked bronchodilating effect, which makes it particularly suitable for patients with chronic bronchitis and asthma.

Halothane is a respiratory depressant. The drug alters the control of respiration and tachypnoea is a feature in patients who have not received opiates. The effect of this is to decrease the tidal volume. Further increases in the inspired concentration of halothane lead to a progressive decrease of volume rather than rate of respiration. This is more marked in the presence of narcotic administration, either as premedication or during operation.

Uterus

Halothane anaesthesia relaxes uterine muscle in direct relationship to the inspired concentration and in vitro studies suggest that this may be due to direct stimulation of the β receptors in the uterus. For this reason it has been recommended that halothane be specifically used for manual removal of the placenta. In common with most other anaesthetics it readily crosses the placental barrier.

Skeletal muscle

Halothane has minimal neuromuscular blocking activity but potentiates the action of the non-depolarising agents, while antagonising the effect of depolarising drugs. Intense muscle spasms are occasionally observed during the early postoperative period. The incidence of shivering after halothane anaesthesia is probably related to the vasodilatory effects of halothane and the ambient temperature.

Central nervous system

Halothane increases cerebral blood flow and decreases cerebral vascular resistance. These changes occur in the presence of normal carbon dioxide tensions, provided there is not a considerable decrease in mean arterial blood pressure. At normal arterial carbon dioxide tensions halothane causes an increase in cerebrospinal fluid pressure and increases the intracranial pressure, particularly in the presence of space occupying intracranial lesions. These increases may be prevented by maintaining moderate hypocapnia before the addition of halothane.

Kidney

Renal effects are transient during anaesthesia and there is no evidence of renal impairment. Initial studies using clearance techniques concluded that, in common with other volatile anaesthetics, halothane reduces renal blood flow. However, later studies using direct measurement techniques concluded that halothane in clinical doses decreases renal vascular resistance without affecting total renal blood flow. Thus autoregulation appears to be maintained during halothane anaesthesia, and at normal blood pressure cortical:medullary distribution of flow is undisturbed. Even when halothane was administered during acute haemorrhagic hypovolaemia in dogs, autoregulation remained intact, maintaining renal blood flow at normal levels. Metabolism of halothane does not produce nephrotoxic intermediate compounds.

Liver

Due to its structural similarity to known hepatotoxins, such as chloroform and carbon tetrachloride, it was not long before anecdotal reports of liver damage following halothane anaesthesia appeared in the literature. In an attempt to clarify some of the controversy surrounding this problem, the United States National Halothane Study was established in 1963 and its findings published in full in 1969. This study, however, posed more questions than answers. Until the mid-1960s it was believed that the inhaled anaesthetics were metabolically inert and were excreted unchanged through the lungs. Various studies indicated that this was not the case and that halothane underwent metabolic conversion to trifluoroacetic acid and bromine and chlorine ions. Further researchers measured the degree of biotransformation of halothane to be about 20%. Animal models provided more detailed knowledge of halothane bioconversion, demonstrating that the overwhelming pathway is an oxidative one depending on the cytochrome P-450 system (P-450 2E1) of the hepatocyte endoplasmic reticulum and that this pathway may be induced by drugs such as phenobarbitone. Although halothane is primarily metabolised via cytochrome P-450 and oxygen-dependent pathways, a non-oxygen-dependent ('reductive') pathway was discovered, associated with an increase in inorganic fluoride and accompanied by the creation of a defluorinated volatile intermediate, 2-chloro-1,1,1-trifluorethane. It was believed that modification of the reductive biotransformation of halothane by enzyme-inducing agents or by depletion of the hepatic antioxidant glutathione might provide the ultimate cause for the severe hepatic necrosis occasionally observed after halothane. However, failure to reproduce a constant animal model of hepatotoxicity has led most observers to agree that the reductive pathway of halothane biotransformation is responsible for the more common, and often subclinical, form of hepatic injury (type I) which may occur in upwards of 40% of patients.

Due to the rarity of severe hepatic necrosis after halothane anaesthesia, research concerning this subject has been difficult but some interesting retrospective work has outlined that repeated exposures, the female gender, obesity and genetics may play varying roles in the genesis of halothane-induced liver damage. The conclusion of several groups of workers was that mild hepatic reactions, manifested only by increases in standard liver tests, might be due to toxic intermediate compounds.

In the context of hepatic necrosis after exposure to halothane, recent data indicate that, in many patients who have been suspected of having 'halothane hepatitis', an antibody to the trifluoroacetyl oxidative metabolite of halothane can be found in high titre in their blood. This antibody is absent in patients with viral hepatitis and cirrhosis and other medical causes of liver disease, and its presence is considered diagnostic. The concept is based on the fact that during oxidative metabolism in the liver a small percentage of incompletely metabolised trifluoroacetic acid (TFA) covalently binds with cytochrome P-450. In some individuals this TFA protein hapten acts as an immunogen, provoking a severe inflammatory response in the liver.

The effects of halothane on the hepatic circulation have been extensively investigated. Most studies have demonstrated that portal blood flow is decreased during halothane anaesthesia and that this decrease is proportional to the decrease in arterial blood pressure and cardiac output. It has been shown that during general anaesthesia with halothane cardiac output is the main determinant of portal blood flow. Blood flow to the liver is under autoregulatory control through the hepatic arterial buffer response. This allows reductions in portal flow to occur without detriment to total hepatic flow because of the ability of the hepatic artery to compensate by increasing its flow. However, during halothane anaesthesia,

this hepatic arterial reciprocity is lost and the net effect is a reduction in total blood flow.

ETHERS

Enflurane

ENFLURANE

Enflurane (Ethrane), like its structural isomer, isoflurane, is a methyl ethyl ether. It was discovered in 1963 and first introduced into clinical anaesthesia by Virtue and colleagues in 1966. Enflurane is commercially available in many countries and is generally regarded as an acceptable inhalational agent for a wide range of surgical specialities. The enflurane molecule differs from its predecessors in being less reactive and is therefore not extensively metabolised (approximately 2.5%). For this reason both it and isoflurane have become the preferred volatile agents for repeat administration.

Chemical and physical properties

Enflurane (CHF_2OCF_2CHFCl) is 2-chloro-1,1,2-trifluoroethyl-difluoromethyl ether. Its chemical structure and some physical properties are given in Table 11.1. Although resembling methoxyflurane chemically, its physical properties are more akin to those of halothane.

Enflurane is a clear volatile liquid with a mild ethereal odour, stable in the presence of metals, alkali, indirect natural light and soda lime. It does not require a preservative. Like halothane it is soluble in rubber, and this may prolong induction and recovery from anaesthesia. It is not flammable in oxygen–nitrous oxide mixtures at clinically used concentrations. Enflurane is a potent drug and should only be administered by means of an agent specific and temperature compensated vaporiser.

The MAC of enflurane in 100% oxygen is 1.68% in adults and the drug is thus only half as potent as halothane (0.8%). In 70% nitrous oxide MAC decreases to 0.6%. Anaesthesia may be induced using 3–5% inspired enflurane, vaporised either in oxygen or nitrous oxide–oxygen, and can usually be maintained using vapour concentrations of 0.4–3.0%. Both 5 and 7% vaporisers are available. The oil:gas solubility coefficient is 98.5. It has a vapour pressure of 184 mmHg at room temperature and a boiling point of 56.5°C.

The blood:gas solubility coefficient of enflurane is 1.8. Thus it is relatively insoluble in blood and under these conditions it allows a relatively rapid induction and recovery from anaesthesia. In clinical practice, induction of anaesthesia does not appear to be any more rapid than an equivalent concentration of halothane. The MAC of enflurane is 1.68.

Cardiovascular system

In common with other halogenated agents, enflurane produces a dose related decrease in systemic arterial blood pressure. The validity of comparing the haemodynamic effects of enflurane with those of halothane is sometimes questionable; variations in species, preanaesthetic medication, MAC values and surgical procedures make true comparisons difficult.

Early clinical reports indicated that circulatory changes were minimal during enflurane anaesthesia, and a study of the inotropic effects of enflurane on cat papillary muscle suggested that this agent caused less myocardial depression than halothane. Subsequent work indicated that the degree of impairment of myocardial contractility during light enflurane anaesthesia was mild or moderate, and that cardiac output was maintained by increased heart rate. When high concentrations are inhaled, however, there may be pronounced depression of cardiac function.

Cardiac output, stroke volume, arterial blood pressure and systemic vascular resistance were markedly reduced in volunteers during controlled ventilation with 1 MAC enflurane in oxygen — 2 MAC inducing unacceptable hypotension. The effects were less marked during spontaneous breathing of 1 MAC with associated hypercarbia. Under these conditions, cardiac output rose due to an increase in heart rate, but both mean arterial blood pressure and systemic vascular resistance decreased by 52 and 38%, respectively. The decrease in arterial blood pressure produced by enflurane may be comparable to or greater than the concurrent decrease in cardiac output, so that total peripheral resistance may be unchanged or decreased.

Heart rate and rhythm

Enflurane causes a modest increase in heart rate, and, although sensitising the myocardium to the effects of catecholamines, it is much less likely than halothane to cause cardiac irregularities when adrenaline is injected. The occurrence of cardiac irregularities during ear, nose and throat or dental procedures is considerably reduced by the use of enflurane rather than halothane. As a result, enflurane is particularly useful when there is likely to be an excess of endogenously produced catecholamines, such as during surgery for phaeochromocytoma.

Respiratory system

Enflurane is non-irritating to the respiratory tract at clinically used concentrations with little excessive salivation, but in high concentrations it can cause coughing and laryngospasm. In particular, enflurane is a profound respiratory depressant and causes apnoea at less than 2 MAC. It is thus a more potent respiratory depressant drug than either isoflurane or halothane. There are considerable decreases in the tidal and minute volumes and increases in $Paco_2$ but no change in the frequency of respiration. Enflurane depresses respiration, both by inhibition of the respiratory centre and by a marked curare-like action on the respiratory musculature. It has a bronchodilating effect comparable to that of halothane, and in common with all volatile anaesthetics it depresses the ventilatory responses to both carbon dioxide and hypoxia.

Central nervous system

A characteristic of enflurane is its capacity to

induce seizure complexes in the electroencephalogram (EEG). Several clinical studies confirm that episodes of paroxysmal activity and periods of burst suppression are features of EEG tracings during deep enflurane anaesthesia, being most marked at low Pa_{CO_2} tensions. These changes are characterised by high voltage, high frequency dome activity alternating with periods of silence or frank 'seizure-like' activity. Tonic–clonic twitching of the facial muscles may also appear at deep levels in the presence of passive hypertension. This response can be rapidly abolished by permitting a return to normocarbia and reducing the enflurane concentration. Patients recover from anaesthesia without any ill-effects, and there is no evidence from animal or human experiments that enflurane causes any permanent upset to the CNS. Enflurane does not exacerbate pre-existing susceptibility to seizure activity in epileptic patients during normocarbia. In children, however, cerebral sensitivity is greater and this, coupled with hypocarbia and the higher concentrations of drug required, may induce generalised epileptic activity of the grand mal type.

Enflurane can alter intracranial haemodynamics. At normocarbia, 1 MAC enflurane abolishes cerebral autoregulation and increases cerebral blood flow. Hypercarbia potentiates these effects, and mask induction of anaesthesia with enflurane in patients with intracranial pathology produces unacceptable increases in intracranial pressure. In general, enflurane increases cerebral blood flow and intracranial pressure except during hyperventilation, when mild hypocarbia is said to reduce the effect.

The ability of the drug to increase intracranial pressure and its epileptogenic potential, particularly during hypocarbia, make enflurane a poor choice both for neurosurgery and for epileptic patients in general.

Liver

The possibility of hepatic damage following the administration of newer inhaled anaesthetics has been reduced but not, unfortunately, to the degree that was anticipated. Enflurane is metabolised by the cytochrome P-450 series, the specific isoform responsible being P-450 2E1. The metabolites of enflurane include trifluoroacetic acid (TFA) and inorganic fluoride ion. Incompletely metabolised TFA can form a protein hapten, which then may act as an immunogen, provoking a severe inflammatory response in the liver. Certain epidemiological factors such as the female gender, obesity, high alcohol intake and middle age support the increased metabolism of enflurane. A series of 24 cases of enflurane 'hepatitis' was reported in 1983, although this was extensively criticised on the grounds of inadequate selection criteria. Cross-sensitisation may occur between all the halogenated anaesthetics, although their toxic potential is a function of the extent to which they are metabolised.

In the intact animal enflurane reduces portal blood flow, mainly by reducing cardiac output. The ratio of cardiac output to hepatic arterial flow is usually increased during enflurane anaesthesia. When enflurane is administered in a dose sufficient to reduce the cardiac output by 33%, hepatic arterial flow is well maintained and only decreases when the cardiac output is reduced to 50% of control. Analysis of the available data suggests that enflurane preserves splanchnic blood flow and liver oxygen supply better than halothane when used in equipotent doses.

Kidney

Biotransformation also results in low plasma concentrations of fluoride ion, averaging 15 μmol l^{-1}. It has been demonstrated that subclinical nephrotoxicity occurs in volunteers receiving 9–10 MAC hours of enflurane anaesthesia, despite plasma fluoride concentrations of only 35 μmol l^{-1}. Higher concentrations of fluoride occur in morbidly obese patients, perhaps due to the larger dose or increased metabolism.

Renal blood flow decreases in direct proportion to the decrease in cardiac output and values rapidly return to normal following cessation of anaesthesia.

Skeletal muscle

Enflurane potentiates the action of the non-depolarising muscle relaxants to a greater extent than halothane in equipotent doses. These effects are less marked with atracurium, the potency of which does not differ during halothane–nitrous oxide and enflurane–nitrous oxide anaesthesia.

Uterus

Enflurane produces a dose related relaxation of uterine smooth muscle. Concentrations of greater than 3% may inhibit oxytocin-induced contractile activity. Several studies have demonstrated the effectiveness of small doses of enflurane or other volatile agents in reducing maternal awareness during caesarean section without any increase in operative blood loss or adverse effects on the baby. Enflurane is a safe drug to use in pregnancy and no teratogenic effects on the fetus have been demonstrated.

Isoflurane

$$F-\overset{\overset{\displaystyle F}{|}}{\underset{\underset{\displaystyle F}{|}}{C}}-\overset{\overset{\displaystyle H}{|}}{\underset{\underset{\displaystyle Cl}{|}}{C}}-O-\overset{\overset{\displaystyle F}{|}}{\underset{\underset{\displaystyle F}{|}}{C}}-H$$

ISOFLURANE

Isoflurane, a structural isomer of enflurane, was first discovered in 1965. Exhaustive testing in animals suggested that isoflurane was an excellent anaesthetic with no significant toxicity and several advantages over existing drugs. However, a pilot study, which was eventually proved to be flawed, suggested that isoflurane administered to mice during gestation and early life caused neoplasia. This delayed its eventual launch until 1979. Isoflurane was introduced into clinical practice in the UK in 1983.

Chemical and physical properties

Isoflurane ($CHF_2OCHClCF_3$) is 1-chloro-2,2,2,-trifluoroethyl difluoromethyl ether, a fluorinated methyl ethyl ether. The three fluorine atoms on the terminal ethyl carbon confer considerable molecular stability and potency.

Isoflurane is a clear, colourless liquid with a pleasant if slightly pungent ethereal odour. It requires no preservative, does not react with metal and is stable in soda lime and in the presence of ultraviolet light. Isoflurane is non-flammable in air, nitrous oxide and oxygen.

Isoflurane has a low blood:gas solubility coefficient (1.4) and this relative insolubility offers the possibility of rapid induction and emergence from anaesthesia. However, the rate of induction is limited by the drug's pungency, requiring it to be introduced at low concentrations. The low blood and lipid solubility permits a rapid clearance at the end of anaesthesia. Approximately 0.2% of isoflurane is recovered as metabolites and this fact, together with a rapid recovery profile, means that isoflurane has a low potential for toxicity.

Isoflurane has a molecular weight of 184.0 and a boiling point of 48.5°C. The saturated vapour pressure is 250 mmHg and the MAC in young patients (aged 18–30 years) is 1.28. The addition of 70% nitrous oxide reduces its MAC to 0.56% in the same age group. As with other inhaled agents, MAC decreases with increasing age and reaches 1.05% (in oxygen) in patients older than 55 years. Maintenance of anaesthesia can usually be achieved with end tidal concentrations of 0.75–2.0%. Recovery from isoflurane anaesthesia is rapid and the drug is suitable for use in the day surgery unit.

Isoflurane is more potent than enflurane although the two drugs have a similar affinity for lipid.

Cardiovascular system

Myocardium and cardiac output. Isoflurane is a direct myocardial depressant. Animal studies have indicated that the mean maximal velocity of shortening (V_{max}) and mean maximal developed force (F_m) are respectively reduced by 36% and 40% of control values during exposure to an isoflurane concentration of 1 MAC. Cardiac output is only slightly affected in young volunteers (Fig. 11.4) but systemic arterial blood pressure and peripheral vascular resistance decreases (Fig. 11.5). In elderly patients the situation is somewhat different, in that cardiac output and

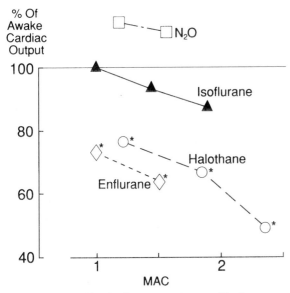

Figure 11.4 Neither isoflurane nor nitrous oxide depresses cardiac output below awake levels in volunteers. In contrast, both halothane and enflurane decrease output significantly (asterisks) and do so to a greater extent at deeper levels of anaesthesia. (Reproduced with permission of Anaquest from Eger 1982.)

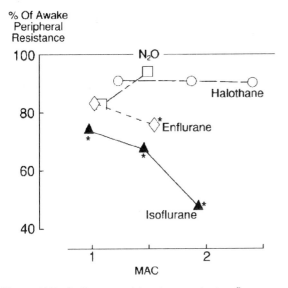

Figure 11.5 Isoflurane and, to a lesser extent, enflurane cause peripheral vasodilatation, while halothane and nitrous oxide do not. Asterisks denote significant change from awake values. (Reproduced with permission of Anaquest from Eger 1982.)

mean arterial blood pressure are both reduced because of the inability of older patients to compensate by increasing heart rate (see Ch. 50). The studies, both in volunteers and older patients, suggest that isoflurane is a less potent depressor of myocardial contractility and left ventricular ejection than halothane.

Heart rate increases in volunteers administered isoflurane, possibly because of more pronounced depression of parasympathetic than sympathetic tone. Studies in clinical situations have produced conflicting data regarding the changes in heart rate seen with isoflurane. These differences may be explained by the concomitant use of premedication, neuromuscular blocking drugs, surgical stimulation, changes in arterial P_{CO_2}, different age groups and underlying cardiovascular disease.

Because it produces considerable peripheral vasodilatation, isoflurane tends to reduce afterload and decrease myocardial oxygen consumption. Patients with coronary artery disease may benefit from a decrease in myocardial work (and hence oxygen demand) and maintained or augmented oxygen supply. These benefits may be offset by an increase in heart rate, which would increase cardiac work and decrease oxygen delivery. In addition, studies in dogs demonstrated that isoflurane in clinical concentrations may divert oxygenated coronary blood from ischaemic and potentially ischaemic myocardial tissue. This 'steal' phenomenon is analogous to that seen in the cerebral circulation where areas of ischaemia due to local vasoconstriction may be further deprived of blood and oxygen by vasodilatation elsewhere in the brain. However, other studies have failed to substantiate this theory. Eger (1984) made a detailed analysis of the arguments for and against this phenomenon and concluded that in practice most patients who have coronary heart disease and who are given isoflurane appear not to suffer from myocardial ischaemia.

Rhythm. Isoflurane anaesthesia produces a stable cardiovascular rhythm and does not sensitise the myocardium to the effects of catecholamines. Slowing of atrioventricular, His–Purkinje and ventricular conduction occurs maximally with halothane and least with iso-flurane, with enflurane in an intermediate posi-tion. Such slowing provides conditions during which re-entry of the cardiac impulse can take place, thereby permitting premature ventricular contractions or supraventricular arrhythmias.

A stable rhythm is more likely when using isoflurane than during halothane or enflurane anaesthesia and this is an important advantage, particularly in the presence of excess circulating plasma catecholamines. In animal and human studies, doses of adrenaline and other sympatho-mimetic drugs needed to trigger dangerous arrhythmias are considerably less with halothane than with isoflurane or enflurane. Isoflurane has been used to provide anaesthesia for patients undergoing surgery for removal of a phaeo-chromocytoma and for induced hypotension.

Respiratory system

As with other potent inhaled anaesthetics, isoflu-rane is a respiratory depressant. It would appear to be slightly more potent than halothane in this regard, although less so than enflurane. The ventilatory response to carbon dioxide is 30% of the awake value at 1 MAC and 14% of the awake value at 1.5 MAC. Isoflurane increases respira-tory rate and decreases tidal volume during light planes of anaesthesia. Increasing concentrations cause further decreases in tidal volume but no change in respiratory rate. Surgical stimulation antagonises the respiratory depression produced by isoflurane. Isoflurane profoundly depresses the ventilatory response to hypoxia. Broncho-motor tone is reduced during isoflurane anaes-thesia, although the effect is less pronounced than with halothane.

Isoflurane produces a decrease in static com-pliance of the total respiratory system and a small decrease in functional residual capacity. Increasing the inspired isoflurane concentration from 1% to 2% does not produce further changes in functional residual capacity or compliance.

The effect of isoflurane on the pulmonary circulation is minimal, with little change in pulmonary artery pressure, pulmonary capillary wedge pressure and pulmonary vascular resis-tance. Isoflurane may be a pulmonary vaso-dilator, as demonstrated by inhibition of hypoxic pulmonary vasoconstriction in dogs.

Muscle

Both depolarising and non-depolarising muscle relaxants produce a more profound neuro-muscular blockade in patients anaesthetised with isoflurane (1.25 MAC) than with halothane (1.25 MAC). Potentiation of neuromuscular blockade by isoflurane is a notable clinical attribute that permits the use of smaller doses of neuromus-cular blocking drugs. The more rapid removal of isoflurane may ensure more rapid reversal of the neuromuscular block and reduce the incidence of partial reversal.

In concentrations approaching or exceeding 2 MAC, the drug can provide sufficient muscle relaxation without recourse to neuromuscular blocking drugs. However, this is achieved at the cost of decreased cardiovascular stability. As with other volatile agents, isoflurane should not be administered to patients suspected of being susceptible to malignant hyperthermia.

Central nervous system

Early animal studies with isoflurane suggested that some spontaneous spike activity might occur with isoflurane; however, no studies in humans anaesthetised with isoflurane show evidence of EEG or overt convulsive activity, in spite of increasing concentrations and/or hypocapnia. Deeper planes of isoflurane anaesthesia produce burst suppression with complete electrical silence.

Isoflurane decreases cerebral metabolism and increases cerebral blood flow by decreasing cerebrovascular resistance. As a result, intra-cranial pressure may increase. This is due to either direct or indirect cerebral vasodilatation. These increases may be offset by passive hyper-ventilation. If an increase in intracranial pressure occurs during the administration of isoflurane, it is possible to reduce this increase by hyperventi-lation, even in patients with space occupying lesions. This contrasts with halothane, where hyperventilation must be applied before the administration of the drug.

Uterus

Isoflurane at a concentration of 1.5 MAC depresses contractility of human uterine muscle to 41% of control, frequency of contraction to 71% of control and developed tension to 58% of control values. In the pregnant ewe model, 2 MAC of isoflurane reduced the maternal blood pressure and cardiac output by more than 35%; uterine vasodilatation and uterine blood flow decreased; and the fetus became hypoxic and acidotic. Neonatal depression occurs at 1–1.5 MAC as a result of the direct narcotising effect of isoflurane.

When used for caesarean section, 0.75% isoflurane in 50% nitrous oxide and oxygen prevents awareness, and at this concentration would appear not to cause appreciable neonatal depression or to increase blood loss during operation.

Kidney

Because of minimal biotransformation to inorganic fluoride, isoflurane would not appear to cause postoperative functional or pathological renal abnormalities in animals or man. Despite higher than expected fluoride concentrations during both prolonged anaesthesia or prolonged subanaesthetic doses for sedation in intensive care patients, renal concentrating ability, tested with vasopressin, is unaffected. Isoflurane produces changes in renal function which revert to normal when anaesthesia is discontinued. Isoflurane decreases glomerular filtration rate by 30–50% and renal blood flow by about 40–60%; urine flow rate decreases to approximately 34% of control values; serum levels of sodium, creatinine and urea as well as serum osmolality remain unaltered, with a small decrease in serum potassium.

Liver

Hepatic toxicity after isoflurane anaesthesia is rare. Two factors suggest that isoflurane is probably much less hazardous than halothane and enflurane. First, because it has a low blood:gas partition coefficient, isoflurane is available for biodegradation for less time than other commonly available inhalation anaesthetics. Second, isoflurane undergoes less biodegradation (0.2% of a given dose is biotransformed) than halothane (25%), enflurane (2.5%) or sevoflurane (3–5%).

Studies in both animals and man support the lack of hepatic toxicity; however, the possibility of hepatic damage following the administration of isoflurane has been reduced but not, unfortunately, to the degree that was expected. Recent work has demonstrated that the metabolic products of the halogenated ethers may act as immunogens capable of inducing hepatic necrosis. Further work has demonstrated that halothane, enflurane and isoflurane are capable of producing metabolite–protein adducts. An ability to demonstrate antibodies to the trifluoroacetyl oxidative metabolite is diagnostic of massive hepatic necrosis ascribed both to halothane and enflurane and occasionally isoflurane. Present evidence suggests that a combination of middle age, female gender, obesity, repeated exposure and relative hypoxaemia contribute to this entity.

Recently, the identification of minor hepatic reactions to inhaled agents has been improved by the development of liver specific tests, in particular an enzyme linked immunosorbent assay (ELISA) method for the determination of hepatic glutathione *S*-transferase (GST) in plasma. Glutathione *S*-transferase concentrations increase with xenobiotic induced liver damage, particularly following paracetamol poisoning and some inhaled anaesthetics. Concentrations of GST during and after isoflurane anaesthesia do not increase; this is in direct contrast to the concentrations seen after both brief and prolonged halothane anaesthesia. This assay is far more specific and sensitive for anaesthetic induced hepatic injury than the standard aminotransferases (aspartate transaminase, alanine transaminase). It will allow the accurate screening of new inhalational anaesthetics for possible hepatotoxic potential.

In common with other inhaled anaesthetics,

isoflurane causes a dose dependent decrease in portal venous blood flow. Unlike halothane, isoflurane in clinical doses maintains hepatic arterial flow because of the preservation of the hepatic arterial buffer response. The net effect is a zero change in total hepatic blood flow.

Desflurane

$$F-\underset{\underset{F}{|}}{\overset{\overset{F}{|}}{C}}-\underset{\underset{F}{|}}{\overset{\overset{H}{|}}{C}}-O-\underset{\underset{F}{|}}{\overset{\overset{F}{|}}{C}}-H$$

DESFLURANE

Desflurane was synthesised by Terrell in the early 1960s. It was the 653rd (hence the original name, I-653) of 700 compounds synthesised in an attempt to identify those that could potentially be useful as inhaled anaesthetics. I-653 was completely halogenated with fluorine and was predicted to be relatively insoluble in blood. However, because of difficulties in chemical synthesis and a vapour pressure close to 1 atmosphere, development of I-653 was not initially pursued. As a result of the pressures on hospitals to increase day procedures, I-653 was re-examined and recently released for clinical use under the name desflurane.

Physical properties

Desflurane ($CF_3CHFOCF_2H$) is a highly fluorinated methyl ethyl ether with a molecular weight of 168. The desirable kinetics of desflurane result from the exclusion of chlorine and bromine in the halogenation process required to produce non-flammability. Desflurane differs solely from isoflurane in the substitution of a fluorine for a chlorine atom on the α-ethyl carbon. Fluorine substitution produces a blood:gas solubility equalling the solubility of nitrous oxide (0.42). As a result it is the least soluble potent inhalational agent. Although two different optical isomers of desflurane exist, the biological activity of each is equivalent. The use of fluorination rather than chlorination increases vapour pressure. Because the vapour pressure of desflurane (680 mmHg)

exceeds 1 atmosphere at 23°C (the boiling point), the vaporiser technology designed for the delivery of halothane, enflurane and isoflurane cannot be applied to desflurane. Desflurane boils literally in the palm of the hand, producing a non-regulable concentration of 100%. A new vaporiser technology addresses this property, producing a regulated concentration by converting desflurane to a gas (by heating), then blending this gas with diluent fresh gas flow. As a result, the required vaporiser is heated and pressurised, with elegant and expensive electronic controls and safeguards. It is probably more accurate than any vaporiser yet produced, owing to the maintenance of a constant temperature and the metering of the agent as a gas. The MAC of desflurane in 30–60-year-old humans has been determined to be 6.0 ± 0.09. As with other potent agents, the MAC of desflurane decreases with age, decreasing body temperature and the concurrent administration of other CNS depressants.

Cardiovascular system

The cardiovascular effects of desflurane can be divided into two parts: the direct effects of the anaesthetic, and a transient, but significant, response involving activation of the sympathetic nervous system. The direct effects of desflurane on the cardiovascular system are remarkably similar to those of isoflurane. There is general consensus that desflurane reduces mean arterial blood pressure, systemic vascular resistance, cardiac output and myocardial contractility in a dose dependent manner. However, the magnitude of these changes is less than those found with equi-MAC concentrations of isoflurane. In dogs, desflurane maintains myocardial blood flow better than halothane or isoflurane but may decrease coronary collateral flow by 20%, in part by a coronary 'steal' mechanism. There is still some doubt as to whether desflurane causes a 'steal' phenomenon in patients with coronary artery disease. Some workers have reported no effects in this regard but there is evidence from a number of well conducted animal studies that 'steal' occurs.

In humans, in contrast to isoflurane, heart rate was not increased in the presence of 1 MAC desflurane. However, a number of workers have reported that induction of anaesthesia with desflurane may be associated with transient, but significant, increases in heart rate and arterial blood pressure. These cardiovascular changes typically occur if concentration is rapidly increased by 0.5 MAC or more from a level that equals or exceeds 1 MAC. The increases in heart rate and arterial blood pressure parallel increases in plasma catecholamines, vasopressin and plasma renin activity. The rapidity of this cardiovascular response is noteworthy, beginning within 30 seconds after the first breath of desflurane concentration. Any proposed mechanism must account for this temporal relationship. The case for the involvement of the baroreceptors in this syndrome is not convincing because the tachycardia is associated with an increase rather than a decrease in arterial blood pressure. The early initial and maximal cardiovascular and adrenaline responses follow the wash-in characteristics of desflurane, suggesting that the afferent limb of this response may be located in the airways, lungs or a very rapidly perfused tissue.

It is possible that an abrupt increase in desflurane concentration stimulates the medullary centres in the brain directly. The resultant heightened medullary activity would transiently increase sympathetic outflow traffic and stimulate the cardiovascular system. A number of recently reported studies have determined that desflurane would indeed appear to stimulate the brain directly, in that intravenous lignocaine in a dose sufficient to obtund airway reflexes and the isolated lung during cardiopulmonary bypass do not prevent the catecholamine increases observed in this syndrome. Similarly, other pharmacological prophylaxis against this sympathetic stimulation has been only partially successful. Clonidine, fentanyl, esmolol and propofol can incompletely block or blunt the response. Etomidate and dexmeditomidine are not effective.

Given the magnitude of this sympathetic stimulation, it may be strongly advisable to avoid the use of desflurane in selected patients where tachycardia and hypertension are particularly undesirable.

Respiratory system

Desflurane causes a dose related respiratory depression similar to that seen with all other volatile agents. In healthy male volunteers, desflurane causes a dose related decrease in tidal volume and the slope of the carbon dioxide response curve. Respiratory rate is increased, but not sufficiently to offset the decreases in tidal volume. The net effect is an increase in Pa_{CO_2}. Apnoea is likely at concentrations exceeding 1.5–2.0 MAC.

Neuromuscular junction

Desflurane is a potent depressant of neuromuscular function. At concentrations greater than 1.5 MAC it may cause a decrease in the train-of-four ratio. This may be due to a prejunctional effect of the drug. Desflurane can produce tetanic fade, which is dose dependent. Like isoflurane, desflurane augments neuromuscular blockade by both depolarising and non-depolarising drugs. Desflurane anaesthesia prolongs the action of vecuronium by 20% and has prolonged 90% response time. Mivacurium also has a prolonged 90% response time in the presence of desflurane.

Desflurane triggers malignant hyperthermia in the susceptible swine model, although the onset may be delayed compared with that seen with halothane.

Central nervous system

Desflurane causes a decrease in the cerebral metabolic rate for oxygen (CMR_{O_2}) similar to that seen with isoflurane. A reduction of approximately 50% in CMR_{O_2} has been observed at concentrations approaching 2 MAC. It causes a significant reduction in cerebral vascular resistance and an increase in cerebral blood flow at doses between 0.5 and 2 MAC. Significant increases in cerebrospinal fluid pressure have been observed in patients, despite the prior establishment of hypocapnia. Desflurane significantly suppresses EEG activity, comparable with equipotent doses of isoflurane. There is no evidence that the drug is associated with epileptiform activity during either normocapnia or hypocapnia. Normal concentrations of desflurane do not abolish somatosensory evoked potentials or cerebrovascular responsiveness to changes in $PaCO_2$. Pupillary dilatation, which can result from sympathetic stimulation, can be blunted by fentanyl before stimulation but not afterwards.

Metabolism and toxicity

The greater strength of the carbon–fluorine bond renders desflurane less vulnerable to biodegradation than its chlorinated analogue, isoflurane. The only evidence of metabolism of desflurane is a finding of measurable concentrations of serum and urinary trifluoroacetate between one-fifth and one-tenth of those produced by the metabolism of desflurane. Prolonged exposure to anaesthetic concentrations of desflurane does not result in increases in serum and urinary fluoride.

Use in low flow and circle rebreathing systems. Desflurane is stable in the presence of soda lime and resists degradation by both strong acids and bases, being even more resistant than isoflurane. Recent concerns associated with the use of soda lime as a carbon dioxide absorbent include the accumulation of nitrogen, methane and carbon monoxide within the breathing system. In particular, the reaction between desflurane and soda lime (or Baralyme) may result in carbon monoxide formation. Desflurane has been shown to produce up to 20 000 p.p.m. of carbon monoxide. Carbon monoxide production is not limited to desflurane. Isoflurane and enflurane produce differing amounts; however, desflurane was found to produce 15 times as much carbon monoxide as isoflurane in the presence of dry carbon dioxide absorbent (particularly Baralyme) and at high temperature.

Most of the reported cases occurred on a Monday morning, leading investigators to propose that carbon monoxide is formed when desflurane reacts with 'dried-out' soda lime. This drying can easily happen if a low flow of oxygen is left running through an unused anaesthetic machine over the course of a weekend. In order to prevent possible carbon monoxide poisoning during anaesthesia it is recommended that all soda lime or Baralyme that has been dormant in the anaesthesia machine for more than 24 hours should be changed and dated and the machine should be flushed continuously with 100% oxygen for a least 1 minute before the first case of the day.

Sevoflurane

$$H-\overset{\overset{\displaystyle H}{|}}{\underset{\underset{\displaystyle F}{|}}{C}}-O-\overset{\overset{\displaystyle H}{|}}{\underset{\underset{\displaystyle CF_3}{|}}{C}}-CF_3$$

SEVOFLURANE

Sevoflurane was synthesised in the early 1970s. Studies at that time in both animals and man demonstrated that this agent produced a rapid and smooth induction of anaesthesia. However, on the debit side, it was observed that sevoflurane anaesthesia resulted in high concentrations of organic and inorganic fluoride and development and commercialisation of the drug was postponed. Interest in the compound reawakened because of its low blood:gas solubility and the need for drugs suitable for day case anaesthesia.

Further studies indicated that when sevoflurane was administered during low flow anaesthesia using conventional carbon dioxide absorbents, a number of breakdown products were released, which had nephrotoxic potential in rats. These findings also delayed the commercial exploitation of the drug. However, sevoflurane was released for clinical use in Japan in 1990. Since its release there it has been extensively used and most of the clinical data are derived from these sources. Phase II and III trials have recently been completed worldwide and sevoflurane is currently available in North and South America, the UK and most other European countries.

Physical and chemical properties

At room temperature and pressure, sevoflurane is a clear, non-flammable liquid with little or no pungent odour. It is an isopropyl methyl ether (empirical formula $H_2FCOCH(CF_3)_2$) with a boiling point of 58.5°C, a saturated vapour pressure of 157 mmHg at 20°C and a molecular weight of 200, which are all within the 'traditional' range of physical characteristics for other volatile anaesthetics (except desflurane). This means that sevoflurane can be administered using conventional vaporiser technology.

The blood:gas coefficient for sevoflurane is 0.6. This compares with 1.41 and 2.40 for isoflurane and halothane respectively. Wash-in and wash-out characteristics of the drug are rapid in human volunteers. In clinical practice it may be not only the blood:gas partition coefficient of sevoflurane but more importantly the tissue:blood partition coefficient of the drug that ultimately determines the speed of emergence from anaesthesia. In this regard, sevoflurane has a relatively high lipid:blood coefficient of 47.5 when compared with the figure for desflurane (27.2).

Sevoflurane is pleasant to inhale and non-pungent, making it easy to breathe. It can be administered using overpressure with no untoward consequences. It is a suitable drug for use during inhalation induction of anaesthesia in children and will undoubtedly succeed halothane in this regard. The MAC of sevoflurane has been stated to be within the range of 1.7% and 2.0% in Japanese and Caucasians, respectively.

Cardiovascular system

Like other volatile anaesthetics, sevoflurane anaesthesia produces a decrease in systolic arterial blood pressure and cardiac output, but to a lesser extent than isoflurane. Coronary blood flow has been shown to increase by 29% in dogs administered 1.2 MAC sevoflurane, a value similar to that seen with equi-MAC concentrations of isoflurane. Sevoflurane dilated coronary arteries, but unlike isoflurane the drug is not a preferential dilator of small coronary arteries.

Sevoflurane does not appear to cause coronary 'steal', and collateral blood flow appears to be well maintained.

Sevoflurane produces a stable heart rhythm but increases in heart rate of the order of 10–15 beats per minute are seen when the concentration exceeds 1.2 MAC. As with other potent inhalational agents, sevoflurane is a systemic vasodilator through endothelium-mediated vascular relaxation. In addition sevoflurane, in contrast to isoflurane, appears to be a pulmonary artery vasodilator.

The dose of adrenaline required to produce dysryzhthmias during sevoflurane anaesthesia in chronically instrumented dogs is considerably greater than that required in the presence of either halothane or enflurane. Sevoflurane causes a decrease in splanchnic and hence portal venous blood flow; however hepatic arterial blood flow is unaffected, with a maintenance of total hepatic flow.

Respiratory system

Again, like all other volatile anaesthetics, sevoflurane produces a dose related respiratory depression. In healthy patients it causes a dose related decrease in tidal volume, a decrease in the slope of the carbon dioxide response curve and a decrease in minute ventilation, despite an increase in ventilatory rate. At lower MAC doses the degree of respiratory depression is equivalent to that seen with halothane, but at 1.4 MAC the respiratory depressant effects of sevoflurane were greater than those observed for halothane at equi-MAC doses.

Sevoflurane produces equivalent bronchodilatation to enflurane and isoflurane and attenuates cholinergic tracheal smooth muscle contraction. Hypoxic pulmonary vasoconstriction is inhibited by sevoflurane in a dose related manner similar to isoflurane and is not mediated by cyclo-oxygenase. Single breath induction of anaesthesia is well tolerated, with a low incidence of coughing and breath-holding. One-lung ventilation has been effectively performed in sheep, although dose dependent right ventricular dysfunction occurred.

Neuromuscular junction

Sevoflurane is a potent depressant of neuromuscular function and adds to established neuromuscular blockade by either depolarising or non-depolarising muscle relaxants. Studies in swine susceptible to malignant hyperthermia indicate that sevoflurane acts as a trigger for malignant hyperthermia and therefore offers no clear advantage over any other inhaled anaesthetic in this regard.

Central nervous system

Sevoflurane decreases the cerebral metabolic rate for oxygen ($CMRO_2$) in a manner similar to that seen with isoflurane. This translates approximately into a 50% reduction at concentrations approaching 2.0 MAC. The effects of sevoflurane on cerebral blood flow have been evaluated in pigs and workers have reported that sevoflurane did not increase cerebral blood flow, in contrast to isoflurane. However, cerebral volume effects and not cerebral blood flow effects are of more concern and it has been suggested that sevoflurane may indeed dilate cerebral blood vessels with the potential to increase intracranial pressure. Sevoflurane suppresses EEG activity and no data exist to suggest that this anaesthetic is associated with seizure activity during either normocapnia or hypocapnia.

The changes caused by sevoflurane on the neurotransmitters dopamine, noradrenaline, MHPG and serotonin have begun to be elucidated, as has the role of excitation and inhibition of dorsal horn wide dynamic range neurones. Sevoflurane lowers the peripheral vasoconstriction threshold, by an unknown mechanism, to impair thermoregulation. Sevoflurane has been shown to reduce damage during focal ischaemia in rats.

Metabolism and toxicity

Approximately 5% of a given dose of sevoflurane undergoes biotransformation in animals and humans. The liver degrades sevoflurane to organic and inorganic fluoride in man. Cytochrome P-450 2E1 appears to be the specific P-450 isoform for the degradation of sevoflurane and, for that matter, all other inhaled anaesthetics. Hepatic degradation of sevoflurane also produces hexafluoroisopropanol, which is rapidly glucuronidated and excreted in the kidney as the glucuronide conjugate. Due to its rapid conjugation, hexafluoroisopropanol has no hepatotoxic effects. Inorganic fluoride increases significantly during anaesthesia with sevoflurane. Studies in human volunteers have demonstrated mean values of between 30 and 35 $\mu mol\ l^{-1}$. The stated nephrotoxic threshold was reported as 50 $\mu mol\ l^{-1}$.

Fluoride has since been shown to inhibit tubular reabsorption, primarily in the medullary portion of the ascending limb of Henle's loop, perhaps by inhibition of an active chloride pump located in this nephron segment. Alternatively, fluoride, with its known inhibitory action on glycolysis, might reduce the energy supply available for active transport processes that are dependent on anaerobic metabolism in the medullary nephron segments.

Although the concentrations of inorganic fluoride above the stated nephrotoxic range are regularly observed after sevoflurane anaesthesia, it is important to note that these increases cease abruptly after the end of surgery. Owing to the low blood:gas solubility of sevoflurane, rapid elimination of the drug occurs at the cessation of anaesthesia and these elevated levels of fluoride decrease over a period of 10 hours. This is quite unlike the situation which occurred with a soluble drug such as methoxyflurane, whose high affinity for body tissues resulted in a slow wash-out.

Furthermore, recent data suggest that methoxyflurane was metabolised within the renal tubular cells, thus intimately exposing these cells to extremely high concentrations of inorganic fluoride. Sevoflurane is not metabolised in the renal tubular cells.

In summary, the increases in serum inorganic fluoride observed after sevoflurane anaesthesia appear relatively benign and the toxicity previously associated with methoxyflurane appears not to occur with sevoflurane.

Use during low-flow and closed circuit anaesthesia. In 1914, Dr D. E. Jackson conceived and built the first machine ever to be used for the closed system of anaesthesia. Jackson used a caustic hydroxide solution for absorbing carbon dioxide in his machine. Since that time various types and mixtures of caustic hydroxides have been used almost exclusively, changing only in physical form.

Despite an interval of 80 years, present-day soda lime or Baralyme still remain the only option; however, there is no denying that these absorbents are far from ideal. The major constituent of soda lime is calcium hydroxide. Sodium hydroxide is added to soda lime and acts as a catalyst for the chemical reactions fundamental to the absorption of carbon dioxide. These chemical reactions are exothermic and as a result the temperature increases within the soda lime. Sevoflurane resists degradation by strong acids. In contrast, several reports indicate that alkalis such as soda lime and Baralyme can degrade sevoflurane and do so in a temperature dependent manner. Five products have been identified: compounds A, B, C, D and E. Only compounds A and B have been found to a measurable degree and, of these two, most attention has been focused on the former. Compound A is an olefin that is produced by the elimination of hydrogen fluoride from the isopropyl moiety of sevoflurane in the presence of alkalis such as sodium and potassium hydroxide. In a low flow system that uses soda lime for the absorption of carbon dioxide, concentrations of the olefin average about 20 p.p.m. When Baralyme is used, the average concentrations are greater because of the higher operating temperature of Baralyme. A peak value of 60 p.p.m. for compound A has been observed in one of eight patients administered sevoflurane. These concentrations are considerably less than the 400 p.p.m. reported by Morio and colleagues to be lethal in rats after a single 3 hour exposure to compound A.

Similarly, in a recent study Eger and coworkers reported that the administration of compound A to rats may injure the brain, liver and kidney. In this study CNS and hepatic damage occurred at higher concentrations (300–400 p.p.m.), whereas injury to corticomedullary renal tubular cells was observed at lower levels (50 p.p.m.) as well as at higher concentrations. These data indicate that the concentrations of compound A produced in clinical practice can reach the threshold for renal injury in young rats. Considerably higher concentrations would be required to produce hepatic injury or death.

The mechanism of compound A metabolism in rats is to glutathione and cysteine conjugates. Such conjugates are known nephrotoxins, metabolised via renal cysteine conjugate β-lyase to ultimately nephrotoxic metabolites. Whether these data are applicable to man has yet to be determined, as renal human β-lyase activity is 10% of that in rat kidney, perhaps suggesting a potential biochemical basis for the differences in the susceptibility of rats and humans to compound A toxicity. Regardless of these perceived differences, certain questions have been posed relating to the potential toxicity and ultimate safety of the administration of sevoflurane to humans during low flow or closed system anaesthesia.

Summary

In conclusion, the low blood:gas solubility of sevoflurane coupled with minimal airway irritation allows for smooth and rapid induction of anaesthesia. Although these properties are of benefit to adult patients, sevoflurane is likely to become an even more popular choice in paediatric practice. By modern standards, sevoflurane undergoes a considerable degree of metabolism but the considerable weight of experimental and clinical data suggests that sevoflurane is safe during normal clinical conditions. However, cost implications demand that the concerns regarding low flow or closed system sevoflurane anaesthesia will require further extensive investigation in humans.

REFERENCES AND FURTHER READING

Aldrete J A, Lowe H J, Virtue R W 1979 Low flow and closed system anaesthesia. Grune & Stratton, New York

Bito H, Ikeda K 1994 Plasma inorganic fluoride and intracircuit degradation product concentrations in long-duration, low-flow sevoflurane anesthesia. Anesthesia and Analgesia 79: 946–951

Cahalan M K, Mangano D T 1982 Liver function and dysfunction with anesthesia and surgery. In: Zakim D, Boyer T D (eds) Hepatology, a textbook of liver disease. Saunders, Philadelphia

Eger E I 1974 Anesthetic uptake and action. Williams & Wilkins, Baltimore

Eger E I II 1984 The pharmacology of isoflurane. British Journal of Anaesthesia 56: 715–995

Fee J P H, Thompson G H. Comparative tolerability profiles of inhaled anaesthetic agents. Drug Safety (in press)

Kenna J G, Van Pelt F N A M 1994 The metabolism and toxicity of the inhalation anaesthetics. Anaesthetic Pharmacology Review 2: 29–42

Kharasch E D, Hankins D C, Thummel K E 1995 Human kidney methoxyflurane and sevoflurane metabolism. Anesthesiology 82: 689–699

McKinney M S, Fee J P H, Clarke R S J 1993 Cardiovascular effects of isoflurane and halothane in young and elderly adult patients. British Journal of Anaesthesia 71: 696–701

12

Anaesthetic gases

H. J. L. Craig

Nitrous oxide, xenon, cyclopropane, ethylene and acetylene possess anaesthetic properties. Although the first four of these have been used in clinical practice, today nitrous oxide is the only one in common use. They have several features in common. All require to be stored in the liquid phase in cylinders under moderate pressure at room temperature (below 10°C for ethylene). By definition, having a vapour pressure above ambient pressure at room temperature, all can be administered in a concentration of up to 100%. They are poorly soluble in blood and so onset and offset of effect is rapid.

NITROUS OXIDE

Nitrous oxide (N_2O) was first prepared by Priestly in 1772, its anaesthetic properties being described by Sir Humphry Davy in 1800. It was first used in clinical practice by Colton and Wells in 1844.

Physical properties

This inorganic natural gas is colourless, slightly sweet smelling and non-irritant, with a molecular weight of 44 and a specific gravity of 1.53. It is readily compressible to a colourless liquid and has a boiling point of –89°C. Its oil:water solubility is 3.2, blood:gas solubility coefficient is 0.47 and it is stable in the presence of soda lime. The gas is neither flammable nor explosive but will support combustion of other agents, even in the absence of oxygen; above 450°C it decomposes into oxygen and nitrogen.

Commercial preparation and storage

Nitrous oxide is prepared by heating ammonium nitrate, impurities being removed by cooling the gas and passing it through water, caustic permanganate and acid scrubbers. The gas is then dried and stored under pressure in metal cylinders. Critical temperature is 36.5°C and below that temperature part of the contents of a full cylinder will be in liquid form, the exact proportion and pressure being dependent on the temperature. At 20°C a full cylinder will have 80% of its contents as liquid (allowing room for expansion with a rise in ambient temperature) at a pressure of 5170 kPa. Latent heat is required for the vaporisation of liquid nitrous oxide and this is obtained from the casing of the cylinder, which rapidly cools and causes freezing of water vapour in the surrounding air. Water must be excluded from the cylinder, otherwise it will freeze as the gas passes through the reducing valve, thus decreasing the rate of flow.

When gas is released the pressure at first reduces but recovers gradually as some of the liquid vaporises. With rapid flows (10 l min^{-1}) there is a sharp linear decrease in pressure due to the temperature drop; with low flows (2 l min^{-1}) there is a small but progressive decrease. Short interruptions to flow allow gas pressure to rebuild as more liquid vaporises. A pressure gauge will not indicate total cylinder contents until all the liquid is exhausted.

A 50% mixture of nitrous oxide and oxygen (Entonox) can be prepared which will remain gaseous under pressure. In these circumstances the nitrous oxide can be considered as being dissolved in the oxygen. Such premixed cylinders usually release a gas of constant composition unless cooled below −5.5°C, when the contents may separate into liquid nitrous oxide and gaseous oxygen, most likely when the cylinder pressure is 117 bar before cooling, less likely at higher or lower pressures. The cylinder could then deliver a high oxygen mixture at first, but later nearly pure nitrous oxide.

Impurities

Impurities created during the manufacture of nitrous oxide include ammonia, nitric acid, nitrogen, nitric oxide, nitrogen dioxide, carbon monoxide and water vapour. It is important that these are removed, particularly the higher oxides of nitrogen. Nitrogen dioxide is highly toxic and in concentrations of greater than 50 p.p.m. causes laryngospasm, reflex inhibition of breathing and pulmonary oedema. Cyanosis is prominent due to altered pulmonary gas exchange and the formation of methaemoglobin. There is combined respiratory and metabolic acidosis, the latter due to nitrous and nitric acids formed by the dissolving of nitrogen dioxide in body fluids. Hypotension may occur as a result of the effects of nitrite and nitrate ions on vascular smooth muscle.

Absorption and fate in body

When nitrous oxide is inhaled the gas is rapidly absorbed from the alveoli. 100 ml plasma can carry up to 45 ml nitrous oxide but it does not combine with haemoglobin. Arterial blood is about 90% saturated after 10 minutes but full equilibrium does not occur for several hours. Elimination is rapid, even after prolonged administration, the gas being rapidly excreted by the lungs, with a small amount diffusing through skin and traces excreted in urine. Although it is not certain that biotransformation takes place in the body there is some evidence that this may occur. The gas is not biologically inert and metabolism of nitrous oxide by human and rat intestinal contents has been demonstrated.

Transfer to closed cavities

Nitrous oxide is about 34 times more soluble in blood than nitrogen and will diffuse into any air-containing cavity more rapidly, in proportion to its partial pressure, than nitrogen molecules will exit. During nitrous oxide anaesthesia any air/gas-filled body cavity will either expand or the gas pressure within it will increase, depending on the compliance of the cavity wall.

Expansion of a pneumothorax or lung cyst may have serious consequences. Air entering the circulation during nitrous oxide anaesthesia will greatly increase in volume, and spaces enclosed by rigid walls, such as the paranasal sinuses and middle ear, in which the normal exits are blocked, may undergo rapid increases in pressure. If the eustachian tube is blocked, pressure changes in the middle ear may cause barotrauma. When nitrous oxide is discontinued the process is reversed, the gas diffusing out more rapidly than nitrogen can enter, with the possibility of a negative pressure in non-compliant spaces.

Cuffs and balloons inflated with air are subject to pressure/volume changes during nitrous oxide anaesthesia, as the walls of tracheal tubes, laryngeal mask airways and pulmonary artery flotation catheters are permeable to gases. There are many variables that determine the rate of change of volume and pressure:

1. time
2. permeability
3. elasticity
4. contents of cuff
5. initial volume and pressure
6. nitrous oxide concentration
7. temperature.

Pharmacology

Central nervous system

Nitrous oxide is a weak anaesthetic with a minimum alveolar concentration (MAC) value of 104%. At normal atmospheric pressure it is possible to render some patients unconscious with 80% nitrous oxide in 20% oxygen. However, surgical anaesthesia cannot be induced with this agent alone without some degree of hypoxia, except at ambient pressures above atmospheric pressure. At twice normal atmospheric pressure 50% nitrous oxide in oxygen is sufficient for surgical anaesthesia. Nitrous oxide is used in combination with more potent volatile anaesthetics where, in concentrations of 66%, it reduces by two-thirds the MAC value of the volatile agent. In addition, because of its rapid uptake, there is a noticeable second gas effect and also a concentration effect, which together hasten the uptake of other agents and speed the induction of anaesthesia.

The gas alters sensory thresholds associated with touch, temperature, light and sound; it also impairs the sense of time and recent memory. Low concentrations lead to dissociation from one's surroundings; higher concentrations cause perseveration, sedation, drowsiness and amnesia. The gas also decreases sensitivity to a stimulus and the ability or willingness of a subject to report a perceived stimulus as painful. The gas has a powerful analgesic effect when used in subanaesthetic doses (usually 50% in oxygen).

Nitrous oxide probably acts primarily by direct suppression of spinal transmission of impulses, although inhibitory supraspinal systems may be activated. There may be a common mechanism of action for opioids and nitrous oxide to explain its analgesic effect. The gas may interact selectively with the opioid receptor–endorphin system. It may stimulate supraspinal centres to activate opioid-releasing spinal cord neurones, which in turn inhibit the transmission of impulses following painful stimuli. This hypothesis is supported by the finding that naloxone usually, but not always, partially reverses the analgesic effect of nitrous oxide. It is probable that other mechanisms of central nervous system depression also play a part in the analgesic action of the gas. Concentrations of 50–70% nitrous oxide dilate cerebral blood vessels and may increase intracranial pressure. Deepening of inhalational or intravenous anaesthesia by the addition of nitrous oxide can increase cerebral blood flow and intracranial pressure dramatically. The effects may be more marked in patients with decreased intracranial compliance.

Cardiovascular system

Nitrous oxide has both a direct depressant and sympathomimetic effect on the myocardium, the latter possibly due to action on suprapontine areas of the brain. The stimulant effect tends to balance the depressant effect, the net effect being very little cardiovascular depression. The depressant action on the myocardium is more evident in subjects with coronary artery disease. Addition of nitrous oxide during high dose morphine or fentanyl based anaesthesia causes a decrease in cardiac output and heart rate because of opioid induced block of centrally mediated adrenergic stimulation. In conditions where there is already strong sympathetic stimulation, such as hypovolaemia, the net effect of nitrous oxide can also be cardiodepressant.

Nitrous oxide usually elevates central venous pressure and, although this follows myocardial depression, it is more likely to be due to an increase in venous tone with a consequent decrease in venous compliance. Increased pulmonary vascular resistance also occurs with nitrous oxide, particularly in the presence of pre-existing pulmonary hypertension, and this may contribute to an increase in right atrial pressure.

Results of studies on coronary artery blood flow are conflicting and, while animal studies (dogs and pigs) have demonstrated epicardial coronary artery constriction, possibly involving inhibition of epicardial dependent noradrenaline turnover, there is no definite evidence of coronary artery constriction in man.

Nitrous oxide, like all anaesthetic agents, depresses the baroreceptor reflexes.

A leftward shift of the oxyhaemoglobin dissociation curve occurs in blood samples exposed to 50% nitrous oxide.

Respiratory system

Nitrous oxide decreases the tidal volume and increases the rate and minute ventilation, arterial carbon dioxide tension tending to remain within normal limits. However, the normal ventilatory response to increased levels of carbon dioxide is markedly depressed, and the response to hypoxia is also reduced.

The greater density of nitrous oxide produces slightly more airway resistance than oxygen or air. Alveolar collapse by absorption of gases in an obstructed lung segment may be more rapid with nitrous oxide than with nitrogen owing to the greater solubility of the former. In addition, nitrous oxide depresses mucociliary flow and neutrophil chemotaxis. All these factors predis-

pose to postoperative respiratory complications. During recovery from nitrous oxide anaesthesia the rapid outpouring of the gas from the lungs will cause dilution of other gases, most importantly oxygen, and this may cause hypoxia (diffusion hypoxia).

Alimentary system

Nitrous oxide is known to cause nausea and vomiting, probably by both a central and a peripheral action, the latter due to distension of the gut by rapid transfer of the nitrous oxide to gas already present in the bowel, particularly likely in the anxious patient in whom air swallowing results in an initial high gut volume. It has been claimed that in bowel surgery better operating conditions and an earlier return of bowel function occur when nitrous oxide is omitted from the anaesthetic technique. However, in intestinal obstruction a poor blood supply to the affected gut segment may render nitrous oxide transfer so slow that the gas may make little practical difference.

Muscular system

Nitrous oxide increases skeletal muscular activity (probably a supraspinal effect) and does not seem to have any effect on the neuromuscular block produced by the non-depolarising neuromuscular relaxants. Potentiation of depolarising block has been demonstrated but has little clinical significance.

Toxic effects

A few hours' exposure to nitrous oxide causes almost total inactivation of methylcobalamin (vitamin B_{12}) by an irreversible oxidation of the cobalt centre converting monovalent cobalamin to its bivalent form. This oxidation prevents the normal function of vitamin B_{12}, which, acting in conjunction with the enzyme methionine synthase, transfers methyl groups from methyl tetrahydrofolate to homocysteine, forming methionine, methyl tetrahydrofolate being converted into tetrahydrofolate. These two products, methionine and tetrahydrofolate, through a series of reactions, are ultimately responsible for the conversion of deoxyuridine to deoxythymidine, an essential component of deoxyribonucleic acid (DNA) synthesis (Fig. 12.2). The eventual consequence would be a decrease in DNA synthesis and, as DNA is a gene carrier and a major component of every cell nucleus, the potential for harmful effects would seem to be unlimited. However, in man the only proven significant effects of this oxidation of vitamin B_{12} are on the bone marrow in the short term and the nervous system in the long term; in rodents fetotoxic effects have been demonstrated.

Exposure to 70% nitrous oxide in some healthy subjects appears to result in abnormal metabolism of folate after as little as 90 minutes (as measured by the excretion of forrniminoglutamic acid in the urine. It is thought that administration for at least 6 hours is needed for this to become significant, and even then the clinical relevance is uncertain. However, ill patients are more susceptible than healthy ones and in these interference with DNA synthesis has been seen after as little as 2 hours' exposure.

Reversible megaloblastic changes can be detected in the bone marrow after 12–24 hours' exposure to the gas, with depression of granulo-

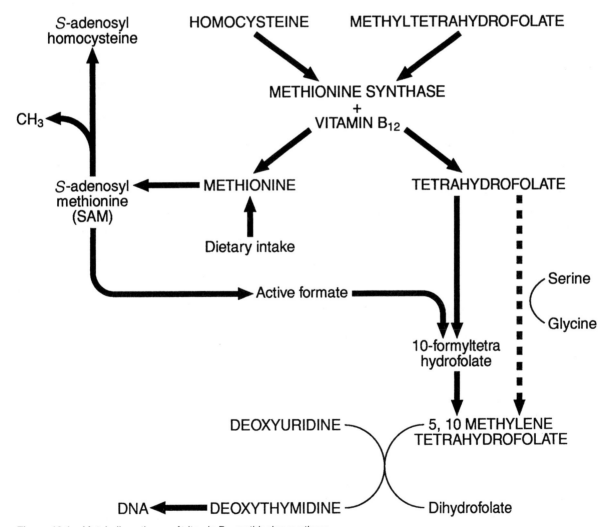

Figure 12.1   Metabolic pathway of vitamin B_{12} methionine synthase.

cyte formation after 24 hours. Peripheral granulo-cytopenia occurs after 3 days exposure to the gas and agranulocytosis within five 5–7 days in healthy subjects.

There would appear to be an absolute contra-indication to the use of nitrous oxide beyond 24 hours, although protection can be obtained in most, but not all patients, by the administration of folinic acid (5-formyltetrahydrofolate), which is converted into 5,10-methylenetetrahydrofolate and restores the metabolic pathway involved in DNA synthesis.

Since inhibition of methionine synthase is rapid and its recovery slow, repeated exposure to nitrous oxide at intervals of less than 3 days may have a cumulative effect, and repeated exposures to short periods of 50% mixtures during physio-therapy have resulted in megaloblastic bone marrow changes.

Neurological effects

A clinical feature of prolonged vitamin B_{12} defi-ciency is a failure to synthesise myelin, resulting in the insidious development of a peripheral neuropathy, which progresses to affect the poster-ior and lateral columns of the spinal cord (sub-acute combined degeneration of the cord). The failure of normal myelin synthesis is thought to be due to a deficiency in formation of S-adenosyl-methionine. Addictive abusers of nitrous oxide have developed neuropathies of this type.

Mutagenic, carcinogenic and teratogenic effects

Interference with DNA synthesis raises the pos-sibility of mutagenic, carcinogenic or teratogenic effects of nitrous oxide. An enormous number of patients are exposed to nitrous oxide in any one year, so even a very low level of mutagenic or carcinogenic activity would be of considerable importance; however, to date, there is no evid-ence of this. The picture is less clear with regard to teratogenicity or other effects on the reproduc-tive system. Animal studies (rats) have demon-strated fetal toxicity of nitrous oxide; however, all studies that have looked for fetal abnormali-ties after nitrous oxide anaesthesia in humans

have been negative. Nevertheless, a potentially dangerous situation could arise if a prolonged nitrous oxide anaesthetic, lasting several hours, was given very early in pregnancy. This is a very uncommon event and it will take a long time to assemble a sufficient number of cases to permit a firm conclusion to be drawn as to the risk. Prophylactic administration of folinic acid might be considered in such circumstances.

There have been many epidemiological studies to try and discover adverse reproductive effects in people exposed to trace concentrations of nitrous oxide for long periods; however, only one study has indicated an increase in spontaneous abortion in women constantly exposed to trace amounts of the gas during pregnancy and recent studies have not been able to confirm this finding.

XENON

Xenon is isolated from liquid air by fractional distillation. This inert gas has similar anaesthetic properties to nitrous oxide and has a MAC value of 71%. It is claimed to produce more stable cardiovascular conditions during surgery with-out any increase in plasma adrenaline concentra-tions, and to be less toxic to the developing fetus. The cost of manufacture is high.

OXYGEN
Manufacture and distribution

Under rigorous quality control medical oxygen is commercially manufactured by the fractional distillation of liquid air from which carbon dioxide has first been removed. As oxygen has a higher boiling point (–183°C) than nitrogen (–195°C), the nitrogen boils off first. Liquid oxygen is taken either directly to hospital liquid oxygen stores or to regional distribution centres for cylinder filling in special transport vessels designed to maintain the liquid under pressure and below the critical temperature. On site the liquid is stored in pressurised (10 bar) vacuum-insulated containers at about –150°C. During storage, heat from the surrounding air passes slowly through the insulated container wall, increasing the tendency to evaporation and elevation of pressure, and when pressure rises above 17 bar a safety valve allows oxygen to escape to the atmosphere. During use the cold gas vaporised inside the container is warmed outside in a copper tubing coil, the consequent increase in pressure being then reduced before the gas is supplied to the hospital. When the supply of oxygen resulting from vaporisation is inadequate, pressure decreases and a valve opens to allow liquid oxygen to pass into an evaporator, from which gas passes into the pipeline system. In normal use the refrigeration of the store is maintained by the continual removal of heat by latent heat of vaporisation of the liquid oxygen. A reserve store of oxygen in large cylinders is required in case of unexpected failure of the system. In the UK, liquid storage is more economical than cylinder storage for hospitals that use more than 50 m^3 (50 000 litres) of gaseous oxygen per week.

Medical gas cylinders are usually made from a chromium molybdenum alloy of carbon steel; however, oxygen cylinders for domestic use are made from a lighter, more expensive, aluminium alloy. Oxygen is supplied in cylinders at a pressure of 137 bar at 15°C (full cylinder), the pressure being dependent on the quantity of oxygen in the cylinder and the ambient temperature. Unfortunately, there is still no worldwide standard colour coding for medical gas cylinders. In the UK, oxygen cylinders are black with a white shoulder (valve end), complying with ISO (International Standards Organization) specification, while in the USA oxygen cylinders are usually green, and in Germany blue.

Oxygen concentrators, which are useful in remote areas and in military surgery, produce oxygen from ambient air by absorption of nitrogen on to certain types of alumina silicates (zeolite crystals). The gas produced contains 6% harmless impurities, mostly nitrogen and argon.

Properties

Oxygen is tasteless, colourless and odourless, has a specific gravity of 1.105, a molecular weight of 32, a critical temperature of –118.4°C, a critical pressure of 50.8 atmospheres and, at atmospheric pressure, liquefies at –183°C. The gas supports combustion; increasing concentrations up to 100% cause a progressive increase in the rate of combustion, with conflagrations or explosions with appropriate fuels.

Pharmacology

Cardiovascular system

An increase in arterial oxygen tension to 30 kPa or higher causes direct vasoconstriction of coronary, cerebral, renal, hepatic and peripheral circulations. This, however, is only likely to be of clinical importance at hyperbaric pressures of oxygen, which also cause direct myocardial depression. In patients with severe cardiovascular disease elevation of arterial oxygen tension to 80 kPa may produce clinically evident cardiovascular depression. Long term exposure to high inspired oxygen concentrations also leads to depression of haemopoiesis and anaemia.

Respiratory system

Inspiration of 100% oxygen may result in rapid absorption atelectasis in as little as 5 minutes in areas of lung distal to airway closure. This is due to the high solubility of the gas in blood. Even small concentrations of nitrogen can have an important beneficial splinting effect. In subjects with severe chronic obstructive airways disease with chronic carbon dioxide retention, a loss of sensitivity of the central chemoreceptors may develop, with consequent reliance, to some degree, on ventilatory drive from peripheral receptors which respond to oxygen tension. Administration of a high oxygen concentration may then diminish hypoxic drive from peripheral receptors, with consequent ventilatory failure.

Prolonged administration (over 30 hours) of high oxygen concentrations (P_iO_2 100 kPa or more) can lead to clinical and radiological appearances similar to those associated with the adult respiratory distress syndrome, notably hyaline membranes, interlobular and alveolar septal oedema, and fibroblastic proliferation.

Loss of pulmonary surfactant encourages absorption collapse. The mechanisms responsible probably include oxidation of —SH groups on essential enzymes (e.g. co-enzyme A), peroxidation of lipids, the resulting peroxides inhibiting cell function, and inhibition of reversed electron transport, possibly by inhibition of flavoproteins.

Central nervous system

Prolonged exposure to high concentrations of hyperbaric oxygen may cause grand mal type convulsions.

Eye

In the neonate a prolonged high retinal artery arterial oxygen tension may damage the eye by inducing arterial retinal vasoconstriction and closure of immature vessels, with subsequent new vessel formation. Leakage of intravascular fluid can cause vitreoretinal adhesions and retinal detachments (retrolental fibroplasia). The condition is most likely to develop in very premature infants with respiratory problems demanding high inspired oxygen concentrations. However, while the triggering threshold of retinal artery oxygen tension for retinal damage is uncertain, umbilical arterial oxygen tension maintained between 8 and 12 kPa is associated with a very low incidence of retinal damage and no evidence of systemic hypoxia.

AIR

Air for medical use is supplied in cylinders, which in the UK are painted grey with black and white shoulder quadrants, compressed to 137 bar. In many hospitals it is also supplied by pipeline. It is used to drive various medical mechanical devices such as ventilators and drills.

FURTHER READING

Armstrong P, Rae P W H, Gray W M, Spence A A 1991 Nitrous oxide and formiminoglutamic acid: excretion in surgical patients and anaesthetists. British Journal of Anaesthesia 66: 163–169

Christensen B, Guttormsen A B, Schneede J et al 1994 Preoperative methionine loading enhances restoration of the cobalamin dependent enzyme methionine synthase after nitrous oxide anesthesia. Anesthesiology 80: 1046–1056

Howell R S C 1990 Medical gases 1: manufacture and uses. In: Kaufman L (ed) Anaesthesia Review 7, pp 87–103. Churchill Livingstone, Edinburgh

Howell R S C 1991 Medical gases 2: distribution. In: Kaufman L (ed) Anaesthesia review 8, pp 195–210.

Churchill Livingstone, Edinburgh

Koblin D D, Tomerson B W 1990 Dimethylthiourea, a hydroxyl radical scavenger, impedes the inactivation of methionine synthase by nitrous oxide in mice. British Journal of Anaesthesia 64: 214–223

Messina A G, Yao E S, Canning N et al 1993 The effect of nitrous oxide on left ventricular pump performance and contractility in patients with coronary artery disease: effect of preoperative ejection fraction. Anesthesia and Analgesia 77: 954–962

Royston B D, Bottiglieri T, Nunn J F 1989 Short term effect of nitrous oxide on methionine and S-adenosyl methionine concentrations. British Journal of Anaesthesia 62: 419–424

13

Intravenous anaesthetic drugs

R. S. J. Clarke

HISTORY

Christopher Wren, the English architect, is credited with the first intravenous injection in man in 1656, in which he administered opium by means of a quill and bladder, resulting in the production of unconsciousness. It was not until 200 years later that the syringe was devised by Alexander Wood of Edinburgh, again for the administration of opiates. Francis Rynd, a Dublin surgeon, had already perfected the hollow needle in 1845, so the technology was available, but only in the 1930s did suitable drugs for the production of anaesthesia become available.

Barbituric acid or malonyl urea was first prepared in 1864 by Adolf von Bayer and many derivatives were prepared before Weese and Scharpff introduced the first rapid acting barbiturate, hexobarbitone. This type of induction satisfied patients, anaesthetist and surgeon, so that intravenous anaesthesia became accepted as the norm, even before thiopentone was launched in 1934 by Ralph M. Waters. These drugs were unfortunately thought of as intravenous anaesthetics rather than induction agents, with disastrous results when they were used on the wounded at Pearl Harbor in 1942. As a result, intravenous anaesthesia was much more popular in the UK than in the USA during the early postwar years. Thiopentone and the very similar alternative agent, thiamylal, remained unchallenged until 1957, in spite of the prolonged recovery with large doses. This delay in achieving full street-fitness after general anaesthesia led to the investigation of many barbiturates in the 1950s but methohexitone was the only one to achieve success. Eventually both their pharmacokinetics and their clinical side-effects indicated that further improvement of the barbiturate molecule was unlikely.

Researchers had been also studying non-barbiturate molecules and the first successful group were derivatives of phenoxyacetic acid, one of which is eugenol. The two main anaesthetics of this group were G 29505 and propanidid, both of which had the advantage of truly rapid breakdown and clinical recovery from anaesthesia. However, they were not water soluble and the former caused a high incidence of venous thrombosis, while the latter, in its solvent Cremophor EL, was soon implicated in anaphylactoid reactions.

CLINICAL GROUPING

It is convenient to classify the intravenous anaesthetic drugs not only by their chemical grouping but by their onset and duration of action.

Regarding *onset*, these drugs can be:

- Rapid acting — that is, having a hypnotic effect within one arm–brain circulation time (10–20 seconds, according to the state of the circulation). This applies to the more widely used induction agents such as thiopentone, methohexitone, propofol and etomidate.
- Slow acting — that is, having a hypnotic effect of slower onset, usually with an onset in 20–30 seconds and a peak effect at 1–3 minutes. This applies to drugs such as diazepam, midazolam and ketamine.

Regarding *duration of action*, most intravenous induction agents (particularly the barbiturates) were classified as long acting, short acting and ultrashort acting. This classification was never completely satisfactory because, while phenobarbitone is truly long acting (elimination half-life 80–120 hours) and amylobarbitone, butobarbitone and cyclobarbitone are short(er) acting drugs of 4–8 hours clinical duration, thiopentone is certainly not ultrashort acting, as it has an elimination half-life of about 11 hours. Even methohexitone has an elimination half-life of about 4 hours and it would appear that no barbiturate that is clinically acceptable can be truly ultrashort acting because they are not rapidly metabolised in the body.

THIOPENTONE

Chemistry

Thiopentone is a derivative of barbituric acid, having a sulphur atom rather than oxygen attached to one of the carbon atoms of the ring. Barbiturates used for induction of anaesthesia are sodium salts, which are freely soluble in water, though of limited stability. Commercial preparations of the powder also contain 5% of anhydrous sodium carbonate, which prevents precipitation of the insoluble free acid and results in a solution of pH 10.5–11.0. It is largely non-ionised at body pH, a fact which facilitates its diffusion through membranes.

Pharmacokinetics

When injected intravenously, thiopentone is 60–80% bound to plasma protein and is therefore non-diffusible. The extent of the binding is influenced by factors such as pH, plasma albumin level and pretreatment with other bound drugs such as probenecid and aspirin, although this last effect is only clinically important for the immediate effects of very large doses. The peak level in vessel-rich tissues is reached in 1–2 minutes and it diffuses rapidly into the brain because of its high lipid solubility. Levels in the brain then begin to fall in a further 60 seconds while the drug is still diffusing into muscle and this rapid redistribution is responsible for the rapid recovery from small doses. Equilibrium with the muscles does not occur for about 15 minutes after administration and thereafter its tissue level parallels that found in plasma. The concentration in adipose tissue rises only slowly, over about 2 hours, in spite of its high solubility, because of the poor blood supply (Fig. 13.1). Thiopentone then diffuses very slowly out of the fat, maintaining a low but clinically significant plasma level for many hours.

Thiopentone is metabolised in the liver and virtually none is excreted unchanged. The hepatic extraction ratio is approximately 0.1–0.2, with a clearance of $3.4 \, \text{ml} \, \text{kg}^{-1} \, \text{min}^{-1}$. The pathways identified are:

1. oxidation of the C_5 side-chains
2. oxidative replacement of the sulphur at C-5 to form pentobarbitone
3. cleavage of the barbiturate ring to form urea and a three-carbon fragment.

Metabolism in the liver and clinical recovery from anaesthesia are virtually unaffected by hepatic dysfunction because of the large capacity of the liver.

The decline in plasma thiopentone level is exponential but is best described by three separate curves, characterised by three half-lives: $t_{\frac{1}{2}}\alpha_1$ of 2–6 minutes, corresponding to diffusion into tissues of high blood flow; $t_{\frac{1}{2}}\alpha_2$ of 30–60 minutes,

corresponding to diffusion into the adipose tissue; and $t_{\frac{1}{2}}\beta$ of 5–10 hours, corresponding to the elimination phase (Fig. 13.2). The effect of this slow elimination is that:

1. Residual effects of a single dose persist for many hours, having an additive effect when other sedative drugs are given.
2. Repeated small doses or infusion of thiopentone result in cumulation in adipose tissue and prolonged residual effects.

Diffusion across the placental barrier is rapid but in fact redistribution to muscular tissues in the mother often means that the baby is more alert than the mother's state would suggest. Certainly the thiopentone concentration in the umbilical vein, which should be similar to that entering the fetal brain, has been shown to be well below that required to produce anaesthesia in adults.

Both hepatic and renal failure lead to hypoproteinaemia with reduced plasma binding and increased clinical effects. However, renal disease does not affect clearance and hepatic cirrhosis

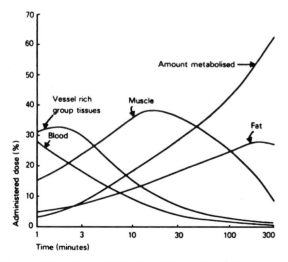

Figure 13.1 Tissue distribution of thiopentone following intravenous injection (according to Saidman and Eger 1966 Anesthesiology 27: 118–126).

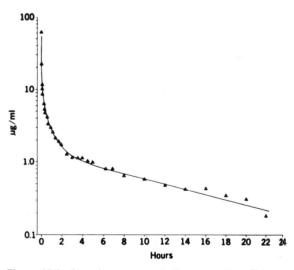

Figure 13.2 Log plasma concentration versus time. Data from a patient given thiopentone $6.4 \, \text{mg} \, \text{kg}^{-1}$ as an intravenous bolus. The solid line represents the triexponential equation determined by non-linear regression. The triangles represent the measured thiopentone plasma concentrations. (Reproduced with permission from Stanski and Watkins 1982 Drug disposition in anaesthesia. Grune & Stratton, New York.)

has no effect on the use of thiopentone for induction of anaesthesia.

Pharmacodynamics

Central nervous system. Thiopentone rapidly diffuses across the blood–brain barrier, causing cortical depression. Loss of consciousness normally occurs within 30 seconds of administration of thiopentone and is unaccompanied by excitatory phenomena such as occur with many intravenous induction agents. The plasma thiopentone level necessary for anaesthesia in fit patients is around 40 µg ml⁻¹.

The electroencephalogram (EEG) pattern shows characteristic changes during induction of anaesthesia, consisting of high amplitude waves of frequency 10–30 Hz or faster. As anaesthesia deepens there is progressive suppression of cortical activity, with occasional bursts of high voltage waves at 10 Hz. Induction doses of thiopentone also have a marked anticonvulsant action.

The cerebral metabolic rate is reduced by thiopentone, especially in areas of high activity. This is accompanied by a corresponding reduction in cerebral blood flow, resulting in cerebral vasoconstriction and a reduction in intracranial pressure. However, the main effects of barbiturates on cerebral blood flow are secondary to those on blood pressure and the usual effect of administering thiopentone is hypotension, fall in cerebral blood flow and a compensatory fall in cerebral vascular resistance.

Thiopentone is not an analgesic and small doses may increase sensitivity to somatic pain. As a result, the depth of anaesthesia under thiopentone depends as much on the surgical stimulus as on the degree of cortical depression.

Acute tolerance is a term applied to the phenomenon of return of consciousness after a single, large dose occurring at a higher plasma concentration than following smaller doses. However, the patient who regains consciousness with a relatively high plasma concentration has more thiopentone in the body stores than one with a lower plasma concentration and full recovery of all mental faculties is therefore slower. Overall

this is an argument for keeping induction doses as low as possible and for using additional drugs in the process of balanced anaesthesia.

Cardiovascular system. Thiopentone, given as a bolus, causes a reduction in arterial blood pressure, left ventricular stroke work index, pulmonary wedge pressure and systemic peripheral resistance. There is a small degree of tachycardia which with lower doses contributes to the maintenance of blood pressure and cardiac output. Cardiac arrhythmias are rare with this as with other intravenous anaesthetics. Higher doses of thiopentone have been given to neurosurgical patients to render the EEG isoelectric and cause increasing myocardial depression and vasodilatation, but apart from the prolonged recovery the only marked disturbances are falls in the left and right ventricular stroke work indices.

The above findings apply specifically to patients with a healthy cardiovascular system. Patients receiving antihypertensive treatment often have no significant rise in heart rate so that the cardiac output falls markedly. Hypovolaemic patients who are already compensating by peripheral vasoconstriction will have a more marked hypotensive response to the drug. A third group at risk is those with fixed cardiac output due to mitral stenosis or cardiac tamponade, who require lower doses and slower administration for safe induction of anaesthesia.

Myocardial oxygen consumption is increased by thiopentone in healthy patients but is reduced by approximately 35% in those with ischaemic heart disease. This effect is due to a reduced oxygen requirement and there is no evidence of any adverse effect on the myocardium.

Respiratory system. Thiopentone has a potent depressant effect on both respiratory rate and depth and depresses the sensitivity of the respiratory centre to carbon dioxide. In deep anaesthesia the hypercapnia is masked because thiopentone may also obtund the usual rise in arterial pressure.

Cough and hiccough are uncommon during administration of thiopentone but laryngeal irritability is heightened. As a result, minor stimuli frequently cause laryngospasm during light thiopentone anaesthesia. Thiopentone may induce bronchospasm in asthmatic patients but many instances of 'bronchospasm' can be reversed by a neuromuscular blocking drug and are probably due to coughing.

Porphyria. This is an inborn error of metabolism in which the level of porphyrins in the plasma increases and porphyrinuria follows. As a result, there are central nervous system, alimentary tract and cutaneous disturbances, leading to psychiatric manifestations, abdominal pain and muscle paralysis. Porphyrins are pigments composed of four pyrrole rings linked by methane bridges and occur particularly in cytochrome and haemoglobin. They are formed in the liver from aminolaevulinic acid (ALA), a process catalysed by ALA-synthetase. It appears that in some patients this progress can be stimulated by certain drugs such as thiopentone and it is particularly important not to exacerbate a spontaneous attack (which may resemble an abdominal emergency) by administration of this drug. It should be said that there are several types of porphyria and not all are adversely affected by thiopentone, but the dangers are so serious that the drug should be avoided in all types.

Local effects. Solutions of thiopentone rarely cause pain on injection or evidence of venous irritation and the incidence of venous thrombosis is approximately 3–4%. However, thiopentone causes pain and tissue damage when injected subcutaneously, particularly in large volumes.

Intra-arterial injection, on the other hand, causes marked local effects which may threaten the circulation to the limb. The sequence following injection is precipitation of crystals of insoluble thiopentone in the smaller vessels, release of adenosine triphosphate (ATP), intimal damage and vascular thrombosis. The patient complains of immediate pain following the injection, loss of consciousness is delayed and the radial pulse may disappear. Avoidance is best achieved by constant awareness of the possibility, and treatment includes the injection of lignocaine and papaverine into the vessel.

Other effects. Thiopentone has no effect on hepatic, renal or adrenocortical function in conventional doses. It has no effect on uterine tone

and it neither causes nor prevents postoperative nausea and vomiting.

METHOHEXITONE

Chemistry

The important differences from thiopentone are largely related to its having a —CH_3 group attached to the N atom, resulting in more rapid recovery but more marked excitatory phenomena. It is, however, an oxy- rather than a thiobarbiturate, which would tend to prolong its action. It is supplied as a powder and usually made up into a 1% solution which is stable in cool conditions for several weeks.

Pharmacokinetics

The uptake of methohexitone is similar to that of thiopentone and its redistribution half-life falls within the same range ($t_{\frac{1}{2}}\alpha_1 = 6$ minutes; $t_{\frac{1}{2}}\alpha_2 = 59$ minutes). However, the elimination half-life is significantly shorter ($t_{\frac{1}{2}}\beta = 4$ hours) than that of thiopentone. This is due to a higher hepatic excretion ratio and the rapid clearance of the drug, which is 10.9 ml kg^{-1} min^{-1} compared with 3.4 ml kg^{-1} min^{-1} for thiopentone.

Pharmacodynamics

The most notable differences from thiopentone consist of a high incidence of spontaneous muscle movements, tremor and hypertonus (20% of cases, compared with about 4% for thiopentone). The incidence is directly dependent on the dose and rate of administration and, while increased by drugs such as hyoscine or droperidol, is decreased by opioid premedication.

The cardiovascular effects of methohexitone are similar to those of thiopentone except for a more marked degree of tachycardia and less hypotension with the former.

Pain on injection is more common with methohexitone than with thiopentone.

ETOMIDATE

CH$_3$CH$_2$O—C
O
N—N
H
C
H$_3$C

Chemistry

Etomidate is water soluble but the solution was not considered sufficiently stable for general distribution. It is also soluble in polyethylene glycol but is marketed as a 0.2% solution in propylene glycol, a solution that is stable at room temperature for 2 years. There are two optical isomers, the dextro isomer having much greater hypnotic activity.

Pharmacokinetics

Etomidate is approximately 76% bound to plasma proteins. There is a rapid distribution and elimination phase, the $t_{\frac{1}{2}}\alpha_1$ being 2.6 minutes, $t_{\frac{1}{2}}\alpha_2$ being 27 minutes and $t_{\frac{1}{2}}\beta$ being 75 minutes. The drug is metabolised mainly in the liver by ester hydrolysis into pharmacologically inactive metabolites, about 75% of the administered dose being excreted in the urine in this form and only about 2% being excreted unchanged. It has been found that the clearance of etomidate is markedly reduced by the presence of a steady-state concentration of fentanyl.

Pharmacodynamics

Central nervous system. The onset of action is within one arm–brain circulation time with the usual clinically effective dose of 0.3 mg kg^{-1} Hypnosis is accompanied by a high incidence of excitatory effects comparable with those with methohexitone, but these can be reduced by prior administration of an opiate (usually fentanyl) or early use of a muscle relaxant. There is no distinc-

tive EEG change to explain these excitatory effects. Recovery after a single dose of etomidate is markedly shorter than after thiopentone.

Cardiovascular effects. Etomidate has less marked effects on the cardiovascular system than any other clinically used anaesthetic. In fit patients 0.3 mg kg^{-1} produces a slight increase in cardiac index, accompanied by a slight fall in heart rate, in arterial pressure (14%) and in peripheral resistance (17%). Cardiac contractility is enhanced as judged by dp/dt_{max}, which rises (9%), with maximum effects occurring about 3 minutes after injection. Myocardial oxygen consumption, which is increased by ketamine (78%), thiopentone (55%) and methohexitone (44%), is not significantly affected by etomidate. In addition, etomidate appears to have a true but weak coronary vasodilator effect. The use of opioids such as fentanyl or alfentanil enables low doses to be used for induction of anaesthesia and these factors have made it the drug of choice with many anaesthetists for poor risk patients.

Histamine release. Unlike other intravenous anaesthetics etomidate does not release significant amounts of histamine, although there are reports of erythema in the upper part of the body in some patients. There is evidence of histamine release synergistically when etomidate is given with suxamethonium, but it still remains one of the safest drugs in terms of anaphylactoid reactions.

Respiratory system. Equipotent doses of etomidate and methohexitone cause a similar shift in the carbon dioxide response curve, but at any given carbon dioxide tension ventilation is greater after etomidate than after the barbiturate. It may therefore have some advantage in patients who are breathing spontaneously, although in clinical practice this will be counteracted by any accompanying opioid.

Adrenocortical function. The pharmacokinetic and pharmacodynamic profile described above made this drug appear to be ideal for prolonged sedation in poor risk patients. However, in a classical study by Ledingham and Watt (1983) it was shown that, over a particular period of time, there was a significant increase in mortality in patients surviving for more than 5 days who had received mechanical ventilation. The only apparent difference in this group accounting for the increased mortality was in the change from a morphine–benzodiazepine regimen to etomidate infusion. The authors suggested that the causative mechanism might be by a direct effect of etomidate on steroid synthesis in the adrenal cortex. This hypothesis has since been confirmed, for we now know that infusion of etomidate will suppress an early stage in steroid formation, affecting aldosterone as well as cortisol formation.

A single bolus dose will inhibit some reactions in the process of steroid synthesis but overall has not been proven to cause significant adrenocortical suppression.

Other systemic effects. No adverse actions have been seen in studies with etomidate on hepatic or renal function. There is, however, a higher incidence of postoperative emesis in patients who have received etomidate compared with other induction agents. Etomidate has been used safely in a known porphyric patient who had developed motor paralysis following a barbiturate anaesthetic. However, studies in rats have shown etomidate to be potentially porphyrogenic, whereas ketamine does not similarly increase porphyrin levels.

Local and haematological effects. Since etomidate is formulated in propylene glycol, it would be expected to cause pain on injection and venous irritation. Venous sequelae have, in fact, been recorded in about 25% of patients and the incidence is dose related. More recently, haemolysis has been seen both on direct examination of the plasma and serially by a fall in the haptoglobin level during the early period after etomidate administration. This effect is related to the high osmolarity of the injected solution rather than to the etomidate itself and is not seen when etomidate is dissolved in a fat emulsion.

KETAMINE

Chemistry

Ketamine is chemically related to phencyclidine and cyclohexamine. It is water soluble, forming a solution of pH 3.5–5.5, and is available in 10, 50 and 100 $mg\ ml^{-1}$ concentrations.

Pharmacokinetics

Ketamine has a high lipid solubility and the pattern of distribution in the body is similar to that of thiopentone. Recovery is due both to rapid breakdown in the liver and to redistribution. The usual induction doses in man are 2 $mg\ kg^{-1}$ and 10 $mg\ kg^{-1}$ by the intravenous and intramuscular routes, and peak plasma levels occur within 1 and 5 minutes, respectively. Initially ketamine is distributed to the highly perfused tissues, including the brain, and then to the less well perfused tissues. The $t_{\frac{1}{2}}\alpha$ is approximately 10 minutes and $t_{\frac{1}{2}}\beta$ is 2–3 hours following single dose administration.

The drug is largely broken down in the liver and excreted in the bile, with 20% appearing in the urine in its various metabolites. The process consists in N-desmethylation by cytochrome P-450 forming norketamine, which can then be hydroxylated to form hydroxynorketamine compounds. Ketamine can also undergo ring hydroxylation but this pathway is of minor importance. Less than 5% appears in the faeces and less than 4% in the urine. The main metabolite, norketamine, has hypnotic properties, with 33–50% the potency of ketamine. This, as well as redistribution and subsequent release, can explain the prolonged recovery phase from ketamine anaesthesia.

Pharmacodynamics

Central nervous system. Loss of consciousness is slow after ketamine administration and may take up to 1 minute, compared with the 15–20 seconds that is common with barbiturates or propofol. It is also difficult to obtain a clear endpoint for onset of sleep as the eyes often remain open with a fixed gaze. The eyelash, corneal and laryngeal reflexes are unimpaired and there is usually increased muscle tone, with some involuntary muscle movement. While the usual induction dose is $2\,mg\,kg^{-1}$, most patients will fall asleep with doses as low as $1\,mg\,kg^{-1}$.

The action of ketamine is on the limbic system, which is dissociated from the thalamocortical systems and explains why the pattern is so different from conventional anaesthesia. It can also be described as catalepsy associated with analgesia but not true anaesthesia. The receptors on which ketamine acts are uncertain but specific interaction with the N-methyl-D-aspartate (NMDA) receptor has been suggested.

Analgesia with ketamine is profound and it has been used for this purpose in subanaesthetic doses with prolonged postoperative effects. The site of this action is thalamic or reticular and is related to blocking the affective-emotional rather than the somatic components of pain perception.

Cerebral blood flow, oxygen consumption ($CMRO_2$) and intracranial pressure are all increased during induction of anaesthesia with ketamine, the blood flow rising by as much as 80% and remaining raised for 30 minutes. These changes make the drug unsuitable for use in patients with intracranial pathology, although they can be reduced by concomitant administration of thiopentone or halothane or by hypocarbia.

Recovery after ketamine anaesthesia is prolonged and difficult to define, with full contact with the environment taking as much as an hour after first signs of awakening. During this period there can be diplopia and patients may think they are blind. Any stimulation causes violent motor activity that is largely purposeless. Sensations vary from a pleasant dream-like state to vivid and terrifying hallucinations. The incidence of unpleasant sequelae with ketamine as the main anaesthetic agent for short procedures is approximately 25% and dose related. However, it is reduced considerably when the drug is used solely as an induction agent followed by surgery lasting for 1 hour or more. Symptoms are more common in women (except in labour) than in men and can be minimised by administration of an opioid, droperidol, a benzodiazepine (notably lorazepam) or thiopentone. There is no evidence of hallucinations in young children

and problems with repeated administration in them are rare. The drug has therefore particular advantages in children, in whom the intramuscular route is often the only practicable route of administration. Similarly, with repetition for burns dressings in adults, sequelae diminish in severity and it may well be the safest intravenous agent.

Cardiovascular system. Unlike almost all other anaesthetic induction agents, ketamine maintains cardiovascular function under most clinical circumstances. The heart rate and systolic blood pressure increase on an average by 30%, and can show peaks of 100%, but there is no significant change in stroke index. There is a rise in plasma catecholamine concentration but this is not clearly related to the haemodynamic changes. The mechanisms of these effects are almost certainly primary direct stimulation of the central nervous system. However, it is known that ketamine is a direct myocardial depressant and this effect is seen particularly in critically ill or traumatised patients. Cardiac arrhythmias are uncommon following ketamine administration and a number of workers have shown that it has an antiarrhythmic action. When ketamine is given by the intramuscular route, anaesthesia and the hypertensive response occur more slowly, requiring 8–10 minutes to reach a peak, and subside more slowly.

Respiratory system. Respiratory depression is minimal and transient after clinical doses of ketamine. However, after opioid premedication there may be depression and even apnoea, especially when ketamine is given rapidly or when given intramuscularly to small children. This can cause a fall in Pa_{O_2} in patients breathing spontaneously on room air and must be remembered when ketamine is given in disaster situations.

Ketamine is a bronchodilator and antagonises the bronchoconstrictor action of histamine, so that it has an advantage in the asthmatic and has even been used in management of status asthmaticus. However, secretions in the tracheobronchial tract are stimulated by ketamine and the use of a drying agent before anaesthesia is to be recommended, particularly in children.

Coughing, hiccough and laryngospasm are also more common with ketamine than after thiopentone.

Laryngeal reflexes are not markedly depressed with ketamine but it is no longer thought that they are intact, as was originally claimed. It can be shown that, after a typical anaesthetic dose of 2 mg kg^{-1}, radiopaque contrast medium can pass from pharynx to lung fields in a patient lying supine. The risks of this are increased by sedative premedication.

Other effects. Intraocular pressure is slightly increased by ketamine. Uterine tone and intra-uterine pressure are also increased in both the non-pregnant and pregnant uterus, effects that may be harmful in abruptio placentae and cord prolapse. An erythematous rash is seen in about 20% of patients given ketamine but this is transient and anaphylactoid/anaphylactic reactions are rare.

Isomers of ketamine

Ketamine occurs in isomers, which have properties differing widely both from each other and from the racemic mixture that is normally used. The (+) isomer has 3.4 times the potency of the (−) isomer and is also a more potent analgesic, as judged by the occurrence of postoperative pain. However, it also causes more psychic emergence reactions. Since the plasma decay curves and patterns of excretion are similar in the isomers, the differences in action can only be explained by pharmacodynamic factors. In spite of its apparent advantages, no attempt has been made to market the (+) isomer of ketamine as a separate product.

MIDAZOLAM

1.   2.

Chemistry

Midazolam is a benzodiazepine but, unlike most drugs of this group, it is water soluble. This is because its formula includes an imidazole ring attached to the diazepam ring. The latter opens at pH values below 4.0, imparting water solubility. At the pH of plasma the ring closes and lipid solubility is enhanced, this closing process having a half-life of about 10 minutes. The absence of organic solvents in the formulation means that the drug lacks the irritant properties of diazepam given as Valium.

Pharmacokinetics

Midazolam is highly protein bound (approximately 95%), although not as highly bound as diazepam. As a result, patients with hypoproteinaemia will have an enhanced response to it. Its distribution follows the usual pattern to vessel-rich tissues and later to those poorly perfused, including fat. Elimination is dependent on hepatic biotransformation, converting it into 4-hydroxymidazolam, a metabolite almost devoid of sedative properties. The initial redistribution phase is shorter than that of diazepam, contributing to the more rapid early recovery from the newer drug. The elimination phase ($t_{\frac{1}{2}}\beta$) is 2–3 hours and also more rapid than seen with diazepam, though slower than with thiopentone or propofol. It is prolonged to as much as double the above figure in elderly patients and following major surgery, probably by effects on hepatic blood flow and metabolism. Placental transmission, as judged by the fetal:maternal ratio in animals, is less for midazolam than diazepam.

Pharmacodynamics

Central nervous system. The benzodiazepines act on specific receptors concentrated in the cerebral cortex, hippocampus and cerebellum. They act by potentiating the depressant interneurones using γ-aminobutyric acid (GABA) as a transmitter. Release of GABA opens the Cl$^-$ channel, resulting in hyperpolarisation of the nerve cell.

The onset of action is slow and, even with a dose of 0.3 mg kg^{-1}, sleep may not occur for 3–5 minutes. As with diazepam the effects are dose related, ranging from tranquillisation to full anaesthesia, but with wide interpatient variation. Even doses of 0.05–1.0 mg kg^{-1} will produce drowsiness and amnesia, which is often all that is required in the clinical situation (e.g. endoscopies). Amnesia, which is an effect common to all benzodiazepines, can be undesirable, but in dental practice, for instance, may be a useful aspect of therapy.

Like other benzodiazepines, midazolam is anticonvulsant (e.g. in status epilepticus) and antihallucinatory (e.g. after ketamine or in delirium tremens).

Cardiovascular system. The benzodiazepines generally have little depressant effect on the heart or circulation, even in large doses. Midazolam causes a fall in systemic vascular resistance rather than the rise seen with thiopentone, thus reducing pre- and afterload. Because of the slow onset of action this effect is often underestimated and may be hazardous in the hypovolaemic patient.

Respiratory system. This group of drugs, when given intravenously, have a depressant effect on the respiratory centre, in contrast to their safety in oral medication. The depression is accentuated by the concomitant use of opioids and is particularly marked in patients with obstructive airway disease. In addition, these drugs cause a central reduction in muscle tone, which may lead to respiratory obstruction if the patient's airway is not being carefully observed.

PROPOFOL

Chemistry and formulation

Propofol is an akyl phenol that is virtually insoluble in water. It is currently solubilised as a 1% emulsion containing 10% soya bean oil, 1.2% egg phosphatide and 2.25% glycerol. The pH is 6–8.5 and pK_a of the drug in water is 11.

The fat emulsion used as solubilising agent is similar to Intralipid, used for parenteral nutrition. It is non-irritant by the intravenous route and is not known to cause hypersensitivity reactions, unlike the solvent Cremophor EL which was studied in early trials. However, its disadvantages include: (1) being an excellent culture medium if bacterially contaminated, and (2) uncertain metabolic effects of high infusion rates administered for long periods. This last has been noted in children being sedated in intensive care units and propofol must be regarded as unsafe for use in this situation, presumably related to the formulation. Finally, the emulsion should be stored below 25°C but must not be frozen and the ampoules should be shaken before use.

Propofol is supplied in 20 ml vials of the 1% emulsion for induction of anaesthesia. The usual induction dose is 1.5–2.5 mg kg^{-1}. It is also supplied in 50 or 100 ml vials for intravenous infusion; these do not contain preservative so they are specifically not for multidose use.

Pharmacokinetics

Propofol is 98% bound to plasma protein and, being highly lipophilic, is rapidly distributed to vessel-rich tissues. Its α-phase half-life is 2.5 minutes and in a two-compartment model its elimination β-phase half-life is 54 minutes. In a three-phase model the β_1 phase has been calculated as 50 minutes and the β_2 phase as 320 minutes, the long terminal phase being due to slow elimination from a poorly perfused fat compartment. Clearance has been estimated as approximately 1.9 l min^{-1} and the volume of distribution (V$_{D_{ss}}$) as 745 litres. Fentanyl modifies this figure, reducing the clearance from 1.9 to 1.3 l min^{-1}, probably because propofol levels are higher in patients pretreated with fentanyl than in a comparable control.

The main metabolite produced in the liver is the glucuronide of propofol, 88% of which is excreted in the urine and 2% in the faeces. As would be expected, renal disease has little effect on the pharmacokinetics of propofol and, because of its high metabolic capacity, moderate degrees of liver damage also have little effect.

Pharmacodynamics

Central nervous system. The onset of anaesthesia with propofol is rapid — that is, occurring in one arm–brain circulation time, as with thiopentone. The frequency of side-effects, such as muscle movements, cough and hiccough, is similar to that with thiopentone. Unlike thiopentone, it does not increase the sensitivity to somatic pain but there is no clear evidence of analgesic properties.

The dose required to induce anaesthesia in healthy adults is about 2 mg kg^{-1} but can be reduced to approximately 1.6 mg kg^{-1} after the age of 60. Opioid premedication and pretreatment with fentanyl also reduce the required induction dose.

Recovery after propofol 2.5 mg kg^{-1}, as judged by reaction times and subjective assessment of coordination, shows a faster return to control values than after thiopentone 5 mg kg^{-1}. Recovery in the early stages is also more rapid than after methohexitone, but this difference is lost by 1 hour (Fig. 13.3). In addition, propofol is not only free from emetic effects but patients are actually keen to have food.

The anticonvulsant action of propofol is less marked than that of thiopentone but it has been shown to be inhibitory against both electroconvulsive therapy (ECT) convulsions and those induced by pentylenetetrazole (an experimental convulsant). Clinically, propofol has also been used to suppress convulsions in a variety of conditions, some of them refractory to the barbiturates and phenytoin. Against these reports, there have been others showing propofol as convulsant and capable of inducing grand mal seizures in patients with no history of epilepsy. The effects of propofol on the EEG do not clarify the issue because they are very similar to those of thiopentone — that is, a general slowing of activity from the α rhythm (8–13 Hz) to the δ activity (<4 Hz), with no epileptiform changes at any stage. On the practical question of whether to use propofol for anaesthesia in ECT, opinion is also divided, but because of considerable doubt as to how the treatment actually acts on the brain, the benefits of propofol as a short acting anaesthetic probably outweigh its anticonvulsant disadvantages.

Cardiovascular system. The most striking feature of the action of propofol is the marked systemic hypotension without tachycardia. This is due mainly to a reduction in peripheral vascular resistance, which is greater than with equivalent doses of thiopentone. It is not accompanied by any increase in heart rate, unlike thiopentone, which accounts for the greater fall in blood pressure. In addition, intubation under thiopentone anaesthesia has been shown to be followed by a greater rise in arterial pressure.

Age affects not only the induction dose of propofol but also the cardiovascular response to the drug, the fall in blood pressure being significantly greater in those over 60 for the same dose. As with other drugs, this effect is also more marked with rapid injection of the drug.

The cardiac output falls during induction of anaesthesia with both propofol and thiopentone, but the decrease is significant after 2 minutes with propofol, whereas it takes 8 minutes to reach statistical significance after thiopentone. The principal factor in the decrease in cardiac output is a decrease in stroke volume for, although there is no tachycardia, there is no significant bradycardia. The cause of this reduction in stroke volume has been attributed by workers using gated nucleotide ventriculography to peripheral pooling of blood (reduction in preload). Others have identified a negative inotropic action on the left ventricle as the cause, in contrast to thiopentone, which caused minimal changes, and etomidate, which had least effect. Overall, this suggests that increased venous capacitance, decreased vascular resistance and depression of contractility all contribute to the propofol induced hypotension. It must also be stressed that, while systemic hypotension in the presence of a low peripheral resistance may be beneficial to the healthy hypovolaemic patient, it may cause a dangerous reduction in myocardial perfusion in the presence of coronary artery narrowing.

Respiratory system. Propofol is more depressant to respiration than thiopentone, often causing apnoea of 30–60 seconds. This is not a

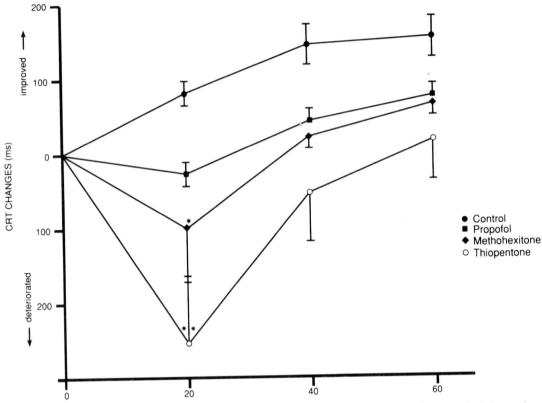

Figure 13.3 Mean (± SEM) changes in choice reaction time (CRT) from baseline, following equivalent doses of propofol (■), methohexitone (◆), and thiopentone (O), and in patients having no anaesthetic, control (●). *Significant difference from propofol. (Reproduced with permission from Milligan et al 1987 Anesthesia and Analgesia 66: S118.)

problem in clinical anaesthesia because ventilation can easily be assisted, but it does cause hypoxaemia and delays the uptake of volatile agents if ventilation is left unaided. Respiratory reflexes appear to be depressed, making tracheal intubation and insertion of the laryngeal mask easier than with thiopentone.

Local effects. Pain on injection has been noted since the first use of propofol in the Cremophor formulation. It is reported most commonly when the drug is injected into the small veins in the back of the hand but is only a problem of practical importance in children. The most effective way of minimising injection pain is to add lignocaine 20–40 mg to the propofol solution or to inject it into the vein immediately before the propofol. The former is the simpler technique and the addition does not appear to affect the stability of the emulsion. Venous thrombosis and phlebitis are uncommon with propofol, the frequency of sequelae being similar to that with most aqueous solutions.

There have now been a number of accidental intra-arterial injections and it appears that propofol has no pathological effect on the endothelium. The patient complains of pain, there is blanching distal to the injection, loss of the peripheral pulse but no harmful long term effects. Even a large dose (60 ml) infused over some hours seems to have no permanent sequelae.

Other effects. No significant abnormality has been noted with propofol anaesthesia regarding adrenocortical, hepatic or renal function. In addition, there is no evidence of histamine liberation, and the frequency of hypersensitivity reactions is similar to that with the barbiturates.

THE STEROIDS

The steroid anaesthetics (Fig. 13.4) have been studied for over 50 years since Hans Selye, in 1941, first reported the occurrence of reversible unconsciousness in rats after the intraperitoneal injection of several steroid hormones. He also commented on their general lack of toxicity — that is, their high therapeutic index. The first actual steroid anaesthetic was hydroxydione

(1955), which was freely soluble in water but had a slow onset and prolonged effect and the available solution was highly irritant to the vein wall.

More successful was the mixture of two steroids, alphaxalone and alphadolone acetate (Althesin), which had a low water solubility but had minimal effects on the cardiovascular and respiratory systems. The formulation that was introduced clinically was solubilised in Cremo-

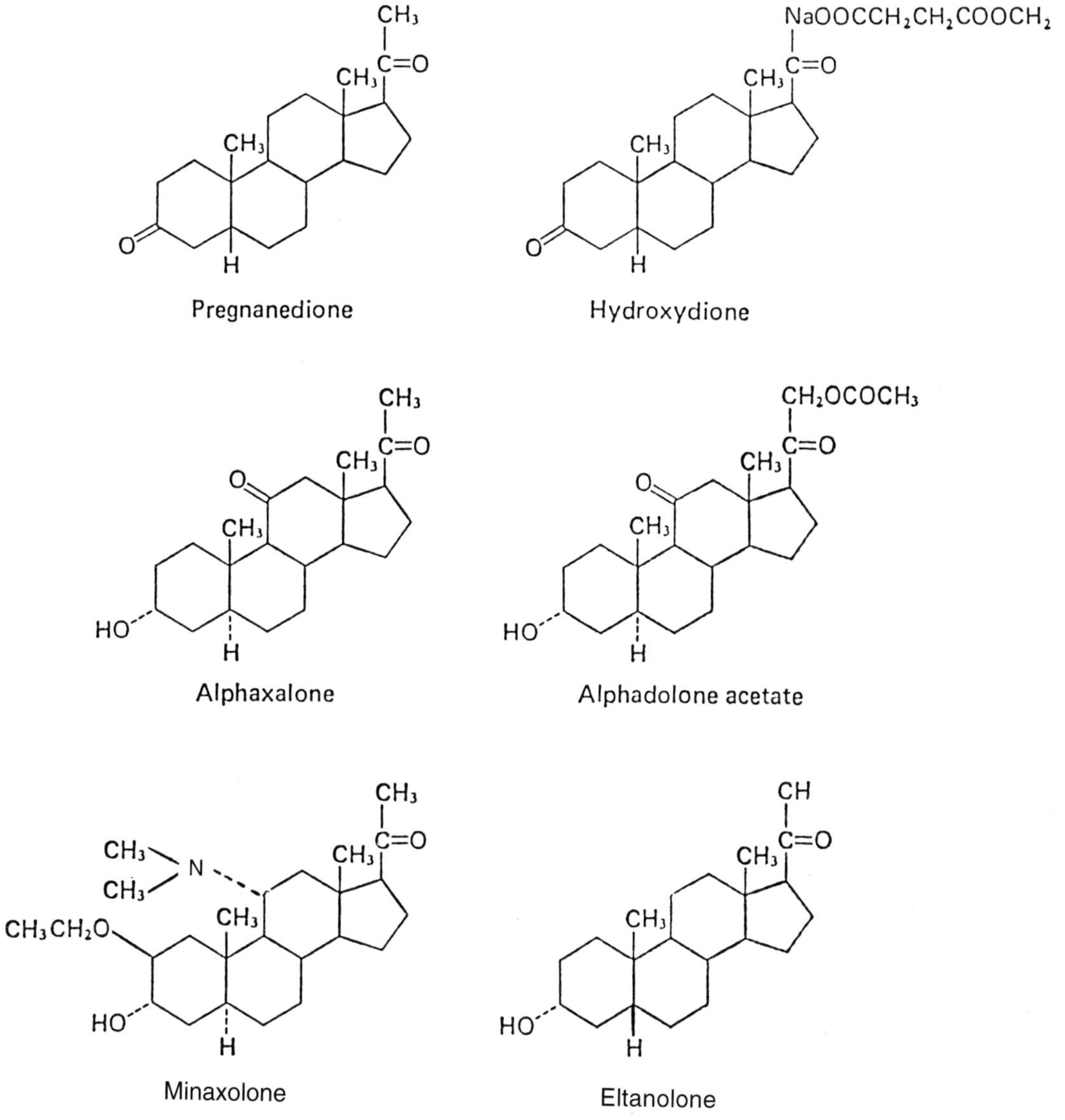

Figure 13.4   Formulae of six anaesthetically active steroids.

phor EL and, as with propanidid, the frequency of anaphylactoid reactions was high. Apart from this problem, over the period 1971–1984 it achieved wide popularity because of its lack of side-effects and the smooth recovery, and many believed that if it had been reformulated it would have continued to be used clinically.

Eltanolone (pregnenolone) has now been studied in man since 1990 and has been shown to have the highest therapeutic index of any of the induction agents studied. It is almost insoluble in water and is currently formulated as an emulsion in soya bean oil. Induction of anaesthesia is similar to that with thiopentone and, with a dose of approximately 0.6 mg kg^{-1}, loss of consciousness occurs within one arm–brain circulation time. Recovery is rapid, with minimal postoperative nausea and vomiting. Anaesthesia is accompanied by a dose-related reduction in arterial pressure and minimal change in heart rate. It causes less respiratory depression than propofol for equipotent doses. It does not cause pain on injection and no venous sequelae have been seen over the subsequent 24 hours. On the whole, eltanolone does appear to be a clinically safe drug but research on it has been slow and detailed comparative studies of its cardiovascular effects and recovery are still required.

REFERENCES AND FURTHER READING

Clarke R S J 1992 Steroid anaesthesia (editorial). Anaesthesia 47: 285–286
Cockshott I D 1985 Propofol (Diprivan) pharmacokinetics and metabolism — an overview. Postgraduate Medical Journal 61: 45–50
Dundee J W, Wyant G M 1988 Intravenous anaesthesia, 2nd edn. Churchill Livingstone, Edinburgh
Ledingham I McA, Watt I 1983 Influence of sedation on mortality in critically ill multiple trauma patients. Lancet 1: 1270
Parke T J, Stevens J E, Rice A S C et al 1992 Metabolic acidosis and fatal myocardial failure after propofol infusion in children: five case reports. British Medical Journal 305: 613–616
Sneyd R 1992 Excitatory events associated with propofol anaesthesia: a review. Journal of the Royal Society of Medicine 85: 288–291
Stanski D R, Watkins W D 1982 Drug disposition in anaesthesia. In: Scurr C F, Feldman S (eds) The scientific basis of clinical anaesthesia. Grune & Stratton, New York
White P F, Ham J, Way W L, Trevor A J 1980 Pharmacology of ketamine isomers in surgical patients. Anesthesiology 52: 231–239

14

Sedative drugs

J. P. H. Fee

Anxiety is a normal human experience, evolved to help heighten alertness in situations of danger and to help the individual manage and escape from these. It may become pathological when it is excessive or inappropriately directed, and management of this is within the domain of the psychiatrist. In anaesthetic practice, anxiety, which is quite appropriate to the patient's situation, is often counterproductive, especially preoperatively, and sedative or tranquillising drugs are prescribed to lessen this. Historically, opioids were used for their euphoriant effect, together with a number of other classes of drug, but currently benzodiazepines are by far the most common drugs used for this purpose in anaesthesia.

For convenience, this chapter will also describe briefly the other classes of drug used in psychiatry to manage anxiety and other mood disturbances, as well as some commonly used drugs with anticonvulsant properties.

BENZODIAZEPINES

The discovery of a hitherto unsuspected group of hypnotic anxiolytic drugs began in 1955 when Leo H. Sternbach synthesised the first benzodiazepine, chlordiazepoxide. Its pharmacological actions were something of a surprise when they were revealed by Randal and his colleagues a few years later. For the first time there was a drug which induced calming without ataxia or somnolence, with marked anticonvulsant properties uncomplicated by toxicity.

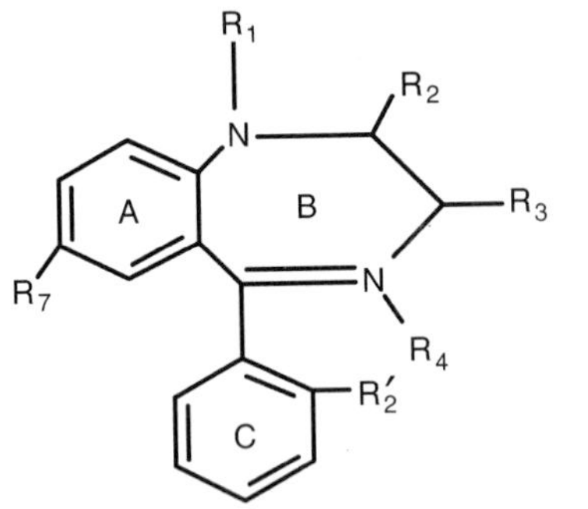

Figure 14.1 General formula of benzodiazepines.

The chemistry of this class of compound was novel and prompted extensive research, leading to the synthesis of a great many compounds. They are based on the benzodiazepine nucleus (Fig. 14.1). Three types of structure exist: (1) 1,4-benzodiazepines, such as diazepam, temazepam and lorazepam — the common feature of these compounds is the position of the Cl group in the 7 position and a phenyl group in the 5 position (Fig. 14.1); (2) substituted 1,4 benzodiazepines, such as triazolam and fosazepam, which tend to be shorter acting; and (3) the 1,5-benzodiazepines, such as clobazepam, which tend to have a more prolonged action.

Towards the end of 1959 Sternbach's group discovered a new compound, diazepam, which was up to ten times more potent than chlordiazepoxide, and this drug was introduced into clinical practice in 1963 (Fig. 14.7).

Although over 2000 1,4-benzodiazepines have been synthesised, only about 25 derivatives are available commercially. Of these only a few are formulated for injection (Table 14.1) and a small number are suitable for use in anaesthetic practice.

Table 14.1 Injectable benzodiazepine agonists

Generic name	Trade name
Diazepam	Valium, Diazemuls, Stesolid
Flunitrazepam	Rohypnol*
Lorazepam	Ativan
Midazolam	Hypnovel, Dormicum, Dobralam
Clonazepam	Rivotril, Clonoptin
Chlordiazepoxide	Librium

*Unavailable in the UK.

Pharmacodynamics

Mode of action

Benzodiazepines possess remarkable similarities in their pharmacological activities and their therapeutic use is perhaps more related to their potency and solubility than any inherent pharmacological differences.

They act on specific receptor sites throughout the central nervous system (CNS) and have a very similar range of actions on the CNS. These receptors are highly dense in the cerebral cortex, less so in the limbic structures, cerebellar cortex, thalamus and hypothalamus, and least dense in the brainstem and spinal cord. White matter is virtually free of specific benzodiazepine binding sites. Benzodiazepines act by potentiating certain inhibitory interneurones which utilise the neurotransmitter γ-aminobutyric acid (GABA; see Ch. 9). Upon release into the synapse, GABA acts on its receptor, which is part of a complex with a chloride channel, and an increase in the flow of Cl^- ions into the target neurone occurs, resulting in hyperpolarisation. The nerve cell is thus made more refractory to any excitatory impulse.

As described in Chapter 9, the chloride channel associated with the $GABA_A$ receptor is composed of (usually) five subunits, including various combinations of α, β and γ subunits. The benzodiazepine receptor is probably situated on the α subunit, and variation in the α and γ subunits leads to variation in benzodiazepine action.

Binding studies have identified three benzodiazepine receptors. Two 'central' benzodiazepine receptor types, BDZ_1 or ω_1 (omega$_1$) and BDZ_2 or ω_2 receptors, are associated with the $GABA_A$ receptor. A third benzodiazepine receptor, BDZ_3 or ω_3, is not related to the $GABA_A$ chloride channel complex; it is also known as the 'peripheral' benzodiazepine receptor, although it does occur in the brain as well as peripherally. The precise roles of the receptor subtypes is not established, but there is some evidence that action at the BDZ_1 receptor is more selective for the sedative or hypnotic effect, and that the BDZ_2 receptor contributes more of the anticonvulsant action and other effects such as ataxia. The BDZ_3

receptor plays no part in the sedative actions of the benzodiazepines.

Agonists acting at the central benzodiazepine receptors do not directly affect chloride conductance, but act by enhancing the response to GABA. This may help explain the high therapeutic ratio of the benzodiazepines, as their activity is limited to the maximal response to GABA. Despite continuing search for an endogenous benzodiazepine ligand, this has not been found, although the β-carbolines, which are endogenous substances with inverse agonist action (i.e. anxiety-promoting activity), have been considered. It is now recognised that a number of other drugs may bind to the GABA–benzodiazepine receptor complex, notably barbiturates (including thiopentone) which bind to a separate site, and some non-benzodiazepine sedatives, such as zopiclone and zolpidem, which act at the benzodiazepine site.

Central nervous system

As a group, the benzodiazepines cause a dose related depression of the CNS. Their effects range from mild daytime sedation to full general anaesthesia, depending on the dosage used and the preparation employed.

Amnesia. When given intravenously, the benzodiazepines are able to produce anterograde — but not retrograde — amnesia. With diazepam (10 mg) and midazolam (5 mg) there is a brief but very intense period of amnesia, which has mainly passed off by 20–30 minutes, while with lorazepam amnesic effect does not reach a peak until about 60 minutes and is still present by 90 minutes (see below for possible reasons for this difference). This amnesic property is useful when the benzodiazepines are used as sedation for endoscopy or for surgical procedures under local anaesthesia. Reliable amnesia is not produced after oral or intramuscular administration.

Anticonvulsant effect. All the benzodiazepines have an anticonvulsant action, although not all are used for this purpose. Differences probably relate to differential BDZ_1 and BDZ_2 receptor affinities of the drugs.

Hypnotic effect. One of the main long term clinical uses of the benzodiazepines is as a night-time hypnotic. Effective doses of these drugs reduce the amount of rapid eye movement (REM) sleep and the amount of time spent in slow wave sleep — normal subjects spend 20–25% of their time in the REM-dreaming state of sleep. The significance of this is not fully understood, but there may be a period of rebound wakefulness following the use, in particular, of very short acting benzodiazepines as hypnotics. Tolerance and dependence occur after long term use of the benzodiazepines, and this has led to clinical and medicolegal problems.

Induction of anaesthesia. Diazepam, midazolam and flunitrazepam have been used as induction agents. The claimed advantage of benzodiazepines is greater cardiovascular stability as compared with, for example, thiopentone, but this is counterbalanced by unreliability of effect and slow recovery. This use is discussed in Chapter 13.

Cardiovascular system

Even in large doses given by injection the benzodiazepines tend not to depress the cardiovascular system. There is a fall in systemic vascular resistance associated with some peripheral vasodilatation and often a slight drop in cardiac output, but this is generally of no clinical significance, although a tendency to postural hypotension could be accentuated.

Respiration

In normal therapeutic doses, oral administration of benzodiazepines does not cause respiratory depression, although in the elderly they may, like other sedatives, predispose to a degree of airway obstruction during sleep.

With intravenous injection, the rate of injection, the concomitant use of opioids and the physical state of the patient have to be taken into account. As consciousness is lost, so is sensitivity to carbon dioxide, and under different circumstances the response to a normal induction dose can vary from no detectable effect to apnoea. The usual effect would be a slight decrease in tidal volume, but this may be compensated for by an increase in respiratory rate. The dose–response curve is different from that of the opioids: while both shift the carbon dioxide response curve to the right, midazolam and diazepam flatten the slopes, indicating a less profound dose–response effect. Nevertheless, in patients with chronic obstructive airways disease the respiratory depressant effect of a benzodiazepine may be greater than in normal subjects. Particular care should be taken with midazolam in the elderly.

Pharmacokinetics

CNS and blood–brain barrier

On entering the brain and cerebrospinal fluid (CSF) the benzodiazepine receptor sites responsible for the activity of the benzodiazepines become exposed to the drug molecule. There is a good correlation between receptor affinity and duration and extent of pharmacodynamic effects.

The onset and duration of action of psychosedative drugs such as the benzodiazepines depend on their capacity to cross the blood–brain barrier — a passive diffusion process, the rate of which is directly proportional to the intrinsic lipid solubility of the drug at physiological pH. The physicochemical properties influencing the rate and extent of drug entry into the CSF and brain are lipid solubility, protein binding and the ionisation constant of the compound. Increasing lipophilicity is associated with more rapid diffusion across this interface. Although relative lipid solubilities differ (Fig. 14.2), all benzodiazepines are highly lipophilic; after a single intravenous dose they rapidly cross the blood–brain barrier and enter brain tissue. The onset of clinical sedation or anxiolysis which follows is fairly rapid, although, unlike standard intravenous induction agents, the peak effects may not occur in one arm–brain circulation time with normal doses. Highly lipophilic derivatives (diazepam, midazolam) act more quickly than those that are less lipophilic (lorazepam, chlordiazepoxide).

Diazepam and desmethyldiazepam have been shown to appear more rapidly in the CSF as compared with slower acting drugs (Fig. 14.3).

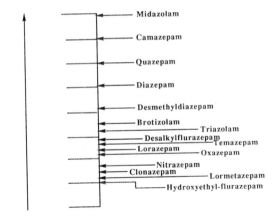

MOST LIPID SOLUBLE

Figure 14.2 Relative lipid solubility of a number of benzodiazepines. Compounds appearing higher on the list have a greater relative lipid solubility.

CSF concentrations of these compounds equilibrate with unbound plasma diazepam and desmethyldiazepam, indicating that there is no accumulation in the CSF or brain, and the half-lives of both drugs in the CSF are the same as their corresponding plasma half-lives, confirming that elimination from CSF and brain is governed by redistribution and the rate of hepatic metabolism. It would seem that CSF elimination of individual benzodiazepines might correlate better with clinical activity than pharmacokinetic values would suggest.

The duration of action varies considerably between members of the group. The more lipophilic the compound the shorter the duration of action, possibly because increasing lipophilicity increases the amount of drug taken up by fat. This, in turn, leads to the movement of drug out of blood and brain, thus diminishing its central effect. Drugs that are less lipophilic may persist in the CNS for longer because of lower intake by peripheral compartments. This has been proposed as an explanation of the apparent paradox that benzodiazepines with a long elimination half-life, such as diazepam, may, when given in a single dose, have a shorter duration of action than derivatives with a shorter elimination half-life, for example lorazepam (Fig. 14.4). The physicochemical properties of lorazepam

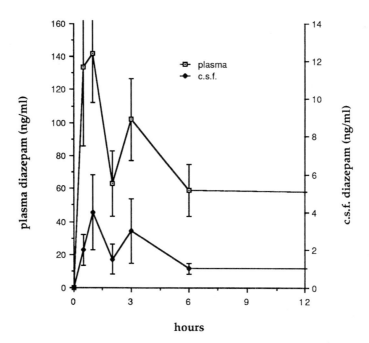

Figure 14.3 Mean (SEM) plasma and cerebrospinal fluid diazepam concentrations after a 10 mg intramuscular dose to 42 patients. (Kanto et al 1975.)

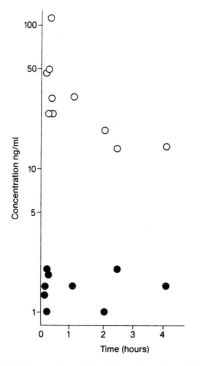

Figure 14.4 Plasma (open circles) and cerebrospinal fluid (closed circles) lorazepam concentration–time profiles. Each point represents the corresponding plasma and cerebrospinal fluid concentrations for one subject. (Aaltonen et al 1980.)

suggest that this drug may cross the blood–brain barrier less rapidly than diazepam, resulting in a slow onset of clinical activity. The CSF data shown in Figure 14.4 indicate that lorazepam may have a longer half-life in CSF than in serum. The half-life of lorazepam in plasma reflects hepatic metabolism, whereas the elimination of lorazepam in CSF may be rate limited by other mechanisms such as receptor binding. This could explain its prolonged clinical effect compared with diazepam.

Thus, traditional pharmacokinetic parameters are of limited value as predictors of onset times or duration of action of single doses of particular benzodiazepines. The elimination half-life of diazepam can range from 20 to 60 hours after a single intravenous injection, whereas the sleep inducing effect may only last for a few minutes. In contrast, the duration of effect of an equipotent dose of lorazepam ($t_{\frac{1}{2}}\beta$ approximately 12 hours), far exceeds that of diazepam. Details of the pharmacokinetic values for some benzodiazepines are given in Table 14.2.

Table 14.2 Pharmacokinetic data for some benzodiazepines (typical figures from a number of studies)

	pK_a	Oral bioavailability (%)	Protein binding (%)	V_D ($l\,kg^{-1}$)	Clearance ($ml\,kg^{-1}\,min^{-1}$)	$t_{\frac{1}{2}}\beta$ (h)
Diazepam	3.4	100	97–99	1.1	0.4	30–50
Lorazepam		93	91	1.3	1.1	14
Midazolam	6.2	48	95	1.1	7	2–2.4
Temazepam		80	97	1.06	0.9	5–15

Transport; protein binding

All the benzodiazepines are bound to plasma albumin, ranging from 40% in the case of flumazenil to almost 99% with diazepam (Fig. 14.5). It is well known that small decreases in protein binding will greatly increase the amount of unbound drug available for receptor binding and thus enhance the clinical effect. This occurs with benzodiazepines in states of hypoalbuminaemia brought about by renal or liver disease or malnutrition. There do not appear to be any serious displacement interactions arising from competition from other drugs for binding sites.

Distribution and metabolism

Following intravenous injection there is the usual initial distribution phase to vessel-rich tissues, including the CNS, kidneys, liver and heart, from where drug is distributed to muscle and later to body fat. The elimination phase is then dependent on hepatic biotransformation. Some degree of 'enterohepatic recirculation' occurs with diazepam: following biliary excretion of the drug into the gastrointestinal tract, there is reabsorption by the intestinal mucosa, which results in a second peak effect that usually occurs within about 4–6 hours after the initial administration and might be accompanied by a period of resedation. There are alternative theories for the cause of this second peak but these are less important than is the realisation that this is a common occurrence.

Biotransformation (Fig. 14.6). It is convenient to consider hepatic biotransformation of benzodiazepines as occurring in two phases: either phase I oxidation mechanisms, utilising the mixed function oxidase (P-450) system of enzymes (*N*-dealkylation or aliphatic hydroxylation); or phase II, glucuronide conjugation. These phases are distinguished by their location in the cells (hepatocytes) where the reaction takes place. Phase I reactions occur mainly in lipid-rich

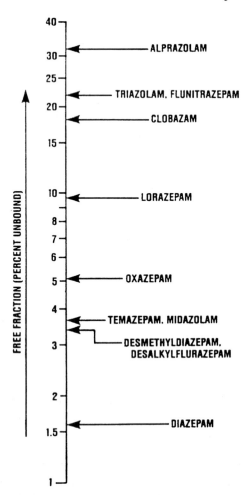

Figure 14.5 Plasma protein binding of a number of benzodiazepines.

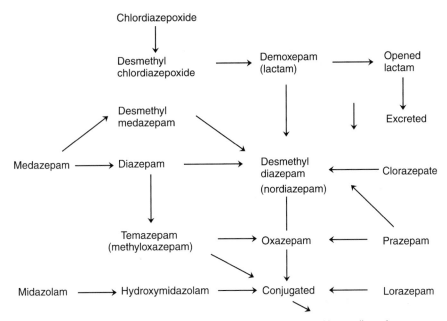

Figure 14.6 Biotransformation pathways of some commonly used benzodiazepines.

membranes such as the endoplasmic reticulum, while phase II reactions take place in the cytoplasm. The two pathways are controlled by different mechanisms. It cannot be assumed that factors which would alter the capacity of one pathway would necessarily have the same effect on the other. Phase I reactions are said to be 'susceptible' as they can be affected by characteristics such as old age and liver disease, or the concomitant use of other drugs which may impair oxidation (cimetidine, oestrogens, disulfiram). Conjugation (phase II), on the other hand, is said to be 'non-susceptible', being far less affected, if at all, by these factors.

It has been proposed, on the basis of 'in vitro' hepatic microsomal studies, that benzodiazepines undergoing conjugation rather than oxidation are the drugs of choice for the old, those with significant hepatic disease and those on drugs likely to interfere with the mixed function oxidase system of enzymes. This proposition has been supported by studies that demonstrate very little or no effect of cimetidine on the disposition of oxazepam, flurazepam and temazepam.

The elimination of the benzodiazepines follows one of the patterns shown in Table 14.3. Drugs

Table 14.3 Classification of benzodiazepines according to their route of metabolism and extraction ratios

Route of metabolism	Low extraction	High extraction
Oxidation	Diazepam Chlordiazepoxide Flunitrazepam	Triazolam Midazolam
Conjugation	Oxazepam Lorazepam Temazepam	
Nitroreduction	Nitrazepam Clonazepam	

can be considered to have a low extraction ratio when the hepatic clearance is lower than hepatic blood flow. With the high extraction drugs, liver blood flow is an important factor in determining alterations in the rate of their metabolism. Biotransformation may produce a compound which itself has some hypnotic activity, such as desmethyldiazepam in the case of diazepam. Metabolites may have longer elimination half-lives than their parent compounds, a feature that can be of great clinical importance during prolonged therapy; for example, very marked cumulation of N-desmethyldiazepam may occur during long term benzodiazepine dosage. This slowly eliminated metabolite may cause prolonged confusion and drowsiness, particularly in elderly patients.

Alterations in liver or kidney function have not been reported after use of the benzodiazepines. There is no evidence that single doses of benzodiazepines cause enzyme induction, as occurs with the barbiturates (although this does not occur with a standard induction dose of thiopentone).

Diazepam and midazolam

Pharmaceutics

A. Diazepam

Diazepam (7-chloro-1,3-dihydro-1-methyl-5-phenyl-2H-1,4-benzodiazepin-2-one) is a colourless crystalline base, insoluble in water with a molecular weight of 285. There are at least three injectable preparations: the established preparation (Valium) contains 5 mg ml^{-1} diazepam in an aqueous vehicle composed of organic solvents, consisting mainly of propylene glycol, ethyl alcohol and sodium benzoate in benzoic acid. This is a slightly viscid solution with a pH in the range 6.4–6.9. A similar preparation, Stesolid, is also solubilised in propylene glycol. An emulsion preparation (Diazemuls) contains 5 mg ml^{-1} diazepam in a lipid emulsion made from soya bean, similar to the fat emulsion used for parenteral nutrition (Intralipid). Intravenous injection of Valium often leads to venous thrombosis or thrombophlebitis, often occurring as late as the 7th–10th day, and for this reason use of the Diazemuls brand of diazepam, or of the aqueous solution of midazolam, is to be preferred for injection.

Biotransformation. Diazepam is broken down mainly to desmethyldiazepam (Fig. 14.8), a metabolite whose duration of action is considerably longer than that of diazepam, which leads to cumulation with prolonged dosing.

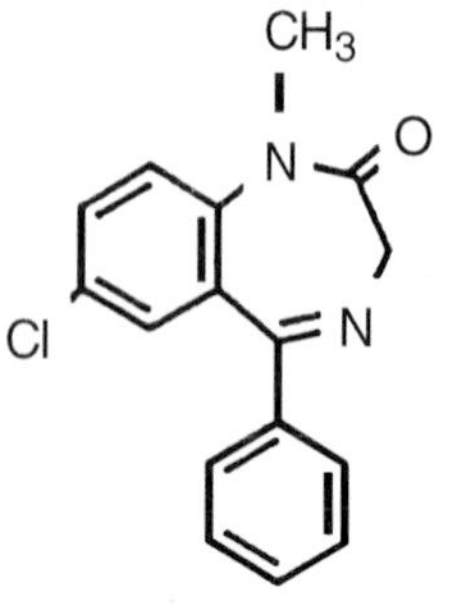

B. Midazolam

Midazolam (8-chloro-6 (2-fluorophenyl)-1-methyl-4H-imidazo [1,5-*a*][1,4] benzodiazepine hydrochloride) is an imidazo benzodiazepine derivative (Fig. 14.9). The nitrogen in the imidazole ring, which is attached to positions 1 and 2 in the diazepine ring, imparts to the molecule a higher basicity and hence water solubility, as well as a shorter duration of action than other injectable drugs. It can be prepared as a water soluble salt with hydrochloric, maleic or lactic acid and is commercially available in a stable aqueous solution as the hydrochloride salt.

Although midazolam is stable in an aqueous solution and freely water soluble, its solubility is pH dependent. As shown in Figure 14.9, the diazepine ring opens reversibly at pH values below 4, imparting water solubility. At the pH of plasma the ring closes and the lipid solubility is enhanced, this closing process having a half-life of about 10 minutes. Midazolam must not be mixed with acidic solutions.

Pharmacokinetics

The pharmacokinetic properties relevant to the fate of diazepam, midazolam, temazepam and lorazepam in the body are summarised in Table 14.2. Their disposition in the body can be described by a two-compartment open model. The greater lipophilicity of diazepam is compensated for by the increased fraction of free drug in the case of midazolam. This is reflected by a similar volume of distribution of the two drugs and by a similar onset time. The initial redistribution ($t_{½}\alpha$) is shorter with midazolam than with diazepam, contributing to a quicker, earlier

Diazepam

Figure 14.7 Structural formula of diazepam.

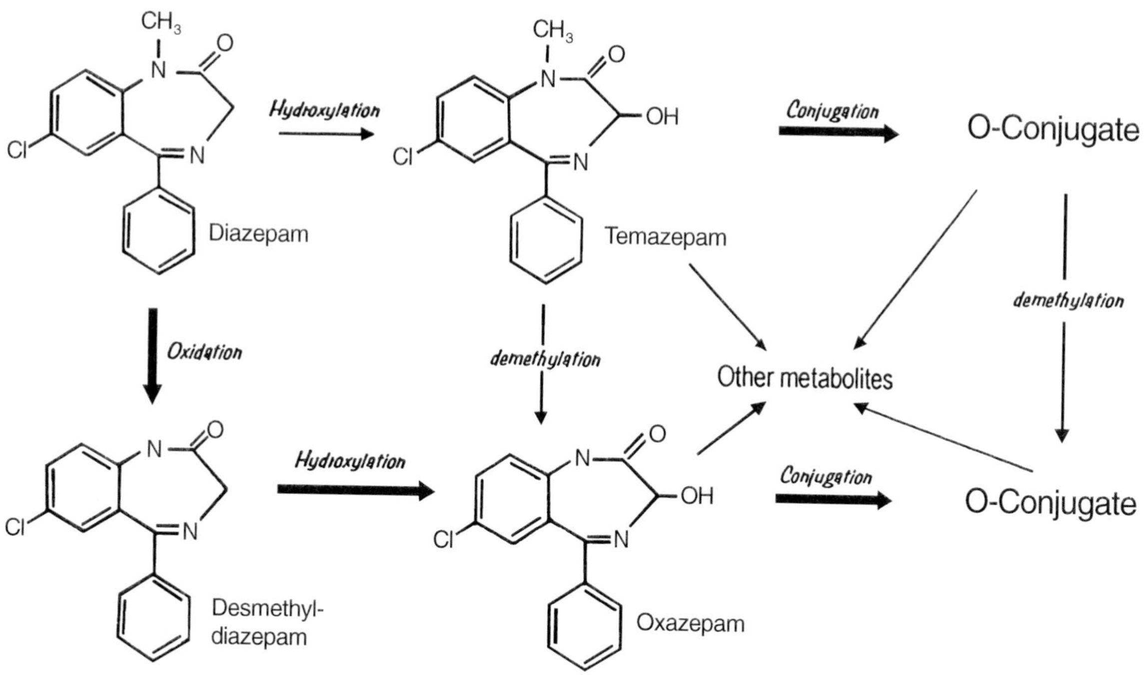

Figure 14.8   Metabolic breakdown of diazepam and temazepam.

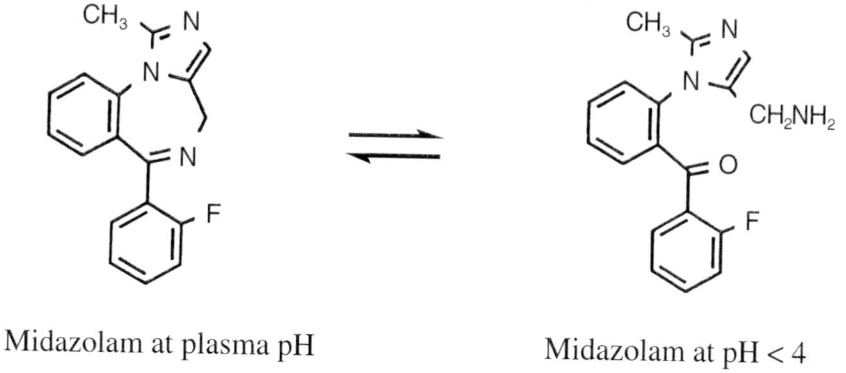

Midazolam at plasma pH

Midazolam at pH < 4

Figure 14.9   Structural formula of midazolam.

recovery with midazolam. The main site of metabolism of both drugs is in the liver; clearance is ten times faster with midazolam than diazepam, resulting in a markedly shorter elimination half life ($t_{\frac{1}{2}}\beta$) of the former.

Systemic bioavailability of midazolam after oral administration averages 44% after a 15 mg dose, although this is reduced with a dose of 7.5 mg, the low bioavailability being a consequence of extensive first pass hepatic extraction. The volume of distribution at steady state (V_{ss}) ranges from 0.8 to 1.5 l kg^{-1}; the value is greater in women than in men and in obese compared with non-obese subjects.

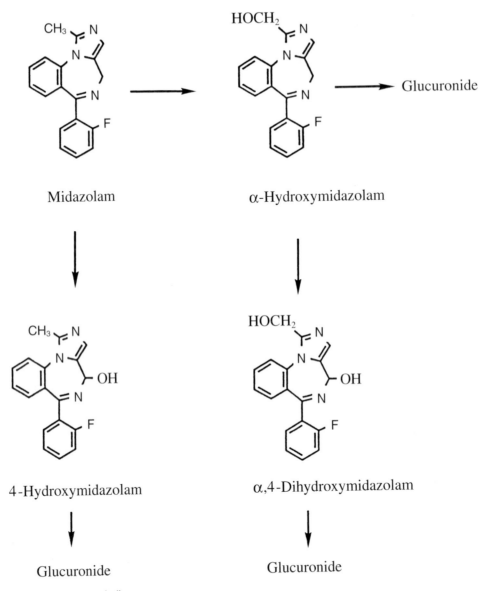

Figure 14.10 Midazolam metabolism.

The breakdown of midazolam is shown in Figure 14.10. The drug is eliminated from the body, mainly by hepatic biotransformation, and the principal metabolite is α-hydroxymidazolam. This metabolite ($t_{½}β$ = 1 hour) is rapidly conjugated by glucuronic acid. Up to 70% of a dose of midazolam is eliminated in the urine as α-hydroxymidazolam within 24 hours of administration. Two other metabolites, 4-hydroxy-midazolam and α-4-hydroxymidazolam, are excreted in very small amounts in the urine.

Plasma clearance ranges from 5.8 to 9.0 ml min^{-1} kg^{-1} in healthy volunteers but is decreased in the elderly. It has also been shown to be altered by ambulation and is increased in the evening. These alterations may be due to changes in hepatic blood flow which occur in the supine position.

The elimination half-life (Table 14.2) of midazolam ranges between 2 and 2.4 hours in healthy subjects, although this may also be considerably prolonged in both the elderly and the obese.

Temazepam

Pharmaceutics

Temazepam (4-hydroxydiazepam) is a 1,4-benzodiazepine and a minor metabolite of diazepam (Fig. 14.8). It is used mainly as a hypnotic or anxiolytic.

The physical characteristics of temazepam are such that it is extremely difficult to solubilise and no commercial preparation suitable for intravenous use has been developed. It has been available commercially in tablet, gel-filled capsule, or elixir preparations, although the capsule formulation has been withdrawn in the UK because of its inappropriate intravenous use by drug abusers. Recent problems with abuse have required it to be reclassified as a Schedule 3 drug which must be stored in a locked cupboard — some hospitals have decided to apply the stricter Schedule 2 controls for drugs such as morphine, to temazepam also.

Pharmacokinetics

The different formulations of temazepam appear to have different absorption characteristics, with higher plasma concentrations 20 minutes after the elixir than after the same dose by gel-filled capsule. Temazepam has a relatively short elimination half-life (Table 14.2) within the range of 5–11 hours in healthy subjects. In the elderly the elimination half-life is prolonged to a mean of about 14 hours.

'In vitro' temazepam is 76% bound to serum albumin and the volume of distribution in man after a single oral dose to healthy subjects has been estimated to be about 57 litres.

Biotransformation. Biotransformation of temazepam in man proceeds mainly by conjugation (Fig. 14.8), with 80% appearing as metabolites in the urine and 12% in the faeces after a single dose. Less than 2% is excreted unchanged in the urine.

Use as premedication

The rapid absorption of temazepam from gel-filled capsules or from the elixir preparation, combined with its relatively short half-life, have made temazepam a popular choice for premedication. It is particularly suitable for the old, those with impaired liver function, day care procedures and those taking other medications. Temazepam elixir is useful as an elixir premedication for children and a dose of 1 mg kg^{-1} offers a safe and reliable alternative to trimeprazine, to which it is to be preferred in this age group. There may be a place for alternative routes of administration: both aerosol and buccal preparations have been investigated.

Benzodiazepine antagonists: flumazenil

Flumazenil is a 1,4-imidazo benzodiazepine and is a competitive antagonist at the GABA/benzodiazepine receptor–chloride channel complex. Drugs that bind to these receptor complexes may have one of three types of effect: agonist, antagonist or inverse agonist. Drugs acting as agonists induce the typical anxiolytic, amnesic, sedative and anticonvulsant properties typical of benzodiazepines. Ligands that produce the opposite effects (anxiety, irritability, convulsions) are inverse agonists and these compounds are also antagonised by flumazenil. In clinical doses flumazenil is therefore a pure benzodiazepine antagonist which is largely devoid of intrinsic activity. It is now appreciated that drugs other than benzodiazepines can bind to the GABA–chloride channel complex. Flumazenil is known to hasten recovery from halothane anaesthesia but the mechanism of this is unclear.

Pharmacokinetics

Flumazenil is commercially available as a water soluble preparation for parenteral use. It is rapidly absorbed after oral administration but undergoes extensive first pass metabolism, reducing its bioavailability to around 16%. It is rapidly redistributed, attaining maximal concentrations in the brain 5–8 minutes after intravenous injection. Unlike the other benzodiazepines, only about 50% of the drug is protein bound, mostly to albumin. Flumazenil is extensively metabolised in the liver and a negligible proportion is excreted unchanged in the urine. The plasma half-life of flumazenil is less than 1 hour and it has a high clearance of about 700 ml min^{-1}.

Clinical usage

Flumazenil may be used to reverse benzodiazepine-induced sedation in circumstances where this is prolonged, for example, in over-dosage or in weaning from ventilation in intensive care. The drug is well tolerated even in very high doses and can be given by infusion for a longer effect. The standard bolus dose is 0.005–0.01 mg kg^{-1} for reversal of midazolam sedation and the drug should be administered in increments of 0.1–0.2 mg. Resedation is unlikely when reversing midazolam as the half-lives of the two drugs are similar. However, the half-lives of the majority of benzodiazepines are considerably more than that of flumazenil and in those circumstances an infusion may be appropriate at the dose of 100–400 μg h^{-1}.

Adverse effects

Side-effects are minor, with a few patients experiencing nausea or transient agitation on reversal of benzodiazepine activity. Flumazenil should not be used for patients with closed head injuries as an increase in intracranial pressure may occur on reversal of sedation. Caution should be used when prescribing the drugs for individuals on long term benzodiazepine medication or who are known to be dependent, as there is a risk of severe withdrawal symptoms.

OTHER SEDATIVES

Chloral derivatives

Chloral (chemical name 2,2,2-trichloroacetaldehyde) is an unstable compound and its derivatives are used as medicines. These include chloral hydrate, dichloraphenazone and triclofos.

The main effects of chloral hydrate are due to trichloroethanol, to which it is very rapidly reduced in the body. Triclofos is rapidly metabolised to chloral hydrate and trichloroethanol. The drugs have a depressant effect on the CNS, causing sedation, but like barbiturates there is little or no analgesic activity. They have some anticonvulsant activity, but are less effective than the benzodiazepines in this respect. They are stated to have relatively little effect on REM sleep.

In normal doses there is little depression of respiration or arterial blood pressure but in over-dose there may be severe respiratory and cardio-vascular depression.

All these compounds are well absorbed after oral administration. Distribution of chloral hydrate is rapid as it is lipid soluble. Triclofos is more hydrophilic but is rapidly metabolised, as described above, and distributes rapidly.

Chloral hydrate is metabolised to trichloroethanol in erythrocytes, liver and other tissues, mainly by alcohol dehydrogenase. Some chloral hydrate and trichloroethanol is oxidised to trichloroacetic acid but the main pathway for excretion is conjugation of trichlorethanol with glucuronic acid and excretion mainly in the urine, with a plasma half-life of around 4 hours. Trichloroacetic acid is excreted more slowly, with a half-life of around 67 hours.

Clinical usage and dosage

Chloral derivatives are considered to be relatively non-toxic hypnotic drugs, and are often recommended for sedation of paediatric and geriatric patients; the usual adult doses are: chloral hydrate 0.5–2 g, triclofos sodium 1–2 g, dichloralphenazone 1.3–2 g by mouth.

Adverse effects

Apart from gastric irritation, the main effects worth noting at normal doses are the occurrence of enzyme induction and the displacement of other drugs from protein binding sites, mainly by trichloroethanol. Thus there may be interactions with other drugs, e.g. oral anticoagulants.

Enzyme inhibition may also occur. Chronic intake of chloral may lead to tolerance, dependence and addiction, similar to alcohol dependence. In toxic doses there is depression of myocardial contractility, and both ventricular and supraventricular tachyarrhythmias may also occur. Supraventricular tachycardias have also been reported with normal doses of chloral hydrate given to children after cardiac surgery.

Zopiclone

Although not a benzodiazepine this drug acts on the benzodiazepine receptor complex and has similar pharmacological properties to the benzodiazepines. The drug is well absorbed after oral administration and it is a useful sedative/anxiolytic with a short duration of action and half-life. It is given by mouth in a dose of 7.5 mg and its main disadvantage is a persistent bitter or metallic taste.

Zolpidem

This is a short acting hypnotic drug, which, although chemically not a benzodiazepine, acts at the benzodiazepine receptor site. Unlike the benzodiazepines themselves, it is selective for the BDZ_1 (ω_1) site, which is claimed to lead to a hypnotic effect divorced from ataxia and other benzodiazepine effects mediated by the BDZ_2 site, and a reduced dependence potential. It is rapidly absorbed and metabolised to inactive breakdown products, with a half-life of 2.4 hours (0.7–3.5 hours). Zolpidem 5 mg produces somewhat less 'hangover' and psychomotor impairment on the next day after use than, for example, temazepam, and one study concluded that it was therefore suitable for use by aircrew.

Meprobamate

Meprobamate belongs to the carbamate group of tranquillisers and, as well as causing anxiolysis, it has some anticonvulsant and muscle relaxant properties. Its central effects may be due to a generalised depression of neuronal excitability.

Meprobamate is a potent inhibitor of adenosine uptake. It may exert its effects by potentiating the effects of endogenously released adenosine by reducing uptake of this inhibitory neurotransmitter.

Pharmacokinetics

Meprobamate is rapidly absorbed from the gastrointestinal tract, with peak concentrations occurring in 1–2 hours, and is widely distributed in body tissues. 90% is excreted in the urine, mainly as a hydroxylated metabolite and its glucuronide conjugate; less than 10% is found in the faeces. The elimination half-life is up to 16 hours, and is prolonged in patients with renal or hepatic insufficiency.

Clinical usage

Meprobamate is used mainly as a tranquilliser in an oral dose of 400 mg three times daily to a maximum of 2.4 g day^{-1}. Its efficacy as a tranquilliser has been questioned.

Adverse effects

These are mostly minor. Hypersensitivity reactions occur occasionally and agranulocytosis rarely. Hepatic enzyme induction occurs and it is contraindicated in acute intermittent porphyria.

ANTICONVULSANT DRUGS

These are used in the treatment and prevention of epileptic seizures. They act to reduce the excitability of abnormal neurones, and thus preventing abnormal discharges, as well as acting to inhibit the spread of such discharges from these abnormal foci. Although an action through GABAergic inhibitory pathways is of major importance, the mechanism of action of many anticonvulsants is incompletely understood. Anticonvulsant drugs include benzodiazepines (described above), barbiturates, hydantoins, carbamazepine, the branched chain carboxylic acid valproic acid, and others.

Phenobarbitone

Phenobarbitone is a long acting barbiturate with an elimination half-life in the region of 80–120 hours. Although once recommended in small (15–30 mg) doses as a daytime sedative and a night-time hypnotic (100 mg), its only therapeutic use now is as an anticonvulsant. A feature of its use is stimulation of liver enzymes (enzyme induction), and in view of the wide implications of this it should be reserved for specific use in epileptics.

Chlormethiazole edisylate

Chlormethiazole is both a hypnotic and an anticonvulsant, and also has antiemetic properties. Available evidence suggests that it enhances GABAergic transmission in the brain, by a mechanism which partly differs from that of the barbiturates and the benzodiazepines. Chlormethiazole appears to act on an allosteric site of the GABA receptor complex, which is closely related to chloride channel function. It also enhances glycine-mediated inhibition. At higher doses chlormethiazole also affects more general functions of GABA, which underlie the hypnotic effects of the drug and its action on other transmitter systems.

Chlormethiazole has little effect on the cardiovascular system, other than causing tachycardia, but in large doses some hypotension may occur. It is also a respiratory depressant at higher doses.

Pharmacokinetics

Chlormethiazole is well absorbed but undergoes extensive first past hepatic metabolism, with a systemic bioavailability of about 15% after oral administration. This effect is markedly reduced in patients with advanced cirrhosis, in whom doses may consequently have to be reduced. After intravenous administration there is rapid redistribution with a biphasic decrease in plasma concentration, with half-lives of about 0.5 and 4 hours. Following prolonged infusion the reduction in plasma concentration is slower, as it is dependent on metabolism, and half-lives of 8–17 hours have been reported.

Clinical usage

Chlormethiazole is used as a night-time sedative, especially in the elderly, in whom its rapid elimination and lack of hangover may be advantageous. Intravenous infusion of 0.8% solution may be used for sedation in the intensive care unit or during regional anaesthetic procedures, and this route is also used in treatment of alcoholic withdrawal states, eclampsia and other convulsive disorders. It may be effective in treatment of status epilepticus resistant to benzodiazepines and barbiturates. A rapid infusion (30–50 ml 0.8% solution) is given at a rate of about 4 ml min^{-1} until the patient is drowsy and the rate is then reduced. Because of its short half-life, treatment may have to be continued by infusion or orally for some time.

Adverse effects include thrombophlebitis, and haemolysis can occur if concentrations greater than 0.8% are used. Chlormethiazole inhibits the hepatic mono-oxygenase system — its effect is 10 times more potent than cimetidine.

Paraldehyde

Paraldehyde is a cyclic polymer of acetaldehyde. It is a colourless or pale yellow liquid (if darker, toxic degradation compounds should be suspected), with a powerful and unpleasant smell.

Paraldehyde is a rapidly acting hypnotic, usually causing sleep within 10–15 minutes of oral administration. In normal clinical dosage it has little effect on respiration or blood pressure, but in large doses or in overdosage, hypotension and respiratory depression occur. In poisoning, respiration is commonly rapid and laboured. Damage occurs to various organs, including the lungs; the lethal dose is probably about 50 g, but is variable. A common feature of paraldehyde toxicity is the occurrence of acidosis, presumably associated with its route of metabolism.

Pharmacokinetics

Paraldehyde is rapidly absorbed and crosses the placenta. Metabolism in the liver, where it is depolymerised to acetaldehyde and then oxidised to acetic acid, accounts for 70–80% of the drug.

The remainder is excreted unchanged, mainly from the lungs together with a small amount in the urine. Elimination is slowed, and the excretion from the lungs becomes more important in hepatic insufficiency.

Clinical usage

Paraldehyde is largely of historic interest. It has been used in treatment of convulsive conditions, including tetanus, eclampsia, status epilepticus, etc., and in management of alcohol withdrawal, and still has a limited use for some of these.

The drug is irritant, whether given orally, intramuscularly or intravenously, and nerve injury or other tissue necrosis may occur. The adult dose is 5–10 ml by deep intramuscular injection (not more than 5 ml at one site) or 4–5 ml, diluted by several volumes of normal saline, given intravenously, or the same dose rectally as a 10% enema diluted in normal saline. It reacts with plastics and must be given in a glass syringe.

Phenytoin

Phenytoin is chemically a hydantoin. It acts as a membrane stabilising agent, inhibiting voltage sensitive Na^+ channels, and probably also having an effect on Ca^{2+} channels. This affects both nerves and also cardiac muscle — its use as an antiarrhythmic drug is described in Chapter 24. Used as an antiepileptic it inhibits seizure activity without causing generalised CNS depression. It is a drug of first choice for treatment of all forms of epilepsy.

Pharmacokinetics

The pharmacokinetic properties of phenytoin are interesting. Absorption is slow and variable. It is 90% bound to plasma protein and is also bound to this extent in the tissues. Approximately 95% is metabolised in the liver. At plasma concentrations below 10 μg ml^{-1}, elimination is a first order process, with a half life of 6–24 hours. However, therapeutic concentrations are usually reached at above 10 μg ml^{-1}, with toxic effects becoming apparent a 20–40 μg ml^{-1}, and at these levels the pattern of metabolism is dose dependent (see Ch. 4), and the half-life increases with concentration and thus with dose, often being 20–60 hours. Metabolism is also subject to both hepatic microsomal enzyme induction and inhibition.

Toxicity

There is a range of toxic effects associated with long term use. When given acutely in management of cardiac arrhythmias or control of seizures, the main adverse effects are cardiac arrhythmias, hypotension and CNS depression. These can be minimised by using dilute solutions and slow injection when the drug is given intravenously.

Carbamazepine

Chemically, carbamazepine is an iminostilbene, and is related to the tricyclic antidepressants. It acts like phenytoin on Na^+ channels, but there are differences in its clinical effect, and there is also evidence of interaction at adrenergic, adenosine, 'peripheral' benzodiazepine and Ca^{2+} channel sites. It is used in management of epilepsy but also has a place in management of chronic pain.

In the pain clinic, carbamazepine is used in management of *tic douloureux* (trigeminal neuralgia), atypical facial pain, phantom limb pain and some other conditions of pathological pain. It appears to be effective in about 50% of cases of trigeminal neuralgia.

Pharmacokinetics

Like phenytoin, absorption is variable. It is metabolised in the liver, initially to an active metabolite, and has a plasma half-life of 10–20 hours, but the rate of metabolism is subject to enzyme induction, both by itself and by other drugs including other anticonvulsants.

Dosage usually starts at 100–200 mg day^{-1}, and increases to up to 1200 or even 1800 mg day^{-1}.

OTHER PSYCHOTROPIC DRUGS

Drugs are very widely prescribed nowadays to modify mental processes — up to a fifth of all prescriptions in the USA; and patients taking some form of psychoactive medication are seen daily in any anaesthetist's practice. They fall into three main groups: antipsychotic drugs used to treat major psychiatric illnesses, antidepressants for mood disorders, and sedative/tranquilliser drugs for anxiety states.

Antipsychotic or neuroleptic drugs

These are used in management of schizophrenia and other psychoses, i.e. psychiatric conditions in which the patient has an impaired grasp of reality, perhaps with delusions or hallucinations. Drugs used for this purpose include the *phenothiazines, butyrophenones* and a number of other groups. They have a wide range of actions on the nervous system, but an antagonism of the neurotransmitter function of dopamine, especially in the forebrain, is believed to be the main underlying mechanism of action. This is also responsible for the main pattern of adverse effects, particularly extrapyramidal or parkinsonism-like effects.

These drugs are described in more detail in Chapter 39, as their main use in anaesthetic practice is related to the antiemetic activity also linked to dopamine antagonism.

Antidepressant drugs

These also depend on influencing the activity of neurotransmitter substances in the brain.

Tricyclic antidepressants (imipramine, amitriptylene, etc.) inhibit the reuptake of noradrenaline into nerve terminals; they also have anticholinergic and α_1-adrenergic blocking properties. Side-effects include antimuscarinic effects, cardiac

toxicity and cerebral intoxication. These are discussed further in Chapters 50 and 51.

Monoamine oxidase inhibitors (MAOIs), which block oxidative deamination of naturally occurring monoamines, including amine neurotransmitters, are less used as they are potentially hazardous. The problems of MAOI interactions are described in Chapter 50. Older MAOIs irreversibly inactivated the MAO enzymes, but newer drugs are selective for the MAO-A subtype, and act reversibly.

Selective serotonin reuptake inhibitors (SSRIs) have become extremely popular in recent years. They include fluoxetine (Prozac) and several others. Unlike tricyclics, which can successfully treat depression but do not elevate mood in normal subjects, SSRIs do seem often to cause a 'supranormal' mood elevation, which may explain their popularity. They are much more selective in their affinity, affecting almost exclusively the neurotransmitter 5-hydroxytryptamine. Their side-effect profile is therefore much better than that of tricyclics or MAOIs. However, they do inhibit hepatic enzymes — in particular, paroxetine and fluoxetine are potent inhibitors of cytochrome $CYP_{450}2D6$, and hence may cause serious interactions with drugs metabolised by this isozyme, notably tricyclic antidepressants, some neuroleptics and some antiarrhythmics. The SSRIs also can interact with MAOIs, leading to a 'serotonin syndrome' (fever, rigidity, decreased level of consciousness).

Antianxiety drugs

These, including the benzodiazepines and other drugs, have been described earlier in this chapter.

15

Sensory function

I. C. Roddie

Human behaviour involves complex physiological responses to complex sensory inputs. Information about the environment is detected by sensory receptors and transmitted by afferent nerves to the central nervous system (CNS). The CNS analyses this information and correlates it with past experience. An appropriate integrated response is then made via efferent nerves to the effector organs, the muscles and glands. This chapter deals with the sensory arm of this complex system.

SENSORY RECEPTORS AS BIOLOGICAL TRANSDUCERS

Sensory receptors are specialised parts of sensory neurones which transduce various forms of external energy (stimuli) into action potentials for transmission to the CNS. Stimuli which excite sensory receptors include deformation, stretch, temperature change, vibration, light, change in salt concentration, etc. These stimuli, regardless of their nature, induce similar electrical potential changes called *generator potentials* in the receptors they excite. Generator potentials are small (about 5 mV) and relatively long lasting (about 5 ms). Localised to the receptor area, they are not propagated along the axon like action potentials. Unlike action potentials, which are all or none, generator potentials can summate in space and time. They induce local currents in the axon adjacent to the receptor. When the induced current is sufficient to depolarise the axon membrane to the threshold for firing, impulses are generated in the axon. These travel along the nerve as afferent impulses in the usual way. Thus generator potentials, which have graded responses, long duration, small amplitude and are localized to one area, differ from action potentials, which are all or none, large in amplitude (about 100 mV), short in duration (about 1.5 ms) and are propagated along the nerve.

Adaptation in sensory receptors

Sensory receptors may be divided into phasic and tonic types, depending on how quickly they adapt to the applied stimulus. *Phasic receptors*, such as those for touch, adapt quickly. When a stimulus is applied, the receptor responds with a train of impulses in the sensory nerve. However, the train does not persist even though the stimulus persists. Phasic receptors give more information about the rate of change of stimulus strength than about the absolute strength of the stimulus. *Tonic receptors* are the opposite. When the stimulus is applied, they generate trains of afferent impulses which persist as long as the stimulus persists. Muscle spindles, which are responsible for conscious sensation of the position of the limbs in space, are tonic receptors. They provide more information about the absolute strength of the stimulus than about its rate of change. Most receptors show mixed phasic and tonic properties.

Specificity of sensory receptors

Sensory receptors are particularly sensitive to one type of stimulus (the 'adequate' stimulus) but can be excited by others if the intensity is sufficiently strong. This means that the threshold sensitivity for their adequate stimulus is lower than for other modalities of sensory stimulus. The receptors in the eye are especially sensitive to light (their adequate stimulus) but a blow to the eye can stimulate retinal receptors and action potentials in the optic nerves. These are interpreted by the brain as light and the recipient may 'see stars'.

The threshold sensitivity of a receptor to its adequate stimulus may change. Lowering the threshold for excitation increases the apparent strength of stimulus. This occurs with respect to pain in injured tissue and is called hyperalgesia. In hyperalgesia, sensory stimuli which do not normally cause pain in healthy tissues evoke pain in injured tissues. This has been attributed to the depolarising effect of chemicals released from injured tissues holding pain receptors closer to their threshold for firing action potentials. The threshold sensitivity of muscle spindles can also be varied. Excitation of γ efferent fibres to the muscle spindles stretches the nuclear bag by contracting intrafusal fibres and brings the sensory nerve endings closer to their threshold for firing. Thus, the receptors become more sensitive to stretch.

Encoding stimulus characteristics in sensory receptors

The nerve impulses generated by a sensory receptor are similar in size and shape regardless of the modality of the stimulus and the intensity of stimulation. However, receptors encode the input and the brain interprets the characteristics of the stimulus from the pattern of impulses it receives.

Strength of the stimulus

Strength of stimulus is signalled in two ways. Stronger stimuli generate higher frequencies of impulses in the sensory nerve. To the brain, higher frequencies mean higher intensity. Another way intensity is signalled is by an increase in the number of nerve endings excited by the stimulus. Stronger stimuli affect greater areas, and thus more sensory nerve endings are recruited to respond, so that more brain cells receive signals.

Type (modality) of the stimulus

The brain interprets incoming sensory impulses which have been generated by a particular sensory nerve ending as indicating a particular type of stimulus. One sensory fibre is thus responsible for only one type of sensation. No matter how its receptor organ is stimulated, by light, heat, touch or whatever, the brain interprets impulses from it as indicating a particular sensory modality.

Location of the stimulus

The location of the stimulus is encoded in a similar way to the modality. The brain interprets incoming impulses from a particular sensory receptor as indicating a particular location. This is a remarkable cerebral accomplishment. Although conscious sensation is generated by cortical cells in the brain, the brain projects the subjective sensation to a particular location inside or outside the body. Sometimes it is projected to the site of the receptors. Skin touch is experienced at the site of receptor stimulation. However, pain generated by the gallbladder can be projected to the shoulder. Sensations may be perceived as coming from parts of the body even after they have been amputated (phantom limb pain). In vision, though the sensory receptors are situated in the retina, the sensations elicited are projected to the field of vision in front of the body. We build up pictures of familiar environments, such as our home, our car, our word processor, and any changes are instantly recognized as 'strange'.

Varieties of sensory receptors

There are many modalities of sensation, some of which enter consciousness and others which do not. All are served by specific sensory receptor organs. The conscious sensations include sight, sound, taste, touch and smell, together with muscle–joint sense, vibration sense, temperature sensation and pain. Unconscious sensory inputs come from cardiovascular stretch receptors, osmo-receptors, muscle–joint proprioceptors, stretch receptors in the lungs and the arterial chemo-receptors. Some of these modalities are served by sensory organs with specific anatomical features, such as the Pacini and Meissner corpuscles, the Ruffini end-organs, Merkel's discs, the retinal rods and cones, the hair cells in the labyrinth and the glomus cells in the arterial chemoreceptors. Others are served by end-organs that look little

more than bare nerve endings. Each sensory receptor has its adequate stimulus, the stimulus to which it is especially sensitive; however, it can be stimulated by other modalities provided stimulus strength is sufficient.

SENSORY PATHWAYS

For most peripheral sensations, three neurones in series are involved in carrying impulses from the peripheral receptors to the cerebral cortex, where sensations enter consciousness. The primary sensory neurones enter the spinal cord via the posterior root and have their cell bodies in the posterior root ganglia. Those serving muscle–joint sense and some touch pass into the posterior columns on the same side and continue up to ganglia at the top of the spinal cord. Here they synapse with the cell bodies of secondary sensory neurones. Axons from the secondary neurones cross to the opposite side of the brainstem and proceed upwards in the medial lemniscus to relay to tertiary neurones in the thalamus.

The primary sensory neurones serving pain, temperature sensation and the rest of touch also enter the spinal cord through the posterior roots but synapse with their secondary sensory neurones in the posterior horns on the same side, not far from the point of entry. The axons from these secondary neurones cross to the opposite side of the cord where they travel up in the spino-thalamic tracts to the thalamus. In the thalamus, secondary sensory neurones serving all sensory modalities, except olfaction, come together. From the thalamus, tertiary sensory neurone axons carry the sensory impulses upwards via the internal capsule to sensory areas in the cerebral cortex, where sensation becomes conscious.

Sensory impulses from different parts of the body are distributed to different parts of the cerebral cortex. Those conveying sight project to the occipital cortex and those for hearing to the temporal lobe. Impulses for touch and temperature go to the postcentral gyrus of the parietal lobe, where there is a spatial representation of the body. The arms, legs and trunk are represented in the upper part of the gyrus and the face, mouth, tongue and pharynx in the lower part. The area allocated to each part of the body is related to the richness of its sensory function rather than to its anatomical dimensions. Thus the face has more cortical area than the thorax and abdomen together.

Effect of damage to the sensory pathway

The pattern of sensory loss can be used to work out where a pathological lesion has interrupted the sensory pathway. If the loss includes all modalities, is associated with pain and paraesthesia and follows the distribution of a peripheral nerve, the lesion is in the peripheral nerve, as in peripheral neuritis. If the sensory loss does not include all modalities, i.e. is dissociated and is not associated with pain and paraesthesia, the lesion is likely to be in the spinal cord. If the sensory loss is confined to one side of the body and all modalities are affected, the lesion is likely to be in the brainstem on the opposite side. If sensation is still present but higher sensory judgement and analysis is reduced, the lesion is likely to be at cortical level on the opposite side. Damage to the cerebral cortex does not eliminate conscious sensation but impairs higher sensory judgements such as two-point discrimination and stereognosis, the ability to recognize an object by its tactile characteristics.

PAIN SENSATION

Pain is the sensation produced when impulses travelling in pain sensory nerve fibres enter consciousness. It has unpleasant qualities that make affected people withdraw from, or remove, the stimulus and teaches them to avoid situations that may cause pain in the future. It is a vital sensation and its purpose is to protect. If pain sensation is lost in a part of the body, failure to care for and protect that part leads to tissue damage. Pain also limits the ability to exercise or move the affected part. This provides injured tissues with the rest needed for repair and recovery.

Pain receptors

Pain does not result from overstimulation of

sensory nerves serving other modalities of sensation. There are specific receptors for pain and their stimulation results in pain, and only pain. Anatomically they are bare nerve endings found in almost every tissue of the body. Their density is high in skin. Discrete pain points can be identified by applying a fine pain stimulator to different areas of skin.

Although the adequate stimulus for eliciting pain varies in different parts of the body, most pain receptors can be stimulated by chemical agents released or formed when tissue is injured. Most stimuli that damage tissue excite local pain nerve receptors if they are present.

Adaptation in pain receptors

Pain receptors tend to be tonic rather than phasic, i.e. they adapt little to the stimulus and keep generating impulses as long as the stimulus persists. This maintains continuing protection for the duration of the stimulus application. In incurable diseases, where pain serves little purpose, failure of the receptors to adapt can be a problem; continuous analgesia may be required.

Threshold levels for stimulating pain receptors

Pain threshold levels vary from place to place in the body and the difference often reflects the susceptibility of the tissue to damage. The cornea has a low threshold. The threshold gets progressively higher in abdominal skin, forearm skin, soles of the feet and skin of the fingers. The threshold level also varies in the same receptor from time to time. Following injury, hyperalgesia lowers the threshold and increases pain sensitivity — for example, a slap on the back, which would hardly hurt in normal circumstances, may cause excruciating pain in skin damaged by sunburn. Hyperalgesia may be due to chemical agents released from damaged tissues persisting at the site of injury. This could hold local pain receptors in a partially depolarised state. Hyperalgesia is useful in protecting injured tissue from further damage. A person takes more care of a hyperalgesic limb than a normal one and is more motivated to rest it.

Pathways for pain sensation

Pain sensory fibres from somatic parts of the body travel in peripheral nerves, enter the spinal cord and synapse with secondary sensory neurones in the substantia gelatinosa at the dorsum of the posterior horn of grey matter. The axons of the secondary neurones cross to the opposite side of the cord and ascend to the thalamus in the spinothalamic tracts. The onward pathway for pain sensory impulses from the thalamus is not certain. Pain may enter consciousness at a subcortical level, as cortical damage does not abolish pain sensation. Collaterals from the pain sensory pathway project to the reticular activating system where they arouse and alert the brain. Other collaterals may stimulate nearby areas to produce reflex effects, such as changes in blood pressure and vomiting. Still others may stimulate the hypothalamus. This may produce the endocrine effects of severe bodily injury, which causes widespread stimulation of pain endings even though the person is unconscious.

Modulation of pain sensation

The synapses in the substantia gelatinosa can be looked on as 'gates' that modulate pain impulse traffic on its way to the thalamus. Simultaneous inputs from other sensory modalities can reduce pain impulse traffic through the synapses — for example, stimulation of touch, vibration or heat receptors over areas generating pain can reduce the apparent intensity of the pain. Counter-irritants are sensory stimulants that alleviate pain when applied to the skin over painful tissues. In acupuncture, small needles introduced and made to vibrate in the skin can also reduce apparent pain.

How these stimuli work is not certain and may involve complex interactions of peripheral and central mechanisms. There are some clues. Sensory fibres travelling in the posterior columns send collaterals to the substantia gelatinosa, where they can inhibit synaptic transmission. Impulses in these collaterals may inhibit synaptic transmission ('close the gates') for impulses running up the pain pathway and so reduce pain sensation.

Recently, endogenous substances have been identified that are ligands for membrane receptors used by morphine. These enkephalins and endorphins are natural opioids. They are polypeptides and can act as neurotransmitters. Receptors for these substances have been identified in the substantia gelatinosa. Synaptic transmission in the pain pathway may be inhibited by enkephalins released by nerve terminals at the substantia gelatinosa synapses or gates.

Substance P may be a neurotransmitter in pain C fibres. It is an 11 amino acid polypeptide found in several tissues of the body, including nerve terminals in the substantia gelatinosa of the dorsal horn. Noxious stimulation may cause substance P to be released at substantia gelatinosa synapses, causing postsynaptic excitation. Conversely, endorphins and enkephalins released from terminals in the substantia gelatinosa may inhibit this excitation, possibly by opening potassium or chloride channels, thereby hyperpolarising neurones in the pain pathway.

Higher centres in the brain can affect the apparent intensity of pain. During stress, especially involving strenuous exercise, body injury may be sustained with little pain sensation. Higher centres may modulate synaptic transmission of pain impulses by inhibition of synapses in the pain pathway by enkephalins and endorphins.

Effects of pain sensation

Withdrawal from the stimulus

The normal response to pain is to withdraw from the painful stimulus. When a noxious stimulus is applied to the foot, there is reflex withdrawal of the injured foot and reflex extension of the opposite leg to remove the hurt foot from the stimulus. This is a spinal reflex. It does not depend on pain entering consciousness; its reflex delay time is too short for that. Subsequent conscious appreciation of pain may reinforce the more primitive spinal reflex but the withdrawal reflex can occur in a spinal animal.

Increase in alertness

Painful stimuli tend to increase alertness and will

wake a person from deep sleep. This effect is the result of activation of the reticular activating system by collaterals from nerves in the pain pathway.

Autonomic side-effects

Pain is associated with various autonomic side-effects such as changes in heart rate and blood pressure which may result in fainting. Sudden vagal slowing of the heart is a characteristic response. Skin pallor, dilatation of the pupils, sweating, vomiting or diarrhoea may also occur. They are seen more commonly with deep or visceral pain than with superficial pain.

Since pain can be frightening and emotionally distressing, some of the autonomic effects could be part of a general emotional response to stress. Some pain fibres project to the cingulate gyrus, which is involved in emotional and autonomic responses, and these connections may mediate the autonomic side-effects.

Varieties of pain

Cutaneous pain

Skin is the body's first line of defence against injury and has a rich and effective pain fibre innervation. Anaesthetists know that skin has a lower pain threshold than deeper tissues. Anaesthesia deep enough to permit the surgeon to cut through the skin without awakening the patient is adequate for exploration of internal organs.

Pain receptors in skin. These are unmyelinated nerve plexuses lying superficially in the skin. They are also found in the cornea, the tooth pulp and tympanic membrane, where pain is the predominant sensation present. Skin biopsied from specific pain points contains these bare nerve plexuses.

Pathways for skin pain. There are two types of pain sensation in skin, each carried by a different type of sensory nerve fibre to the spinal cord. When skin is pricked with a needle, the first pain experienced is immediate, short, sharp and well localised. It is called fast pain and the impulses for it are carried in well myelinated Aδ fibres at a rate of about 30 m s^{-1}. Fast pain is followed by slow pain, in which the sensation is slow to develop, burning in character, relatively long in duration and less well localised. The impulses for this are carried in small unmyelinated C fibres that conduct impulses at about 1 m s^{-1}. Substance P may be involved as a chemical mediator for excitation and as a neurotransmitter in these slower nerves. When substance P is injected into the skin it causes the pain, redness and swelling characteristic of the triple response when the skin is injured.

Stimulation of pain receptors in skin. Most stimuli causing pain in the skin are noxious stimuli that injure the tissues. Chemical agents released at the site of injury are the likely adequate stimulus for the receptors. Some chemical agents elicit pain when applied to a blister base or injected into the skin. These include histamine, bradykinin, potassium ion, 5-hydroxytryptamine, substance P and nitric oxide.

Projection of skin pain sensation. Skin pain sensation is projected quite accurately to the point of stimulation — more so for fast than for slow pain. When skin is grafted to the arm from the trunk with its nerve supply intact, sensations elicited in the grafted skin are still perceived as coming from the trunk, suggesting that this projection is a learned phenomenon.

Deep somatic pain

Pain elicited from pain nerve endings in deep somatic structures differs from skin pain in being less well localised, less sharp, more prolonged and associated with local muscle contraction and autonomic side-effects.

Receptors for deep pain. The receptors for pain in deep somatic tissues, such as fascia, bone, muscle, connective tissue, periosteum, joint capsules, parietal pleura and peritoneum, blood vessels, etc., are bare nerve endings that are similar anatomically to those in skin but more scantily distributed.

Stimulation of deep pain receptors. The mechanism of excitation is not well understood. As in skin, a common denominator for excitation may be chemical agents released or formed by injured tissues. Deep pain is caused by factors that raise tissue pressure, such as an intramuscular injection. Tissue swelling causes more pain in anatomically restricted sites than in lax tissues.

In skeletal muscle, pain is elicited when muscle is exercised with inadequate blood supply, as in intermittent claudication. This pain is due to accumulation of pain-producing metabolites (the 'P factor') in ischaemic muscle. Pain gradually dies away when exercise stops as the metabolites are slowly cleared from the tissues. The nature of the pain-producing metabolites involved is not known. Potassium released from the muscle during exercise is a possible factor. Injection of potassium salts into muscle elicits pain.

Deep pain is also elicited by irritation of the parietal pleura or peritoneum by an inflamed viscus. Here the stimulus is probably a chemical formed or released as a product of the inflammation. Similar irritation of the visceral pleura or peritoneum does not cause pain. Prostaglandins probably play an important part in muscle and joint pain, which is relieved by inhibitors of prostaglandin synthesis such as aspirin.

Nerve pathways for deep somatic pain. Not much is known of the specific fibre types or pathways involved in transmitting deep somatic pain but they are probably similar to those involved in transmitting slow skin pain.

Projection of deep somatic pain. Deep pain is usually projected as a dull, diffuse ache to the general area where the impulses are generated but it may be referred to nearby skin. Deep pain causes contraction of nearby skeletal muscles, which limits movement of the tissues in the area. Irritation of the parietal peritoneum causes muscle rigidity over the site of the pain. Pleural pain limits chest movements on that side. Bone fracture causes local muscle contraction, which pulls the broken ends of the bone together. Severe deep pain is accompanied by autonomic side-effects such as sweating, nausea and cardiovascular changes.

Visceral pain

Pain arising from visceral structures is poorly localized and may be referred to distant sites. It has unpleasant qualities and is associated with autonomic disturbances.

Receptors for visceral pain. The receptors are thought to be the bare nerve plexuses scantily distributed in the walls of the intestines, mesentery and elsewhere.

Stimulation of visceral pain receptors. The exact mechanism is not clear. Normally people have little conscious awareness of what their viscera are doing. Consciousness of visceral events takes place when the tissues are made hyperalgesic by tissue damage. Electric shocks applied to the healthy gastric mucosa do not elicit pain or other sensation; however, they elicit pain and discomfort when the mucosa is inflamed or irritated. Normally, intestines can be palpated through the abdominal wall without causing discomfort, but palpation causes pain ('local tenderness') when the intestines are injured or inflamed.

When the abdomen is opened under local anaesthesia, healthy intestines may be cut, cauterised or nipped without eliciting any pain. This applies to many viscera, such as the liver and kidney. Nevertheless, in abnormal conditions, these structures can cause pain. In the intestines, pain may result from ulceration of the mucosa or distension of the bowel. The pain of peptic ulceration is closely related to the acidity of the luminal fluid bathing the ulcer. The vigorous peristaltic contractions behind an obstruction in the gut, biliary or urinary tract elicit colic pain. Pain can also be elicited by pulling on the gut mesentery.

The pain associated with myocardial ischaemia is due to the accumulation of pain-producing metabolites (the P factor) when blood supply is inadequate. Cell damage in the ischaemic tissue may also contribute.

In the cranium, the brain substance does not give rise to pain, but headache can be elicited by traction on the meninges, dilatation of the intracranial vessels or a rise in intracranial pressure. Headache, of course, can also arise from extracranial structures. Dilatation of extracranial blood vessels is important in migraine, and tension headaches have been attributed to spasm, or prolonged contraction, of the neck muscles.

Nerve pathways for visceral pain. Pain impulses from the viscera are carried to the spinal cord with the autonomic nerves. Most are carried with sympathetic nerves. Parasympathetic nerves carry those from viscera above the segmental level of the oesophagus and below that of the sigmoid colon.

Surgical interventions to cut sensory pathways are used to alleviate intractable pain — for example, cutting the splanchnic (abdominal sympathetic) nerves abolishes most of the pain sensation arising from the viscera. All pain fibres pass through the posterior roots into the spinal cord. Section of these roots (posterior rhizotomy) has been used for the relief of chronic pain at the cost of cutting off all other sensory input to the cord. Another technique is to make cuts in the anterolateral aspects of the spinal cord to sever the anterior spinothalamic tracts.

Projection of visceral pain. Pain from viscera is often felt as a diffuse ache in the midline but may be referred to somatic structures in other parts of the body. The pain in appendicitis is felt first as a colicky ache in the region of the umbilicus. Only when the parietal peritoneum is involved does it become localized to the right iliac fossa. Pain from the kidney can be felt as a dull heavy ache on the affected side or in the groin. Pain from the heart may be a midline, crushing substernal pain or be referred to the neck, left arm or abdomen. Gallbladder trouble, when it involves the diaphragm, may be referred to the right shoulder. The physiological basis of pain referral is a subject of controversy. Referred pain is usually experienced in somatic structures served by the same spinal cord segments as the viscus. It has been suggested that a sensory input from a diseased viscus increases the 'central excitatory state' in the segment of cord that it enters and that this hyperexcitability can cause impulse traffic in somatic pain sensory pathways.

FURTHER READING

Bonica J J (ed) 1990 The management of pain, 2nd edn. Lea & Febiger, Philadelphia
Cervero F 1994 Sensory innervation of the viscera; peripheral basis of visceral pain. Physiological Reviews 74: 95–138
Melzack R 1990 The tragedy of needless pain. Scientific American 262 (Feb): 27–33
Munglani R, Fleming B G, Hunt S P 1996 Remembrance of times past; the significance of c-fibres in pain. British Journal of Anaesthesia 76: 1–4

Perl E R 1984 Pain and nocioception. In: Handbook of physiology, sect 1, vol 3, part 2. American Physiological Society, Bethesda
Sinclair D 1981 Mechanisms of cutaneous sensation. Oxford University Press, Oxford
Swerdlow M (ed) 1986 The therapy of pain, 2nd edn. MTP Press, Lancaster
Wall P D 1995 Inflammatory and neurigenic pain: new molecules, new mechanisms. British Journal of Anaesthesia 75: 123–124

16

Pharmacology of pain management

J. G. Bovill

In order to understand the pharmacology of pain treatment it is necessary to appreciate the patho-physiological mechanisms underlying the pain process. Pain is the most basic and primitive of the somatic senses. It is important to understand the distinction between pain and nociception. Nociception refers to the reception and process-ing in the central nervous system (CNS) of signals originating from specialised sensory receptors (nociceptors), which provide informa-tion about stimuli that are harmful or potentially harmful to the organism. Pain is the conscious perception of a nociceptive stimulus and thus is highly subjective. While someone who is uncon-scious cannot experience pain, he or she can react to a noxious stimulus by a reflex, protective with-drawal of the stimulated part, or by increased autonomic activity.

NOCICEPTION

Receptors and peripheral nerve pathways

The primary afferent nociceptor is a bipolar neurone, with its peripherally directed axon innervating the tissues and its centrally directed axon entering the dorsal horn of the spinal cord to synapse with a variety of secondary neurones, interneurones and projection neurones. Noci-ceptors in the skin are the simplest of the sensory receptors — naked, unmyelinated nerve endings in the dermis and deeper layers of the epidermis. Two types of nerve fibres are associated with nociception, Aδ and C fibres. Aδ fibres are thin, myelinated fibres with a conduction velocity of 5–30 m s^{-1}, while C fibres are unmyelinated and slowly conducting (0.5–2 m s^{-1}). Each carry distinctive nociceptive signals. Cutaneous Aδ nociceptors are high threshold receptors that discharge only when an intense mechanical (but not chemical or thermal) stimulus is applied. This is 'first' or 'rapid' pain, a sharp or pricking pain that is felt immediately and is well localised, e.g. a skin incision or local burn. The subsequent dull, diffuse and poorly localised sensation referred to as 'second' pain is carried by C fibres. C nociceptors can be activated by mechanical and thermal stimuli and also by chemical mediators released after tissue injury or inflammation (Table 16.1). Aδ and C fibres are widely distributed in the skin and other tissues, except the brain and spinal cord. C fibres make up 80% of nociceptive primary afferents.

Tissue damage results in the release of substances that are potent activators of nociceptors (Table 16.1). Important among these is bradykinin, the most potent endogenous algogenic agent known. Bradykinin stimulates nociceptive nerve terminals directly and also sensitises them to other stimuli. Others substances released by tissue injury or produced during inflammation, including prostanoids such as PGE$_2$ and PGI$_2$ and the leukotriene LTB$_4$, sensitise nociceptors, either by lowering their threshold or rendering them more responsive to other agents. Nociceptors themselves release peptides, including substance P, which stimulate the release of histamine and serotonin. Histamine is a potent inflammatory

mediator. Serotonin (5-HT) activates nociceptors via 5-HT$_3$ receptors and also induces direct sensitisation via 5-HT$_1$ and 5-HT$_2$ receptors. Cell membrane damage results in the liberation of arachidonic acid, which is converted to prostaglandins and leukotrienes. Inhibition of prostaglandin synthesis is the basis for the analgesia and anti-inflammatory actions of the nonsteroidal anti-inflammatory drugs (NSAIDs).

Spinal pathways

Aδ and C fibres enter the spinal cord via the lateral division of the dorsal horn root. Non-nociceptive sensory information carried in Aβ fibres enters through the medial division (Fig. 16.1). Within the dorsal horn, the terminals of all three types of fibres synapse at different layers with projection neurones and interneurones. Aδ and C nociceptive fibres bifurcate upon entering the spinal cord, and branches ascend and descend for a few segments in Lissauer's tract before synapsing with neurones in the superficial dorsal horn. The dorsal horn consists of several layers or laminae, known as the laminae of Rexed. Aδ fibres terminate in lamina I and lamina V. C fibres terminate mainly in the substantia gelatinosa (lamina II). Aβ fibres terminate in lamina IV. Lamina I contains high threshold neurones that respond only to high intensity noxious stimuli and a class of projection neurones that receive input from low threshold mechanoreceptors in addition to input from nociceptors. These are the wide dynamic range (WDR) neurones which respond to increasing stimulus intensity with increasing firing frequency. A second major population of WDR neurones is found in laminae V and VI. High threshold neurones respond exclusively, and WDR neurones respond preferentially with a much greater firing frequency, to noxious stimuli.

From the dorsal horn several ascending tracts bring nociceptive information to supraspinal systems. The spinothalamic and spinoreticular tracts originate mainly from WDR neurones in laminae I, V and VI. The spinomesencephalic tract contains the axons of neurones that have their origins in laminae I and V, and projects to

Table 16.1 Endogenous substances that activate or sensitise primary afferent neurones

Substance	Source	Effect
Potassium	Damaged cells	Activation
Serotonin	Platelets	Activation
Bradykinin	Plasma kininogen	Activation
Histamine	Mast cells	Activation
Prostaglandins	Arachidonic acid/ damaged cells	Sensitisation
Leukotrienes	Arachidonic acid/ damaged cells	Sensitisation
Substance P	Primary afferent	Sensitisation

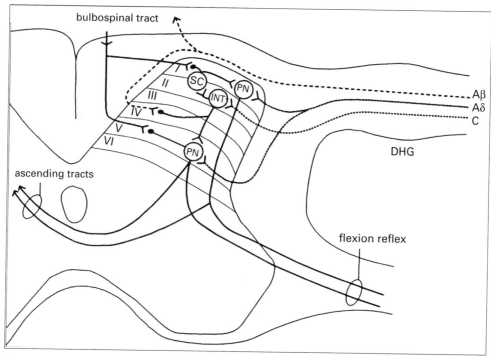

Figure 16.1   Dorsal horn of the spinal cord showing connections of afferent neurones involved in nociception. Roman numerals indicate the laminae of Rexed. PN, projection neurone; SC, stalk cell; INT, interneurone; DHG, dorsal horn ganglion.

the midbrain reticular formation, the periaqueductal grey (PAG) and other midbrain sites. The two divisions of the spinothalamic tract form the main pathway for nociceptive transmission. The neospinothalamic tract, containing fibres that have synapsed with afferent Aδ fibres, ascends directly to the ventral posterolateral nucleus of the thalamus. From there it projects to the somatosensory cortex, providing information about the quality, intensity and location of the originating noxious stimulus. By contrast the paleospinothalamic tract, which carries 'second pain' information, is polysynaptic, with numerous connections to medullary and midbrain centres. It terminates in several thalamic nuclei and then projects diffusely to limbic and subcortical areas. The projections to the limbic areas are responsible for the emotional aspects of nociception.

The dorsal horn is the primary site for the modulation and processing of nociceptive in-

formation. It is not a simple relay station but consists of a complicated set of neuronal circuits, comprising projection cells and interneurones (Fig. 16.2). Most cells in the substantia gelatinosa are locally connecting interneurones containing enkephalin and dynorphin. The dorsal horn also receives descending modulatory signals from centres in the brainstem and medulla. μ-Opioid receptors are located presynaptically on the terminals of the primary afferents and on the dendrites of postsynaptic neurones, and descending inhibition of spinothalamic neurones is mediated in part by activation of these interneurones. The interneurones of laminae I, II and III also contain a variety of neurotransmitters and neuromodulators, including noradrenaline, 5-HT, γ-aminobutyric acid (GABA), calcitonin gene related peptide (CGRP), glutamate and the peptides substance P, somatostatin and cholecystokinin (CCK).

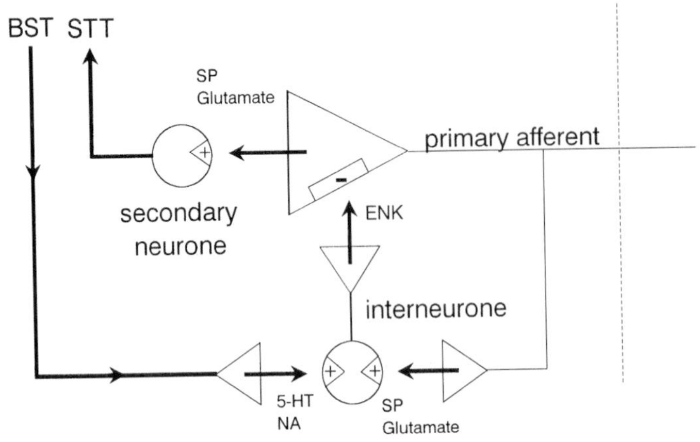

Figure 16.2 Interconnections in the dorsal horn of the spinal cord between primary nociceptive afferent fibres, enkephalinergic interneurones, descending inhibitory fibres carried in the bulbospinal tracts (BST) and the secondary neurones which transmit nociceptive information to the brain via the spinothalamic tract (STT) and other ascending tracts. ENK, enkephalin; SP, substance P; 5-HT, serotonin; NA; noradrenaline.

Neurotransmitters and neuromodulators

The primary afferent fibres release substance P, CGRP, CCK and the excitatory amino acids, glutamate and aspartate. These evoke excitation of second order neurones. Within the primary synapses glutamate excitation is mediated by non-NMDA (N-methyl-D-aspartate) receptors, most likely AMPA (α-amino-3-hydroxy-5-methyl-4-isoxazole propionate) receptors. However, the excitation of second order neurones by glutamate released by interneurones is mediated by NMDA receptors. NMDA plays a pivotal role in multi-synaptic local circuit nociceptive processing in the spinal cord.

The majority of opioid terminals in the dorsal horn are derived from local interneurones. Enkephalin neurones are mainly found in laminae I, II and V but some are also distributed in the non-nociceptive regions of inner laminae II and III. In contrast, dynorphin neurones and terminals are found almost exclusively in laminae I and V. Opioid interneurones are important in the descending control of nociceptive processing. Opioid receptors are also located presynaptically on the terminals of the primary afferents and on the dendrites of postsynaptic

neurones, and descending inhibition of spino-thalamic neurones is mediated in part by activation of these interneurones. Opioids modulate nociceptive transmission by a combination of pre-synaptic and postsynaptic actions. Presynaptically they inhibit the release of substance P, glutamate and other neurotransmitters from the sensory neurones. Enkephalins are localised in interneurones in close proximity to afferent terminals containing substance P. Substance P and opioid peptide-containing nerve terminals functionally interact in the dorsal horn as two opposing systems in the regulation of the nociceptive pathway, and endogenous opioids regulate substance P receptor activity in the spinal cord. Postsynaptically opioids decrease the amplitude of the evoked excitatory postsynaptic potentials (EPSPs) and hyperpolarise the cell (Fig. 16.3). These mechanisms are responsible for the analgesia produced by spinal opioids.

THE GATE-CONTROL THEORY OF PAIN

The inhibitory interneurones of the dorsal horn also synapse with terminals of Aβ fibres. Although Aβ receptors respond maximally to

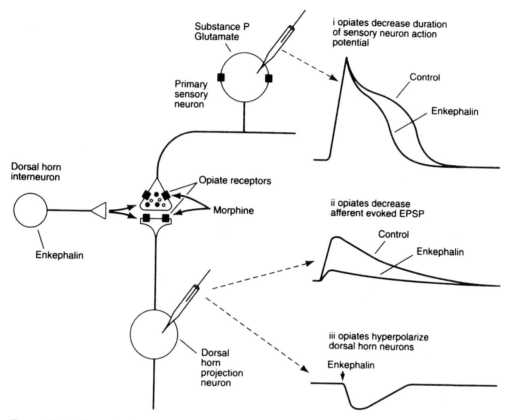

Figure 16.3 Electrophysiological analysis of the actions of opioids on sensory and dorsal horn neurones. A primary afferent neurone makes contact with a postsynaptic dorsal horn neurone. Opioids decrease the duration of the sensory neurone action potential, probably by decreased Ca^{2+} influx. Opioids may have a similar action at the terminals of the sensory neurone. Opioids hypolarise the membrane of dorsal horn neurones by activating a K^+ conductance. Stimulation of the sensory neurone normally produces a fast excitatory postsynaptic potential in the dorsal horn neurone; opioids decrease the amplitude of the postsynaptic potential. (Reproduced with permission from: Jessel T M, Kelly J P. Pain and analgesia. In: Kandel E R, Schwartz J H, Jessel T M (eds) Principles of neural science, 1991 3rd edn. Elsevier, New York.)

innocuous stimuli, they are also activated by noxious stimuli and can modulate nociceptive transmission. This is the reason why pain often can be relieved by gently massaging the skin around the injured area. The gate-control theory of pain, proposed by Melzack and Wall in 1965, was an attempt to explain this phenomenon. The essence of this theory was that the interneurones acted as 'switches' or 'gates', controlling the transmission of nociceptive information through the dorsal horn. Whether the gate was open (pain) or closed (analgesia) depended on the balance between inputs to interneurones from C fibres and Aβ fibres. Supraspinal influences on the

spinal gate were proposed but there was little evidence for the existence of descending control of nociception in 1965. This theory, although incorrect in some details, stimulated the extensive research that has resulted in our current understanding of nociceptive processing.

The effects of Aβ afferents in modulating nociceptive transmission in the dorsal horn appears to be under the control of GABA and/or glycine. GABA acts via the GABA receptor, whereas glycine binding sites are present on the NMDA receptor. GABA, the major inhibitory neurotransmitter in the CNS, is present in approximately 30% of the synapses in the CNS. GABA receptors are found pre- and postsynaptically on GABA and non-GABA terminals, including those also containing NMDA receptors. GABA is present in high concentrations in the dorsal horn of the spinal cord, in particular in the substantia gelatinosa, and $GABA_A$ receptors may play an important role in spinal nociceptive processing. Intravenous midazolam suppresses noxiously evoked activity of spinal WDR neurones, an action mediated via the $GABA_A$ receptor. Intrathecal midazolam produces analgesia in animals and humans.

DESCENDING NOCICEPTIVE CONTROL

As the sensory tracts ascend to the brain, they give off numerous collaterals to structures in the medulla and brainstem involved in supraspinal analgesia. These, in turn, send descending fibres to the dorsal horn. The main sites involved in supraspinal analgesia are the PAG located in the upper brainstem, the rostral ventromedial medulla (RVM), which includes the nucleus raphe magnus, the dorsolateral pontomesencephalic tegmentum (DLPT) and the locus ceruleus. Activation of these supraspinal systems results in descending inhibitory signals passing to the inhibitory interneurones in the dorsal horn (Fig. 16.2). The neurotransmitters primarily implicated in descending antinociception in the dorsal horn are noradrenaline and serotonin (5-HT), although many of the spinally projecting 5-HT and noradrenaline neurones contain other neurotransmitters. Among these are enkephalin, substance P and GABA.

Periaqueductal grey

The PAG plays a major role in supraspinal nociception modulation. In addition to major projections arising from lamina I neurones of the dorsal horn, it receives input from the hypothalamus, thalamus and frontal cortex. These rostral inputs are critical for initiating the powerful descending control on spinal nociceptive neurones. Major inputs to the PAG also originate from adjacent brainstem nuclei, including the locus ceruleus and other catecholaminergic nuclei. The PAG is a

main site by which higher cerebral activity can influence nociceptive responses. Electrical stimulation of the PAG produces total body analgesia without motor, sensory or autonomic block.

The PAG contains significant quantities of opioid peptides. Neurones containing enkephalins and dynorphin are intrinsic to the PAG, while β-endorphin is derived exclusively from cells in the hypothalamus. Direct administration of morphine into the PAG produces analgesia and it is likely that a significant contribution to the supraspinal analgesia produced by opioids is mediated in this area. Most of the PAG descending analgesia is not direct, but relayed via the RVM. When opioids are applied to the PAG they change the firing not only of nociceptive-modulating cells in the dorsal horn but also those in the RVM.

Rostral ventromedial medulla

This area in the lower brainstem is the major source of brainstem axons that project to the spinal cord. It receives input from the PAG and hypothalamus as well as a significant noradrenergic input from the A5 and A7 cell groups in the rostral medulla and pons. There is also a limited input from the locus ceruleus. Most of the descending fibres from the RVM are serotonergic and release 5-HT from their presynaptic endings in the dorsal horn. RVM neurones also contribute to descending noradrenergic controls, via direct projection from the RVM to noradrenergic cell groups which project to the dorsal horn. Destroying these serotonergic and noradrenergic neurones, or applying 5-HT antagonists to the dorsal horn of the spinal cord, reduces or abolishes the analgesia produced by systemic morphine. Enkephalin-containing interneurones in laminae I and II of the dorsal horn synapse with terminals of serotonergic neurones, which most likely derive from the RVM. The RVM contains many enkephalinergic neurones and microinjection of μ-opioids produces intense analgesia.

The RVM contains cells that respond in a specific manner to nociceptive signals. 'On-cells' are excited and 'off-cells' are inhibited by noxious stimuli. Both types of cells project to the dorsal horn. On-cells, which may facilitate nociceptive transmission in the dorsal horn, are inhibited by opioids administered systemically or micro-injected into the PAG or RVM. Off-cells, when stimulated, inhibit nociceptive transmission. Surprisingly, they are excited by morphine, although unaffected by direct iontophoresis of opioids, suggesting that their activation by systemic opioids is an indirect effect, secondary to inhibition of an inhibitory neurone. It is thought that opioids inhibit a GABAergic neurone that tonically inhibits the off-cell. RVM on-cells receive a significantly greater density of enkephalinergic contacts than off-cells. On- and off-cells are also present in the PAG and the DLPT.

Locus ceruleus

The locus ceruleus, located in the dorsal brainstem, and the related subceruleus nuclei are the primary origins of fibres belonging to the noradrenergic descending inhibitory system. This area receives input from the PAG and projects to the nucleus raphe magnus and the dorsal horn. Analgesia produced by stimulation of the locus ceruleus appears to be mediated by release of noradrenaline activating α_2 adrenoceptors in the substantia gelatinosa. The analgesic properties of epidural clonidine, an α_2 agonist, are explained by an interaction with spinal α_2 receptors. There are also important interactions between opioids and the descending adrenergic system. Supraspinally, opioids may activate the adrenergic system in the locus ceruleus. A synergistic antinociceptive interaction between spinally administered opioids and α_2 agonists has been demonstrated in animals, although the evidence for this in humans is less convincing.

Dorsolateral pontomesencephalic tegmentum

The DLPT lies adjacent to the PAG and shares many of its anatomical features. It receives input from lamina I of the dorsal horn and the RVM and projects to the RVM and directly to the dorsal horn. It includes the A7 region of noradrenaline-containing neurones, many of which project to the

dorsal horn. Like the RVM and PAG, activation of the DLPT by opioids or by electrical stimulation causes a reduction in the firing of nociceptive dorsal horn neurones and analgesia, as well as inhibiting nociceptive spinal reflexes.

HYPERALGESIA, CENTRAL SENSITISATION AND NEURONAL PLASTICITY

Hyperalgesia is a consistent feature of tissue injury and inflammation. In hyperalgesic regions the pain threshold is lowered and the response to suprathreshold stimuli is enhanced, so that pain is evoked by normally innocuous stimuli, such as light touch. Hyperalgesia occurs at the site of injury (primary hyperalgesia) and also in the surrounding uninjured tissues (secondary hyperalgesia). Primary hyperalgesia is characterised by enhanced pain to heat and mechanical stimuli, whereas secondary hyperalgesia is evoked only by mechanical stimuli. The increased sensitivity of nociceptors is caused by the release of chemical mediators. In addition to changes induced in the primary nociceptors, other receptor types that are normally associated with the sensation of touch acquire the capacity to evoke pain. Secondary hyperalgesia is also associated with changes induced in the CNS by continuing nociceptive input. The afferent barrage from peripheral nociceptors results in a sensitisation of second order neurones in the dorsal horn, such that input from low threshold receptors is augmented. This response can be blocked by blocking the peripheral nerve with local anaesthesia prior to the tissue damage. Preventing this central sensitisation and the subsequent cascade of changes within the CNS induced by peripheral injury underlies the concept of pre-emptive analgesia.

The hyperexcitability induced following local tissue injury or inflammation is accompanied by profound changes in synaptic activity, synaptic plasticity and neuronal modulatory processes in the dorsal horn. These changes occur over a time scale varying from milliseconds to hours or days. The initial response to injury occurs within 100 ms and in the dorsal horn involves the excitatory amino acids, glutamate and aspartate, the primary neurotransmitters of the primary nociceptive afferents. They activate the AMPA receptor, leading to the release of substance P, neurokinin A and CGRP, which are colocalised in the central terminals of primary afferent neurones. These enhance the excitatory action of excitatory amino acids, causing activation of NMDA receptors. Substance P produces a prolonged enhancement of the responses of dorsal horn neurones to glutamate or NMDA. In addition, substance P, neurokinin A and CGRP increase the release of glutamate and aspartate in the dorsal horn. The result is a persistent depolarisation of local circuit neurones. A few seconds of C-fibre input can result in several minutes of postsynaptic depolarisation. The induction and maintenance of central sensitisation is dependent on NMDA receptor activation, as is the development of neuronal plasticity associated with chronic pain, tissue injury and inflammatory states. Nitric oxide is involved in NMDA related neuronal plasticity in the dorsal horn.

In animals subjected to repeated peripheral nerve stimulation of sufficient intensity to activate C fibres, the firing frequencies of dorsal horn neurones increase with each subsequent stimulus. This phenomenon is referred to as 'wind up' and is associated with facilitation of spinal nociceptive reflexes or hyperalgesia. Repeated C-fibre stimulation can result in a sudden 10-fold increase in the response of dorsal horn neurones to a constant peripheral stimulation. Wind up is closely associated with the NMDA receptor and is selectively reduced by NMDA antagonists such as ketamine. Temporal summation of second pain in humans, the correlate of wind up in animals, is selectively attenuated by ketamine. NMDA receptor-mediated neuronal responses such as wind up are poorly responsive to opioids, although these may be amenable to increased doses or opioid administration given before the nociceptive insult (pre-emptive analgesia).

Persistent nociceptive input over many minutes or hours activates the expression of intermediate early genes (proto-oncogenes) and the expression of dynorphin and κ-opioid receptors. If the nociceptive stimulus persists for hours or days, slower processes of long term potentiation and long term alterations in the cellular architecture of the CNS structures involved in pain processing occur (structural plasticity). The activation of NMDA receptors by glutamate, and tachykinin receptors by substance P and neurokinin A, results in an increased calcium entry through ligand and voltage gated ion channels and activation of G proteins. This changes the level of second messengers in the spinal neurones. These, in turn, alter protein kinase activity, which results in a positive feedback effect on NMDA receptors, increasing their efficacy.

Increases in intracellular Ca^{2+} and activation of protein kinases result in the increased expression of proto-oncogenes such as c-*fos* and c-*jun*. These control downstream genetic programmes. The protein products of these proto-oncogenes, such as fos, are expressed in postsynaptic dorsal horn neurones after noxious stimulation. There is also an increased expression of fos in other CNS structures involved in nociceptive transmission, including the PAG, thalamus and the somatosensory cortex. They act as 'molecular switches' or 'third messengers' and are involved in the transcriptional control of genes that encode a variety of neuropeptides, including enkephalins, dynorphin and tachykinins. The fos protein couples transient intracellular signals to long term changes. Morphine pretreatment produces a dose dependent suppression of fos expression and this correlates with its analgesic effects. Neurones in the dorsal horn showing increased fos proteins after injury also have increased levels of dynorphin and enkephalin. The changes induced by c-*fos* in dynorphin synthesis may be important in the changes in spinal cord hyperexcitability. Prodynorphin-derived peptides also have a prominent function in the neuronal plasticity in the spinal cord associated with chronic pain or inflammatory processes. Dynorphin may contribute to the spinal hyperexcitability seen during peripheral inflammation by a specific facilitation of NMDA receptor activity.

A proposed sequence of events leading to dorsal horn hyperexcitability is shown in Figure 16.4. The release of excitatory amino acids from nociceptive afferents is facilitated by substance P

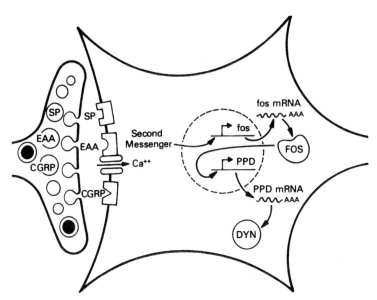

Figure 16.4 A proposed sequence of events leading to dorsal horn hyperexcitability and possible excitotoxicity (see text for a detailed explanation). SP, substance P; EAA, essential amino acids; CGRP, calcitonin gene related peptide; DYN, dynorphin; PPD, prodynorphin-derived peptides. (Reproduced with permission from Dubner R, Ruda M A 1992 Trends in Neural Science 15: 96–100.)

and CGRP, and leads to the activation of NMDA receptor sites on local circuit neurones, including those that express dynorphin peptide. The actions of substance P and CGRP at their postsynaptic receptors can result in further depolarisation. Persistent stimulation leads to activation of immediate-early genes, such as c-*fos*. The protein product of c-*fos*, fos, may be involved in the regulation of dynorphin gene transcription. Although unconfirmed, NMDA antagonists have been shown to reduce fos expression in the dorsal horn. Thus, an increase in dynorphin gene expression and peptide synthesis would occur, leading to the release of dynorphin peptide locally. Dynorphin-containing neurones have direct synaptic connections with spinal cord projection neurones, with neurones at supraspinal sites and possibly with inhibitory local circuit neurones. Dynorphin potentiation of excitatory amino acid activity at NMDA receptor sites, and substance P and CGRP facilitation of excitatory amino acid activity at presynaptic and postsynaptic sites, would affect projection neurones

and local circuit neurones and lead to dorsal horn hyperexcitability and expansion of receptive fields.

Pre-emptive analgesia

Noxious stimulation-induced neuroplasticity can lead to the persistence of pain symptoms long after the initiating stimulus has been removed. This is a characteristic of neuropathic pain, and is also relevant to postoperative pain. Surgery is associated with two phases of nociception. During surgery there is direct nociceptive input from the damaged tissues. Postoperatively, nociceptive stimuli are produced by the inflammatory reactions to the damaged tissues. The central hypersensitivity and neuroplasticity induced by this second phase can alter the patient's perception of pain in such a way that nociceptive input from the surgical wound is perceived as more painful than it would otherwise have been, and innocuous inputs may give rise to frank pain (allodynia). Sensitisation accounts for a major part of the pain experienced by patients after surgery. Central to the concept of pre-emptive analgesia is that blocking the intense afferent input to the spinal cord before surgery can prevent the occurrence of central sensitisation and reduce the impact and discomfort of postoperative pain. Further, adequate pain relief after acute trauma, by preventing the initialisation of the longer term neuronal plasticity, may help to prevent the subsequent development of the chronic neuropathic pain that some patients develop.

The effectiveness of pre-emptive analgesia has been convincingly demonstrated in animal studies. Numerous clinical trials have attempted to show the benefits of pre-emptive analgesia for surgical patients. A variety of approaches have been used, including preoperative administration of opioids, NSAIDs and regional blocks with local anaesthetics, or combinations of these. The findings of these studies have not been consistent, although most have shown that pre-emptive analgesia does provide some benefit.

Capsaicin

Capsaicin is the alkaloid that makes red chilli peppers hot. It is an irritant and algogenic substance that has been used topically as a counterirritant for a least a century, and many proprietary topical analgesic preparations still contain capsaicin or capsicum extracts. The pharmacological importance of capsaicin lies in its highly selective effects on sensory neurones, and in particular polymodal C-fibre neurones and warm thermoceptors. When capsaicin is applied to the skin or mucous membranes it causes a transient burning pain and hyperalgesia by activating and sensitising primary afferent C and probably also $A\delta$ neurones. After the initial neuronal activation, however, capsaicin can also produce a paradoxical inactivation of these same afferent neurones. It is this selective blocking of sensory neurones that has aroused recent interest in the substance for the treatment of local pain syndromes.

The mechanisms of capsaicin-induced antinociception is unclear. It acts on a subpopulation of primary sensory neurones, whose peripheral afferents are widely distributed to the skin and mucosal surfaces, inducing the release of substance P and CGRP. This accounts for the initial pain when capsaicin is applied, while the subsequent analgesia may be due to depletion of neuronal stores of substance P and a functional block of nociceptive fibres. Capsaicin causes a depolarisation of nociceptive neurones, accompanied by an increase in the permeability of the cell membrane to cations, particularly calcium and sodium ions. The membrane ion channel activated by capsaicin is unique and is insensitive to conventional calcium and sodium ion channel blockers.

Topically capsaicin is used for the management of pain caused by a diverse range of medical conditions, including postherpetic neuralgia and peripheral neuropathies, such as those due to diabetes, stump pain and trigeminal neuralgia. It is also used for some dermatological disorders, in particular psoriasis. Intranasal capsaicin relieves non-allergic rhinitis, and intravesical capsaicin has a beneficial effect on patients with neurogenic bladder dysfunction. However, while capsaicin appears to be effective, many of the reports have been poorly controlled and often involved small numbers of patients. Although treatment with capsaicin seems to be devoid of major side-effects, the initial pain when therapy is started can deter some patients from persisting with treatment.

Antidepressants and pain management

It has long been recognised that antidepressant drugs can be beneficial in the management of patients with chronic pain. The most common drugs used for this purpose are the tricyclic antidepressants. Agents such as amitriptyline are effective in the treatment of migraine, postherpetic neuralgia and painful peripheral neuropathies. Not surprisingly, many patients who suffer from chronic pain become depressed, and the changes in mood produced by these drugs contribute to their ability to ameliorate the impact of the patient's pain. Additionally, tricyclic antidepressants and monoamine oxidase inhibitors (MAOI) have direct analgesic properties independent of their antidepressant effects, although the mechanisms underlying both are probably similar. Analgesic effects are seen with doses below the antidepressant range and the onset of analgesia is faster than their antidepressant action. The mechanism of the analgesic action of the tricyclic antidepressants is not fully understood but is likely to involve 5-HT and possibly also noradrenaline. The tricyclic antidepressants act primarily by inhibiting the cellular reuptake of biogenic amines, but there is a varying degree of selectivity between the drugs for inhibition of noradrenaline compared with 5-HT. Both amines are important in nociceptive processing, and blockade of their uptake by presynaptic neurones will increase the pain threshold. The analgesic properties of MAOI is due to suppression of noradrenaline metabolism. Because of the high potential for side-effects they are seldom used in the treatment of chronic pain states.

Peripheral opioid analgesia

Traditionally, opioid-mediated analgesia has been considered to be exclusively central in origin, in the spinal cord or brain. Recently, however, it has become apparent that opioid peptides and opioid receptors are also involved in peripheral antinociception. In particular, the opioid system appears to have a novel role in peripheral inflammation, rather than direct tissue injury. Several immune cells, namely T and B lymphocytes, monocytes and macrophages, found in inflamed tissue contain significant amounts of β-endorphin and Met-enkephalin. It is likely that these peptides are synthesised within these cells. The membranes of immune cells also possess opioid binding sites, although it is unlikely that these are involved in opioid-mediated analgesia. It is more likely that opioids act via receptors on the peripheral terminals of the primary afferent sensory neurones. It is well established that opioid receptors are synthesised in the sensory neurone cell body and transported in both central and peripheral directions. All three opioid receptor types (μ, δ and κ) are likely to be present in the periphery. It is likely that inflammation increases the synthesis and the peripherally directed transport of opioid receptors.

Two explanations have been proposed for opioid-mediated analgesia in the periphery. One is that activation of the opioid receptors either attenuates the excitability of the nociceptive input terminal or inhibits propagation of the nociceptive action potentials. The second possibility is that the release of excitatory neurotransmitters such as substance P from either central and/or peripheral endings of primary afferents is inhibited. Consistent with this latter hypothesis is the observation that substance P receptors are not localised, as are most other receptors, but are distributed over most of the surface of subpopulations of CNS neurones. While most of the evidence for peripheral opioid antinociception comes from animal studies, peripherally administered opioids are being used increasingly to treat pain in human patients. In particular, the intra-articular administration of morphine appears to be effective in treating pain after knee arthroscopy.

FURTHER READING

Agnati L F, Zoli M, Biagini G, Bjelke B, Fuxe K, Benfenati F 1993 Neurophysiological aspects of pain. Anaesthetic Pharmacology Review 2: 101

Coderre T J, Katz J, Vaccarino A L, Melzack R 1993 Contribution of central neuroplasticity to pathological pain: review of clinical and experimental evidence. Pain 52: 259

Fields H L, Heinricher M M, Mason P 1991 Neurotransmitters in nociceptive modulatory circuits. Annual Review of Neuroscience 14: 219

Meller S T, Gebhart G F 1993 Nitric oxide (NO) and nociceptive processing in the spinal cord. Pain 52: 127

Pockett S 1995 Spinal cord synaptic plasticity and chronic pain. Anesthesia and Analgesia 80: 173

Schaible H-G, Grubb B D 1993 Afferent and spinal mechanisms of joint pain. Pain 55: 5

Woolf C J 1989 Recent advances in the pathophysiology of acute pain. British Journal of Anaesthesia 63: 139

Woolf C J, Chong M 1993 Preemptive analgesia — treating postoperative pain by preventing the establishment of central sensitization. Anesthesia and Analgesia 77: 362

17

Opioid drugs

J. G. Bovill

The pharmacological effects of opium, derived from the juice of the unripe seed heads of the poppy plant, *Papaver somniferum*, have been recognised for about 4000 years. Raw opium contains at least 50 active alkaloids, of which only three — morphine, codeine and papaverine — remain in clinical use. The opium alkaloids and the opioid drugs produce their pharmacological effects by interacting with one or more of the opioid receptors, mimicking the actions of the endogenous opioid peptides. Various terms are used to describe these compounds. They are often referred to as opiates, i.e. opium-like drugs. However, many of the newer synthetic compounds, although having pharmacological properties similar to that of the opium alkaloids, have chemical structures that bear little resemblance to them. For this reason the term 'opioid' is preferable for describing this class of drugs and will be used throughout this chapter. An 'opioid' has been defined as any substance, whether derived from opium, or of synthetic origin, or produced within the body, having morphine-like actions that are potently and competitively blocked by naloxone.

Structure–activity relationships

Despite an apparently wide diversity in chemical structure among the opioids, there are many basic similarities (Fig. 17.1). There are two basic opiate structures, the rigid molecules of the morphine-like alkaloids and the more flexible molecules of the phenylpiperidine drugs.

Morphine has a skeleton of five, rigidly interlocked rings bearing several peripheral functional groups. Certain portions of this pentacyclic molecule are important for pharmacological activity, whereas others play no role in activity and can be removed without altering receptor binding. The essential part of the morphine molecule is the phenylpiperidine structure (a phenyl ring connected to a six-membered ring containing five carbon atoms and one nitrogen atom). An important class of opioids is the phenylpiperidines, which includes pethidine and the fentanyl analogues.

The basic amino site in the piperidine ring is essential for opioid activity and substitution at this site profoundly alters activity. Substitution of a phenylethyl group increases agonist activity. Fentanyl is 600 times as potent as pethidine, which has a similar structure but without the phenylethyl group. Replacing the nitrogen methyl with short chain alkyl groups results in drugs that are either partial agonists or antagonists. The most effective substitutions have three-carbon chains, e.g. allyl ($—CH_2—CH=CH_2$). Substitution of an alkyl group alone results in compounds that have partial agonist properties. Nalorphine, for example, is *N-allyl*-morphine. When substitution with an alkyl group is combined with hydroxylation at the C-14 position, pure antagonists are formed — for example, naloxone differs from oxymorphone only in the *N*-allyl substitution at the C-14 position (Fig. 17.5).

A structural similarity also exists between the opioids and the opioid peptides. The enkephalins contain amino acid sequences in which tyrosine and phenylalanine are separated by two glycine molecules. Morphine is synthesised by the poppy plant from two molecules of tyrosine, and the skeletal backbone of tyrosine is evident in the morphine molecule. The structure of phenylalanine, which differs from that of tyrosine by the absence of a hydroxyl group in the phenyl ring, can be recognised in the phenylpiperidine molecule.

OPIOID RECEPTORS

Most of the original knowledge about opioid receptors derives from the work of Martin and his colleagues, who studied the behavioural effects of a variety of opioid compounds on non-dependent chronic spinal dogs. They found that morphine and allied opioids produced three distinct syndromes, which they attributed to separate receptors. They named these after the prototype agonist producing the distinct physiological effect: μ (mu) for morphine, κ (kappa) for ketocyclazocine and σ (sigma) for SKF-10 047 (*N*-allylnormetazocine). A fourth, the δ receptor, was described soon after from in vitro studies.

There is now unequivocal evidence for the existence of three opioid receptor types, μ, δ and κ. The σ receptor, proposed by Martin to explain the dysphoric effects of nalorphine, is not an opioid receptor, as actions mediated by it are not reversed by naloxone and it shows a preferential affinity for dextro rather than laevo isomers of some benzomorphans.

The opioid receptors, which are widely distributed within the central nervous system, are members of the family of guanine nucleotide binding protein (G protein)-coupled receptors. μ Receptors are most dense in those regions of the central nervous system (CNS) associated with the regulation of nociception and sensorimotor integration. The distribution of δ receptors is less extensive that μ receptors. Within the brain, κ receptors are located mainly in areas associated with nociception, such as the periaqueductal grey (PAG), and regulation of water balance and food intake. Human brains contain 29% μ receptors, 34% δ receptors and 37% κ receptors. In contrast, rat brain has 41% μ receptors, 50% δ receptors and only 9% κ receptors.

The μ receptor has two subtypes, a high affinity $μ_1$ receptor and a low affinity $μ_2$ receptor. The supraspinal mechanism of analgesia produced by μ-opioid agonist drugs is thought to involve the $μ_1$ receptor, whereas spinal analgesia, respiratory depression and the effects of opioids on gastrointestinal function have been associated with the $μ_2$ receptor. Two subtypes of the δ receptor and three subtypes of the κ receptor have been described. The full physiological significance of these various subtypes remains to be elucidated. Selective κ agonists which produce antinociception in animals may have therapeutic potential as analgesics in humans, lacking the adverse side-effects produced by the μ-receptor agonists. Unfortunately, all of the κ agonists identified until now also produce a spectrum of side-effects, including locomotor impairment, sedation, CNS disturbances and diuresis.

A major problem in studying the pharmacological specificity of the individual opioid receptors is that most tissues coexpress several classes of receptors. The recent availability of cloned opioid receptors will allow each receptor type to be examined independently. Since 1992 all three opioid receptors have been successfully cloned. The first of these was the δ receptor. This was soon followed by cloning of the κ and μ receptors. The human μ and δ receptors have also been cloned very recently. The human μ receptor contains a 409 amino acid sequence and appears to be associated with chromosome 6. The human δ receptor is a 372 amino acid protein. The human κ receptor has been isolated and partially characterised.

Endogenous opioid peptides

The natural ligands for the opioid receptors are the endogenous opioid peptides, which belong to one of three peptide families, the endorphins, the enkephalins or the dynorphins. All share a common N-terminal tetrapeptide fragment, Tyr-Gly-Gly-Phe- . . . extended with either methionine or leucine. This terminal appears to have a messenger or signal function. β-endorphin binds primarily to μ-opioid receptors whereas Met- and Leu-enkephalin bind to both μ and δ receptors, although more so to δ than μ receptors. The dynorphins appear to be the natural ligand for the κ receptors. Each of the opioid peptides is derived from distinct precursors, pro-opiomelanocortin (POMC), proenkephalin and prodynorphin, which are translation products of separate genes whose structures have been determined using recombinant DNA techniques. POMC, predominantly expressed in the pituitary but also in peripheral tissues such as the adrenal medulla, is the precursor of β-endorphin as well as several other biologically active peptides including adrenocorticotrophic hormone (ACTH) and

various melanocyte stimulating hormone (MSH) peptides.

The proenkephalin gene is expressed in the CNS and several peripheral tissues, particularly the adrenal medulla. Neurones containing proenkephalin-derived peptides can be found at virtually all levels of the CNS, from the cerebral cortex down to the spinal cord. Proenkephalin-derived peptides are involved in a variety of CNS functions, including pain modulation, processing of sensory information, motor function and endocrine modulation. Human proenkephalin contains four copies of Met-enkephalin, one copy of Leu-enkephalin and several other short peptides. The human proenkephalin gene is about 5200 base pairs long and has been localised to chromosome 8.

Prodynorphin is a precursor of several opioid peptides that contain Leu-enkephalin at the N-terminus, in particular dynorphin A and B. It is synthesised throughout the CNS, with a distribution intermediate between that of POMC and proenkephalin. The complete structural organisation of the human prodynorphin gene is known. It is localised on chromosome 20. Prodynorphin-derived peptides appear to be particularly involved in the modulation of pain associated with inflammation and tissue injury and to have a prominent function in the neuronal plasticity in the spinal cord associated with chronic pain. In the spinal cord prodynorphin messenger ribonucleic acid (mRNA) levels are markedly increased by acute or chronic inflammatory processes.

MECHANISMS OF ACTION

The endogenous opioid system has extensive physiological functions. In the CNS, it is involved in the response to stress, sexual function, water balance and autonomic control, in addition to the modulation of nociception and pain responsiveness. Endogenous opioid peptides are also involved in the control of pituitary and adrenal medulla hormone release and activity, the regulation of the immune system and cell growth. They play a distinct role in the early development of the nervous system, acting as neuromodulators and neurotrophic agents.

The actions of opioids are primarily inhibitory, brought about by altering the regulation of K^+ and Ca^{2+} ion channels. Activation of μ and δ receptors increases K^+ conductance by opening K^+ channels whereas κ-opioid receptor agonists cause N-type calcium channels to close, reducing Ca^{2+} conductance. Both result in hyperpolarisation of the cell and a reduced excitability of the postsynaptic neurone or a shortening of the action potential and then a secondary decrease in Ca^{2+} conductance. It is probable that opioid-mediated inhibition of neurotransmitters such as substance P is regulated via changes in intracellular free calcium.

Activation of an opioid receptor does not lead directly to changes in ion channels but is mediated via regulatory G proteins. These transmit the signal to effectors, which transduce the binding of an agonist to the receptor into an intracellular signal, such as changes in the concentration of a second messenger (e.g. cyclic adenosine-3',5'-monophosphate (cAMP)) or the gating of an ion channel. One result of G-protein activation by opioids is a decrease in adenylyl cyclase activity and thus a decrease in the intracellular concentration of cAMP. Adenylyl cyclase enzymatically facilitates the conversion of adenosine triphosphate (ATP) to cAMP. cAMP serves as an intracellular 'second messenger', activating and regulating specific protein kinases that catalyse the phosphorylation of various protein substrates, which may be enzyme or ion channels. However, while opioid-induced alterations in cAMP can account for modulation of neurotransmitter release (e.g. substance P), the actions on potassium and calcium channels may be mediated via a direct coupling between G protein and the ion channels or via second messengers other than cAMP, one of which may be calcium.

The inhibitory effects of opioids are mediated by G_i and possibly G_o proteins. By contrast, the G_s protein, responsible for stimulation of adenylyl cyclase activity, mediates the excitatory effect of low, nanomolar concentration of opioids on certain neurones. This excitatory effect may account for some aspects of opioid pharmacology, such as paradoxical hyperalgesia and pruritus.

Opioids and analgesia

Two anatomically distinct sites exist for opioid receptor-mediated analgesia: supraspinal and spinal. Systemically administered opioids produce analgesia at both sites. The dorsal horn of the spinal cord is the primary site for modulation of nociceptive input and involves multiple receptor types. Opioids selectively modulate 'second pain' sensation carried by C fibres but have little effect on 'first pain' carried by Aδ fibres. Opioid receptors are located presynaptically on the terminals of the primary sensory afferents entering the dorsal horn and on the dendrites of postsynaptic interneurones. Descending inhibition of spinothalamic neurones is mediated in part by activation of these interneurones. Presynaptically, opioid peptides and opioid drugs inhibit the release of substance P, glutamate and other neurotransmitters from the sensory neurones (this topic is discussed in more detail in Chapter 16). Opioids also act postsynaptically, decreasing the amplitude of the afferent evoked excitatory postsynaptic potentials and hyperpolarising the cell. Substance P and opioid peptide-containing nerve terminals functionally interact in the dorsal horn as two opposing systems in the regulation of the nociceptive pathway, and endogenous opioids regulate substance P receptor activity in the spinal cord. The effectiveness of the analgesia produced by epidurally and intrathecally administered opioids to patients is largely due to direct spinal action by opioids.

The PAG is a major site of the supraspinal component of opioid analgesia. Electrical stimulation of this area or microinjection of opioids results in profound analgesia that is reversed by naloxone, both in animals and in humans. The PAG has a very high density of μ receptors. The finding of analgesia after microinjection of morphine into the PAG was initially difficult to explain, as the PAG is not involved in the relay of afferent nociceptive stimuli to the brain. It is now appreciated that the mechanism involved is not one of ascending, but of descending, inhibition. The PAG receives an inhibitory, β-endorphinergic projection from neurones in the hypothalamus. By means of a complex interaction between various inhibitory neurones and interneurones, in the medulla and in the substantia gelatinosa of the spinal cord, afferent nociceptive transmission can be inhibited at virtually every synapse of its ascending pathway.

μ Receptors play a central role in the modulation of nociceptive stimuli and μ agonists are effective against all nociceptive modalities, such as thermal, pressure or chemical, while δ agonists produce analgesia primarily against thermal pain and κ agonists are active against chemical but not thermal noxious stimuli. Because the naturally occurring enkephalins are rapidly inactivated by peptidases they have little analgesic activity, even when injected into the cerebral ventricles. Enzyme resistant analogues such as D-Ala-2-methionine enkephalin are, however, potent analgesics. β-endorphin is more resistant to enzymatic degradation and is a potent analgesic when injected into the cerebral ventricles.

Respiratory depression

All pure μ-agonist opioids produce a dose related respiratory depression. High densities of opioid receptors are present in the lower medulla and the floor of the fourth ventricle. The primary respiratory effect of opioids is a reduction in the sensitivity of the respiratory centre to carbon dioxide so that initially respiratory rate is affected more than tidal volume, which may even increase. Slowing of the respiratory rate is largely due to prolongation of the expiratory time. With increasing doses, respiratory rhythmicity and reflexes are also disturbed, resulting in the irregular, gasping breathing characteristic of opioid overdose. Patients who have been given large doses of morphine will often breathe on command, but when left unstimulated are indifferent to respiration and become apnoeic. Other stimuli, especially pain, are also effective in counteracting opioid induced depression. In addition to retention of carbon dioxide, opioids also depress the hypoxic drive to ventilation.

Elderly patients are more sensitive to the respiratory depressant effects of opioids than younger patients and the dose used needs to be adjusted accordingly. It is also important to remember that other CNS depressants, such as barbiturates, benzodiazepines and inhalational anaesthetics, will potentiate the respiratory effects of opioids.

Cardiovascular system

The endogenous opioid system is involved in cardiovascular regulation within the CNS, in the peripheral circulation and possibly also within the heart. Opioid receptors and endogenous opioid peptides are involved in autonomic function, including the control of blood pressure, possibly via the vagus nerve and its brainstem nuclei. The afferent fibres of the vagus and the nucleus tractus solitarius and nucleus commissuralis have very high densities of opioid receptors. This also accounts for the bradycardia that may be induced by opioids.

Most of the haemodynamic effects of opioids in humans can be related to their influence on sympathetic outflow from the CNS, specific vagal effects or, in the case of morphine and pethidine, histamine release. Fentanyl and its analogues do not cause histamine release. Depression of baroreceptor reflexes by opioids may also contribute to the overall haemodynamic response.

Gastrointestinal tract

The gastrointestinal tract is the only system outside the CNS with significant concentrations of opioid receptors. This reflects the common embryonic origins of these two systems. In the gastrointestinal tract the opioid system has an important function in the regulation not only of peristalsis but also of water and electrolyte in the gut. Opioids increase the tone of the intestinal wall, while decreasing propulsive peristalsis. This results in a delay in gastric emptying and constipation or ileus. Opioids also influence gastrointestinal function via a central effect. Both mechanisms appear to be mediated via μ_2 rather than μ_1 receptors. In the biliary system, opioids increase the tone of the bile duct and decrease bile production and flow, primarily as a result of spasm of the sphincter of Oddi.

Emetic effects

Nausea and vomiting are common side-effects of opioids. Opioids initiate the vomiting reflex by stimulating the chemoreceptor trigger zone (CTZ), a specialised area of the brain located in the area postrema. This in turn leads to activation of the 'vomiting centre' located in the reticular formation of the medulla close to the area postrema. Nausea and vomiting are more common in ambulatory patients, due to vestibular stimulation of the CTZ. Opioids depress the vomiting centre, and with increasing plasma concentrations this effect overcomes the CTZ stimulant effect.

Muscle rigidity

Muscle rigidity is commonly associated with the administration of opioids. Rigidity involving the thoracic and abdominal muscles can seriously interfere with ventilation — sometimes to an extent that manual ventilation is impossible without the use of a muscle relaxant. It is most commonly observed when an opioid is given during induction of anaesthesia, e.g. during high dose opioid anaesthesia for cardiac surgery, but may manifest itself at other times, including the postoperative period. Catatonic movements of the limbs are frequently observed in patients given high doses of opioids. Delayed postoperative rigidity, interfering severely with ventilation, several hours after the end of surgery under high dose opioid anaesthesia has been reported. Muscle rigidity is reversed by naloxone and by neuromuscular blocking drugs. It is also attenuated by concomitant administration of a barbiturate or a benzodiazepine.

The exact mechanism of opioid induced muscle rigidity remains unresolved, but may involve inhibition of dopamine release in the striatum. Preoperative treatment with amantadine, a drug that stimulates release of dopamine within the basal ganglia, prevents muscle rigidity in patients given a high dose of fentanyl, suggesting a similarity between this effect and parkinsonism. The mechanism has a central rather than peripheral origin. Electromyographic studies in humans have confirmed a similar pattern of marked rigidity in all muscle groups, including not only intercostal and abdominal muscles but also forearm flexors and gastrocnemius.

Tolerance and physical dependence

Drug tolerance is a state of decreased responsiveness to the pharmacological effect of a drug as a result of prior exposure to that drug or a related drug. Physical dependence is a state, sometimes associated with drug tolerance, that comes about as a consequence of sustained exposure to a drug whereby adaptive changes occur, leading to the required presence of the drug for normal function. Withdrawing the drug or antagonising its action elicits various pathophysiological disturbances collectively known as a 'withdrawal syndrome'. In humans, opioid withdrawal initially results in restlessness and an intense craving for the drug, accompanied by yawning, running nose, lacrimation, perspiration and aches and pains. The pupils become dilated and there are associated signs of hyperactivity of the sympathetic nervous system such as hypertension and pilomotor stimulation.

It has been suggested that acute tolerance may be the result of receptor downregulation, whereas chronic tolerance may be due to a decoupling of the opioid receptor from an inhibitory G protein, which disconnects the receptor from downstream enzymatic regulation of adenylyl cyclase. Receptor uncoupling would lead to an opioid that is not functional, i.e. binding to the receptor would have no consequence for the cell. This hypothesis, however, cannot account for the profound withdrawal syndrome that is produced by administration of an opioid antagonist such as naloxone. Naloxone has no intrinsic activity; all it does is displace opioids from the opioid receptor. The marked response to naloxone in tolerant animals is evidence that the state of tolerance is one in which the opioid is still functional and the receptor remains coupled to a G protein. A more rational explanation is that the continued presence of the opioid results in the cell developing a compensatory response to opioid inhibitory effects. Tolerance to opioids after chronic receptor stimulation by agonists may cause compensatory, slowly developing increases in adenylyl cyclase activity and elevations in cellular cAMP. The overshoot produced by naloxone in tolerant animals can be explained by the sudden failure of the counterbalancing of this compensatory response by opioid inhibitory effects. This hypothesis also explains the physical dependence induced by opioids.

PHARMACOLOGY OF INDIVIDUAL OPIOID AGONISTS

Morphine

Morphine is the most abundant of the alkaloids present in opium and constitutes about 10% by weight of raw opium. The structure of morphine is shown in Figure 17.1. Morphine was first isolated in 1806 by Sertürner, who named it after the Greek god of dreams, Morpheus. Many semisynthetic derivatives, e.g. heroin (diacetylmorphine), can be readily prepared by simple modifications of the morphine molecule. Codeine (methylmorphine), hydromorphone, oxymorphone and hydrocodone are obtained by

substitution of side-chains at the C-3, C-6 or C-17 position of the morphine molecule. Morphine is an almost pure μ-receptor agonist and is the yardstick against which all other agonist opioids are measured. It is available either as the sulphate or hydrochloride salt.

Morphine is an amphoteric molecule, i.e. it has both basic and acidic properties, with pK_a values of 7.87 and 9.85, respectively. At physiological pH, however, it acts as an acceptor of protons and can therefore be considered as a basic drug. At pH 7.42 and 37°C, approximately 76% of the drug is in the ionised form. Morphine is poorly lipid soluble, with an octanol:water partition coefficient of 1.42. This is related to the presence of two hydroxyl groups that confer polar characteristics to the molecule. The low lipid solubility means that morphine cannot easily cross the blood–brain barrier. This can account for a slow onset of analgesia after intramuscular injection; however, with bolus intravenous administration influx to the brain may be almost as rapid as with more lipid soluble drugs because the drug is forced down a steep concentration gradient. As the concentration gradient dissipates, efflux from the brain becomes dependent on factors such as lipid

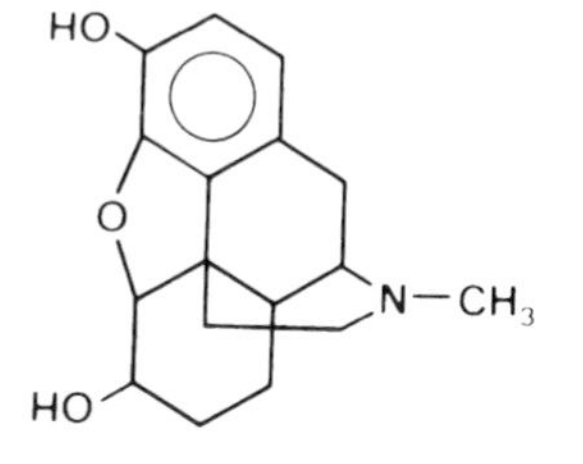

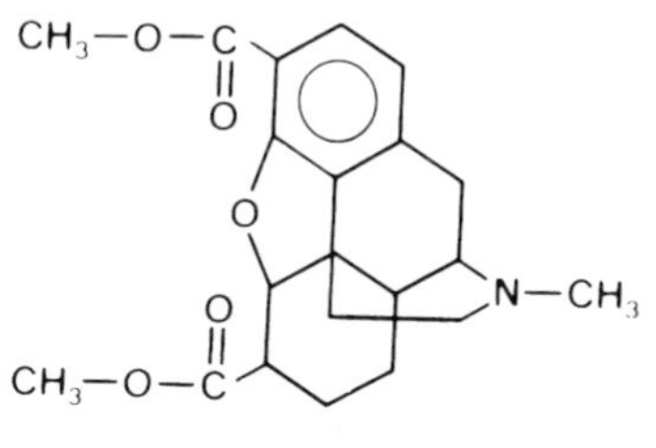

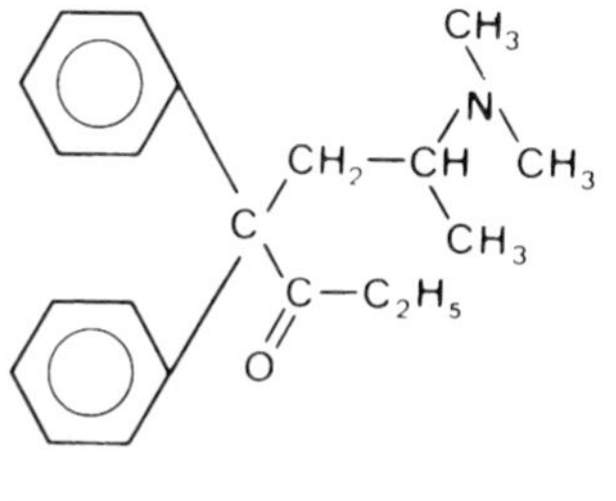

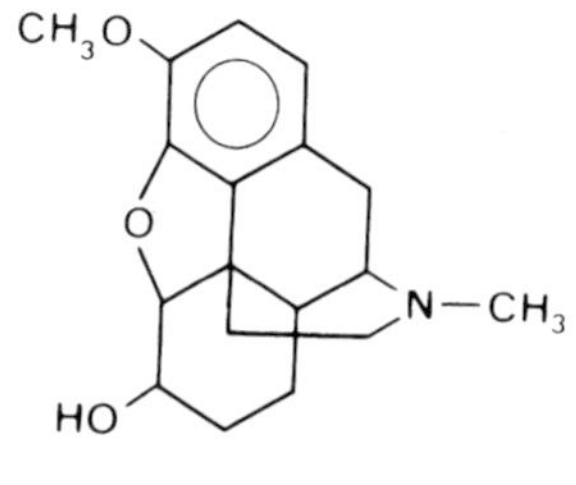

Figure 17.1 Chemical structure of morphine and allied opioids.

solubility, and so will be slower. Morphine binds for 30–35% to plasma proteins, mainly albumin.

Morphine is well absorbed from the gastro-intestinal tract, although significant presystemic metabolism occurs. The analgesia is also more variable than with parenteral administration. The oral route is useful in the management of patients with chronic cancer pain. Morphine is rapidly and completely absorbed after subcutaneous and intramuscular injection, with peak plasma concentrations reached after about 15 minutes. The usual adult intramuscular dose is 10–15 mg, which will produce analgesia reaching a peak in about 30 minutes and lasting from 4 to 5 hours. With larger doses the incidence of side-effects increases out of proportion to the increase in analgesia. The oral dose is about 50% higher than the intramuscular dose. For severe pain, for example postoperatively, it is preferable to titrate small doses, e.g. 1–2 mg, intravenously until adequate analgesia is achieved.

Cardiovascular system

Clinical doses of morphine produce minimal effect on the cardiovascular system of normal subjects in the supine position. Morphine causes release of histamine in humans, and this may be responsible for decreased systemic vascular resistance. Hypotension may be severe in hypo-volaemic patients, in whom morphine, if required, should be titrated slowly intravenously. The intramuscular administration of morphine is potentially dangerous in shocked patients because absorption can be slow and unpredictable as a result of low muscle blood flow. Subsequent resuscitation and improvement in muscle blood flow may then result in a sudden increase in plasma morphine concentration.

Morphine is a valuable drug in the management of patients with acute left ventricular failure. Part of this beneficial effect is due to the sedation and alleviation of fear that it produces. More important, however, may be its peripheral vascular effects. Reduction in systemic vascular resistance, and particularly the increase in venous capacitance, by reducing both preload and afterload, will allow the left ventricle to function more efficiently.

Central nervous system

Central nervous system depression is the usual effect of morphine, and sedation and drowsiness are frequently observed with therapeutic doses. Euphoria, an unrealistic sense of well-being, a manifestation of a limbic system effect, is common and may be largely responsible for the abuse potential of morphine-like drugs. An important aspect of morphine's pain relieving ability is the alteration that it produces in the subject's attitude to pain — it is still perceived but fails to elicit the former unpleasant response. When given in the absence of pain, morphine may sometimes produce dysphoria — an unpleasant sensation of fear and anxiety. Some animals, e.g. cats, pigs and horses, react to morphine by excitation leading to convulsion rather than depression. Excitatory effects are rare in humans given even large doses of morphine, but are seen with pethidine. The most important stimulatory effects of morphine in humans are emesis and miosis. Miosis occurs with all morphine-like drugs and is due to stimulation of the Edinger–Westphal nucleus of the third nerve. The combination of pinpoint pupils, coma and respiratory depression are classical signs of morphine overdosage. Stimulation of the solitary nuclei may also be responsible for depression of the cough reflex (antitussive effect).

Epidural and subarachnoid morphine

The realisation that opioid receptors and enkephalin-containing neurones in the spinal cord played a major role in opioid analgesia led to a widespread interest in the intrathecal and epidural administration of morphine. Intrathecal administration has the advantage that the drug is deposited close to its site of action. This reduces the total dose required (about one-tenth of the epidural dose) and the time to maximum effect. The optimal dose appears to be 0.5–1 mg, although doses as low as 0.1–0.5 mg can provide excellent postoperative analgesia. The onset of analgesia is slow, 20–30 minutes. The limiting factor is the speed of penetration from the water phase of the cerebrospinal fluid (CSF) to the lipid phase of the neural tissue. Morphine, being poorly lipid soluble, tends to remain in the CSF. The duration of the analgesia produced by intrathecal administration of opioids is, in contrast, inversely related to lipid solubility. Drugs such as morphine cross lipid barriers with difficulty — i.e. they take a long time to enter neural cells but once they have arrived also have difficulty in leaving. The duration of analgesia with spinal morphine is 14–20 hours.

Morphine administered via the epidural space has an extra barrier to cross before it reaches the CSF. Larger doses are therefore required than with intrathecal administration. Commonly used doses are 2.5–10 mg, diluted in 10 ml normal saline. The latency of onset of analgesia is about 35–45 minutes. Systemic uptake can result in blood morphine concentrations similar to those seen with intramuscular injections of the same dose. Some of the reported adverse effects of intrathecal and epidural morphine, and other opioids, such as nausea, vomiting, sedation and early respiratory depression, are dose related and in part are a consequence of systemic vascular uptake of the opioid.

The side-effects and complications tend to be higher with the intrathecal than the epidural route. One of the most common side-effects is pruritus, the incidence of which is higher with morphine than with other opioids, and is higher with intrathecal than with epidural administration. It is dose dependent, with an incidence of about 10% after epidural morphine 5 mg. The risk of severe, distressing itching is about 1%. Pruritus most commonly affects the head and trunk region initially, but may spread to all areas of the body and begins about 3 hours after injection. It may be related to cephalad spread of morphine within the CSF. Prophylactic naloxone infusion at a rate of 5 μg kg^{-1} h^{-1} will reduce the frequency of pruritus without reversing analgesia. A small, 10 mg, intravenous dose of propofol may be equally effective.

Rostral spread is largely responsible for emetic symptoms and respiratory depression. Nausea and vomiting has a reported incidence of up to 75% and again is worse with intrathecal than epidural morphine. The incidence of respiratory depression is low (0.25–0.5%) with epidural morphine but is potentially the most serious complication with these routes and is frequently delayed until several hours after drug administration. It can be profound and long lasting. The other important side-effect is urinary retention, with an overall incidence of about 40%. It can develop insidiously and, as bladder sensation is partially or wholly lost, may not be reported by the patient until gross overdistension of the bladder has occurred. Although administration of parasympathetic agents has been recommended as the first line of treatment of retention, there is a high failure rate. Naloxone, 0.4 mg intravenously, will immediately restore normal micturition but will also reverse analgesia.

There has been speculation that pruritus after epidural morphine may reactivate herpes simplex in pregnant patients. Epidural pethidine has also been reported to reactivate herpes simplex. Most cases occur around the nose and mouth. The aetiology is unclear but may be due to the virus being reactivated as a consequence of mechanical irritation of sensory nerves in response to facial itching. Alternatively it may be related to rostral spread of morphine in the CSF and consequent high concentrations of morphine in the substantia gelatinosa of the trigeminal nerve. Herpes simplex after delivery is potentially dangerous because of the risk of herpes encephalitis in the infant. Spinal opioids should therefore be avoided in the parturient with a history of recurrent herpes simplex.

Pharmacokinetics and metabolism

Morphine undergoes extensive hepatic biotransformation and less than 10% of a parenterally administered dose is excreted unchanged in the urine. Because of the high hepatic first pass effect the dose of oral morphine required to produce a therapeutic effect is about 50% larger than with parenteral administration. The terminal elimination half-life of morphine is relatively short (2–4 hours) in comparison to fentanyl or pethidine.

Table 17.1   Pharmacokinetic parameters for the opioid agonists

	pK_a	Unionised (%)	Lipid solubility (λ_{ow})	Protein binding (%)	Bound to AAG (%)	Cl (ml min^{-1})	V_{dss} (litre)	$t_{\frac{1}{2}\lambda z}$ (h)
Morphine	7.9	24	1.4	35	<20	1200	200	1.7
Methadone	8.3	5.9	57*	85	80	178	410	35
Pethidine	8.6	7.4	39	70	60	1020	260	48
Fentanyl	8.4	9.1	816	84	44	1530	335	3.6
Alfentanil	6.5	88.8	128	92	92	238	27	1.6
Sufentanil	8.0	19.7	1757	93	83	900	123	2.8

λ_{ow}: octanol-water partition coefficient. A measure of lipid solubility. $t_{\frac{1}{2}\lambda z}$: terminal elimination half-life. Cl, clearance; V_{dss}, volume of distribution at steady state; *l isomer; λ_{ow} of the d isomer is 28.

Unlike fentanyl or pethidine, plasma morphine concentrations are poorly correlated with pharmacological response, owing to the very low lipid solubility. The most important pharmacokinetic parameters for morphine and other agonist opioids are reproduced in Table 17.1.

The major metabolic route for morphine biotransformation is by phase II conjugation. About 70% undergoes conjugation to morphine-3-glucuronide (M3G), the major metabolite, 5–10% to morphine-6-glucuronide (M6G), and the remainder undergoes sulphate conjugation. About 1–2% is excreted by the kidneys as unconjugated drug. Although the liver is the primary organ of conjugation, extrahepatic metabolism of morphine

may occur. Conjugation of morphine to glucuronide has been demonstrated in the kidneys.

M3G has no analgesic activity but may antagonise the analgesic effects of morphine. M6G is pharmacologically active, with a potency higher than morphine. Despite its polarity M6G can cross the blood–brain barrier, and is found in the CSF within 2 hours of a parenteral dose of morphine. It is eliminated more slowly than morphine from the CSF, with an average half-life of 10.5 hours. M6G occurs in significant quantities after administration of morphine and its concentration in plasma exceeds that of the parent drug by a factor of 9 within 30 minutes of intravenous administration of morphine (Fig. 17.2). It

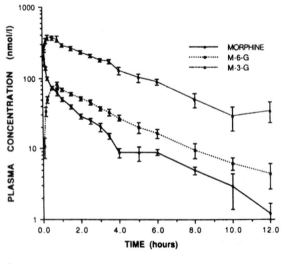

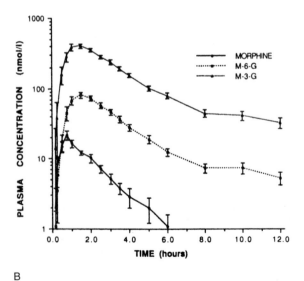

A

B

Figure 17.2   Mean (SEM) plasma concentrations of morphine, morphine-3-glucuronide (M3G) and morphine-6-glucuronide (M6G) after administration of (A) morphine 5 mg intravenously or (B) 11.7 mg orally. (Reproduced with permission from Osborne R et al 1990 Clinical Pharmacology and Therapeutics 47: 12.)

contributes to the analgesic effect of morphine. M6G is a ventilatory depressant with a potency substantially in excess of that of free morphine. Even allowing for its slower penetration into the brain, it may be that 50% or more of the respiratory depression observed by 1 hour after systemic administration of morphine is due to this metabolite, and this contribution will subsequently increase with time. Patients with renal insufficiency have relatively normal metabolism and elimination of morphine, but they do have impaired elimination of morphine glucuronides. M6G makes a significant contribution to morphine intoxication in patients with renal failure.

Use in neonates

Morphine is a popular analgesic for paediatric patients, including neonates. Neonates are considered to be more sensitive to the respiratory depressant effects of morphine. This is partly related to the higher plasma concentrations required for analgesia and sedation than in older children, as well as age related differences in the development of opioid receptors. It is equally likely that impaired clearance and thus higher morphine concentrations also contribute. Additionally, the mechanism for glucuronide conjugation is poorly developed in neonates, and especially in premature infants. At the same time renal function (both glomerular filtration and tubular secretion) is also very inefficient. Not surprisingly, therefore, the pharmacokinetic profile of morphine in neonates is markedly different from that in older children and adults.

Papaveretum

Papaveretum (Omnopon) is a mixture of the water soluble alkaloids of opium standardised to contain 50% anhydrous morphine. Since, in papaveretum, morphine is in the anhydrous form, while available preparations of morphine contain the alkaloid combined with five molecules of water of crystallisation, it thus contains more than 50% effective alkaloid — papaveretum 20 mg contains morphine alkaloid equivalent to that contained in 13.3 mg morphine sulphate. Papaveretum is claimed to be more sedative than morphine, possibly due to the non-morphine alkaloids that it contains. It has been popular as a premedication drug, often given in combination with hyoscine (scopolamine). The side-effects are similar to those with morphine. Papaveretum is well absorbed after oral administration.

Codeine phosphate

Codeine, one of the principal alkaloids of opium, has an analgesic efficacy much lower than other opioids, due to an extremely low affinity for opioid receptors. It is approximately one-sixth as potent as morphine. It has a low abuse potential and does not fall under the Control of Drugs Act. In contrast to other opioids, with the exception of oxycodone, codeine is relatively more effective when administered orally than parenterally. This is due to methylation at the C-3 site on the phenyl ring (Fig. 17.1), which may protect it from conjugating enzymes, and also because a small proportion (approximately 2–7%) is metabolised to morphine and M6G. (Metabolism to morphine is less in patients deficient in cytochrome CYP2D6 — poor metabolisers of debrisoquine — and codeine may be less effective in these). It is used in the management of mild to moderate pain, often in combination with non-opioid analgesics such as aspirin or paracetemol. It is valuable as an antitussive and for the treatment of diarrhoea. Side-effects are uncommon and respiratory depression, even with large doses, is seldom a problem.

Diamorphine

Diamorphine (3,6-diacetylmorphine, heroin) is a semisynthetic derivative of morphine. The chemical structure is shown in Figure 17.1. It is a prodrug, and does not bind to the opioid receptors, nor has it any opioid activity itself. All its pharmacological activity derives from hydrolysis products formed in the blood. It is a potent analgesic with a high potential for addiction, and its manufacture and use, even for medical purposes, is illegal in many countries, including the USA. Although it is claimed that diamorphine produces more sedation and less nausea and vomiting than morphine, it is likely that the incidence of side-effects with equianalgesic doses is similar to other opioids. A dose of 5 mg diamorphine is equipotent with 10 mg morphine, but the duration of action is shorter, about 2 hours. Because diamorphine in solution rapidly undergoes deacetylation, injections should always be freshly prepared. Diamorphine undergoes rapid deacetylation in the plasma and tissues to monoacetylmorphine (MAM) and then to morphine. The latter may account for a major part of its activity. Both diamorphine and MAM are more lipid soluble than morphine and may act as carriers to facilitate the entry of morphine into the CNS. Interest in the use of diamorphine by the epidural or intrathecal routes has recently become more evident owing to its greater lipid solubility in comparison with morphine.

Methadone

Methadone is a synthetic opioid belonging to a chemical series known as 3,3-diphenylpropyl-amines. Its chemical structure is shown in Figure 17.1. Although the two-dimensional structure does not resemble that of other opioids, in three dimensions the molecule has an opioid-like pseudopiperidine configuration. Methadone is commercially available as a racemic mixture but almost all of the activity resides in the $R(-)$-isomer, which is up to 50 times more potent than the $S(+)$-isomer. The pharmacological properties of methadone are qualitatively similar to those of morphine. It produces less sedation and euphoria but in other respects the side-effects are the same. Its high bioavailability after oral administration (80%) and its long half-life make it useful in the management of severe chronic pain, e.g. that due to cancer. It is widely used in the treatment of withdrawal symptoms in opioid addicts. Methadone is equipotent with morphine when given orally or intramuscularly, but may be somewhat less potent when given intravenously. In addicts, 1 mg methadone is equivalent to 1 mg heroin or 3 mg morphine.

Pharmacokinetics and metabolism

About 85% in the plasma is protein bound, preferentially to α_1-acid glycoprotein. The terminal half-life is very long, with a mean value of 35 hours. Despite the much longer half-life, the duration of a single dose is comparable with that of morphine. With repeated doses accumulation occurs so that there need to be either lower doses or longer intervals between doses to avoid overdosage. Methadone undergoes hepatic biotransformation by N-demethylation to form pyrrolidines.

Pethidine

Pethidine (meperidine) was the first totally synthetic opioid to be introduced. The chemical structure of pethidine is shown in Figure 17.3. Pethidine was synthesised in 1939 for its possible smooth muscle relaxant properties. However, when given to mice it produced a Straub phenomenon (erection of the tail due to anal sphincter spasm), a characteristic of morphine-like drugs, and this attracted attention to its analgesic properties. Pethidine is less potent than morphine, 75 mg pethidine being approximately equivalent to 10 mg morphine. It is well absorbed from the gastrointestinal tract, but bioavailability is low (47–73%) owing to presystemic metabolism. Peak plasma concentrations after oral administration occur after about 1 hour. Pethidine is moderately lipid soluble and plasma protein binding is about 70%, with binding to albumin, lipoprotein and α_1-acid glycoprotein. The elimination half-life is 3–5 hours. Pethidine is metabolised mainly by the liver and only about 7% of unchanged pethidine is excreted in the urine. This amount is, however, markedly influenced by urinary pH. Acidification of the urine reduces the excretion of unchanged pethidine to less than 1%, whereas with urinary alkalinization this is increased to 20–25%.

Cardiovascular system

Doses of pethidine 0.5–1 mg kg^{-1} cause minimal cardiovascular disturbances, but higher doses

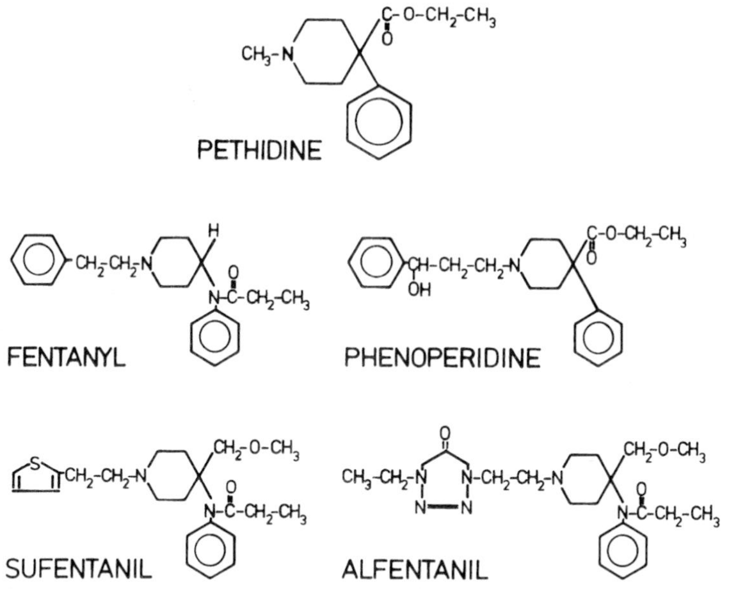

Figure 17.3 Chemical structure of the phenylpiperidine opioids.

can cause hypotension. This is in part due to histamine release, but is also related to pethidine's negative inotropic effect. In contrast to other opioids, pethidine administration often results in tachycardia. This may be related to its atropine-like structure.

Central nervous system

The incidence of sedation and euphoria is similar to that observed after equianalgesic doses of morphine. Pethidine differs from morphine, however, in that, with increasing doses, signs of CNS excitation — tremors, muscle twitching and eventually convulsions — predominate over CNS depression. Norpethidine, a major metabolite of pethidine, may be the principal mediator of those CNS excitatory effects.

CNS toxicity is most likely to occur in patients taking pethidine for long periods, in patients with renal failure and where the oral route is used. The last is due to the significant presystemic metabolism, which results in rapid accumulation of norpethidine. Norpethidine toxicity has been reported in patients receiving pethidine by PCA for several days after surgery. Toxic CNS symptoms should be treated by withdrawal

of pethidine (substituting another analgesic if required), supporting respiration and controlling convulsions. It may take several days for normal neurological function to return. Naloxone may exacerbate rather than antagonise the convulsions caused by toxic doses of pethidine.

Interaction with monoamine oxidase inhibitors

Pethidine should be avoided in patients taking monoamine oxidase inhibitors (MAOIs) because the combination can cause serious adverse reactions. MAOI–pethidine interactions have two distinct forms. The excitatory form is characterised by sudden agitation, delirium, headache, hypo- or hypertension, rigidity, hyperpyrexia, convulsions and coma. It is thought to be caused by an increase in cerebral 5-hydroxytryptamine (5-HT) concentrations as a result of inhibition of monoamine oxidase. This is potentiated by pethidine, which blocks neuronal uptake of 5-HT. The depressive form, which is frequently severe and fatal, consists of respiratory and cardiovascular depression and coma. It is the result of the inhibition of hepatic microsomal enzymes by the MAOI, leading to accumulation of pethidine. With the possible exception of phenoperidine, other opioids appear safe to use in combination with MAOIs.

Pharmacokinetics and metabolism

Pethidine undergoes extensive hepatic metabolism by N-demethylation to norpethidine and hydrolysis to pethidinic acid. Norpethidine, the predominant metabolite, is pharmacologically active and is thought to be responsible for most of the excitatory effects of pethidine overdosage. Norpethidine's binding affinity for opioid receptors is similar to that of pethidine. It has a long plasma half-life in normal patients (14–21 hours) and even longer in those with diminished renal function. Pethidine and norpethidine can readily cross the placental barrier and accumulate in the fetus. Both compounds are weak bases (the pK_a of pethidine is 8.5 and that of norpethidine higher) and ion trapping in the fetal plasma occurs. The elimination of pethidine in neonates is also longer than in adults, with half-lives prolonged up to 6 days.

Phenoperidine

Phenoperidine is an N-phenylpropyl derivative of norpethidine (Fig. 17.3). It is almost totally restricted to use as a supplement to inhalational anaesthesia and in patients requiring prolonged mechanical ventilation. As a supplement during anaesthesia the usual dose is 0.5–1 mg intravenously in spontaneously breathing patients, and up to 5 mg in those where intermittent positive pressure ventilation is used. For postoperative pain relief 2 mg phenoperidine is equipotent with 10 mg morphine. Phenoperidine undergoes hepatic biotransformation, with pethidine, norpethidine and pethidinic acid the most important metabolites. Phenoperidine is probably best avoided in patients taking MAOIs in view of its metabolites, pethidine and norpethidine.

Fentanyl

Fentanyl is a phenylpiperidine of the 4-anilopiperidine series (Fig. 17.3). It is a basic amine with a pK_a of 8.43, so that at physiological pH only 8.4% of the drug is in the unionised form. Fentanyl is highly lipid soluble with an octanol:water partition coefficient of 816. At pH 7.4, fentanyl is 80–85% bound to plasma proteins. The acute phase protein, α_1-acid glycoprotein, accounts for about 44% of the protein binding. Fentanyl is rapidly transferred across the blood–brain barrier, resulting in a peak effect within 5 minutes after intravenous injection. The properties that enable fentanyl to cross the blood–brain barrier also ensure rapid penetration across the placental barrier. Fentanyl is commercially available as the citrate salt in an aqueous solution containing 50 μg fentanyl base per millilitre.

In humans, fentanyl is 60–80 times more potent than morphine on a milligram basis. At the opioid receptor, however, this potency difference becomes less obvious and the intrinsic affinities of fentanyl and morphine differ only by a factor of 2–3. The differences between the receptor affinities and clinical potency ratios arise from the different physicochemical and pharmacokinetic properties of these drugs, and in particular the differences in lipid solubility.

Respiratory system

Delayed respiratory depression in the postoperative period has been reported after small intravenous doses of fentanyl given during anaesthesia. This biphasic respiratory depression is probably related to secondary peaks in the plasma fentanyl concentration during the elimination phase. There is enterohepatic recirculation of fentanyl, with sequestration of fentanyl in the stomach and subsequent reabsorption from small intestine. Partitioning into gastric juice occurs as a result of the difference between gastric pH and the high pK_a of fentanyl. As much as 16% of an administered dose of fentanyl may accumulate in the stomach. However, since the average volume of gastric juice is small (25–100 ml), the amount of fentanyl that will reach the small intestine for reabsorption is likely to be negligible. Furthermore, because of its high first pass hepatic metabolism, little of the reabsorbed fentanyl will reach the systemic circulation. Enterohepatic recirculation is therefore unlikely to account for the secondary peaks. A more likely explanation is release of fentanyl from body stores, especially muscle, as a result of increased patient activity in the postoperative period. Because of its large mass, muscle can store up to 55% of fentanyl present in the body.

Cardiovascular system

Clinical doses of fentanyl, even those used in cardiac anaesthesia, have little or no direct effect on myocardial function or direct actions on peripheral vessels. It can cause hypotension in some patients, particularly if they are hypovolaemic, as the result of a decrease in sympathetic tone. Fentanyl appears to exert a protective effect on the heart during periods of ischaemia, by decreasing myocardial energy demand. This is mainly as a result of its negative chronotropic effect.

Central nervous system

Fentanyl produces less sedation than equianalgesic doses of morphine, although electroencephalogram (EEG) changes can be observed with doses as low as $2 \mu g kg^{-1}$ in human volunteers. None the less, large doses of fentanyl will cause unconsciousness in ventilated subjects, and doses greater than $5 \mu g kg^{-1}$ are regularly used in anaesthesia for cardiac surgery. With doses of this magnitude very striking EEG changes are produced, characterised by large increases in the amplitude of the very low frequencies in the δ band (0.5–3.5 Hz) and virtual disappearance of frequencies above about 6 Hz. Convulsions are seen in dogs given doses 20 times the highest dose given to humans. Epileptic activity has never been proven to occur with the doses used clinically in humans.

Low doses of fentanyl ($5 \mu g kg^{-1}$) are effective in blocking the hypertensive responses to endotracheal intubation. This may be simply an analgesic effect, but may also be due to a more specific blockade of afferent nerve impulses from the pharynx and larynx. There are high concentrations of opioid receptors in the solitary nucleus and the nuclei of the ninth and tenth cranial nerves. These nuclei are associated with visceral afferent fibres originating in the pharynx and larynx.

Epidural fentanyl produces a more consistent and intense analgesia than morphine, with a faster onset. The incidence of side-effects is also less, although nausea, sedation and itching occur. Epidural fentanyl $100 \mu g$ will produce analgesia lasting 2–4 hours. The short duration of action and the low incidence of side-effects is probably related to the high lipid-solubility of fentanyl, which results in rapid uptake by epidural blood vessels and nervous tissue. Although late-onset respiratory depression is rare, early respiratory depression within 30 minutes of injection can occur as a result of extensive uptake into the systemic circulation.

Pharmacokinetics and metabolism

Fentanyl is rapidly and extensively metabolised by the liver to inactive metabolites. The primary metabolic pathway in man is *N*-dealkylation, which converts fentanyl to the inactive norfentanyl. Hepatic clearance of fentanyl is flow dependent and is thus sensitive to reduction in liver perfusion. The elimination half-life is 3–5 hours. After bolus intravenous injection, plasma fentanyl concentrations decrease rapidly owing to distribution from the plasma to tissues. This rapid distribution explains why, after moderate (up to $10 \mu g kg^{-1}$) doses, fentanyl has a short duration of action. However, attempts to increase the intensity of effect by giving a larger initial dose converts fentanyl from a short acting to a long acting drug. With the larger dose, the distribution phase is completed before the fentanyl concentration declines to theshold levels, so that the duration of action now becomes dependent on the decrease in concentration during the much slower elimination phase. Distribution to the tissues increases the likelihood of accumulation with regularly repeated doses of fentanyl.

Clinical application

Fentanyl is commonly used intraoperatively to provide the analgesic component of anaesthesia.

When given in appropriate doses at induction of anaesthesia it reduces the dose of induction agent required and contributes to suppression of the cardiovascular responses associated with laryngoscopy and intubation of the trachea. Opioids also reduce the minimum alveolar concentration (MAC) of inhalational anaesthetics. Typical doses of fentanyl given at induction of anaesthesia range from 0.7 to 5 µg kg^{-1}, depending on the nature of the procedure and the clinical condition of the patient. Lower doses are obviously indicated for short procedures or when the patient will be breathing spontaneously during anaesthesia, and in patients who are elderly, debilitated or in shock.

A single intravenous bolus of fentanyl 50 µg (1 ml) will produce a peak plasma fentanyl concentration of 3–5 ng ml^{-1} and the concentration will fall below 1 ng ml^{-1} by about 4 minutes. A fentanyl concentration of 1 ng ml^{-1} is associated with moderate analgesia and minimal respiratory depression. Note, however, that because of the delay in fentanyl crossing the blood–brain barrier ($t_{1/2}k_{e0}$ = 5–6 minutes), the peak concentrations in the effect site will only be reached after about 3.5 minutes. It is, therefore, advisable to administer fentanyl before the induction agents to ensure that peak effect coincides with the stimulus of laryngoscopy and intubation. When higher bolus doses of fentanyl are given, the duration of analgesia and ventilatory depression will be prolonged. After fentanyl 150 µg (3 ml), it will take about 12–15 minutes for the plasma concentration to decrease to 1 ng ml^{-1}, and after 350 µg (7 ml) it will take 50–75 minutes. These figures refer to healthy patients and will be longer in patients with cardiovascular, renal or hepatic disease. The much longer time needed for a decrease in concentration with the higher dose is because now the decay in plasma concentration occurs during the elimination phase rather than as a result of distribution.

For fentanyl administered in combination with nitrous oxide and a volatile agent, plasma concentrations of about 2 ng ml^{-1} are associated with adequate analgesia for most types of surgery. After a single dose of 350 µg this level will be reached after 20–30 minutes. When indicated by patient responses, additional boluses of fentanyl 50–150 µg can be given, depending on the anticipated intensity of the surgical stimulus and duration of the procedure. An alternative to repeated boluses is to follow an initial loading dose with a continuous infusion of fentanyl. For example, an initial dose of 350 µg followed by an infusion of 0.5 µg kg^{-1} min^{-1} will result in plasma concentrations of 2–3 ng ml^{-1}. The pharmacokinetics of fentanyl are such, however, that for infusions longer than about 2 hours the rate of decrease of plasma concentration becomes markedly slower as the infusion duration increases (Table 17.2). In the example above, it takes about 50–60 minutes for the concentration to fall to 1 ng ml^{-1} when the infusion is stopped at 120 minutes. If the infusion is continued to 180 minutes the comparable time becomes 85–90 minutes. In comparison with fentanyl, sufentanil and alfentanil are more appropriate drugs for administration by intravenous infusion (Table 17.2).

Much higher doses of fentanyl are often used for patients undergoing cardiac surgery. Doses vary from 10 to 50 µg kg^{-1}, although on occasions doses as high as 150 µg kg^{-1} have been given. An advantage of these moderate to high doses of fentanyl in cardiac surgical patients is the associated cardiovascular stability. However, opioids are not capable of producing complete anaesthesia on their own. Fentanyl is thus combined with a hypnotic, such as propofol or midazolam, or with a low concentration of a volatile anaesthetic.

Table 17.2 Time for plasma concentration of opioids to decrease by 50% after infusions of different durations. Values are derived from computer simulations using the program PK-SIM (Specialized Data Systems, Jenkintown, USA)

Infusion duration (min)	Fentanyl	Sufentanil	Alfentanil	Remifentanil
60	20	20	33	5.4
90	28	24	42	5.4
120	39	28	50	5.4
180	82	34	55	5.4
240	148	38	58	5.4
360	230	43	60	5.4

In recent years there has been an increasing use of epidural fentanyl for postoperative analgesia and pain associated with labour. The recommended dose of epidural fentanyl for postoperative pain is 30–50 μg diluted in 10–15 ml saline. This will give adequate pain relief for 1.5–3 hours. Increasing the dose prolongs the duration but often will also result in a disproportionate increase in side-effects, especially respiratory depression, urinary retention and nausea and vomiting. To overcome the short duration of epidural fentanyl, it may be given as a continuous epidural infusion at a rate of 50–100 μg h^{-1}.

Although epidural opioids will provide adequate analgesia during the early stage of labour, they are usually ineffective in controlling pain during the final stages of labour. For this reason it has become common practice to combine low concentrations of an opioid such as fentanyl with the local anaesthetic bupivacaine. A frequently used combination is bupivacaine 0.125% with fentanyl 1 μg ml^{-1}. An initial epidural bolus of 10 ml of this solution is followed by an epidural infusion at a rate of 8–10 ml h^{-1}. This will provide good analgesia throughout labour with minimal side-effects.

Alfentanil hydrochloride

Alfentanil is a phenylpiperidine analogue of fentanyl (Fig. 17.3). It is supplied as an aqueous solution containing 500 μg alfentanil base per millilitre. In humans, alfentanil is between 5 and 10 times less potent than fentanyl when single intravenous boluses are compared; however, when comparing steady-state concentrations the potency is 20–40 times less than that of fentanyl. The apparent volume of distribution of alfentanil in the brain is about 20 times less than that of fentanyl and thus the brain compartment will fill more rapidly than with fentanyl. The half-time for plasma–brain equilibration is 1.1 minutes for alfentanil, compared with 5.8 minutes for sufentanil and 6.4 minutes for fentanyl. When given by bolus injection its effects are also of short duration, making it a versatile opioid for use in anaesthesia.

Respiratory system

As with fentanyl, there have been several reported occurrences of delayed, life threatening respiratory depression after the intraoperative use of alfentanil given by continuous infusion. The decline in plasma concentration when an infusion is stopped is less rapid than from a comparable concentration after a single bolus injection. This is because redistribution is less marked because the tissues are already partially saturated. Administration of alfentanil by infusion can convert a short acting drug into a relatively long acting one. When administering alfentanil by infusion it is important, therefore, to terminate the infusion in good time, before the end of surgery, to allow for this effect.

Pharmacokinetics and metabolism

After bolus intravenous administration alfentanil is very rapidly distributed from the plasma to the tissues. The terminal half-life is about 1.5 hours. The short half-life is the result of a low volume of distribution (approximately 0.9 l kg^{-1}) and a moderate plasma clearance. Alfentanil has a lower lipid solubility than fentanyl or sufentanil and is highly protein bound, mainly to α_1-acid glycoprotein. Alfentanil differs from other opioids in having a pK_a value below physiological pH (pK_a = 6.8). At pH 7.4, 85% of alfentanil will be present in plasma in the unionised form. Since only the unionised form of a drug can readily cross cell membranes, this may explain why, despite a moderate lipid solubility, alfentanil has such a rapid onset of effect.

Total hepatic clearance of alfentanil in humans is lower than with fentanyl or sufentanil, with a hepatic extraction ratio of approximately 0.5. As with fentanyl, oxidative N-dealkylation at the piperidine nitrogen is the major metabolic pathway to noralfentanil. Less than 1% of a dose of alfentanil is eliminated unchanged by the kidneys.

Clinical applications

Alfentanil is particularly indicated in those situations where a rapid and short opioid effect is wanted, e.g. outpatient surgery or short procedures. A single bolus of alfentanil 15 µg kg^{-1} (approximately 1000 mg or 2 ml) will provide analgesia lasting about 10 minutes, with respiratory depression less than 2 minutes. Doses of alfentanil 30–50 µg kg^{-1} will substantially attenuate the haemodynamic responses to laryngoscopy and intubation of the trachea. Because of its relatively short duration, alfentanil is well suited to administration as a continuous intravenous infusion. Various infusion regimens have been published. One that has proved clinically useful in the author's hospital is a loading dose of 50 µg kg^{-1} followed by an infusion of 10 µg kg^{-1} min^{-1} thereafter. This will result in steady-state plasma concentrations of around 200 ng ml^{-1}, which are sufficient for most types of surgery under anaesthesia with nitrous oxide and a volatile anaesthetic. If the infusion is stopped after 2 hours, plasma concentrations will fall to levels at which most patients will have satisfactory spontaneous ventilation within 20–30 minutes of stopping the infusion. Although alfentanil is effective when given epidurally, the duration of analgesia is short: 40–80 minutes after a single bolus of 15 µg kg^{-1}. For this reason alfentanil has never achieved the popularity associated with epidural fentanyl or sufentanil.

Sufentanil citrate

Sufentanil is a thienyl derivative of the 4-anilinopiperidine series chemically related to fentanyl (Fig. 17.3). Sufentanil is 8–10 times more potent than fentanyl in humans. It is supplied as the aqueous solution of the citrate salt containing 50 µg ml^{-1} sufentanil base; in a limited number of countries it is also available in a concentration of 5 µg ml^{-1}. Sufentanil is a basic amine, with a pK_a of 8.01. At physiological pH 20% of the drug in solution is in the unionised form. It is extremely lipid soluble with an octanol:water partition coefficient of 1757.

Central nervous system

At low doses sufentanil may produce more drowsiness than fentanyl. Epidural sufentanil

has been used for the treatment of postoperative pain. The onset of analgesia is rapid and lasts 3–5 hours. Respiratory depression can occur within the first 30 minutes after epidural injection and may be related to systemic vascular uptake. The combination of sufentanil and low concentrations of bupivacaine (0.125% or 0.0625%) has proven valuable in obstetric analgesia.

Pharmacokinetics and metabolism

Sufentanil is highly bound to plasma protein (93%), primarily to α_1-acid glycoprotein, which accounts for 83% of the total binding. Sufentanil is rapidly distributed after intravenous administration so that within 30 minutes 98% of the injected dose will have left the plasma. The terminal half-life is about 165 minutes. It is metabolised almost exclusively in the liver, principally by N-dealkylation. Oxidative O-demethylation is a minor metabolic pathway, although its end-product, desmethylsufentanil, is pharmacologically active, with a potency about one-tenth that of sufentanil. Since the concentration of desmethylsufentanil is very low, even after large doses of sufentanil, this is unlikely to be clinically significant. The hepatic intrinsic clearance of sufentanil is greater than liver blood flow so that the first pass effect will be almost total. The clearance of sufentanil in children is similar to that of young adults; however, clearance of sufentanil in neonates is only about 40% of the value in infants and older children. In neonates the activity of the enzyme cytochrome P-450, responsible for the biotransformation of many opioids, is only 25–50% of that in adults.

Clinical applications

The indications for sufentanil in anaesthesia are similar to those of fentanyl. For use in balanced anaesthesia doses are approximately one-tenth those of fentanyl. Although the pharmacokinetic profile of sufentanil suggests that it would be superior to fentanyl for use by continuous intravenous infusion (Table 17.2), there is currently little experience with this technique. Sufentanil has become especially popular in neurosurgery and in cardiac surgery, where doses of 5–15 µg kg^{-1} are common. A technique that the author has found to produce good anaesthesia for patients undergoing cardiac surgery is induction of anaesthesia with sufentanil 5 µg kg^{-1} given over 3–5 minutes, followed by an infusion of sufentanil 150–250 µg h^{-1}. This is combined with either midazolam or propofol to ensure complete anaesthesia.

Sufentanil epidurally is popular in many obstetric centres for analgesia for labour. As with fentanyl, sufentanil is usually combined with bupivacaine. The technique used in the author's department is to add 1 ml (50 µg) sufentanil to 49 ml bupivacaine 0.125% or 0.0625%. An initial epidural bolus of 10 ml of this solution is followed by an epidural infusion at a rate of 8–10 ml h^{-1}. The lower concentration of bupivacaine is adequate for the first stage of labour, while the 0.125% solution is used for delivery. A similar regimen has also proved very successful for providing pain relief after major surgery, including orthopaedic and thoracic surgery.

Remifentanil

Remifentanil is a new µ-agonist opioid characterised by a rapid onset and a very short duration of action. It is the hydrochloride salt of 3-[4-methoxy carbonyl-4[(1-oxypropyl)phenyl amino]-1-piperidine] propanoic acid, methyl ester. It has an analgesic potency similar to that of fentanyl. Its molecular structure and metabolic pathways are shown in Figure 17.4. Remifentanil is structurally unique among currently available opioids because of its ester linkage. The ester linkage makes remifentanil susceptible to rapid hydrolysis by non-specific esterases in the blood and tissues, resulting in very rapid degradation to inactive metabolites. The β-adrenoreceptor antagonist esmolol is metabolised by a similar mechanism. The elimination half-life is 10–20 minutes and the clearance is 3–4 l min^{-1}. Clearance is not affected by the presence of a cholinesterase inhibitor such as neostigmine. Remifentanil is not a good substrate for butyrylcholinesterase (pseudocholinesterase). Its pharmacokinetics are thus not likely to be different in patients with

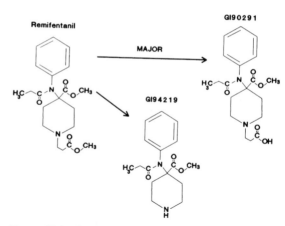

Figure 17.4 Structure of remifentanil and its metabolic pathways. The primary metabolic pathway is by de-esterification by non-specific plasma and tissue esterases to the carboxylic acid metabolite, G190291, which has only 1/300th–1/1000th the potency of the parent compound. N-dealkylation of remifentanil to G194219 is a minor metabolic pathway.

cholinesterase deficiency. The rapid elimination of remifentanil from the blood suggests that it is most likely to be administered by intravenous infusion, rather than by intermittent boluses, for all but the shortest procedures. Even after a 3 hour infusion, plasma concentrations of remifentanil fall by 50% within 5–7 minutes (the so-called context-sensitive half-time), compared with 55–60 minutes for alfentanil (Table 17.2). In other respects remifentanil possesses essentially similar pharmacological properties to the other phenylpiperidine opioids. It does not cause release of histamine and has minimal effects on the cardiovascular system.

PURE ANTAGONISTS

Naloxone

Naloxone is the N-allyl derivative of oxymorphone (Fig. 17.5). It is by itself virtually devoid of pharmacological activity, but will precipitate withdrawal symptoms in opioid addicts and has been used for the detection of addiction. When given to patients who have had an excessive perioperative dose of an opioid, naloxone will reverse not only the respiratory depression but also analgesia. There have been reports of intense

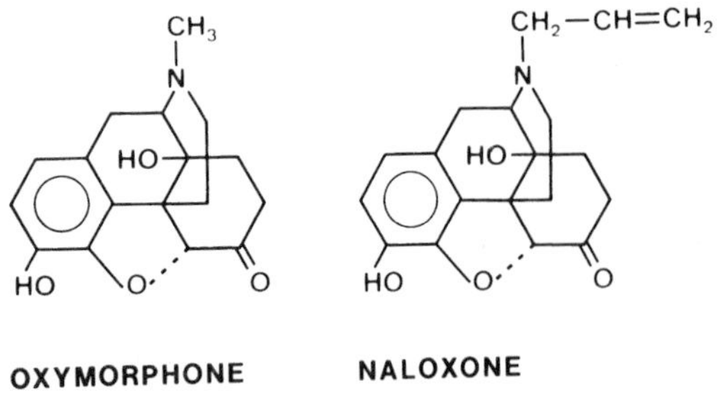

Figure 17.5   Chemical structure of oxymorphone, a full μ-agonist, and naloxone, a pure antagonist.

pressor responses, tachycardia and severe pulmonary oedema occurring when naloxone has been used to reverse the effects of large doses of an opioid.

Recently attention has focused on the therapeutic use of naloxone in patients with hypovolaemic endotoxic shock. There is considerable animal evidence to support this therapeutic approach, which is thought to work by antagonising the high levels of circulating β-endorphin produced by endotoxins. The results of naloxone treatment of shock in humans remain controversial.

A dose of 0.2–0.4 mg is effective in reversing opioid induced respiratory depression, although it is better to titrate naloxone in increments of 0.04 mg. The plasma half-life of naloxone (1.0–1.5 hours) is considerably shorter than most opioids, and on occasions repeated doses or a continuous intravenous infusion may be required.

Naltrexone and nalmefene

Naltrexone and nalmefene are analogues of naloxone created from oxymorphone by the substitution on the nitrogen atom. They have similar pharmacological properties to naloxone but longer durations of action, with elimination half-lives in excess of 8 hours. Naltrexone is used mainly in the management of addicts. Nalmefene has been used in anaesthesia to reverse opioid induced respiratory depression. Its prolonged effect could make it potentially useful, given prophylactically to prevent respiratory depression due to spinal opioids.

PARTIAL AGONISTS

The history of this class of drugs dates from 1914 when Pohl, in an attempt to improve the analgesic properties of codeine, synthesised N-allylcodeine, which he found could antagonise respiratory depression produced by morphine. This discovery remained almost unnoticed by the medical fraternity until Weijland and Erickson synthesised N-allylmorphine (nalorphine) in 1942. Nalorphine is an example of how minor structural changes to an existing opioid can give compounds with very different pharmacological properties. Nalorphine is equipotent with morphine as an analgesic and in causing respiratory depression. Unfortunately, nalorphine's severe psychotomimetic activity, including unpleasant visual hallucinations, precludes its clinical use as an analgesic. Until the discovery of naloxone it was widely used for its antagonist properties in the treatment of opioid overdose.

The term 'mixed agonist-antagonist drugs' is often used to describe this class of drugs. It was thought that they were agonists or partial agonists at the κ receptor and antagonists at the μ receptor. Although this explained rather neatly the phenomenon that they could act as analgesics and yet antagonise the effects of morphine, it is now generally accepted that they are partial agonists at both receptors. When a partial agonist is combined with a low concentration of a full agonist, so that few of the receptors are occupied by the agonist, the partial agonist can occupy the free receptors and complement the analgesic effect of the full agonist. However, when a partial agonist is introduced in the presence of a high concentration of full agonist, the latter will be displaced from the receptor by the partial agonist, resulting in a reduction in the response (Fig. 17.6). The dysphoric side-effect of some of this class of drugs is thought to be due to binding to the non-opioid σ receptor.

Pentazocine

Pentazocine, the N-dimethylallyl derivative of phenazocine (Fig. 17.7), was the first member of the so-called agonist-antagonist opioids to be

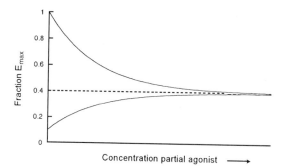

Figure 17.6 Hypothetical concentration–response curves for the combined effects of a partial opioid agonist with a maximum effect (intrinsic activity) of 0.4 and a full agonist. The lower curve shows the response when increasing concentrations of the partial agonist are added to a low concentration of the full agonist; the combined response increases asymptotically to the E_{max} of the partial agonist. When increasing concentrations of the partial agonist are added to a high concentration of the full agonist, the combined response decreases asymptotically to the E_{max} of the partial agonist.

clinically successful. Its analgesic potency is approximately one-third to one-fifth that of morphine. Pentazocine is a racemic mixture and analgesia resides exclusively in the L-isomer. Peak blood concentrations after oral administration are reached by 1–3 hours, and between 15 and 45 minutes after intramuscular administration. The oral bioavailability is about 20%.

Respiratory system

In equianalgesic doses pentazocine causes the same degree of respiratory depression as morphine. However, as with other partial agonists, the response curves for both respiratory depression and analgesia are plateau shaped, with the plateau being reached at a dose of approximately 60 mg for the average adult.

Cardiovascular system

Pentazocine causes an increase in blood pressure, heart rate and plasma catecholamines. This is associated with increased systemic vascular resistance, pulmonary artery pressure and myocardial workload, and decreased myocardial contractility. Pentazocine is contraindicated in the treatment of patients with acute myocardial infarction.

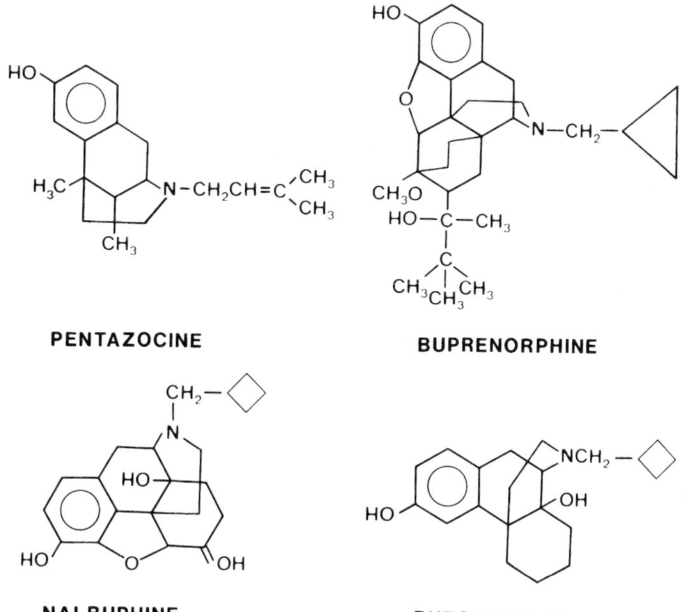

PENTAZOCINE

BUPRENORPHINE

NALBUPHINE

BUTORPHANOL

Figure 17.7 Chemical structure of the partial opioid agonists currently available for clinical use.

Central nervous system

Psychotomimetic side-effects, such as hallucinations, bizarre dreams and sensations of depersonalisation, occur in about 6–10% of patients. They are more common in elderly patients, in those who are ambulatory and when doses above 60 mg are given. Nausea occurs in approximately 5% of patients, although vomiting is less common. Other commonly reported side-effects are dizziness and drowsiness. Euphoria is less common than with pure agonist drugs, which may account in part for the lower risk of physical dependence and 'drug seeking' behaviour, although repeated use of pentazocine will result in physical dependence.

Butorphanol tartrate

Butorphanol tartrate is a fully synthetic morphinan derivative (Fig. 17.7), 3.5–5 times as potent as morphine. It is a weak partial μ-receptor agonist and is relatively ineffective at reversing the effects of full agonists. The relatively low incidence of psychotomimetic effect in humans compared with pentazocine suggests a lack of significant σ-receptor action. The recommended doses are 1–4 mg intramuscularly every 3–4 hours, or 0.5–2 mg intravenously. The onset of analgesia occurs within 10 minutes after intramuscular administration and peak analgesic activity is reached within 30–45 minutes. Given intravenously, peak analgesia is reached in less than 30 minutes. Butorphanol is metabolised mainly in the liver to inactive metabolites, hydroxy- and norbutorphanol. The terminal half-life is 2.5–3.5 hours. Butorphanol is about 80% bound to plasma proteins.

Respiratory system

Respiratory depression produced by butorphanol 2 mg i.v. is similar to that of 10 mg morphine; however, unlike morphine, a ceiling effect for respiratory depression is seen with increasing doses of butorphanol. Clinically, near maximum depression occurs after 4 mg in normal adults.

Cardiovascular system

In healthy volunteers, butorphanol 0.03–0.06 mg kg^{-1} produces no significant cardiovascular changes. However, in patients with cardiac disease, progressive increases in cardiac index and pulmonary artery pressure occur. These changes are similar to those produced by pentazocine, and butorphanol is therefore best avoided in patients with recent myocardial infarction.

Nalbuphine hydrochloride

Nalbuphine hydrochloride is structurally related to oxymorphone and naloxone (Fig. 17.7). It is approximately equipotent with morphine. The onset of analgesia is within 2–3 minutes of intravenous administration and 15 minutes after intramuscular injection, and lasts 3–6 hours with an adult dose of 10 mg. With equianalgesic doses, similar degrees of respiratory depression to that of morphine occur up to a dose of approximately 0.45 mg kg^{-1}. With higher doses a 'ceiling effect' is seen in the carbon dioxide response curve.

Cardiovascular system

Intravenous nalbuphine causes minimal haemodynamic changes in patients with cardiac disease. Nalbuphine does not increase cardiac workload or pulmonary artery pressure, and is thus safe in the management of patients after acute myocardial infarction.

Central nervous system

Sedation, possibly mediated by κ-receptor activation, occurs in one-third of subjects given doses of 10–20 mg. The incidence of psychotomimetic side-effects is lower than with pentazocine. Chronic administration can result in physical dependence, which resembles that seen with pentazocine rather than morphine, although the abuse potential would seem to be low. Nalbuphine causes withdrawal symptoms in opioid dependent subjects. Nalbuphine in doses of up to 0.2 mg kg^{-1} is an effective antagonist of opioid induced respiratory depression. Its use is sometimes associated with a number of side-effects, including nausea, hypertension, tachycardia and confusion. Larger doses also tend to antagonise analgesia. However, by careful titration of small incremental doses, it is possible to achieve satisfactory reversal of respiratory depression without precipitating pain and haemodynamic side-effects.

Pharmacokinetics and metabolism

Nalbuphine is metabolised in the liver to inactive metabolites, which are excreted mainly in the bile. About 7% of adminstered nalbuphine is excreted in the urine as unchanged drug or conjugates. The plasma terminal half-life is approximately 5 hours in humans.

Buprenorphine

Buprenorphine is a semisynthetic derivative of thebaine, one of the most chemically reactive of the opium alkaloids (Fig. 17.7). It has significant μ-receptor agonist activity, although its intrinsic activity is low. Buprenorphine binds to and dissociates from the μ receptor very slowly, which may account for its low potential for physical abuse. This stable interaction with the μ receptor is also likely to be the explanation for the difficulty with which naloxone will reverse the agonist effects of buprenorphine once these have been established, although the agonist effects can be blocked by naloxone given before buprenorphine.

Buprenorphine is approximately 30 times as potent as morphine. A dose of 0.3 mg intramuscularly has a duration of analgesic action of 6–18 hours. Buprenorphine is also effective sublingually. The average bioavailability by this route is about 55%, but absorption is slow and the time to achieve peak plasma concentrations is variable, with a range of 90–360 minutes. The onset of action is rather slow (5–15 minutes) after both intramuscular and intravenous administration, possibly due to slow receptor association.

In animals there is a bell-shaped response curve for respiratory depression with buprenorphine, rather than the typical flattened dose–response curve of the partial antagonists. There

is some evidence for a similar effect in humans, with the response curve peaking at doses between 0.3 and 0.6 mg intramuscularly. When respiratory depression occurs, it is important to realise that no satisfactory antagonist exists: naloxone, even with doses as large as 14–16 mg, may only partially reverse this side-effect. Doxapram may in some situations prove a useful alternative.

Drowsiness and dizziness are the most common side-effects, although they rarely constitute a major problem. In comparison with other opioids buprenorphine appears to have a very low abuse potential. This may be due to the lack of euphoria and the nature of the drug interaction with the opioid receptor.

Buprenorphine is lipophilic and extensively bound to plasma proteins — protein binding is 95–98%. Its pK_a is 9.24. There are no data on oral bioavailability in humans but in the dog it is only 3–6%. In humans the hepatic extraction ratio is 0.85, so that oral systemic availability would be expected to be about 15% or less. Buprenorphine is almost completely metabolised in the liver by N-dealkylation and conjugation. The terminal half-life is approximately 5 hours. Because of slow receptor binding there is no direct relationship between plasma concentration and clinical effect.

MISCELLANEOUS DRUGS

Meptazinol

Meptazinol is a hexahydroazepine derivative structurally related to pethidine (Fig. 17.8). It is approximately equipotent with pethidine. It is moderately selective for the $μ_1$ receptor and clinically it behaves as a partial μ agonist. It has low affinity for κ receptors. Meptazinol induced analgesia can be almost completely reversed by naloxone, although higher doses are needed than for pure opioid agonists. Meptazinol will also reverse the signs of acute morphine overdosage and precipitate withdrawal symptoms in morphine dependent animals. A component of meptazinol's analgesic activity is mediated by an effect at central cholinergic synapses, a mode of action different from all other conventional analgesics. Unlike opioids, each of the isomers of

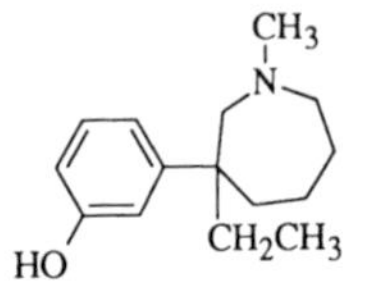

Figure 17.8 Chemical structure of meptazinol.

meptazinol possesses equal analgesic potency, although its cholinergic-mediated analgesia is stereospecific.

Meptazinol in clinically effective analgesic doses appears to be almost devoid of respiratory side-effects. It has minimal effect on haemodynamics after intramuscular administration. It may have mild positive inotropic activity, and increases in blood pressure and heart rate lasting up to 20 minutes have been reported after meptazinol 1.6 mg kg^{-1} given intravenously. The incidence of nausea and vomiting associated with meptazinol seems to be higher than with morphine or other opioids.

Meptazinol is a basic lipophilic drug with a low (23%) protein binding. It is rapidly conjugated in the liver to the glucuronide. The terminal half-life in adults is approximately 2 hours.

Dezocine

Dezocine is a partial μ agonist approximately equipotent to morphine with respect to analgesia. Its chemical structure is shown in Figure 17.9. It has proved at least as effective an analgesic as morphine in moderate to severe postoperative pain. It produces sedation and dysphoria in humans, suggesting that it has κ activity. As with some other partial agonist analgesics, a 'ceiling' effect to dezocine-induced respiratory depression occurs with increasing dosage, beyond which further depression has not been observed. Maximum depression occurs at a dose of about 2.3 mg kg^{-1} given intravenously. In single doses, however, dezocine is a slightly more potent respiratory depressant than morphine. Clinically important haemodynamic changes have not been observed with usual analgesic doses. Dezocine produces euphoria and increased drug-liking scores in individuals without histories of drug abuse, and produces subjective effects in human ex-addicts that are similar to those of morphine. The drug can produce substantial cardiovascular depression in dogs, but cardiovascular effects are not found in humans given analgesic doses.

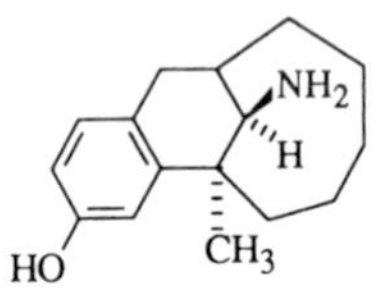

Tramadol hydrochloride

Tramadol (Fig. 17.10) is a centrally acting analgesic that acts at opioid receptors and also modifies nociceptive transmission by inhibition of noradrenaline and serotonin. It has a low affinity for opioid receptors, comparable with that of codeine. It is approximately equipotent to pethidine. It may be administered orally, rectally or intravenously. Oral tramadol has proved effective for the treatment of patients with cancer pain. The tolerance and dependence potential of tramadol is low, even during treatment for up to 6 months. It can cause respiratory depression, although this is considerably less than with the classical opioid agonists, when it is given in the recommended dose. It is generally well tolerated, with dizziness, nausea, sedation, dry mouth and sweating the most common side-effects.

The mean oral availability of tramadol is 68%, with peak plasma concentrations achieved by 1.5–2 hours. It is extensively metabolised by the liver and the elimination half-life is about 5–6 hours. The metabolite o-desmethyltramadol has 2–4 times the analgesic potency of tramadol in mice and rats. Tramadol should not be given to patients taking monoamine oxidase inhibitors.

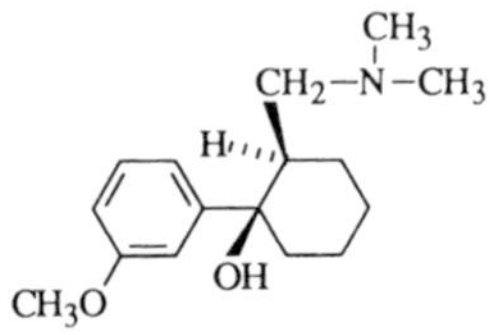

Figure 17.9 Chemical structure of dezocine.

Figure 17.10 Chemical structure of tramadol.

FURTHER READING

Bernards C M, Hill H F 1992 Physical and chemical properties of drug molecules governing their diffusion through the meninges. Anesthesiology 77: 750

Bovill J G 1993 Pharmacokinetics and pharmacodynamics of opioid agonists. Anaesthetic Pharmacology Review 1: 122

Bowdle T A 1993 Partial agonist and agonist-antagonist opioids: basic pharmacology and clinical applications. Anaesthetic Pharmacology Review 2: 135

Gourley G K, Wilson P R, Glynn C J 1982 Pharmacodynamics and pharmacokinetics of methadone during the postoperative period. Anesthesiology 57: 458

Hanna M H, Peat S J, Woodham M et al 1990 Analgesic efficacy and CSF pharmacokinetics of intrathecal morphine-6-glucuronide: comparison with morphine. British Journal of Anaesthesia 64: 547

Lee C R, McTavish D, Sorkin E M 1993 Tramadol: a preliminary review of its pharmacodynamic and pharmacokinetic properties and therapeutic potential in acute and chronic pain states. Drugs 46: 313

Mazoit J X, Sandouk P, Scherrmann J-M, Roche A 1990 Extrahepatic metabolism of morphine occurs in humans. Clinical Pharmacology and Therapeutics 48: 613

Osborne R, Joel S, Trew P, Slevin M 1990 Morphine and metabolite behaviour after different routes of morphine administration: demonstration of the importance of the active metabolite morphine-6-glucuronide. Clinical Pharmacology and Therapeutics 47: 2

Pleuvry B 1993 Opioid receptors and their relevance to anaesthesia. British Journal of Anaesthesia 71: 119

Rawal N 1993 Spinal and epidural opioids. Anaesthetic Pharmacology Review 2: 168

Shafer S L, Varvel J R 1991 Pharmacokinetics, pharmacodynamics and rational opioid selection. Anesthesiology 74: 53

18

Non-steroidal anti-inflammatory analgesics

J. G. Bovill

Non-steroidal anti-inflammatory analgesics (NSAIDs) are a heterogeneous group of compounds with analgesic, anti-inflammatory and antipyretic properties (Table 18.1 and Fig. 18.1). Many, e.g. phenylbutazone, have a high toxicity that restricts their use to the treatment of chronic inflammatory conditions such as rheumatoid arthritis. Other less toxic compounds, e.g. paracetamol, diclofenac and ketorolac, are increasingly being used for the treatment of postoperative pain. NSAIDs are weak organic acids (pK_a 3–5) that bind extensively to plasma albumin (Table 18.1). An exception is paracetamol, which has a pK_a of 9.3 and negligible protein binding. Most are completely absorbed from the gastrointestinal tract. Their hepatic clearance, and consequently first pass metabolism, is low so that they have high bioavailability after oral administration. An exception is diclofenac, which has a high hepatic metabolism and an oral bioavailability of 54%. Aspirin also undergoes significant hepatic metabolism. Because of their very high protein binding, NSAIDs have the potential to displace other drugs from plasma proteins. Warfarin is displaced from its albumin binding site by NSAIDs. The binding of phenytoin to plasma proteins is reduced by salicylates.

MECHANISMS OF ACTION

Analgesia and anti-inflammation

Arachidonic acid is a major component of cell membrane phospholipids. The enzyme cyclo-

253

Table 18.1 Pharmacokinetic characteristics of some commonly prescribed NSAIDs classified according to their chemical classes

NSAID	pKa	Protein binding (%)	Urinary excretion (%)	Clearance (ml min^{-1} kg^{-1})	Volume of distribution (l kg^{-1})	Elimination half-life (hours)
Carboxylic acids						
Aspirin	3.5	85–90	< 2	93	0.15	0.25 ± 0.03
Salicylates	3	80–95	2–30*	0.1–0.9	0.17	2–19†
Arylacetic acids						
Diclofenac		99.5	< 1	3.7	0.12	1.1 ± 0.2
Arylpropionic acids						
Ibuprofen	4.4	> 99	< 1	0.6–1.4	0.1–0.15	2.1 ± 0.3
Heterocyclic acetic acids						
Indomethacin	4.5	> 99	16	1–2	0.3–1.6	4.6 ± 0.7
Ketorolac		> 99	58	0.4–0.6	0.1–0.25	4–6
Enolic acids						
Piroxicam	6.3	> 99	4–10	< 0.1	0.15	57 ± 22
Para-aminophenols						
Paracetamol	9.3	0‡	3	5 ± 0.4	0.95	2 ± 0.4

* Dependent on urinary pH; increases as urinary pH increased.
† Increases as plasma concentration increases.
‡ By therapeutic doses less than 2 g; by toxic concentrations protein binding can increase to 20–50%.

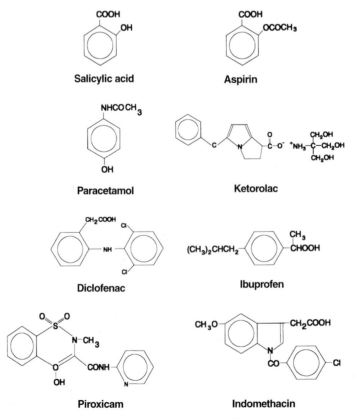

Figure 18.1 Chemical structures of the NSAIDs discussed in detail in this chapter.

oxygenase (prostaglandin endoperoxide synthase) converts arachidonic acid to the cyclic endoperoxides PGG_2 and PGH_2, which are then further metabolised to various prostaglandins, prostacyclin (PGI_2) and thromboxanes (Fig. 18.2). The prostaglandins PGE_2 and PGI_2 and the leukotriene LTB_4 are produced during inflammation and tissue damage and either excite nociceptors or, more usually, produce hyperalgesia by sensitising them so that mechanical or chemical stimuli that would normally be painless produce pain. Inhibition of prostaglandin synthesis from arachidonic acid by cyclo-oxygenase is considered the principal mode of action of NSAIDs in the relief of pain secondary to tissue injury or chronic inflammation. Cyclo-oxygenase is inhibited irreversibly by aspirin and reversibly by other NSAIDs. The effect on prostaglandin synthesis is not selective for inflamed tissue, and the widespread inhibition of cyclo-oxygenase is responsible for several of the adverse effects of these drugs. In addition, the lipoxygenase pathway, which converts arachidonic acid to leukotrienes, is inhibited by some NSAIDs (e.g. indomethacin and diclofenac), but not by salicylates. A component of the analgesic action of NSAIDs is also due to a central action by reduction of prostaglandin production within the central nervous system (CNS). This is the main action of paracetamol. Because they act indirectly, NSAIDs have a latent period during which their effects are minimal, and so have a slow onset of action, requiring up to 40 minutes for the onset of effective analgesia.

Cyclo-oxygenase exists in at least two isoforms. Type I, which is the constitutive form, is responsible for the production of prostaglandins involved in cellular 'house-keeping' functions, such as the regulation of vascular homoeostasis and coordinating the actions of circulating hormones. Type II cyclo-oxygenase is induced in cells activated by exposure to mediators of inflammation, such as cytokines and endotoxin, and may be responsible for the production of prostanoids that mediate inflammation, pain and fever. There are wide differences in the selectivity of NSAIDs for the isoforms. Some, such as aspirin, indomethacin and ibuprofen, are more potent inhibitors of type I than type II. Diclofenac, paracetamol and naproxen are equipotent inhibitors of both types (Table 18.2). The therapeutic effects of the NSAIDs may be due to their

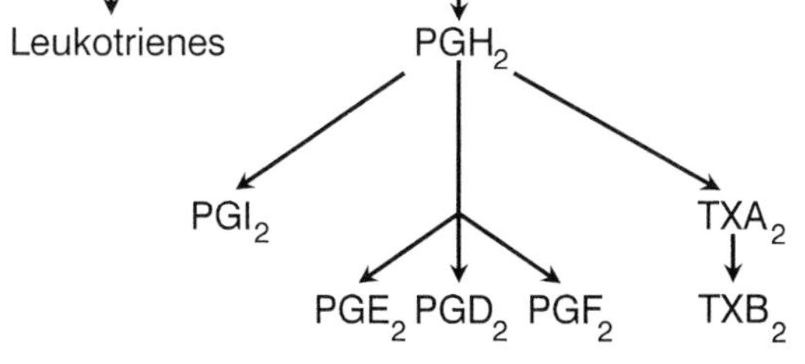

Figure 18.2 Metabolic pathways in the conversion of arachidonic acid to prostaglandins, thromboxanes and leukotrienes. N.B. The activity of phospholipase A_2 is increased by angiotensin II, bradykinin and thrombin and inhibited by steroids. 5-HPETE, 5-hydroperoxyeicosatetraenoic acid; TXA, thromboxane A; TXB, thromboxane B.

Table 18.2 Potencies of several NSAIDs for inhibition of cyclo-oxygenase isoform activity in bovine aortic endothelial cells (COX-1) and murine macrophages (COX-2)

NSAID	IC_{50} ($\mu g\ ml^{-1}$)		
	COX-1	COX-2	Ratio
Aspirin	0.3 ± 0.2	50 ± 10	166
Indomethacin	6.01 ± 0.001	0.6 ± 0.08	60
Ibuprofen	1.0 ± 0.07	15 ± 5.3	15
Paracetamol	2.7 ± 2.0	20 ± 12	7.4
Sodium salicylate	35 ± 11	100 ± 16	2.8
Diclofenac	0.5 ± 0.2	0.35 ± 0.15	0.7
Naproxen	2.2 ± 0.9	1.3 ± 0.8	0.6

Data are mean ± SEM for 3–5 determinations.
IC, inhibitory concentration.
Potency is expressed as the IC_{50} except for paracetamol, for which IC_{30} values are shown because 50% inhibition of COX-2 was not achieved at concentrations up to 1 mg ml^{-1}. The ratio in the final column is the ratio of the IC_{50} values for the NSAID on COX-2 relative to COX-1. (From Mitchell J A et al 1993 Selectivity of nonsteroidal antiinflammatory drugs as inhibitors of constitutive and inducible cyclooxygenase. Proceedings of the National Academy of Sciences of the USA 90: 11693–11697.)

ability to inhibit the type II isoenzyme, while the side-effects, such as gastric and renal damage, correlate with their ability to inhibit type I.

Acute pain, such as postoperative pain, as well as chronic inflammatory pain involve both peripheral and central sensitisation of nociception pathways. The central sensitisation, in the dorsal horn, involves substance P and N-methyl-D-aspartate (NMDA) receptors. Among the intracellular processes that these spinal receptors activate is prostaglandin synthesis, and in animals intrathecally administered NSAIDs reduce the hyperalgesia produced by the spinal actions of substance P and NMDA. It is probable that the clinical response to NSAIDs involves a direct effect on spinal nociceptive processing, in addition to a peripheral effect. NSAID-induced analgesia may also involve serotonergic and GABAergic descending pathways. NSAIDs interfere with a variety of membrane associated processes, including the activity of NADPH oxidase in neutrophils and the activity of phospholipase C in macrophages. Some NSAIDs are thought to inhibit cellular processes by uncoupling protein–protein interactions within the lipid bilayer of the plasma membrane, including the processes regulated by G proteins. The effects appear to be a direct interaction with the G protein, probably at the α site.

Antipyretic effect

The antipyretic effect of the NSAIDs is also a consequence of central prostaglandin inhibition. Temperature regulation is controlled by the hypothalamus, which sets the point at which body temperature is maintained. In fever this is adjusted upwards, under the influence of pyrogens and prostaglandins released from the inflammatory process. Aspirin also prevents the release of endogenous pyrogens from white cells. NSAIDs in normal doses have no effect on temperature regulation in subjects with normal body temperature. However, toxic doses of salicylates produce hyperpyrexia as a result of intracellular uncoupling of oxidative phosphorylation, which inhibits a number of adenosine triphosphate (ATP) dependent reactions. The increased energy

released by this abnormal cellular respiration is dissipated as heat, instead of being used to convert inorganic phosphate and adenosine diphosphate (ADP) to ATP. There is a concomitant rise in oxygen consumption and carbon dioxide production. These effects can be measured with the large doses used in the treatment of rheumatoid arthritis.

Platelet function

Platelets occupy a primary role in haemostasis, maintaining vascular integrity and contributing to the complex process of coagulation. They have also been implicated in the promotion of arteriosclerotic lesions. NSAIDs can interfere with platelet function by several mechanisms involving inhibition of cyclo-oxygenase. This blocks the formation not only of platelet activating eicosanoids, such as PGG_2, PGH_2 and thromboxane A_2, but also of the platelet inhibitors PGD_2 and PGI_2. PGI_2 causes an increase in platelet cyclic adenosine monophosphate (cAMP), which prevents them from aggregating but not from adhering to the endothelium, thus allowing minor endothelial injury healing. In health there is a balance between PGI_2 and thromboxane A_2. Aspirin is the only NSAID that is used therapeutically for its antiplatelet effects.

For most NSAIDs, except aspirin, the antiplatelet effect is present only while the drug is present in the body in sufficient concentration. In the case of aspirin the effect lasts for the 5–11 days of the life of the platelet because of the irreversible acetylation of platelet and megakaryocyte cyclo-oxygenase coupled with the inability of platelets to synthesise new enzyme. With the exception of the therapeutic antiplatelet effect of the NSAIDs in patients with cardiovascular disease, the antiplatelet effect is of no or minimal clinical significance in haematologically normal patients. Despite numerous studies on NSAIDs and surgical bleeding, no firm conclusions can be drawn as to an increased risk of haemorrhage in patients taking NSAIDs. Even the impact of peroperatively administered NSAIDs on blood loss is unclear. Several studies have reported no significant blood loss compared with placebo in patients given indomethacin or diclofenac. Aspirin and other NSAIDs should be avoided, where possible, during pregnancy. NSAIDs can cross the placenta and have been associated with significant neonatal bleeding. The mother may also have excessive intrapartum blood loss. In some pregnancies aspirin may, however, have a therapeutic indication, specifically in the prevention of pre-eclampsia.

ADVERSE EFFECTS

Gastrointestinal tract

A major limitation to the use of NSAIDs is their detrimental effects on the mucosa of the gastrointestinal tract, in particular the stomach. The bleeding and ulceration induced in the stomach by NSAIDs, commonly referred to as 'NSAID gastropathy', are linked to suppression of gastric prostaglandins, although other factors also play a role. A particularly troublesome feature of NSAID gastropathy is that the ulceration is often asymptomatic, the initial presentation frequently being severe haemorrhage or perforation. Bleeding ulcers and perforations are more common in patients over 60 years. Women are at greater risk than men to develop NSAID induced gastric ulcers and ulcer related complications. This may reflect the fact that rheumatoid arthritis is three times more common in women than in men, so that there is a higher exposure in women. Conventional antiulcer therapy, such as antacids, histamine H_2-receptor antagonists or proton pump inhibitors, are relatively ineffective in preventing NSAID induced ulceration. The concomitant administration of the PGE_1 analogue, misoprostol, is more effective but is expensive and associated with an appreciable incidence of side-effects, notably diarrhoea.

Several NSAIDs, including aspirin, phenylbutazone and indomethacin, produce direct mucosal injury and alter the structure of the gastric mucosa. At a pH below its pK_a (3.5), aspirin greatly reduces the surface hydrophobic, non-wettable layer of surface active phospholipids that cover the gastric mucosa and prevent the passage of H^+ ions, to the point where cellular injury can occur. This hydrophobic layer is maintained by prostaglandins. NSAIDs reduce gastric mucosal blood flow at sites that eventually ulcerate, and injury to the vascular endothelium of the gastric mucosa occurs early after their administration.

Aspirin, in particular, undergoes ion trapping within the cells of the gastric mucosa. In the acid medium of the stomach aspirin is non-ionised and is rapidly absorbed by passive diffusion. However, in the more alkaline milieu of the cell, salicylate ions are released. Salicylates inhibit cellular energy production by impairing mitochondrial phosphorylation, leading to increased cell membrane permeability and a cascade of events that result ultimately in cell death, focal erosions and bleeding. Other NSAIDs, especially indomethacin, can also cause focal lesions by increasing the permeability of the cell membrane, but the mechanism is not fully understood.

Renal system

Adverse reactions involving the renal system are uncommon in patients with normal kidneys but rarely can present as life threatening acute renal failure. Acute renal failure is the most common form of NSAID associated renal impairment. The renal medulla is one of the most active prostaglandin-producing tissues, and prostaglandins modulate renal blood flow and glomerular filtration rate, although they are not essential to maintaining renal function in the unstressed kidney. Any reduction in the renal circulation causes a homeostatic increased production of catecholamines and activation of the renin–angiotensin system. The resulting renal vasoconstriction is counterbalanced by a compensatory release of prostaglandins to maintain adequate renal perfusion. It is therefore not surprising that inhibition of prostaglandin synthesis by NSAIDs can result in renal dysfunction. Dehydration, haemorrhage, congestive heart failure, cirrhosis with ascites and excessive diuresis may reduce the effective circulating volume to the extent that prostaglandins become operative in the maintenance of renal perfusion. Under these circumstances NSAIDs will decrease renal blood flow and glomerular filtration rate. This is reversible if the

NSAID is discontinued, but if not recognised can lead to prolonged renal ischaemia, acute tubular necrosis and permanent renal damage. While administration of NSAIDs to healthy patients will reduce renal blood flow by less than 10%, in patients in whom the renin–angiotensin system has been activated (e.g. those with congestive heart failure) the reduction may be up to 60% and lead to clinical renal failure. NSAIDs can also cause acute renal insufficiency in patients with pre-existing chronic renal insufficiency because in these patients prostaglandins are essential to maintain renal function.

Acute interstitial nephritis is a rare but severe form of NSAID nephrotoxicity. It differs from acute ischaemic renal insufficiency in onset, severity and duration. Although it can occur within 1 week of NSAID administration, it usually occurs between several months and 1 year after the start of NSAID therapy. Many of the patients are elderly, but the disease also occurs in children receiving NSAIDs for the treatment of juvenile rheumatoid arthritis. Most patients respond to discontinuation of the NSAID within 1–3 months.

The most severe and often irreversible form of NSAID induced renal toxicity is analgesia associated nephropathy. Patients who develop this syndrome have typically been using analgesic mixtures, often containing aspirin, phenacetin and caffeine, for many years. The syndrome is characterised by papillary necrosis and many patients present with end-stage renal failure and hypertension. It appears that a requisite for the development of the syndrome is the use of a drug that selectively concentrates in the renal papillae. Both aspirin and paracetamol selectively distribute to the renal medulla, but phenacetin, which has been frequently implicated, does not. There have been no reports of this syndrome associated with ingestion of phenacetin alone. The mechanism is unknown, but may be related to an oxidised metabolite of paracetamol produced in the kidney. Phenacetin is almost completely metabolised to paracetamol after absorption in the gut.

Some diuretics, e.g. thiazides, stimulate prostaglandin production, and the action of loop diuretics such as fruseamide is prostaglandin dependent. Interactions between these agents and NSAIDs are common. All NSAIDs, and indomethacin in particular, can interfere with the pharmacological control of hypertension and congestive heart failure in patients receiving β-adrenoceptor antagonists, diuretics or angiotensin converting enzyme inhibitors. Although the average effect on blood pressure control may be small, there is substantial variability between individuals. Inhibition of the renal excretion of digoxin and lithium may increase the plasma concentrations of these drugs and increase the risk of toxicity.

Hypersensitivity reactions

In susceptible individuals NSAIDs may precipitate acute bronchospasm, a clinical syndrome referred to as aspirin induced asthma. It affects between 10 and 20% of adults with asthma but is rare in asthmatic children. The mechanism is related to cyclo-oxygenase inhibition, with shunting of arachidonic acid metabolism from the prostaglandin pathway to the biosynthesis of leukotrienes, with resulting bronchospasm, increased mucosal permeability and secretion and neutrophil influx to the tissues. Patients susceptible to this syndrome should obviously avoid NSAIDs that inhibit cyclo-oxygenase, as the bronchospasm may be severe and has been fatal. Paracetamol in doses up to 1000 mg daily will be tolerated by most patients. Non-acetylated salicylates, because they are relatively weak cyclo-oxygenase inhibitors, may be tolerated, but patients taking these drugs should be monitored carefully.

True type I allergic reactions to NSAIDs, with specific immunoglobulin (IgE), are rare, but an anaphylactoid reaction with cardiovascular collapse has occasionally been described. It is more likely to occur in patients with a history of allergy or atopy, bronchial asthma or in patients with nasal polyps. Zomeperic seems to be the NSAID most frequently involved in anaphylactic shock. Many of the rare but serious haematological reactions to NSAIDs, such as aplastic anaemia, agranulocytosis and thrombocytopenia, are likely to have an immunological basis.

INDIVIDUAL DRUGS

Aspirin

Aspirin (acetylsalicylic acid) is a derivative of salicyclic acid, the bitter principle of the willow bark, which was first introduced in 1875 as an antiseptic, antipyretic and antirheumatic. The usual dose for mild pain is 300–600 mg orally. In the treatment of rheumatic diseases, larger doses, 5–8 g daily, are often required. Peak plasma levels are reached within 2–3 hours although appreciable concentrations are found within 30 minutes. Aspirin is rapidly hydrolysed in the plasma, liver and erythrocytes to salicylate, which is responsible for some, but not all, of the analgesic activity. Approximately 70% of an oral dose of aspirin is absorbed into the systemic circulation intact, the remainder being absorbed as salicylate. The absorbed aspirin is rapidly hydrolysed to salicylate, which is more slowly eliminated than aspirin. Both the unchanged drug and its metabolites are excreted in the urine — in normal circumstances 10% appears as free salicylic acid and 75% as salicyluric acid. Excretion is facilitated by alkalinisation of the urine, when up to 85% of the ingested drug is eliminated as salicylate. In acidic urine this proportion may be as low as 5%. Metabolism is normally very rapid and aspirin has a plasma half-life of only 2–3 hours; however, liver enzymes that form salicyluric acid and phenolic glucuronide are easily saturated and after multiple doses the terminal half-life may increase to 10 hours.

Aspirin, like other NSAIDs, causes gastric irritation, ulceration and haemorrhage. In patients who are regular users of aspirin the faecal blood loss can amount to 8 ml daily, and result in iron deficiency anaemia. The incidence of gastric irritation can be reduced by using buffered preparations of aspirin. Because of gastrointestinal irritation, oral aspirin is not used for the treatment of postoperative pain. A soluble salt, lysine acetylsalicylic acid, with similar pharmacological properties to aspirin, has been used by parenteral administration for postoperative pain.

Aspirin in low doses is widely used in patients with cardiovascular disease to reduce the incidence of myocardial infarction and strokes. The usual recommended dose is 80–160 mg daily, although some physicians recommend 325 mg daily. Even doses as low as 40 mg per day can produce maximal inhibition of thromboxane and prostacyclin synthesis. The use of aspirin can reduce the risk of myocardial infarction by 25% and reduce the risk of a fatal infarction significantly. Aspirin, with or without dipyridamole, has been found clearly to be effective for preventing acute occlusion in patients undergoing percutaneous transluminal coronary angioplasty and in patients after coronary artery surgery. Dipyridamole is a compound with antithrombotic and vasodilatatory properties. The exact mechanism of its actions is unknown.

With plasma concentrations over $350 \, \mu g \, ml^{-1}$, such as occur with overdose, salicylates directly stimulate the respiratory centre, resulting in marked hyperventilation, with increases in both rate and depth. The respiratory changes induced by aspirin are accompanied by changes in acid–base and electrolyte balance. Most commonly observed with full therapeutic doses is a compensated respiratory alkalosis. However, when toxic doses are ingested, particularly by infants and children, metabolic acidosis occurs as a result of accumulation of acids caused by salicylate acid derivatives, circulatory collapse and renal impairment. Respiratory acidosis will also occur if plasma salicylate concentration becomes high enough to cause medullary depression of respiration. This stage of intoxication is accompanied by dehydration, hypernatraemia and hypokalaemia.

Aspirin is the NSAID most commonly involved in adverse hypersensitivity reactions. Aspirin intolerance is strictly defined as the presence of acute urticaria, angioneurotic oedema, bronchospasm, severe rhinitis or shock occurring within 3 hours of aspirin ingestion. The first case of aspirin intolerance, acute angioneurotic oedema, was reported in the literature only 3 years after the drug was introduced. In the normal population the incidence is between 0.3 and 0.9%, and in asthmatic patients 4%; however, patients suffering from chronic urticaria have an incidence of 23%. In this last group, intolerance is mostly manifested by urticarial-type reactions, while in asthmatic patients bronchospastic symptoms predominate. These two types of manifestation seem to be mediated by different mechanisms.

Paracetamol

Paracetamol (acetaminophen *USP*) is the major active metabolite of phenacetin, an analgesic that has been withdrawn from the UK market because of renal toxicity. Its analgesic and antipyretic effects are similar to those of aspirin, but it has negligible anti-inflammatory activity. Like aspirin, it is a potent prostaglandin inhibitor, but this activity is mainly restricted to within the CNS. The adult dose of paracetamol is 0.5–1 g orally.

Paracetamol is widely used in the treatment of mild to moderate pain, and is incorporated as an ingredient of many proprietary compounds together with aspirin, codeine or other mild analgesics. It is well absorbed from the gastrointestinal tract and does not cause the gastric irritation or blood loss seen with aspirin. Indeed, side-effects with paracetamol are uncommon with normal doses. Occasional haemolytic anaemia has been reported in patients with glucose-6-phosphate dehydrogenase deficiency in the erythrocytes.

In contrast to the lack of toxicity with therapeutic doses, overdosage with paracetamol is extremely dangerous and potentially fatal, due to liver damage. This hepatotoxicity is due to the *N*-hydroxyl metabolite, which binds covalently to essential macromolecules in hepatic cells, particularly those with sulphydryl (—SH) groups. With normal doses this toxic metabolite is excreted as the harmless conjugates of sulphur-containing amino acids, such as glutathione or methionine; however, after ingestion of toxic doses this process becomes swamped, resulting in free metabolite in the plasma, which causes cellular damage. Liver damage has been reported after a single dose of 5 g paracetamol, and deaths have occurred after 15 g (30 tablets). Since the hepatic damage is caused by a metabolite, signs of liver failure may not become apparent for many hours after an overdose has been taken. The treatment of paracetamol poisoning is dealt with in Chapter 52.

Ibuprofen

Ibuprofen is a propionic acid derivative with analgesic properties similar to aspirin. It is rapidly absorbed after oral administration, with peak analgesia being reached within 1–2 hours. The usual dose for mild to moderate pain is 400 mg every 4–6 hours. It is better tolerated than aspirin, mainly due to less severe gastrointestinal disturbances, which occur in about 10–15% of patients. There have been a few reported cases of toxic amblyopia, and any patient developing ocular symptoms should discontinue ibuprofen treatment immediately.

Ibuprofen and other arylpropionic acids have an asymmetric carbon atom; each therefore exists as two distinct optical isomers or enantiomers. Only naproxen is marketed as the pure $S(-)$ enantiomer; the remainder of this group are available only as the racemic mixtures. The cyclo-oxygenase inhibitory activity resides in the $S(-)$ enantiomer. Interestingly, an oral dose of racemic ibuprofen results in higher blood concentrations of the $S(+)$ enantiomer, due to chiral inversion from the inactive $R(-)$ to the active $S(+)$ enantiomer. Approximately 60% of the inactive enantiomer of ibuprofen is converted to the active enantiomer.

Indomethacin

Indomethacin, a methylated indole derivative, is a potent anti-inflammatory drug but less effective as an analgesic for pain of non-inflammatory origin than aspirin. In addition to inhibition of prostaglandin synthesis, indomethacin is also an inhibitor of leucocyte motility.

Indomethacin is rapidly and almost completely absorbed from the gastrointestinal tract after oral administration. The recommended dosage is initially 25 mg three times a day, gradually increasing to about 100 mg a day. To diminish gastrointestinal disturbances it should be taken with food. Owing to a high incidence of side-effects, indomethacin is reserved for the treatment of rheumatoid and osteoarthritis and ankylosing spondylitis. It is also useful in the management of acute attacks of gout, and can be of value in relieving the pain and inflammation of uveitis after ophthalmic surgery. Troublesome side-effects occur in approximately 30–35% of patients, and in 20% are severe enough to require reduction of dosage or complete withdrawal of the drug. The most common complaints are headache and gastrointestinal disturbances. Corneal deposits and retinal disturbances have been reported and patients on long term indomethacin therapy should undergo routine ophthalmic examination.

Indomethacin has been used in neonates in the treatment of cardiac failure caused by a patent ductus arteriosus. PGE causes dilatation of the ductus arteriosus, and inhibition by indomethacin may allow the ductus to close, thereby reducing the load on the heart. Successful closure can be expected in 70% of neonates.

Piroxicam

Piroxicam is the most commonly used of the oxicam derivative, a class of enolic acid NSAID. It is approximately equivalent to aspirin and indomethacin for the treatment of rheumatoid arthritis. It is also recommended for the treatment of acute gout. It has occasionally been used for postoperative pain, but appears not to have any distinct advantage over other NSAIDs. It can be administered orally, rectally or intramuscularly. Like most NSAIDs, it is well absorbed after oral administration, and peak plasma concentrations are reached within 2–4 hours. The elimination half-life varies between 30 and 70 hours and neither the age of the patient nor renal or hepatic dysfunction seems to have any major effect on the pharmacokinetics of piroxicam. The long half-life is a principal advantage for patients, permitting therapy with a single daily dose. The usual dose is 20 mg and is the same by all routes of administration. The drug reduces the renal excretion of lithium to a clinically significant extent. In addition to inhibition of cyclo-oxygenase, an additional mode of anti-inflammatory activity of piroxicam and other oxicams is modulation of various cytokines, including interleukin 2, interleukin 6 and tumour necrosis factor α.

Diclofenac

Diclofenac is a derivative of phenylacetic acid, with anti-inflammatory and analgesic activity, and is a potent inhibitor of prostaglandin synthesis. Its anti-inflammatory activity is similar to that of indomethacin and greater than that of aspirin. This may be due to the ability of diclofenac to decrease the production of leukotrienes by inhibiting lipoxygenase activity. In addition to prostaglandin inhibition, a central analgesic action of diclofenac mediated by endogenous opioid peptides has been demonstrated. A further mechanism for the analgesia produced by diclofenac may be a functional downregulation of sensitised, peripheral nociceptors. This seems to be the result of stimulation of the cyclic guanosine monophosphate (cGMP) system via the arginine–nitric oxide pathway.

Diclofenac can be administered orally, intramuscularly or intravenously in a dose of 75–150 mg. Diclofenac administered orally is almost completely absorbed, with peak plasma concentrations reached in 10–30 minutes, but these times may be greatly prolonged when there is food in the stomach. With most anti-inflammatory drugs the ability to cause peptic ulceration is related to the degree of reduction in gastric prostaglandin. However, diclofenac is an exception, in that it has a higher therapeutic ratio than most, while having high potency for prostaglandin inhibition. Nevertheless, gastric irritation and occult blood loss is also a feature of diclofenac.

Several studies have shown that diclofenac is effective as a postoperative analgesic. When given in combination with an opioid, opioid consumption may be reduced by up to 60%. The analgesic efficacy of diclofenac may be improved by commencing administration of the drug preoperatively. Diclofenac does not appear to increase blood loss during or after surgery.

Ketorolac tromethamine (trometamol)

Ketorolac, a recent addition to the NSAID group, has been widely investigated as an analgesic for postoperative as well as chronic pain. It is a chiral compound marketed as the racemate. Like other chiral NSAIDs, the cyclo-oxygenase inhibitory activity resides in the S enantiomer. However, unlike other chiral NSAIDs, the S enantiomer has the (−) rather than the (+) optical rotation. The tromethamine salt possesses sufficient water solubility to allow for parenteral administration. It appears to have a greater analgesic than anti-inflammatory or antipyretic activity. It does not inhibit lipoxygenase activity. When administered orally or intramuscularly, ketorolac is rapidly and well absorbed, with peak plasma concentrations attained between 30 and 50 minutes. The bioavailability after oral administration is 80–90%. There is relatively little transfer across the placenta or the blood–brain barrier.

Ketorolac is extensively metabolised to inactive or mainly inactive metabolites. The major metabolite is the acylglucuronide, which accounts for 70–75% of the amount of an oral dose excreted in the urine. The other major metabolite is *p*-hydroxyketorolac, which has about 20% of the anti-inflammatory and 1% of the analgesic activity of the parent compound. Ketorolac has a low hepatic extraction ratio (< 0.1) and thus under-goes negligible hepatic first pass metabolism. Unlike some other arylpropionic acid derivatives, chiral inversion does not occur, and the pharmacokinetics of ketorolac do not appear to be stereoselective. Like other NSAIDs, it is extensively bound to plasma proteins (99%). The protein binding may be non-linear, i.e. saturable, at higher plasma concentrations.

Ketorolac has been extensively investigated for its efficacy in the control of postoperative pain. In doses of 10–30 mg intramuscularly it is reported to be comparable or superior to morphine or pethidine in patients with moderate or severe pain after surgery; however, there is little evidence that ketorolac 30 mg provided any better analgesia than 10 mg. Indeed the Committee on Safety of Medicines in the UK has recently recommended that the starting dose of ketorolac be reduced from 30 mg to 10 mg i.m. or i.v. The usual precaution applicable to all NSAIDs should be observed when using ketorolac in the perioperative setting. Current evidence is that the incidence of adverse effects with ketorolac is similar to that found with other NSAIDs.

FURTHER READING

Borda I T, Koff R S 1992 NSAIDs: a profile of adverse effects. Mosby-Year Book, St Louis

Brocks D R, Jamali F 1992 Clinical pharmacokinetics of ketorolac tromethamine. Clinical Pharmacokinetics 23: 415

Brooks P M, Day R O 1991 Nonsteroidal anti-inflammatory drugs — differences and similarities. New England Journal of Medicine 24: 1716

Camu F, Van Lersberghe C, Lauwers M H 1992 Cardiovascular risks and benefits of perioperative nonsteroidal anti-inflammatory drug treatment. Drugs 44 (suppl 5): 42

Code W 1993 NSAIDs and balanced analgesia. Canadian Journal of Anaesthesia 40: 401

Day R O, Graham G G, Williams K M 1988 Pharmacokinetics of non-steroidal anti-inflammatory drugs. Baillière's Clinical Rheumatology 2: 363

McCormack K 1994 Non-steroidal anti-inflammatory drugs and spinal nociceptive processing. Pain 59: 9

Mather L E 1992 Do the pharmacodynamics of the nonsteroidal anti-inflammatory drugs suggest a role in the management of postoperative pain. Drugs 44 (suppl 5): 1

Murray M D, Brater D C 1993 Renal toxicity of the nonsteroidal anti-inflammatory drugs. Annual Review of Pharmacology and Toxicology 32: 435

Simons L S 1994 Actions and toxic effects of the nonsteroidal anti-inflammatory drugs. Current Opinion in Rheumatology 6: 238

19

Skeletal muscle

D. F. Goldspink
V. M. Cox

In most mammals at birth, including man, approximately 20–25% of the body weight is attributable to the musculature. During postnatal growth the proportion of skeletal muscle increases so that in the adult it represents 40–45% of the body's weight and protein content. By virtue of being the largest tissue in the body, muscle contains the largest reserve of amino acids, both free and covalently bound in proteins. The movement of these amino acids between the muscle and plasma is important in the normal, everyday homeostatic regulation of plasma nutrients, and it is essential for survival during crises such as starvation and situations of hormone deficiency (e.g. diabetes) or excess (e.g. Cushing's syndrome or hyperthyroidism). Muscle protein is also used for survival in the metabolic response to major surgery and severe trauma. So, while the main emphasis here will be placed on the contractile properties and mechanical functions of skeletal muscle, the musculature is also extremely important to the individual in metabolic terms.

MYOGENESIS AND REGENERATION

At a very early stage in embryonic development the different stem cells within the somites are committed to different pathways, e.g. becoming either myoblasts (precursors of muscle fibres) or fibroblasts. After a period of proliferation under the influence of growth factors, such as fibroblast growth factor, the myoblasts aggregate and fuse with one another, initially forming myotubes (at

7–9 weeks of gestation in man). The addition of more myoblasts then turns the myotube into a multinucleate fibre, attached by tendons to the developing skeleton. This fusion of myoblasts represents specific mutual recognition, as they will not fuse with adjacent non-muscle cells. By secreting certain factors the fusing myoblasts appear to encourage other myoblasts to engage in fusion, thereby reinforcing the process. Fusion itself results in the nuclei ceasing to replicate, although a few inactive myoblasts are retained within the adult muscle (see below). Fusion also represents the onset of muscle cell differentiation, which is believed to be triggered by one or a small number of master gene regulatory proteins, such as myoD1. MyoD1 appears to be involved in specifying which stems cells will become myoblasts, and in the coordinated activation of a battery of muscle specific genes whose proteins give rise to the contractile apparatus (see below), creatine phosphokinase for the specialised metabolism of muscle fibres, and acetylcholine receptors for neuromuscular transmission. All of these changes occur on myoblast fusion.

Once formed, a muscle fibre normally exists throughout the life span of the organism. Hence, the adult number of muscle fibres in mammals is fixed around the time of birth. The enormous postnatal increase in muscle bulk involves enlargement of these existing fibres, without fibre proliferation (see below).

A few myoblasts (satellite cells) persist in adult muscle as small, flattened cells lying in close contact with the mature fibres, just beneath the basement membrane but outside the plasma membrane. These satellite cells can be reactivated to proliferate in response to muscle elongation or repair after damage. The growth in muscle fibre length needed to keep pace with elongation of the skeleton involves the addition of more sarcomeres at the ends of the fibre, new nuclei being added through the division and incorporation of satellite cells. Proliferation of satellite cells also occurs in damaged, but otherwise nongrowing, muscle fibres. The progeny of the satellite cells fuse to form a new fibre to replace the degenerating one. Satellite cells therefore represent a small proportion of myoblasts, normally quiescent but held in reserve in adult muscle. If needed, they act as a cell-renewing source of terminally differentiated cells to maintain the appropriate fibre numbers. Unlike the large loss of neurones in the brain, normal ageing is not accompanied by an appreciable loss of muscle fibres; however, in inherited diseases, such as Duchenne muscular dystrophy, attempts to regenerate viable fibres within the degenerating muscle fail because the nuclei of the satellite cells also carry the same genetic defect, a deficiency of dystrophin.

INNERVATION AND FIBRE TYPES

Skeletal muscle is responsible for practically all movements under voluntary control. The individual fibres are cylindrical in shape and in adult humans can often be very long, up to 0.5–1.0 cm in length and 100 μm in diameter (Fig. 19.1A). Each fibre is a syncytium possessing many nuclei, which tend to be peripherally located within a common cytoplasm (sarcoplasm).

During perinatal development each fibre will be supplied by several motor neurones. All but one of these will be subsequently withdrawn, to leave each adult muscle fibre innervated by only one motor neurone. That same motor nerve fibre will however innervate several muscle fibres, bringing these together as a functional unit (a *motor unit*) under the control of that one motor neurone. The size of the motor unit can vary substantially, ranging from as few as 1–5 fibres in some muscles (e.g. fingers or eyes) to as many as 200 fibres or more in some trunk or leg muscles; the fewer the number, the finer the control over movements. Although the muscle fibres can be classified into different types (see below), a motor unit will only contain fibres of one particular type. Different motor units possess different thresholds of activation, this being determined by the threshold of the motor neurone. Hence the progressive recruitment of more motor units can influence the overall speed of contraction and the amount of force developed, this being maximal when all motor units are activated simultaneously.

The different muscles within the musculature vary considerably in their contractile profiles.

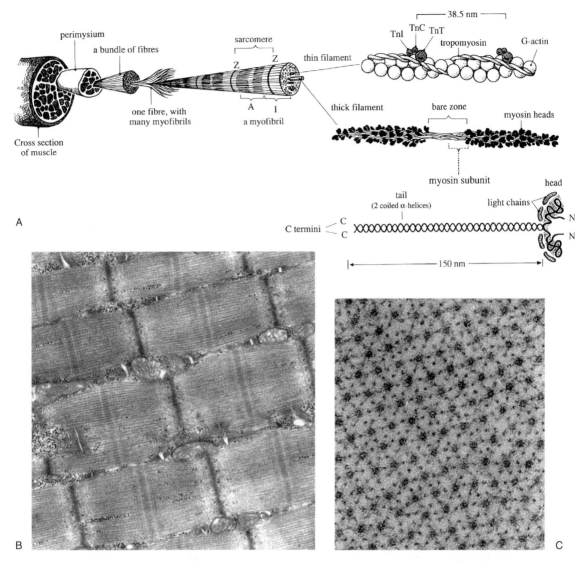

Figure 19.1 (A) Basic structure of thick and thin filaments within a myofibril of an individual muscle fibre. Electron micrographs (courtesy of Dr P. E. Williams, University of Hull) show (B) sarcomeres within the myofibril (×26 000), and (C) the spatial relationship between the overlapping thick and thin filaments as seen in a cross-section of the A band (×120 000).

Such differences arise from the fact that every muscle consists of more than one type of muscle fibre, with the predominant fibre type tending to characterise the muscle as a whole. Muscle fibres are mainly classified with respect to their biochemical and/or physiological properties, e.g. fast or slow twitch fibres, with the fast fibres further subdivisible into 2–3 categories. Such classifications have been largely developed from a variety of histochemical techniques but principally those relating to the staining for the myosin ATPase (Fig. 19.2A) and the mitochondrial enzyme succinate dehydrogenase. The myosin heavy chain contains an adenosine triphosphate (ATP) splitting enzyme that varies in its specific activity and pH stability depending on the type or isoform of the heavy chain being expressed. This variable stability of the enzyme has been well exploited. For example, using a preincubation pH of 4.6, three distinct fibre types are

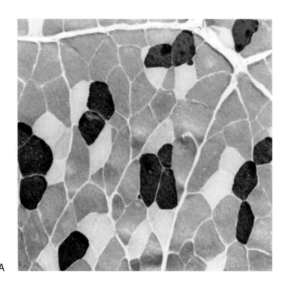

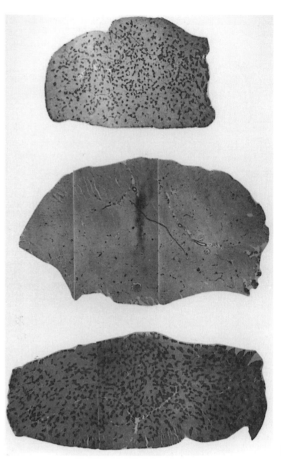

Figure 19.2 (A) Standard myosin ATPase stain (acid preincubation) revealing three fibre types: slow oxidative (dark), fast oxidative glycolytic (pale) and fast glycolytic (intermediate staining intensity) (Courtesy of H. Wright and V. M. Cox.) (×250) (B) Transverse sections of the entire soleus muscle of the rat showing large increases in size despite a fixed number of fibres. Note the conversion of a mixed fibre-type profile at 7 weeks of age (top) to a totally slow muscle (middle; 91 weeks) and back again in senescent (bottom; 121 weeks) muscle. (Courtesy of C. A. G. Boreham and D. F. Goldspink.) (Lower magnification)

clearly discernible, the dark staining fibres are *slow fibres* expressing the type I myosin heavy chain (Fig. 19.2A). The two remaining fibres are fast, with these subdivided into *fast oxidative glycolytic* (with type IIa myosin heavy chain) and *fast glycolytic* (with either type IIb or IId myosin heavy chain) fibres (Table 19.1). The relative proportions and cross-sectional areas of these fibres can be counted or measured using an image analyser. In serial sections of the same muscle both the slow and some fast oxidative glycolytic fibres stain strongly for succinate dehydrogenase and are therefore more oxidative than the pale fast glycolytic fibres, which depend more heavily on glycolysis to generate their ATP. These and other features of the three fibre types are summarised in Table 19.1.

In functional terms the *slow oxidative* fibres are more economical in their use of ATP and fatigue

only slowly, properties which make them ideally suited for maintaining posture and carrying out movements of a slow repetitive nature. Fast fibres usually possess more myofibrils and hence have a greater cross-sectional area. They are therefore adapted to provide a high power output. *Fast glycolytic fibres* are only used when very rapid movements are required. In contrast, *fast oxidative glycolytic* fibres possess intermediate properties to those of the *slow oxidative* and *fast glycolytic fibres* (Table 19.1) and are probably recruited after motor units composed of slow fibres. *Fast oxidative glycolytic* fibres are suited for fast movements of a repetitive nature.

Each muscle will have a different proportion of these fibre types, reflecting different metabolic and contractile characteristics. Although fibre number remains constant, the proportions of these three fibre types are not stable with age

Table 19.1 Muscle fibre types

Feature	Slow oxidative	Fast oxidative glycolytic	Fast glycolytic
1. Fibre diameter	Smallest	Larger	Largest
2. Speed of shortening	Slow	Faster	Fastest
a. type of myosin	I	IIa	IIb or IId
b. specific activity of myosin ATPase	Low	High	Highest
3. Relaxation	Slow	Faster	Fastest
a. specific activity of SR Ca^{2+} ATPase	Low	High	Highest
b. volume of SR	Small	Large	Large
4. Metabolism			
a. oxidative phosphorylation	High	Moderate	Low
b. glycolysis	Moderate	Moderate	Moderate
c. capillary:fibre ratio	High	Low	Low
d. fatigue resistance	High	Moderate	Low
5. Colour	Red	White	White
a. myoglobin	High	Moderate	Low
b. cytochromes	High	Moderate	Low
c. blood supply	High	Low	Low
6. Innervation, motor neurone			
a. diameter	Smallest	Larger	Largest
b. threshold	Lowest	Higher	Highest

Sarcoplasmic reticulum

(Fig. 19.2B); hence, fibre type proportions, as well as fibre size, can and do vary during development through to old age. Some research workers believe that all mammalian muscles are developmentally programmed to be fast twitch muscles. Only when the activity level is substantially increased, as in postural muscles, do the slow oxidative and fatigue resistant properties become 'stamped' on a muscle. Certainly when a postural muscle is rendered less active than normal through some form of injury, the slow oxidative properties are lost and fast glycolytic properties become more strongly expressed.

All of this points to the tremendous flexibility, or plasticity, of muscles in responding to the varying physiological needs of the organism, all of which is accomplished through changes in size or in gene expression to modify the phenotypic properties of a fixed number of fibres. The ability to understand and manipulate gene expression is currently being exploited in medical research to enable muscles to perform new functions within the body, e.g. in recreating anal or urethral sphincters from the gracilis muscle to treat incontinence, or in providing an auxiliary pump from the latissimus dorsi muscle to assist a failing heart. Under such circumstances muscles need to be trained to acquire more appropriate properties (e.g. fatigue resistance) for the new function that they are called upon to perform within the body.

In vertebrates, coordinated voluntary movements, such as walking, running, flying or swimming, all depend on the ability of skeletal muscles to contract and pull against various parts of the skeleton. To fulfil such functions skeletal muscle fibres have become highly specialised, expressing large quantities of specific proteins that are assembled into highly organised units which comprise the contractile machinery.

About two-thirds of the dry weight of a muscle fibre is made up of contractile proteins. These are arranged into cylindrical elements, myofibrils, which are approximately 1 or 2 μm in diameter and usually run the whole length of the fibre (Fig. 19.1A). Individual myofibrils consist of repeated contractile units, called sarcomeres, which possess prominent light and dark refractive bands that, under the microscope, give the classical striated appearance of muscle (Fig. 19.1A,B).

MUSCLE STRUCTURE AND CONTRACTILE MECHANISM

The sarcomere

Each sarcomere represents the distance (usually about 2.5 μm) between two Z discs and is repeated along the length of the myofibril (Fig. 19.1A,B). Within each sarcomere there are two sets of parallel and partially overlapping filament structures. The thick filaments (mainly composed of myosin, see below) span the dark A band, while the thin filaments (mainly actin) extend throughout the region of each light or I band and part of the way into the two neighbouring dark bands (Fig. 19.1A). A cross-section taken through the region of the dark band, where both thick and thin filaments overlap, is shown in Figure 19.1C. The thick filaments are clearly arranged in a regular hexagonal lattice, with the thin filaments positioned between them. This region of overlap increases in length, at the expense of the light band, as the sarcomeres shorten during muscle contraction. The thin filaments are pulled over the thick filaments, and as each sarcomere shortens this is reflected as a shortening of the myofibril and muscle as a whole. This shortening movement is described as the sliding filament model, which is better understood after a more detailed examination of the proteins that are contained within, and interact between, the thick and thin filaments.

Thin filament

Although actin is the principal protein found in the thin filament, it is not the only one (Fig. 19.1A). The actin filaments arise from the polymerisation of globular subunits of actin (G-actin monomers), which consist of single polypeptides of 375 amino acids, derived from a highly conserved gene. These G-actin molecules are packed into the tight helix structure of the actin filament, with about two monomers per turn and a width of approximately 8 nm. This gives the overall appearance of two helical strands of actin molecules twisting around each other every 37 nm. It may be helpful to visualise two strands of beads in a necklace twisted around each other, with a regular repeat sequence.

Thick filament

Next to collagen, myosin is the most abundant protein in the body. Much of it is associated with the skeletal musculature, and the thick filament of the sarcomeres in particular. Although it is the dominant protein found here, it is not the only one present.

Each molecule of myosin (Fig. 19.1A) consists of six polypeptide chains: two heavy chains and two pairs of light chains. The latter can be stripped off a heavy chain by simple chemical treatments. The heavy chains consist of long (150 nm) helical rod-like regions (the myosin tail) and two globular heads. The latter are responsible for interacting with neighbouring actin filaments to form cross-bridges through which force is generated and the actin moved relative to the myosin. The tail filament is made up of two individual heavy chains that form a stable α helix through hydrophobic interactions. Many similar tailed filaments are packed together within the thick filament, with these tail regions arranged in a bipolar manner, leaving a bare central support region where the two sets of oppositely orientated myosin tails come together. These same myosin heavy chain molecules are staggered so that as their globular heads point towards the ends of the thick filament, they rotate and project out in a repeating pattern, which enables them to interact with the surrounding six thin filaments (Fig. 19.1C) and form cross-bridges where appropriate.

Molecular mechanisms associated with cross-bridge formation

The presence of other proteins in addition to actin in the thin filament of the sarcomere is crucial for the regulation of muscle contraction.

One of these accessory proteins is the rod-shaped tropomyosin molecule, which is a dimer of two identical α-helical chains, which wind around each other. The tropomyosin molecules bind along the length of an actin filament, helping to provide strength and stability (Fig. 19.1A).

The other major accessory protein is troponin (Tn), which is a complex of three polypeptide subunits. These subunits are named troponin T, I and C in recognition of their roles in tropomyosin binding (Tn-T), inhibitory binding to actin (Tn-I) and Ca^{2+} binding (Tn-C). Unlike the tropomyosin

molecule, only one molecule of the Tn complex is present in every seven actin monomers along the actin filament.

In a resting muscle the Tn-I binds to actin, such that the tropomyosin molecule along the actin filament is moved into a position that sterically inhibits the myosin heads from interacting with the actin (Fig. 19.3A). The presence of Tn-C makes this complex acutely sensitive to changes in the concentration of cytosolic Ca^{2+}. When a Ca^{2+} transient is triggered (see below), each Tn-C can bind up to four molecules of Ca^{2+}. In so

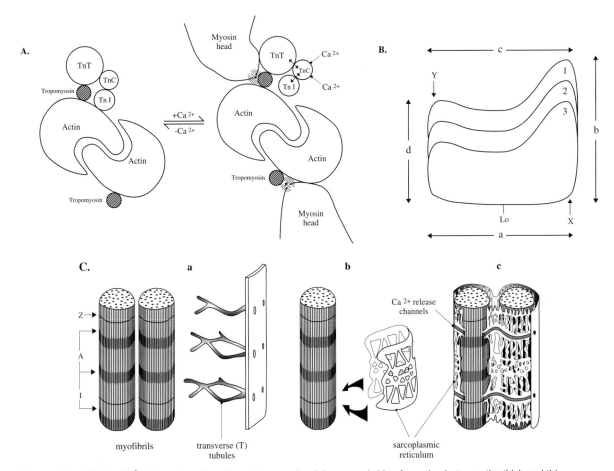

Figure 19.3 (A) The Ca^{2+}-induced conformational changes involving cross-bridge formation between the thick and thin filaments. (B) Oscillatory work loops. Stage (a) is the passive extension phase, (b) the rapid rise in force in response to muscle activation (at X), (c) the decline in force during muscle shortening, and (d) the fall in tension following de-activation (at Y). The amount of work (i.e. area within each loop) is seen to decline in progressing from the first (1) to the 20th (2) and 25th (3) consecutive loops, indicating some fatigue. (C) The intimate relationships between the transverse tubule invaginations of the plasma membrane and the network of the sarcoplasmic reticulum with the myofibrils of a muscle fibre.

doing, a conformational change occurs in the Tn complex. The Tn-I subunit releases its inhibitory hold on the actin and allows movement of the tropomyosin molecule such that the myosin head and actin can now interact and form a cross-bridge. The rapid withdrawal of cytosolic Ca^{2+} by the sarcoplasmic reticulum will subsequently reverse this process, leading to relaxation (see below).

Energetics of muscle contraction

The projecting globular heads of a myosin molecule bind to neighbouring actin filaments, causing movement of the actin relative to the myosin. This process involves the hydrolysis of ATP. The ATP splitting enzyme is associated with the myosin head, and the specific activity of this enzyme varies with the type, or isoform, of myosin present. This correlates with the speed of contraction, with the adult slow myosin isoform having a lower ATPase activity than fast myosin heavy chain isoforms (Table 19.1).

Usually a free myosin head binds a molecule of ATP (stage 1). This is then hydrolysed and, while the adenosine diphosphate (ADP) and inorganic phosphate products remain bound to it, the head interacts with an actin molecule (stage 2). The myosin head then releases the inorganic phosphate and binds even more tightly to the actin filament (stage 3). The head now undergoes a large but poorly understood conformational change which, in a ratchet-like manner, pulls the actin over the myosin molecule (stage 4). ADP is now released and ATP takes its place. This causes a loss of affinity between the myosin head and the actin and the cross-bridge dissociates. At the end of this cycle the actin filament has now moved relative to the myosin. A new cycle of cross-bridge formation and detachment can now take place. Each of the two heads on a myosin molecule is thought to cycle independently of the other.

Each thick filament has approximately 500 myosin heads, and each head cycles about 5 times a second in the course of a rapid contraction, the thick and thin filaments sliding past each other at a rate up to 15 μm s^{-1}.

MECHANICAL PROPERTIES OF SKELETAL MUSCLE

Traditionally, muscle function has been measured using two types of mechanical recording. Isometric recordings measure tension development while muscle length is kept constant. Isotonic measurements are of muscle shortening while tension is kept constant. In fact, these recordings represent the two extremes of muscle function, as most muscles *in situ* seldom contract in either a purely isometric or isotonic manner. Similarly, muscles seldom contract in the classical form of a single twitch in response to one stimulus, or tetanically in response to rapid repeated stimuli. Usually muscle contraction is carefully coordinated, with smooth movements arising from time-related modifications in the number and types of motor units recruited.

Isometric recordings have, however, been useful in establishing that:

- The development of tension or force (in Newtons per square metre of cross-sectional area) is directly proportional to the number of cross-bridges formed; maximum force production occurs at a sarcomere length that provides optimal overlap between the thick and thin filaments.
- The connective tissue elements in a muscle offer resistance to passive stretching.
- Tetanic tension is several times greater than that of a single twitch. In part this represents the internal stretching of elastic elements (e.g. collagen fibres) within the muscle. With each twitch, in response to a single supramaximal stimulus, the elastic fibres in series (e.g. in the tendons) and in parallel (the endomysium and perimysium; Fig. 19.1A) are stretched out fully. This necessitates a largish component of internal work. When the muscle relaxes these stretched elements recoil. This cycle of events has to be repeated with each twitch. During a fused tetanic contraction, in response to multiple stimuli, the muscle remains in a contracted state and the elastic elements continuously stretched. Hence, a much larger proportion of the muscle's overall energy is expressed as external, rather than internal, work.

Isotonic recordings have indicated that:

- The faster a muscle contracts and shortens, and hence recycles its cross-bridges, the less external work it is capable of performing, i.e. force generation and velocity of shortening are inversely related.
- Each muscle in situ usually works most efficiently (i.e. around its maximum power output) by combining muscle shortening with force generation. The precise proportions of these will depend upon the anatomical location and the type of work required in the body. For example, the deltoid muscle is a relatively short, bulky and powerful muscle, its fibres having a large cross-sectional area packed with myofibrils. In contrast, other muscles, e.g. the quadriceps in the thigh, have much longer fibres with many more sarcomeres in series. When this muscle contracts it provides a great deal of shortening, moving the lower leg through the large angle provided by the knee joint.

The oscillatory work loop technique, used on muscles either in vitro or in situ, more closely simulates muscle function in vivo. In this technique (Fig. 19.3B) the muscle is extended beyond its resting length, as would be accomplished in the body by antagonist muscles. The muscle is then electrically stimulated, and as it is activated there is a rapid rise in force development. The muscle is allowed to shorten and as it does so the force declines, as more cross-bridges are in a state of recycling. Deactivation is accompanied by a sharp fall in force before the passive lengthening phase recommences. The area inside this loop represents the net work undertaken, i.e. the positive work performed by the muscle minus the negative work that has to be done on the muscle to passively extend it. The muscle's resistance to stretching will increase with any increase in its connective tissue content, e.g. in association with repair of damaged fibres. The power output (in watts) is calculated from: (work performed per loop) × (number of loops performed per unit time).

Work loop measurements are more useful than the isotonic or isometric recordings in defining muscle performance *in vivo* because they in-

corporate all of the major phases of muscle function, activation, shortening, deactivation and extension (Fig. 19.3B).

MUSCLE FIBRE GROWTH

Increases in fibre cross-sectional area (muscle girth)

Postnatal growth (i.e. accumulation of protein) of bodily tissues, and in particular skeletal muscle, is extremely rapid. This is associated with high rates of protein synthesis and degradation, which progressively decline with increasing age. Although it is not known what precisely regulates the number of fibres in a muscle, it is at least partly under genetic control. Once determined (around birth) there is no further increase in fibre number. Growth occurs as an enlargement of these fibres, mainly by increasing the myofibrillar material within each fibre — for example, in some muscles the number of myofibrils may increase from approximately 50 in a myotube to over 1000 in a fully mature fibre. The volume of the sarcoplasmic reticulum and transverse tubular systems, which are involved in for the activation of the myofibrils, increases at a similar rate. Three types of factor can influence muscle size and the amount and type (isoforms) of the proteins found within the contractile apparatus: genetic, systemic (e.g. hormones and nutrients) and mechanical.

Genetic factors

Some individuals are genetically predisposed to be better at certain types of sport than others; training simply fine tunes the phenotypic properties most suited for a particular type of activity.

Systemic factors

Hormones and growth factors. These chemical agents can either act systemically or in a local paracrine/autocrine manner to alter muscle size by modifying either the rates of protein synthesis, protein degradation, or both. In some instances hormones can also change the muscle's phenotypic properties and mechanical perform-

Table 19.2 Hormonal effects on skeletal muscle protein turnover

Hormone	Protein synthesis	Protein breakdown	Change in phenotype
Anabolic (net effect)			
Insulin	+	−	
IGF-1 and IGF-2	+	−	
Thyroid	+	+	+
Growth hormone	+	0	+
Catabolic (net effect)			
Glucocorticoids	−	+ or −	
Glucagon	−	0	
Catecholamines	Unclear		

IGF, insulin-like growth factor.

ance (Table 19.2). Clearly these chemical signals are important in promoting generalised growth throughout the musculature.

In adolescent boys testosterone appears to act as an additional stimulus for growth, leaving the male more heavily muscled. After the fifth decade there can often be a marked loss of muscle mass and strength, this being particularly noticeable in postmenopausal women. However, even in the adult, when muscle growth is slow and protein turnover rates low, regionalised adaptive growth is still possible.

Nutrients. After surgery, elevated levels of stress hormones, possibly exacerbated by reduced activity levels, cause patients to exhibit a marked negative nitrogen balance. The same is true with sepsis and cachexia. Certain amino acids, particularly the branched chain amino acids, like leucine and valine, are known to stimulate protein synthesis and inhibit protein degradation in skeletal muscle. Hence, these branched chain amino acids represent crucial components in mixtures of amino acids, which, when infused, minimise the muscle wasting. A variety of anabolic steroids and β agonists (e.g. clenbuterol) have also been used in an attempt to either slow atrophy or increase muscle mass; β agonists can, however, cause undesirable side-effects, such as tremor.

Contractile activity. There is a strong link between muscle activity, rates of protein turnover, muscle size and strength. After birth, as an animal becomes active and heavier, more muscle fibres will be recruited and some will be overtaxed. More myofibrils are produced to generate more force to meet the greater work demands imposed on these muscles. Once myofibrils reach a certain critical size, through the addition of more filament proteins, they split longitudinally, producing daughter myofibrils. These in turn can enlarge to the same maximum size, while providing the extensive sarcoplasmic reticulum and transverse tubular systems the opportunity to infiltrate and assume close proximity with the contractile apparatus.

The reverse is also true: situations that decrease muscle activity will cause muscle wasting — for example, bed rest, denervation, limb immobilisation due to a fracture or joint disease, and space travel, all reduce muscle activity. Inactivity leads to a decrease in the rate of protein synthesis and an increase in protein degradation, complementary changes leading to reductions in muscle fibre cross-sectional area and hence muscle mass. Reduced activity, with a muscle operating at a shorter length than normal, also causes a loss of sarcomeres in series and hence shorter myofibrils and muscle fibres. The reverse occurs when muscles are stretched (see below).

Exercise. Different types of activity influence muscle fibre size and/or its metabolic profile. Endurance activities, e.g. long distance running or cycling, are known to cause hypertrophy of slow oxidative fibres. Even so, the overall muscle mass may remain unchanged because of a small degree of atrophy in some of the fast fibres. This type of exercise usually results in a more noticeable metabolic adaptation, leaving the muscle more oxidative and hence resistant to fatigue. This metabolic adaptation involves the proliferation of mitochondria, thus enabling the fibres to produce ATP more effectively through oxidative phosphorylation. The repetitive nature of this type of exercise often causes the muscle to become slower in its contraction and relaxation.

In contrast, short bursts of high intensity exercise (e.g. weight lifting and athletic field events) increase the cross-sectional area of all types of muscle fibre, but with a disproportionately greater effect on the fast fibres. Such exercise usually induces large increases in muscle mass without changing either the metabolic or contractile properties. The aim of this type of exercise is to retain fast movements, but with more explosive power.

Increases in muscle length

Muscle lengthening must occur in concert with the elongation of the skeleton. This is achieved by increasing the number of sarcomeres in series along the length of each myofibril. In mammalian muscles the de novo synthesis of the new sarcomeres takes place in the myotendonous regions of each fibre. Mechanical stretching of the muscle appears to be a potent signal for muscle elongation. This has been shown in animal models where the lower hindlimb muscles have been immobilised in a lengthened, stretched position by placing a plaster cast around the ankle. In the stretched position the overlap between the actin and myosin is no longer optimal for cross-bridge formation and hence the development of tension. The muscle adapts to the stretch stimulus by rapidly adding more sarcomeres along its length, effectively eliminating the overstretching. If, however, the stretch stimulus is applied incrementally, e.g. at weekly intervals after the muscle has adapted to each prior stimulus, the muscle may become up to one-third longer. More myonuclei are obtained within these longer fibres through satellite cell division, thereby retaining an appropriate nuclear:sarcoplasmic ratio. The additional sarcomeres gained in response to stretch are rapidly shed if the cast is removed and normal muscle and joint function restored.

Summary

Any anaesthetic, therapeutic drug or surgical intervention that modifies dietary intake or the level of circulating hormones, or restricts the activity patterns or operating lengths of either individual muscles or the musculature as a whole, will inevitably modify muscle mass and length and hence force and power generation.

NEUROMUSCULAR JUNCTION AND EXCITATION CONTRACTION COUPLING

The physical continuity between the motor neurone and muscle fibre is interrupted by the neuromuscular junction, a synaptic gap of approximately 50–100 nm. Chemical transmission across this synapse is accomplished by the release of acetylcholine, which acts as an amplifying system, charging up the capacitance of the much larger muscle cell. The integration of all inhibitory and excitatory inputs via the central and peripheral nervous system has been accomplished prior to the motor neurone. Hence, under normal circumstances, for every action potential that is transmitted down the motor neurone, an action potential will be generated and propagated across, and within, each skeletal muscle fibre — that is, the neuromuscular junction is an excitatory synapse, and activation of one motor neurone will cause contraction of that particular motor unit.

Most of the acetylcholine is synthesised in the nerve terminals, from choline and acetyl coenzyme A, in a reaction catalysed by choline acetyltransferase in the presence of ATP and glucose. The acetylcholine is then stored in large numbers of minute vesicles, each some 30–60 nm in diameter.

As each action potential sweeps across the nerve terminal, it depolarises the membrane, opens voltage gated calcium channels and hence causes Ca^{2+} to move down its concentration gradient into the nerve terminal. The influx of Ca^{2+} causes several of the numerous vesicles storing acetylcholine to exocytose, liberating the transmitter substance into the synaptic gap. Upon interacting with the acetylcholine receptors, which are concentrated in the highly folded membrane systems of the muscle end-plate region, depolarising potentials (miniature end-plate potentials, MEPPs) are set up. The MEPPs arise from an increased membrane permeability to Na^+. In response to each action potential sufficient acetylcholine is released so that the summation of the MEPPs always depolarise the end-plate membrane beyond its threshold, causing the initiation of an action potential in the muscle fibre. This electrical excitation then spreads rapidly into a series of membranous invaginations, the transverse tubules. The transverse tubular system (Fig. 19.3C) extends inwards from the plasma membrane into the fibre and around each myofibril, giving rapid access to the interior as well as the periphery of the large muscle cell. The electrical signal is then transmitted from the transverse tubular system to the sarcoplasmic reticulum, an adjacent flattened anastomosing sheath of vesicles that surrounds each fibril like a net stocking (Fig. 19.3C). Where the transverse tubule meets the sarcoplasmic reticulum, the two membranes are very closely associated, but their two lumina are not continuous. Excitation of the transverse tubular system causes Ca^{2+} channels to open in the membrane of the sarcoplasmic reticulum and Ca^{2+} escapes from this storage site into the sarcoplasm. A resultant rise in cytosolic Ca^{2+} (from approximately 10^{-7} to 10^{-5} mol l^{-1}) initiates contraction (see below). Ca^{2+} is therefore acting as the crucial link that effectively couples electrical excitation and mechanical contraction.

Unlike smooth and cardiac muscle, where extracellular Ca^{2+} can enter the cell across the plasmalemma and contribute to the Ca^{2+} transient, in skeletal muscle the sarcoplasmic influx of Ca^{2+} is derived solely from the large reserve in the sarcoplasmic reticulum. The precise mechanisms surrounding Ca^{2+} release from the sarcoplasmic reticulum are unclear. Possibilities include depolarisation of the membrane of the sarcoplasmic reticulum, cytosolic Ca^{2+}-induced release of Ca^{2+} as occurs in cardiac muscle, and electron dense structures, called 'feet', which are seen in the triad region and possibly act as Ca^{2+} channels. The plant alkaloid ryanodine increases Ca^{2+} release via the ryanodine receptor (RYR1), which is a large protein similar in shape to, and possibly a part of, the 'feet' structure. Whatever the mechanism(s) involved, at appropriate doses ryanodine, caffeine and procaine are able to induce Ca^{2+} release, while dantrolene sodium blocks it.

The acetylcholine in the synaptic gap and on the receptors is rapidly broken down by acetyl-choline esterase, clearing the system in readiness for the next incoming action potential. After hydrolysis of this neurotransmitter, choline is taken up into the nerve terminals by active transport, where it is reused to synthesise more acetylcholine. This transport of choline back into the nerve terminal can be blocked by hemicholium. The very rapid transmission (milliseconds) of the action potential through the transverse tubular system to the release of Ca^{2+} from the sarcoplasmic reticulum enables all of the sarcomeres in each myofibril, including those deep in the interior of the large muscle cells, to contract synchronously. For relaxation to occur, the increased cytosolic Ca^{2+} has to be rapidly pumped back into the sarcoplasmic reticulum (Fig. 19.3C). Ca^{2+} is accumulated in the centrally located longitudinal vesicles before being stored in terminal cisternae at a concentration of about 1 mmol l^{-1}. As this sequestration is against a concentration gradient, it involves active transport and a Ca^{2+}-ATPase enzyme in the membrane of the sarcoplasmic reticulum. The activity of this ATP splitting enzyme depends on whether it has been derived from a 'fast' or 'slow' gene. Like the myosin ATPase, the fast isoform of the Ca^{2+}-ATPase has a higher specific activity than that of the slow isoform. This, together with the greater volume of sarcoplasmic reticulum, enables more rapid relaxation to occur in fast fibres (Table 19.1). Although this time scale is variable, typical resting levels of sarcoplasmic Ca^{2+} are restored within 30 ms, enabling all myofibrils to relax.

MUSCLE METABOLISM

Skeletal muscle converts chemical energy (ATP) into mechanical work. Approximately 30–50% of this energy is lost as heat. Although this may appear to be an inefficient conversion ratio, it is actually considerably better than most petrol driven engines, with 80–90% wastage. The heat generated during contraction also contributes to the homeostatic maintenance of body temperature.

The ATP that is available (approximately 4 mmol kg^{-1} of muscle) has an appreciable 'back-up' (20 mmol kg^{-1}) of high energy phosphates in the form of creatine phosphate. This means that, regardless of the level of muscular activity, the ATP concentrations will not fall until the creatine phosphate stores have almost been exhausted, which is usually prevented by the creatine phosphate store being replenished by oxidative metabolism via the ATP-producing tricarboxylic acid cycle (Fig. 19.4). However, during severe exercise the muscle may work faster than the blood can deliver oxygen and nutrients to the muscle fibres. Under such conditions the muscle will break down its own glycogen stores and the ATP supply will be regenerated through anaerobic glycolysis. The major disadvantages of anaerobic metabolism are: (1) glycolysis produces only two ATP molecules from each glucose molecule, compared with 36 ATP molecules via oxidative phosphorylation; and (2) the build up of lactic acid has to be cleared by the bloodstream. If muscles are worked to exhaustion, two ADP can regenerate one ATP and adenosine monophosphate (AMP) (catalysed by myokinase) as part of an 'emergency system'.

As discussed above, most muscles are composed of different types of fibres (Table 19.1). Some of these (e.g. slow oxidative and fast oxidative glycolytic) have adapted by acquiring more mitochondria. This enables them to use the more efficient oxidative form of metabolism and highly economical fuels such as lipids. Others (e.g. fast glycolytic fibres) can supply ATP very rapidly, but more expensively, through anaerobic glycolytic metabolism.

Bearing in mind the general recruitment patterns of motor units within a muscle, free fatty acids from the circulation are the preferred fuel (via mitochondria in slow oxidative fibres) for low levels of muscular activity. Further increases in activity will involve more of the faster motor units, and hence the utilization of glucose, derived either from the circulation or internal stores of glycogen. During very vigorous activity anaerobic glycolysis will predominate.

As far as the whole person is concerned, the proportions of the energy expenditure drawn from the two substrates will vary between indi-

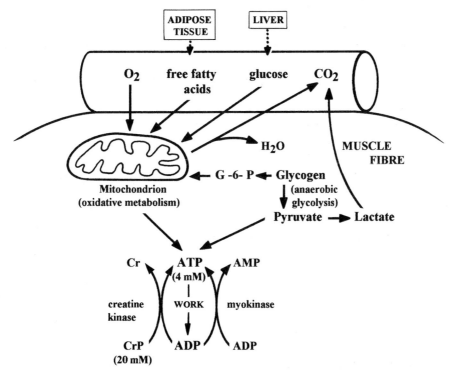

Figure 19.4 Different pathways of producing energy (ATP) in relation to skeletal muscle activity.

viduals, depending on their normal activity/ working patterns, level of training and fitness and diet. For example, in the equivalent of a marathon race, an untrained individual will metabolise and use stored fatty acids, but this will only make a significant contribution to total energy expenditure after about 1 hour, i.e. when the glycogen stores have been depleted. In contrast, in the elite athlete fat reserves are mobilised and oxidised much earlier, helping to spare carbohydrate. Caffeine, in coffee, taken immediately before the exercise will stimulate lipolysis and mobilise fatty acids earlier in the race. Glycogen stores can be increased before such endurance exercise by the consumption of a diet high in carbohydrate.

The ATP generated within the muscle is also used to maintain appropriate ion concentration gradients, for example Na^+ and K^+ across the plasmalemma, Ca^{2+} sequestration across the sarcoplasmic reticulum, the synthesis of new proteins and cross-bridge cycling.

ANAESTHESIA AND MUSCLE PATHOLOGY

Most of the inherited diseases of skeletal muscle carry an increased risk with anaesthesia. Some of them, e.g. central core disease, are also associated with an increased incidence of *malignant hyperthermia* (see below).

In all myotonias depolarising agents and anticholinesterases should be avoided as they tend to trigger generalised myotonia. This can cause weakness for several days after surgery. In McArdle's disease (an inherited disorder of glycogen storage) any impairment of blood, and hence oxygen, supply to muscles, e.g. by the use of a tourniquet, can cause ischaemia and permanent muscle damage. McArdle's sufferers can also respond to suxamethonium by releasing large quantities of myoglobin into the blood. Diuresis is then necessary.

In familial periodic paralysis mental or physical trauma may cause an attack of paralysis and this can persist for several days after operation. In these disorders serum K^+ can be abnormally low or high, and this must be monitored to prevent generation of arrhythmias. Some of the inherited muscle diseases, such as dystrophia myotonica and Duchenne dystrophy, directly involve cardiac muscle. Heart block and heart failure (preceded by tachycardia) are both common. Respiration can also be impaired, either by involvement of intercostal muscles (e.g. in Duchenne dystrophy) or by thoracic deformity (e.g. congenital myopathy). Dystrophia myotonica and sometimes Duchenne dystrophy involve the oropharyngeal muscles, which means that swallowing reflexes are impaired and inhalation pneumonitis may occur.

MALIGNANT HYPERTHERMIA
Discovery and incidence

The disease now known as malignant hyperthermia (MH) or hyperpyrexia was first reported in 1960 by Denborough and Lovell. They described a patient with a badly broken leg who would not undergo anaesthesia because 10 of his relatives had died following the use of ether. He was persuaded to accept halothane anaesthesia instead; however, within a few minutes of the operation beginning he became very hot and slipped into a coma. He subsequently recovered and investigations into his family history were initiated Almost certainly other reports of 'ether convulsions' and 'heat stroke during surgery' can now be attributed to MH.

Exact incidence figures for MH vary, between 1:6000 in Japan and 1:200 000 in the UK, but may be higher in some relatively isolated communities where a single mutation has been able to spread. A lower incidence in children probably reflects the use of different anaesthetic regimens. Briefly, during anaesthesia with trigger agents, the patient undergoes massive muscle contraction and shivering. This leads to the generation of an enormous amount of heat and other secondary effects such as hyperkalaemia and myoglobinaemia. If untreated, the body temperature will continue to rise and the patient will die.

Clinical management

This is discussed in Chapter 51. Most important

is early recognition or suspicion of the condition, and immediate discontinuation of the triggering agent, followed by symptomatic management including cooling and treatment of the hyperkalaemia, which can be the fatal event. Specific treatment includes *dantrolene sodium*, which has a specific action on skeletal muscle (see below and Ch. 51), and corticosteroids, which stabilise cell membranes. Dantrolene treatment should be started immediately.

Screening

Blood enzyme levels

Patients are usually asymptomatic before exposure to a triggering agent. Many attempts have been made to find a test that will identify MH individuals before they undergo anaesthesia — for example, blood levels of the muscle enzyme creatine kinase were found to be high in MH patients but the existence of low serum creatine kinase in family members does not mean they are clear of the disorder, so the test is of limited value, and in fact such false negative results are potentially extremely dangerous. Other tests based on the measurement of other substances in the blood, such as pyrophosphate and cholinesterase, have also been abandoned.

Contracture tests

It has been shown that a 2 cm × 1 mm strip of muscle (from an MH positive patient) in Ringer's solution will contract if exposed to either caffeine or halothane — the contracture test. Some more elaborate variations first apply passive stretch to the muscle and then allow it to contract.

In 1984 the European Malignant Hyperthermia Group established a standard protocol for conducting these tests. The two trigger substances, halothane and caffeine, are given separately. If the muscle contracts in the presence of each substance the subject is classified as having malignant hyperthermia syndrome (MHS); if the muscle contracts in the presence of only one of these triggers the patient is equivocal (MHE); and if no contracture occurs at all the patient is normal (MHN). In North America an alternative test is used, in which caffeine and halothane are administered to the muscle simultaneously; however, this combined test is known to give false positive results.

The contracture tests that are currently used are known to have some quite serious limitations. They require a sizeable biopsy, for which suitable non-trigger anaesthesia must be provided, and there are known to be both false positive and false negative results. The test is also technically complex and is only offered in a few specialist centres. Obviously the contracture test can only be used in close family members of a known MH patient and could not be applied for population screening of everyone about to undergo surgery. Perhaps the largest limitation therefore is that over half of all MH patients present with no family history.

Genetics

Porcine stress syndrome

There is a very similar condition to MH in pigs, known as porcine stress syndrome (PSS). Stress of any type (including changes in external temperature) leads to a rapid rise in temperature, muscle spasm and death. Rigor mortis sets in almost immediately and the meat is described as soft exudative pork. This cannot be sold and the condition can have severe effects in the meat industry.

MH is transmitted as an autosomal dominant in both pigs and humans. In pigs a single gene defect has been localised in 450 animals from six different lean, heavily muscled breeds. This suggests the existence of a single ancestral animal with the defect. This condition has probably been bred in by farmers searching for lean pigs, as heterozygotes for the condition have 2–3% increased dressed carcass weight.

The defect isolated in PSS is in the ryanodine receptor (RYR1) and is a single amino acid substitution of cysteine for arginine at amino acid 615. As explained above, this protein is involved in the movement of Ca^{2+} from the sarcoplasm into the sarcoplasmic reticulum. A defect in this system will therefore result in an increase in cellular free Ca^{2+}.

Human genetic studies

The human situation appears to be more complex than that in the pig. An identical amino acid substitution in RYR1 has been shown, but only in one MH family out of 50 studied in Canada. However, in a European study 8 of 15 families had their genetic defect mapped to a region on chromosome 13, identified as 19q13.1–13.2. This is the location of the RYR1 receptor gene in humans, but these families did not have the same amino acid substitution found in the MH pigs. These families could therefore be examples of mutations at other sites in the RYR1 gene. Hence, in about 50% of European MH families, a defective RYR1 gene might be responsible for the disorder.

Clearly, some other gene must be responsible for causing the condition in the other families. Other possible candidate genes involved in Ca^{2+} regulation are the calcium pump and the DHP (dihydropyridine) sensitive Ca^{2+} channel. It has also been suggested that there may be a link between some cases of MH and fatty acid or inositol 3-phosphate metabolism. MH pigs have an abnormal fatty acid and lipid composition in the cell membranes of their muscles.

The complex genetic picture in humans means that genetic counselling based on linkage markers can only be offered to those families where the 19q13.1–13.2 region has been shown to be the site of the defect.

MH, a spectrum of disorders?

It seems that MH may be part of a whole spectrum of disorders with qualitatively and quantitatively different responses to trigger substances being found during in vitro testing. In vivo responses also seem to be very variable. For example, some patients undergo several anaesthetics with trigger substances before showing an MH response. A trigger anaesthetic may not even be necessary to initiate an attack. There are some reports of relatives of MH patients exhibiting MH-like symptoms without any anaesthetic being administered. The common factor in all these cases seemed to be some form of emotional stress. A 'human familial stress syndrome' has been proposed, a spectrum of disorders of which classic MH is a part.

Mechanism of MH muscle damage

The way in which trigger substances initiate an MH response is poorly understood. Volatile gases such as halothane can pass through cell membranes, and so may have a direct effect on the Ca^{2+} channels. Succinylcholine may exert its effect by causing depolarisation of the sarcolemma. However, the normal influence of nerves on muscles during exercise has a similar effect, yet these patients tend to tolerate exercise well, and indeed may even excel at sport.

The way in which muscle damage occurs during an episode of MH is not yet clearly understood but it does seem likely that an increase in intracellular Ca^{2+} occurs. This could arise from a defect in one of the Ca^{2+} transporting proteins or secondary to changes in other Ca^{2+} chelating proteins in the cell. This situation could lead to a stimulation of calcium-induced calcium release, which is a form of positive feedback. High levels of intracellular Ca^{2+} can activate certain proteinase enzymes, which leads to an acceleration of protein degradation. Dantrolene prevents the release of Ca^{2+} from the sarcoplasmic reticulum. Presumably this is the explanation of its effect in vivo.

Muscles of MH patients go into contractures when exposed to trigger substances in vitro. This leads to a sustained force production and the generation of heat. Substrates are rapidly used up and lactic acid begins to accumulate. Such changes in vivo could lead to membrane damage and the release of K^+ and proteins into the blood. It may be that the muscle membranes in these patients are initially abnormal and so more prone to damage.

REFERENCES AND FURTHER READING

Ball S P, Johnson K J 1993 The genetics of malignant hyperthermia. Journal of Medical Genetics 30: 89–93

Denborough M A, Lovell R R H 1960 Anaesthetic deaths in a family. Lancet ii: 45

Ellis F R 1981 Malignant hyperpyrexia; D. W. Wingard Familial stress syndrome; muscle disease. In Ellis F R (ed) Inherited disease and anesthesia, monographs in anesthesia, 9th edn. Elsevier North Holland, Amsterdam

Goldspink D F 1991 Exercise-related changes in protein turnover in mammalian striated muscle. Journal of Experimental Biology 160: 127–148

Jones D A, Round J M 1992 Skeletal muscle in health and disease: a textbook of muscle physiology. Manchester University Press, Manchester

Josephson R K 1993 Contraction dynamics and power output of skeletal muscle. Annual Review of Physiology 55: 527–546

20

Neuromuscular blocking drugs

C. C. McLoughlin
R. K. Mirakhur

HISTORY

Sixteenth century explorers to South America carried back reports of paralysis induced by 'woowara paste', an arrow poison used by natives. While this phenomenon produced fascination in Europe, it was not until the nineteenth century that scientists obtained sufficient quantities of this extract, containing crude curare, to study its effects. There were many reports of its ability to paralyse skeletal muscle, but it was Claude Bernard in 1856 who first identified the site of action of curare as the neuromuscular junction.

Early medical uses of the drug in the twentieth century were in the treatment of tetanus and epilepsy in doses insufficient to produce complete paralysis, but as there was no convenient technique for the control of ventilation in the event of inadequate respiration, there were obvious limitations in its application. Nevertheless, by the early 1940s, curare had been administered to approximately 30 000 patients. Curare was administered during the course of an anaesthetic for the first time in Montreal Homeopathic Hospital by Harold Griffith and Enid Johnson on 23 January 1942 — to a 20-year-old patient having an appendicectomy. Although it was noted that abdominal muscle relaxation occurred, allowing a reduction in the quantity of cyclopropane administered, it was not appreciated immediately that the drug could form an integral part of a general anaesthetic allowing surgery to be conducted at lighter planes of anaesthesia than hitherto possible. Instead, doubts over the safety of curare led to it being seen as an adjunct to anaesthesia to supplement relaxation in difficult cases. It was only in the 1950s and 1960s in Britain, when the drug was used in much larger doses and with controlled ventilation in the so-called 'Liverpool technique' developed by Gray and Halton, that the role of muscle relaxation in balanced anaesthesia became established.

While the introduction of tubocurarine represented a very major advance in anaesthesia, the limitations of the drug were only too apparent. It is a drug with slow onset and prolonged recovery and at neuromuscular blocking doses it has significant cardiovascular effects. This is related to inhibition of central and peripheral autonomic nicotinic receptors, muscarinic receptors to a lesser extent, and to the release of histamine from tissue mast cells.

The search for muscle relaxant drugs free of significant side-effects has led to the development and frequent discarding of a large number of drugs in the last 50 years. There have, however, been a number of significant milestones. Decamethonium was the first depolarising relaxant drug to be introduced. It enjoyed only brief clinical usage and was superseded in 1951 by suxamethonium, which for the first time allowed for rapid onset of short duration muscle paralysis, a property that has secured its continued use ever since. Pancuronium, introduced in the late 1960s, was the first of a new generation of quaternary ammonium steroid compounds with muscle relaxant properties. As the first non-depolarising relaxant drug which did not produce ganglionic blockade or histamine release, it was a major step in the development of 'cleaner' relaxant drugs. Like many contemporary relaxant drugs, however, it did show muscarinic receptor blocking action contributing to tachycardia. In addition, this agent showed a sympathetic stimulating effect, frequently producing hypertension. From the mid-1980s onwards, a significant number of new relaxant drugs belonging to both steroid and benzylisoquinolinium series of compounds have been introduced into clinical practice. Vecuronium and atracurium are almost completely devoid of muscarinic effects and for the first time

offered muscle relaxation without significant side-effects. Later developments have produced mivacurium, with the shortest duration of action of current non-depolarising drugs, and rocuronium, which produces a rapid onset of action almost rivalling that of suxamethonium.

PHYSIOLOGY OF NEUROMUSCULAR TRANSMISSION AND BLOCKADE

The physiology of neuromuscular transmission in skeletal muscle has been described in detail in Chapter 19 but some salient aspects are summarised here.

Nicotinic cholinoceptors are divided into two basic kinds: receptors at the autonomic ganglia and at the neuromuscular junction. In addition to the well characterised postjunctional receptors at the neuromuscular junction, there is putative evidence for the existence of prejunctional receptors on the nerve cell membrane. Postjunctional cholinoceptors lie in clusters on the crests of junctional folds, which are the shoulders of invaginated pockets on the muscle fibre membrane within the neuromuscular junction. The receptor density at these points is of the order of 5000–10 000 μm^{-2}. In normal adult muscle, nerve fibre activity appears to increase the stability of these receptors and to inhibit their extension to extrajunctional sites. If a skeletal muscle is denervated, however, this inhibition is removed and extrajunctional receptors develop, which leads to an extension of chemosensitivity to the entire muscle fibre membrane. Chronically denervated muscle thus becomes more sensitive to agonists such as acetylcholine and suxamethonium.

Structurally, the postjunctional receptor consists of five protein subunits held together within the cytoskeleton around a central pore or ion channel. In adult skeletal muscle there are two α subunits and one each of β, γ (or ε in mature age) and δ (Fig. 20.1). The α units carry the so-called recognition sites for acetylcholine. Activation of the cholinoceptor requires a conformational change in the protein structure and a resultant transient opening of the central ion channel. While this may result from binding to one α subunit, the probability of activation is enhanced

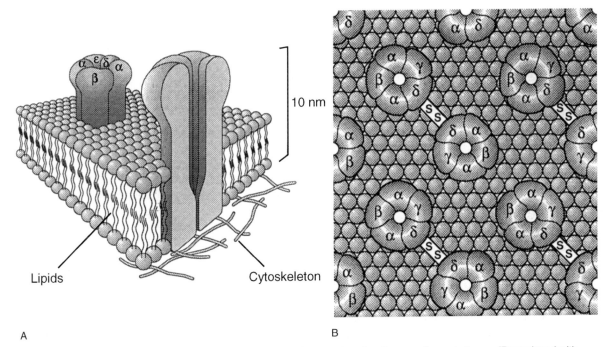

10 nm

Lipids

Cytoskeleton

A

B

Figure 20.1 Structure of the neuromuscular junction illustrating protein subunits around a central pore. (Reproduced with permission from Bowman W C 1990 Pharmacology of neuromuscular function, 3rd ed. Wright, London.)

when binding occurs at both units. In the 1 ms that the receptor opens (when acetylcholine is the agonist), approximately 10^4 sodium and potassium cations cross in opposite directions to produce a small end-plate potential (EPP). If the summation of EPPs exceeds a threshold level, a spreading wave of depolarisation or action potential is generated in the muscle fibre. As individual ion channels close, acetylcholine molecules dissociate and are rapidly inactivated by acetylcholinesterase.

As stated previously, there is evidence that acetylcholine may also activate prejunctional cholinoceptors located on the nerve ending. These so-called autoreceptors act in a positive feedback loop to increase mobilisation of acetylcholine, to keep pace with requirements in sustained muscle contraction. Although these receptors have not been structurally demonstrated, their presence is implied and they are invoked to explain the various fade phenomena associated with repetitive and high frequency stimulation in the presence of non-depolarising relaxant drugs.

Although the normal process of neuromuscular transmission may be interfered with in vitro by a number of mechanisms, we confine ourselves in the clinical setting to drugs that interfere with normal receptor function. These are broadly classified as depolarising or non-depolarising agents.

Suxamethonium chloride is the only depolarising muscle relaxant drug in clinical use. Structurally it appears like two acetylcholine molecules joined together, which gives it a linear and flexible structure. Its mode of action is similar to acetylcholine, and in fact acetylcholine may produce a similar kind of paralysis if delivered to the neuromuscular junction in sufficiently high concentrations, such as by arterial injection. In the clinical setting, onset of depolarising blockade or phase I block is heralded by fasciculations, which are random asynchronous muscle contractions. These are thought to represent a presynaptic stimulation of nerve endings with antidromic propagation of the action potential, which then proceeds orthodromically along nerve fibres in the same motor unit. Unlike acetylcholine, suxamethonium is not inactivated rapidly at the neuromuscular junction but rather its metabolism is dependent on the drug being drawn back into the central circulation where it is broken down by the enzyme plasma cholinesterase. The persistence of suxamethonium at the neuromuscular junction means that depolarisation is prolonged. In effect the postjunctional membrane repolarises some time before recovery of phase I block occurs. However, the neuromuscular junction is surrounded by a zone of inexcitability, through which an action potential will not propagate. This appears to be related to local electrical currents which induce closure of membrane sodium channels. During the period of depolarisation, however, there may be considerable efflux of potassium ions sufficient to raise serum concentrations.

While phase I or depolarising block is the one usually observed with suxamethonium administration, the character of block may change into what is commonly known as phase II block. Clinically this is seen in man when suxamethonium is used in doses in excess of 3–5 mg kg^{-1}, as might be seen if the drug is infused over a period of time. The nature of phase II block is poorly understood but it shares many of the characteristics of a non-depolarising blockade and may persist for many minutes or even hours. Unlike phase I block, when high frequency stimulation is associated with approximately constant, albeit reduced, muscle twitch response, phase II block shows fade in response to such stimulation. Characteristically a train-of-four ratio less than 0.4 is seen. Established phase II block can frequently be reversed using anticholinesterase drugs, but this may be unreliable, particularly in the presence of atypical cholinesterase. The aetiology of this block is not known but suggested mechanisms include an inhibition of acetylcholine synthesis or receptor ion channel blockade.

Suxamethonium is therefore capable of producing at least two different kinds of block, each with distinct characteristics. In reality, there is considerable species variation in response to suxamethonium and between different muscles of the same species. Thus the soleus muscle of the rat is very resistant to depolarisation by suxamethonium, while the chick biventer cervicis muscle shows marked depolarisation.

The normal pattern of stimulation and relaxation seen with suxamethonium is usually not seen in chronically denervated muscle or in muscle fibres innervated by multiple nerve endings. In both these situations, a large part of the muscle fibre membrane is chemosensitive, and its stimulation produces simultaneous depolarisation of the fibre, such that the contractile mechanism is directly activated. In this situation the muscle develops a sustained shortening or contracture. Contracture responses to depolarising blockade may also occur in the congenital myotonias, and in myasthenia gravis, a reduction in receptor density produces 'resistance' to suxamethonium.

Non-depolarising blockade

Non-depolarising muscle relaxants (NDMR), like acetylcholine, have a high affinity for the recognition site on the α subunits of the nicotinic receptor, but unlike acetylcholine are devoid of intrinsic activity. By reducing the access of acetylcholine to the receptors, the number of ion channels opened is reduced and the ability to transmit a muscle action potential limited. In healthy muscle there is a very large excess of receptors over those required for normal muscle function. More than 70% of receptors need to be occupied by an NDMR before any diminution in muscle tone occurs. The competitive blockade essentially consists of two components: reduction in twitch height amplitude, and fade in response to repetitive stimulation. The first component is assumed to represent a postsynaptic effect — a simple blockade of cholinoceptors on the muscle fibre. The fade component, represented clinically as a poorly sustained tetanic contraction or fade following train-of-four stimulation, is thought to represent a frequency dependent reduction of acetylcholine release. It is assumed, as previously suggested, that this relates to a blockade of prejunctional cholinoceptors causing impaired mobilisation of acetylcholine. This impairment can be temporarily overcome after a tetanic stimulation, when subsequent stimulations result in muscle

Table 20.1 Characteristics of depolarising and non-depolarising blockade

Depolarising blockade	Non-depolarising blockade
Fasciculations	No fasciculations
Partial blockade associated with uniform reduction in twitch height during train-of-four stimulation	'Fade' in twitch height with train-of-four
Absence of post-tetanic facilitation	Post-tetanic facilitation
Block deepened by anticholinesterases	Block reversed by anticholinesterases

contractions of increased amplitude. This effect persists for about 1 minute after a 5 second tetanus and, caused by increased mobilisation of acetylcholine, is referred to as *post-tetanic facilitation*. This facilitation is characteristic of non-depolarising block (Table 20.1).

Structure–activity relationships

Most of the currently used NDMRs are based on the steroid nucleus or belong to the benzylisoquinolinium series of compounds. The gradual accumulation of knowledge about the structure of NDMRs and the way in which it affects the profile of activity and side-effects means that chemists can now produce drugs with greater predictability. It was originally assumed that muscle relaxant properties required a bisquaternary ammonium structure with an interonium distance (between quaternary nitrogens) of 12–14 Å (1.2–1.4 nm). We now know that these constraints are not correct and many NDMRs have interonium distances considerably less than this. In fact, tubocurarine and vecuronium are more accurately described as monoquaternary molecules. The modification of compounds has been effected to produce agents of short, medium or long duration of action or with a rapid onset of action. In the ideal situation, muscle relaxation is achieved without autonomic side-effects or release of histamine. Antimuscarinic properties resulting in vagolysis are prominent in trisquaternary molecules such as gallamine. In steroid molecules the removal of the methyl group in position 2 of the A ring in the conversion of

pancuronium to vecuronium also dramatically reduces vagolytic property. Benzylisoquinoline compounds (tubocurarine, atracurium, mivacurium and doxacurium) release histamine and, while this occurs at about one effective dose (ED_{95}) with tubocurarine, it occurs at about three times the ED_{95} with atracurium and mivacurium, but only at very high doses with doxacurium.

There is an inverse relationship between potency of NDMR and time to onset of maximum block. Thus doxacurium, the most potent relaxant drug in use, has a very long onset time. Modification of the D ring of the vecuronium nucleus produced rocuronium, a relaxant drug with about 15% of its potency but with a much faster onset time. This relationship between potency and onset time may be explained on the basis of occupation of receptors at the neuromuscular junction. Irrespective of potency, drug molecules must bind to a critical number of receptors to produce paralysis. When a less potent agent is employed, a considerably greater number of molecules are administered and consequently gain access to the synaptic cleft in a shorter time. Similarly the potency of a drug may affect recovery independent of metabolism. A potent drug with a high receptor affinity will diffuse slowly from the neuromuscular junction into the circulation as it is effectively *buffered* by the receptor, such that the amount of free drug available for diffusion is reduced.

Factors affecting the quality of non-depolarising blockade

Non-depolarising blockade is enhanced in a number of clinical situations and by some drugs administered concurrently. The first group includes a fall in body temperature, acidosis and hypokalaemia. Additionally, patients with poorly controlled myasthenia gravis or myasthenic (Eaton–Lambert) syndrome are often sensitive to NDMRs. The latter condition is distinguished from the former by also exhibiting sensitivity to suxamethonium.

Drugs that are known to enhance neuromuscular blockade include aminoglycoside antibiotics, barbiturates, calcium channel blocking

Table 20.2 Interactions involving muscle relaxants

Potentiation	Antagonism
Hypothermia	Hyperkalaemia
Acidosis	Anticonvulsants
Volatile agents: isoflurane	Aminophylline
> enflurane > halothane	Steroids?
Hypokalaemia	
Hypocalcaemia	
Magnesium	
Aminoglycosides	
β Blockers: prolong duration of suxamethonium	
Anticholinesterase eye drops: prolong duration of	
suxamethonium	
Calcium antagonists	
Local anaesthetics	

drugs and local anaesthetics (Table 20.2). Although the precise mechanisms of these interactions is not known, and in some cases may be related to inhibition of acetylcholine release, there is considerable speculation on a form of non-competitive blockade known as *open ion channel blockade*. This relates to the process whereby the receptor ion channel, opened by agonist action, is occupied by the molecule so the channel is 'plugged' before closing, preventing current flow across the post-junctional membrane and thereby inactivating the receptor. As this process is dependent on an agonist first opening the channel, it is more likely to occur with increasing frequency of channel opening. An alternative form of synergism known as *closed ion channel blockade* may explain the synergism caused by some tricyclic anti-depressant drugs. These drugs may combine with the closed form of the receptor complex and prevent ion channel opening. Volatile anaesthetic agents may enhance non-depolarising blockade by increasing the normal rate of desensitisation of the acetylcholine receptor to agonist activity. Thus the receptor becomes relatively resistant to agonist action. The potentiation of NDMRs by volatile agents is of the order of 20–40% and is greatest in the order: isoflurane > enflurane > halothane.

MONITORING OF NEUROMUSCULAR BLOCKADE

The degree of neuromuscular blockade is conventionally assessed by stimulating a peripheral nerve and measuring the strength of contraction of an innervated muscle. In the clinical situation, this approach is used not only to assess the adequacy of surgical relaxation but also to predict the time to recovery from profound neuromuscular blockade and to assess the adequacy of recovery of neuromuscular function at the end of surgery. The latter is particularly important because residual neuromuscular paralysis may adversely affect the ability of the patient to protect the integrity of the airway. Stimulation of the ulnar nerve at the wrist and monitoring of the adductor pollicis muscle is conventionally employed. While manual assessment is most commonly used in the clinical setting, more precise information on the mechanical response of the thumb is obtained if it is attached to a force transducer (mechanomyography). Alternatively, devices are available for measuring the evoked compound muscle action potential (electromyography).

Train-of-four (TOF) stimulation is the stimulation mode most commonly employed. It consists of four square-wave impulses each of 0.2 ms duration given over 2 seconds. For non-depolarising relaxant drugs partial neuromuscular blockade is associated with a fade in response from T1 to T4 and increasing blockade produces progressive disappearance of twitch responses starting with T4. With recovery from complete paralysis, T1 recovers first, followed by T2, T3 and T4. Partial depolarising blockade, in contrast, shows twitch responses of reduced but equal amplitude. TOF stimulation is used to assess various aspects of muscle paralysis. Complete absence of mechanical response is taken to represent adequate surgical relaxation. In addition, while no single test specifically predicts adequate return of muscle tone at the end of surgery, a TOF ratio (T4:T1) of 0.7 is considered a minimum requirement. This finding should be taken in conjunction with a number of clinical signs, such as adequacy of respiration, strength of hand squeeze or ability to sustain head lift. In reality, accurate assessment of fade with TOF stimulation is difficult without proper recording facilities. An alternative stimulation mode for assessing minor degrees of neuromuscular blockade is *double-*

burst stimulation. This consists of two sequential minitetanic bursts separated by 750 ms. Fade between the two contractions is more readily appreciated using this mode of stimulation and can be detected at a level of neuromusculer block equivalent to a TOF ratio of about 0.6.

During profound muscle relaxation, when there is no response to conventional stimulation, the block may still be assessed by a process known as *post-tetanic count* (PTC). This consists of application of a 5 second 50 Hz tetanus, followed 3 seconds later by repetitive stimulation at a frequency of 1 Hz. The number of palpable twitch responses following the tetanus is counted and can be used to predict the time to return of the first twitch of the TOF. A PTC of 4 for atracurium predicts this will occur on average in about 4 minutes, while for pancuronium it will be about 25 minutes.

Pharmacokinetics

While different muscle relaxant drugs may differ chemically, they share many similarities in the way they are handled by the body. They are essentially polar molecules and therefore the volume of distribution is related primarily to the size of the extracellular fluid volume. As this is frequently increased in liver disease, a given dose of relaxant drug is distributed in a greater volume and the plasma concentration is reduced, making the patient apparently resistant to the drug. With the exceptions of atracurium and mivacurium, however, most non-depolarising relaxant drugs rely on hepatic metabolism and/or renal excretion for termination of action. Thus, while larger doses of relaxant drugs may be required in liver disease to achieve a desired effect and a set plasma concentration, they may show significant prolongation of action if the elimination half-life is increased. Similarly, in renal disease an increased volume of distribution may produce 'resistance' to the relaxant drug but the effects of agents that are highly dependent on renal excretion will be prolonged. As renal clearance of many drugs also reduces with age, elderly patients frequently exhibit slower spontaneous recovery. Prolonged paralysis may also occur when the route of elimination of metabolites is compromised, as in a few notable cases metabolites of the parent drug may have intrinsic muscle relaxant properties.

It should also be noted that as the neuromuscular junction is the site of action of these drugs, their duration of effect is not always related to elimination half-life, $t_{1/2}\beta$, from the plasma (Table 20.3).

NON-DEPOLARISING RELAXANT DRUGS

For comparative purposes the potency of NDMRs is defined in terms of their ED_{50} or ED_{95} at the adductor pollicis muscle of the thumb. This is the dose of drug calculated to produce 50% and 95% suppression respectively of twitch response;

Table 20.3 Pharmacodynamic and pharmacokinetic parameters of non-depolarising relaxant drugs

Drug	ED_{95} (mg kg^{-1})	Clinical duration ($2 \times ED_{95}$ dose) (min)	Elimination half-life (min)	Route of excretion (%)	
				Kidney	Liver
Vecuronium	0.05	30–40	62	30	70
Atracurium	0.25	30–45	20	Hydrolysis/Hofmann elimination/organ uptake	
Rocuronium	0.3	30–45	95	30	70
Mivacurium	0.08	15	3–6	Hydrolysis by plasma cholinesterase	
Pancuronium	0.06	60–120	145	90	10
Tubocurarine	0.5	120+	239	90	10
Pipecuronium	0.045	60–120	118	90	10
Doxacurium	0.03	90–150	99	Predominantly kidney	
Gallamine	2.5	90	163	100	—

for intubation a dose in the order of $2 \times ED_{95}$ is commonly used. Clinical classification of non-depolarising drugs is frequently based on their duration of action. This *clinical duration* conventionally refers to the time to recovery of the twitch response (T1) to 25% of control. Thus we can divide drugs into:

1. Short duration. The only member of this group is mivacurium.
2. Intermediate duration. This refers to drugs with clinical duration of about 30–40 minutes and includes atracurium, vecuronium and rocuronium.
3. Long duration. Drugs in this group have a clinical duration of greater than 60 minutes and include pancuronium, tubocurarine, alcuronium, pipecuronium, doxacurium and gallamine.

Short duration NDMRs

Mivacurium

2 Cl⁻

Mivacurium chloride is a bisquaternary benzyl-isoquinolinium drug with a structure similar to atracurium and doxacurium and, in the pharmaceutical preparation, exists in three isomers. The drug has an ED_{95} of 0.06–0.08 mg kg^{-1}, with an onset time to maximum block of 2–2.5 minutes and a clinical duration of about 15 minutes. Cardiovascular effects related to histamine release are more frequently observed if the drug is administered rapidly or in doses exceeding 0.15 mg kg^{-1}. Short lived but moderate hypotension with associated increases in heart rate may be seen but can be reduced by slow administration of the drug.

Mivacurium is metabolised by plasma cholinesterase at a rate of about 75% that of suxamethonium and spontaneous recovery occurs in 25–30 minutes. In theory reversal with an anti-cholinesterase drug will inhibit its metabolism, but in practice recovery time is shortened by about 5 minutes when neostigmine is administered. The short duration of action means that mivacurium may be used conveniently by infusion. Maintenance requirements under balanced anaesthesia in adults are 3–15 µg kg^{-1} min^{-1}. The duration of action of mivacurium may be lengthened in renal failure or severe liver disease, probably as a result of decreased pseudo-cholinesterase activity.

Intermediate duration NDMRs

Atracurium

Atracurium is a benzylisoquinolinium diester and is one of the most commonly administered muscle relaxant drugs. It consists of 10 isomers, of which one, cisatracurium, is now in clinical use as a relaxant by itself. Atracurium has an ED_{95} of 0.25 mg kg^{-1} and at twice this dose produces muscle paralysis in 3–5 minutes, with a clinical duration of 30–45 minutes. When used by infusion, a dose of 4–12 µg kg^{-1} is required. It represents one of the newer and 'cleaner' NDMRs introduced into clinical practice in the 1980s, with minimal cardiovascular effects. The dose ratio for ganglion and neuromuscular blockade is 50:1. At doses in excess of 0.5 mg kg^{-1} administered rapidly, histamine release may occur, causing cutaneous flushing and a transient decrease in arterial pressure. This effect can be ameliorated by giving the drug slowly or with prior treatment with H_1- and H_2-receptor blockers.

One of the most notable features of atracurium is its novel method of metabolism, which consists of ester hydrolysis in the plasma and liver and a process known as Hofmann elimination. This eponymous process was first described by a German chemist in 1851, and is a pH and temperature dependent conversion of atracurium from a quaternary ammonium to a tertiary ammonium structure. Although the reaction, as originally described by Hofmann, occurred at high temperature and pH, in the example of atracurium it occurs at a pH of 7.4 and at body temperature. The stability of the drug is, however, well maintained by refrigeration.

While little is known about the precise site of breakdown of atracurium, less than 10% is excreted unchanged in the urine. The most notable major metabolite is laudanosine, a tertiary amine compound that has known convulsant properties in dogs. Although there is concern that this metabolite may accumulate when atracurium is used for prolonged muscle paralysis in intensive care, there have been no confirmed reports of high laudanosine concentrations, even in patients with hepatic or renal disease. Elimination of the drug is little affected by age and the presence of renal or hepatic dysfunction, and the predictability of clinical effects makes it the drug of choice in these conditions.

the fewest side-effects, as it is free from histamine release and both vagal or ganglion block. When used with opioid drugs, bradycardia and asystolic arrest have been reported, but this is attributed to unopposed opioid action.

20–30% of vecuronium is excreted unchanged in the urine. The remainder is deacetylated and hydroxylated in the liver to its 17-, 3,17- and 3-hydroxy metabolites, and these are excreted in urine and bile. The last of the three, 3-desacetyl-vecuronium, is the major derivative and has intrinsic muscle relaxant properties, with a potency of about 70% of the parent compound. The relative importance of hepatic and renal mechanisms for the excretion of this metabolite is not known, but it has been implicated in prolonged paralysis of a number of patients with renal failure receiving long term administration of vecuronium in intensive care units. The duration of action of vecuronium is prolonged in the elderly, in neonates and in patients with hepatic or renal dysfunction.

Vecuronium

Rocuronium

Vecuronium is a synthetic steroid molecule formed by the demethylation of pancuronium to form a monoquaternary structure. It is stable in solution for only 24 hours and is therefore supplied as a freeze dried powder for reconstitution. The ED_{95} of vecuronium is 0.05 mg kg^{-1} and at a dose of 2 × ED_{95} has an onset time of 2–3 minutes and a clinical duration of 30–40 minutes. Onset time can be further reduced by increasing the dose administered, but with a dose dependent increase in duration of relaxation. Infusion requirements are 0.8–2.0 µg kg^{-1}min^{-1}.

Vecuronium is possibly the relaxant drug with

Rocuronium is a recently introduced steroid muscle relaxant drug with a potency of about 15% of that of vecuronium. It has an ED_{95} of about 0.3 mg kg^{-1}, which, with the exception of gallamine, makes it the least potent of NDMRs in common usage. As discussed earlier, this low potency allows for the possibility of a rapid onset of action. A dose of 0.6 mg kg^{-1} produces maximum blockade in 1.8 minutes, with a clinical duration of about 45 minutes. Good intubating conditions are frequently present at about 60 seconds after administration and before onset of maximum block. Thus rocuronium may be used to facilitate rapid tracheal intubation, especially in situations when suxamethonium is contraindicated. When used by infusion, requirements are $8–12 \, \mu g \, kg^{-1} \, min^{-1}$.

Rocuronium is free of major side-effects. The ratio of vagal to neuromuscular blockade is 3.0, which is considerably less than that of vecuronium. The heart rate may therefore show a small increase when doses of $0.6–1.0 \, mg \, kg^{-1}$ are administered.

Rocuronium appears to undergo little metabolism, and although significant amounts of the drug are excreted in the urine, the liver would appear to be the main route of elimination. The duration of action is modestly increased in patients with renal failure (elimination half-life 97 versus 71 minutes) but may be prolonged in severe hepatic dysfunction.

Long duration NDMRs

Tubocurarine

Tubocurarine, as previously mentioned, was the first muscle relaxant introduced but is rarely used now. It belongs to the benzylisoquinolinium group of compounds and, although originally thought to be a bisquaternary compound, it is now known to be better represented as a monoquaternary structure. The ED_{95} of tubocurarine is $0.5 \, mg \, kg^{-1}$ and this dose produces surgical relaxation lasting 60–100 minutes. Onset of block is slow and takes 5–7 minutes to produce maximum blockade. As with most long acting NDMRs, repeated administration of the drug causes cumulation, leading to a prolonged block.

The most noteworthy side-effect of tubocurarine is histamine release, which occurs even at doses below its ED_{95}. This can be reduced if the drug is administered slowly. The large increase in histamine concentrations is frequently accompanied by skin flushing and occasionally bronchospasm. Significant falls in blood pressure of 30–50% can occur secondary to histamine release and ganglion blockade. This property once made it a muscle relaxant suitable for use in controlled hypotension during anaesthesia.

Tubocurarine is not metabolised to a significant extent and is excreted unchanged in bile and urine. The kidney is the major route of elimination, with only 10% excreted via the liver. This is increased, however, in the presence of renal impairment. With the introduction of better alternatives, it would not be considered wise to use tubocurarine in either hepatic or renal disease. Its use in modern practice is restricted to pretreatment against suxamethonium-induced muscle pains.

Gallamine

Gallamine was the first synthetic muscle relaxant drug released into clinical practice and is now, like tubocurarine, chiefly of historical interest because limitations in its clinical profile have reduced its usefulness. It has a trisquaternary structure and an extremely low potency. Gallamine is not, however, as rapid acting as rocuronium. The ED_{95} is approximately $2.5 \, mg \, kg^{-1}$ and an intubating dose produces maximum block in 4–7 minutes, with a duration of about 90 minutes. Gallamine has a potent vagolytic effect even at low doses and its use is associated with dose related tachycardia and a small increase in blood pressure. It does not, however, exhibit ganglion blocking properties, nor does it produce a direct histamine release.

The notable features of gallamine's termination of effect are that it undergoes minimal metabolism and relies exclusively on renal excretion of the unchanged drug; thus the presence of renal impairment profoundly affects its duration of action. Like tubocurarine, its use in modern practice is largely confined to pretreatment of suxamethonium.

Alcuronium

Alcuronium was introduced into clinical practice in 1961 as an alternative drug to tubocurarine with fewer side-effects. It is a semisynthetic diallyl derivative of toxiferine with a bisquaternary structure. The ED_{95} of alcuronium is 0.25 mg kg^{-1} and this dose produces maximum block in about 4–6 minutes, with a duration of 60–90 minutes. Although it causes less direct histamine release than tubocurarine, mild hypotension may be seen in hypovolaemic patients as a result of weak ganglion blockade. A slight increase in heart rate (5–10%) usually occurs as a result of minor vagolysis. A relatively high incidence of allergic reactions has been reported, with a cross-sensitivity with suxamethonium.

Alcuronium is 40% protein bound and undergoes negligible metabolism. Renal excretion is the predominant route of elimination, with a small amount of biliary clearance of the unchanged drug. The clearance of the drug is significantly impaired in elderly patients with a concomitant prolongation of action.

Pancuronium

Pancuronium represented a major milestone in muscle relaxant pharmacology, as not only was it the first steroid muscle relaxant introduced, paving the way for future drugs, but it also had significant benefits over contemporary drugs with respect to cardiovascular side-effects. Muscle relaxant activity was conferred to the steroid nucleus by the introduction of acetylcholine-like moieties into the A and D rings. Pancuronium is a potent drug with an ED_{95} of 0.06 mg kg^{-1} and a dose of $2 \times ED_{95}$ produces full paralysis in 2–3 minutes, with a clinical duration of 60–20 minutes. Pancuronium is free of autonomic ganglion blockade and does not release histamine. Cardiovascular parameters are well maintained and in fact it produces a small increase in blood pressure, heart rate and cardiac output secondary to a sympathomimetic action and moderate vagolytic effect.

Clearance of the drug and its metabolites is predominantly by the renal route, with about 10% recovered from the bile. About 20% is deacetylated by the liver in the 3 and 17 positions to give 3-hydroxy, 17-hydroxy and 3,17-dihydroxy derivatives. As with vecuronium, the 3-desacetylpancuronium metabolite possesses muscle relaxant activity, with a potency of about 40% of the parent compound. Not surprisingly, plasma clearance is reduced by 60–70% in renal failure, with significant prolongation of action. In hepatic impairment, an increase in volume of distribution leads to apparent resistance to pancuronium, but the terminal elimination half-life may be considerably prolonged (up to 80%), such that recovery from block may be very slow.

Pipecuronium

Pipecuronium is a steroidal drug derived from pancuronium. Substitutions at the 2 and 16 positions on the steroid nucleus effectively increase the separation between the quaternary nitrogens and this effect reduces vagolytic activity by a factor of 10. Although used predominantly in Eastern Europe in the 1980s and released in the USA in the 1990s, pipecuronium has still to be made available in the UK.

The ED_{95} of pipecuronium is 0.045 mg kg^{-1} and an intubating dose produces maximum block in about 3 minutes. As expected, dose dependent prolongation of action is seen. $1 \times ED_{95}$ and $2 \times ED_{95}$ doses will produce surgical relaxation for 40–60 and 60–120 minutes, respectively.

The notable feature of pipecuronium is an absence of cardiovascular side-effects, even with high doses. It does not release histamine, nor does it appear to act at autonomic ganglia or the vagus nerve. The drug does not appear to undergo significant metabolism and is excreted predominantly by the kidney. In the presence of renal impairment, the liver may be a secondary route of elimination, but the terminal half-life may still be doubled in renal failure. Hepatic disease does not appear to significantly influence duration of action. Although considerable variation in duration exists between individuals, the drug has similar pharmacokinetic properties in elderly and young patients.

Doxacurium

H$_3$CO, H$_3$CO, H$_3$CO, CH$_2$, CH$_3$ $^+$N—(CH$_2$)$_3$—OC—(CH$_2$)$_2$—CO—(CH$_2$)$_3$—N$^+$ OCH$_3$, OCH$_3$, H$_3$C, CH$_2$, OCH$_3$ • 2 Cl$^-$ H$_3$CO, OCH$_3$, OCH$_3$ H$_3$CO, OCH$_3$, OCH$_3$

Doxacurium is a bisquaternary benzylisoquinolinium drug which was introduced into the USA in 1991. It is the most potent muscle relaxant drug currently available, with an ED_{95} of 0.03 mg kg^{-1}, but, as might be expected, onset of block is exceedingly slow. A dose of $1 \times ED_{95}$ may take up to 10 minutes to produce block, with a variable duration of 30–90 minutes. Although onset time can be reduced by increasing the dose employed, it is at the expense of a considerably increased duration of action. A $2 \times ED_{95}$ dose produces relaxation for 90–150 minutes. As might be

expected with such a long acting agent, antagonism of its effects with neostigmine is only satisfactory if significant spontaneous recovery has taken place.

Doxacurium has an extremely 'clean' cardiovascular profile and has no vagolytic or ganglion blocking effects. Histamine release may occur at doses unlikely to be used in clinical practice ($>4 \times ED_{95}$).

Doxacurium is not metabolised to any significant extent and the unchanged drug is recovered in urine and bile. Renal excretion is the major route of elimination, and consequently the drug action is prolonged in chronic renal impairment. Hepatic impairment does not produce significant alteration in its pharmacokinetic indices. Although potency is similar in elderly patients, plasma clearance is reduced and clinical relaxation may be prolonged by about 25%.

New relaxant drugs

Cisatracurium is a stereoisomer of atracurium and is four times more potent than its parent drug (ED_{95} 0.05 mg kg^{-1}). It has only recently been released into clinical usage. Like atracurium it undergoes Hofmann elimination. It is less likely, however, to provoke histamine liberation and has weaker autonomic effects. Heart rate and blood pressure are little altered with doses within the clinical range, and at doses up to 0.25 mg kg^{-1} no adverse cardiovascular, pulmonary or cutaneous effects are seen. The drug appears to be slightly slower in onset and longer in duration of action when compared with atracurium.

A number of other new relaxant drugs are currently undergoing clinical assessment.

ORG 9487 is a new steroidal muscle relaxant drug with a rapid onset and possibility of early reversal. Onset time of a standard intubating dose is around 1 minute, with complete recovery in 24 minutes; however, administration of neostigmine accelerates recovery to about 12 minutes.

ANQ 9040 is another steroidal drug with low potency (ED_{95} 1.3 mg kg^{-1}) and rapid onset, with medium duration of action. Initial data suggest onset of complete paralysis after a standard intubating dose in 28–67 seconds. The main disadvantage of the drug would appear to be histamine liberation with marked tachycardia and some reduction in blood pressure in clinically useful concentrations. The drug is unlikely to be used in clinical practice.

SUXAMETHONIUM

$$CH_3-\overset{\overset{\displaystyle CH_3}{|}}{\underset{\underset{\displaystyle CH_3}{|}}{N}}-CH_2-CH_2-O-\overset{\overset{\displaystyle}{||}}{\underset{\underset{\displaystyle O}{}}{C}}-CH_2-CH_2-\overset{\overset{\displaystyle}{||}}{\underset{\underset{\displaystyle O}{}}{C}}-O-CH_2-CH_2-\overset{\overset{\displaystyle CH_3}{|}}{\underset{\underset{\displaystyle CH_3}{|}}{N}}-CH_3$$

Suxamethonium was first administered to human volunteers in 1949 and is the only depolarising relaxant drug used in clinical practice. Structurally it is a bisquaternary compound consisting of two acetylcholine molecules joined at their acetyl groups. Despite a variety of side-effects it is still considered the agent of choice to facilitate tracheal intubation during a rapid sequence induction. The ED_{95} of suxamethonium has been estimated as $0.28–0.49 \, \text{mg kg}^{-1}$. A dose of $1.0 \, \text{mg kg}^{-1}$ produces profound relaxation and excellent intubating conditions within 1 minute and return of normal muscle tone occurs within 5–10 minutes. The most common cardiovascular effect on administration is bradycardia as a result of stimulation of cardiac muscarinic receptors. This may occur on the first dose in children but in adults is more commonly seen on repeat administration. Nodal rhythm or ventricular arrhythmias are also occasionally produced. Administration of the drug may be associated with an increase in masseter muscle tone lasting 1–2 minutes. This increase is modest and can easily be overcome by the laryngoscopist.

With the advent of new short or intermediate NDMRs, the use of suxamethonium by infusion has largely declined. The development of phase II block was a frequent complication of this technique, and its onset was associated with tachyphylaxis, i.e. the need to give increasing doses to achieve the same clinical effect. Onset of phase II block is enhanced by concurrent administration of volatile agents. As previously described, the characteristics of phase II block resemble relaxation with NDMRs with fade, post-tetanic facilitation and reversal of block with anticholinesterase drugs.

Suxamethonium is metabolised in the plasma in a two-stage reaction to succinic acid and choline by the enzyme plasma cholinesterase. While the activity of this enzyme may be reduced in a number of conditions, such as pregnancy, hepatic dysfunction or uraemia, this rarely results in clinically significant prolongation of action. Synthesis of the normal enzyme is governed by two allelic genes at the E1 locus and the usual genotype is E1u E1u. Genetic variants producing an atypical cholinesterase occur in about 1 in 2500 individuals in the population. While a variety of abnormal genes are known (*atypical, fluoride resistant, silent*), a heterozygous or homozygous atypical gene (E1a) pattern is the most common abnormality presenting clinically. The activity of plasma cholinesterase in most cases is defined in terms of a dibucaine number (DN). Dibucaine produces about 80% inhibition of activity of normal plasma cholinesterase (DN 80), while atypical cholinesterase is resistant to this inhibition. The E1a E1a gene pair classically gives rise to a DN of about 20, while E1u E1a produces a DN of about 60.

Side-effects

Muscle pains occur in 40–50% of patients who receive suxamethonium. The predominant sites are neck and shoulders, abdomen and limbs, and pain is usually evident within 24–48 hours of administration. The aetiology of this problem is not consistently explained. It is known to be common in young adults and is particularly associated with early mobility after surgery, but the incidence is low in children and the obstetric population. Asynchronous muscle contraction associated with fasciculations has been suggested as a possible mechanism, but the severity of pain does not correlate with severity of fasciculations or biochemical indices of muscle damage. This notwithstanding, damage to muscle spindles is a likely mechanism. A variety of techniques have been employed to reduce the severity of pain:

- pretreatment with low doses of NDMRs, e.g. tubocurarine, gallamine

- i.v. lignocaine
- pretreatment with oral or i.m. NSAID drugs, e.g. aspirin, diclofenac
- vitamin C
- vitamin E
- i.v. chlorpromazine
- i.v. diazepam
- i.v. magnesium
- preoperative stretch exercises
- oral dantrolene.

By far the most common technique is pretreatment with a small dose of an NDMR. While extremely effective, it should be borne in mind that this reduces the effectiveness and speed of onset of suxamethonium and the dose of drug should be increased by 50%.

Suxamethonium produces a transient increase in serum potassium concentrations of the order of 0.3–0.5 mmol l^{-1}, returning to normal within about 5 minutes. The source of this potassium is assumed to be muscle. The increase is particularly marked when induction with halothane precedes administration of suxamethonium. Exaggerated increases in potassium may occur in the presence of denervated muscle, muscle trauma, abdominal sepsis, prolonged immobility or after major burns. The changes in sensitivity to suxamethonium after trauma and burns take place within a few days of the injury and persist for an indeterminate period of several months. Hyperkalaemic cardiac arrest may also explain sudden deaths following administration of suxamethonium to patients with Duchenne muscular dystrophy.

A short term increase of 5–10 mmHg in intraocular pressure is seen with suxamethonium administration, thought to be due to a contracture of extraocular muscles and to an increase in choroidal blood flow. This effect is not reliably prevented by pretreatment with NDMRs. While this has been cited as a reason for avoiding suxamethonium in anaesthetic management of the penetrating eye injury, it should be borne in mind that this change is modest with respect to changes related to laryngoscopy in a poorly paralysed patient or if anaesthesia is light.

An increase in intragastric pressure proportional to the intensity of fasciculation of abdominal muscles has been noted. While this was felt to increase the risk of regurgitation of gastric contents, it is generally accepted that it is accompanied by a parallel increase in lower oesophageal pressure, such that the pressure gradient across the lower oesophageal sphincter is actually well maintained.

Suxamethonium is a recognised trigger agent for the rare syndrome of malignant hyperpyrexia (MH) which complicates about 1 in 50 000 anaesthetics and carries a high mortality if not recognised and treated promptly. Muscle rigidity is present in 75% of cases where suxamethonium is the stimulus, and rigidity of the masseter muscle (MMR) in particular has been taken to herald onset of MH. Reported cases of MMR occur most commonly when the depolarising agent is administered after inhalational induction with halothane. The difficulty arises with the recognition that suxamethonium produces an increase in masseter muscle tone as a normal pharmacological effect, and it is argued that many so-called cases of MMR were simply extreme examples of this effect. This has produced two schools of opinion. The first advocates an expectant approach to the management of isolated cases of MMR, with continuation of the anaesthetic and close monitoring of end-tidal carbon dioxide, temperature, etc. The second approach is to discontinue the anaesthetic immediately and assess the need for further investigation of the patient.

Adverse reactions to suxamethonium are more common than with other relaxants in common use and these vary from cutaneous histamine release to severe anaphylaxis. Immunoglobulin (IgE) antibodies to suxamethonium are the most commonly encountered in the population. It is possible, however, that these may actually represent autoantibodies to acetylcholine which cross-react with suxamethonium.

On the basis of the incidence of side-effects to suxamethonium, there has been considerable decline in its usage within recent decades. It still remains the drug of choice if there is a high risk of aspiration, particularly in obstetric general anaesthesia. It remains to be seen, however, if new NDMRs with rapid onset of action will reduce further the indications for its use.

FURTHER READING

Bowman W C 1990 Pharmacology of neuromuscular function, 3rd edn. Wright, London

Brull S J 1994 Monitoring of neuromuscular function. Seminars in Anesthesia 13: 297–309

Donati F, Meistelman C 1991 A kinetic-dynamic model to explain the relationship between high potency and slow onset time for neuromuscular blocking drugs. Journal of Pharmacokinetics and Biopharmaceutics 19: 537–552

Ellis F R 1980 Inherited muscle disease. British Journal of Anaesthesia 52: 153–164

Enbæk J, Østergaard D, Viby-Mogensen J 1989 Double burst stimulation (DBS): a new pattern of nerve stimulation to identify residual neuromuscular block. British Journal of Anaesthesia 62: 274–278

Harper N J N, Pollard B J (eds) 1995 Muscle relaxants in anaesthesia. Edward Arnold, London.

Meistelman C, McLoughlin C 1993 Suxamethonium — current controversies. Current Anaesthesia and Critical Care 4: 53–58

Mirakhur R K 1992 Newer neuromuscular blocking drugs. Drugs 44: 182–199

Savarese J J, Kitz R J 1975 Does clinical anaesthesia need new neuromuscular blocking agents? Anesthesiology 42: 236–239

Viby-Mogensen J, Howardy-Hansen P, Chræmmer-Jørgensen B et al 1981 Posttetanic count (PTC): a new method of evaluating an intense nondepolarizing neuromuscular blockade. Anesthesiology 55: 458–461

Whittaker M 1980 Plasma cholinesterase variants and the anaesthetist. Anaesthesia 35: 174–197

21

Anticholinergic and anticholinesterase drugs

G. McCarthy
R. K. Mirakhur

ANTICHOLINERGICS

Both cholinergic agonists and antagonists have been known to man for centuries, in one form or another. Muscarine, found in small amounts in the mushroom *Amanita muscaria*, was noted by Nordic shamans to produce hallucinogenic 'out of body' experiences that are now known to result from cholinergic agonist activity. In the twentieth century Sir Henry Dale named a new class of receptors after muscarine, producing the familiar division of cholinergic receptors into the muscarinic and nicotinic families. The muscarinic receptors have now grown into at least five muscarinic subtypes, M_1–M_5 which are found in many cell types, including cholinergic postganglionic sites and cardiac and smooth muscle cells. The effects of blockade of these receptors are widespread and are summarised in Table 21.1

The best known of the antagonists to muscarinic receptors are the belladonna alkaloids, atropine and hyoscine. Atropine is commonly found in plants of the family Solanaceae, which includes deadly nightshade (*Atropa belladonna*). Its toxic reputation led the drug to be called after Atropos, one of the Greek fates who cut short the lives of men. Nowadays atropine is commercially extracted from an Australian genus, *Duboisia*. Hyoscine, found in henbane (*Hyoscyamus niger*), is also popular with ethnopharmacologists for its widespread use in folk remedies.

Structure–activity relationships

Both atropine and hyoscine are competitive

Table 21.1 The main effects of muscarinic receptor inhibition

Tissue or organ system	Effect
Brain	Sedation or excitation; ataxia; memory loss; antiemesis
Heart	Bradycardia in small doses, tachycardia in large ones
Blood vessels	Vasodilatation — flushing in the 'blush' area
Respiratory tract	Decrease in secretions; bronchial dilatation
Urinary tract	Relaxation of the ureter; relaxation of the detrusor muscle
Gastrointestinal system	Reduction in salivation; reduced gut tone; reduced gastric, pancreatic, biliary and intestinal secretions
Ciliary muscle	Relaxation of ciliary muscle
Sphincter pupillae muscle	Relaxation of pupillae muscle — pupil dilatation; possible rise in intraocular pressure
Skin	Inhibition of sweating

antagonists of acetylcholine at the muscarinic receptor. Either a tertiary or quaternary ammonium group is required for this action, which depends on obstructing a vital anionic site in the muscarinic receptor. The actual tertiary or quaternary amine structure is important because the former are small enough to cross the blood–brain barrier, while the latter are not. It is this access to central cholinergic receptors that helps to explain the differential effects of the various naturally occurring and synthetic antagonists. Thus both atropine and hyoscine (tertiary amines) can result in delirium, a side-effect not shared by glycopyrronium (quaternary amine). Similarly, anticholinergic drugs that enter the brain have some antiemetic actions, an effect shared by some H_1-histamine receptor blockers, which actually owe their antiemetic actions to antimuscarinic effects. Figure 21.1 shows the structures of the common anticholinergic compounds used in anaesthesia.

Atropine

Historically, atropine was used, either alone or with pethidine, in premedication, to reduce salivary and bronchial secretions and so facilitate the induction of anaesthesia with irritant inhalational agents. Other beneficial effects of atropine lay in its weak antiemetic properties and smooth muscle relaxant effects, especially on the bronchial musculature. Unfortunately in routine use it also inhibited sweating, which could induce hyperthermia, especially in small children. The introduction of more potent and less irritant inhalational agents led to a decline in the routine use of anticholinergic premedication in adults.

Although atropine is chemically the racemic mixture of dl-tropyl-tropate, it is the laevorotatory isomer which is pharmacologically active at muscarinic receptors. Several studies have failed to show any significant activity at nicotinic receptors.

Atropine can cross intact skin and mucous membranes and is well absorbed orally. About 30% of a dose is recovered unchanged in the urine, although hepatic first pass metabolism does occur, with the drug undergoing N-demethylation and glucuronidation. The terminal elimination half-life is between 2 and 5 hours.

Atropine is used in anaesthesia for its antimuscaric properties, either alone or to counter the muscarinic effects of anticholinesterases used to antagonise neuromuscular blockade. The dose for premedication (i.v. or i.m.) in adults is 0.4–1 mg; in children 10–20 µg kg^{-1}. (When given orally 30 µg kg^{-1} is required.) A typical dose for controlling the muscarinic side-effects of neostigmine or edrophonium is 10–20 µg kg^{-1}.

The cardiac effects of the drug are dose related; although large doses accelerate the heart rate, smaller amounts can produce slowing, even in animals with a vagotomy, from which it is inferred that atropine has a weak peripheral muscarinic receptor agonist activity. Because of these associated cardiovascular effects, atropine itself is not used for its effects on gastrointestinal motility or secretions, although anticholinergic agents such as dicyclomine are used for this purpose. Furthermore, atropine administration decreases the tone of the lower oesophageal sphincter and reduces gastric motility, thereby increasing the likelihood of gastric reflux, despite a reduction in gastric acidity. It should be noted that the decrease in lower oesophageal sphincter tone is not overcome by the administration of metoclo-

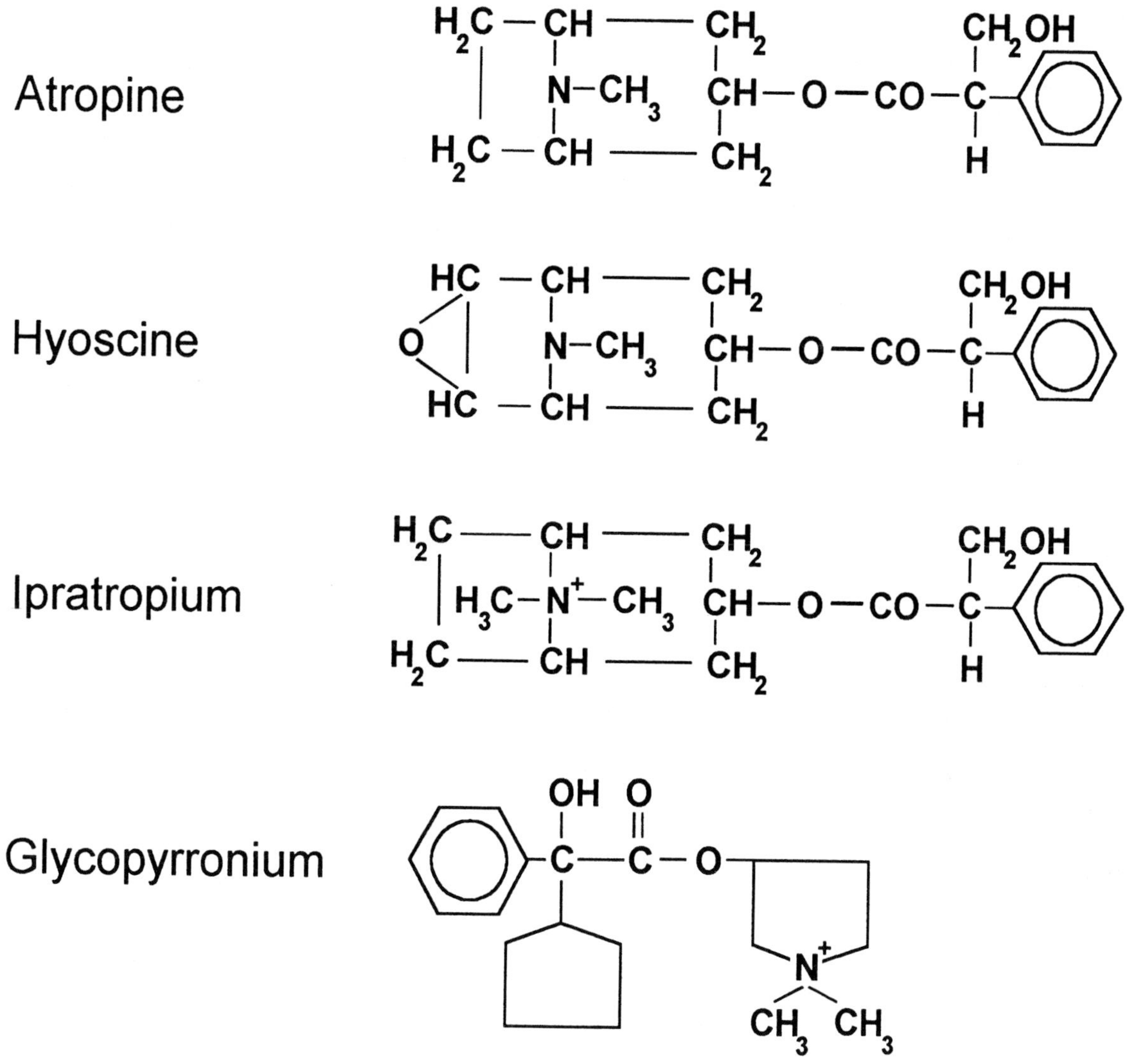

Figure 21.1 Structures of the common anticholinergic agents.

pramide. Atropine, whether administered before or with an anticholinesterase, does not seem to prevent changes in smooth muscle tone that are induced by anticholinesterase administration. (This unrestricted rise in intraluminal pressure may theoretically result in the disruption of a bowel anastomosis, especially in the presence of an epidural block).

In the eye the antimuscarinic effects of atropine result in mydriasis, blurred vision and an increase in intraocular pressure. From an anaesthetic viewpoint, the key consideration is the route of administration of the agent and the dose. The topical application of atropine is contraindicated in patients with narrow angle glaucoma, because mydriasis impairs the drainage of aqueous fluid. When, however, atropine is administered in routine doses intramuscularly for premedication, this effect is not significant. Topical use of atropine and related compounds is indicated for the treatment of uveitis. Relaxation of the ciliary body and iris, in this case, leads to pain relief and limits the occurrence of adhesions to the iris or lens. The duration of action here can be prolonged. The effects on the eye after intramuscular administration are delayed in onset and last longer.

The relaxant properties of atropine are also apparent in the urinary tract where urinary retention can be precipitated in patients with prostatic disease. On the other hand, pethidine is often preferred for the treatment of renal colic precisely because of its atropine-like antispasmodic properties.

The ability of atropine to cross the blood–brain barrier leads to a number of central effects. In normal clinical doses it has insignificant sedative effects, although memory and concentration may become impaired. Larger doses can result in the central anticholinergic syndrome, with agitation, confusion, hallucinations and even coma. This type of effect limits the use of many anticholinergic agents in the treatment of Parkinson's disease, where they are indicated to control rigidity and tremor.

Hyoscine

Hyoscine hydrobromide is the *l* isomer of tropylscopate. Well absorbed across the gut and blood–brain barrier, it can be administered transdermally, orally or parenterally. The terminal half-life is approximately 2 hours after intramuscular administration, with 50% of the dose excreted unchanged in the urine. The dose intravenously or intramuscularly is 0.2–0.6 mg. A transdermal patch is available containing 1.5 mg, and delivering about 5 μg h^{-1} for 72 hours; this is mainly used for antiemetic purposes (see Ch. 39).

Hyoscine is similar to atropine in many of its properties. It is, however, more potent than atropine in its actions on the iris, ciliary body and secretory glands and less potent in its effects on the heart, bronchial smooth muscle and gut. Like atropine it has central effects, but these are much more pronounced, resulting in sedation, amnesia, fatigue and occasionally euphoria. The sedative-amnesic effects were exploited in obstetrics as an ingredient of 'twilight sleep'. It is contraindicated in the elderly because of the ease with which it produces the central anticholinergic syndrome. The antiemetic properties of

hyoscine result from both a direct effect on the emetic centre and an action on vestibular input to the brain, which makes it particularly useful for motion sickness. This activity has been exploited in the transdermal drug delivery system, which has been used in anaesthesia to control postoperative nausea in children (see also Ch. 39).

Glycopyrronium (glycopyrrolate USP)

This semisynthetic quaternary ammonium compound is highly polar and does not exhibit central cholinergic effects, such as sedation or antiemesis.

The drug is largely excreted unchanged in the urine with a terminal half-life of over 75 minutes. The dose when used to counter the muscarinic effects of neostigmine is 0.2 mg per milligram of neostigmine; in other situations 0.2–0.4 mg is administered intravenously.

It is more a more potent and long acting antisialagogue than atropine. It exhibits typical antimuscarinic effects on the bronchi, causing relaxation, while in the gut inhibition of acid secretion and general decrease in motility occurs. It shares the ability of atropine to decrease heart rate in very small doses, while it is vagolytic in larger doses. Overall it is about five times as potent as atropine as an antisialagogue, but only about twice as potent with regards to effects on the heart rate.

Ipratropium

This is a muscarinic receptor blocker used for the treatment of reversible chronic obstructive airways disease. It is another quaternary amine compound, which is poorly absorbed, allowing it to be administered by inhalation so that a local effect in the bronchial tree can be produced (see Ch. 31).

ANTICHOLINESTERASES

Acetylcholine is hydrolysed by enzymatic activity to choline and acetate. In the synaptic cleft it is acetylcholinesterase that provides this function. In the plasma and liver (and some nervous tissue not associated with the synaptic cleft) it is broken down by pseudocholinesterase (butyrylcholin-esterase or plasma cholinesterase). A single mole-cule of acetylcholinesterase contains six active sites, each containing two subsites: the anionic and the esteratic. The former becomes associated with the quaternary ammonium 'head' of acetyl-choline so that the molecule's ester bond lies at the esteratic site, which catalyses hydrolysis of the molecule. This is a two-step process: acetyl-choline is first broken down to choline and acety-lated enzyme, followed by hydrolysis to liberate acetic acid and the original enzyme. Each acetyl-choline molecule is destroyed in 80–100 μs. The different anticholinesterases all decrease acetyl-choline metabolism, which will therefore prolong the life of acetylcholine at all parasympatheti-cally innervated sites, at nicotinic receptors and of course at cholinergic receptors in the brain if the compound can cross the blood–brain barrier.

Figure 21.2 depicts acetylcholine at the anionic and esteratic sites and summarises the reaction between acetylcholine and acetylcholinesterase.

In chemical terms, the monoquaternary amines, the bisquaternary amines (the carbamates), and the organophosphates are the three broad classes of anticholinesterases. Edrophonium is a mono-quaternary amine, while neostigmine and pyri-dostigmine are representatives of the carbamates. Physostigmine is also in this group but is not used for reversal of neuromuscular blockade (see Ch. 14). To produce inhibition of the enzyme the inhibitor must simply block either the anionic or esteratic site. In the case of edrophonium the drug is not metabolised by the enzyme but is active principally at the anionic site, where it is a reversible competitive inhibitor with a dissocia-tion half-life of less than 30 seconds. Neostigmine and pyridostigmine, however, make a non-covalent bond to the anionic site; a carbamated intermediate is formed (instead of an acetylated one), which then is slowly hydrolysed. In the case of neostigmine the half-life for this hydrolysis is of the order of 1 hour.

Anticholinesterases were first used in medi-cine to control the effects of atropine. As early as

Acetylcholine

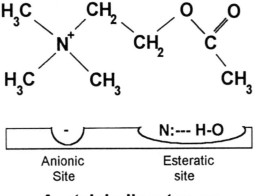

Acetylcholinesterase

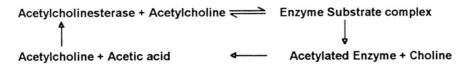

Figure 21.2 Acetylcholine, cholinesterase and the hydrolysis of acetylcholine by cholinesterase.

1900, however, in animal experiments on gut motility it was observed that cholinesterase inhibition antagonised the paralytic effects of curare. These actions remained a curiosity until utilised to treat myasthenia gravis, when it was appreciated that raising acetylcholine concentrations resulted in a restoration of muscle power. Overdosage with anticholinesterase gives rise to a 'cholinergic crisis', which is characterised by nausea, vomiting, bradycardia, salivation, sweating, bronchospasm, and also weakness and paralysis. A small dose of edrophonium (Tensilon test) is used to distinguish between the two states.

Anticholinesterases are used to raise the concentration of acetylcholine at the neuromuscular junction, an effect augmented by a variable contribution from enhanced acetylcholine release from nerve endings and depolarisation of the end-plate. It should be remembered that this shift in concentration in favour of acetylcholine does nothing to accelerate the disappearance of the muscle relaxant, which continues at its underlying spontaneous rate secondary to redistribution and metabolism. By implication, if the concentration of relaxant does not decrease to a subparalytic level by the time the period of cholinesterase inhibition is over, the neuromuscular block may reappear. Figure 21.3 illustrates the structures of the common anticholinesterases.

Neostigmine

This is a quaternary ammonium molecule originally used for treatment in myasthenia gravis. When administered without pre-existing nondepolarising neuromuscular blockade, neostigmine can itself induce a depolarising neuro-

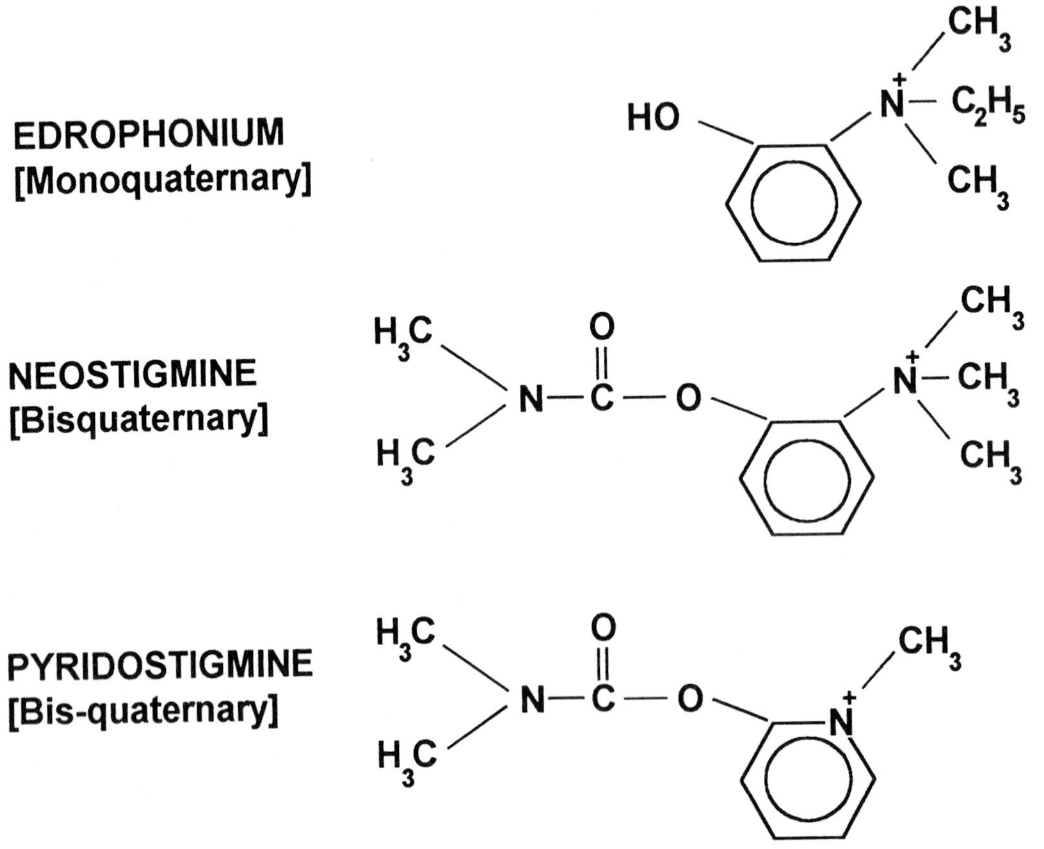

Figure 21.3   Structures of the common anticholinesterases.

muscular block. In clinical practice, however, this is not significant with single doses of the drug, although prior neostigmine administration does prolong the duration of action of suxamethonium.

Neostigmine is partly metabolised and partly eliminated by urinary excretion, with a reported half-life ranging from 24 to 80 minutes. Renal impairment therefore prolongs the duration of action of the drug.

The dose of neostigmine required to reverse neuromuscular block may range from 0.02 to 0.07 mg kg^{-1}. In infants and children, however, the dose requirement is only 50% of that recommended for adults About 3 minutes are required before neostigmine induced reversal of neuromuscular block becomes apparent, with the peak effect being seen in about 7 minutes. The duration of action is about 1 hour. The actual muscle relaxant used and degree of neuromuscular blockade are, however, critical factors in determining the rate of reversal of block. If the degree of blockade is profound and the underlying spontaneous rate of recovery slow, then neostigmine induced recovery will be partial at best. The physiological state of the patient and background anaesthesia used also influence the rate of reversal. Respiratory acidosis and metabolic alkalosis are reported to impair the action of neostigmine, while enflurane anaesthesia in particular slows neostigmine induced recovery from non-depolarising neuromuscular blockade.

Pyridostigmine

This is the pyridine analogue of neostigmine. It has a longer elimination half-life than neostigmine, with reported times of 46–112 minutes. It is also metabolised by cholinesterases in the liver and elsewhere, but differs from neostigmine in having an even greater renal clearance.

Pyridostigmine is about one-fifth as potent as neostigmine and the dose to reverse neuromuscular block is in the range 0.18–0.35 mg kg^{-1}, given intravenously. The onset of effect is slower than that of neostigmine, with a time to peak effect of 12 minutes, but it is about a third longer acting; otherwise pyridostigmine is similar to neostigmine in its effects.

Edrophonium

This drug has pharmacokinetics similar to those of neostigmine; the elimination half-life is reported to be between 33 and 110 minutes. Glucuronidation in the liver provides a metabolic route of elimination, but again about 70% of clearance is renal.

The potency of edrophonium is between 1/12 and 1/35 that of neostigmine. In a dose of 0.5–1 mg kg^{-1} it has a time to peak effect of 1–2 minutes and a duration of action only marginally shorter than that of neostigmine. Because the dose–response curves for the two agents are not parallel, and the degree of cholinesterase inhibition does not correlate well with the degree of antagonism of blockade, it is often suggested that edrophonium has a greater prejunctional activity. Unfortunately it cannot reliably reverse profound degrees of neuromuscular blockade. Consequently it is indicated to antagonise intermediate acting non-depolarising agents in situations where some spontaneous recovery has already occurred. The advantages offered by the drug lie in its speed of action and less intense muscarinic effects, although these differences are less obvious with the use of larger doses.

Because the onset of action of edrophonium is rapid, it may be necessary to administer a slower acting anticholinergic agent like glycopyrronium well before the onset of the muscarinic side-effects of edrophonium.

Organophosphate compounds

These represent a class of long lasting anticholinesterase compounds. These agents have been mainly used as insecticides or as 'nerve gas' in warfare. *Sarin* and *Soman* are examples; being highly lipid soluble they can easily penetrate both intact skin and the blood–brain barrier. Irreversible enzyme inhibition results in unrestricted acetylcholine activity. At central cholinergic sites the result is seizure activity, at nicotinic sites muscle weakness, while action at muscarinic sites leads to bronchospasm, salivation, bradycardia and hypotension.

Pyridostigmine orally has been used to protect against these agents because cholinesterase combined with it is resistant to the action of the irreversible cholinesterase inhibitors. When the pyridostigmine has been metabolised it leaves uncontaminated enzyme free to function normally, so that a reservoir of enzyme can be protected from the organophosphate agent. This is called the 'nerve agent pretreatment' regimen.

Ecothiopate is the only organophosphate compound used clinically. It is administered topically for the treatment of glaucoma. The topical application of cholinesterase inhibitors results in miosis by enhancing cholinergic transmission, but accommodative spasm may also occur. There is, however, a reluctance to use long acting agents because of an association with cataract formation. Anaesthetists know ecothiopate better for its ability to potentiate the action of suxamethonium by inhibiting pseudocholinesterase.

FURTHER READING

Ali-Melkkila T, Kanto J, Iisalo E 1993 Pharmacokinetics and related pharmacodynamics of anticholinergic drugs. Acta Anesthesiologica Scandinavica 37: 633–642

Bevan D R, Donati F, Kopman A F 1992 Reversal of neuromuscular blockade. Anesthesiology 77: 785–805

Bonde J, Viby-Mogensen J 1994 Evoked reversal of neuromuscular block. In: Pollard B J (ed) Applied neuromuscular pharmacology, pp 123–139. Oxford University Press, New York

Karalliedde L, Senanayke N 1989 Organophosphorus insecticide poisoning. British Journal of Anaesthesia 63: 736–750

Millard C B, Broomfield C A 1995 Anticholinesterases; medical applications of neurochemical principles. Journal of Neurochemistry 64: 1909–1918

Mirakhur R K, Dundee J W 1993 Glycopyrrolate pharmacology and clinical use. Anaesthesia 38: 1195–1204

Mirakhur R K, McCarthy G J 1993 Basic pharmacology of reversal agents. In: Partridge B L (ed) Anesthesiology clinics of North America, pp 237–250. Saunders, Philadelphia

Stephens R, Spurgeon A, Calvert I A et al 1995 Neuropsychological effects of long term exposure to organophosphates in sheep dip. Lancet 354: 1135–1139

22

Autonomic nervous system

R. Hainsworth

GENERAL FEATURES OF THE AUTONOMIC NERVOUS SYSTEM

The name 'autonomic nervous system' was introduced by J. N. Langley in the early part of the twentieth century to describe those nerves that are largely concerned with the control of bodily functions. The autonomic system is predominantly unconscious and involuntary, although this distinction from somatic nerves is not absolute because, for example, some pain sensation is mediated through autonomic nerves and some individuals have learnt voluntary control of some autonomic nervous activity. Other terms for the autonomic nervous system have included the involuntary, vegetative and visceral systems. These, however, are rarely used now.

Although autonomic nerves and ganglia can be identified as discrete structures, they are integrated with the rest of the central nervous system so that afferent activity in autonomic nerves can also influence activity in some somatic nerves and vice versa. Many regions within the brain, particularly the hypothalamus, are known to influence autonomic activity.

Autonomic nerves comprise parasympathetic and sympathetic nerves and both divisions convey both afferent and efferent impulses along myelinated and non-myelinated fibres. The motor effects of the two divisions tend to be opposite. Thus, for example, activity in sympathetic nerves increases heart rate, whereas parasympathetic stimulation slows it; sympathetic impulses decrease intestinal motility and constrict smooth muscle sphincters, whereas parasympathetic impulses stimulate gland secretion, increase gut motility and relax sphincters. Not all structures, however, are innervated by both divisions, and control of visceral functions is not competitive but by subtle and often discrete changes in activity in one part of the system.

Anatomical features

The autonomic nervous system is conveniently divided into the parasympathetic system (cranial and sacral outflow) and the sympathetic system (thoracolumbar outflow).

Parasympathetic nerves

The nervous origins, principal structures supplied and the responses to stimulation are summarised in Table 22.1.

The efferent preganglionic parasympathetic cell bodies lie in nuclei within the central nervous system. Preganglionic fibres are generally long and synapse in ganglia situated near to the effector organs. Preganglionic nerves are cholinergic (nicotinic). Postganglionic nerves are also cholinergic (muscarinic) but they also release a number of peptide cotransmitters which may modulate the effects of the acetylcholine.

Many parasympathetic nerves are afferent and convey information from a variety of mechanoreceptors and chemoreceptors to relay in cerebral nuclei (cranial nerves) and spinal centres (pelvic nerves). Afferent parasympathetic fibres may be myelinated, but far more are non-myelinated and much less is known about the function of those.

Sympathetic nerves

The motor neurones of the sympathetic system originate in the lateral grey horn cells of the spinal cord between the upper thoracic and second or third lumbar segments of the spinal cord. The preganglionic fibres are myelinated and are therefore the white rami communicantes. The postganglionic fibres do not have a myelin sheath and are therefore grey rami. The arrangement of these rami is shown in Figure 22.1. The segmental thoracolumbar outflow that forms the sympathetic system may run up or down the sympathetic chain for two or three segments before running to supply the various structures. Table 22.2 summarises the segmental levels, the structures supplied by the sympathetic nerves and their responses to stimulation.

Table 22.1 Parasympathetic nerves

Nerve	Structure supplied	Effect
Cranial III	Eye — iris circular muscle Ciliary muscle	Contraction (miosis) Contraction (for near vision)
Cranial VII	Lacrimal gland Submaxillary and sublingual glands	Secretion Secretion
Cranial IX	Parotid gland	Secretion
Cranial X	Heart — sinoatrial node Atrioventricular node Atrial muscle Bronchi Stomach, gallbladder, pancreas, small intestine, glands Pancreatic islets	Bradycardia Slow conduction, block Negative inotropism Constriction, mucus secretion Increase motility, contract gallbladder, relax sphincters, gland secretion Increase insulin
Sacral S1, S2	Large intestine Bladder detrusor Bladder sphincter Penis	Increase motility, secretion Contraction Relaxation Vasodilatation and erection

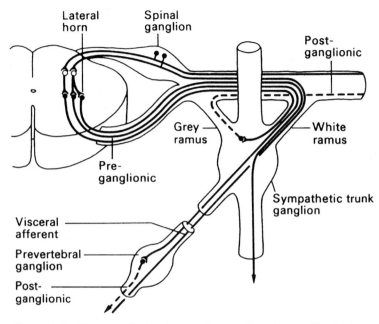

Figure 22.1   The sympathetic reflex arc. Sensory fibres have cell bodies in the spinal ganglia and synapse with intermediate neurones in the dorsal horn. Motor neurones originate in the lateral horn of the thoracolumbar outflow and form the myelinated white rami. Some synapse in the sympathetic ganglia to form the grey rami (non-myelinated fibres). Some synapse in visceral ganglia. (Reproduced with permission from Bannister and Mathias 1992 Autonomic Failure)

Table 22.2 Sympathetic nerves

Segmental level	Structure supplied	Effect
T1–2	Eye — iris radial muscle	Contraction (mydriasis)
	Cerebral blood vessels and face and neck	Vasomotor, sudomotor and pilomotor
T3–4	Heart	Positive inotropic and chronotropic effects
T5–9	Arm	Vasomotor, sudomotor, pilomotor
T6–L2	Gastrointestinal tract	Decrease motility, contract sphincters, vasoconstriction
	Liver	Glycogenolysis
	Pancreatic islets	Decrease insulin, increase glucagon
T10–L2	Leg	Vasomotor, sudomotor, pilomotor
L1–2	Bladder detrusor	Relax
	Bladder sphincter	Contract
	Penis and sex glands	Ejaculation

Many sympathetic nerves do not relay in the spinal ganglia but, like the parasympathetic nerves, relay in ganglia much closer to the organ that they innervate. Like parasympathetic nerves, the preganglionic fibres are cholinergic (nicotinic). However, with the notable exception of the cholinergic (muscarinic) innervation of sweat glands, sympathetic motor fibres are adrenergic, releasing noradrenaline at their terminals. Recent work has demonstrated the release of cotransmitters, particularly adenosine triphosphate (ATP) and neuropeptide Y, which may modulate the actions of noradrenaline.

In addition to the well known motor effects of the sympathetic system, there are also sensory fibres, both myelinated and non-myelinated. Some of these effectively behave as somatic nerves and relay sensation, for example cardiac or visceral pain, to the higher centres. Afferent nerves in the sympathetic system may also participate in segmental reflex responses. These reflexes seem generally to be excitatory and it has been proposed that sympathetic–sympathetic reflexes may act as positive feedback mechanisms. An example of this is where some cardiac or vascular receptors, which are stimulated by increases in blood pressure, evoke reflex vasoconstriction, which further increases blood pressure. This contrasts with most parasympathetic reflexes, which function as negative feedback mechanisms and thereby act to control or stabilise the system.

The adrenal medulla

The adrenal medulla is essentially a sympathetic ganglion. Because of this, it is unlike other glandular tissue in that it is innervated by preganglionic sympathetic nerve fibres. Activity in these fibres acts upon the chromaffin cells to result in release into the blood of the twin hormones adrenaline and noradrenaline. The ratio of the hormones secreted is about 70% adrenaline to 30% noradrenaline. This contrasts with sympathetic nerve endings, which release only noradrenaline. Adrenal medullary secretion is very low at rest but increases in response to various stimuli, including emotional stress, exercise, cold, anaesthesia and trauma. Secretion increases in response to various reflexogenic stimuli, which cause widespread increases in sympathetic nervous activity, including hypotension, hypoxia and hypoglycaemia. Because more adrenaline is secreted than noradrenaline, adrenal medullary stimulation causes effects that are subtly different from those resulting from sympathetic activity elsewhere. Adrenaline stimulates glycogen breakdown in the liver to form glucose. It also dilates blood vessels in skeletal muscle, while constricting vessels elsewhere, thereby diverting more of the cardiac output to muscle. This forms part of the 'fright and flight' response.

INNERVATION OF THE CARDIOVASCULAR SYSTEM

Although to some extent the cardiovascular system can function after loss of the autonomic innervation, reflexes involving sympathetic and parasympathetic afferent and efferent nerves play important roles in the responses to various stresses, including postural changes and exercise. Autonomic efferent activity may also be influenced by somatic afferent inputs, as seen by the increases in heart rate and blood pressure that occur in response to painful stimuli.

Motor innervation

The heart

Heart rate is determined by the rate of depolarisation of the cardiac pacemaker, normally the sinoatrial node. In the absence of neural or hormonal influences, the heart rate in humans is 100–120 beats min^{-1}. The maximal heart rate achieved during high levels of sympathetic activity, usually provoked by maximal exercise, is about 200 beats min^{-1} in young people and rather less in older subjects. As a rule of thumb, the maximal age related heart rate can be taken as 220–age (years). Heart rate at any time is determined by the balance of vagal and sympathetic activity and, at rest, because heart rate is below the intrinsic rate, vagal activity must predominate. Vagal activity results in hyperpolarisation of the cardiac pacemaker cells and decreases the rate of their spontaneous depolarisation. Activity in the sympathetic nerves, on the other hand, increases the rate of depolarisation of the pacemaker cells. High levels of vagal activity can cause a profound bradycardia or even aystole. In animal experiments it has been possible to compare the effects of separate stimulation of right and left autonomic nerves. These have shown little difference between the effects of the two vagi but the right sympathetic nerves have a much larger effect on heart rate than the left (Fig. 22.2).

The relationship between the frequency of stimulation of the autonomic nerves and the heart rate is not linear: a change in activity at low frequencies causes a much larger response than the same change at a higher frequency. This nonlinearity disappears if, instead of determining changes in heart rate, we express the cardiac

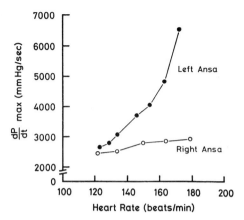

Figure 22.2 Comparison of inotropic and chronotropic responses to stimulation of right and left sympathetic nerves in anaesthetised dog. Inotropic responses expressed as maximal rate of change of left ventricular pressure (dP/dt max at paced heart rate and controlled aortic pressure). Increasing frequency of stimulation to right sympathetic nerves (ansa subclavia) cause large increases in rate but only a small inotropic change. Left sympathetic stimulation induces both inotropic and chronotropic changes. (Reproduced with permission from Furnival C M, Linden R J, Snow H M 1973 Chronotropic and inotropic effects on the dog heart of stimulating the efferent cardiac sympathetic nerves. Journal of Physiology 230: 137–153.)

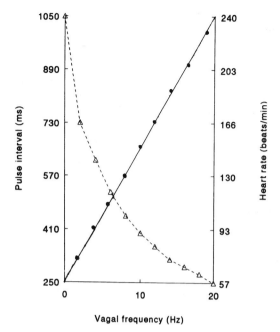

Figure 22.3 Chronotropic effects of vagal stimulation in anaesthetised rabbit. Responses expressed as heart rate (△) and as pulse interval (●). Note that heart rate does not change linearly with vagal stimulation; low frequencies induce much larger changes. Pulse interval, by contrast, does change linearly. (Reproduced with permission from Hainsworth R 1995 The control and physiological importance of heart rate. In: Malik M, Camm A J (eds) Heart rate variability. Futura, New York.)

response as the effect on pulse interval (Fig. 22.3). This implies that it is the interval between beats rather than the heart rate that is actually controlled by the autonomic nerves. In addition to the effect on the rate of depolarisation of the sinoatrial node, the autonomic nerves also influence the velocity of the spread of the cardiac impulse, with sympathetic stimulation increasing the velocity and vagal stimulation slowing it and possibly even inducing heart block.

Autonomic nerves control the force of contraction of cardiac muscle. Sympathetic stimulation causes the myocardium to contract more rapidly, more powerfully and for a shorter duration. Thus at any end-diastolic volume the heart empties more completely and, because systole is shortened, more time is available for diastolic filling. Activity in the left cardiac sympathetic nerves has a greater effect on the force of contraction (inotropic effect) compared with the right, which mainly affects heart rate (Fig. 22.2).

Vagal stimulation has a negative inotropic effect on the atrial myocardium, which reduces its force of contraction at given fibre lengths. However, whether vagal activity also directly affects the ventricular muscle is more controversial, and in mammalian hearts, if there is any effect, it is very small. There may be an indirect effect on the ventricle owing to reduced filling from the atrium due to the negative inotropic effect. On the other hand, the negative chronotropic effect causes a greater cardiac distension and consequently a greater stroke volume.

Blood vessels

Arteries, arterioles, venules and veins in many parts of the body are innervated by sympathetic nerve fibres. These are almost exclusively α-adrenergic and vasoconstrictor in effect. The only possible exception is that cutaneous vessels are affected by cholinergic sympathetic vasodilator fibres. However, cutaneous vasodilatation may be secondary to increased activity in sweat glands and the consequent release of metabolic factors. The question of the existence of sympathetic cholinergic vasodilator fibres supplying blood vessels in skeletal muscle has been controversial. They have been shown to exist in several subprimate species, such as cat, but there is no anatomical or physiological evidence for their existence in several types of primate that have been studied and it is most unlikely that they are present in humans.

At rest there is a low level of activity in sympathetic efferent nerves and this enhances arteriolar smooth muscle 'tone' and causes contraction of venous smooth muscle. It is the degree of constriction of resistance vessels (mainly arterioles) that is responsible for controlling vascular resistance and for maintaining arterial blood pressure. Constriction of the capacitance vessels (mainly veins) enhances the return of blood to the heart and thereby contributes to the maintenance of cardiac output. Low levels of activity in peripheral sympathetic nerves cause a relatively high degree of constriction of capacitance vessels but have little effect on the arteriolar resistance. As impulse frequency increases, the resistance vessels also constrict more powerfully (Fig. 22.4). This implies that moderate stresses which stimulate sympathetic activity result in reflex capacitance changes before there are marked changes in resistance and, therefore, in blood flow.

Parasympathetic nerves do not generally play a role in the control of blood vessels but they do control various secretory glands, and vasodilatation in glands occurs largely as a consequence of the increased metabolic demand as the gland becomes active. However, there is evidence that some parasympathetic fibres may also directly cause vasodilatation by non-adrenergic non-cholinergic transmitters, because it is possible to block the secretory response and still retain some degree of vasodilatation.

Parasympathetic nerves do cause vasodilatation in erectile tissue, hence the name nervi erigentes.

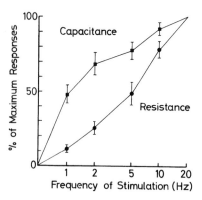

Figure 22.4 Responses of vascular resistance and capacitance in splanchnic circulation of anaesthetised dogs to graded splanchnic sympathetic nerve stimulation. Responses are expressed as percentages of those at 20 Hz. Note that at low stimulus frequencies capacitance responses are a much greater proportion of maximal than the corresponding resistance responses, which require higher stimulus frequencies. (Reproduced with permission from Hainsworth R and Karim F 1976 Responses of abdominal vascular capacitance in the anaesthetized dog to changes in carotid sinus pressure. Journal of Physiology 262: 659–677.)

Sensory innervation and reflex responses

Baroreceptors

The name baroreceptor implies a sensory receptor responsive to pressure; however, although this is essentially true, baroreceptors are actually stretch receptors that are stimulated when the transmural pressure increases across the relevant vessel wall.

The best known and most widely studied baroreceptors are those in the carotid sinuses. These are dilated sections at the origins of the internal carotid arteries. In humans, their location is just behind and below the angle of the jaw (with the neck extended). Their afferent innervation is in the sinus nerve which is a branch of the glossopharyngeal (IXth cranial) nerve. The fibres of the sinus nerve, some of which are myelinated and many non-myelinated, arborise in the adventitia of the carotid sinus.

Although carotid baroreceptors may be particularly important, in that they respond to changes in pressure in the arteries perfusing the brain, there are other baroreceptor areas in other regions of the cardiovascular system. In addition to those in the aortic arch, which are well known, baroreceptors have also been described in the subclavian, coronary and mesenteric arteries, although much less is known about these.

Baroreceptors do not merely detect changes in the level of mean arterial blood pressure: they also have important phasic properties. During normal pulsatile blood pressure the receptors are active during the rising phase of pressure and silent during the falling phase. The reflex response to baroreceptor stimulation is importantly influenced by the degree of pulsatility. A reduction in pulse pressure, even when mean pressure does not change, provides a smaller reflexogenic stimulus (Fig. 22.5). Thus baroreceptors are able to respond to changes in cardiac stroke volume because it is this that is mainly responsible for determining pulse pressure.

The reflex responses to changes in the baroreceptor stimulus function as part of a negative feedback system. Thus a fall in pressure evokes responses which cause pressure to increase again. These responses are an increase in sympathetic activity and decrease in vagal activity. The sympathetic response leads to constriction of resistance vessels in most regions of the body, causing an increase in vascular resistance. There is also evidence that there is constriction of capacitance vessels, at least in the splanchnic region, and this enhances venous return and consequently increases cardiac output and arterial pressure. In the heart the decrease in vagal activity and increase in sympathetic activity result in positive chronotropic and inotropic changes.

The responses to changes in baroreceptor pressure occur very rapidly and are limited mainly by the speed of response of the effector organ. Because of the rapidity of the cardiac responses to changes in vagal stimulation, a rapid change in baroreceptor pressure may actually result in the subsequent heart beat being delayed. Sympathetic responses are rather slower, but may be seen in 5–10 seconds.

Although there is no doubt that baroreceptors are able to respond to small changes in mean arterial pressure or pulse pressure, their role in determining the actual level of the blood pressure is uncertain. Animal experiments have shown

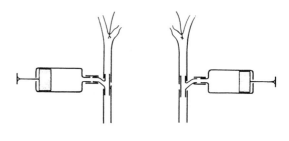

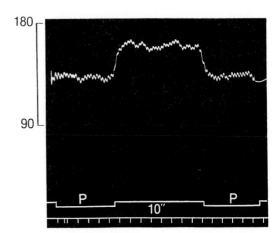

Figure 22.5 Importance of pulse pressure in carotid sinus reflex. Top shows method of changing carotid pulse pressure without affecting mean pressure. Using 'T'-shaped connectors, air filled syringes damp down the carotid pulse. The damping effect can be prevented by clamping the connecting tubes leading to the damping chambers. Lower part shows effects on blood pressure of changing from pulsatile pressure (P) to less pulsatile pressure. The pulsatile stimulus is stronger, resulting in a marked decrease in blood pressure despite the fact that then the mean pressure to the sinus would also be less. (Modified with permission from Ead H W, Green J H, Neil E 1952 A comparison of the effects of pulsatile and non-pulsatile blood flow through the carotid sinus on the reflexogenic activity of the sinus baroreceptors in the cat. Journal of Physiology 118: 509–519.)

that after baroreceptor denervation there is little change in the average level of blood pressure, although the fluctuations in pressure are much greater.

The characteristics of baroreceptors can be defined in terms of their threshold — that is, the lowest pressure at which afferent baroreceptor discharge can be detected or the lowest pressure to induce a reflex change; the inflexion or the midpoint of the range; and the saturation pressure — the pressure above which no further responses can be obtained. Baroreceptors overall tend to operate about the mean level of arterial pressure — that is, the inflexion of the response curve is close to mean arterial pressure. It has, however, been suggested that carotid baroreceptors have their inflexion point below the resting level of arterial pressure, and are therefore more sensitive to decreases rather than increases in pressure. Aortic receptors, on the other hand, may have higher operating ranges and thus be more sensitive to pressure increases.

Baroreceptors 'reset' if changes in blood pressure persist for any length of time. The resetting occurs in two phases: a partial resetting occurs in less than 30 minutes and more complete resetting occurs with chronic hypertension. In resetting there is a shift in the curve so that the inflexion remains close to the operating pressure. In hypertension, in addition to a shift of the curve to the right, i.e. to operate at higher pressure, there is also a decrease in the sensitivity of the baroreceptors.

Atrial receptors

Atrial receptors are the endings of large myelinated vagal fibres found mainly at the junctions of the great veins with the atria and in the atrial appendages. The receptors are situated in the subendocardium and form complex unencapsulated endings. Their principal stimulus is stretch and consequently they signal the degree of atrial filling. The activity of the receptors is phasic in relation to the cardiac cycle. Their discharge pattern has been classified into type B, which occurs during the filling phase of the atrium ('v' wave); intermediate, which discharges both during filling and during atrial systole; and the much less common type A, which discharges only during atrial systole. These discharge patterns are not fixed and may change depending on circumstances. Atrial receptor discharge is linearly related to atrial pressure and the receptors detect the degree of filling of the heart. Because filling is dependent amongst other things on blood volume, atrial receptors are sometimes referred to as volume receptors.

The reflex responses to stimulation of atrial receptors have the effect of decreasing cardiac volume as well as decreasing blood and extracellular fluid volume. The most immediate response is an increase in heart rate (Fig. 22.6). This is caused by an increase in the discharge in efferent sympathetic nerves to the sinoatrial node and, unless filling is enhanced, it reduces cardiac volume. There seems to be no increase in activity in other sympathetic nerves to the heart or to blood vessels. Renal nerves, however, show a decrease in their discharge. Stimulation of atrial receptors also influences the hypothalamus and results in a decrease in secretion of antidiuretic hormone (ADH). The decrease in ADH secretion and the decrease in renal nerve activity lead to increased secretion of water and salt and, therefore, to a decrease in extracellular fluid volume.

The activity of atrial receptors becomes depressed in heart failure and this may partly explain the observed increase in extracellular fluid volume.

It should be mentioned that increases in atrial volume causing stretch of the myocytes results in the release into the circulation of atrial natriuretic peptide (ANP). This causes vasodilatation and increased sodium excretion. It is important to note that ANP release is from the direct effect of stretch on the atrium. It is not a reflex and does not involve the autonomic nerves.

Ventricular receptors

The left ventricle has a much greater afferent innervation than the right, and most of the afferent fibres are non-myelinated and run in the vagal and, to some extent, sympathetic nerves. These nerves may be excited by mechanical events, usually abnormally high volumes or pressures, chemical stimuli, or both. Chemical stimulation of ventricular receptors, by injection of various chemicals into the coronary circulation, can induce very powerful reflex depressor responses characterised by a profound vagally induced bradycardia and intense vasodilatation resulting from sympathetic withdrawal (Fig. 22.7). This is called the Bezold–Jarisch reflex and is probably not elicited during normal physiological conditions but may occur if chemical

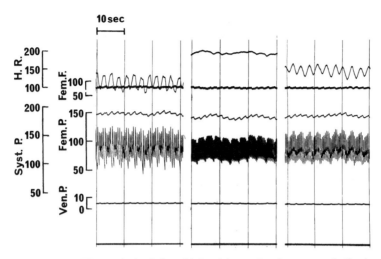

Figure 22.6 Effects of stimulation of left atrial receptors in an anaesthetised dog. Atrial receptors were distended by small balloons at the pulmonary vein–atrial junctions, which simulates an increase in atrial filling. Traces are of heart rate (HR in beats per minute); femoral flow (Fem. F.) held constant to perfused limb; femoral perfusion pressure (Fem. P.), which, at constant flow, is proportional to vascular resistance; systemic arterial blood pressure (Syst. P.) and central venous pressure (Ven. P.). All pressures are in millimetres of mercury. Panels show traces before, during and after atrial receptor stimulation. Note that during atrial receptor stimulation (middle panel) there is a reflex increase in heart rate but no change in limb vascular resistance. (Reproduced with permission from Carswell F, Hainsworth R, Ledsome J R 1970 The effects of distension of the pulmonary vein — arterial junctions upon peripheral vascular resistance. Journal of Physiology 207: 1–14.)

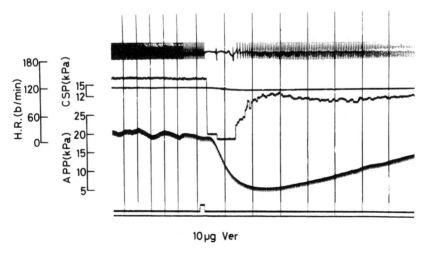

10 μg Ver

Figure 22.7 Effects of stimulation of ventricular or coronary chemosensitive afferents (Bezold–Jarisch reflex). Traces from anaesthetised dog of ECG, heart rate (HR), carotid sinus pressure (CSP) (held constant), and hind limb perfusion pressure (APP) (flow constant). Stimulation by injection of veratridine into coronary circulation results in profound bradycardia (5 s asystole) and vasodilatation. Vertical lines are 10 s time markers. (Reproduced with permission from McGregor K H, Hainsworth R, Ford R 1986 Hind-limb vascular responses in anaesthetized dogs to aortic root injections of veratridine. Quarterly Journal of Experimental Physiology 71: 577–587.)

irritants, such as ionic radiopaque contrast media, are injected into the coronary circulation. They may also be excited during myocardial ischaemia or infarction.

Other cardiovascular reflexogenic areas

Stimulation of a vast number of afferent nerves induces reflex changes in autonomic nervous activity to the cardiovascular system. Some changes occur during normal physiological events; others seem to be more related to pathological processes.

Cushing response. Cerebral hypotension, hypoxia or compression elicits the Cushing response. This is a very powerful excitation of the sympathetic drive to the heart and blood vessels and leads to very high levels of arterial blood pressure. There may also be an associated baroreceptor-mediated bradycardia.

Carotid body chemoreceptors. Chemoreceptors are stimulated by hypoxia, hypercapnia and acidaemia and, in addition to their role in stimulating respiration, may also lead to vasoconstriction and bradycardia. However, the bradycardia may not be apparent during spontaneous respiration because the increased rate and depth of breathing results in a reflex tachycardia that masks the primary chemoreceptor induced bradycardia. Hypoxia during artificial ventilation is likely to lead to bradycardia because the secondary respiratory effects are prevented.

'Diving' reflex. Stimulation of trigeminal afferents by cold facepacks or immersion results in a diving response of apnoea, bradycardia and vasoconstriction.

Lung inflation. Pulmonary stretch receptors are responsible for the Hering–Breuer reflex, which causes inhibition of inspiration. They also cause reflex tachycardia by inhibition of the baroreceptor reflex and thus are partly responsible for the respiratory sinus arrhythmia.

Muscle metaboreceptors. Exercising muscle forms metabolic products which activate chemoreceptors attached to somatic afferent nerves. These nerves influence the cardiovascular centres and lead to vasoconstriction and therefore hypertension.

Painful stimuli. Many thoracic and abdominal viscera are innervated by sympathetic fibres. Many of these are nociceptors and mediate pain sensations. The reflex responses tend to be excitatory, resulting in increases in sympathetic efferent activity. The net reflex response to myocardial ischaemia depends on whether it is predominantly the vagal or sympathetic afferent fibres that are excited. Inferolateral wall ischaemia excites mainly vagal afferents and causes bradycardia and vasodilatation; anterior wall ischaemia tends to stimulate mainly sympathetic afferents, causing tachycardia, vasoconstriction and a susceptibility to arrhythmias. Responses are also influenced by psychological factors and the degree of sedation.

Painful stimuli at the surface of the body usually result in an increase in blood pressure. Deep visceral pain, however, frequently results in bradycardia and vasodilatation. Surgical procedures can thus lead to quite large changes in blood pressure — for example, skin incisions may elevate blood pressure by 20 mmHg or more.

Some complex events involving cardiovascular reflexes

Valsalva manoeuvre

The Valsalva or straining manoeuvre involves making a forced expiratory effort against a closed glottis or obstruction. The pressure generated may be maximal or may be controlled using a manometer to, typically, 40 mmHg. It is important to realise that, because the pressure is generated by contraction of abdominal as well as thoracic muscles, the thoracoabdominal circulation is relatively unaffected because there is no change in the pressure gradients in those regions. Venous return to the heart is reduced due to blood being impeded from entering from the head and neck and limbs. There are four phases to the Valsalva manoeuvre and these are illustrated in Fig. 22.8. Firstly, the pressure generated in the thorax and abdomen compresses the large arteries and this results in an immediate increase in arterial blood pressure. Secondly, blood is impeded from entering the pressurised region,

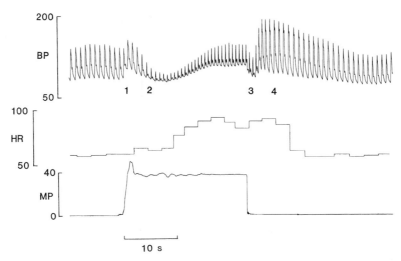

Figure 22.8 The Valsalva manoeuvre. Traces show finger arterial blood pressure (BP) (from FINAPRES photoplethysmograph, mmHg), heart rate (HR) (beats per minute) and mouth pressure (MP) (mmHg). Four phases of Valsalva are seen: 1, increase in blood pressure; 2, decrease in pressure followed by restoration of pressure and tachycardia; 3, transient decrease in pressure following expiration; 4, overshoot with associated fall in heart rate.

resulting in a fall in cardiac output and therefore in blood pressure. This is detected by baroreceptors and the consequent reflex vasoconstriction largely restores the mean pressure but, due to the stroke volume being lower because of the decreased cardiac output and increased heart rate, pulse pressure is less and it is this which sustains the lower stimulus to the baroreceptors. The third phase is the transient fall in blood pressure when the Valsalva is released, due to the reduction in the external compression of the arteries. Finally, there is an overshoot of blood pressure as the blood re-enters the central circulation from the periphery and is pumped out into a constricted circulation. There is also often a reflex bradycardia in this phase.

The Valsalva manoeuvre is often used as a test for autonomic neuropathy. If the reflexes are ineffective, blood pressure continues to fall during the strain and the tachycardia is reduced or absent. The overshoot of pressure on release of the strain is also not seen.

Positive pressure breathing

During normal negative pressure ventilation, the subatmospheric intrathoracic pressure, particularly during inspiration, enhances the return of blood into the thoracic vessels. In positive pressure breathing the pressure gradient is reversed and venous return is impeded, leading to a decrease in the cardiac output. The baroreceptor reflex maintains mean pressure but pulse pressure is reduced. It is the reduction in pulse pressure, despite the unchanged mean pressure, that provides the signal for the baroreceptors. The stress induced is similar to that in the Valsalva manoeuvre. However, there is one important difference — during lung inflation blood is retained in the abdominal circulation as well as in the limbs, head and neck. This is important because the abdominal veins are very distensible and can readily accommodate large volumes of blood. It has been estimated that the compliance of the abdominal circulation is as great as the whole of the rest of the body.

Postural changes

In the supine position, there are only small pressure gradients between the various arteries and between the various veins. In the upright posi-

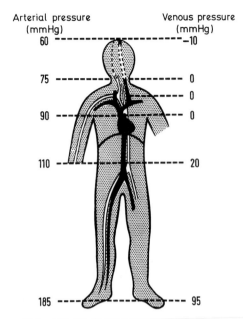

Arterial pressure (mmHg) / Venous pressure (mmHg)

Figure 22.9 Effects of posture on arterial and venous pressures. Gravity causes decreases in arterial and venous pressures above heart level and increases below. The high venous pressures result in venous distension and increased capillary transudation. (Reproduced with permission from Hainsworth R 1985 Arterial blood pressure. In: Enderby G E H (ed.) Hypotensive anaesthesia. Churchill Livingstone, Edinburgh.)

tion, gravity imposes large gradients (Fig. 22.9). The effect on the arterial system is that it is the cerebral circulation that is most susceptible to hypotension, although cerebral perfusion pressure actually falls less — because of the negative venous pressure. On the venous side, the increases in pressure result in distension of the blood vessels in the dependent regions. The effect is to shift 0.5 litre or more of blood from the central circulation to the dependent vessels. Furthermore, because venous pressure increases, capillary pressure also increases, thereby causing a decrease in the plasma volume by capillary filtration. The overall effect of this is to reduce venous return and consequently cardiac output. Mean blood pressure, however, is normally unchanged because of the reflex responses.

It is instructive to examine in some detail the sequence of events occurring when a person actively stands up, then remains standing motionless.

The act of standing involves muscular work. Initially, as part of the response to voluntary exercise, there is an increase in heart rate due to withdrawal of vagal tone. Muscle contraction compresses veins and venous return is initially enhanced, and this transiently increases cardiac output and may increase blood pressure. Muscle contraction, however, also produces vasodilator metabolites and muscle resistance vessels dilate. Thus, immediately after standing, gravity causes blood to pool in dependent vessels, reducing venous return. This and the initial muscle vasodilatation often leads to a transient fall in blood pressure. The subject may feel momentarily dizzy at this stage. Next, due to a reduction in the stimulus to baroreceptors there is a reflex increase in sympathetic vasoconstrictor activity, leading to the restoration of mean blood pressure. In the steady state, mean pressure at heart level is restored or may even be a little increased. Usually systolic pressure is unchanged and diastolic pressure is raised. The decrease in pulse pressure provides the decrease in the baroreceptor stimulus, which causes the mean pressure to be maintained (cf. Fig. 22.5). Note, however, that although mean pressure is controlled, cardiac output remains typically 20–25% lower than in the supine position. If muscular activity ensues, however, muscle pump mechanisms result in venous return being enhanced and cardiac output increased. Standing still also results in loss of blood volume from capillary transudation at the high hydrostatic pressures. The loss of capillary fluid slows after about 5–10 minutes standing. This is the result of the marked vasoconstriction, reducing capillary pressure, and the increased capillary oncotic pressure in the legs from the loss of fluid, which opposes filtration.

Prolonged standing still causes a progressive decrease in venous return. The point may be reached at which vasoconstriction is unable to maintain the normal blood pressure. At this point the sympathetic drive abruptly ceases and there may also be an associated vagally mediated bradycardia (Fig. 22.10). This is the vasovagal response. Its trigger mechanism is unknown but the inhibition of vasoconstrictor discharge results

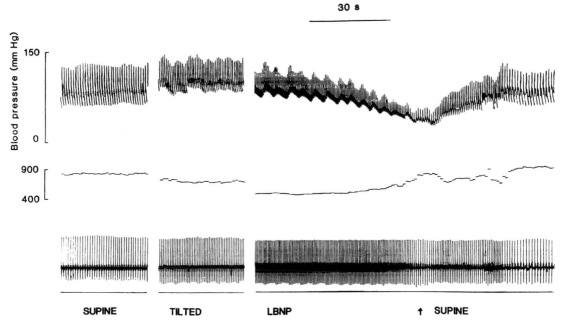

Figure 22.10 An experimentally induced vasovagal reaction in a healthy subject. Traces are of blood pressure (FINAPRES), pulse interval and ECG. Subject was initially tilted head-up by 60°, which resulted in increases in diastolic and mean blood pressures and tachycardia. Imposition of lower body negative pressure (LBNP), which further decreases venous return, initially caused a small decrease in blood pressure and increase in heart rate. Blood pressure then quite rapidly decreased, followed by bradycardia. At this point the subject developed symptoms of impending syncope. (Reproduced with permission from El-Bedawi K H, Hainsworth R 1994 Combined head-up tilt and lower body suction: a test of orthostatic tolerance. Clinical Autonomic Research 4: 41–47.)

in an abrupt fall in blood pressure and loss of consciousness.

INNERVATION OF THE LUNG

The two main components of the lung are the airways and the pulmonary circulation. Both receive motor innervation from the autonomic nervous system and may give rise to reflexes when appropriately stimulated. In addition, the lung contains bronchial glands and a bronchial circulation which partly anastomoses with the pulmonary vessels.

Motor innervation

Airways

Bronchial smooth muscle relaxes in response to β-adrenergic agonists. In people there appears to be little if any direct sympathetic innervation so bronchodilatation would occur only as the result of increases in concentrations of circulating catecholamines. In resting healthy subjects β_2 blockade has no effect on airways calibre. In asthmatic subjects, however, even at rest there is evidence of β_2 mediated bronchodilatation, and β blockade in these people may precipitate an acute asthmatic attack. In normal subjects, increases in circulating catecholamines which occur with exercise induce bronchodilatation and thereby facilitate the ventilatory response.

The parasympathetic supply to the lungs is from the vagus nerves. Increased activity in these nerves excites airways muscarinic receptors and induces bronchoconstriction. At rest, there is a degree of vagal tone, which decreases with exercise, contributing to the bronchodilatation.

Pulmonary circulation

The pulmonary circulation is a low pressure system and any resting tone in the pulmonary blood vessels is very low. The pulmonary vessels, nevertheless, are innervated by both divisions of the autonomic nervous system. Activity in sympathetic adrenergic nerves elicits vasoconstriction, and stimulation of vagal muscarinic receptors leads to vasodilatation. Unlike the systemic circulation, where the greatest innervation is to the small arteries and arterioles, in the lung the innervation is greatest in the large vessels and the supply to the peripheral vessels is less. The effects of the autonomic nerves on the pulmonary vessels are probably minor under most conditions but may be relevant during stresses, including exercise and hypoxia.

Sensory innervation and reflex responses

Pulmonary stretch receptors

Pulmonary stretch receptors are from myelinated vagal fibres ending in the airways smooth muscle. They have low thresholds and some receptors are still active at the end of expiration. Their discharge frequency increases with the depth of breathing. As for other reflexogenic areas, pulmonary receptors have a variety of operating ranges and, as inspiration increases, not only is there an increase in discharge frequency but more receptors become recruited.

The primary reflex effect from pulmonary stretch receptors is to inhibit inspiration. It has been suggested that their role is to regulate the depth and rate of breathing to an optimal level. Other reflex responses to stimulation of these receptors are to cause bronchodilatation and to increase heart rate, both effects being mediated through decreases in efferent vagal activity. The effect on heart rate is partly responsible for the respiratory sinus arrhythmia. Most of the conclusions concerning the role of pulmonary stretch receptors have been derived from experiments on animals and work on humans suggests that they may be less important.

Lung irritant receptors

Myelinated vagal fibres ramify in the epithelium of the airways from the trachea as far as the respiratory bronchioles. Activity in these fibres is elicited from a variety of stimuli but, unlike the pulmonary stretch receptors, their discharge rapidly adapts. Irritant receptors, as their name implies, are stimulated by chemicals and dusts on the epithelial surface. They are also excited by bronchial spasm, for example in response to histamine inhalation. They may also become transiently stimulated during maximal inspiration.

The reflex responses to stimulation of irritant receptors include hyperpnoea and bronchospasm. They may also be responsible for the unpleasant sensation felt when irritants are inhaled.

Pulmonary 'C' fibres

Non-myelinated vagal afferents terminate in the region of the alveoli and pulmonary capillaries. They are sometimes refered to as 'J' receptors or juxtapulmonary capillary receptors because of their accessibility to noxious chemicals in the pulmonary circulation. Experimentally, they have been strongly excited by chemicals either in the alveolar gas or in the circulating blood. They may also be excited by overdistension or collapse of the lungs. Inhalation anaesthetics may not only stimulate the C fibres but they also have the effect of lowering their thresholds to distension so that they can then be excited by normal levels of inspiration. They are also excited in a variety of pathological conditions, including pulmonary embolism, oedema and inflammation.

The reflex responses to stimulation of pulmonary C fibres include apnoea, followed by rapid shallow breathing. They also may influence the cardiovascular system to cause bradycardia and vasodilatation.

INNERVATION OF THE DIGESTIVE SYSTEM

Several other chapters in this book deal with

related topics: nutrition (Ch. 37), gastrointestinal physiology (Ch. 38), vomiting (Ch. 39) and the liver (Ch. 41). This section contains a summary of the innervation of the alimentary system and an account of some of the principal reflexes involving autonomic nerves.

Motor innervation

As summarised in Tables 22.1 and 22.2, all parts of the alimentary system are innervated by both divisions of the autonomic nervous system. In general, activity in the parasympathetic nerves causes glandular secretion, increases in gut motility and relaxation of sphincters. Activity in sympathetic nerves, on the other hand, decreases gut motility and contracts sphincters.

Gastric secretion is initiated by efferent vagal activity. Stimulation of the vagus nerve, initially in response to the sight or smell of food, results in secretion of acid and pepsin. It also stimulates the release of gastrin and this further enhances acid secretion. Vagal activity also provokes gastric contractions. After vagotomy both gastric secretion and motility are reduced and gastric distension is liable to occur.

Vagal stimulation also initiates pancreatic secretion to produce an enzyme-rich fluid. This response occurs within minutes of ingestion of food. The pancreatic secretion is sustained and modified by humoral agents.

In the liver, bile secretion is provoked by vagal activity. Vagal stimulation also causes contraction of the gallbladder and relaxation of the sphincter of Oddi.

The intestine as far as the transverse colon is supplied with parasympathetic nerves from the vagus nerves; the remainder comes from the pelvic nerves. Parasympathetic ganglia are found in the myenteric (Auerbach's) and submucosal (Meissner's) plexuses and in the hypogastric ganglia. The sympathetic innervation of the gut originates from segments T6 to L2, with many of the synapses in the superior mesenteric, coeliac and hypogastric ganglia. The postganglionic fibres terminate in the submucosal and myenteric plexuses. Intestinal motility is controlled mainly by the intrinsic neurones which form the plex-uses in the intestinal walls. Consequently intestinal function, secretion, motility and absorption, continue in absence of external innervation; however, activity in the autonomic nerves is able to modify this function and allow various reflex responses to occur.

Reflexes

Local reflexes are involved in control of intestinal motility. Distension of a segment of intestine results in relaxation of the segment in front and contraction of the segment behind. Excessive distension of part of the intestine results in reflex relaxation of the rest of the intestine. The gastroileal and gastrocolic 'reflexes' occur in response to distension and secretion in the stomach. The response is to increase movement of the terminal ileum to accelerate filling of the colon and to increase colonic motility. These 'reflexes' are thought to be partly caused by humoral factors.

Defecation. This is a complex procedure that is partly under autonomic control and partly voluntary. Normally the rectum is empty. Colonic motility, often following gastric distension, results in the propulsion of faeces into the rectum. Rectal distension stimulates stretch receptors which transmit impulses to the pelvic nerves and are appreciated centally as the desire to defecate. Under most circumstances continence is maintained by contraction of the external anal sphincter.

The internal sphincter is smooth muscle and under the control of autonomic nerves and this relaxes when the rectum is distended. The external sphincter is striated muscle controlled by pudendal nerves, and contracts as the internal sphincter relaxes and thereby continence is maintained. The fundamental defecation reflex is that stimulation of rectal stretch receptors excites pelvic afferent nerves and this results in efferent parasympathetic stimulation, which increases colonic and rectal motility and inhibits the internal sphincter. The external sphincter remains closed unless defecation is permitted to occur.

Defecation involves causing an increase in abdominal pressure, essentially by the Valsalva manoeuvre (see above). The longitudinal muscles of the rectum and distal colon contract and this has the effect of shortening and straightening the segments. The levator ani muscles pull the anal canal upwards and relaxation of the external sphincter allows the faeces to be expelled. Afferent impulses from the anal canal form the afferent pathway of a reflex which augments the colonic contractions. They also enable the distinction to be made between distension by flatus or by faeces.

Defecation may occur purely as a spinal reflex and functions as such in infants. Following spinal transection, defecation again becomes a spinal reflex.

INNERVATION OF THE URINARY SYSTEM

The kidney

Renal nerves are sympathetic postganglionic fibres originating mainly from segments T10–12 and relaying in the coeliac ganglion. Activity in renal nerves causes vasoconstriction in the kidney and enhances tubular sodium absorption. This is involved in the atrial receptor reflex where distension of atrial receptors selectively decreases renal nerve activity and thereby increases sodium excretion. It should be noted that the kidney functions quite adequately in the absence of a nerve supply (for example, transplanted kidneys). Autoregulation of renal blood flow is pronounced and is not dependent on its innervation.

Renal nerves also supply the juxtaglomerular apparatus. This apparatus includes the macula densa of the thick ascending limb, the extra-glomerular mesangial cells and the granular cells of the afferent and efferent arterioles. The granular cells form renin, secretion of which is stimulated when blood pressure falls in the afferent arteriole, when sodium chloride concentration falls, and when renal sympathetic nerves are stimulated. The neural mechanism involves β-adrenergic transmission. Renin results in the formation of angiotensin I, and consequently of angiotensin II and aldosterone, and thus promotes an increase in blood pressure and retention of sodium.

The bladder and urethra

Innervation

The bladder is supplied with sympathetic nerves originating in the first two lumbar segments. The fibres from each side converge to form a nerve in front of the sacrum, the presacral nerve. These divide to form the hypogastric nerves running to the hypogastric ganglia where they mingle with parasympathetic fibres originating from the pelvic nerves from the upper sacral segments. The internal sphincter of the bladder is supplied by autonomic nerves, whereas the urethra and external sphincter are innervated by the pudendal nerves, which are somatic. Activity in efferent sympathetic nerves results in relaxation of the detrusor muscles of the bladder and contraction of the internal sphincter. Activity in parasympathetic nerves relaxes the internal sphincter and contracts the detrusor.

Several neurotransmitters have been implicated in the control of the bladder. Bladder contraction is stimulated not only by cholinergic (muscarinic) receptors but also by purinergic and substance P-sensitive receptors. Bladder relaxation, in addition to β-adrenergic receptors in the body of the bladder, is stimulated by vasoactive intestinal peptide (VIP) receptors. In the sphincter region and urethra, purinergic, VIP and neuropeptide Y receptors have also been described; they are thought to modulate the effects of the classical neurotransmitters.

Bladder reflexes and micturition

The sensory input from the bladder is mediated through both divisions of the autonomic system. Both small myelinated and non-myelinated nerves run in the pelvic nerves to the spinal cord. Pelvic afferents are most important for bladder control, although afferents in the sympathetic system are mainly responsible for the pain sensations that occur with overdistension or inflammation. Both passive distension and active bladder contractions result in afferent discharge in nerves from the bladder. The threshold for discharge is about 10 mmHg and it is at about this level that humans start to become aware of bladder distension. As the bladder becomes more filled, periodic reflex contractions occur and these increase the desire to micturate. The bladder can accommodate quite large volumes of fluid before pressure increases steeply. This is partly due to a reflex that increases sympathetic efferent discharge.

Micturition is a complex process involving afferent and efferent autonomic nerves as well as somatic nerves (Fig. 22.11). It is normally partly inhibited by control from higher centres, which maintains contraction of the external sphincter and inhibits the micturition reflex. Also, during moderate bladder filling, afferent pelvic nerve fibres are stimulated, increasing the sympathetic discharge to the bladder base as well as contracting the external sphincter and inhibiting the parasympathetic motor activity. When the bladder pressure reaches a critical level the micturition reflex may be initiated. The micturition response involves reflex contraction of the detrusor muscle and relaxation of the bladder neck and sphincters. Urine flowing through the urethra elicits another reflex which enhances the parasympathetic outflow and ensures that the bladder is completely voided. In addition to reflex contraction of the bladder, expulsion of urine may also be aided by increases in intrabdominal pressure effected by the Valsalva manoeuvre.

The major pathways in the micturition reflex involve parasympathetic nerves. Sympathetic supply is not essential, although, because sympathetic activity causes bladder relaxation, sympathetic denervation is associated with smaller bladder volumes and increased frequency of micturition. If the spinal cord is transected, voluntary control is lost. Initially detrusor muscle tone disappears but sphincter tone soon returns and acute retention of urine is an early problem. If the patient is catheterised to avoid bladder damage and infection, the micturition reflex becomes re-established as a simple spinal reflex

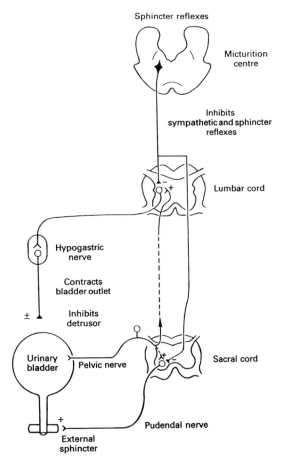

Figure 22.11 Reflex control of bladder. During storage phase, low level of afferent activity in pelvic nerves stimulates sympathetic efferent discharge (relaxes bladder wall muscle, contracts neck muscle) and stimulates pudendal nerve discharge to external sphincter. Micturition is initiated by central descending discharge which inhibits the storage reflexes and excites parasympathetic activity (not shown). (Reproduced with permission from de Groat W C 1992 Neural control of the urinary bladder and sexual organs. In: Bannister and Mathias, Autonomic Failure)

response. Spontaneous evacuation may occur when bladder pressure increases to a critical level. The patient may be able to initiate this response before the critical level of bladder distension is reached by procedures such as increasing intra-abdominal pressure or stroking the region of the urethral orifice.

FURTHER READING

Bannister R, Mathias C J 1992 Autonomic failure. A textbook of clinical disorders of the autonomic nervous system. Oxford University Press, Oxford.

Eckberg D L, Sleight P 1993 Human baroreflexes in health and disease. Oxford Medical Publications, Oxford.

Hainsworth R 1990 The importance of vascular capacitance in cardiovascular control. News in Physiological Sciences 5: 250–254

Hainsworth R 1991 Reflexes from the heart. Physiological Reviews 71: 617–658

Hainsworth R, Mark A L 1993 Cardiovascular reflex control in health and disease. Saunders, London

Zucker I H, Gilmore J P 1991 Reflex control of the circulation. CRC Press, Boca Raton

Cardiovascular system

SECTION CONTENTS

23

Physiology of the heart

J. D. Allen

CELLULAR BASIS OF CARDIAC FUNCTION

The functions of the heart express the special features of the different cell types of which it is comprised. The primate heart differs in myocardial structure and coronary circulation from that of most other animals, and these differences are a major factor limiting the application of experimental studies to clinical practice.

The branching cells are separated from each other by *intercalated discs*, where there are specialised connections to link adjacent cells. Mechanical links are provided by the desmosomes, where fibrillar connections bridge the gaps between cells, and the membrane is apparently reinforced. Adjacent gap junctions (or nexuses) give low resistance electrical connections to join the cells in a functional syncytium. Protein channels (connexons), with a central pore size of 2 nm, have been identified at these points. These electrical couplings enable the remarkable spread of activity from the sinoatrial node to the last cells activated, near the pulmonary conus.

Striated myofibrils occupy about half of the cell volume. The orderly arrangement of actin and myosin fibrillar proteins in the *sarcomeres* (length 1.5–2.5 μm) is similar but not identical to that in skeletal muscle. Action potentials at the outside membrane of the cylindrical cells activate the myofibrils by a system of t or transverse tubules, invaginations of the cell membrane which are located at the Z lines (or end) of the sarcomeres. The contiguous *sarcoplasmic reticulum* then releases calcium into the sarcoplasm to initiate contraction. Termination of contraction follows the reaccumulation of calcium ions in the sarcoplasmic reticulum. The calcium concentration inside the cell fluctuates from 10^{-7} M or less at rest, to 5×10^{-6} M or more during contraction. The variation in strength of contraction is due to modulation of the intracellular calcium concentration and the responsiveness of the myofibrils to it.

Between the myofibrils lie many mitochondria, some 35% of cell volume, providing adenosine triphosphate (ATP) for contraction. The capillary network is extensive, with an overall ratio of one capillary per cell. Since there is no possibility of a rest in cardiac activity to repay an extensive oxygen debt, the supply of oxygenated blood must be continuous, and is capable of major increases as cardiac output or work rises by fivefold or more on exercise.

Electrical activity

The myocardium is an excitable tissue, and shares many properties with other excitable tissues, nerve and skeletal muscle. In general, the resting membrane potential of cardiac muscle has a similar basis to that of skeletal muscle. Cardiac cells contain many large non-diffusible anions, proteins and phosphates. Hence there are few diffusible anions (Cl^-, HCO_3^-) in the sarcoplasm. The concentration of K^+ ions in the cell (some 150 mM) is high with respect to the extracellular concentration (some 5 mM). Thus these freely diffusible cations will tend to leave the cell, causing an accumulation of negative charges (unbalanced, non-diffusible anions) in the cell. If this process proceeded to equilibrium, at a certain electrical potential within the cell (E_K) the tendency of K^+ to diffuse out along its concentration gradient ($RT \times \log_e [K^+]_o / [K^+]_i$, where $[K^+]_o$ is the concentration of K^+ outside the cell and $[K^+]_i$ is the concentration inside the cell; R is the gas constant; T is the absolute temperature) would be balanced by the negative charge accumulated by the loss of the same amount of K^+ from the cell (zF per mole of the ion; where z is the valency of the ion and F is the Faraday,

or electrical charge per electron lost from 1 mole of the cation). This is the basis of the Nernst equation:

$$E_K = (RT/zF) \log_e ([K^+]_o / [K^+]_i) = 61.5 \log_{10} (5/150)$$
$$= -90.8 \text{ mV at } 37°C.$$

The figure found for E_K is very close to the actual resting membrane potential of the atrial and ventricular muscle and the specialised conducting tissue. The small pacemaker and nodal cells of the sinoatrial node and atrioventricular node show lower resting potentials, indicating that the situation is more complex in those tissues.

The negative resting potential of the cardiac cells would soon be lost, but for two additional factors. Firstly, the permeability of the resting membrane to Na^+ ions is low, so that the inward diffusion of sodium is restricted. Secondly, when Na^+ ions enter they are extruded by the sodium-potassium pump. This keeps the internal concentration of Na^+ low. The pump also contributes slightly to the resting membrane potential, since it extrudes 3 Na^+ ions for each 2 K^+ ions pumped into the cell. This unbalanced movement of positively charged ions by the pump is the basis for its *electrogenic* behaviour. By preventing the accumulation of Na^+ in the cell the pump also maintains the osmotic balance across the cell membrane, and prevents the accumulation of water which would make the cell swell.

The excitable nature of cardiac cells is due to the fast Na^+ channels (protein structures) in the sarcolemma. As in nerve and skeletal muscle these channels open when the cell is depolarised to a threshold voltage (some –70 mV). The opening of some channels, and the rapid influx of positive current, depolarises the cell further, so opening more fast Na^+ channels in a rapid spike of depolarisation, the *all-or-none response*, which ends in 1–2 ms when the fast Na^+ channels close again. The upstroke of the action potential is so brief that relatively few ions enter the cell. Rather like the many bright flashes from the battery of an electronic flashgun, the cell can produce many large action potentials of some 120–130 mV before the cellular battery becomes discharged.

If the Na^+ channels remained open for longer, the influx of sodium ions from the extracellular space (some 145 mM) into the cell (some 14.5 mM) could proceed to an equilibrium potential (E_{Na}) at which the tendency of Na$^+$ to enter the cell, due to the high extracellular concentration [Na$^+$]$_o$, is balanced by the positive potential inside the cell repelling the entry of Na$^+$. This can be evaluated by the Nernst equation for Na$^+$ ions:

$$E_{Na} = (RT/zF) \log_e ([Na^+]_o/[Na^+]_i)$$
$$= 61.5 \log (145/14.5)$$
$$= +61.5 \text{ mV at } 37°C.$$

Since this equilibrium potential (+61 mV) is not achieved, the influx of Na$^+$ does not reach equilibrium. The fast Na$^+$ channels close before the equilibrium is achieved, and hence the cell is depolarised to only +30 to +40 mV. The initial fast phase of depolarisation (phase 0) and the decline in potential after the spike (phase 1) are due to the opening and closing of these fast Na$^+$ channels (Figure 23.1). An influx of Cl$^-$ ions may occur at this time, into the positively charged cell.

The prolonged plateau (phase 2), so characteristic of the cardiac action potential, is due to the influx of calcium ions through slow inward channels. These voltage-dependent Ca^{2+} channels open at −40 mV, at a higher potential than that needed to open the fast Na$^+$ channels, and stay open for much longer (100–200 ms) — the L-type (long lasting) channels. The slow inward drift of positive current keeps the cell depolarised to near 0 mV. This influx of Ca^{2+} ions never reaches the equilibrium potential for Ca^{2+}, theoretically greater than +150 mV as the ratio of Ca$_o$:Ca$_i$ is more than 300. Modulation of this slow inward current by autonomic nerves is important in the regulation of cardiac function. Sympathetic agonists increase the inward current in all heart muscle cells, emphasising the plateau of the action potential and increasing contractile force. Acetylcholine reduces the influx of Ca^{2+} in atrial and nodal tissues, and reduces the force of atrial contraction.

Repolarisation to resting membrane potential (phase 3) is caused by the closure of the slow inward current channels, and the opening of specific K$^+$ channels leading to the outward K$^+$ current. Since the inside of the cell membrane is less negative, there is less charge to hold the

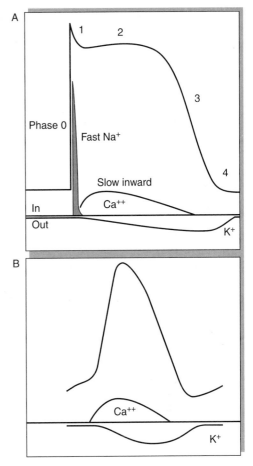

Figure 23.1   Action potentials from (A) cardiac muscle and (B) sinus node cells. In A: rapid depolarisation (phase 0) is due to the entry of Na$^+$ ions through the voltage dependent (fast) channels for 1–2 ms. Early repolarisation follows closure of these Na$^+$ channels (phase 1), and is delayed by the prolonged opening of voltage dependent (slow, L-type) Ca^{2+} channels to give the plateau of the action potential (phase 2). Later K$^+$ channels open with outward ion flow (phase 2–3). In B: the smaller, rounded action potential is initiated by the pacemaker current, running smoothly into the upstroke of the action potential. The low membrane potential of the cell inactivates fast Na$^+$ channels, so that the main currents are the slow inward Ca^{2+} and the outward K$^+$ currents.

K$^+$ ions, and they leave through these voltage dependent K$^+$ channels.

In non-pacemaker tissues the period between the action potentials (phase 4) is characterised by little change in membrane potential. However, as a result of these varied ion fluxes the cell has gained Na$^+$ and Ca^{2+}, and lost K$^+$. Since the heart must keep beating throughout life, the cells have developed complex mechanisms to restore ionic balance. Na^+ is extruded and K^+ pumped into the cell by the sodium-potassium pump. These pumps do not stop during the action potential. However, their small capacity is swamped by the large and rapid changes in membrane conductance during the action potential.

It is essential to maintain low concentrations of Ca^{2+} in the cell, as muscle relaxation depends on low concentrations of Ca^{2+}. Large concentrations of this ion are toxic and cause cell death. Hence Ca^{2+} is extruded by the Na^+-Ca^{2+} exchanger. The inward diffusion of 3 Na^+ ions along their concentration gradient is used to pump out 1 Ca^{2+} ion. The Na^+ ions are then extruded by the sodium-potassium pump, which pumps more Na^+ out than K^+ in, and maintains the ionic gradient for Na^+-Ca^{2+} exchange. This is a good example of secondary active transport, i.e. the expenditure of energy on the active pumping of Na^+ provides a source of potential energy which is used for the extrusion of Ca^{2+}. This Na^+-Ca^{2+} exchanger has a high capacity, and can prevent the excessive accumulation of Ca^{2+} at heart rates over 200 per minute. The effectiveness of the exchanger is less when the intracellular $[Na^+]$ is high. This may be the basis of the therapeutic effects of the digitalis glycosides, which block the Na^+-K^+ pump and raise intracellular $[Na^+]$: the subsequent intracellular accumulation of Ca^{2+} increases the force of cardiac contraction. As an exchanger this mechanism can work equally well in either direction. Reversal would bring Ca^{2+} into the cell and extrude Na^+ when intracellular Na^+ is high.

Atrial and ventricular myocardium

The branched cylindrical muscle cells of the atrium and ventricle are linked at the intercalated discs. The low resistance gap junctions allow the easy movement of K^+ ions from cell to cell, providing an internal path for ionic currents.

When action potentials leave the sinoatrial node they do so by cell to-cell conduction. The local depolarisation of the action potential causes depolarisation of the adjacent cell by currents in the intracellular pathway. At the site of the action potential the inside of the cell is less negatively (or more positively) charged than the interior of the adjacent cell. Hence positively charged K^+ ions will flow forward to the more negative non-active area, through the gap junctions. Large non-diffusible anions cannot move easily. Outside the cell the polarised, non-active cell membrane is more positively charged than the area of active membrane at the action potential. Hence return currents will occur in the extracellular space. The adjacent cell will be depolarised and brought to threshold, to fire off an action potential and conduct the excitation.

Due to the efficiency of the gap junctions in the intercalated discs this process is comparable to the spread of the action potential along an unmyelinated nerve fibre (see Ch. 6). These cell-to-cell connections are not fixed structures. Under certain conditions (low extracellular Ca^{2+}, or the intracellular accumulation of Ca^{2+}) the gap junctions may disconnect and the myocardium fails to conduct from cell to cell.

The long action potential duration and refractory period of normal cardiac muscle prevents previously activated muscle from being re-excited by the randomly spreading wavefronts as the myocardium is excited.

Sinoatrial node

The nodal tissues of the heart are specialised in both appearance and function with respect to the ordinary atrial and ventricular muscle. The cells of the sinus node are small, with few myofibrils. Cell-to-cell connections are poor, and the maximum resting membrane potential is low (-50 to -60 mV). Transitional cells are seen between the pacemaker cells and the ordinary atrial myocardium. The sinus node is the dominant pacemaker of the normal heart. Not only does it beat faster than possible lower sites but, under the influence of autonomic nerves, it has the widest range of possible rates (normally around 50–200 per minute). Lower pacemakers tend to have a slower intrinsic rate of firing, and also are suppressed by being driven at a faster rate (overdrive suppression).

The Ca^{2+} dependent *action potentials* of the sinoatrial node are due not to the opening of fast Na^+ channels, but to the slower opening of the transient T-type and long-lasting L-type inward Ca^{2+} channels (Figure 23.1). Hence sinoatrial rate is more sensitive to a drug which blocks these slow inward L-channels (e.g. verapamil; Ch. 24) than to a drug which blocks fast Na^+ channels, such as lignocaine.

However, the cardiac rhythm is caused by the spontaneous, gradual depolarisation of the *pacemaker potential*, which follows each action potential (Figure 23.2). When the membrane potential reaches threshold level (–40 to –50 mV) a new action potential is produced, and the cycle is repeated. The ionic basis of the pacemaker potential remains controversial. Since the contribution of anions can be ignored, either the cells are losing fewer positive ions or gaining additional positive ions. Hence possibilities include a gradual reduction in the out flow of K^+ ions, or an inward leakage of Na^+ ions (I_f or 'funny' current) or Ca^{2+} ions (I_t or T 'transient' Ca^{2+} channels).

The heart rate is slowed by vagal nerve activity, as acetylcholine increases the permeability of the cell membrane to potassium ions; more K^+ ions leave the cell, which is then more negative. Acetylcholine also reduces influx of Ca^{2+} ions. The threshold does not change but the slope of the pacemaker potential is reduced. The second messenger appears to be an increase in cyclic GMP (guanosine monophosphate) in the pacemaker cells.

Conversely noradrenaline, adrenaline and other β-adrenoceptor agonists increase heart rate, increasing both cyclic adenosine monophosphate (cAMP) and the slope of the pacemaker potential. The pancreatic hormone glucagon binds to different receptors to increase cAMP and heart rate.

Autonomic nerves provide the effector mechanism for the changes in heart rate due to diverse reflexes, such as the Valsalva manoeuvre, the Bezold–Jarisch reflex and raised intracranial pressure; however the dominant factor on a minute-to-minute basis is the baroreceptor reflex.

Heart rate can also be altered by the direct effects of myocardial temperature on the slope of the pacemaker potential. Myocardial cooling (hypothermic perfusion or whole body hypothermia) reduces heart rate. In fever the rate is faster by some 10 beats per minute per °C of pyrexia.

Atrioventricular node

The atrioventricular (AV) node lies in the right atrium between the coronary sinus and the fibrous valve ring of the tricuspid valve. Again the cells are small, with few myofibrils. The slow conduction through this area is due to the small size of the cells, the low resting membrane potential and the scarcity of cell-to-cell connections (gap junctions). These combine to slow the speed of conduction from 1 m s^{-1} in the atria to some 0.1 m s^{-1}. The delay in conduction permits the ventricles to fill with blood from the atrial contraction before the ventricular contraction is activated. The other feature of this tissue is the prolonged refractory period which follows, and lasts beyond the duration of each action potential. The action potential in this tissue, as in the sinus node, is dependent on slow inward calcium current, and not fast sodium channels. Thus AV conduction is especially sensitive to blockade with verapamil and other drugs that block voltage sensitive Ca^{2+} channels in the myocardium.

The autonomic nerves in this tissue serve to adjust the timing of ventricular contraction after

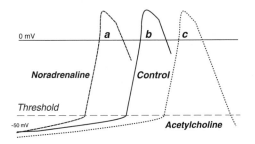

Figure 23.2 Pacemaker potentials (from –50 mV) give rise to action potentials in sinoatrial node cells when depolarisation reaches threshold potential, as in the control action potential (b). Sympathetic stimulation (a) increases the slope of the pacemaker potential and heart rate. Acetylcholine (c) increases the negativity of the membrane potential and decreases the slope of the pacemaker potential to slow heart rate.

atrial contraction. Vagal activity slows conduction in the atrioventricular node and prolongs the PR interval of the ECG. Sympathetic activity, as in exercise, speeds conduction in the node and shortens the PR interval.

The long refractory period of the AV node protects the ventricle from rapid atrial firing rates which could disrupt ventricular pump function. The vagus prolongs the refractory period, while the sympathetic nerves shorten the refractory period. Hence in a rapid atrial arrhythmia the proportion of atrial beats conducted to the ventricles can fall due to vagal activity, or rise due to sympathetic activity, and seriously compromise cardiac output.

While the AV node can also conduct in a retrograde direction, from ventricle to atrium, its long refractory period tends to prevent this from occurring. An expectation that true nodal tissue should show pacemaker activity has not always been confirmed. Adjacent cells in the atrium are often the site of origin of nodal rhythm and coronary sinus rhythm. The principal function of the AV node is to provide an appropriate delay between atrial and ventricular contraction.

Conducting tissue

From the AV node the action potentials pass down the bundle of His, bundle branches, and Purkinje fibre network at some 2 m s^{-1} — faster than some small unmyelinated nerves. Once the action potentials have entered ventricular muscle the conduction velocity falls to 0.5 m s^{-1}, as the excitation front moves transversely across the myocardial cells to excite the thick wall of the ventricles.

The Purkinje cells are specialised for rapid conduction of action potentials, with a large diameter, scanty myofibrils, many gap junctions in the intercalated discs, a resting membrane potential of −90 mV, and tall action potentials (to +30–40 mV). The long action potential duration and long refractory period in these cells close to the ventricular muscle act as a one-way gate, preventing normal electrical activity in ventricular muscle from regaining entry to the conducting system. The U wave sometimes seen in the ECG may represent the delayed repolarisation of these Purkinje fibres, after repolarisation of the bulk of ventricular muscle (T wave).

Myocardial contraction

Contraction of the myocardial cell is initiated by the action potential at its surface. The transverse or t tubules provide a route from the cell surface throughout the cytoplasm of the cell. The calcium-containing cisterns of the sarcoplasmic reticulum lie adjacent to this tubular network. It is attractive to think of the action potential being conducted into the heart of the cell by the t tubules, but their narrow diameter causes such a high electrical resistance that this simple concept is unlikely to be true. The exact nature of the link between the action potential and the release of Ca^{2+} from the sarcoplasmic reticulum (excitation–contraction coupling) is not clear. However, there is good evidence that the entry of Ca^{2+} ions into the cell during the action potential — *activator calcium* — initiates the release of more Ca^{2+} from the sarcoplasmic reticulum. It is the rise in intracellular Ca^{2+} concentration from 10^{-7} M or less in the relaxed state, to 5–10 × 10^{-6} M that causes contraction. Calcium antagonist drugs, such as verapamil, and other agents, including fluothane, can reduce this influx of activator Ca^{2+}.

The termination of myocardial contraction and the diastolic relaxation of the muscle cell are due to the return of Ca^{2+} into the sarcoplasmic reticulum, caused by the Ca^{2+}-ATPase of the reticulum membrane. This membrane pump binds Ca^{2+} and ATP and moves the Ca^{2+} into the lumen of the sarcoplasmic reticulum. While additional amounts of Ca^{2+} can be stored in the mitochondria and other sites within the cell, these are relatively unimportant in heart muscle. Cellular overload of Ca^{2+} can occur with severe hypercalcaemia; with no relaxation the heart arrests in a sustained contracture.

As in smooth muscle the strength of contraction varies from minute to minute in cardiac muscle. This variability depends on two factors: firstly, the final concentration of Ca^{2+} in the cell; and, secondly, the responsiveness of the contractile proteins to this Ca^{2+}. Variable contractile force is not seen in skeletal muscle, as the sarcoplasmic reticulum contains adequate stores of Ca^{2+} for maximal contraction, and the action potential is brief. Changes in the activity of the channels releasing Ca^{2+} from the sarcoplasmic reticulum and of the Ca^{2+}-ATPase pump give two major mechanisms for alterations in systolic or diastolic performance with changes in the physiological, pathological and pharmacological environment of the cardiac cell.

Ca^{2+} binds to the myofilament protein, troponin C, to initiate contraction, as in skeletal muscle (see Ch. 19). The resultant sliding of the actin and myosin filaments is energised by the splitting of ATP by the myosin ATPase. As a muscle the dark red, myoglobin-containing myocardium behaves like the slow postural muscles, with low ATPase activity.

The individual sarcomeres of the cell shorten simultaneously to approximate the intercalated discs at each end of the cell, and thus reduce the length of the cell. Force production depends not just on intracellular Ca^{2+} concentration, but also on the initial, resting length of the fibre before the muscle contracts. Careful studies have been made of the force of contraction produced at different resting sarcomere lengths, when the contracting muscle is not allowed to shorten but remains *isometric*. With stretching of the resting cell the force generated rises to a plateau (Figure 23.3A). Further stretch results in a decline in the force of contraction. The optimum force production occurs at sarcomere lengths of some 2.2 µm, and must represent an optimum initial overlap of the actin (length some 1 µm) and myosin (length 1.5 µm) myofilaments. These in vitro studies have established a cellular basis for Starling's law of the heart. However, the heart normally operates at sarcomere lengths close to the optimum for force generation. Despite these changes in initial muscle length or *preload*, the peak force is developed at a similar time after the start of the contraction.

Additional insights into force production come from studies of the relation between the load on the muscle and the velocity of contraction in muscle preparations which shorten, but remain under the same load throughout — *isotonic*. As

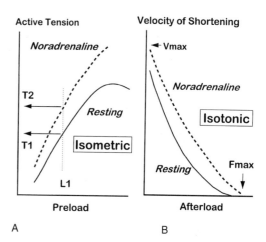

Figure 23.3 Force of contraction is shown under two conditions, before and after noradrenaline. In (A) the resting length of the muscle before contraction is varied (the end-diastolic length, or preload, abscissa) and the muscle is not allowed to shorten, but contracts internally to generate tension which is measured — an isometric contraction. For the same initial length of muscle (L1), sympathetic stimulation increases the contractile force produced (contractility). In (B) the muscle is allowed to shorten to lift a fixed load (the afterload), and the velocity of contraction is measured — an isotonic contraction. Sympathetic stimulation increases both the maximum velocity of contraction (Vmax) and the maximum force of contraction (Fmax).

may be expected, the bigger the load or force to be generated, the more slowly the muscle contracts (Figure 23.3B). The maximum velocity of contraction occurs at the theoretical point of zero load, or complete unloading of the muscle. Hence the cross-bridges between actin and myosin filaments break and reform at maximum velocity when the load on the filaments is least. Maximum force develops with minimal breakage of actin–myosin cross-bridges. Sympathetic stimulation and positive inotropic agents increase both the maximum velocity of contraction and the maximum force produced by the muscle.

However, these simple muscle preparations are only of limited help in understanding the complex events of contraction in the intact ventricle. The initial build-up of pressure in the ventricles is isometric, but after the aortic or pulmonary valve opens the muscle shortens to eject blood and generate the peak systolic pressure in a near-isotonic state.

The actions of autonomic neurotransmitters on muscle contraction have been studied in isolated preparations. Acetylcholine reduces force production in atrial tissues only. As cyclic GMP increases in the cell, the influx of Ca^{2+} in the action potential is reduced, with a loss of plateau of the action potential, and peak force declines. Noradrenaline increases the influx of Ca^{2+} through slow inward channels, and the plateau becomes more positive in both atrial and ventricular muscle. The speed of muscle contraction increases, with a higher peak tension and quicker relaxation, indicating widespread effects in the cell.

Other regulatory hormones and paracrine substances can modulate the force of myocardial contraction. In health, nitric oxide (NO; endothelial derived relaxing factor or EDRF) is formed mainly in the endothelial cells of the coronary circulation. However, in disease (septic or endotoxic shock; cardiomyopathy), NO is produced in the myocardial cells by inducible NO synthase enzymes, and causes weaker contraction. In contrast endothelial derived endothelin increases the force of contraction of cardiac muscle and constricts vascular smooth muscle. Pharmacological doses of glucagon can increase the force of contraction as well as heart rate.

Thyroid hormones can alter the contractility of the heart in a number of ways. Sympathetic activity may be facilitated by an increase in response to β-adrenoceptor agonists. Contractile proteins are also altered, as excess thyroid hormones increase the proportion of the α form of myosin heavy chain, which has more ATPase activity. The activity of Ca^{2+}-ATPase in the sarcoplasmic reticulum is also increased. Hence tension is developed more quickly, and the durtion of contraction is shorter as the sarcoplasmic reticulum reaccumulates Ca^{2+} faster. Conversely in hypothyroidism the β form of myosin heavy chain is predominant, and contraction is slower.

Cardiac metabolism

The oxygen consumption of the heart is largely determined by heart rate and left ventricular systolic pressure (peak wall tension). The myocardium relies on oxidative metabolism to provide the energy for contraction. Within a few minutes of occlusion of a local artery the unperfused muscle has stopped contracting and shows paradoxical movement (bulging) with each heart beat. While the muscle is rich in myoglobin, giving the dark red colour of the heart, the oxygen released from it is inadequate for any prolonged period of anoxia. The production of ATP is closely matched to the oxygen consumption of the heart.

The main substrates for normal metabolism are the free fatty acids, glucose and lactate. Glucose enters the myocardial cell through an insulin controlled transporter, to be metabolised or stored as glycogen granules. Hence it tends to be used more after a recent meal. Complete aerobic oxidation gives 38 bonds of ATP. Anaerobic glycolysis to lactic acid results in only about 5% of this energy production:

glucose + 2 ATP → 2 lactic acid + 4 ATP — a gain of 2 ATP molecules *Anaerobic*
glucose + 2 ATP + 6 O_2 → 6 CO_2 + 6 H_2O + 40 ATP — a gain of 38 ATP *Aerobic*.

Free fatty acids provide a readily accessible source of energy in the presence of adequate oxygenation and intracellular glucose, as after a fat meal or when fasting. Blood levels remain fairly constant except in prolonged fasting, when they rise. The citric acid cycle of the mitochondria couples the orderly metabolism of these substrates to ATP production. In the absence of adequate oxygen the cell relies more on glucose than free fatty acids as a substrate for metabolism. There is some evidence that high concentrations of free fatty acids are toxic to the ischaemic heart, causing cardiac arrhythmias and myocardial depression.

The metabolism of the heart may be considered as 'pay as you go'. There is no oxygen debt in the normal heart in exercise. The normal heart removes available lactate from the coronary blood, converts it to pyruvate, and metabolises it to carbon dioxide and water. Low blood levels of lactate at rest (< 1 mM) limit its use as substrate. However, in exercise lactate is available at higher concentration (e.g. 5 mM in moderate exercise; 10 mM in severe exercise). Lactate production by the heart itself, with a higher lactate concentration in the coronary sinus (venous) blood than in the arterial blood, is the definitive indicator of myocardial ischaemia, usually due to narrowed coronary arteries. Occasionally such lactate production can occur in the presence of apparently normal coronary arteries (syndrome X).

The entry of amino acids to the cardiac cells is stimulated by insulin. Protein synthesis is required throughout life for growth of the heart and replacement of old protein. A physiological increase in muscle mass can follow high levels of athletic achievement (athlete's heart). Pathological hypertrophy results from increased cardiac work (pressure or volume load) or the effects of hormones (acromegaly). While the effects of growth hormone are presumably similar to those in other organs, the exact signal stimulating hypertrophy in response to increased work load (wall tension) is not known. Breakdown of myocardial proteins is relatively suppressed in the presence of prolonged malnutrition. Severe thyrotoxicosis can cause cardiomyopathy.

The regulation of coronary blood flow further emphasises the important role of a maintained oxygen supply for myocardial function. Oxygen lack and accumulated myocardial metabolites (such as adenosine and carbon dioxide) have a dominant role in dilating small arterioles and precapillary sphincters to increase coronary blood flow. The coronary flow and oxygen supply are adjusted to fulfil the demands of myocardial metabolism on a minute to minute basis. In circumstances where the flow is restricted (arterial stenosis) or oxygen carriage is reduced (anaemia), ischaemic anginal pain can develop. During a prolonged period of myocardial hypoxia (anaemia, life at high altitude) more and larger anastomotic vessels develop in the coronary bed.

Ischaemic myocardium

With the sudden cessation of coronary arterial flow, in either the heart as a whole, or in the territory of a local branch artery (ischaemic heart disease), the stores of oxygen, glycogen and high energy phosphates are rapidly exhausted in the affected muscle. Contraction stops, and H^+ ions

and compounds of adenosine accumulate. This rise in H^+ and loss of high energy phosphates can now be monitored by nuclear magnetic resonance cardiography (MRI, magnetic resonance imaging), elegantly confirming earlier biochemical analyses of biopsied tissue. The Na^+-K^+ pump no longer functions efficiently, and K^+ accumulates in the narrow clefts between the myocardial cells. The duration of the action potential shortens, and the ischaemic tissue repolarises before the adjacent normal muscle. Between QRS complexes, the loss of resting membrane potential in the ischaemic zone causes current to flow between it and the adjacent resting muscle, which is more polarised. This current flow is recognised as ST elevation in the ECG, although it really represents depression of the baseline of the ECG between the T wave and the next QRS complex. Normally there is sufficient ATP in the myocardium to block specific ATP-sensitive K^+ channels in the muscle cells. The reduction in ATP concentration in the ischaemic muscle allows these ATP-sensitive K^+ channels to open, contributing to the shortening of the duration of the action potential and helping to maintain resting membrane potential in the damaged tissue. Cardiac action potentials are conducted slowly in the acutely ischaemic tissue. Soon areas develop where conduction is blocked. With the fragmented and irregular spread of the electrical activity in the ischaemic zone and the shortening of the action potential, adjacent muscle is reactivated to cause ventricular arrhythmias — *re-entrant* arrhythmias. With injury of myocardial cells *abnormal pacemaker activity* can develop, particularly on the endocardial surface of ventricular aneurysms, and act as a source of recurrent ventricular arrhythmias.

These ventricular arrhythmias and ectopic beats can deteriorate to ventricular fibrillation. The absence of a cardiac output, due to the uncoordinated myofibrillar contractions, can be corrected by internal or transthoracic electrical direct current (DC) countershock. Large shocks across the chest (some 2000–3000 V as 300 J stored energy) terminate electrical activity in the heart by depolarising and hyperpolarising cells, and prolonging the refractory period. In the electrical silence which follows the shock, the sinus node should succeed in capturing the heart. Because of the interposition of the skin, chest wall and lungs, only a small fraction of the total transthoracic current (30–40 A) passes through the heart, perhaps 5%. Internal shocks of some 20–40 J by transcardiac paddles or an implanted internal defibrillator are equally effective. While it is not necessary to defibrillate all of the heart, the arrhythmia can be re-established if a small fraction receives an inadequate distribution of the shock energy.

Simple uncomplicated ventricular fibrillation responds well to such shocks. However, patients who require multiple shocks for recurrent arrhythmias have a poor rate for successful resuscitation. While there is experimental evidence that multiple or very large shocks can cause obvious myocardial injury, with cell death, there is little clinical evidence of such gross effects.

The mechanism of contractile failure in acutely ischaemic muscle is not fully understood. The fall in creatine phosphate, and accumulation of inorganic phosphate and H^+ (lactate and carbon dioxide) may contribute to the decreased responsiveness of the contractile myofilaments to Ca^{2+} seen after 5 minutes of ischaemia. In the sarcoplasmic reticulum the Ca^{2+}-ATPase shows decreased uptake of Ca^{2+}, after 10 or more minutes of ischaemia, and the gradual accumulation of free Ca^{2+} in the cell causes sustained contracture and contributes to cell injury.

The duration of complete ischaemia determines the effects on the cells. Irreversible contractile failure and cell death occur after long periods of ischaemia (> 15–20 minutes). Myocardium reperfused after less than 15 minutes of ischaemia can survive, but may show delayed restoration of contractile function over the next 1–7 days — *stunned* myocardium. Recently it has been shown that brief periods of ischaemia (more than 2 minutes) can protect the myocardium from lethal injury caused by further ischaemia in the next hour or so — *preconditioning* of the myocardium. These phenomena may occur in the acutely ischaemic heart when the coronary circulation resumes after occlusion (e.g. after thrombolysis). While their bases and clinical importance are not clear, study of these phenomena may lead to improved treatment of ischaemic myocardium.

Cardioplegia and myocardial protection

During unmodified cardiopulmonary bypass the heart is usually ischaemic and may be fibrillating. On cessation of bypass, attempts to restart the normal cardiac pumping action may be unsuccessful owing to a number of factors. The heart may have deteriorated during the period of warm ischaemia. While removal of Ca^{2+} from the myocardial circulation seems a logical way to reduce contraction, it is particularly injurious because the return of normal Ca^{2+} to the heart may cause a sustained contracture — 'stone heart'. Cardiac injury may also be caused by the readmission of oxygenated blood to the coronary tree — reperfusion injury. This may be related to the generation of highly reactive free radical species which damage cardiac cells.

To prevent these problems cardioplegic solutions are infused through the coronary arterial tree, at a temperature of 26–28°C after cross-clamping of the aorta, and additional amounts may be given intra-arterially or topically to the heart. There is good experimental, electron microscopic and clinical evidence that their use has reduced problems after cardiopulmonary bypass. Initial efforts to protect the myocardium resulted in the development of ionic solutions such as the St Thomas's cardioplegic solutions, with normal total osmolality and high K^+ (16–20 mM) to depolarise the cardiac cells. High Mg^{2+} concentrations (16 mM) oppose the actions of Ca^{2+} (1.2 mM) and maintain diastole. More recent developments include the addition of energy sources (ATP, creatine phosphate) and putative myocardial protectants, or the use of blood cardioplegia.

Similar problems are faced in preserving a donor heart for transport to a distant hospital for subsequent transplantation. The cold ionic cardioplegic solution is perfused through the coronary arterial system via the aortic root, and the myocardium is immersed in additional cold solution at 4°C. Viability can be maintained for 4–5 hours.

PUMPING FUNCTION OF THE HEART

Cardiac cycle

The function of the cardiac pump, as of any pump, is critically dependent on the orderly and adequate filling and emptying of its chambers. The flow of blood through the heart proceeds from areas of high pressure to those of lower pressure. Valves open and close, depending on the pressure gradient across them. During contraction the cardiac muscle of both atria and ventricles shortens towards the rigid fibrous skeleton of the heart, where lie the four valves. The fibrous chordae tendineae of the closed mitral valve provide additional anchorage for the contracting left ventricle as the mitral valve descends towards the apex.

The atria act as distensible collecting chambers. When the pressure in the right and left ventricles is lower than that in the corresponding atrium the AV valve opens. Most (some 70%) of the blood filling the ventricles during diastole is carried across the tricuspid and mitral valves by the elasticity of the distended atria. The *third heart sound* is caused early in this period of passive filling of the heart by rapid stretch of the healthy ventricle behind a youthful chest wall, or of the less compliant, failing ventricle in the elderly. The increase in pressure with contraction of the atria finally stretches the ventricles before systole begins. In cardiac disease this atrial ejection of blood may be more prominent, and sudden tensing of the ventricles is heard as the *fourth heart sound.*

With ventricular systole a rapid increase in intraventricular pressure is initiated by contraction spreading from the apex of the heart up towards the pulmonary and aortic valves. The atrioventricular valves shut as the ventricular pressure exceeds the low atrial pressure (*first heart sound*). At slow heart rates the cessation in blood flow from the atria may allow the leaflets to drift into the closed position before systole develops. Isometric contraction builds up the pressure in the ventricles to open the pulmonary and aortic valves. Once the semilunar valves have opened, blood flows out into the pulmonary artery and aorta and pressure rises to a systolic peak.

With the end of ventricular contraction blood continues to flow out under inertia acquired from the rapid contraction of healthy ventricles. However, the rapid relaxation of the myocardium results in a drop in intraventricular pressure, and the flow in the pulmonary artery and aorta reverses to catch and close the light cusps of the semilunar valves. The high frequency of the *second heart sound* is due to the higher pressures and smaller resonant mass of the aortic (which normally closes first) and the pulmonary valves.

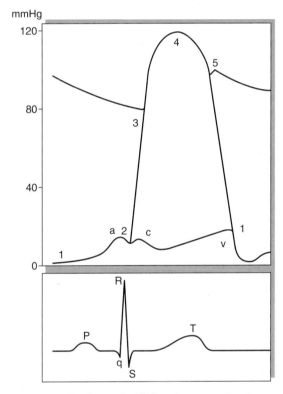

Figure 23.4 Cardiac cycle. ECG and pressure–time traces for aorta (120/80 mmHg), Left ventricle (LV; points 1–5–1) and left atrium (LA *a, c, v* waves). At point 1 the LV fills passively from the LA. Atrial depolarisation (ECG P wave) initiates LA contraction (*a* wave), and ventricular depolarisation (ECG QRS complex). At point 2 the mitral valve closes (first heart sound; LV end-diastolic pressure). Isometric ventricular contraction (2–3) ends as the aortic valve opens (3). Blood is ejected from the LV into the aorta to give a peak systolic pressure (4). The ventricle starts to relax (ECG T wave) and pressure falls in LV. The aortic valve closes (second heart sound; point 5) with the dicrotic notch. Isometric ventricular relaxation (points 5–1) is followed by opening of the mitral valve (1) when the pressure in LA (*v* wave) exceeds that in LV. This cycle then resumes.

The *duration of systole* is measured from the time between the first heart sound and the second sound due to closure of the aortic valve and the pulmonary valve. The lower pressure in the pulmonary artery is associated with a longer duration of systole in the right ventricle.

The changes in pressure during the cardiac cycle are traditionally represented by the pressure–time, volume–time and other traces for each chamber, related to each other in the standard diagram of Carl Wiggers (Figure 23.4).

The sequential changes in pressure and volume in the ventricles can be represented graphically as a plot of ventricular volume against pressure (Figures 23.5 and 23.6). Intraventricular pressure is measured by an intraventricular catheter-tip pressure transducer, or less accurately by a fluid filled intraventricular cardiac catheter and external transducer. It is much more difficult to determine the volume of the ventricle. Typical methods include ultrasonography, ventricular catheterisation and biplane cineangiography, or by a catheter to measure ventricular conductance (which increases with intraventricular blood volume).

These plots are valuable in emphasising not just the volume of blood ejected in systole but also the diastolic volume and the compliance or elasticity of the ventricle. Hence both the *ejection fraction*, widely accepted as an index of ventricular performance, and the adequacy of ventricular filling can be assessed. For a given contractile state the ejection fraction (stroke volume/end-diastolic volume) depends on *pre-*

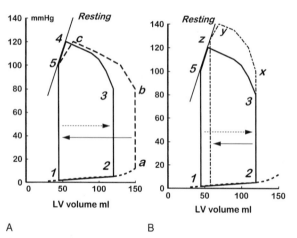

A   B

Figure 23.5 Stylised pressure–volume curves for the left ventricle, with pressure (mmHg) on the ordinate, and volume (ml) on the abscissa. The width of the trapezoid indicates stroke volume, and the height peak systolic pressure. Points 1–5 are as in pressure–time curve (Figure 23.4). A: End-diastolic pressure (filling pressure) rises as the ventricle fills with blood (120 ml; 1–2). Isometric ventricular contraction (2–3) increases pressure to 80 mmHg before ejection (stroke volume 75 ml; 3–5, dotted arrow). The cycle resumes after isometric relaxation (5–1). Increased filling or preload (to 150 ml; 1–a) results in a stronger contraction, and the ejection of more blood (b–5, solid arrow; stroke volume 105 ml). B: An acute increase in afterload results in a higher pressure before the aortic valve opens (100 mmHg; x), a higher peak systolic pressure (140 mmHg; y) and earlier valve closure (z), compared with the resting cycle (1–5). Less blood is ejected on this beat (solid arrow; 62 ml). As there has been no change in inotropic state, end-systolic pressures (5, z) lie on the regression line marked 'Resting'. The LV now starts to fill from a higher starting volume and pressure. With the same volume of blood filling the LV the stroke volume will return towards initial values over the next few beats (not shown) due to more forceful contraction (Starling mechanism; Figure 23.5A).

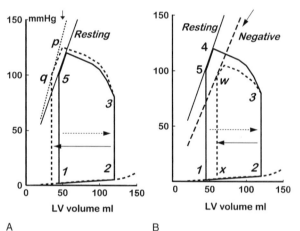

A   B

Figure 23.6 Stylised pressure–volume curves for the left ventricle. A: End-diastolic (or filling) pressures rise with increased ventricular filling. For contractions at different filling pressures the end-systolic pressures (at closure of the aortic valve) tend to lie on a line ('Resting'). Positive inotropic effects increase the slope of this line (vertical arrow). The resting cardiac cycle (1–5) has a stroke volume of 75 ml and an ejection fraction of 63%. A positive inotrope (e.g. adrenaline) increases myocardial contractility so that more blood is ejected (3–q; 85 ml) and ejection fraction rises to 70%. B: Negative inotropic effects reduce the slope of the end-systolic pressure–volume relationship (dotted regression). An acute fall in contractility results in earlier valve closure and the ejection of less blood (3–w, solid arrow; 60 ml). Ejection fraction fell from 63 to 50%.

load (filling pressure and end-diastolic volume) and *afterload* (systolic pressure as a measure of peripheral resistance).

Cardiac output and its measurement

The measurement of cardiac output can be achieved by a number of procedures, ranging from the classic Fick and indicator-dilution methods to newer gated radioisotope scans, Doppler flow probes and ultrasonography.

The *Fick principle* simply states that the amount of a substance taken up or excreted by an organ must equal the difference between the amount going to the organ in the arterial blood and the amount leaving the organ in the venous blood, provided the organ does not store, synthesise or metabolise the substance, i.e. the substance is stable. Hence the uptake of oxygen by the lungs can be used to determine pulmonary blood flow (a close approximation to cardiac output and not to be confused with bronchial flow):

amount removed or added = organ blood flow
$$\times \{[\text{arterial blood}] - [\text{venous blood}]\}.$$

Cardiac output is estimated by measuring the uptake of oxygen by the lungs, the content (free and bound to haemoglobin) of oxygen in the pulmonary arterial blood, and the content of oxygen in pulmonary venous blood. At rest, oxygen uptake reduces oxygen in inspired air from 21% to some 16% in mixed expired air. This difference can be measured accurately by a good paramagnetic analyser and used with the measured volume of expired air to determine oxygen uptake. Since some minutes of collection are required to obtain a stable sample of mixed expired air, the Fick principle can only be used in a steady state of rest or exercise. Pulmonary arterial blood samples must be obtained anaerobically in a heparin-loaded syringe, stoppered and kept on ice until analysis. Since pulmonary venous samples cannot be obtained percutaneously, systemic arterial blood samples are collected instead, simultaneously with the pulmonary arterial samples, in similar syringes. Typical values at rest would be:

$$O_2 \text{ uptake} = 5000 \text{ ml min}^{-1} \times 5\% \ O_2 \text{ difference}$$
by lungs
$$= 250 \text{ ml min}^{-1}$$
$$= \text{pulmonary blood flow} \times (200 \text{ ml } O_2 \text{ per litre arterial} - 150 \text{ ml } O_2 \text{ per litre venous blood}).$$

Hence:

$$\text{cardiac output} = 250/50$$
$$= 5 \text{ litres min}^{-1}.$$

There is a small error due to the shunting of blood from systemic arteries to the left heart without oxygenation in the pulmonary capillaries. Some cardiac thebesian veins may drain directly to the left (and not the right) atrial and ventricular cavities. Some bronchial venules may empty into pulmonary veins. Due to these shunts the P_{O_2} of systemic arterial blood (95 mmHg) is less than that of pulmonary venous blood (100 mmHg). This physiological shunt is some 5% of total lung flow. While the estimation of the oxygen content of blood is best achieved by chemical analysis (van Slyke method), it is more usual to use spectrophotometry to estimate the proportions of different forms of haemoglobin in the blood. The overall error in such determinations of cardiac output is of the order of ± 10%.

Indicator-dilution methods rely on determining the blood concentration of a stable indicator substance. The principle is shown by the measurement of a volume (V) of fluid by adding a known weight (W) of dye to the fluid, mixing the fluid homogeneously, and determining the final concentration (C) of the dye, since $W = V \times C$. In the indicator-dilution methods a known amount of the dye or indicator (W) is added to the circulation, mixes with a volume of flowing blood (V), and the concentration (C) is determined over a period of time (t). Here the volume in which the dye is mixed is not static, but moving, and the concentration varies with time. If the mean concentration is determined from the integration of the variable concentrations over time t then the volume of blood flowing through the mixing site in time t can be estimated.

W = flow in t seconds $\times \int_0^t C\, dt$ = flow in t seconds $\times$ mean concentration over t seconds.

If volume of flow V in t seconds = F, then volume of flow in 1 minute = 60 F/t.

With stable indicators this simple integration is complicated by recirculation of dye-containing blood by shorter paths back to the mixing site, before complete removal of the dye from this site has occurred, causing artefactual increases in values for the concentration–time curve (Figure 23.7). Algorithms to control for the effects of such recirculation artefacts rely on determining the rate of washout of the dye from the mixing site before recirculation develops. The Stewart–Hamilton method uses a simple replotting of the concentration data on a logarithmic scale to estimate the decline before recirculation as a monoexponential process, extrapolate to baseline concentration, and determine the period t seconds of mixing in the absence of recirculation.

The most commonly used dye, indocyanine green, is harmless and is excreted by the liver. Arterial puncture is required. Blood is steadily withdrawn from the aorta or a major artery through a carefully calibrated cuvette spectrophotometer into a syringe. When green light is passed through the withdrawn blood the absorp-

tion is a function of the concentration of the dye (Beer's law). Unlike the use of a blue dye with blue light, the relative proportions of oxygenated and deoxygenated haemoglobin do not affect the absorption of green light. This is important when measuring cardiac output in critically ill and hypoxic patients. The dye accumulates with repeated determinations, and so the baseline rises progressively.

The use of an indicator which is removed in one passage round the circulation will prevent recirculation from occurring. The standard *thermodilution method* of Swan and Ganz uses ice-cold 5% dextrose solution as the indicator, and an integrated two-port catheter with inflatable balloon. After injection into the central venous port of the catheter the indicator should mix homogeneously with blood flowing through the right atrium and ventricle, and the fall in blood temperature is determined by the catheter thermistor in the pulmonary artery. There will be no appreciable change in the baseline temperature after repeated determinations of cardiac output. Repeated determinations with isotonic saline could result in fluid overload in compromised patients. The same principles are used in the 'continuous' cardiac output monitor, which instead of injecting a cold solution uses a pulse of electrical current to heat a coil of thin film around the proximal part of the catheter, thus creating a 'bolus' of warmed blood. The temperature rise is again sensed by a distal thermistor.

The shape of the curve changes with cardiac output. High outputs give rapid flow through the heart and low, sharp curves of brief duration. Low outputs with slow flow generally give taller curves with a longer duration, as the indicator is diluted less. However, small stroke volumes may cause erroneously low, broad, slurred curves, which cannot be analysed. Thermodilution methods may overestimate very low cardiac outputs, which are small by the Fick method, especially if < 2.5 l min⁻¹. Presumably this is due to heat gain in the heart at slow flow rates. A number of precautions should be taken to ensure more reproducible data. The injection should be by gas powered piston rather than manually. Since the cool indicator can gain heat from the

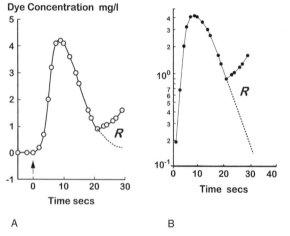

Dye Concentration mg/l

A

B

Figure 23.7 The concentration data in trace (A) show the effects of recirculation (R) on the indicator dilution curve. The data are replotted (B) as the logarithm of the dye concentration against time to give a straight line which is extrapolated to estimate the effects of recirculation (R).

initially warm catheter and cardiac structures before reaching the pulmonary artery, the data from the first two injections should be discarded, as the catheter is cooling down. The final decline in temperature to baseline is slow, so the computer system may be programmed to stop integration once 70% fall from maximum temperature change has occurred; an estimate is then given for the uncollected data. Respiration causes fluctuations in basal temperature of the pulmonary arterial blood. Variation in values for output is reduced if estimations are made at end-expiration. Positive pressure ventilation tends to impede pulmonary indicator flow, and where possible should be stopped during output determination.

In *equilibrium radionuclide* methods the isotope (technetium-labelled red cells) is added to venous blood and the radioactivity determined over the heart at a series of time intervals linked to the phases of the cardiac cycle, or 'gated' by the QRS complex of the electrocardiogram (ECG). After several hundred cardiac cycles the image of the left ventricle is demarcated for ventricular systole and diastole by subtracting background radioactivity in adjacent structures. Stroke volume is (end-diastolic volume – end-systolic volume). The ejection fraction % can be calculated from the ratio of (stroke volume)/(end-diastolic volume). The cardiac output is the product of heart rate and stroke volume. Multiple measurements can be made over a period of time. Data collection requires the patient to lie still for a prolonged period. While the method is not as accurate as the standard radiographic method of biplane cinecardiography, the non-invasive determination of ejection fraction provides clinically valuable information.

Echocardiographic determination of the end-diastolic and end-systolic volumes of the ventricle should give the stroke volume, which could be multiplied by the heart rate to indicate the cardiac output. However, the assumptions made about the irregular shape of the ventricles, particularly in disease, reduce the accuracy of this method.

There has been interest in the use of *impedance methods* to determine cardiac output continu-

ously and non-invasively in critical care units. Two electrode bands with conductive gel are placed around the neck at least 3 cm apart, one around the lower thorax, and one around the abdomen. A small oscillating current (40–100 kHz frequency; < 4 mA) of constant amplitude is passed between the outer pair of electrodes (abdomen–neck), and the resultant voltage drop is recorded from the inner electrode pair (neck–thorax) to give the transthoracic impedance. Inspiration of non-conducting air increases impedance. In the absence of respiration impedance varies with the phase of the cardiac cycle, falling as blood is ejected by the ventricles into the large arteries of the chest. Despite this attractively simple theory the accuracy of change or rate of change in impedance in estimating the stroke volume is low. Determination of relative changes in stroke volume over a period may be more successful.

Control of cardiac function

The cardiac output is the product of the heart rate (pump cycles per minute) and the stroke output from the pump (volume ejected per beat). The right ventricle ejects against a relatively low pressure in the pulmonary artery, compared with the much higher pressure in the aorta opposing ejection by the left ventricle. By Laplace's law pressure and radius determine wall tension, and hence the structures of the two ventricles. Thus the thin-walled right ventricle is best thought of as a low pressure volume pump, and the thick-walled left ventricle as a high pressure pump.

The wide range of heart rates (50–200 per minute) seen in young fit people reflects the uniquely variable rate of the sinus node. This capacity to change rate is almost entirely due to the effects of parasympathetic and sympathetic neurotransmitters and hormones on the pacemaker potential of these cells. The upper limit to the effectiveness of further increases in heart rate in increasing cardiac output is related to the shorter duration of diastole for filling the ventricles with blood, and for perfusing the coronary arteries to supply the increased myocardial need for oxygen. In diseased hearts in older people ventricular pacing rates greater than 90–100 beats per minute may cause no further increase in cardiac output.

Increases in stroke volume occur as a consequence of changes in any of three main groups of factors: firstly, changes in ventricular filling, *preload* or venous return; secondly, changes in *myocardial contractility*; and, thirdly, alterations in the forces which oppose ventricular ejection, *afterload* or aortic impedance (Figure 23.8).

The simple response to increased end-diastolic stretch or *preload* was described for an isolated cardiac muscle preparation — the Starling mechanism (see above). As the filling of the ventricle

increases (the end-diastolic volume or preload) so also does the stroke work (the integral of the volume and the pressure of the ejected blood during the cardiac beat). In the isolated muscle the force of contraction falls with overstretch. However, it is impossible to establish that such a deterioration in output occurs in the intact heart on the basis of sarcomere overstretch, as expected by the classical Starling mechanism. This is because of the many curves that describe the relation between end-diastolic function and stroke work, and the inability to exclude a shift to another curve as the basis of the decline in function.

For a spherical or cylindrical lumen Laplace's law states that in equilibrium the wall tension will be proportional to the product of lumen pressure and radius. This indicates that in the intact ventricle a greatly increased wall tension, or force of contraction, will be required to achieve the same increase in pressure in a larger volume of blood. The dilated ventricle will require additional oxygen for this increased tension. Hence deterioration in ventricular performance can occur in the overstretched ventricle on the basis of inadequate oxygen supply, myocardial sarcomere overstretch, or overstretch of the AV valve rings to the point of incompetence.

At a set end-diastolic volume (fixed fibre and sarcomere lengths) an increase in *myocardial contractility*, with a faster rate of force production and higher peak force, causes either the ejection of more blood from the ventricle (a bigger stroke volume and ejection fraction) or a higher peak systolic pressure and rate of ejection. In either case more stroke work is done for the same initial stretch of the fibres of the heart. Many alterations in cardiac contractility are due to factors that increase or reduce the intracellular availability of Ca^{2+}, such as the increase in contractility that follows sympathetic nervous or hormonal stimulation of the heart.

The effects of *afterload* (or aortic impedance) on the ejection of blood from the left ventricle are complex. The use of the term impedance may seem pedantic, as much of the afterload is due to the initial level of aortic diastolic pressure. However, the ejection of blood from the ventricle, which is a near sinusoidal phenomenon, is then

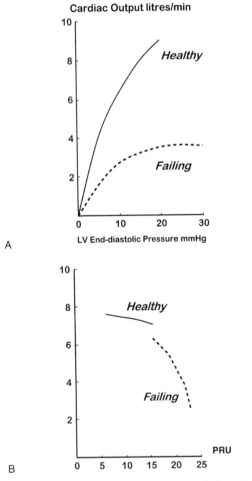

Figure 23.8 Effects of filling pressure (end-diastolic pressure or preload; A) and systemic vascular resistance (afterload; B) on the cardiac output of a healthy and a failing ventricle. PRU, peripheral resistance units (mmHg per litre cardiac output per minute; see text).

opposed by the elasticity of the aorta, the runoff of blood into the arterial tree (peripheral resistance), and the resultant increase in pressure in the aorta (systolic pressure). Little effect of increased afterload is observed in the normal heart until very high levels of resistance to the ejection of blood are achieved. Starling also observed this in the isolated heart–lung preparation, where an increase in aortic resistance resulted in less complete emptying of the heart for a few beats, but the resulting increase in end-diastolic volume restored stroke output.

The failing heart, however, is very sensitive to the adverse effects of increases in aortic impedance (Figure 23.8). By Laplace's law the generation of the same systolic blood pressure will require a bigger wall tension (pressure × radius) in a large ventricle than in a normal ventricle. Hence increasing afterload and arterial blood pressure by the use of vasoconstrictor agents will cause much greater deterioration in the performance of a large, poorly emptying ventricle than a healthy ventricle. Reduction in ventricular afterload is associated with increased exercise tolerance and cardiac output in many patients with heart failure. Some patients with hypotension and peripheral vasoconstriction (shock) may also benefit from a reduction in the resistance to ventricular ejection.

Atrial natriuretic hormone

For some 40 years it has been known that stretch of the atria and great vessels results in a diuresis of water and salt. A number of mechanisms contribute to this effect. Stretch of low pressure baroreceptors in the walls of the atria and great vessels relays action potentials to the hypothalamus to inhibit the release of ADH (arginine vasopressin) from the posterior pituitary. Stretch of these receptors also reduces the activity of renal sympathetic vasoconstrictor nerves. Nervous reflexes cause only part of the response. The realisation that atrial muscle cells contain granules resembling those seen in endocrine organs, and that atrial extracts cause diuresis, has been followed rapidly by the determination of the structure of the human peptide hormone (atrial

natriuretic hormone, ANP; 28 amino acids), and of the sequence of the responsible gene.

This peptide hormone dilates blood vessels, opposing the actions of vasoconstrictors such as noradrenaline and angiotensin II, with more effect on arteries than veins. It also opposes the effects of the renin–angiotensin–aldosterone system, by reducing renin release from the juxtaglomerular apparatus, and by reducing aldosterone release from the zona glomerulosa of the adrenal cortex.

Thus the natriuresis and diuresis caused by ANP is due in part to direct effects on the kidney, increasing blood flow to the glomeruli, in part to antagonism of the release and effects of both renin and aldosterone, and in part to inhibition of the reabsorption of Na^+ in the collecting duct.

The only known stimuli for the release of ANP act through stretch of the atria. The hormone appears to be responsible for the well recognised diuresis that follows paroxysmal atrial tachyarrhythmias, or rapid atrial pacing. ANP release and diuresis also follow stretch of the atria by increased central blood volume, caused by a reduction in the effects of gravity on the circulation, or by intravenous salt loading. Immersion of a normal subject in water to neck height causes an increase in both central blood volume and ANP secretion — a simple experiment to demonstrate the mechanism.

However, it is difficult to assign a significant role to this hormone in cardiac disease. Despite high blood levels of ANP, both salt and water are still retained to excess in oedematous congestive cardiac failure. Indeed blood levels of the hormone or of the related peptide, brain natriuretic peptide, have been used as indicators of ventricular dysfunction. Very high blood concentrations of ANP also occur in renal failure, due in part to reduced metabolism by the kidneys, and may help to reduce blood pressure.

Assessment of cardiac function

Having discussed some of the problems in making measurements of cardiac function, the purpose of this section is to indicate some of the basic normal values and calculations that can be used in monitoring patients. The use of pulmonary artery flotation catheters for measurements of cardiac output may be supplemented by the use of transducers for measurements of pressures at the catheter orifices in the great veins and pulmonary artery. Recognition of these pressure traces is essential for the safe passage of a central venous or cardiac catheter (Figure 23.9). When wedged in the distal pulmonary arterial circulation the brief inflation of the catheter balloon prevents the onward flow of blood through that branch pulmonary artery. The pressure then drops to that at the venous end of the capillaries, the pulmonary artery wedge pressure (PAWP) or pulmonary capillary wedge pressure, which is an index of the left atrial pressure, and hence of the filling presure of the left ventricle. However, the use of pulmonary balloon catheters is more hazardous (pulmonary infarction, arrhythmias, branch artery rupture) than the use of simple central venous catheters, and confers little advantage in most patients with normal right ventricles. When pulmonary vascular resistance is normal, with little pressure drop across the pulmonary circulation, then the end-diastolic pressure in the pulmonary artery is a practical and safer index of left atrial pressure than PAWP, avoiding the hazards of repeated balloon inflation and replacement of catheters with burst balloons.

For normal pressures refer to Table 23.1. Using the measured values for mean systemic arterial (AP), mean right atrial (RAP), mean pulmonary

Table 23.1 Normal upper limit of pressures in cardiac chambers and great vessels

Chamber/vessel	Pressure (mmHg)
Right atrium	Mean 6
Right ventricle systolic/diastolic	30/5
Pulmonary artery	30/15
Pulmonary capillary wedge	Mean 12
Left ventricle	140/12
Aorta	140/90
Pulmonary vascular resistance	3 mmHg per litre blood per minute
Systemic vascular resistance	18 mmHg per litre blood per minute

arterial (PAP) and mean pulmonary artery wedge (PAWP) pressures the *perfusion pressures* through the pulmonary circuit (mean PAP − PAWP) and the systemic circuit (mean AP − RAP) may be calculated. From Ohm's law ($V = I \times R$) the *vascular resistance* of a circuit may be estimated, e.g:

pulmonary vascular resistance = (pulmonary perfusion pressure) / (cardiac output).

While peripheral resistance units are often used clinically (mmHg min litre^{-1}), it is more correct to multiply these values by 80 to give units of dynes s cm^{-5}. Increased pressure in the pulmonary artery, if due to pulmonary arteriolar constriction during *alveolar hypoxia*, will give a high value for pulmonary vascular resistance which reverses with adequate alveolar ventilation.

The pressure in a central venous catheter indicates the pressure in the great veins and right atrium, and hence represents the end-diastolic or filling pressure of the right ventricle, if errors due to a kinked or blocked catheter are eliminated. It is a complex function of central blood volume and other factors. Central venous pressure will rise with increases in intrathoracic pressure (positive pressure ventilation). Constriction of systemic peripheral veins may maintain central venous pressure in the presence of a low blood volume.

The PAWP generally represents left atrial, and hence end-diastolic or filling pressure in the left ventricle. Pulmonary oedema is likely to develop if PAWP is elevated above 20 mmHg. However, the PAWP can be greater than left ventricular

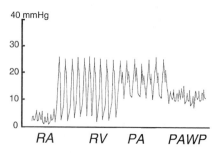

Figure 23.9 Pressure traces in the right heart. The catheter is advanced from right atrium (RA), through right ventricle (RV) and pulmonary artery (PA) to wedge in the pulmonary arterial tree (PAWP). (Redrawn from Hopkinson R B 1983 In: Peters J L (ed) A manual of central venous catheterization and parenteral nutrition. Wright, Bristol.)

filling pressure if there is mitral valve stenosis or obstruction. When the left ventricle is stiff (e.g. severe hypertrophy), or the end-diastolic pressure in the left ventricle is very high (> 25 mmHg), the high compliance (stretch) of the left atrium and pulmonary veins may reduce the PAWP below the left ventricular diastolic pressure. In the presence of raised intrathoracic pressure (positive pressure ventilation, tension pneumothorax) or intrapericardial pressure (cardiac tamponade) the PAWP and RAP do not represent filling pressures for the respective ventricles. In positive pressure ventilation the raised intra-alveolar pressure will give a PAWP higher than left atrial pressure, unless left atrial pressure is already high (> 20 mmHg). Hence pressures should be measured in end-expiration in these patients.

On each side of the heart the ventricle raises the stroke volume of blood from atrial pressure to systolic ventricular (or systolic arterial) pressure. Hence for the left ventricle:

stroke work (gram.metre) = (stroke volume) × (mean arterial BP − PAWP) × (0.0136).

Here stroke volume is measured in millilitres, and pressures in millimetres of mercury. Division by the body surface area of the patient will give the stroke work index for the left ventricle (normally > 30 g.m m^{-2}). Graphing the cardiac performance (stroke work index) against the filling pressure (left ventricular end-diastolic pressure or pulmonary artery wedge pressure) can indicate poor cardiac function as depressed contractility with adequate ventricular filling (increased filling pressure; Figure 23.10). Changes in the stroke work index in relation to filling pressure are useful in monitoring changes in left ventricular function with therapeutic interventions (infusions to increase ventricular filling, or inotropic agents).

The ejection fraction is a useful measure of contractile performance, which correlates well with survival after acute myocardial infarction, cardiac surgery and heart failure. Ejection fractions of 0.6 or greater are regarded as normal, values of 0.5–0.6 as borderline, and lower values as depressed cardiac function (0.5–0.4 mildly, 0.4–0.3 moderately, and less than 0.3 severely).

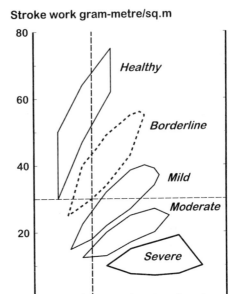

Stroke work gram-metre/sq.m

Mean PA wedge pressure mmHg

Figure 23.10   The stroke work per square metre of body surface has been plotted against the mean pulmonary artery (PA) wedge pressure, which in the absence of mitral valve obstruction is an indicator of left ventricular filling pressure. This relationship gives a series of families of curves, represented by the areas above. Progressive deterioration in myocardial contractility causes lower stroke work despite a higher filling pressure. Sudden severe deterioration would be recognised clinically as cardiogenic shock. Normal values should lie in the upper left quadrant, defined as stroke work more than 30 g.m m^{-2} at a mean PA wedge pressure less than 12 mmHg. The lower left quadrant indicates reduced work due to either poor ventricular filling or reduced contractility. Data values in the lower right quadrant show poor ventricular contraction despite adequate filling.

Hence the normal left ventricle ejects two thirds (66 %) of the blood filling it at the end of diastole.

The heart in exercise

As the body does physical work, the active skeletal muscles consume oxygen. Increases in cardiac output are related to increases in whole body oxygen consumption, and hence the level of physical exertion. The cardiac output can rise from resting values of some 5 l min^{-1} to a maximum of some 25 l min^{-1} in the sedentary or up to 35 l min^{-1} in the athlete. The controlling mechanisms responsible are far from clear.

Some increase in skeletal muscle blood flow may occur prior to exercise, due to increased sympathetic cholinergic vasodilator nerve activity, and/or reductions in sympathetic noradrenergic vasoconstrictor nerve activity. However, with exertion the fall in tissue oxygen and accumulation of vasodilator metabolites soon cause large reductions in vascular resistance in the active skeletal muscle. This metabolic-induced relaxation of arteriolar and precapillary sphincter smooth muscle is aided by the effects of these metabolites in antagonising sympathetic vasoconstrictor nervous activity in the exercising skeletal muscles, and by flow-induced increases in the release of NO from the arterial and arteriolar endothelium.

The overall fall in peripheral resistance tends to reduce aortic and carotid blood pressure, with a reduction in stretch of the high pressure baroreceptors of the aortic arch and the carotid sinus. The reduction in inhibitory action potentials in the vagus and glossopharyngeal nerves permits the vasomotor centre of the medulla to become more active. Sympathetic noradrenergic vasoconstrictor nerve activity is increased to the arterioles of the skin, inactive skeletal muscle and abdominal viscera. Vagal tone is withdrawn from the heart so the heart rate rises. With more cardiac sympathetic nerve activity, there is a further increase in heart rate and in the force of contraction of both atria and ventricles, with a rise in cardiac output.

This increase in cardiac output can only be sustained if there is adequate venous return to the heart. Increased venous return is aided by the greater movements of the diaphragm and chest wall, with lower intrathoracic pressures, and by the active contractions of skeletal muscles (in isotonic work) pressing on the peripheral veins and lymphatics to speed the flow of fluid through their valves towards the right atrium. Although it would be expected that venous constriction should accompany increased sympathetic vasoconstrictor activity to arterioles, this is disputed in man. Only in the gastrointestinal circulation does this seem to be true, mobilising blood volume towards the central venous pool.

An increase in venous return will tend to stretch the ventricles more, increasing stroke volume by the Starling mechanism. This does not occur at moderate levels of exercise, where the increase in heart rate and in ventricular ejection is sufficient to maintain the increased cardiac output. At maximal levels of exercise the Starling mechanism may contribute to an increase in stroke volume. The relative unimportance of the Starling mechanism was established many years ago. The proponents of the Starling mechanism in exercise argued that in exercise the diastolic size of the heart should increase. However, radiographic screening of the exercising heart showed that the heart became smaller. Rushmer confirmed by direct measurement that the end-diastolic ventricular diameter of the exercising dog became smaller. Any increase in stroke volume under these circumstances would be due to more complete ejection of blood from the ventricle by increased myocardial contractility, with the ejection fraction rising from 60 to 80 %.

The central role of the sympathetic nervous sytem in the cardiovascular response to exercise is shown by the effects of blockade of β adrenoceptors. General blockade of β adrenoceptors with propranolol or similar drugs reduces exercise capacity in general, and the maximal heart rate in particular. More cardio-specific blockade of β adrenoceptors (e.g. with atenolol) similarly reduces both exercise tolerance and the heart rate response to increased activity.

The cardiac response to exercise is altered after cardiac transplantation. The transplanted donor heart has no autonomic nerve supply from the recipient, beyond the suture lines. Hence the heart rate cannot be increased by changes in vagal or sympathetic nervous activity, and any bradycardia does not respond to atropine. Indeed the resting heart rate tends to be faster as there is no vagal tone. Some slow increase in heart rate can occur in exercise and other stresses, due to an increase in catecholamines circulating in the blood. These catecholamines also tend to increase the force of contraction and stroke volume. However, the main factor responsible for the near-normal increase in cardiac output on exercise in these patients is a large increase in stroke volume due to the Starling response to an increased venous return. This reserve mechanism appears to be largely responsible for the increased activity (e.g. golf, tennis) which is possible after a successful cardiac transplant. Some patients have competed successfully in marathons.

This description appears to explain many of the factors responsible for the increase in cardiac output during exercise. However, experimental studies in dogs have shown that the arterial baroreceptors are not essential for increased cardiac performance in exercise. During exercise there is a multiplicity of inputs to the cardiovascular control centres in the cortex, hypothalamus and brainstem. Past experience and training should indicate not just the skeletal muscle effort required to undertake a task but may alert the sympathetic nervous system in a more general or specific fashion. Competitive athletic events produce major activation of the sympathetic nervous system before exercise. It is well established that input from muscle–joint receptors increases respiratory performance in exercise, and may contribute to cardiovascular adaptations.

The above description refers to isotonic exercise, where the skeletal muscles are allowed to shorten, as in running or cycling. In isometric exercise, as in lifting weights, the rise in heart rate and cardiac output is accompanied by a rise in both systolic and diastolic arterial blood pressure, and sweating. The posture of the body must also be considered when evaluating published reports of measurements of cardiac output in exercise. Exercise in the supine position is easily arranged in a catheter laboratory; however, stroke volume is large at rest. In the erect position the stroke volume is small at rest. Hence changes in stroke volume are more dramatic as the erect subject exercises to a higher level of oxygen consumption.

DISTURBED CARDIAC FUNCTION

Cardiac arrhythmias and cardiac output

Cardiac arrhythmias can interfere with the pumping function of the heart by loss of control of heart rate, and by abnormalities in the timing of the sequence of atrial and ventricular contraction.

An abnormally slow heart rate, such as severe sinus bradycardia (< 50 min^{-1}) or complete AV block with an idioventricular pacemaker (35–40 min^{-1}), greatly limits cardiac output at rest and particularly on exercise. In some patients increases in stroke volume by the Starling mechanism can maintain adequate cardiac output, but this may not occur in the presence of a damaged heart. Simple ventricular pacing can restore a normal cardiac output at rest and greatly improve the health of the patient.

Rapid tachycardias compromise cardiac pumping by reducing the time available in diastole for passive filling of the ventricles, or for filling the coronary arteries and perfusing the endocardial areas of the heart. Reduction in coronary blood flow will further impair cardiac function.

The beneficial effect of atrial contraction in stretching the ventricles at the end of diastole is lost with atrial fibrillation, and reduced in other supraventricular tachyarrhythmias. However, restoration of sinus rhythm by elective DC conversion of atrial fibrillation increases the cardiac output at rest by only 5–10%. Despite this apparently small impairment of cardiac output these arrhythmias can cause serious deterioration in a critically ill patient. In more healthy patients cardiac output at rest is adequate, but output on exercise, and hence exercise capacity, is severely compromised.

In ventricular tachycardias the normal spread of ventricular contraction is disrupted, and so inefficiency of ventricular contraction is added to the loss of effective atrial pumping. Electrical instability in the ventricles can easily deteriorate to ventricular fibrillation.

The failing heart

Cardiac failure is best defined as an output of oxygenated blood which is inadequate for the needs of the body as a whole. Most commonly the cardiac output is less than normal, and cannot supply normal body needs. On some occasions the cardiac output is high but remains inadequate to supply the increased needs of the body tissues, as in thyrotoxic storm. In left ventricular failure the main features are a reduced ejection fraction, a high left ventricular end-diastolic pressure (PAWP), often with pulmonary oedema, and a relative lack of inotropic response to sympathetic stimulation (see Figure 23.8). Indeed the onset of overt cardiac failure appears to be associated with this attenuation of the normal response of the myocardium to the cardiac sym-pathetic nerves. Tissue P_{O_2} falls with the reduction in blood flow. The extraction of oxygen from the blood is more complete. Mixed venous oxygen saturations may fall to 35%, and AV oxygen difference rises to give some three times the normal resting oxygen removed per litre of blood. This partially compensates for a fall in cardiac output. However, a cardiac output one-third of the normal value is not compatible with survival.

FURTHER READING

Baim D F, Grossman W 1996 Cardiac catheterization, angiography and intervention, 5th edn. Williams & Wilkins, Baltimore

Levick J R 1996 An introduction to cardiovascular physiology, 2nd edn. Butterworth, London

McPhee S J, Lingappa V R, Ganong W F, Lange J D 1995 Pathophysiology of disease. Prentice-Hall International, Fort Lee

Moylan J A (ed) 1994 Surgical critical care. Mosby, St Louis

Priebe H-J, Skarvan K 1995 Cardiovascular physiology. BMJ Publishing Group, London

West J B (ed) 1991 Best and Taylor's physiological basis of medical practice, 12th edn. Williams & Wilkins, Baltimore

24

Antiarrhythmic drugs

J. P. Alexander

ORIGINS OF ARRHYTHMIAS

Cardiac arrhythmias may be due to disorders of impulse formation or disorders of conduction. Sinus tachycardia is the most common example of enhanced impulse formation due to release of circulating catecholamines or β-adrenergic stimulation. Hypoxia, hypokalaemia, hypomagnesaemia and myocardial stretch all change the permeability to K^+ and Na^+ which can lead to spontaneous cellular depolarisation. The increase in intracellular Ca^{2+} concentrations may lead to oscillation in the resting membrane potential. When oscillations are of sufficient magnitude, cell depolarisation will occur.

Cardiac conduction disorders are common causes of clinical arrhythmias, and arise when the heart becomes electrically unstable due to increased automaticity and the development of re-entry. Increased automaticity refers to accelerated phase 4 spontaneous depolarisation. Since the arrhythmia will depend on the area of the heart which is affected, it can explain a sinus tachycardia, atrial or ventricular premature beats and atrial and ventricular tachycardias.

Re-entry depends upon unidirectional block with slow conduction through a depressed area of the myocardium. An impulse travelling through the conducting system finds part of its pathway blocked, while the other conducts normally. The impulse which conducts normally is capable of slowly depolarising the blocked pathway in a retrograde direction. The impulse arrives back at the area which conducts normally to find it repolarised and capable of conducting another impulse (circus movement). Patients with ischaemic heart disease are prone to tachyarrhythmias. Electrical instability is indicated by single premature ventricular contractions (PVCs), multiple PVCs, multifocal PVCs and ventricular tachycardia, which may be followed by ventricular fibrillation. Patients with valvular disease are likely to develop sinus tachycardia, atrial fibrillation and atrial flutter. The Wolff–Parkinson–White syndrome involves a circus movement of impulses through the atrioventricular (AV) node with retrograde conduction back along the accessory bundle of Kent, thereby again reaching the atrioventricular node. The circus movement may be initiated by either atrial or ventricular extrasystoles, and therapy is directed to prevention of supraventricular tachycardia, verapamil being the drug of choice. In a less common version of the syndrome, anterograde conduction occurs down the accessory bundle from rapid atrial fibrillation or flutter, and there is a danger of ventricular fibrillation. Here amiodarone or disopyramide may be of value, while digoxin should be avoided because it may accelerate the anterograde conduction.

CLASSIFICATION OF ANTIARRHYTHMIC DRUGS

Vaughan Williams proposed the first antiarrhythmic classification in 1970 and with minor modifications this is still in use. It was based on the electrophysiological action that appropriate drugs exercised on isolated cardiac fibres. Four types of basic activity are recognised (Table 24.1). Although some drugs have more than one action, a dominant effect can usually be recognised. Class I antiarrhythmics have local anaesthetic properties that exhibit membrane stabilising activity and affect conduction, refractoriness and the action potential. Depolarisation of the cardiac cell membrane is slowed by restricting entry of the fast sodium current so that the maximum rise of phase 0 of the action potential is reduced, as is the rate of phase 4 diastolic depolarisation (Fig. 24.1). Spontaneous automaticity is reduced. Class I is further subdivided into a, b and c. Class Ia agents have a moderate effect on phase 0 depression, slow conduction and prolong repolarisation. Class Ib drugs have little effect on phase 0 depolarisation, slow conduction and shorten repolarisation. Class Ic antiarrhythmics are characterised by a marked effect on sodium conductance, prolonging conduction but not affecting repolarisation.

Class II agents reduce the response to catecholamines. They are the β-adrenergic antagonists ('blockers') which depress automaticity and increase the effective refractory period of the atrioventricular node, perhaps by blocking the potential arrhythmogenic effect of cyclic adenosine monophosphate (cAMP).

Class III agents prolong the duration of the

Table 24.1 Classification of antiarrhythmic agents by effects on action potential

Class	Action	Additional classification		Prototype agent	Other agents
I	Membrane stabilising agents (fast sodium channel blockers)	Ia	Slows dV/dt of phase 0 Prolongs repolarisation Prolongs PR, QRS, QT	Quinidine	Procainamide Disopyramide
		Ib	Limited effect on dV/dt of phase 0 Shortens repolarisation Shortens QT Elevates fibrillation threshold	Lignocaine	Mexilitine Tocainide
		Ic	Markedly slows dV/dt Little effect on repolarisation Markedly prolongs PR, QRS	Flecainide	Propafenone Moracizine (Encainide)
II	β-Adrenoceptor blockade			Propranolol	All β blockers
III	Prolongs repolarisation, alters membrane response			Amiodarone	Bretylium Sotalol (mixed II and III)
IV	Calcium channel blockers			Verapamil	Diltiazem

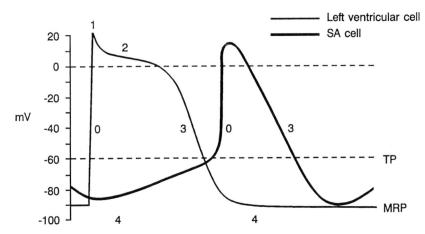

Figure 24.1 The action potential of a left ventricular myofibril and of a cell in the sino-atrial node. Spontaneous depolarisation of the sino-atrial node during phase 4 is characteristic of automatic cells within the heart. TP = threshold potential; MRP = transmembrane resting potential.

action potential so that the effective refractory period is prolonged. They also have important antifibrillatory effects.

Class IV antiarrhythmics are the calcium channel antagonists ('blockers') which inhibit the slow inward calcium-mediated current and depress phase 2 and phase 3 of the action potential. These actions are of particular importance in the atrioventricular node where re-entry circuits can occur.

A clinically useful classification categorises drugs according to the cardiac tissues that each affects (Table 24.2) and may be of use when an appropriate choice of drug to treat a specific arrhythmia has to be made.

Class Ia agents

Quinidine

Quinidine is the prototype of class Ia agents and is an isomer of the alkaloid quinine. It slows phase 0 of the action potential but leaves the resting potential unaltered. Conduction through atrial, ventricular and Purkinje fibres is slowed, while its antivagal action may accelerate atrioventricular nodal conduction. It also possesses α-adrenergic blocking activity. There is no suitable parenteral formulation in the UK so its use is restricted to prophylaxis after cardioversion

Table 24.2 Classification of antiarrhythmic drugs by site of action

Site of action	Drugs
Sinoatrial node	β Blockers Class IV drugs Digoxin
Atrioventricular node	Class Ic drugs β Blockers Class IV drugs Digoxin Adenosine
Ventricles	Class I drugs Class III drugs
Atria	Class Ia drugs Class Ic drugs β Blockers Class III drugs
Accessory pathways	Class Ia drugs Class III drugs

or after acute administration of lignocaine. It is active against both atrial and ventricular arrhythmias.

Pharmacokinetics. Clearance and protein binding is reduced in liver disease. Interaction with digoxin may precipitate digoxin toxicity.

Dosage and administration. The oral dose is 200–400 mg three or four times daily, or 500 mg 12-hourly by slow release preparation.

Adverse effects. High plasma concentrations

(which should be monitored) cause myocardial depression, vasodilatation and hypotension. Conduction defects, prolongation of QRS and QT interval and re-entry arrhythmias may be seen. There is a risk of paroxysmal ventricular fibrillation or of *torsade de pointes* (polymorphic or atypical ventricular tachycardia). Nausea, vomiting, diarrhoea, cinchonism and hypersensitivity reactions can occur.

Procainamide

Procainamide exerts similar electrophysiological effects as described for quinidine. Procainamide is closely related to procaine, the CO.O ester grouping being replaced by CO.NH. It may be effective in the treatment of atrial, junctional and ventricular arrhythmias.

Pharmacokinetics. Procainamide is metabolised to an active metabolite, *N*-acetylprocainamide. The rate of metabolism in the population has a bimodal distribution so that patients are classified as being fast or slow acetylators. The latter require require smaller doses in long term therapy. High plasma levels of the drug and its metabolite can occur in renal or cardiac failure.

Dosage and administration. The standard intravenous dose is 100 mg every 2 minutes, repeating this to a total of 1000 mg in the first hour. The oral dose is 250 mg every 4–6 hours or 1.0–1.5 g of a slow release preparation 8-hourly.

Adverse effects. Rapid intravenous administration may lead to reduced cardiac output, hypotension and vasodilatation. Heart block and QRS and QT prolongation may occur. Long term use may be associated with a drug-induced lupus erythematosus syndrome, more likely to be seen in slow acetylators, and usually reversible.

Disopyramide

The electrophysiological properties of disopyramide are similar to those of quinidine, with some class III activity. The range of activity includes action against both atrial and ventricular ectopics.

Pharmacokinetics. Disopyramide is available as either the base compound or as the phosphate salt. The main metabolite is the *N*-dealkylated form, which has some antiarrhythmic action and is also excreted by the kidneys. Dosage is reduced in severe renal failure. Protein binding sites can be saturated by both the drug and its metabolite. This means that drug clearance will vary depending on whether it is given by mouth or by intravenous injection.

Dosage and administration. Intravenous dose is 2 mg kg^{-1}, up to 150 mg, administered over 5 minutes. A maintenance infusion of 20–30 mg h^{-1} can be given to a total dose of 800 mg in 24 hours. The oral dose is 300–800 mg daily in divided doses; slow release preparations are available.

Adverse effects. Disopyramide has considerable negative inotropic potential and heart failure is a contraindication to the use of the drug. Sinus node depression and QT prolongation predisposing to ventricular re-entry arrhythmia may occur. Disopyramide may precipitate ventricular fibrillation and torsade de pointes. Urinary retention, dry mouth, blurred vision and precipitation of glaucoma are related to the anticholinergic activity of the drug and a metabolite.

Class Ib agents

Lignocaine (Lignocaine hydrochloride BP; lidocaine hydrochloride USP)

Lignocaine has typical class Ib electrophysiological effects. It is an aminoacyl amide and a derivative of acetanilide. It is the first line drug used for treating ventricular arrhythmias after myocardial infarction and cardiac surgery.

Pharmacokinetics. Lignocaine is hydrolysed in the gastrointestinal tract and is subject to extensive first pass metabolism in the liver. Absorption after intramuscular injection is erratic. Clearance is related to hepatic blood flow and hepatic function and to liver microsomal activity. Clearance is prolonged in liver disease and heart failure, and in the elderly, so that infusion rates require appropriate adjustment. Speed of injection may be important in precipitating toxic reactions that are related to the free drug concentration, which is particularly determined by the concentration of acute phase proteins, notably α_1-acid glycoprotein. The latter increases after myocardial infarction, so that although long term infusion may lead to increasing lignocaine concentrations, the free drug level may remain relatively constant.

Active metabolites are monoethylglycylxylidine and glycylxylide, which are weaker antiarrhythmics but have CNS excitatory effects, while 4-hydroxyxylidine is inactive.

Dosage and administration. Lignocaine is given as an intravenous bolus of 1–2 mg kg^{-1} (100–150 mg) and then an intravenous infusion at 4 mg min^{-1} for 30 minutes, 2 mg min^{-1} for 2 hours and 1 mg min^{-1} thereafter will usually maintain steady therapeutic levels. Ideally an exponential infusion rate would maintain plasma levels in the therapeutic range.

Adverse effects. High concentrations may cause hypotension, bradycardia or asystole. Apart from nausea and vomiting, central nervous system (CNS) effects including paraesthesiae and twitching, and grand mal seizures can occur. Hepatic clearance is reduced in patients receiving cimetidine, propranolol or halothane. As with other class I agents, hypokalaemia must be corrected for maximum efficacy.

Mexiletine

Mexiletine is a primary amine and has similar structure and electrophysiological effects to lignocaine. It has been described as an 'oral lignocaine'.

Pharmacokinetics. The half-life is prolonged in heart failure and myocardial infarction. Primary elimination is by hepatic metabolism. About 85% is metabolised to inactive compounds. The remainder is excreted by the kidneys, and alkalinisation of the urine increases reabsorption in the distal tubule.

Dosage and administration. The intravenous dose is 100–250 mg given slowly over 5–10 minutes, followed by an infusion of 250 mg in the first hour, 250 mg over the next 2 hours and then 0.5–1 mg min^{-1} until oral therapy is established. The oral loading dose is 400 mg followed by maintenance doses of 200 mg 6–8-hourly. A slow release formulation is available.

Adverse effects. Hypotension, bradycardia and atrioventricular block can occur, and neurological

side-effects include tremor, nystagmus, diplopia, dizziness, dysarthria, paraesthesiae, ataxia and confusion. Nausea and vomiting also occur.

Tocainide

Tocainide is a primary amine with similar electrophysiological properties to those of lignocaine, and is another oral lignocaine analogue, used to treat acute and chronic ventricular arrhythmias.

Pharmacokinetics. Bioavailability approaches 100%. Hepatic clearance is low, about 25% is excreted as the inactive N-carboxytocainide, 35% is excreted unchanged and elimination half-life is doubled in severe renal failure.

Dosage and administration. Tocainide can be administered intravenously or orally. The intravenous dose is 0.5–0.75 mg kg^{-1} min^{-1} for 15 minutes (500–750 mg), followed immediately by 600–800 mg by mouth and then 400 mg 8-hourly or 600 mg twice daily.

Adverse effects. These include anorexia, nausea, vomiting, constipation, abdominal pain, effects on the CNS similar to those with mexiletine, rashes and rarely interstitial pulmonary alveolitis. A high incidence of blood dyscrasias makes this drug unsuitable for prolonged therapy of benign arrhythmias.

Class Ic agents

Flecainide

Flecainide is a fluorinated aromatic hydrocarbon and is the prototype of class Ic agents. It is used to suppress ventricular arrhythmias. Dizziness, visual disturbances, nausea and vomiting may occur. Occasionally proarrhythmic effects are seen and caution should be observed in administering the drug to patients with pacemakers because it increases endocardial pacing thresholds.

Dosage and administration. The intravenous dose is 1–2 mg kg^{-1} and oral doses of 100–300 mg twice daily are recommended.

Adverse effects. The potentially serious proarrhythmic effect requires that this drug is used under careful observation. Ventricular arrhythmias may be aggravated in 5–12% of patients.

CNS effects are common. The Cardiac Arrhythmia Suppression Trial (CAST) showed that patients receiving flecainide are at greater risk of dying than those taking placebo.

Propafenone

Propafenone is an orally active sodium channel blocking agent with β-adrenoceptor antagonist and weak calcium antagonist activity. It also prolongs action potential duration and thus appears to have mixed class I, II, III and IV antiarrhythmic activity. The drug is indicated only for the treatment of life threatening ventricular arrhythmias.

Pharmacokinetics. Propafenone is completely absorbed after oral administration. Due to high first pass metabolism, bioavailability is low but can be increased with high doses. The principal metabolites are 5-hydroxypropafenone and *N*-dipropylpropafenone, the former of which is active. Approximately 90% of the population are genetically determined fast metabolisers of propafenone, while 10% are slow metabolisers.

Dosage and administration. The standard oral dose range is 150–300 mg 8-hourly.

Adverse effects. These are similar to those noted for flecanide. Proarrhythmia effects are variously reported as between 5 and 20%. The weak non-selective β-blocking activity may exacerbate symptoms in asthmatic patients.

Moracizine

Moracizine is a class Ic antiarrhythmic originally developed in the former USSR. A phenothiazine derivative, its principal electrophysiological effects are caused by a concentration dependent blockade of the sodium channels. Moracizine decreases the maximum upstroke velocity of the action potential and increases the rate of membrane repolarisation. It is effective against ventricular arrhythmias.

Pharmacokinetics. After oral administration, moracizine undergoes rapid absorption and first pass metabolism. About 35% of the total dose is absorbed. Hepatic metabolism is complex, and at least nine metabolites have been identified, two of which have significant antiarrhythmic activity. Because of this complexity, plasma concentrations are not helpful in correlating with antiarrhythmic efficacy.

Dosage and administration. Moracizine is available in 200, 250 and 300 mg tablets. Daily dosage ranges from 600 to 900 mg day^{-1}.

Adverse effects. These are attributed to its phenothiazine structure and include dizziness, nausea, headaches, and elevation of liver enzymes. The second limb of the Cardiac Arrhythmia Suppression Trial (CAST II) reported an initial higher mortality in the moracizine treatment group than in the placebo treated group, causing the study to be stopped.

Encainide

Encainide was available in the USA but its use is now restricted to patients whose arrhythmia cannot be controlled with other drugs. Along with flecainide and moracizine, it was the third class Ic antiarrhythmic to undergo trial in the CAST study. Like flecainide, it produced an excess in sudden deaths as compared with placebo when used to suppress premature ventricular contractions in patients who had sustained a myocardial infarction. This proarrhythmic effect varied from 3 to 16% and appeared to be dose dependent.

Class II agents

β-Adrenergic receptor antagonists

β-Adrenergic receptor antagonists or β blockers have been in clinical use for 30 years, and have an accepted role in the treatment of hypertension, angina, the secondary prevention of myocardial infarction and the treatment of arrhythmias. Some β blockers are, to a greater or lesser extent, cardioselective and have a greater effect on the β$_1$ adrenoceptors of the heart than the β$_2$ adrenoceptors of the bronchi. They may, in theory, be safer to administer to patients with respiratory diseases in whom bronchoconstricition would be hazardous. However, cardioselectivity is not complete and asthmatic patients are always at risk if exposed to β blocking drugs. Some drugs have partial agonist activity or intrinsic sympathomimetic activity and patients treated with

Table 24.3 Properties of β-adrenergic-blocking drugs

Drug	Relative β selectivity	ISA	MSA	Absorption (%)	Bioavailability (%)	Elimination half-life	Major route of elimination
Acebutolol	+	+	+	70	50	3–4 h	R
Atenolol	+	−	−	50	40	6–9 h	R
Betaxolol	+	−	+	100	90	16–20 h	H+R
Bisoprolol	+	−	−	90	90	12–24 h	H+R
Carvedilol	± + α_1	−	−	100	25	2–8 h	H
Celiprolol	+	+	−	50	50	4–5 h	R
Esmolol	+	−	−	—	—	9–10 min	H
Labetalol	− + α_1	−	−	90	50	3–5 h	R
Metoprolol	+	−	−	90	50	3–4 h	H
Nadolol	−	−	−	30	30	14–24 h	R
Oxprenolol	−	+	+	80	40	1–3 h	H
Pindolol	−	++	+	90	90	3–4 h	R+H
Propranolol	−	−	++	90	30	3–4 h	H
Sotalol	−	−	−	70	60	8–10 h	R
Timolol	−	−	−	90	75	4–5 h	R+H

ISA, intrinsic sympathomimetic activity; MSA, membrane stabilising activity, R, renal; H, hepatic.

these drugs are less likely to exhibit profound bradycardia or falls in cardiac output (Table 24.3). The antiarrhythmic effects of the β blockers are chiefly related to their capacity to inhibit the β receptor. Some drugs, in particular propranolol, the prototype of the β blockers, have 'quinidine-like' membrane stabilising effects that may play a small part in the antiarrhythmic properties, in addition to causing slow conduction and increased atrioventricular nodal refractoriness. The method of elimination from the body seems to be related to their degree of lipid solubility. The lipid soluble group, given orally, undergo first pass liver metabolism and are eliminated by this route. The non-lipid soluble drugs are unaffected by the liver and are excreted unchanged by the kidneys (Table 24.3).

Clinical use. The β blockers are of value in the prevention and treatment of supraventricular arrhythmias, especially those due to the Wolff–Parkinson–White Syndrome. They are also effective in arrhythmias related to excessive cardiac adrenergic stimulation, such as those associated with thyrotoxicosis, phaeochromocytoma, exercise, emotion and anaesthesia with halothane. The β blockers are effective in preventing exercise-induced ventricular ectopics in patients with coronary artery disease, in treating arrhythmias associated with mitral valve prolapse, and in reducing the number and complexity of ventricular ectopics after myocardial infarction. They appear to reduce the incidence of sudden death after myocardial infarction by attenuating sympathetic stimulation.

Adverse effects. Although severe hypotension, bradycardia and reduction in cardiac output can occur, the most common adverse effects are not cardiovascular. These include exacerbation of asthma and chronic obstructive pulmonary disease, fatigue, insomnia, impotence, nightmares and depression. CNS effects are more common with the lipid soluble drugs. Cardiac effects can include worsening of left ventricular function, congestive cardiac failure, sinus node dysfunction, atrioventricular block, worsening of compromised limb blood flow with claudication, and Raynaud's phenomenon. In general, β blockers are contraindicated in patients with heart block. In addition, a β-adrenoceptor blocker withdrawal syndrome has been described. In patients on chronic treatment with β-blocking drugs, abrupt withdrawal of the drug 10–48 hours before major surgery (elective coronary artery bypass grafting) produced much greater sympathetic responses to intubation and surgery compared with those patients who continued to take their medication up to the time of surgery. The explanation seems to be that in patients on chronic treatment there is an increase in the number of β adrenoceptors. When the β blocker is suddenly withdrawn, an increased pool of sensitive receptors becomes open to endogenous catecholamine stimulation. The result may be unstable angina, myocardial infarction, hypertension and stroke, or lethal arrhythmia.

At the time of writing (1996), there are 15 β blocking drugs listed in the *British National Formulary*. The following discussion is limited to those drugs considered to be of most interest to anaesthetists.

Propranolol

Propranolol is the prototype of the β blocking drugs, and most of the information on the antiarrhythmic actions of β blockers comes from studies with propranolol. It is non-cardioselective and has high lipid solubility and protein binding. Extreme caution is required where it is used in combination with clonidine, class I antiarrhythmics or Ca^{2+} blocking drugs such as verapamil.

Dosage and administration. Oral dosage may vary from 10 mg twice daily to 320 mg day^{-1}, depending on whether arrhythmia or severe systemic hypertension is being treated. Sustained release preparations are available. Intravenous doses of 0.25–5 mg are used to control blood pressure, heart rate and arrhythmia during anaesthesia.

Metoprolol

Metoprolol is a cardioselective drug used in the treatment of hypertension, angina, arrhythmias, thyrotoxicosis and postmyocardial infarction. In the latter use it may reduce infarct size. It is contraindicated in atrioventricular block and in heart failure refractory to digitalis. Insulin dosage may require adjustment in diabetic patients. It is relatively safe in asthmatics.

Dosage and administration. Oral dosage may vary from 100 to 400 mg daily. The intravenous dose for control of arrhythmias is up to 5 mg at a rate of 1–2 mg min^{-1}, repeated after 5 minutes, total dose 10–15 mg.

Acebutalol

Acebutalol is cardioselective and possesses in-

trinsic sympathomimetic activity which tends to balance the negative chronotropic and inotropic effects of the drug. It accumulates in renal failure.

Dosage and administration. Oral dosage is 200–400 mg twice a day.

Atenolol

Atenolol is relatively cardioselective and therefore has a lesser effect on airways resistance. It is water soluble and thus less likely to enter the brain and cause sleep disturbance and nightmares. Atenolol is excreted by the kidneys and may accumulate in renal failure.

Dosage and administration. Oral dosage is 50–100 mg daily. By intravenous injection the dosage is 2.5 mg at a rate of 1 mg min^{-1} to a maximum of 10 mg.

Oxprenolol

Oxprenolol has some partial agonist activity (intrinsic sympathomimetic activity) which helps to balance the negative chronotropic and inotropic effects of the drug. It is used in the treatment of angina, hypertension, sympathetic-induced arrhythmias, anxiety and anxiety-induced tachycardia. It is also used in the treatment of hypertrophic obstructive cardiomyopathy, thyrotoxicosis and arrhythmias associated with anaesthesia.

Dosage and administration. Oral dosage is 40–100 mg three times a day.

Esmolol

Esmolol is a recently introduced drug whose unique properties should guarantee an essential place in anaesthesia and intensive care medicine where a rapidly controllable effect is required. Esmolol's ester linkage is rapidly hydrolysed by plasma and erythrocyte esterases (not pseudocholinesterase), so that the half-life is only 9 minutes. The carboxylic acid metabolite has 1/500 the potency of the parent compound but has a half-life of 4 hours and is excreted by the kidneys. The peak effect of esmolol occurs within 6 minutes of the loading dose and disappears within 20 minutes of stopping the drug. It is very effective in controlling tachycardias resulting from noxious stimuli. Hypotension may occur. Fatal cardiac arrest was reported where the drug was used to control stress tachycardia in a patient suffering from multiple trauma.

Dosage and administration. An intravenous loading dose of 500 μg kg^{-1} over 4 minutes has been suggested, followed by an infusion of 50 μg kg^{-1} min^{-1}. If the desired effect is not achieved, the loading dose is repeated and the infusion increased to 100 μg kg^{-1} min^{-1}. This can repeated to a maximum infusion rate of 300 μg kg^{-1} min^{-1}. This requires caution and clinical judgement. Titration of the loading dose in 10 mg bolus increments may be preferred. The safety of prolonged infusions has not been established.

Class III agents

Amiodarone

Amiodarone prolongs the duration of the action potential and the refractory period in both atria and ventricles. High dose may lead to a β blocking action and effects similar to those with quinidine. Good results are obtained with both ventricular and supraventricular arrhythmias, in the latter particularly if associated with the Wolff–Parkinson–White syndrome (aberrant atrioventricular conduction). Use of amiodarone is limited to those arrhythmias resistant to standard antiarrhythmic compounds, but it is now the drug of choice in such circumstances, and is a first line drug in perioperative and critical care situations.

Pharmacokinetics. Onset of action is slow, taking 6 days with oral treatment. The drug is very lipid soluble and antiarrhythmic activity after intravenous administration is variable in onset. The drug molecule is deiodinated and leads to a rise in serum tri-iodothyronine levels by blocking conversion of thyroxine. Plasma concentrations of the main metabolite, desmethyl-amiodarone, which is active, are similar to that of the parent drug. Elimination is by hepatic excretion.

Dosage and administration. The intravenous dose is 5 mg kg^{-1} given by infusion over a period of 20 minutes to 2 hours, in an emergency it can be given slowly, 150–300 mg over 1–2 minutes. The usual oral dose is 200–800 mg daily, 5–7 days a week.

Adverse effects. Vasodilatation, hypotension or bradycardia may occur after intravenous administration, particularly if given rapidly. Corneal microdeposits, photosensitisation, skin discoloration (grey or blue pigmentation), hypo- or hyperthyroidism, liver dysfunction, interstitial pulmonary infiltration and muscle weakness may all occur but are usually reversible. Simultaneous administration of amiodarone and quinidine is dangerous. Warfarin and digoxin dosage may require reduction.

Bretylium

Bretylium has adrenergic nerve-blocking properties and accumulates in sympathetic ganglia, decreases noradrenaline release and in high dosage produces a chemical sympathectomy. There may be an initial sympathomimetic effect from transient discharge of noradrenaline from adrenergic postganglionic terminals.

Bretylium is effective against ventricular fibrillation refractory to lignocaine and direct current shocks. It may also be used in other ventricular arrhythmias refractory to more conventional therapy.

Pharmacokinetics. Onset of action after intramuscular injection is slow and erratic. Plasma concentrations are of no value in predicting efficacy or toxicity.

Dosage and administration. The drug is only used in resuscitation. The intravenous dose is 5–10 mg kg^{-1} given slowly over 10–30 minutes with blood pressure and electrocardiogram (ECG) monitoring. Dilute solutions of 10 mg ml^{-1} can be given to a total dosage of 30 mg kg^{-1}. Intramuscular injections of 5 mg kg^{-1} 6–8 hourly may cause muscle necrosis.

Sotalol

Sotalol is a non-selective β-adrenoceptor antagonist which also prolongs cardiac repolarisation — in other words it has class III antiarrhythmic properties. The class III effects predominate, and the drug exhibits a broader antiarrhythmic profile than other β blockers. It is devoid of intrinsic sympathomimetic action, is lipid insoluble, has negligible first pass metabolism and is minimally metabolised, accumulates in renal failure, and has a low proarrhythmic effect. Its use in hypokalaemia or with other drugs likely to prolong the QT interval is hazardous.

Dosage and administration. The oral dose is 80–300 mg twice a day, while the intravenous dose is 20–60 mg given over 2–3 minutes with ECG monitoring; this can be repeated.

Class IV agents

Calcium channel blockers

The calcium channel blockers, sometimes less correctly called calcium antagonists, interfere with the inward displacement of calcium ions through the slow channels of active cell membranes (Fig. 24.2). Increased free intracellular calcium increases smooth muscle contractility, peripheral resistance and blood pressure. Calcium blocking drugs lower intracellular calcium levels and cause vasodilatation. Large arteries are less affected than peripheral resistance vessels, and cerebral, coronary and mesenteric arteries. Endogenous catecholamines stimulate α_2 receptors, an effect mediated by an influx of calcium ions which may be inhibited by calcium blockers. All of these drugs are effective in treating essential hypertension and the coronary vasodilating properties make them useful in treating angina. Diltiazem and verapamil depress sinoatrial node automaticity and slow atrioventricular node conduction and are therefore useful in treating supraventricular arrhythmias. There are three chemical classes of calcium channel blockers: phenylalkylamines, benzothiazepines and dihydropyridines. They are all well absorbed from the gut but undergo extensive first pass metabolism, so their bioavailabilities range from 10 to 50%. The drugs are hightly protein bound, and the main route of elimination is the liver. They are rapidly metabolised and have short half-lives. Slow release preparations are available for some. At the time of writing, nine drugs are listed in the British National Formulary. Only those of

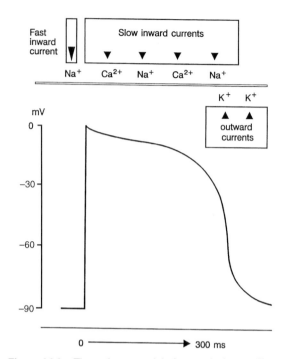

Figure 24.2 The action potential of a ventricular myofibre and associated ion fluxes. The fast inward current is carried by sodium and is followed by a plateau due to a second, slower inward current carried by calcium. The outward current in carried by potassium.

particular interest to anaesthetists are discussed here.

Verapamil

Verapamil is a diphenylalkamine. It exerts its antiarrhythmic effect by blocking the transmembrane movement of calcium ions within the myocardium. Its greatest effects are observed in the sinoatrial and atrioventricular nodes by inhibiting depolarisation. Electrocardiographically, verapamil prolongs the AH interval and the effective refractory period of the atrioventricular node. On the surface ECG, the PR interval is prolonged. Verapamil is very effective in the treatment of supraventricular arrhythmias. It is not as effective in the treatment of ventricular ectopic beats or ventricular tachycardias, although occasional success has been seen.

Pharmacokinetics. After oral administration, the drug is rapidly absorbed. First pass metabolism is extensive so that bioavailability is only 10–20%. Protein binding is approximately 90%. The principal metabolite, norverapamil, is active, with about 20% of the antiarrhythmic activity of verapamil. The elimination half-life is 4–5 hours.

Dosage and administration. The recommended oral dose is 240–480 mg day^{-1} in divided doses. A sustained release formulation is available. The intravenous dose is 5–10 mg given over 1–3 minutes and repeated in 5–10 minutes if necessary.

Adverse effects. Transient hypotension after intravenous injection is common. Bradycardia or atrioventricular block may occur, particularly if the patient is receiving β-blocking therapy. It should not be used in patients with the sick sinus syndrome, second or third degree heart block or poor left ventricular function. Severe adverse effects may be countered by calcium salts.

Nifedipine

Nifedipine is the prototype of the dihydropyridines. It has no effect on atrioventricular conduction and therefore no antiarrhythmic effect. It can rapidly lower blood pressure when given sublingually or orally. It is widely used in the treatment of hypertension and of angina and can be used in the emergency treatment of acute hypertension. It is also used in the treatment of Raynaud's phenomenon. Although an intravenous preparation has been prepared, it is very unstable in light, and is not available in the UK. Intranasal administration has been described.

Dosage and administration. The usual dose is 10–20 mg (1–2 capsules) every 6–8 hours.

Diltiazem

Diltiazem is a benzothiazepine which has been extensively used in the treatment of angina and hypertension. Its mechanism of action is similar to that of other calcium channel blocking agents. It also slows atrioventricular nodal conduction and prolongs refractoriness and therefore has a significant antiarrhythmic effect, although less so than verapamil. However, diltiazem has less effect on left ventricular function than verapamil,

so it may have some advantage. An intravenous formulation has been made available in the USA.

Pharmacokinetics. Diltiazem is 90% absorbed after oral administration. First pass metabolism is rapid. N-monodesmethyl diltiazem is the principal metabolite and possesses 20% of diltiazem activity. Protein binding is 80–90% and the elimination half-life is 2–11 hours.

Dosage and administration. Oral dosing is 120–360 mg daily. Sustained release preparations are available.

Adverse effects. The drug is usually well tolerated. Atrioventricular block may occur, particularly if the patient has received β-blocking drugs.

Nimodipine

Nimodipine is a dihydropyridine calcium channel blocker which acts particularly on cerebral blood vessels. It is used in the prevention and treatment of ischaemic neurological deficits caused by arterial vasospasm following subarachnoid haemorrhage. When taken by mouth, nimodipine is rapidly absorbed from the gastrointestinal tract. First pass metabolism is extensive and the bioavailability is about 13%. It readily crosses the blood–brain barrier. It is extensively metabolised in the liver. Elimination half-life is 1–2 hours and protein binding is 95%.

Dosage and administration. Oral dosage for prophylaxis of neurological deficit is 60 mg 4-hourly. Once cerebral ischaemia occurs, the drug is infused into a central vein at a rate of 1 mg h^{-1} increasing to 2 mg h^{-1}. The infusion is continued for at least 5 days and not more than 14 days. The solution is light sensitive and incompatible with some plastics, including polyvinylchloride.

Adverse effects. Severe hypotension may occur, particularly where other antihypertensive agents, diuretics or β blockers are being used.

Miscellaneous agents

Adenosine

Adenosine is an endogenous purine nucleoside which is active on the myocardium through stimulation of cAMP and the adenosine receptor. Two adenosine receptors (A$_1$ and A$_2$) have been identified. Adenosine causes arterial vasodilatation and coronary vasodilatation. The principal electrophysiological effect is prolongation of atrioventricular refractoriness and conduction. Adenosine slows the heart by a dose dependent increase in AH conduction with atrioventricular block. It is administered intravenously and has an ultrashort half-life of 0.6–1.5 seconds and a duration of effect of 1–2 minutes. Adenosine is effective in the termination of supraventricular tachycardias and Wolff–Parkinson–White syndrome tachycardias and in diagnosis of wide complex tachycardia as against supraventricular tachycardia. Its use with ventricular tachycardia has led to profound collapse and cardiac arrest. Its use in any form of heart block should be avoided.

Dosage and administration. The recommended dose is 3 mg given rapidly intravenously over 1–2 seconds. This can be repeated at a dose of 6 mg if the tachycardia is not terminated in 1–2 minutes, and again at a dose of 12 mg, but if still ineffective should not be tried further.

Adverse effects. Facial flushing, nausea, dizziness and syncope are common. Hypotension and bradycardia may occur. Dipyridamole may potentiate the action of adenosine, by inhibiting degradation, and may lead to prolonged atrioventricular nodal block, and their combined use should be avoided.

Digoxin

Although the cardiac glycosides have been around for over 200 years, the precise mechanism for their action is still a matter for debate. Digitalis glycoside or digoxin binds to the enzyme Na^+,K^+-ATPase on the cardiac cell membrane. This binding is reversible and associated with enzyme inhibition, thus leading to an increase in intracellular sodium and a decrease in intracellular potassium. The increase in sodium reduces calcium exchange by reducing the transmembrane sodium gradient and depressing the Na^+,Ca^{2+} ion countertransport system. The net effect is thus an increase in sodium and calcium inside the cell, and the latter is thought to be responsible for the positive inotropic effect.

Digoxin also exerts its cardiovascular effects partly through cholinergic stimulation. The principal electrophysiological effect is slowing of the atrioventricular node conduction and prolonging of the refractory period. Sinus node automaticity is also slowed, an effect mediated through the vagus nerve. The PR interval is prolonged and there may be ST and T changes. Digoxin is primarily used to treat atrial fibrillation and paroxysmal supraventricular tachycardia. It is said to be as effective as the β blockers or the calcium channel blockers. It is ineffective in the Wolff–Parkinson–White syndrome.

Pharmacokinetics. Bioavailability for digoxin tablets is 60–80%. Approximately 20–25% is protein bound. The volume of distribution is 7 l kg^{-1}. The elimination half-life is 20–30 hours in healthy volunteers. In renal failure and in the aged, the elimination half-life increases. Therapeutic serum concentrations range from 0.9 to 2.0 ng l^{-1}. Patients with a serum concentration > 2 ng l^{-1} usually show some signs of toxicity.

Dosage and administration. Digoxin is available in oral and intravenous formulation: for rapid digitalisation by mouth 1–1.5 mg in divided doses over 24 hours; less urgent digitalisation 250–500 μg daily. The maintenance dose is 62.5–500 μg daily, according to renal function. When very rapid control is needed, digoxin may be given intravenously in a dose of 0.75–1 mg, preferably as an infusion over 2 hours or more. This is followed by normal maintenance therapy.

Adverse effects. These are usually a sign of toxicity. Cardiac effects include atrial or ventricular premature beats, ventricular tachycardia, bigeminy, trigeminy, junctional rhythm and heart block. Non-cardiac effects include nausea, vomiting, anorexia, malaise, fatigue, delerium and seizures. Digoxin toxicity is occasionally seen in the elderly. Treatment of toxicity is usually supportive, although lignocaine and phenytoin have been used to treat arrhythmias. Rapid reversal of acute toxicity can be achieved with the use of digoxin specific antibodies (Fab fragments).

Phenytoin

Phenytoin by slow intravenous injection was

formerly used in ventricular arrhythmias, particularly those caused by cardiac glycosides, but this use is now obsolete. The dose was 3.5–5 mg kg^{-1} by slow intravenous injection at a rate not exceeding 50 mg min^{-1}, with blood pressure and ECG monitoring.

Magnesium (Magnesium sulfate USP)

Magnesium has electrophysiological effects similar to those of class III agents and has been compared to amiodarone. Magnesium slows the conduction through the atrioventricular node and prolongs the refractory period in the atria and ventricles. It may be effective in patients with ventricular tachycardia or torsade de pointes unresponsive to other agents. It may also protect against sudden death after myocardial infarction.

Dosage and administration. Magnesium salts are poorly absorbed from the gut. The usual dose for treating arrhythmia is 8 mmol (200 mg) of the sulphate given intravenously over 10–20 minutes.

Adverse effects. The major adverse effect after bolus injection or infusion of magnesium is hypotension. Haemodynamic collapse can be fatal. Magnesium is excreted by the kidneys and accumulates in renal failure.

GENERAL ANAESTHESIA AND ANTIARRHYTHMIC DRUGS

Halothane (and trichlorethylene and cyclopropane) strongly sensitises the myocardium to the action of adrenaline, which accelerates phase 4 depolarisation and thus increases automaticity. Halothane prolongs atrioventricular nodal conduction time and can probably set up re-entry mechanisms in the atrioventricular node. The lesser effect of enflurane on atrioventricular conduction makes such disturbances less likely. Isoflurane has no demonstrable effect on atrioventricular conduction. The cardiovascular effects of sevoflurane and desflurane are similar to those of isoflurane. Hypercarbia provokes ventricular arrhythmias during halothane anaesthesia, presumably due to increased endogenous secretion of adrenaline. Exogenous adrenaline will have the same effect.

Specific α-adrenergic receptors are thought to exist in the heart, which respond to adrenaline in the presence of halothane. Pancuronium, gallamine and alcuronium all increase heart rate. Suxamethonium frequently causes bradycardia in children or after repeated doses, but where a sudden increase in serum potassium is caused, as in severe burns or in patients with paralysed muscles, a variety of tachyarrhythmias occur. Sympathetic stimulation during laryngoscopy and intubation, and surgical stimulation during light anaesthesia, are other frequent causes of tachyarrhythmias.

Treatment

In general, supraventricular tachyarrhythmias are benign, while ventricular tachyarrhythmias are more likely to be malignant. This must be qualified by stating that patients with severe coronary artery disease, the elderly and the ill may tolerate any tachycardia badly.

Sinus tachycardia often responds to increasing the depth of anaesthesia. Paroxysmal supraventricular tachycardia may involve a re-entry process within the atrioventricular connection in parallel with the node. Termination of an attack of tachycardia may be effected by any manoeuvre which will alter autonomic tone and block atrioventricular conduction. Thus carotid sinus pressure, the Valsalva manoeuvre, digoxin or intravenous edrophonium (up to 10 mg) may all be effective, but a β-adrenergic blocking drug is preferable as specific therapy for slowing atrioventricular node conduction. Verapamil may also be useful, but should not be used after β blockade because a synergistic effect on myocardial function may precipitate heart failure. Atrial fibrillation or flutter is usually treated with intravenous digoxin with rapid short term control by β blockade. Esmolol may be useful in this situation. Premature ventricular contractions that occur singly and are unifocal, do not require treatment. Premature ventricular contractions that occur in salvos, more than five per minute, are multifocal or exhibit an R on T phenomenon usually require urgent treatment as they herald ventricular tachycardia or ventricular fibrillation. Occasionally simple measures to increase the depth of anaesthesia while increasing ventilation are sufficient. Malignant ventricular ectopic beats and ventricular tachycardias are an indication for antiarrhythmic drug therapy. Lignocaine is usually effective in a 100 mg bolus (or 1 mg kg^{-1}). Some arrhythmias considered to be ventricular in origin may be supraventricular and these respond best to a β blocker, as will sinus tachycardias which cause ST depression in patients with severe myocardial ischaemia. Ventricular fibrillation, and in many instances, ventricular tachycardia are indications for immediate electrical direct current countershock and the antiarrhythmic drugs are used to prevent the patient converting back to the arrhythmia. Cardioversion may also be indicated to terminate some episodes of supraventricular tachycardia, and to convert atrial flutter or fibrillation to normal rhythm. In deciding which antiarrhythmic drug to use, one appropriate to the arrhythmia and its site of origin must be selected (Tables 24.2–24.5). Thus digoxin, propranolol, esmolol, intravenous potassium and bretylium suppress enhanced automaticity of the sinus node. Digoxin increases — while quinidine, procainamide and lignocaine reduce — the automaticity of the Purkinje system. Patients are more sensitive to the hypotensive effects of calcium channel blockers when inhalational agents are being used. Ca^{2+} infusions will reverse the haemodynamic depressive effects of calcium blockers on the myocardium and vasculature, although a β agonist may be required to oppose unwanted conduction effects. When deciding between a β-blocking drug or a calcium blocker it should be appreciated that verapamil is highly efficacious (close to 90%) in the treatment of paroxysmal atrial tachycardia. Both β blockers and verapamil will slow the ventricular response to atrial flutter and fibrillation. The β blockers are effective in treating some types of ventricular arrhythmia, while the role of verapamil is somewhat unclear. The latter would be preferable in a patient with asthma or bronchospasm but verapamil and β blockers must not be used together. Amiodarone is becoming more and more a first line drug in the treatment of both ventricular and supraventricular arrhythmias in the perioperative period.

Tachyarrhythmias: causes and treatment

Outside the operating theatre, the place where arrhythmias are most commonly found is in the intensive care unit. Here, inadequate sedation can result in a marked sinus tachycardia, often accompanied by hypertension. Heart disease and various medical disorders, sepsis, electrolyte disturbances or digoxin toxicity may be responsible for a variety of supraventricular and ventricular arrhythmias. Atrial and ventricular ectopics may be due to inotropes, theophylline, hypoxia and other factors, where antiarrhythmic drugs may not be the treatment of choice. Where the patient is haemodynamically compromised, verapamil, flecainide, class Ia agents and β blockers should be avoided and synchronised direct current (DC) cardioversion may be the treatment of choice. Multiple organ dysfunction will affect drug clearance and increase the risk of drug interactions. In the treatment of supraventricular tachycardia, adenosine in an initial bolus of 3 mg through a large vein followed by a saline flush may be effective. It can be very effective in the treatment of paroxysmal junctional re-entrant tachycardias but should be used with caution in patients with asthma or chronic obstructive airways disease. Other drugs commonly used in supraventricular tachycardia are β blockers, digoxin, amiodarone and solatol; other drugs which should not be used where there is impaired left ventricular function are verapamil, flecainide, disopyramide and procainamide. Esmolol may be the drug of choice in the treatment of rapid atrial fibrillation. If given via a peripheral vein, it requires dilution and can result in a substantial fluid load: higher concentrations can be given via a central vein. Hypotension is common but 95% of patients become normotensive within 30 minutes of the infusion being stopped. Esmolol is contraindicated in patients who are dependent on β-adrenergic stimulation, which rather limits its use. Digoxin is no longer recommended as the drug of first choice in atrial fibrillation due to its slowness and uncertainty of action, amiodarone is more effective and may cardiovert or maintain normal rhythm, as may sotalol. The class Ic agents flecainide or propafenone have also been used to cardiovert and to prevent recurrence of atrial fibrillation. Flecainide should not be used where there is left ventricular dysfunction due to the high risk of proarrhythmia. The class Ia agents quinidine and disopyramide have been in use for many years. If the situation is urgent and atrial fibrillation of recent onset, DC cardioversion may be the treatment of choice.

In atrial flutter, slowing the ventricular rate with atrioventricular nodal blocking drugs, such as verapamil, β blockers or digoxin, may be difficult. Synchronised DC cardioversion with low energy shocks is the treatment of choice and class Ic, III or Ia agents can be used as prophylaxis against recurrence. Occasionally right atrial pacing will be required. Class Ia or Ic agents should not be used in flutter unless atrioventricular nodal blocking drugs have also been administered, as there is a risk of a 1:1 ventricular response. Atrial tachycardias are notoriously difficult to treat and are often refractory to both drugs and cardioversion. Atrial tachycardia with atrioventricular block is often due to digoxin toxicity and associated with potassium or magnesium deficiency.

Ventricular tachycardias are usually associated with significant ischaemic myocardial disease or hypertrophic cardiomyopathy. Cardioversion may be the safest treatment, although if the haemodynamic consequences of the arrhythmia are not serious, an intravenous lignocaine infusion is still the treatment of choice. Procainamide is an effective alternative, and high dose amiodarone may be used as second line therapy in resistant cases. Occasionally ventricular pacing is required.

Polymorphic ventricular tachycardia, of which *torsade de pointes* is a specific form, is often a manifestation of a proarrhythmic effect of either antiarrhythmics or other drugs, often associated with an electrolyte upset. Prompt cardioversion is required and antiarrhythmics must be avoided, as further proarrhythmic effects may be seen. Electrolyte correction with potassium and magnesium is required, and either atrial, ventricular or atrioventricular sequential dual chamber pacing may be required.

Bradyarrhythmias: causes and treatment

The bradyarrhythmias are due to decreased automaticity of the sinoatrial node or to a block in the atrioventricular conduction system. A rate of under 60 beats per minute is considered to be a bradycardia, although this is common in athletes and is also a feature of pathological conditions such as myxoedema, jaundice and raised intracranial pressure and occurs secondary to adrenergic blocking drugs and digoxin. Rates below 40 beats per minutes are usually symptomatic. A latent pacemaker may or may not assume dominance. High vagal tone slows impulse formation in the sinoatrial node and slows conduction through the atrioventricular node. The vagus nerve does not affect conduction through the His–Purkinje system. Block occurring in the His–Purkinje system (infranodal block) is usually permanent and may be progressive. Patients with right bundle branch block and left posterior hemiblock were at one time thought to run a high risk of developing trifascicular or complete heart block and to require pacing; it is now thought that only about 1% of patients progress to complete heart block each year and that the remainder tend to be reasonably stable. Treatment of sinus bradycardia is with oxygen and either lightening or deepening of anaesthesia according to circumstance, and the use of atropine 0.3–2.0 mg, glycopyrrolate 0.2–0.6 mg, isoprenaline 1 mg diluted to 250 ml with saline or 5% dextrose (giving 4 μg ml^{-1}) and infused beginning at 0.01 μg kg^{-1} min^{-1} and adjusted to attain the required response, or in resistant cases, cardiac pacing.

Sick sinus syndrome

This refers to rhythm disturbances resulting from failure of normal impulse formation in the sinoatrial node. These rhythm disturbances may include:

- persistent sinus bradycardia
- intervals of sinus arrest

- paroxysmal or chronic atrial fibrillation
- tachycardia alternating with bradycardia.

The most common cause for the sick sinus syndrome is ischaemic heart disease.

Heart block

Heart block may have organic or functional causes. Reasons for organic lesions are fibrotic degenerative disease of the conduction system (Lenègre's or Lev's disease), ischaemic heart disease, cardiomyopathies, myocarditis, surgical operations or congenital abnormalities. These lesions tend to be permanent. Functional causes are increased vagal tone, and drug therapy with digoxin, quinidine, procainamide, propranolol or potassium, all of which are usually reversible. The different degrees of heart block are tabulated in Table 24.4.

Proarrhythmia

Drug treatment of cardiac arrhythmias is not always effective and may cause side-effects. The Cardiac Arrhythmia Suppression Trial (CAST) was instituted in 1986 and patients convalescing from myocardial infarctions who had asymptomatic ventricular ectopic beats that were suppressed by encainide or flecainide were randomly assigned to long term drug therapy or placebo. The mortality rate in the patients receiving either

drug was two to three times higher than that in the patients receiving placebo. CAST was designed to test the hypothesis that suppressing ventricular ectopic beats reduces mortality, which it clearly does not. The mechanisms responsible for these results are unclear, but a likely explanation for the increase in mortality was an increase in fatal arrhythmias due to a proarrhythmia effect of the drugs. A third drug, moracizine, was tested more recently in CAST II. Overall, the mortality rate was similar among patients treated with moracizine and those given placebo, but there was significantly greater mortality during the initial two-week period among the patients treated with moracizine. All these drugs belong to class Ic and block cardiac sodium channels, and it has been suggested that sodium channel blockade may activate, rather than suppress, potential circuits for ventricular tachycardia. No other antiarrhythmic drugs have been as rigorously tested as those in the CAST trials, but there is evidence to suggest that therapy with lignocaine, procainamide, quinidine, sotalol, disopyramide and amiodarone all increase long term mortality. The last five named are all capable of markedly prolonging the QT interval and this can set the scene for the polymorphic ventricular tachycardia known as *torsade de pointes*. Most episodes of *torsade de pointes* are self-limiting or associated with syncope but they can progress to ventricular fibrillation, the incidence of which is unknown. No one would question that patients with sustained tachycardias benefit from termination of their arrhythmia; the risks associated with intravenous administration of adenosine or verapamil in patients with supraventricular tachycardia, or lignocaine or cardioversion in those with ventricular tachycardia, are small and the benefits of therapy are self-evident. Long term therapy to prevent recurrences depends on an understanding of the underlying problem. Re-entry within the atrioventricular node or involving an accessory atrioventricular bypass tract can be prevented with atrioventricular blocking drugs such as digoxin or verapamil, provided there is no pre-excitation on the sinus rhythm ECG. Flecainide could be considered if there is no

Table 24.4 Heart block

Type of heart block	Description
First degree	PR interval > 0.21 s
Second degree	
Mobitz type I	Progressive lengthening of PR prior to dropping of the QRS complex (Wenckebach phenomenon)
Mobitz type II	No progressive lengthening of PR, but sudden drop of QRS — serious prognosis, often progression to third degree block
Third degree	Atrial and ventricular rate independent, may be infranodal (slow rate, QRS wide, cardiac output decreased) or AV nodal (QRS normal width, faster rate, adequate cardiac output

underlying heart disease. Catheter ablation may be considered for those with pre-excitation (the Wolff–Parkinson–White syndrome). The most common cause of sustained ventricular tachycardia is re-entry at the border zone of an old myocardial infarct. Sotalol or amiodarone seem to have the most efficacy. The role of implantable cardioverter defibrillators is being examined, although their effect on long term survival (beyond 5 years) may be small.

Preoperative care

Bradyarrhythmias, particularly if profound or associated with dizziness or syncope, are usually managed with pacemakers. Very rarely does chronic bifascicular block (right bundle branch block with left anterior or posterior hemiblock) progress to complete heart block and sudden perioperative death. However, these patients have a high 5 year mortality (30–40%) and most

Table 24.5 Antiarrhythmic drug therapy

Drug	Indication	I.v. dose regimens	Comments
Adenosine	Supraventricular tachycardia WPW syndromes	3–6–12 mg over 1–2 s followed by saline flush	Avoid in heart block Avoid after dipyridamole
Amiodarone	Atrial, re-entrant junctional, ventricular tachycardias Atrial flutter/fibrillation	300 mg infused over 20–30 min followed by infusion of 1000 mg over 24 h	If possible use central vein to avoid phlebitis
Bretylium	Ventricular tachycardia and fibrillation	5 mg kg^{-1} i.m. 6–8-hourly or bolus 500 mg i.v. diluted	RF. May cause hypotension after initial sympathomimetic effects
Digoxin	Atrial flutter/fibrillation*	0.5–1.0 mg by slow i.v.i. or infusion	RF
Disopyramide	Atrial, re-entrant junctional tachycardias	2 mg kg^{-1} over 5 min to max 150 mg Maintenance infusion up to 800 mg 24 h^{-1}	Risk of heart failure, urinary retention. RF
Esmolol	Supraventricular tachycardia WPW syndrome, PVCs	500 μg kg^{-1} over 4 min then 50 μg kg^{-1} min^{-1} by infusion	Contraindicated in LVF, CCF, heart block, asthma
Flecainide	Atrial, re-entrant junctional and ventricular tachycardias Atrial fibrillation	2 mg kg^{-1} over 10 min or longer. Max bolus 150 mg. Infusion 1.5 mg kg^{-1} in first hour, then 0.25 mg kg^{-1} h^{-1}	May precipitate heart failure Not in AV block unless pacing available. RF
Lignocaine	Ventricular tachycardia	100 mg bolus, then infusion 4 mg min^{-1} for 30 min; maintenance 2–3 mg min^{-1}	Avoid in AV block. HF
Metoprolol	Sinus, re-entrant junctional tachycardias Atrial fibrillation*	5 mg bolus, max. dose 15 mg	As for esmolol. Avoid concomitant therapy with verapamil
Mexiletine	Ventricular arrhythmias	100–250 mg in 5–10 min, then infusion 250 mg in first hour 250 mg in next 2 h, then 0.5 mg min^{-1}	CNS and gastrointestinal side-effects, bradycardia, hypotension
Procainamide	Atrial, junctional and ventricular arrhythmias	100 mg every 2 min to total 1000 mg in 1 h	May cause hypotension, heart block
Sotalol	Supraventricular and ventricular arrhythmias, PVCs, WPW syndrome	20–60 mg over 2–3 min. Can be repeated	Monitor ECG. As for esmolol, metoprolol
Tocainide	Ventricular tachycardia	250 mg in 2 min, 500 in 15 min, then 500 mg every 6 h for 48 h	As for lignocaine. Dose dependent CNS, gastrointestinal effects. RF
Verapamil	Multifocal atrial tachycardia Re-entrant junctional tachycardia Atrial flutter/fibrillation*	5 mg bolus, repeat after 5–10 min to max. 15–20 mg	May cause hypotension, heart failure. Avoid if β blocker has been given

WPW, Wolff–Parkinson–White; PVCs, premature ventricular contractions; RF, reduce dose in renal failure; HF, reduce dose in heart failure; LVF, left ventricular failure; CCF, congestive cardiac failure.
* Slows ventricular response.

of the deaths are due to myocardial infarction or tachyarrhythmias, events usually not preventable by pacemakers. The anaesthetist should be aware that patients with bifascicular block on ECG may have associated coronary artery disease or left ventricular dysfunction. Although prophylactic insertion of temporary pacing wires is thought to be unnecessary, it would seem reasonable to establish central vein access in case a temporary pacemaker is required. Premature ventricular ectopics of more than five per minute on preoperative examination correlate with perioperative morbidity. Premature atrial contractions may also indicate that cardiac reserve is poor but careful management through the perioperative period is more important than specific antiarrhythmic therapy (Table 24.5). Similarly, management of the patient with the pre-excitation syndrome to avoid techniques that may stimulate the sympathetic nervous system to release catecholamines may be more important than any particular drug regimen.

Although there is insufficient evidence available to warrant changing the dosage of antiarrhythmic drugs during the perioperative period, the pharmacological properties of some drugs can affect anaesthetic management. Disopyramide may produce anticholinergic effects, including tachycardia, urinary retention and psychosis. Hepatitis may also occur. Chronic therapy with bretylium has been associated with hypersensitivity to vasopressors. Quinidine can have vagolytic effects that can decrease atrioventricular block. Most of the antiarrhythmic agents enhance non-depolarising neuromuscular blockade; this has been confirmed for quinidine, phenytoin, lignocaine, procainamide and propranolol. Amiodarone can cause peripheral neuropathy, hypertension, bradycardia and decreased cardiac output. With a half-life of 29 days, its pharmacological effects persist for over 45 days after discontinuance.

Pacemakers

More than 90% of pacemakers are inserted for bradyarrhythmias. The most common pacemakers used are the multiprogrammable, ventricular

Table 24.6 Code for pacemaker modes

Chamber paced	Chamber sensed	Mode of response
V = ventricle	V = ventricle	I = inhibited
A = atrium	A = atrium	T = triggered
D = double (atrium and ventricle)	D = double (atrium and ventricle)	D = double (atrium triggered and ventricle inhibited)
	O = none	R = reserve
		O = none

A fourth character refers to pacemaker programmability.
A fifth character refers to antitachycardia capability.

inhibited or dual chamber types. Three-letter pacemaker codes are listed in Table 24.6. Lithium batteries have a 5–10 year life span. Atrial or ventricular pacemakers are used to terminate appropriate arrhythmias. Thus, in addition to knowledge of the patient's physical problems and drug therapy, detailed information should be obtained concerning the type and method of functioning of the pacemaker. Demand pacemakers can sense electrocautery, which sometimes inhibits pacemaker firing and leads to asystole. Most pacemakers can be converted to a fixed rate for the period of the operation. Diathermy and cardioversion should be done with the electrodes at least six inches (15 cm) away from the pacing box, or a bipolar form of electrocautery can be used. Since electrocautery may interfere with ECG monitoring and mask asystole, some form of flow detection should be employed, that is, diathermy-proof pulse oximetry, an intra-arterial line or a Doppler flow detector. The most common reason for pacemaker malfunction is loss of contact between the electrode and the endocardium. Treatment consists of advancing the electrode until it captures, administering isoprenaline, external pacing or cardiopulmonary resuscitation. Advances in the technology of implantable cardioverter defibrillators have increased the applicability of this potentially life saving device, but the impact on overall outcome has not been thoroughly tested and total mortality from cardiac causes remains substantial (30% at 5 years). Several large studies are underway to compare implantable devices with drug treatment, particularly amiodarone, sotalol and β blockade.

25

Inotropic drugs

T. J. McMurray
G. G. Lavery

A positive inotrope is a drug that, by a direct effect on the myocardium, increases cardiac contractility. This group of drugs does not include those that improve contractility solely by indirect mechanisms such as reducing afterload. In order to reflect common usage, the terms positive inotrope and inotrope are used synonymously.

Positive inotropic agents are widely used in critical care settings for a variety of problems, including cardiogenic and septic shock, chronic and acute congestive heart failure, coronary artery disease and postoperative deterioration of circulatory function.

Indications in cardiac surgery

There is invariably a mild to moderate depression of myocardial contractility after cardiac surgery. This reversible depression is due to manipulation of the heart, ischaemia during bypass, the presence of myocardial depressant drugs and the underlying preoperative myocardial pathology. The altered contractile state necessitates higher than normal filling pressures for optimal cardiac performance, and cardiac output is more sensitive to changes in preload and afterload.

Traditionally the treatment of low cardiac output associated with a cardiac operation has concentrated on the left ventricle and the systemic vasculature. Efforts are directed towards optimising left ventricular function, improving oxygen supply and demand, and allowing time for the ventricle to recover. This has been achieved largely with pharmacological enhancement of the contractile (inotropic) state of the myocardium in conjunction with the use of vasodilators.

Indications in intensive care

Inotropes are used for the treatment of hypoperfusion, tissue hypoxia, hypotension, acute cardiac failure, cardiogenic shock and the attainment of target parameters for oxygen transport.

Many intensive care patients will have systemic sepsis and/or multiple organ dysfunction. As described below, the need to improve either arterial blood pressure and/or tissue perfusion will dictate the choice of inotrope. The most controversial indication for inotropic support is the improvement of oxygen transport.

Oxygen transport encompasses oxygen delivery to the tissues and oxygen consumption by the tissues, and the relationship between them. The ratio of oxygen consumption to delivery (oxygen extraction ratio) is normally in the range 20–32%, averaging approximately 25%. Thus when oxygen delivery decreases there is some scope for compensation by increasing oxygen extraction to 40% or greater, but as this increases the tissues have increasing difficulty removing oxygen molecules from haemoglobin. At this point the factor limiting oxygen consumption is oxygen delivery, i.e. oxygen consumption is supply dependent.

In the late 1980s several groups investigated the haemodynamic profiles of critically ill patients. It appeared from these studies that patients who could spontaneously achieve a supranormal cardiac index, and thus high levels of oxygen delivery and consumption, had a significantly lower mortality rate than those who could not. Thus the concept of *supranormal goals* evolved and these were arbitrarily defined as cardiac index $> 4.5 \, l \, min^{-1} \, m^{-2}$, oxygen delivery $> 400 \, ml \, min^{-1} \, m^{-2}$ and oxygen consumption $> 170 \, ml \, min^{-1} \, m^{-2}$. Later, it was shown that *non-achievers* could be helped to attain these supranormal goals by the use of intravenous fluids and/or inotropes and that, if this occurred, their chances of survival were increased. The preferred

inotrope was usually dobutamine, although dopexamine may also be suitable.

CLASSIFICATION OF INOTROPIC DRUGS

Although there is increasing recognition that all inotropic agents are not alike, they continue to be viewed in the generic sense because of a lack of a classification system. Feldman (1993) proposed a classification system (Table 25.1) based on their mode of action, which is analogous to the classification system used for antidysrhythmic drugs by Vaughan Williams.

Myocardial stimulus–response coupling

A rational discussion of the classification of inotropes requires an understanding of the myocardial stimulus–response coupling process. Contraction of a myocyte is initiated by inward movement of calcium across the cell membrane through voltage dependent calcium channels. This inward flow of activator calcium triggers the release of calcium from the sarcoplasmic reticulum; the released calcium combines with troponin C, which induces a change in tropomyosin, thereby allowing the sliding of actin and myosin filaments and thus contraction. Therefore

Table 25.1 Classes of inotropic drugs by mechanism of action (after Feldman 1993)

Class	Definition
I	Agents that increase intracellular cyclic adenosine monophosphate *cAMP* β-Adrenergic agonists Phosphodiesterase inhibitors Glucagon
II	Agents that affect sarcolemma ion pumps/channels Digoxin
III	Agents that modulate intracellular calcium mechanisms by either: (a) release of sarcoplasmic reticulum calcium (IP$_3$), or (b) increased sensitization of the contractile proteins to calcium α$_1$-agonists; phenylephrine
IV	Drugs having multiple mechanisms of action Vesnarinone

the contractile state of the myocyte is closely related to the intracellular calcium concentration.

The modulation of intracellular calcium is controlled by the levels of cyclic adenosine monophosphate (cAMP), which can be increased by either stimulating the enzyme adenylate cyclase or averting its destruction by inhibiting the enzyme phosphodiesterase III. Adenylate cyclase can be stimulated by the binding of agonists to β_1 and β_2 receptors on the cell surface.

An increase in cAMP levels stimulates protein kinases, producing phosphorylation of membrane calcium channels. This augments calcium influx and thus contractility. Relaxation is induced by the sequestration of calcium into the sarcoplasmic reticulum, which is also an energy consuming process driven by adenosine triphosphate (ATP) dependent calcium pumps on the sarcoplasmic reticulum. Phosphorylation of phospholamban, a regulatory protein, by cAMP in cardiac cells leads to the enhanced extrusion of ionised calcium into the sarcoplasmic reticulum. This results in an increased rate of relaxation (lusitropy). Thus agents that increase cAMP can stimulate both increased force of contraction (inotropism) and increased relaxation (lusitropy).

CLASS I

These are agents that increase intracellular cAMP.

Catecholamines

Sympathomimetic drugs contain a benzene ring with an ethylamine side-chain; they mimic the effects of activation of the sympathetic nervous system. A catecholamine is a sympathomimetic drug whose benzene ring portion has hydroxyl group substitutions at positions 3 and 4 (catechol).

Both β-adrenergic receptor agonists and phosphodiesterase inhibitors increase cardiac contractility by increasing intracellular levels of cAMP. Whenever acute inotropic support is necessary, the agonists adrenaline, isoprenaline, dobutamine and noradrenaline are the mainstay of drug therapy. This is because of their favourable pharmacokinetic profile, predictable pharmaco-

dynamic response and a wide range of possible haemodynamic actions. These drugs (also called catecholamines) act by binding to different adrenergic receptors, which additionally are divided into different subtypes with distinct pharmacodynamic actions (Table 25.2). The physiological effect can be considered to be the algebraic sum of their relative action on the α, β and dopamine (DA) receptors. Each drug has a distinctive effect qualitatively and quantitatively on the myocardium and peripheral vasculature (Table 25.3).

In discussing the individual drugs it is essential to understand the following basic relationships:

$$\text{stroke volume } \alpha \text{ preload, contractility, afterload} \tag{1}$$

$$\text{cardiac output} = \text{heart rate} \times \text{stroke volume} \tag{2}$$

$$\underline{\text{arterial pressure} = \text{cardiac output} \times \text{peripheral resistance}.} \tag{3}$$

Therefore, from 2 and 3:

$$\underline{\text{arterial blood pressure} = \text{heart rate} \times \text{stroke volume} \times \text{peripheral resistance}.} \tag{4}$$

The pharmacodynamic effects of catecholamines are directly and, over the usual dose range, linearly related to their plasma concentrations, which directly depend upon the infusion rate. The plasma half-lives of the commonly used agents are short, ranging from 2 to 3 minutes, permitting steady-state plasma concentrations to be achieved within 10–15 minutes. Similarly, discontinuing the drug will end its haemodynamic effects within a similar period.

Adrenaline

Adrenaline is synthesised in sympathetic nerve endings and in the adrenal medulla, where it makes up 80% of the catecholamines present. It is derived from the amino acid phenylalanine, and the pathway also leads to the synthesis of dopamine and noradrenaline. Adrenaline is metabolised either by oxidation by monoamine oxidase or conjugation by catechol O-methyl transferase. This combined degradation pathway ensures fairly rapid elimination, although slower

Table 25.2 Adrenergic receptors

Receptor	Anatomical site	Action	LV function and stroke volume
α_1	Peripheral vascular smooth muscle	Constriction	Decreased
	Renal vascular smooth muscle	Constriction	
	Coronary arteries	Constriction	
	Myocardium (20–40% resting tone)	Positive inotropism	Improved
α_2	Peripheral vascular smooth muscle	Inhibits NA $\rightarrow$ dilatation	Improved
	Coronary arteries (endocardial)	Constriction	Decreased
β_1	Myocardium	Positive inotropism	Improved
	SA node	and chronotropism	
	Ventricular conduction		
β_2	Presynaptic (NA sensitive) myocardium	Accelerates NA release	Improved
	SA node		
	Postsynaptic (Adr sensitive) myocardium	Positive inotropism and chronotropism	Improved
	Vascular smooth muscle	Dilatation	
	Bronchial smooth muscle	Dilatation	Improved
	Renal vessels	Dilatation	Improved
DA_1	Blood vessels (renal, mesenteric, coronary)	Dilatation	
	Renal tubules	Naturesis, diuresis	
DA_2	Postganglionic sympathetic nerves	Inhibits NA release $\rightarrow$ vasodilatation	Improved
	Renal, mesenteric vessels	?Vasoconstriction	

LV, left ventricle; SA, sinoatrial; NA, noradrenaline; Adr, adrenaline

Table 25.3 Receptor activity of different adrenergic agonists

Drug	α_1	α_2	β_1	β_2	DA_1	DA_2	Dose dependence (α, β, or DA)
Phenylephrine	++++	?	+/−	0	0		+
Noradrenaline	++++	++++	+++	0	0		+++
Adrenaline	++++	+++	++++	++	0		++++
Isoprenaline	0	0	++++	++++	0		0
Dopamine	+ to ++++	?	++++	++	++++	+++	++++
Dobutamine	0 to +	?	++++	++	0		++
Dopexamine	0	0	+	++++	++	++	++
Ephedrine	++	?	+++	++	0	0	++

than circulating acetylcholine, and most adrenaline is excreted in the urine as vanillylmandelic acid.

Cardiovascular effects. Adrenaline has predominant actions at α and β_1 adrenoceptors and moderate activity at β_2 receptors. Its cardiovascular effects are complex and sometimes variable due to the spectrum of receptors upon which it acts. Its agonist action at β_1 receptors has positive inotropic and chronotropic effects. Arteriolar vasodilatation occurs in skeletal muscle and splanchnic and hepatic vascular beds, whereas arterioles supplying the skin and mucous membranes are constricted. Systemic vascular resistance is reduced or unchanged but cardiac output tends to increase. Low dose infusions (< 0.01 μg kg^{-1} min^{-1}) may decrease blood pressure through skeletal muscle vasodilatation (β_2 action), while moderate doses ($0.04–0.1\ \mu g\ kg^{-1}\ min^{-1}$) increase the heart rate, contractility and cardiac output, with little change in peripheral vascular resistance (β_1 action). If the dose exceeds $0.2\ \mu g\ kg^{-1}\ min^{-1}$ α effects predominate, resulting in increased peripheral vascular resistance and elevated systolic and diastolic pressure. At moderate doses vasoconstriction is seen in renal and musculocutaneous vascular beds, presumably because of their predominant population of α receptors. The standard measures of preload, central venous pressure and pulmonary artery occlusion pressure will therefore be increased. At higher doses or infusion rates, adrenaline produces generalised vasoconstriction and this increase in afterload may ultimately increase both systolic and diastolic blood pressures and reduce cardiac output.

Although adrenaline dilates myocardial arterioles and venules, the increases in heart rate and contractility may cause imbalance in the myocardial oxygen supply:demand ratio and predispose to ischaemia. Adrenaline also has a direct accelerating effect on the sinoatrial node and ectopic foci, shortens the ventricular refractory period and thereby possesses a significant proarrhythmic potential that limits its therapeutic potential. However, its usefulness lies in its greater efficacy than other β agonists and it is indicated in the treatment of patients with life threatening congestive heart failure, anaphylactic shock and status asthmaticus.

Other effects. Adrenaline is a neurotransmitter and has slight excitatory effects on the central nervous system (CNS). In high doses, however, it can cause tremors, agitation and headache. It has a powerful relaxant effect on bronchial smooth muscle and is widely used for treating severe bronchospasm. It has a central role in the management of anaphylaxis on account of its vasoconstricting (α_1) and bronchodilating (β_2) properties. The decrease in mucosal blood flow due to arteriolar vasoconstriction reduces mucosal swelling and bronchial secretions.

Since adrenaline is the major catecholamine, it is hardly surprising that it has many effects on general metabolism. It promotes glucagon secretion, while inhibiting insulin release. Glycogenolysis is increased in most tissues and peripheral glucose uptake is reduced. This produces a significant increase in plasma glucose concentrations. Free fatty acids and glycerol are increased in the plasma because of increased activity of triglyceride lipase in adipose tissue. In addition, serum cholesterol, phospholipid and low density lipoproteins are increased.

Clinical use. Adrenaline is available for intravenous administration as a 1:1000 ($1\ mg\ ml^{-1}$) or 1:10 000 ($100\ \mu g\ ml^{-1}$) aqueous solution of adrenaline hydrochloride. This may be administered as a slow bolus or, after further dilution, as a continuous infusion. Since the early 1980s, in many clinical situations, it has been supplanted by the newer synthetic agents such as dopamine and dobutamine. More recently, however, the use of adrenaline has been increasing. Sometimes it will produce a haemodynamic response when other inotropic agents have ceased to have any effect.

Noradrenaline

Noradrenaline is a naturally occurring neurotransmitter at postganglionic neurones and in the brain and is secreted by the adrenal medulla.

Cardiovascular effects. Noradrenaline is a powerful agonist at α_1 and α_2 adrenoreceptors and has similar β_1 effects to adrenaline. It has very little β_2 activity. Infusions of $<0.05\ \mu g\ kg^{-1}\ min^{-1}$ increase myocardial inotropy and heart rate due to stimulation of β_1 receptors. If the dosage exceeds $0.1\ \mu g\ kg^{-1}\ min^{-1}$, α-adrenergic activity predominates, with increased peripheral resistance, elevated systolic and diastolic pressures and a reflex reduction in heart rate. Both the increased inotropy and peripheral vascular resistance cause an increase in myocardial oxygen demand. Furthermore, the combination of a decreased heart rate and increased afterload may lead to a reduction in cardiac output. Coronary arterial blood flow is often increased as a result of increased aortic root pressure, increased diastolic filling time (due to a reduction in heart rate) and coronary vasodilatation (due to increased myocardial oxygen consumption and accumulation of vasodilatory metabolites).

Like adrenaline, noradrenaline increases pulmonary vascular resistance and causes vasoconstriction in the mesenteric and renal vascular beds. Although noradrenaline increases renal vascular resistance, it may increase renal blood flow and glomerular filtration pressure by elevating arterial blood pressure in hypotensive patients.

Other effects. Unlike adrenaline, the cerebral cortex is not stimulated by noradrenaline and so it does not produce anxiety, agitation or sweating. Cutaneous pallor can occur as a result of widespread arteriolar vasoconstriction and, if extravasated from a peripheral intravenous line, noradrenaline will frequently cause significant skin necrosis requiring skin grafting. Although it has an inhibitory effect on some types of smooth muscle, this is less marked than with adrenaline and so there is no clinically useful bronchodilatation with noradrenaline. In contrast, during late pregnancy, noradrenaline stimulates uterine contractions.

Clinical use. Noradrenaline is administered as a controlled infusion into a central vein at a rate of 2–10 µg min^{-1} initially. Its cardiovascular effects last only a few minutes after stopping the infusion and there is a tendency for patients to become unresponsive after prolonged treatment.

The haemodynamic effect of noradrenaline depends on the balance between increased afterload and increased contractility. The main indication for noradrenaline is to maintain perfusion pressure in states of uncontrolled vasodilatation, such as systemic sepsis, systemic inflammatory response syndrome, neurogenic shock and, possibly, drug toxicity. In sepsis/systemic inflammatory response syndrome, noradrenaline is used to counteract the generalised vasodilatation thought to be due to the overproduction of nitric oxide, an extremely potent substance which causes smooth muscle relaxation. In such cases the use of noradrenaline, usually in conjunction with another inotrope, will increase systemic vascular resistance and (possibly) filling pressures. Cardiac output, which is usually significantly elevated due to decreased afterload, may be reduced modestly. The dose of noradrenaline should be titrated to achieve an acceptable arterial pressure or a reduction in the infusion rate of another inotrope (e.g. dopamine) if this is viewed as desirable.

Noradrenaline may also be used after surgical removal of tumours that secrete vasoactive substances e.g. phaeochromocytoma (see Ch. 27). In this case, exogenous noradrenaline replaces tumour secreted catecholamines and maintains arterial blood pressure by continuing α-adrenoreceptor stimulation. Gradually this may be withdrawn as the circulating blood volume is increased (usually from a contracted state) and as the circulation readjusts to a change in receptor activity. The requirement for noradrenaline and the duration of the infusion is dictated by profile of vasoactive substances secreted by the tumour and the degree of receptor blockade administered in the preoperative period.

Isoprenaline

Isoprenaline, a synthetic catecholamine, has potent β_1- and β_2-agonist effects without α activity.

Cardiovascular effects. Infusions of 0.025 µg kg^{-1} min^{-1} increase myocardial contractility and cause a significant increase in heart rate, thereby increasing cardiac output. Systolic and diastolic blood pressures are decreased, with diversion of blood flow from vital organs to muscle and skin. This combination of increased myocardial oxygen demand in the presence of a potential reduction of myocardial oxygen supply predisposes to myocardial ischaemia and arrhythmias.

Isoprenaline has an effect on the conducting system of the heart, reducing the QT interval on the electrocardiogram. This property is used therapeutically in *torsade de pointes,* a condition in which recurrent ventricular fibrillation or tachycardia occurs in association with excessive use of (usually several) antiarrhythmic drugs.

Other effects. Since it relaxes smooth muscle, it is not surprising that isoprenaline is a bronchodilator. In some forms of bronchoconstrictive disease the therapeutic effect of isoprenaline is further augmented by an inhibition of histamine liberation from mast cells. However, its vasodilating effect on the pulmonary circulation may worsen pre-existing ventilation/perfusion mismatches and increase the functional right-to-left shunt.

Clinical use. Isoprenaline is administered

diluted in either normal saline or 5% dextrose. Its inotropic effect occurs at an infusion rate of up to $0.015 \mu g \, kg^{-1} \, min^{-1}$. At rates of greater than $0.02 \mu g \, kg^{-1} \, min^{-1}$, tachycardia, ventricular irritability, tachyarrhythmias, excessive peripheral dilatation and hypotension may occur.

In general, isoprenaline has been superseded by other agents and is now rarely used in intensive care units. Dopamine and dobutamine have superior inotropic effects, with a lower incidence of tachycardia and/or tachyarrhythmias. However, isoprenaline is of use in the treatment of bradycardia and atrioventricular block, and is particularly useful in denervated hearts. Pulmonary vasodilator properties make it effective in the treatment of pulmonary hypertension and right ventricular failure.

Dobutamine

Dobutamine, a synthetic catecholamine, was modified from isoprenaline. The clinically used preparation is a racemic mixture — the stereoisomers having different receptor affinity and/or activity. Dobutamine is a powerful inotrope with weak chronotropic and vascular effects, reflecting its predominant β_1 activity (and weak β_2 and α effects). Increases in cardiac output are primarily through direct inotropism and, secondarily, by reduced afterload. Onset of action occurs within 2 minutes, with peak effects occurring 10–12 minutes after any change in the infusion rate. The plasma half-life is less than 3 minutes and is due to both redistribution and metabolism by catechol O-methyl transferase. This results in two inactive metabolites, which are excreted in urine.

Dobutamine produces a lesser increase in heart rate per unit gain in cardiac output than either isoprenaline or dopamine but may cause tachycardia in sensitive or hypovolaemic patients. Whereas dobutamine may decrease diastolic coronary filling pressure, many studies have indicated an improvement in myocardial ischaemia and increased coronary blood flow. These studies have indicated that, despite an increase in inotropism, dobutamine produces an overall favourable metabolic environment for the ischaemic myocardium and should be considered as the preferred drug in patients with acute myocardial infarction. However, tachyphylaxis can occur after 72 hours administration.

The net haemodynamic effects of dobutamine include: (1) increased cardiac output, (2) decreased left ventricular filling pressure, (3) decreased systemic vascular resistance. Like its parent drug, isoprenaline, dobutamine is of benefit in patients with right ventricular failure.

Cardiovascular effects. Dobutamine has β_1 effects and increases myocardial contractility. It also acts at the β_2 and α receptors, causing peripheral vaso- and venodilatation and reducing both preload and afterload. These effects are thought to be due to the (+) isomer; the (–) isomer is an α agonist. The overall effect is to increase cardiac output (due to increased contractility and reduced afterload), with a variable/unpredictable effect on peripheral vascular tone. Arterial blood pressure may either increase or decrease.

Dobutamine does not liberate noradrenaline from sympathetic fibres and does not have any activity at renal dopaminergic receptors.

Other effects. Dobutamine has few side-effects. By enhancing atrioventricular conduction, it may precipitate atrial fibrillation in susceptible individuals. Unlike the other inotropes it may be administered into a peripheral vein, as inadvertent extravasation is unlikely to produce significant cutaneous vasoconstriction or necrosis.

Clinical use. Dobutamine is administered as a controlled continuous infusion of a dilute solution (1 g in 250 ml isotonic saline or 5% dextrose). It is an excellent drug for increasing global perfusion but often has no effect on hypotension. Since it reduces both afterload and preload and does not (usually) increase arterial pressure, it helps preserve the balance between myocardial oxygen delivery and demand. It is frequently the inotrope of choice after myocardial infarction, cardiac surgery or cardiogenic shock. Since it improves left ventricular performance and reduces left sided filling pressures, it may be of benefit in either left ventricular or acute congestive cardiac failure.

In the shocked state associated with severe sepsis or the systemic inflammatory response syndrome, tissue production of potent vasodilating agents (e.g. nitric oxide) results in a hyperdynamic circulation, with high cardiac output, uncontrolled peripheral vasodilatation and capillary leak, which leads to both real and relative hypovolaemia. In this situation hypotension is frequent. Since the main problem is excessive peripheral vasodilatation, an α agonist, e.g. noradrenaline or moderate/high dose dopamine, is indicated. Dobutamine is often used in conjunction with one or both of these because it is better to preserve cardiac output and increase systemic vascular resistance rather than use a vasoconstrictor alone, which will increase systemic vascular resistance, reduce cardiac output and decrease tissue perfusion.

Dobutamine is the inotrope most frequently used to improve oxygen transport. After prolonged infusion, especially in severe sepsis, there may be receptor desensitisation and this may necessitate a significant increase in the rate of infusion. If no rhythm disturbances ensue, there is no upper limit and doses of $200\ \mu g\ kg^{-1}\ min^{-1}$ have been employed.

Although global perfusion is usually improved with dobutamine, it is unclear how this improvement in perfusion is distributed. It has no specific effect on renal blood flow except secondary to improved cardiac output. It may, however, improve creatinine clearance. Adequate splanchnic flow may be crucial to survival in critical illness but some studies, using gastric tonometry, suggest that dobutamine does not improve splanchnic flow despite increased cardiac output.

Dopamine

Dopamine is the naturally occurring precursor to noradrenaline and produces dose related effects at all three types of adrenoceptors.

Cardiovascular effects. Dopamine is said to have a dose related effect on the circulation. As dopaminergic, then β adrenoreceptors and finally α adrenoreceptors are stimulated, it may act as a renal vasodilator, an inotrope and a peripheral vasoconstrictor with increasing dose. Although these effects are to some extent dose

related, individuals may exhibit increased or decreased dose responsiveness.

While there is considerable interpatient variability, it can be generally stated that low doses (0.5–$3\ \mu g\ kg^{-1}\ min^{-1}$) predominantly stimulate DA receptors, leading to increased renal, mesenteric and coronary perfusion. In normovolaemic patients this dosage produces a diuresis and natuResis, possibly due to a combination of increased renal blood flow, inhibition of aldosterone secretion and inhibition of tubular Na^+,K^+-ATPase activity. At higher doses (3–$5\ \mu g\ kg^{-1}\ min^{-1}$) β_1 (and to a lesser degree β_2) stimulation leads to increased chronotropism and contractility, with a slight reduction in systemic vascular resistance. This dose would appear to be the most appropriate for the management of congestive heart failure.

At 5–$15\ \mu g\ kg^{-1}\ min^{-1}$ dopamine stimulates myocardial β receptors, increasing contractility and therefore cardiac output and stroke volume. There is little peripheral effect and so afterload (systemic vascular resistance) is relatively unaffected. The clinical effect will be an increase in systolic pressure and a modest increase in heart rate. As the infusion rate reaches the upper end of this dosage band and beyond, α receptor stimulation becomes more prominent and noradrenaline release from myocardial stores is more marked. The result is generalised vasoconstriction, increased systemic vascular resistance, increased diastolic and systolic pressure — similar to the effect of noradrenaline. Tachycardia and ventricular irritability may also occur at high doses.

Dopamine increases filling pressures (increased central venous pressure and pulmonary capillary wedge pressure) and so increases myocardial wall tension at any given intraventricular pressure (law of Laplace). This will increase myocardial oxygen demand, as will the increase in systemic vascular resistance and heart rate. Since the increase in wall tension and the decrease in diastolic filling time (associated with tachycardia) reduce myocardial oxygen delivery, dopamine, at least in high dosage, is likely to impair myocardial oxygen balance.

Other effects. Dopamine does not cross the

blood–brain barrier and so has no CNS side-effects when administered intravenously. As a naturally occurring catecholamine, it is perhaps surprising that the metabolic and endocrine effects of exogenous dopamine infusion have only recently been appreciated. In healthy volunteers, at a moderate infusion rate ($10\,\mu g\,kg^{-1}\,min^{-1}$) it has been shown to increase basal metabolic rate by up to 15%. This was associated with significant increases in plasma glucose, insulin and free fatty acid concentrations.

A more unexpected and potentially worrying finding is that exogenous dopamine causes a rapid, potent but reversible reduction in pro-lactin secretion. Hypoprolactinaemia has been associated with inhibition of macrophage activation and T-lymphocyte function, thus compromising cell mediated immune function. This would, if proven, have implications for immuno-compromised patients, including patients in intensive care.

In addition, dopamine suppresses pulsatile secretion of human growth hormone and reduces plasma concentrations of insulin-like growth factor I. These effects may partially explain, in some patients, the profound catabolic state in critical illness despite optimal or excessive nutritional support.

Dopamine has also been found to aggravate or induce the euthyroid sick syndrome, as evidenced by reduced tri-iodothyronine concentrations. Luteinising hormone and testosterone concentrations in the blood are also decreased. Dopamine would appear to accentuate hypopituitarism associated with critical illness.

Clinical use. Dopamine, administered at 2–$3\,\mu g\,kg^{-1}\,min^{-1}$, is used to increase urinary flow and improve renal function. There is little convincing evidence that it will prevent acute renal failure, although it is often used clinically for this purpose. If, however, it results in high output rather than oliguric renal failure, it may still be beneficial in terms of ultimate outcome. As an inotrope it is particularly useful when both inotropic and pressor effects are required, e.g. cardiogenic shock/systemic sepsis. However, when the rate of dopamine infusion has reached a level at which α-adrenoreceptor stimulation is the major effect, a change to another inotropic regimen is indicated.

Dopexamine

Dopexamine is a synthetic catecholamine with pronounced β_2 activity (60 times more potent than dopamine), minor β_1-activity, no α activity, significant DA_1 activity (one third the potency of dopamine) and mild DA_2-receptor activity. In addition, it is a potent reuptake inhibitor of neurally released catecholamines.

The summated effects of dopexamine are due to afterload reduction by renal and mesenteric vasodilatation (DA_1 and β_2 activation), positive inotropism (myocardial β_2- and reduced noradrenaline reuptake) and naturesis (DA_1). It has been described as an 'inodilator' because its main effects are vasodilatation and inotropy. Regional blood flow may be influenced by dopexamine. Vasodilatation occurs in the lungs and will inhibit the normal (protective) pulmonary vasoconstrictive reflex, and there may be an increased shunt. The increase in renal blood flow with dopexamine is greater than the coexisting increase in cardiac index, indicating specific renal vasodilatation. Although it is claimed that dopexamine is as effective as dopamine in preserving renal function in patients undergoing liver transplantation, its efficacy in preventing renal failure is unproven.

The infusion rate for effective doses of dopexamine ranges from 0.5 to $6\,\mu g\,kg^{-1}\,min^{-1}$, depending on the pathology. Dopexamine has a plasma half-life of 6–7 minutes in health and 11 minutes in low output states. Clearance from the circulation is by tissue uptake and the drug is metabolised by monoamine oxidase and catechol O-methyl transferase.

Clinical use. Dopexamine is normally infused at 0.5–$6.0\,\mu g\,kg^{-1}\,min^{-1}$, the dose being carefully titrated because many patients respond to very low infusion rates. Cardiac surgical patients generally exhibit the optimum response at $2\,\mu g\,kg^{-1}\,min^{-1}$, whereas those with chronic heart failure require higher infusion rates. Dopexamine has been used for treatment of acute cardiac failure after cardiac surgery but infusions of

>6 µg kg^{-1} min^{-1} can produce unacceptable tachycardia and angina in patients with ischaemic heart disease.

Whereas the increase in left ventricular contractility is less than that seen with dobutamine, dopexamine produces a greater reduction in pulmonary and systemic vascular resistance and has proven beneficial in short and long term management of pulmonary hypertension.

Xamoterol

Xamoterol is a cardioselective β$_1$-adrenoceptor partial agonist which has approximately 40% of the agonist activity of isoprenaline, causing positive inotropic and chronotropic effects. β-adrenoceptor antagonists with partial agonist activity confer different haemodynamic properties following acute administration. When endogenous sympathetic tone is low (e.g. at rest), xamoterol exerts a moderate inotropic effect, but when it is high (e.g. during exercise), it acts as an antagonist, reducing exercise induced tachycardia. Xamoterol therefore appears to modify the responses of the heart to underlying sympathetic influences and prevent excessive swings in sympathetic activity.

Resting studies in patients with mild to moderate heart failure have shown that both intravenous and oral administration produce an increase in inotropy, as indicated by increased systolic blood pressure, cardiac output, myocardial contractility and relaxation. However, some patients with poor ventricular function experience a further deterioration in function and xamoterol is best reserved for patients with mild heart failure.

Phosphodiesterase inhibitors

Progress in research is continuously shedding new light on the physiology and pharmacology of the cardiovascular system. In patients with severe heart failure, positive inotropic response to β sympathomimetic agents is diminished, owing to downregulation of β$_1$ receptors. Diminished sensitivity of these receptors may also be associated with advancing age and with the stress of surgery.

Treatment with catecholamines is also known to induce desensitisation of β$_1$ adrenoceptors, reducing responsiveness to further stimulation by receptor dependent inotropes. Downregulation can develop within 72 hours of dobutamine administration.

Phosphodiesterase (PDE) inhibitors act through non-receptor mediated inhibition of the vascular and cardiac PDE isoenzyme, causing an increase in intracellular cAMP. This, in turn, causes a net influx of Ca^{2+} in cardiac muscle (inotropy) and a net outflux of Ca^{2+} in vascular smooth muscle (vasodilatation). PDE inhibitors have a unique beneficial effect on the diastolic function of the left ventricle that includes relaxation, compliance and filling — this has been termed a 'lusitropic' effect. In contrast to catecholamines, this lusitropic effect occurs at doses lower than those required for inotropy.

Many forms of PDE isoenzymes have been identified. That fraction responsible for cardiac inotropy and vasodilator activity is referred to as PDE-III and has previously been termed peak IIIc, type IV, F3 and PIII (Table 25.4).

PDE inhibitors increase myocardial inotropy, improve myocardial performance and, following rapid administration, can significantly reduce arterial blood pressure. Venous capacitance is also increased and this reduces venous return and myocardial wall tension.

When treating patients with impaired myocardial function it is essential to use drugs that will improve myocardial performance without jeopardising the ischaemic myocardium. Administration of PDE inhibitors, e.g. amrinone, enoxi-

Table 25.4 Actions of PDE-III inhibitors

Cardiac
  Positive inotropy
  Positive lusitropy
  Coronary vasodilatation
  Positive chronotropy
  Positive dromotropy

Vascular
  Peripheral vaso/venodilatation
  Decreased pulmonary vascular resistance

mone, can improve myocardial performance without increasing myocardial oxygen consumption, provided there is no significant increase in heart rate. However, PDE inhibitors have positive chronotropic effects, enhance sinoatrial conduction and decrease atrioventricular refractoriness, and are therefore proarrhythmic in nature.

These cardiotonic drugs also significantly reduce pulmonary vascular resistance and are a rational choice for treatment of patients with mitral valve disease or those with pulmonary hypertension awaiting heart–lung transplantation.

The available PDE inhibitors share similar haemodynamic properties. Amrinone, a bipyridine derivative, was the first PDE inhibitor to be introduced into clinical practice (for intravenous administration), in 1984. However, its inotropic effects have been questioned and its beneficial effects in the management of congestive heart failure have been attributed to its vasodilator properties. The imidazole derivative, enoximone, is currently available for intravenous administration. It has similar haemodynamic actions although, unlike amrinone, it does not alter platelet function. Milrinone, another bipyridine derivative, appears to be 20–30 times more potent than amrinone. In addition, it possesses more favourable pharmacokinetic properties, in that it has a more rapid onset and shorter duration of action.

Unlike catecholamines, PDE inhibitors are not subject to tachyphylaxis. Additionally, the beneficial effects of PDE inhibitors appear to be augmented when β-receptor agonists are administered. This synergistic inotropy is particularly important in patients with severe pre-existing heart failure.

From a haemodynamic viewpoint, there are three major risks associated with the use of these drugs: (1) reduction in arterial blood pressure, (2) increase in heart rate and/or induction of arrhythmia, and (3) critical increase in myocardial oxygen consumption. Some of these negative effects appear to be highly dependent on the dosage and rate of administration. Choosing the appropriate dose of PDE-III inhibitors is of fundamental importance (Table 25.5).

Table 25.5 PDE-III inhibitor dosage and inotropy:vasodilatation ratio

Drug	Dosage	Inotropy:vaso-dilatation ratio
Amrinone	0.75–1.0 mg kg^{-1} loading dose 5–10 µg kg^{-1} min^{-1} maintenance	1:4
Enoximone	0.5–0.75 mg kg^{-1} loading dose 5–10 µg kg^{-1} min^{-1} maintenance	1:2
Milrinone	50 µg kg^{-1} loading dose 0.375–0.75 µg kg^{-1} min^{-1} maintenance	1:20

Glucagon

Glucagon is a polypeptide hormone, produced by the pancreas, which binds to the myocyte cell surface, activates adenylate cyclase and increases intracellular cAMP. As the glucagon receptor is distinct from the β receptor, β antagonists do not block its actions. Glucagon (1–5 mg intravenously) is a positive inotrope with positive chronotropy, while having a variable effect on peripheral vascular resistance. However, the drug causes a significant incidence of nausea and vomiting, hyperglycaemia and rebound hypoglycaemia, which limits its use to the emergency management of β-antagonist overdose.

CLASS II

These agents affect sarcolemma ion pumps/channels. The prototype of the group is the cardiac glycoside, digoxin.

Digoxin

The substance, digitalis, originally used by Withering in the eighteenth century because it 'had a power of motion of the heart to a degree yet unobserved in any other medicine', is found in the purple foxglove (*Digitalis purpurea*) and is a mixture of cardiac glycosides particularly rich in digitoxin. Digoxin, another cardiac glycoside, is obtained from the dried leaves of the species

Digitalis lanata. This plant is also a source of other glycosides: lanatoside C and digitoxin. Another member of the group is ouabain, which is obtained from *Strophanthus gratus*. None of these compounds has been synthesised commercially and they are still prepared from the dried leaves of the appropriate plant.

Digoxin is the only member of the cardiac glycosides in common usage and will be the only one considered in detail. In common with others in the group, it is composed of a 23-carbon steroid nucleus with an unsaturated lactone ring at position 17 and a sugar based side-chain.

Digoxin is readily absorbed from the gastrointestinal tract but bioavailability varies from 40 to 90%, depending on the preparation. It is 25% bound to plasma proteins and is significantly tissue bound. Myocardial digoxin concentrations are 30% greater, and skeletal muscle concentrations 30% lower, than plasma. Elimination is 85% renal, with both glomerular filtration and tubular secretion occurring. The mean half-life is 36 hours but this is dependent on renal function and glomerular filtration rate. Digoxin cannot be removed in appreciable amounts by dialysis.

Cardiovascular effects. A major effect of digoxin is to enhance myocardial contractility in all chambers. The mechanisms suggested for this effect are both controversial and complex but there is no doubt that all the cardiac glycosides bind reversibly to Na^+,K^+-ATPase and cause enzyme inhibition. This leads to an increase in intracellular Na^+, which reduces the transmembrane sodium gradient and thus reduces extracellular movement of Ca^{2+}. The resultant increase in intracellular Ca^{2+} is responsible for the inotropic effects of digoxin. Hypokalaemia increases binding of digoxin to the Na^+,K^+-ATPase and increases toxicity, whereas hyperkalaemia decreases binding. At concentrations below those required to inhibit Na^+,K^+-ATPase, however, it seems that digoxin may also exert an inotropic effect by decreasing neuronal reuptake of catecholamines. However, digoxin is not simply a positive inotropic agent. The drug also restores the inhibitory effect of cardiac baroreceptors on sympathetic outflow from the CNS and thus reduces the activation of both the sympathetic nervous system and the renin–angiotensin mechanism.

The negative chronotropic effect of digoxin is also multifactorial but is due predominantly to its actions on the parasympathetic system. These include: sensitisation of central baroreceptors, increased efferent activity due to stimulation of vagal nuclei, increased cardiac sensitivity to vagal stimulation, and release of myocardial stores of acetylcholine. At low doses digoxin contributes to myocardial irritability by prolonging the action potential and decreasing the threshold potential. At higher doses, the action potential is shortened, and repolarisation accelerated. The tendency towards spontaneous depolarisation is accentuated when K^+ concentration is low. This explains the increased frequency of ventricular irritability when patients on digoxin become hypokalaemic.

Digoxin also slows depolarisation in the atrioventricular node. This reduces the ability of the ventricular conducting system to respond to high rates of supraventricular or nodal depolarisation.

Other effects. The therapeutic index of digoxin is low (<2) and it would appear that around 25% of patients show signs of toxicity. Signs of overdose include anorexia, nausea, vomiting, lethargy, confusion, visual disturbances, neuralgia and convulsions. Digoxin may also cause gynaecomastia because its molecular structure is similar to that of the female sex hormones. It may cause arrythmias related to sinoatrial node dysfunction (sick sinus syndrome, bradycardia, paroxysmal atrial tachycardia), junctional rhythm, atrioventricular block and ventricular ectopic foci.

A large number of cardioactive and other drugs may interact with digoxin. Some of these, such as verapamil, amiodarone and quinidine, may often be given concurrently. The interactions may be caused by reductions in renal clearance and alterations in the volume of distribution of digoxin (quinidine, verapamil, captopril, cyclosporin), whereas others may be due to increased absorption (erythromycin, omeprazole) or pharmacodynamically related (inotropes, diuretics, β blockers, calcium channel blockers).

Suggested treatment of digoxin toxicity includes: correction of electrolyte imbalance, treatment of arrhythmias (phenytoin, lignocaine), correction of bradycardia with atropine, minimising absorption (cholestyramine/activated charcoal), and reduction of plasma digoxin concentrations by antidigoxin immunotherapy using purified ovine fragmented digoxin antibodies (Fab fragments).

Clinical use. Digoxin may be administered orally or parenterally. Onset of action is 90 minutes after oral administration, with maximum plasma concentrations occurring after 3 hours and peak pharmacological effect after 4–6 hours. Therapeutic plasma concentrations are said to be 0.5–2.0 ng ml^{-1}. Digoxin therapy is normally commenced with a 1 mg loading dose administered over a 2–12 hour period. Without this strategy, four half-lives (6 days) would be required to reach steady-state plasma concentrations.

Digoxin is used for the treatment of atrial fibrillation, atrial flutter and cardiac failure, particularly when this is associated with accumulation of oedema fluid within the pulmonary or systemic vascular beds. Although plasma concentrations are helpful in confirming toxicity, they are of limited value in monitoring therapy because they do not mirror myocardial concentrations. It is usual, however, to aim for plasma concentrations of about 1 ng ml^{-1}.

Although digoxin has been administered to patients with congestive heart failure for more than 200 years, its use remains controversial. Several recent multicentre clinical trials demonstrated that low dose digoxin improved the ejection fraction, decreased the incidence of worsening heart failure and improved exercise tolerance in patients with congestive heart failure receiving concomitant therapy with either a diuretic or angiotensin converting enzyme inhibitor. It has been postulated that the beneficial effects of low dose digoxin are primarily due to neurohumoral effects rather than inotropism.

The use of digoxin in intensive care units has diminished as other inotropic drugs have become available. It still has a place, however, in the medium to long term enhancement of myocardial performance and/or rhythm control.

Since hypokalaemia and decreased renal function are common findings in patients in intensive care, the regular measurement of plasma digoxin concentration is prudent if toxicity is to be avoided or diagnosed early.

'Prophylactic digoxin' to reduce the incidence of arrhythmias in patients scheduled for thoracotomy was a common practice that has, for the most part, ceased. The findings of Chee and colleagues (1982) suggest that it is of value.

Digoxin is contraindicated in patients with hypertrophic obstructive cardiomyopathy because it exacerbates the outflow obstruction. It should be used with caution in patients with aberrant atrioventricular conduction (e.g. Wolff–Parkinson–White syndrome) because there is an increased incidence of tachyarrhythmias.

CLASS III

These agents modulate intracellular calcium mechanism.

Although the inotropic role of β adrenoceptors has been well established for many years, the role of α_1 adrenoceptors has been recognised only recently. In contrast to the β adrenoceptor response, the inotropic response induced by α_1 agonists such as phenylephrine is not accompanied by an increase of myocardial cAMP, and adrenoceptors are not downregulated in heart failure. The main role of the α_1 adrenoceptor is the activation of phopholipase C, which enhances the hydrolysis of phosphatidyl inositol biphosphate (PIP$_2$), leading to activation of two second messengers: diacyl glycerol, which activates protein kinase C, and 1,4,5-inositol triphosphate (IP$_3$). IP$_3$ increases the concentration of intracellular calcium through increased release from the sarcoplasmic reticulum, thus increasing the sensitivity of contractile proteins in the cardiac muscle, especially in patients with severe heart failure. Phenylephrine is as potent as noradrenaline at the α_1 receptor but is almost devoid of activity at other adrenoceptors. When combined with enoximone, this drug has been shown to provide a reliable pharmacological 'bridge to transplantation' in patients awaiting cardiac transplantation.

Calcium

While calcium salts (5 mg kg^{-1}) cause significant vasoconstriction and blood pressure elevation, they do not reliably improve cardiac output or tissue oxygen delivery in normocalcaemic or mildly hypocalcaemic patients undergoing or recovering from cardiac surgery. Doses larger than 5 mg kg^{-1} may produce several toxic effects. A high [Ca^{2+}] is toxic to the atrioventricular node, sometimes causing heart block, arrhythmia and hypotension. Calcium may also worsen cellular dysfunction and increase mortality rate during ischaemia and shock. Excess intracellular calcium, seen in low perfusion states and sepsis, can activate destructive cellular processes (proteases, lipases, free radical production) and injure the cell. There is also some evidence that calcium salts may reduce the efficacy of β-adrenergic agonists.

CLASS IV

These agents with multiple mechanisms of action form a fourth group of inotropic agents that augment cardiac contractility by utilising two or more metabolic pathways.

Vesnarinone

This is a quinolinone derivative that has unique mechanisms of action: (1) it decreases the outward and inward rectifying potassium current (electrophysiologically resembling a class III anti-arrhythmic agent); (2) it increases intracellular sodium by prolonging the opening of sodium channels; and (3) it exhibits modest inhibition of PDE. In marked contrast to agents that increase intracellular cAMP, vesnarinone slows heart rate and prolongs the action potential. In a recent randomised placebo controlled trial, low dose vesnarinone demonstrated a substantial reduction in the risk of death and worsening heart failure, with a significant improvement in quality of life. This drug combines inotropy with vasodilatation, negative chronotropy and anti-arrhythmic properties.

REFERENCES AND FURTHER READING

Chee T P, Prakash N A, Desser K B, Benchimol A 1982 Postoperative supraventricular arrhythmias and the role of prophylactic digoxin in cardiac surgery. American Heart Journal 104: 974–977

Doyle A R, Achal K D, Moors A H, Latimer R D 1995 Treatment of perioperative low cardiac output syndrome. Annals of Thoracic Surgery 59: S3–11

Feldman A M 1993 Classification of positive inotropic agents. Journal of the American College of Cardiology 22(4): 1223–1227

Kulka P J, Tryba M 1993 Inotropic support of the critically ill patient. A review of the agents. Drugs 45(5): 654–677

Packer M 1993 The development of positive inotropic agents for chronic heart failure: how have we gone astray? Journal of the American College of Cardiology 2(4) (suppl A): 119A–126A

Penefsky Z J 1994 The determinants of contractility in the heart. Comparative Biochemistry and Physiology 109(1): 1–22.

Skarvan K (ed) 1944 Vasoactive drugs. Baillière's Clinical Anaesthesiology 8: 1

26

Peripheral circulation

I. C. Roddie

FUNCTIONAL DIFFERENTIATION OF BLOOD VESSELS

The pulmonary and systemic circuits of the circulation consist of different types of blood vessel arranged in series. Each type of vessel is adapted anatomically and physiologically to serve particular functions.

Large arteries damp out the pressure fluctuations generated by the heart to create a fairly steady head of pressure to perfuse the tissues. Because of this, arterial vessels are sometimes called *damping vessels*. They are designed to deliver blood at high velocity with little energy cost.

The *arterioles* are the main site of vascular resistance in the circulation and because of this are sometimes called *resistance vessels*. Arterioles regulate the rate of blood flow to the tissues by altering the resistance they offer to blood flow. They can be thought of as the 'taps' which control outflow from the constant pressure arterial system. They are also important in the regulation of arterial pressure because they determine the level of the total peripheral resistance.

The *capillaries* have thin walls and are designed for exchange of nutrients, respiratory gases and waste products between the blood and the cells of the tissues. Because of this, they are sometimes called *exchange vessels*.

Venules and *veins* return blood from the capillaries to the heart at relatively high velocity and low energy cost. They contain most of the circulating blood volume and because of this are sometimes called *capacitance vessels*. The vessels can alter their capacity to hold blood by contraction and relaxation of the smooth muscle in their walls.

The *lymphatics* drain the tissue spaces of excess tissue fluid. Most of the fluid filtered from the capillaries into the tissue spaces is returned to the circulation across capillary and venular walls. However, the rest is returned via lymphatics. Lymphatics are thin walled vessels that can absorb fluid from the tissue spaces and return it to the circulation via the thoracic duct. Functionally, they are *tissue drainage vessels*.

HAEMODYNAMICS IN THE PERIPHERAL CIRCULATION

Laminar and turbulent flow

Blood flow through tubes can be laminar or turbulent. Normally flow in most of the blood vessels in the human circulation is laminar. This means that it travels in concentric layers which flow over one another at different velocities. The layers in the centre of the stream flow more quickly that those close to the wall. The layer in contact with the wall flows at zero velocity. It is the friction, or lack of slipperiness, between these layers flowing over one another that is responsible for resistance to flow in the circulation.

When flow is turbulent, blood does not flow in regular straight concentric laminae but irregularly, with eddy currents carrying fluid from one part of the lumen to another. Normally, flow is not turbulent in the human circulation. The tendency to turbulence increases with (1) increasing flow velocity, (2) increasing vessel diameter, and (3) increasing fluid density. The tendency decreases with increasing fluid viscosity. These factors are summarised in the formula for *Reynolds number*, which estimates the tendency to turbulence. When the number exceeds a critical value (2000), turbulence may occur.

$$\text{Reynolds number} = \frac{VDd}{\eta},$$

where V is velocity, D is diameter, d is density and η is viscosity.

Turbulence in the circulation

In the human circulation turbulence may occur in anaemia. The increase in flow velocity and decrease in fluid viscosity raise Reynolds number. Turbulence is also seen when there is a sudden change in vascular diameter, as when blood passes from a narrow vascular segment to a dilated one. This may occur when blood enters an aneurysm, passes a stenosed valve or emerges from an artery partly collapsed by a pneumatic cuff (Korotkoff sounds during blood pressure measurement).

Effects of turbulence

In energy terms, turbulent flow is less efficient than laminar flow, as energy is dissipated in the eddy currents and vibrations set up in the fluid. Thus resistance to flow is greater for turbulent than for laminar flow because more energy is required to drive the same amount of blood.

The eddy currents set up vibrations in the walls of the vessels, which can be heard as murmurs or bruits or felt as thrills on the surface of the body. The systolic murmur and thrill detected over a stenosed aortic valve result from such turbulence.

Rate of volume flow

The rate of flow along a tube (measured in volume per unit time) is related to (1) the pressure gradient driving it and (2) the fourth power of the radius of the tube. It is inversely related to (1) the length of the tube and (2) the viscosity of the fluid. These relationships are summarised in *Poiseuille's equation*, which states that flow ($\dot{Q}$) is related to these as in:

$$\dot{Q} = \frac{\pi}{8} \times \frac{(P_1 - P_2) \times r^4}{L \times \eta}$$

where $(P_1 - P_2)$ is the pressure gradient, r is the radius, L is the length and η is the viscosity. In the circulation, vessel length and blood viscosity are relatively constant so the pressure gradient and the vessel radius are the most important factors in regulating flow.

Pressure gradient

There is a direct relationship between pressure gradient and flow. All other things being constant, halving the perfusion pressure gradient halves blood flow, and doubling the perfusion pressure doubles it. In the body the relationship is not so simple. Poiseuille's equation applies to flow in rigid tubes but the walls of blood vessels are not rigid. As intravascular pressure rises and falls, vascular radius increases and decreases because to a variable degree, the vessels are distensible.

Although flow is directly related to perfusion pressure over a wide range of pressures, it has been observed that flow through vascular beds may cease when the perfusion pressure falls below a certain critical level. This phenomenon has been attributed to an instability of the vessel walls at low transmural pressures that causes them to collapse shut. It is referred to as 'critical closure'.

Vessel radius

Radius is a most important factor in determining flow because of the fourth power relationship. Halving the radius decreases flow to 1/16 of its former rate; doubling it increases flow 16-fold. The vessels best designed to vary their radii are the arterioles and they are therefore important in regulating flow rates.

Blood viscosity

Viscosity is due to friction (lack of slipperiness) between the adjacent layers of blood as they flow in concentric laminae at different velocities through the vessels. Blood viscosity can be measured by timing its flow though a narrow tube (viscometer) and comparing its rate with that of water. Normal blood is about four times as viscous as water and this is due mainly to its red cell content. Thus viscosity is raised in polycythaemia and reduced in anaemia. Plasma proteins, especially fibrinogen, also contribute to blood viscosity.

The apparent viscosity of blood in small blood vessels in the body is reduced by axial steaming, the tendency of flowing red cells to move away from the wall to form a core of cells towards the centre of the vessel. Friction between layers is reduced as the central core of cells slides over a cushion of plasma lining the inner walls of the vessels.

Peripheral resistance

Peripheral resistance is the frictional resistance encountered by blood flowing round the circulation. The energy needed to overcome it can be calculated using the hydraulic equivalent of Ohm's law. This states that resistance in a circuit is directly related to the pressure gradient around the circuit and inversely related to the flow rate through it:

$$\text{resistance} = \frac{(P_1 - P_2)}{\dot{Q}},$$

where $(P_1 - P_2)$ = the pressure gradient and $\dot{Q}$ = flow rate.

To measure total peripheral resistance in the systemic circuit, it is necessary to measure mean arterial and central venous pressures to determine the pressure gradient, and cardiac output to determine the flow. With a mean arterial pressure of 100 mmHg, a central venous pressure of 0 mmHg and a cardiac output of 5 l min⁻¹, total peripheral resistance would be 20 mmHg l⁻¹ min⁻¹. In the pulmonary circuit, with a pulmonary artery pressure of 20 mmHg, a pulmonary vein pressure of 0 mmHg and a flow rate of 5 l min⁻¹, total resistance would be 4 mmHg l⁻¹ min⁻¹, one-fifth of that in the systemic circuit.

The relative resistance offered by different segments of the circulation can be estimated if the pressure drop across each segment is measured. Flow through each segment must be the same per unit time, i.e. the cardiac output. The segments where the largest pressure drops occur must offer the greatest resistance, and vice versa. In the circulation, the greatest pressure drop occurs across the arteriolar segment. This indicates that the arteriolar segment offers greater resistance than the others.

Individual large vessels offer less resistance to flow than individual small ones; from a rearrangement of Poiseuille's equation, resistance is inversely related to the fourth power of the radius. This is because the wall effect is relatively greater in small radius vessels, in which relatively more of the flowing blood makes contact with the wall where flow velocity is zero.

Velocity of blood flow

Blood velocity depends on the total cross-sectional area of the bed through which it flows. In a stream, fluid must flow faster through narrow than through wide sections because the same volume flow must pass any particular point in unit time.

Though the aorta is a wide vessel, there is only one aorta. Total arterial cross-sectional area at this point is relatively small. In the capillaries the cross-sectional area is huge. Although individual capillaries have small cross-sectional areas, there are so many capillaries in parallel that the total cross-sectional area of the capillary bed is enormous. Thus blood flows more rapidly in the aorta than in the capillaries. In the arterial bed, the mean blood velocity of about 25 cm s^{-1}, whereas in the capillary it is about 0.5 mm s^{-1} — 500 times slower than in arteries. In veins, where total cross-sectional area is a little greater than in the arteries but much smaller than in the capillary bed, the mean velocity is about 15 cm s^{-1}.

LARGER ARTERIES (damping vessels)

The main functions of the arterial system are (1) distribute blood to the tissues at relatively high velocity and low energy cost, (2) to damp out the large pressure fluctuations generated by the ventricles to create a fairly steady pressure head for the tissues and (3) limit deviation from the normal arterial pressure level when other factors tend to change it.

Arterial structure

Arteries have the usual three vascular coats, intima, media and adventitia, but the walls are thick and tough. This gives arteries the low compliance (distensibility) needed to withstand high pressures; they show little change in volume with change in distending pressure. Near the heart, the media coat is predominantly elastic, but towards the periphery smooth muscle becomes the predominant tissue.

Role of elastic tissue. The elastic tissue is mainly responsible for damping pressure fluctuations. During ventricular systole, when blood is ejected into the arterial system, the rising pressure stretches the elastic tissue and some of the energy of contraction is stored. Because of this, aortic pressure does not rise as much as it would in a more rigid system. During diastole, the elastic recoil feeds energy back into the system so diastolic pressure does not fall as much as it would in a more rigid system. When the arteries harden with age, systolic pressures tend to rise and diastolic pressures tend to fall — to give a larger pulse pressure. Conversely, in babies, where the arterial elastic is in pristine condition, pulse pressures are relatively small.

Role of smooth muscle. In more peripheral arteries, smooth muscle replaces elastin as the predominant tissue in the media. By contracting in response to stretch, it limits arterial distension when arterial pressure rises sharply. Smooth muscle tends to contract when stretched (the myogenic response). When a subject stands up, blood pressure in foot arteries rises by about 100 mmHg, the hydrostatic equivalent of the column of blood between the heart and the feet. The sudden doubling of intravascular pressure tends to distend the arteries. The myogenic response helps them resist such distension.

Another function of the smooth muscle is to limit haemorrhage when arteries are severed. Smooth muscle in arteries tends to go into spasm when the walls are traumatised. Spasm is induced more readily by coarse injury than by fine cuts with sharp instruments. Thus bleeding is more copious from an artery cut with a sharp scalpel than with a blunt saw.

Arterial resistance

As mentioned earlier, vascular resistance is inversely related to the fourth power of the vessel's radius. Because arterial radii are relatively large, the resistance they offer to flow is relatively small. This allows blood transport from the heart to the periphery at low energy cost. There is little pressure drop along the arterial system. Blood leaving the heart with a mean pressure of about 100 mmHg reaches the peripheral arteries with a mean pressure only 5–10 mmHg lower.

Because arterial resistance is relatively small, small changes in arterial diameter make relatively little difference to the total peripheral resistance of the circuit and therefore to the flow rate round the circuit.

Arterial flow velocity

Mean velocity in arteries is high, about 25 cm s^{-1}. This is higher than in any other vessels and is due to the fact that the arterial bed has a small total cross-sectional area. The flow velocity is phasic, especially near to the heart where it changes with the phases of the pulse pressure.

Arterial pulse

With each beat of the heart, stroke output generates a pressure wave which travels down the arteries, where it can be felt by palpation. It travels towards the periphery at a velocity of 5 m s^{-1}, about 20 times faster than the blood velocity (0.25 m s^{-1}). Pulse velocity is related to the stiffness of the arterial walls. It is slower in babies with very elastic arteries and faster in elderly subjects whose arterial systems are hardened by arteriosclerosis.

The shape of the pulse depends on the point at which it is measured. Pulse amplitude is greater at the periphery than close to the heart. This is because the reflected pulse pressure wave from the end of the arterial tree sums with the descending wave of the subsequent pulse in the peripheral arteries.

Arterial blood pressure

Arterial blood pressure is measured indirectly using pneumatic cuffs applied to the upper arm while auscultating or palpating an artery distal to the cuff. More precise measurement is made by introducing a needle or catheter into an artery and connecting it to an electrical manometer. The pressure wave is described in terms of the highest pressure in the cycle (systolic pressure), the lowest pressure in the cycle (diastolic pressure), the difference between systolic and diastolic pressure (pulse pressure) and the average pressure over the cycle (mean pressure).

Although the normal pressure is usually taken as 120 mmHg in systole and 80 mmHg in diastole, there is considerable normal variation. Mean blood pressure also tends to rise with age. The body's physiological control systems are adept at keeping mean arterial pressure fairly constant despite large changes in cardiac output and peripheral resistance. Nevertheless, systolic pressures persistently over 140 mmHg and diastolic pressures persistently over 100 mmHg in a young adult suggest that blood pressure is abnormally high.

Determinants of arterial pressure. Mean arterial pressure depends on two factors — the amount of blood flowing into the system (the cardiac output) and the amount flowing out (an inverse function of peripheral resistance). If the cardiac output or the peripheral resistance rise, arterial pressure will rise, and vice versa.

Regulation of arterial pressure. Arterial blood pressure is held within a set range in any individual, and homeostatic mechanisms maintain it within that range despite the changes in cardiac output and peripheral resistance that tend to shift it. One mechanism is reflex. It works through the arterial baroreceptor system and provides rapid correction of sudden changes in arterial pressures. Another mechanism is hormonal. It uses the renin–angiotensin system and is more important in long term homeostasis.

Reflex regulation. When mean pressure rises, stretch receptors in the aortic arch and carotid sinus are stretched. This increases impulse traffic in the sensory nerves that travel from these receptors in the vagus and glossopharyngeal nerves to centres in the medulla. Here, the impulses inhibit impulse outflow in the sympathetic vasoconstrictor nerves to peripheral blood vessels. The resulting vasodilatation decreases peripheral resistance. The impulses also stimulate the cardiac centre to increase impulse traffic in the vagus nerves to the heart. The resulting vagal slowing of the heart reduces cardiac output. Thus a rise in blood pressure reflexly triggers a fall in cardiac output and a fall in peripheral resistance, which drive arterial pressure back again into its normal range.

Hormonal regulation. A fall in arterial pressure is also detected by the juxtaglomerular cells in the kidney. They respond by increasing output of the hormone, renin, which is carried away in the renal venous blood. In the blood, it acts on the plasma protein, angiotensinogen, breaking it down into angiotensin I which has little physiological action; however, angiotensin I is converted by angiotensin converting enzyme in the pulmonary vascular bed into angiotensin II which has vasopressor effects. It raises peripheral resistance by a direct vasoconstrictor effect on arteriolar smooth muscle. It also raises cardiac output. It does this by stimulating the release of aldosterone from the suprarenal glands. This mineralocorticoid leads to increased reabsorption of sodium chloride and water from the renal tubules. The resulting expansion of the extracellular fluid and blood volume compartments increases the filling pressure of the heart and, through this, cardiac output by the Frank–Starling mechanism. Thus, when arterial pressure falls, the hormonal mechanism triggers a sequence of changes which raise cardiac output and peripheral resistance and thereby raise arterial pressure back to its normal range. Another hormone thought to be involved in blood pressure regulation is atrial natriuretic peptide. Stretch of the atria is thought to be the stimulus for its release. It increases sodium excretion in the kidneys and thus tends to lower blood pressure. Its effects, therefore, oppose those of renin–angiotensin.

Whereas the reflex nervous mechanism makes corrections in a matter of seconds, the hormonal mechanism may take hours or days to correct the change. If the change in arterial pressure is persistent, the baroreceptor system adapts to the change and loses its effectiveness in blood pressure regulation. Then the body must rely on hormonal mechanisms for blood pressure homeostasis.

SMALL ARTERIES AND ARTERIOLES (resistance vessels)

The arteries divide and subdivide into smaller and smaller vessels, and when the lumen diameter falls to less than 0.5 mm they are referred to as arterioles. The arteriolar segment of the circulation is of great functional importance. It is the dominant vessel in the regulation of (1) local blood flow, (2) total peripheral resistance and (3) tissue fluid formation.

Structural features of arterioles

Though arterioles have a small lumen (diameters of 0.5 mm or less), they have a well developed muscular coat, giving them a wall to lumen ratio of about 1:1. The smooth muscle is highly reactive with a rich autonomic innervation. When the smooth muscle contracts in response to humoral or nervous stimuli, it can cause a large reduction in, or even obliterate, the lumen of the arteriole.

Arteriolar resistance

As mentioned above, the pressure drop across a segment of a circuit is an index of the relative resistance offered by that segment in the circuit. We have seen that the small pressure drop across the arterial segment of the circulation (5–10 mmHg) indicates that it offers only a small proportion (5–10%) of the total vascular resistance in the systemic circuit. In contrast, blood enters the arterioles with a pressure of about 90 mmHg and leaves with a pressure of about 30 mmHg at the arterial end of the capillaries. Thus about 60% of the pressure head generated by the heart (100 mmHg) to drive the blood around the circulation is used up driving blood past the short arteriolar segment.

The arteriolar bed offers about four times the resistance offered by the capillary bed. In capillary beds the pressure drop is only 15 mmHg. This may appear confusing because arterioles have larger radii than capillaries and resistance is inversely related to the fourth power of the radius. The explanation is as follows. Although a single capillary vessel offers more resistance than a single arteriole, there are many more capillaries in parallel than there are arterioles in parallel. When resistances are in series the total resistance is the sum of the individual resistances. When they are in parallel, the reciprocal of the total resistance (R_T) is the sum of the reciprocals of the individual resistances:

$$\frac{1}{R_T} = \frac{1}{R_1} + \frac{1}{R_2} + \frac{1}{R_3} + \frac{1}{R_4}, \text{etc.}$$

Thus total resistance is much less than each of the component parallel resistances. Since conductance is the reciprocal of resistance, total conductance (C_T) is the sum of the parallel conductances:

$$C_T = C_1 + C_2 + C_3 + C_4, \text{etc.}$$

Thus the total resistance offered by the capillary bed is less than that offered by the arteriolar bed, and total capillary conductance is correspondingly greater.

Effect of change in arteriolar resistance

The arterioles are well adapted to vary the resistance they offer because of their high wall:lumen ratio and the reactivity of their vascular smooth muscle. They alter their radii by smooth muscle contraction and relaxation. Changes in the radii of the arterioles serve three important functions.

Regulation of local blood flow. If changes are localised to one part, the effect is to increase or decrease blood flow to that tissue without much effect on total peripheral resistance and, therefore, mean arterial pressure. Because arteriolar resistance is high, small changes in their radii cause large changes in local resistance and therefore local blood flow. Local blood flow to tissues rises and falls to serve their individual metabolic needs. This is brought about by local factors which dilate the vessels (open the taps) when there is increased demand for blood, and vice versa.

Regulation of total peripheral resistance. If arterioles constrict all over the body, total peripheral resistance and hence the level of arterial

blood pressure will be raised correspondingly but there will be little change in the relative blood flow to the different tissues. Because the arteriolar system normally offers such a high proportion of total peripheral resistance, generalised changes in the calibre of arteriole vessels cause large changes in the total resistance of the circuit. Such changes are used in the regulation of arterial blood pressure, as mentioned in the section on arterial pressure above.

Regulation of tissue fluid formation. Local and generalised changes in arteriolar resistance cause local and generalised changes in the rate of formation of tissue fluid. Arteriolar dilatation allows higher pressures to be transmitted through to the capillary vessels. This increases filtration of plasma to the interstitial spaces. Conversely, generalised resistance vessel constriction lowers the pressure in the capillaries and leads to net movement of fluid from the tissue spaces to the blood.

Central control of resistance vessels

Most resistance vessels are innervated with sympathetic vasoconstrictor fibres. These are noradrenergic and their activity is coordinated by the vasomotor centre in the medulla. The centre normally sends several impulses per minute to resistance vessels, holding them in a state of tonic vasoconstriction. Cutting the sympathetic nerves to a limb increases blood flow to the limb by release of vasoconstrictor tone. The vasomotor centre modulates peripheral resistance by increasing or decreasing vasoconstrictor tone by varying the impulse discharge rate in vasoconstrictor nerves.

Tissues with a rich vasoconstrictor nerve supply include the gut, the kidneys, the skin and skeletal muscle. The heart and brain have a poor sympathetic vasoconstrictor nerve supply and are little affected by vasoconstrictor reflexes.

Sympathetic vasoconstrictor reflexes. These include the baroreceptor reflexes which help to maintain a steady blood pressure. Falls in arterial pressure are detected by stretch receptors in the walls of the carotid sinus and aortic arch. The information, carried to the reflex centres in the brain in the glossopharyngeal and vagus nerves, triggers a range of responses designed to raise the blood pressure. One of these responses in an increased outflow of impulses in the sympathetic vasoconstrictor system, which raises peripheral resistance. It is worth noting that the heart and cerebral vessels are little affected because of their poor sympathetic innervation. This allows diversion of blood from the splanchnic area, kidneys and skin to more vital organs, such as the heart and brain. Sympathetic vasoconstrictor fibres are also involved in the reflex dilatation of skin resistance vessels when body temperature rises. The rise in temperature is detected by cells in hypothalamic temperature regulating centres. They respond by reducing the outflow of sympathetic vasoconstrictor impulses to skin. The resulting increase in skin blood flow raises skin temperature and facilitates heat loss from the skin. Sympathetic vasoconstrictor tone is also modulated reflexly in response to inputs from the chemoreceptors, respiratory centre, cerebral cortex, etc.

Autonomic vasodilator reflexes. Some resistance vessels are supplied with autonomic vasodilator fibres. These are fibres which, when stimulated, cause relaxation of the smooth muscle in the vessels they innervate. The chemical mediators involved are uncertain but may include nitric oxide, acetylcholine, bradykinin, etc. Vasodilator innervations have been described in skin, skeletal muscle, erectile tissue, exocrine glands, etc. They may be involved in the skin vasodilatation during body warming, the flight or fight responses in skeletal muscle, and the functional vasodilatation accompanying gland secretion and penile erection.

Circulating hormones. Adrenaline and noradrenaline released from the suprarenal medulla in times of emotional stress have widespread effects on the body to adapt it for fight or flight. They cause constriction of resistance vessels in skin, splanchnic area and kidney but vasodilatation in skeletal muscle. This helps divert blood to skeletal muscle to prepare the body for flight or fight. Angiotensin II is a hormone that causes widespread vasoconstriction in the body. Renin, released from the kidney in states of hypotension, results in the formation of angiotensin II.

The ensuing generalised vasoconstriction raises total peripheral resistance as part of the response to restore the arterial pressure.

Local control of resistance vessels

Normally blood flow to a tissue is matched to its metabolic needs. Local metabolic activity causes the local production of vasoactive substances, which adjust local blood flow to meet local metabolic needs. A number of these vasoactive substances are listed below.

Metabolites. When products of metabolism accumulate, they cause dilatation of the resistance vessels. These increase local flow to clear the excess metabolites from the tissue. This accounts for the *exercise hyperaemia* that occurs in a limb after it is exercised. When exercise ceases, the blood flow rises to several times its resting value and then falls exponentially as the vasodilator metabolites are washed away and the vessels return to their resting condition. It also accounts for the *reactive hyperaemia* that occurs after blood flow to a limb is temporarily occluded. Products of metabolism accumulate during occlusion and dilate the resistance vessels. Therefore, when occlusion stops, blood flow rises immediately to high levels and falls off again exponentially as the accumulated metabolites are cleared from the tissues.

Respiratory gases. Most systemic resistance vessels dilate in response to a rise in local P_{CO_2}, a fall in local P_{O_2} and a fall in local pH. This helps increase blood flow to areas where metabolic activity is increased. Cerebral resistance vessels are especially sensitive to changes in P_{CO_2}. Cerebral blood flow is increased in the hypercapnia of respiratory failure and decreased in the hypocapnia of hyperventilation.

The resistance vessels in the lung are exceptional in their response to respiratory gas pressures. Hypoxia in the lungs leads to pulmonary vasoconstriction, not vasodilatation as in systemic vessels. This response helps divert pulmonary flow away from poorly ventilated alveoli to better ventilated parts where P_{O_2} is higher.

Local vasoactive substances. Many vasoactive substances have been described which are released in certain circumstances and affect local blood flow. These include *5-hydroxytryptamine* (serotonin), which is released from blood platelets when they aggregate during haemostasis. Serotonin contracts vascular smooth muscle in cut vessels and so limits blood loss. *Histamine,* released from damaged tissue and mast cells in certain antigen–antibody reactions, results in local vasodilatation. *Bradykinin,* a potent vasodilator released when certain exocrine glands are active, may account for the rise in local blood flow that accompanies secretion. *Prostaglandins,* a family of vasoactive substances involved in the inflammatory response, may be responsible for some of the vascular reactions in inflammation. The endothelium is a rich source of vasoactive substances, which are important in the local control of resistance blood vessels. These include *endothelium derived relaxing factor* (EDRF) and *endothelin.* EDRF, which is now accepted to be nitric oxide, is a potent vasodilator that is released when acetylcholine is applied to the endothelium. It may also be released in response to many other stimuli, including deformation of the endothelium. Damage to the endothelium may be a cause of hypertension by reducing its ability to produce EDRF. Endothelin is a vasoconstrictor substance produced by the endothelium but its physiological role has yet to be settled.

Local physical factors. Locally applied heat and cold dilate and constrict resistance vessels respectively. A hand put in water at 45°C will feel comfortable if the circulation is intact because the rise in local blood flow keeps tissue temperature cool and prevents tissue damage. However, if the circulation to the limb is occluded, immersion of the hand in water at 45°C will result in pain and tissue damage. Similarly, immersing the hand in freezing water causes periodic large vasodilatations (the hunting reaction), which keeps tissue temperature warm and protects the fingers from frostbite.

CAPILLARIES (exchange vessels)

Capillary walls consist of a single layer of endothelium surrounded by basement membrane and a fine fibrous sheath. They permit exchange of respiratory gases, nutrients and excretory products between the blood and the tissues.

Topography of capillary beds

Capillaries are organised in capillary beds. The true capillary arcades open off metarterioles (or through-going vessels), which are continuations of the true arterioles. Metarterioles have some smooth muscle in their walls and the entrance to each capillary arcade is surrounded by a ring of smooth muscle arranged as a precapillary sphincter. Not all capillaries are open at the same time. Vasomotion in the precapillary sphincters results in periodic opening and closure of different arcades at different times. The number open at any one time depends on the metabolic activity of local tissues.

Capillary porosity

Capillary endothelium has varying degrees of porosity, which determines its hydraulic conductivity. The least porous (*continuous endothelium*) is found in capillaries in brain, skin and skeletal muscle, where no gaps or pores can be detected in the endothelial cytoplasm. Fluid crosses continuous endothelium via the tight junctions between adjacent endothelial cells. In *fenestrated endothelium*, which occurs in renal glomerular and gut mucosal capillaries, there are small gaps or pores in the attenuated endothelial cytoplasm. The most porous endothelium is *discontinuous endothelium*, which occurs in the capillaries of liver and spleen. It has large gaps or slits between adjacent endothelial cells, through which even cells may pass.

Capillary surface area

Although an individual capillary has a small surface area available for exchange purposes, they are so numerous that, together, they offer an enormous surface area for fluid exchange. This area is about 300 m^2 at rest in the systemic circuit and 60 m^2 in the pulmonary circuit.

Capillary fragility

Although the walls of capillaries are extremely thin and fragile, they can stand distending pressures of over 100 mmHg without bursting. The ability to withstand high pressures can be explained by the law of Laplace for cylindrical tubes which states that:

$$T = Pr,$$

where T is the tension in wall, P is the internal pressure and r is the radius.

Tension in the wall depends on the radius of the vessel as well as the distending pressure. The capillary radius is so small that very large distending pressures are needed to raise tension in the walls to a level where bursting occurs. Nevertheless, small capillary leaks occur spontaneously and regularly and this becomes apparent when the small ruptures cannot be plugged adequately because of platelet deficiency. This results in thrombocytopenic purpura. Another type of purpura can occur even when platelet counts are normal. In these conditions, capillary fragility is increased and the vessels rupture easily at normal capillary pressures to give petechial haemorrhages.

Capillary haemodynamics

Capillary vessels are small, about 5 μm wide and 750 μm long. Red cells, which have a 7 μm diameter, have to be deformed into bullet-shaped cylinders as they pass through the vessels. Blood flows through capillaries at slow velocity, 0.5 mm s^{-1}. This means that a red cell spends 1–2 seconds passing through the capillary, allowing time for exchange to occur. The explanation of the slow flow is the large cross-sectional area of the capillary bed. The fact that there are so many capillaries in parallel accounts for their low vascular resistance. Blood enters the capillaries with a pressure of about 30 mmHg at the arterial end and falls to 15 mmHg at the venous end, a pressure drop of 15 mmHg across the capillary bed.

The haematocrit of capillary blood is about 25% lower than that in the arteries as the result of 'plasma skimming'. Relatively more plasma than cells is skimmed off when daughter vessels branch sideways from parent trunk vessels.

Capillary reserve

In the resting state, most capillary vessels are closed, but open up when metabolic activity increases. This increases the capillary surface area available for exchange in the systemic circuit from about 300 m^2 at rest to about 1000 m^2 when the vessels are maximally dilated. For the pulmonary circuit the corresponding figures are 60 m^2 at rest to 100 m^2 when maximally dilated.

Capillary contractility

There is argument about whether the capillary wall has intrinsic contractility. The vessels do not have a smooth muscle coat but the endothelial cells contain fibrils of actin and myosin which may contribute to capillary opening and closing. However, it is likely that most capillary opening and closing is a passive consequence of change in intravascular pressure. When precapillary sphincters relax, blood flowing into the capillaries raises intravascular pressure and passive distension results. When the sphincters close, blood runs out of the capillaries and the fall in intravascular pressure leads to their passive collapse.

Capillary exchange

Four processes contribute to movement of material across the capillary wall: (1) filtration–reabsorption, (2) diffusion, (3) pinocytosis and (4) diapedesis.

Filtration–reabsorption. In this process about 20 litres of fluid per day are filtered into the tissues at the arterial end of the capillary system where blood hydrostatic pressure is higher. This fluid perfuses the tissue spaces and 80–90% is reabsorbed back into the blood at the venous end of the capillaries and in small venules, where capillary hydrostatic pressure is lower. The factors involved in the filtration–reabsorption process are given in the filtration equation for solvent flow:

$$F = h(P_i - P_o) - r(C_i - C_o),$$

where F is the net fluid filtered, h is the hydraulic conductivity, P_i is the hydrostatic pressure inside the capillary, P_o is the hydrostatic pressure outside the capillary, r is the reflection coefficient, C_i is the colloid osmotic pressure inside the capillary and C_o is the colloid osmotic pressure outside the capillary. Fluid is driven out of the capillaries by the hydrostatic pressure gradient $(P_i - P_o)$ between capillary blood and tissue fluid. The amount filtered for a given pressure gradient depends on the *hydraulic conductivity* of the capillary wall, which varies in different capillaries. In capillaries with continuous endothelium (where h is small), fluid moves out through the limited areas afforded by the intercellular clefts. In fenestrated and discontinuous capillaries (where h is larger), fluid is also filtered through the pores and intercellular gaps.

The factors responsible for reabsorption are given by $r(C_i - C_o)$ in the filtration equation. About 18 of the litres filtered is reabsorbed back into the capillaries, mainly at their venous ends. The force for this is the colloid osmotic pressure gradient $(C_i - C_o)$ across the capillary wall. The colloid osmotic pressure is greater in blood than in tissue fluid because plasma proteins are retained in the circulation.

The effectiveness of the osmotic gradient in moving fluid depends on the impermeability of the wall to the colloids concerned. This is described by the *reflection coefficient, r*. The impermeability of the wall to colloids is due mainly to a glycocalyx layer applied to the endothelial side of the capillary wall. If the layer is damaged so that it becomes leaky to colloid, or if the size of the colloid particles falls, the colloid osmotic gradient is less effective in reabsorbing fluid, and oedema results.

Many factors can influence the filtration–reabsorption process. These include the levels of capillary and tissue hydrostatic pressure, the levels of blood and tissue fluid colloid osmotic pressure, the hydraulic conductivity of the endothelium and the reflection coefficient for colloids

at the capillary wall. An understanding of these factors is necessary for understanding the causes of oedema.

Diffusion. The movement of some substances across the capillary wall can be explained by simple diffusion. Substances move down their concentration gradients at a rate that depends on the diffusion distance, the area available for diffusion, the concentration gradient and the diffusion coefficient for the substance. Diffusion is responsible for the movement of respiratory gases across the capillary walls and other, especially fat soluble, substances.

Pinocytosis. In pinocytosis, macromolecules are engulfed into the cytoplasm on one side of the capillary endothelium to form vesicles. These vesicles move across the cell to fuse with the opposite endothelial wall where they release their contents by exocytosis. Quantitatively, this is not an important means of capillary exchange but explains how large macromolecules such as antibodies can cross capillary walls.

Diapedesis. This describes the process by which certain white cells move from the blood to the tissue spaces. First they attach themselves to the capillary wall and then insinuate themselves by amoeboid movement through the intercellular clefts in the endothelium.

VENULES AND VEINS (capacitance vessels)

Although all vessels hold blood, veins and venules hold more than the other vessels, as can be seen from the figures below that show the percentages of the blood volume in different parts the circulation:

- systemic circuit   80%
  - — systemic arteries   10%
  - — systemic capillaries   5%
  - — systemic veins and venules 65%
- pulmonary circuit   12%
- heart   8%.

Structure of capacitance vessels

Veins have the usual three tissue layers in their walls: intima, media and adventitia. There are intimal folds forming valves which prevent the retrograde flow of blood. Compared with arteries, the media is thin and its smooth muscle has a rich sympathetic vasoconstrictor innervation. Veins are more compliant than arteries and this increases their capacity to hold blood. When fluid is injected into a closed arterial segment, there is little increase in volume before intra-arterial pressure rises rapidly. In closed venous segments, injected fluid is first accommodated with little pressure rise until the elastic limit of the vessel is reached. Then the pressure rises rapidly.

Venous haemodynamics

Veins permit rapid return of blood from the tissues to the heart at little energy cost. The high velocity of flow is due to the venous system's relatively small total cross-sectional area. Although larger than that of arteries, it is much smaller than that of capillaries. Veins offer relatively little resistance to flow because of their relatively large radii. Thus blood can travel back to the heart with a pressure gradient of 10–15 mmHg.

Problems due to gravity

The compliance of the venous system causes problems during change in posture. On standing up, blood tends to accumulate in the distensible vessels in the lower half of the body and may compromise venous return to the heart. One way the body copes with this problem is the *muscle pump*. When skeletal muscles contract, they compress the veins that lie between them. Because of the orientation of the valves, the contained blood cannot be driven retrogradely. Instead it is pumped in the direction of the heart. When veins become varicose, the valves in the lower extremity may become incompetent and this makes the muscle pump less effective.

Breathing assists in the return of blood from the lower parts of the body when standing. During inhalation, the compression of the abdominal contents by the diaphragm, together with the development of negative pressure in the thorax, results in a pressure gradient driving blood back to the heart.

Capacitance function of the veins

The pressure in the great veins entering the heart is the filling pressure for the heart. Through the Frank–Starling mechanism, this pressure determines the diastolic distension and therefore the work done by the heart when it contracts. This in turn influences cardiac output. Central venous pressure should be kept at levels that provide satisfactory outputs. Relaxation of the veins causes central venous pressure, and thus cardiac output, to fall. Contraction of the venous system has the opposite effect. The venous system contracts reflexly to raise central venous pressure in the baroreceptor response to a fall in arterial pressure. In shock, veins may be so constricted that venepuncture is difficult.

The venous system also constricts when adrenaline and noradrenaline are released from the adrenal glands in times of stress. Again the response assists in raising cardiac output.

LYMPHATICS (tissue drainage system)

Although the lymphatic system returns excess tissue fluid to the circulation, it is also involved in immune surveillance, production of immunity and in fat transport from gut to blood.

Structure of lymphatics

The lymphatic system begins as blind-ended lymphatic capillaries whose walls consist of a single layer of endothelial cells. There are large slits between the edges of adjacent cells and the cells are attached to surrounding structures by anchoring filaments. Lymphatic capillaries join together to form larger vessels which carry lymph to the lymph nodes in afferent lymphatics. Afferent lymphatics have innervated smooth muscle in their walls and valves which allow lymph to flow in one direction only — towards the heart. In the nodes, lymph is filtered and surveyed for foreign antigens. From the nodes, lymph is carried back to the great veins by efferent lymphatics, whose structure is similar to afferent lymphatics.

Lymph formation

The mechanism of lymph formation is not well understood but is likely to be, at least in part, a mechanical process. One theory suggests that tissue movements pull the overlapping lips of the adjacent endothelial cells apart by pulling on the anchoring filaments. This creates a negative pressure inside the terminal lymphatics and draws tissue fluid down the pressure gradient into the lymphatic. When movement stops, the sequence is reversed. Elastic recoil of the tissues takes tension off the anchoring filaments, raises pressure in the lymphatic and the overlapping intercellular slits close. The contained fluid cannot escape back into the tissues and is driven downstream. Rhythmic massage of the tissues increases lymph formation greatly. Lymph is similar in composition to plasma except that its protein content is lower (about 4%). It also contains some white cells.

Lymph transport

The lymphatic system does not have a heart to generate the pressure head needed to drive fluid from the lymphatic capillaries to the great veins. The energy required comes from two other mechanisms. One is the lymphatic analogy of the muscle pump for veins. When muscles contract they squeeze the lymphatics that lie between the muscle bellies. Because of the orientation of the valves the lymph is driven in one direction only — towards the great veins. Additionally, the lymphatics have intrinsic contractility. When distended with lymph, they beat in a heart-like fashion, which drives lymph centripetally. The contractility is modulated by sympathetic nerve activity which increases the rate and force of the lymphatic contractions.

Lymphatic obstruction

Lymphatic obstruction results in lymphoedema. The tissues drained by the blocked vessels become swollen and the swelling does not pit on pressure, as in ordinary oedema. One of the reasons for this is the accumulation of protein in the tissues.

SPECIAL CIRCULATIONS
Pulmonary circulation
Pulmonary vascular resistance

The pulmonary circuit is a low resistance circuit. Whereas it needs about 100 mmHg pressure to drive blood round the systemic circuit, it requires only 20 mmHg to drive blood round the pulmonary circuit. This is because pulmonary arterioles offer relatively little resistance to flow. When cardiac output rises, pulmonary vascular resistance falls. Thus there is little rise in pulmonary arterial pressure during exercise. This is not due to baroreceptor reflexes in the pulmonary circuit. The increase in cardiac output may lead to passive distension of the pulmonary resistance vessels. It has been suggested that the increase in flow stimulates endothelial cells to release of nitric oxide (EDRF), which dilates the vessels.

Vascular responses to Po_2 changes

Ventilation of the lungs with air is normally matched to pulmonary capillary perfusion with blood to give a fairly constant ventilation:perfusion ratio. One of the factors responsible for this is the vascular response of pulmonary resistance vessels to Po_2. Whereas oxygen lack causes vasodilatation in the systemic circuit, it causes vasoconstriction in the pulmonary circuit. This tends to divert perfusion from underventilated areas of the lung to well ventilated parts. However, if the hypoxia is widespread in the lungs, as in respiratory failure and at high altitudes, the generalised vasoconstriction that results leads to *pulmonary hypertension*.

Pulmonary capillary pressure

The low capillary hydrostatic pressure in the lungs protects against pulmonary oedema. In systemic capillaries, mean capillary hydrostatic pressure (25 mmHg) is similar to the capillary colloid osmotic pressure. A rise in hydrostatic pressure results in net movement of fluid into the tissues. In pulmonary capillaries, the mean capillary hydrostatic pressure is about 5 mmHg and the colloid osmotic pressure is the same as in the systemic circuit (25 mmHg). Thus there is a large safety margin before rises in capillary pressure exceed colloid osmotic pressure levels and push fluid into the alveoli.

Dual blood supply to the lungs

The lungs receive blood from both pulmonary and bronchial arteries. This allows the pulmonary circuit to act as a filter removing small emboli and other material from the circulating blood with reduced danger of infarction of lung tissue.

The pulmonary circuit is also capable of modifying the activity of certain substances passing through it. For example, angiotensin I is converted to angiotensin II by enzymes in the pulmonary vascular endothelium. The endothelium can partially inactivate or remove serotonin, prostaglandins, noradrenaline and acetylcholine passing though the lungs to limit their passage to the systemic circuit.

Renal circulation

Blood is sent in large amounts to the kidneys for processing. One-quarter of the cardiac output is sent to the kidneys, although they account for only 0.5% of body weight. Thus renal blood flow (1.25 l min^{-1}) is greatly in excess of the kidney's metabolic needs and renal venous blood has a high oxygen content.

The renal vascular bed has a double capillary bed (a 'portal' system). Blood flows in afferent arterioles to the glomerular capillaries, where about one-fifth of the plasma flow is filtered into the renal tubules. The glomerular capillaries lead into a second set of arterioles (the efferent arterioles), which in turn open into the tubular capillary network.

The glomerular capillaries filter a greater proportion of delivered blood plasma than other capillary beds in the body. This is due to the unusually high hydrostatic pressure in the glomerular capillaries, which in turn is due to the unusually low resistance offered by the afferent arterioles. The glomerular capillary hydrostatic

pressure greatly exceeds the colloid osmotic pressure of the plasma proteins. Pressure in the glomerular capillaries can be modulated by modulating the relative resistances of the afferent and efferent arterioles.

Autoregulation

Autoregulation results in blood flow to an organ staying relatively constant despite changes in its perfusion pressure. Most vascular beds exhibit autoregulation but it is especially well developed in the renal circulation. There is no agreement on what mechanisms are responsible for autoregulation in the kidney. However, it is important for maintaining renal function in hypotensive states.

Vasomotor innervation

Renal resistance vessels have a well developed sympathetic vasoconstrictor system. These nerves are activated in baroreceptor reflexes and in fight or flight reactions. This helps to divert the kidneys' high blood flow to the heart and the brain in emergency situations.

Renin mechanism

As mentioned above, the kidneys detect falls in arterial pressure and respond by releasing renin into the circulation. This sets up responses that tend to raise arterial pressure by increasing cardiac output and peripheral resistance.

Coronary circulation

The coronary circulation is affected by the contractions of heart muscle. Ventricular systole obstructs blood inflow and aids outflow by squeezing the vessels. As a result, coronary vessel perfusion occurs mainly in diastole. Factors that shorten the diastolic period limit the time available for coronary inflow.

Blood flow to heart muscle is regulated mainly by metabolites and therefore has a close relationship to the work done by the heart. The metabolites involved include falls in tissue P_{O_2} levels and rises in adenosine, potassium, lactate, hydrogen ion concentration and P_{CO_2}. The oxygen extraction rate is high in the coronary circulation and coronary venous blood has a relatively low Po_2. When the rate or strength of the heart contractions is increased, the increased production of metabolites decreases coronary vascular resistance to a level where the increased blood flow can clear the metabolites from the tissues.

Vasomotor nerves play little part in the regulation of coronary blood flow. Although coronary resistance vessels have some vasoconstrictor innervation, the effect of their activity is normally outweighed by the metabolic response of the heart to sympathetic stimulation. Thus the coronary vessels are little affected in the generalised vasoconstrictor responses to systemic hypotension.

There are few anastomotic connections between the small coronary arteries. They are referred to as *functional end-arteries*. When a small artery becomes obstructed, the tissue served by that artery is not supplied by collaterals from neighbouring arteries and may become infarcted.

Cerebral circulation

The cerebral circulation is a critical one because cerebral tissues are very intolerant of hypoxia. Cessation of circulation for a few minutes can produce permanent damage to the brain. Not surprisingly, the cerebral circulation shows good autoregulation, and anastomotic connections are available through the circle of Willis. Carbon dioxide is an important metabolite for flow regulation. Cerebral resistance vessels are dilated by rises in Pco_2, and vice versa. Cerebral vessels have relatively thin walls, perhaps because they are protected from large transmural pressure changes by being enclosed in the cranium. The smooth muscle has little vasomotor innervation so, like coronary resistance vessels, cerebral resistance vessels play little part in baroreceptor reflexes.

The walls of the cerebral exchange vessels prevent or limit the entry of certain substances to brain tissues from the blood. This is known as the *blood–brain barrier*. The mechanism of the barrier is not well understood but it prevents substances such as bilirubin being deposited in the adult brain.

Being enclosed in a rigid cranium, the cerebral circulation is affected by intracranial pressure. Large increases in intracranial pressure decrease cerebral perfusion by compressing cerebral vessels.

Skeletal muscle circulation

Exercise hyperaemia

The circulation to skeletal muscle is determined mainly by metabolic factors. It can rise about 40-fold during exercise, despite the periodic compression of the vessels during muscle contractions. Nevertheless, demand for oxygen can outstrip oxygen delivery in severe exercise and the muscle acquires an oxygen debt. Thus blood flow remains high after exercise, as the accumulated metabolites keep the resistance vessels dilated until the metabolic debt is paid off.

Vasomotor nerves

Skeletal muscle blood vessels are supplied with sympathetic vasoconstrictor nerves and are held in tonic vasoconstriction. Release of vasoconstrictor tone can double blood flow, and increased sympathetic tone can reduce resting flow to almost zero. These nerves are involved in the baroreceptor reflexes but not in exercise hyperaemia. A system of vasodilator nerves to skeletal muscle has been described, the activity of which is coordinated through centres in the hypothalamus. They are not active at rest, but may cause vasodilatation in muscle vessels in fight or flight reactions.

Skin circulation

The metabolic requirements of skin are small. Blood flow to the skin is normally in excess of these requirements and the oxygen content in blood draining skin is high. Blood flow to skin is mainly concerned with temperature regulation. Local application of cold or heat to the skin causes local vasoconstriction and dilatation respectively. Skin resistance vessels have a constrictor innervation maintaining tonic vasoconstriction. When hypothalamic thermoreceptors detect a rise in body temperature, sympathetic vasoconstrictor tone in skin is reflexly reduced. The resulting rise in skin temperature allows more heat to be lost to the environment. The greatest increases in flow are seen in the extremities, where there are numerous arteriovenous anastomoses and the surface to volume ratio favours heat dissipation.

Splanchnic circulation

Like the kidneys, the splanchnic circulation has two capillary beds in the circuit, forming a 'portal' circulation. The first capillary bed is in the walls of the gut. The veins draining the gut pass to the liver in the portal vein, where they enter a second capillary bed in the liver. Obstruction of this bed by cirrhosis or similar pathology causes pressure to rise in the portal vein. The back pressure in capillaries in the walls of the intestines increases fluid exudation, causing ascites.

The splanchnic circulation has a rich sympathetic vasoconstrictor innervation and reduces splanchnic blood flow in the baroreceptor responses to hypotension.

Most changes in splanchnic blood flow are related to secretory activity in digestive glands and absorption of food from the gut. This vasodilatation is due in part to metabolites produced by local metabolic activity. Vasoactive polypeptides such as bradykinin, vasoactive intestinal peptide and neurotensin may also be involved, especially in the vasodilatation that accompanies secretion in exocrine glands.

CIRCULATORY ADAPTATION TO HAEMORRHAGE

Effects of haemorrhage

Haemorrhage that causes a significant fall in the blood volume can lead to death. The fall in blood volume reduces the venous return to the heart and thus the filling pressure of the heart. The reduced filling results in reduced strength of myocardial contraction, a fall in stroke volume and hence cardiac output, and a lowering of arterial pressure. If the body does not compensate for this, there is underperfusion of the tissues. The most serious consequences arise from underperfusion of the vital structures, the brain and the heart. In the brain, cerebral ischaemia leads to depression of consciousness followed by coma and death. Myocardial ischaemia weakens myocardial contractility further, so that a vicious circle is set up. The myocardial weakness reduces cardiac output further, which in turn reduces myocardial blood flow, and so on. In the kidneys, the fall in glomerular filtration pressure may result in cessation of urine formation. In the gut, ischaemia can impair the digestion and absorption of food. There is evidence that prolonged ischaemia in the gut in circulatory failure may damage the mucosa, allowing entry of bacteria and endotoxins. In skeletal muscle, ischaemia leads to a metabolic acidosis because lactic acid accumulates if oxygen delivery is insufficient. Ischaemia in skin results in pale, cold extremities, and gangrene in severe cases.

The healthy body attempts to prevent tissue ischaemia after haemorrhage by triggering physiological adaptations to overcome the effects of blood loss.

Early adaptation

After haemorrhage, the body takes measures to raise blood pressure to a level where tissue perfusion, especially that of the vital organs, is sufficient to maintain life despite the reduction in blood volume. Early adaptation occurs within a few seconds or minutes following the haemorrhage. It is mainly a reflex response to the fall in arterial pressure detected by the baroreceptors in the proximal arterial tree. The response is widespread.

In the heart there is reduction in vagal tone and an increase in sympathetic nerve activity, giving an increase in the rate and strength of contraction of the heart. This tends to raise arterial pressure. In the less essential tissues, such as skin, skeletal muscle, gut and kidneys, intense sympathetic vasoconstriction raises total peripheral resistance and thus blood pressure. The reduction in flow to less vital tissues diverts more blood to the heart and the brain circulations, which are little affected by reflex vasoconstrictor activity. These effects are augmented by reflex release of adrenaline and noradrenaline from the adrenal glands. Reflex venoconstriction is also a part of the response to baroreceptor stimulation. This contraction of the veins raises central venous pressure, which causes greater cardiac filling and myocardial performance.

Intermediate adaptation

Within about 15 minutes of the haemorrhage, the body takes measures to raise blood volume to levels that can support adequate cardiac outputs and to restore blood content to normal by mobilisation of tissue fluid. Constriction of resistance vessels reduces capillary hydrostatic pressure in the non-vital tissues. Since the colloid osmotic pressure of blood is initially unchanged, the fall in fluid filtration results in a net inward shift of fluid from the tissues to the blood, which helps to restore blood volume. Later this process is augmented by the renin–angiotensin and antidiuretic hormone (vasopressin) systems, which decrease the urinary output of water and salt. This becomes effective 2–3 days after the haemorrhage. The fall in blood pressure after haemorrhage is detected by receptors in the juxtaglomerular apparatus in the kidneys as well as by the arterial baroreceptors. The former leads to the production of renin and later angiotensin II. By its action on the kidneys to increase the reabsorption of salt and water from the glomerular filtrate, it expands blood volume and hence venous return to the heart. Angiotensin II also increases total peripheral resistance by its direct vasoconstrictor action on arterioles. Antidiuretic hormone released in response to signals from low pressure receptors in the circulation also reduces water loss via the kidneys and so helps in expanding blood volume. The restoration of volume without a corresponding increase in red cell content is responsible for the low blood haematocrit seen after haemorrhage.

Long term adaptation

The fall in oxygen carrying capacity in the blood is detected by cells in the kidney and results in the formation of erythropoietin. This stimulates bone marrow to increase erythropoiesis until the haemoglobin level is restored to normal. This final adaptation takes place over a period of about 6 weeks.

FURTHER READING

Guyton A C 1991 Blood pressure control — special role of the kidneys and body fluids. Science 252: 1813–1816

Haynes W G 1995 Endothelins as regulators of vascular tone in man. Clinical Science 88: 509–517

Miller J D 1995 Editorial: Ensuring adequate cerebral perfusion during aneurysm surgery. British Journal of Anaesthesia 75: 518–519

Niemann J T 1992 Cardiopulmonary resuscitation. New England Journal of Medicine 327: 1075–1080

Rowell L B 1993 Human cardiovascular control. Oxford University Press, Oxford

Shepherd J T, Abboud F M (eds) 1983 Peripheral circulation and organ blood flow. In: Handbook of physiology, sect 2, vol 3, parts 1 & 2. American Physiological Society, Bethesda

27

Control of arterial blood pressure

G. D. Johnston
T. J. McMurray
W. B. Loan
J. P. H. Fee

This chapter covers aspects of the control of arterial blood pressure which are of importance to the practising anaesthetist. The first section reviews normal control and should be read in conjunction with Chapter 22. This section also covers some of the mechanisms underlying essential hypertension and its pharmacological control in the long term. Perioperative pharmacological control of blood pressure in special circumstances is also reviewed.

REVIEW OF NORMAL CONTROL

Control of blood pressure (haemodynamic aspects)

According to the non-pulsatile flow model of the circulation, mean blood pressure is directly proportional to the product of the blood flow (cardiac output) and resistance to the movement of blood through the precapillary arterioles (peripheral vascular resistance):

$$\text{Arterial blood pressure} = \text{cardiac output} \times \text{peripheral vascular resistance.}$$

Blood pressure is maintained by beat-to-beat regulation of cardiac output and peripheral vascular resistance at three sites within the cardiovascular system: arterioles capacitance vessels and the heart. The kidney is also involved in the maintenance of blood pressure by regulating the extravascular fluid volume. Baroreflexes, mediated by the sympathetic nervous system, act with a variety of humoral mechanisms especially the renin–angiotensin system to coordinate the control sites and regulate blood pressure in normal and hypertensive individuals; however, regulation in hypertensive patients differs from that in normal individuals in that the baroreceptor and renal blood volume pressure control seem to be set at a higher level.

The determinants of pressure that exist at any moment within the arterial system cannot be evaluated with great precision and the constant flow model of the circulation has major limitations. The pressure in all systemic arteries fluctuates due to the pumping action of the heart. The systolic and diastolic pressures represent the limits of the pressure fluctuations during the cardiac cycle (Fig. 27.1). More information about the interaction of the heart and systemic circulation can be obtained by measuring the mean arterial pressure and considering the systolic and diastolic blood pressures as the upper and lower limits of periodic oscillations about the mean. The mean arterial pressure is obtained by measuring the area under the arterial pressure wave tracing and dividing this area by the time interval involved. An approximation to this value can be obtained by adding one-third of the pulse pressure to the diastolic blood pressure. As previously discussed, the mean arterial pressure depends only on the cardiac output and the peripheral resistance. The pulse pressure, by contrast, is principally a function of stroke volume and arterial compliance. In general, an increase in stroke volume or a decrease in arterial compliance will produce an increase in pulse pressure, although the level of the mean arterial blood pressure also has an impact on arterial compliance. Arterial compliance, i.e. the amount of stretch in the vessel wall for a given pressure, is important for a variety of reasons. Arterial compliance decreases with age and is an important factor in the development of systolic hypertension. In isolated systolic hypertension in the elderly, little change in mean arterial blood pressure occurs, while arterial compliance is significantly reduced. Recent clinical trials have demonstrated that systolic blood pressure is as important a risk factor as diastolic blood pressure and that reducing isolated systolic blood pressure in elderly patients decreases the risk of stroke and heart disease. In addition, in patients with hypertension and diabetes, relatives of hypertensive patients and those with borderline hypertension, arterial compliance is reduced.

Baroreflex mechanisms

Baroreceptor reflexes are responsible for moment-to-moment adjustments of blood pressure such as changes in posture (Fig. 27.2). Sympathetic neurones arising from the vasomotor centre in the medulla are tonically active. Carotid baroreceptors are stimulated by the stretch of the blood vessel walls, which is largely dependent on the

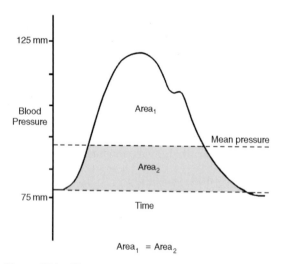

Figure 27.1 Changes in blood pressure with time during one cardiac cycle. The line representing mean blood pressure divides the area under the curve into two equal parts.

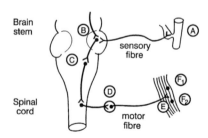

Figure 27.2 Basic components of the baroreceptor reflex arc. A, Baroreceptor in the carotid sinus; B, nucleus of the tractus solitarius; C, vasomotor centre; D, autonomic ganglion; E, sympathetic nerve ending; F_1, β adrenoceptor; F_2, α adrenoceptor.

pressure exerted by the blood within the vessel. Baroreceptor activation inhibits central sympathetic discharge and a reduction in stretch inhibits baroreceptor activity. When the body assumes an upright position baroreceptors detect the reduction in blood pressure, which results from venous pooling, and sympathetic discharge is increased. The reflex increase in sympathetic outflow through the nerve endings results in an increase in peripheral resistance and cardiac output by constricting the resistance and capacitance vessels and increasing the force of contraction of the left ventricle. The baroreflex acts in response to any event which lowers blood pressure, in particular peripheral vasodilatation and fluid loss.

Role of the kidney

The kidney is primarily responsible for the long term regulation of blood pressure. A reduction in renal perfusion pressure causes intrarenal distribution of blood flow and increased reabsorption of salt and water by the renal tubule. Reduced pressure in the renal arterioles combined with increased sympathetic nerve activity stimulates renin and angiotensin II production through the β receptors (Fig. 27.3). The two main actions of angiotensin II are direct constriction of the resistance vessels and increased aldosterone production by the adrenal cortex. These effects increase renal sodium absorption and intravascular blood volume.

Disturbed mechanisms in essential hypertension

The cause of essential hypertension is unknown, although hereditary factors, excessive intake of alcohol and salt, obesity and cigarette smoking all have a role to play. In patients with long standing hypertension peripheral vascular resistance is elevated, the cardiac output is normal, plasma volume is normal or slightly decreased and the baroreceptor function is reset at a higher level. Renal vascular resistance is increased, with a decrease in renal blood flow and an increase in the filtration fraction due to efferent arteriolar

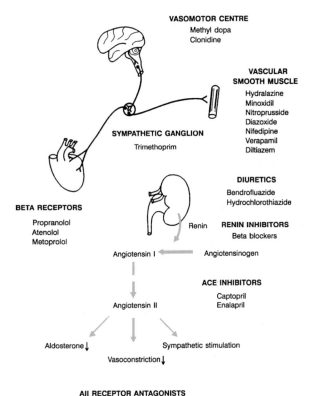

Figure 27.3   Sites of action of the major classes of antihypertensive agents.

vasoconstriction. The most consistent feature of hypertension is reduced diameter of the resistance vessels due to vasoconstriction and hypertrophy of vascular smooth muscle. Despite these changes the system usually continues to regulate itself satisfactorily and further increases in blood pressure result in prompt counterregulatory mechanisms such as increased excretion of salt and water by the kidney and reduced sympathetic responses through the baroreceptor mechanism. There is considerable disagreement about the initiating events, which may have been present since the time of birth. The theories can be broadly divided into three groups: renal autoregulatory, neurogenic and sodium transport hypotheses.

Autoregulatory hypothesis

It is proposed that the initiating event is increased cardiac output and the enhanced flow to the tissues results in reflex vasoconstriction in the resistance and renal vessels. Cardiac output then returns to normal but the peripheral vasoconstriction persists. With time, there is hypertrophy of the small resistance vessels, which helps to maintain the elevated blood pressure despite normal cardiac output. The most popular theory is that the increased cardiac output occurs secondary to a renal defect which causes sodium and water retention and increased plasma volume. The ensuing elevated pressure produces a pressure natriuresis and a return of the plasma volume towards the normal. There are some animal data to support the hypothesis.

Neurogenic hypothesis

This hypothesis is somewhat similar but it is proposed that the primary defect is increased neurogenic activity rather than a renal abnormality. This leads to increased venous tone, vascular resistance and heart rate. The increased venous tone moves blood from the capacitance vessels to increase volume in the central system. This increase in central blood volume causes an increase in cardiac output and heart rate and increased sympathetic activity to the kidney results in sodium retention and volume expansion. In keeping with this hypothesis is the observation that young labile hypertensive patients with normal peripheral resistance and a high cardiac output change to a normal cardiac output and a high peripheral resistance pattern over a period of 10 years.

Defect in sodium transport

This theory suggests that the primary defect is an abnormality of sodium transport in vascular smooth muscle. This results in an increase in intracellular sodium and a secondary increase in intracellular calcium as extracellular calcium is exchanged for intracellular sodium. Increased calcium results in contraction of vascular smooth muscle and increases peripheral resistance and blood pressure. There is little to confirm that this is the primary defect in hypertension, and impaired sodium excretion by the kidney could cause these abnormalities by causing volume expansion and secretion of a natriuretic hormone, which in turn inhibits the enzyme sodium potassium ATPase.

Hereditary aspects

There is a general consensus that the predisposition to high blood pressure has a strong hereditary basis. This is based on records of single families, studies of family histories and investigations in identical and non-identical twins. Epidemiological studies confirm that the distribution of blood pressure values in the relatives of hypertensive patients is significantly higher than in the relatives of normotensive control populations. The genes involved have not been accurately identified in man but restriction fragment length polymorphism for the renin and angiotensinogen gene have been described in hypertensive rats and links between the angiotensin converting enzyme (ACE) gene and atherosclerosis have been identified.

PHARMACOLOGICAL CONTROL OF BLOOD PRESSURE

Antihypertensive drugs produce their effects on blood pressure by interacting at one or more of four anatomical control sites, illustrated in Figure 27.3. They can be divided into four groups: drugs that alter sodium and water balance; those that alter sympathetic nervous system function; agents that directly relax vascular smooth muscle; and substances that decrease the production or action of angiotensin II.

Drugs that alter sodium and water balance

Diuretics

Diuretics differ in structure and major sites of action within the nephron. Thiazide diuretics principally act on the cortical diluting segment of the distal tubule, the loop diuretics on the thick ascending part of the loop of Henle and the potassium sparing diuretics on the distal tubule and collecting ducts (see Fig. 35.1). They are discussed more fully in Chapter 35.

Thiazide diuretics

Thiazide diuretics act by inhibiting sodium and chloride cotransport across the luminal membrane in the cortical diluting segment of the distal convoluted tubule, where 5–10% of the filtered sodium load is reabsorbed. The precise mechanisms underlying the antihypertensive effects of thiazide diuretics have not been clearly defined. A negative sodium balance is probably involved in the early stages of treatment. Thiazide diuretics may also exert weak potassium channel opening activity and some of the antihypertensive activity could be related to peripheral vasodilatation and reduced peripheral vascular resistance and/or reduced vascular sensitivity to circulating pressor hormones. With conventional doses of diuretics, plasma and extracellular fluid volumes decrease initially but return to normal within a few weeks as a result of humoral and intrarenal counterregulatory mechanisms. Sodium intake and excretion are usually balanced within 3–9 days and peripheral resistance increases. Within 4–8 weeks, peripheral resistance declines and the blood pressure lowering effect is maximum. Commonly used thiazides include bendrofluazide, hydrochlorothiazide and cyclopenthiazide.

Loop diuretics

Loop diuretics block chloride reabsorption by inhibiting the $Na^+K^+2Cl^-$ cotransport system of the luminal membrane in the thick ascending limb of the loop of Henle (see Fig. 35.1), where 35–45% of the filtered sodium load is reabsorbed. They have a more rapid onset of action in terms of their diuretic activity than the thiazides, and increasing the dose produces increasing diuresis. They have no clear advantages over thiazide diuretics in terms of efficacy or adverse effects in the treatment of hypertension. Their major role is in patients with renal insufficiency or in combination with vasodilator drugs in resistant hypertension. Examples include frusemide and bumetanide.

Potassium sparing diuretics

This group of drugs acts on the distal tubule to prevent potassium loss and facilitate sodium excretion. They either work by directly inhibiting sodium-potassium exchange mechanisms (triamterene and amiloride) or antagonising the effects of aldosterone on the exchange of sodium and potassium within the tubule. All three are relatively weak diuretics and their main role is to reduce the hypokalaemia induced by thiazide and loop diuretics.

Drugs that alter sympathetic nervous system function

This constitutes the largest group of antihypertensive agents. It includes the α- and β-adrenoceptor antagonists and the centrally acting antihypertensive drugs.

β-Adrenoceptor antagonists

The precise modes of action of β-adrenoceptor antagonists in lowering blood pressure has been the subject of controversy since their introduction for the treatment of hypertension almost 30 years ago. All currently available agents act on the β_1 receptor and those that are selective for the β_2 receptor have no significant antihypertensive activity. Despite this, β_1-selective agents, such as atenolol, metoprolol and bisoprolol, are no more effective than non-selective drugs such as propranolol and sotalol. Most evidence suggests that β-adrenoceptor antagonists lower blood pressure by renal and cardiac mechanisms (Fig. 27.3). Reductions in plasma renin activity probably play a part but the decrease in blood pressure is mostly related to decreases in heart rate and cardiac output, although there is no direct relationship between these two measures and blood pressure reduction. Total peripheral resistance increases initially to compensate for the fall in cardiac output but returns to normal or near normal levels as baroreceptor activity declines. With time, cardiac output also tends to increase to near pretreatment levels. The antihypertensive action of β-adrenoceptor antagonists therefore depends on at least two mechanisms: reduced renin release and a cardiovascular mechanism triggered by reductions in heart rate and cardiac output.

α-Adrenoceptor antagonists

α Adrenoceptors can be divided into two subtypes, α_1 and α_2. This classification is based on the affinity of selective agonists and antagonists for these two subtypes. Adrenoceptors are also defined in terms of their localisation within the synapse. Presynaptic receptors are located on the sympathetic nerve endings and postsynaptic on the target organ, e.g. blood vessels (Table 27.1 and Fig. 27.4).

Stimulation of the α_1 adrenoceptors at the postsynaptic sites causes vasoconstriction, increased peripheral resistance and hence increased blood pressure. Drugs that selectively antagonise the α_1 adrenoceptors are therefore effective peripheral vasodilators and antihypertensive agents. Nonselective α blockers such as phenoxybenzamine and phentolamine are of little value in the long term management of hypertension because they increase heart rate and blunt the antihypertensive effect resulting from α_1 adrenoceptor blockade. Noradrenaline released from the sympathetic nerve endings stimulates the postsynaptic α_1 receptors to increase blood pressure and the α_2 presynaptic receptor to inhibit further release of noradrenaline. By antagonising the α_1 and α_2 receptors, blood pressure decreases but the continued release of noradrenaline stimulates the postsynaptic β_1 receptors to increase heart rate (Fig. 27.4). Drugs such as prazosin and doxazosin selectively block the postsynaptic α_1 receptor but do not facilitate the release of endogenous noradrenaline from the sympathetic nerve endings. As a result they are more effective as antihypertensive agents and do not induce reflex tachycardia.

Table 27.1 Distribution of α adrenoceptors and the effect of stimulation.

Receptor subtype	Organ/system	Response to stimulation
α_1 (postsynaptic)	Blood vessels Heart Eye Central nervous system	Contraction Increased force of contraction Mydriasis, increased intraocular pressure Inhibition of afferent inputs to the baroreceptor
α_2 (presynaptic)	Sympathetic neurones	Inhibition of noradrenaline release
α_2 (postsynaptic)	Central nervous system Eye Pancreas	Hypotension, bradycardia Increased intraocular pressure Inhibition of insulin secretion

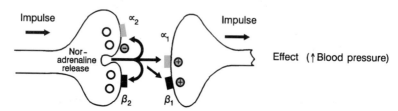

Figure 27.4 Proposed mode of action of α antagonists. Non-selective: block α_1 and α_2 resulting in increased noradrenaline release. Selective: block postsynaptic α_1 without preventing the inhibitory effect of the α_2 receptor on noradrenaline release.

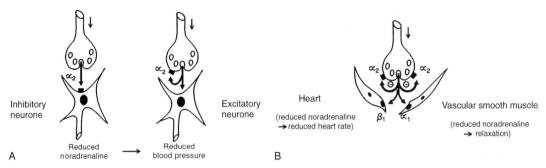

Figure 27.5 Possible sites of action of centrally acting antihypertensive drugs. A: Central nervous system. B: Peripheral nervous system.

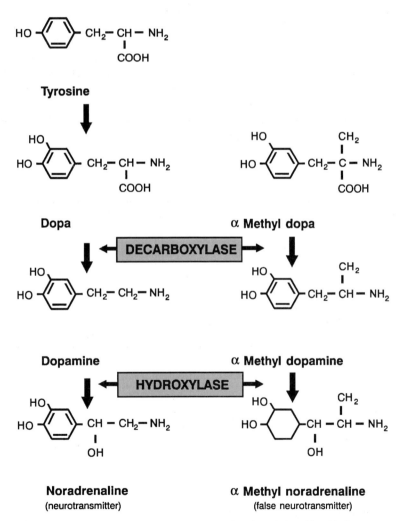

Figure 27.6 Metabolism of methyldopa showing the relationship with the biosynthetic pathway for noradrenaline.

Centrally acting inhibitors of the sympathetic nervous system

Clonidine and methyldopa act by similar mechanisms. They stimulate the α_2 adrenoceptors in the vasomotor centre of the medulla oblongata reducing sympathetic outflow from the brain (Fig. 27.5). Clonidine produces its effect directly but methyldopa requires conversion within the brain to α-methylnoradrenaline (Fig. 27.6). Stimulation of the presynaptic α_2 receptors by clonidine and α-methylnoradrenaline in the peripheral nervous system probably makes a contribution to their antihypertensive activity (Fig. 27.5).

Direct acting vasodilators

The direct acting vasodilator antihypertensive drugs are heterogeneous groups of compounds that relax vascular smooth muscle by a variety of mechanisms. The most important group are the calcium channel antagonists, which have largely replaced the other direct acting vasodilator drugs in the management of hypertension.

Calcium channel antagonists

This group of compounds acts by inhibiting postexcitation influx of calcium through the L-calcium channels of the cell membrane into myocardial and smooth muscle cells. This in turn interferes with the action of calcium-dependent ATPase required for the contraction of these cells. The overall effect is a reduction in myocardial contractility and dilatation of vascular smooth muscle. These agents appear to selectively block the calcium channels and leave the sodium channels unaffected. Myocardial contractility is therefore reduced, with no effect on cell depolarisation (Fig. 27.7).

Different groups of calcium channel antagonists recognise different binding sites. The relative binding to the different sites determines which agents have the greatest effects on vascular smooth muscle, cardiac muscle or conducting tissue. Therefore, although these drugs have a common mode of action, they differ with respect to myocardial contractility, systemic vascular resistance, coronary artery dilatation,

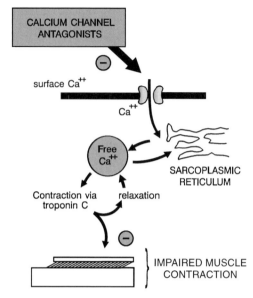

Figure 27.7

venomotor tone and antiarrhythmic activity (Table 27.2).

Other direct acting vasodilator drugs

In this group of antihypertensive drugs two orally active agents, minoxidil and hydralazine, and two parenteral vasodilators, nitroprusside and diazoxide, are included. All four drugs relax arteriolar smooth muscle and so reduce systemic vascular resistance. Decreased arteriolar resistance and decreased blood pressure elicit compensatory responses mediated by baroreceptors, sympathetic and renin–angiotensin–aldosterone systems. These effects on heart rate, blood volume and inotropic activity tend to oppose the antihypertensive effects of vasodilators (Fig. 27.8) but can be largely prevented by coadministration of diuretics and β-adrenoceptor antagonists.

Hydralazine appears to produce its vasodilator effect by interfering with the cellular calcium movements responsible for initiating or maintaining muscle contraction. Minoxidil prevents the uptake of calcium by the cell membrane of vascular smooth muscle cells and may enhance the opening of the potassium channels. The observation that endogenously pro-

Table 27.2 Calcium channel antagonists

Type	Group	Example	Principal action
I	Phenylalkylamines	Verapamil	*Cardiac:* Depressed AV conduction (+++) Depressed myocardial contractility (+++) *Vascular:* Vasodilatation (++)
II	Dihydropyridines	Nifedipine Amlodipine Nicardipine	*Cardiac:* Depressed myocardial contractility (+) *Vascular:* Vasodilatation (+++)
III	Benzothiazepine	Diltiazem	*Cardiac:* Depressed AV conduction (+++) Depressed myocardial contractility (+) *Vascular:* Vasodilatation (++)

* Slight effect; (++) moderate effect; (+++) marked effect.

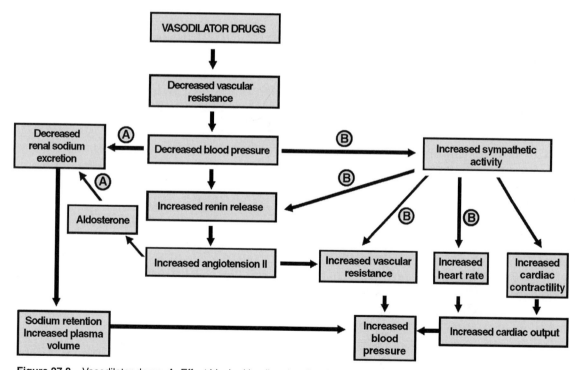

Figure 27.8 Vasodilator drugs. A, Effect blocked by diuretics; B, effect blocked by β-adrenoceptor antagonists.

duced nitric oxide from the vascular endothelium is a potent vasodilator suggests that sodium nitroprusside may mimic this action in vascular smooth muscle. Diazoxide acts directly on smooth muscle by opening potassium channels and exerts its effect on all circulatory beds. Diazoxide, hydralazine and minoxidil act principally on the resistance arterioles, while sodium nitroprusside has combined arteriolar and venodilator activity.

Drugs affecting the renin–angiotensin system

Angiotensin converting enzyme inhibitors

Angiotensin converting enzyme inhibitors block the conversion of the inactive decapeptide angiotensin I to the active vasoconstrictor octapeptide angiotensin II. Reductions in angiotensin II levels decrease circulating aldosterone concentrations, facilitating sodium loss and potassium retention. ACE inhibitors also prevent the breakdown of kinins, locally formed vasodilator peptides which stimulate the formation of vasodilatory prostaglandins by acting on cell membrane phospholipase (Fig. 27.9). These additional vasodilator effects may be involved in the antihypertensive effects of ACE inhibitors. Unlike most other peripheral vasodilators, ACE inhibitors do not cause reflex increases in heart rate, and this is possibly related to reduced sympathetic and/or increased parasympathetic activity. In uncomplicated hypertension, renal perfusion is unaffected or slightly improved, but in patients with reduced renal perfusion due to renal artery stenosis and heart failure, renal function can decline to critical levels. Examples include captopril, a short acting agent which works as the parent compound, a series of longer acting drugs which require conversion to the active form in the liver, enalapril, quinapril. perindopril and ramipril, and a long acting ACE inhibitor, lisinopril, which does not require conversion in the liver.

MANAGEMENT OF HYPERTENSION

Non-drug therapy

All patients with hypertension should be advised about lifestyle modification if appropriate, whether or not they receive drug therapy.

Stopping smoking

Until recently it was widely stated that cigarette smoking had little effect on blood pressure and the main reason for recommending that patients should stop smoking was that it represented a powerful independent risk factor for the development of coronary heart disease and stroke. Recent evidence suggests that there is a 15–30 minute elevation in blood pressure each time an individual smokes a cigarette. These pressor effects have been described during 24 hour blood pressure monitoring and, although not proven, it is possible that the rises in blood pressure contribute to the increased incidence of vascular events in smokers and their apparent resistance to the effects of antihypertensive medication.

Reduced alcohol intake

Several population studies have confirmed that there is a positive association between blood pressure and regular alcohol consumption. Blood pressure is higher in patients who consume more than three units daily and the risk of developing hypertension is two to three times more common in heavy drinkers. A mean decrease in alcohol consumption from 452 to 64 ml per week resulted in a mean decrease of 5 mmHg in systolic pressure and a mean decrease of 3 mmHg in diastolic blood pressure, independent of changes in weight in treated hypertensive patients. Alcohol reduction is of proven benefit in hypertensive patients.

Weight reduction

Obesity is associated with increased blood pressure. On average a decrease of 1 kg body weight is associated with a decrease of approximately 1% in systolic and diastolic blood pressures, and this decrease is independent of changes in salt and alcohol intake.

Salt restriction

Modest salt restriction by about one third has been shown to reduce systolic blood pressure by 5 mmHg and diastolic blood pressure by almost. 3 mmHg. Elderly patients and those with the highest initial blood pressure show the greatest responses. Moderate sodium restriction would seem to be a desirable goal for individual hypertensives and for the population at large.

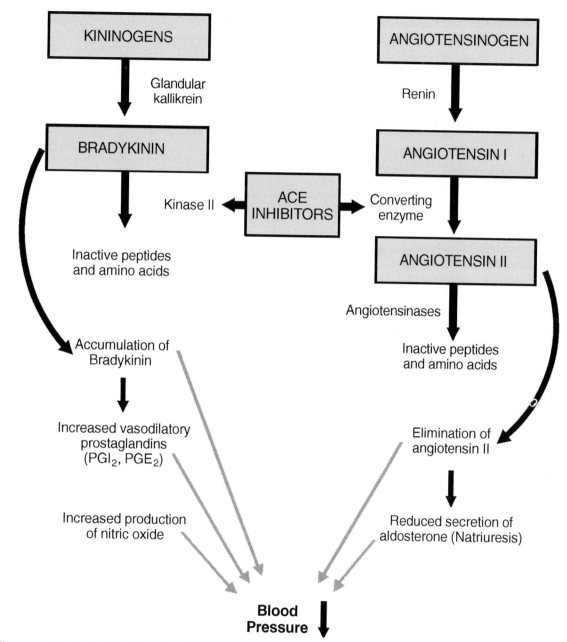

Figure 27.9 Mechanisms by which ACE inhibitors lower blood pressure.

Increased potassium intake

Some of the benefits observed with salt restriction are probably related to increased potassium intake in the diet and epidemiological evidence suggests an inverse relationship between potassium intake and blood pressure. An adequate intake of potassium, especially in patients receiving thiazide or loop diuretics, is therefore recommended but a high intake of potassium cannot be recommended as routine, especially in elderly patients and those with poor renal function.

Other non-pharmacological interventions

Several other non-pharmacological measures have been investigated in hypertensive populations but the majority are of no proven value in reducing blood pressure in the long term. These include reduced intake of dietary calcium, increased magnesium, biofeedback and relaxation. There is limited evidence that increased exercise and a vegetarian diet may prevent increases in blood pressure, with small but significant decreases in normotensive and hypertensive populations.

In conclusion, there is sound evidence that weight reduction, moderate salt restriction and alcohol reduction will lower blood pressure, at least in short term studies. Although all patients should receive advice on lifestyle modification, there remains the danger that prolonged non-pharmacological treatment will result in suboptimal treatment. This form of therapy should be regarded as a useful supplement to antihypertensive drug treatment and not an alternative to it.

Choice of antihypertensive agent

New antihypertensive drugs are being continually introduced into clinical practice. There is little evidence that any of these newer agents have major advantages over diuretics and β-adrenoceptor antagonists in terms of efficacy and adverse effects, provided appropriate doses are chosen. Almost all orally active drugs lower blood pressure by about 10% in patients with mild-to-moderate hypertension. When direct comparisons between various drugs are made, they almost always show similar efficacy for periods up to 5 years. However, some patients will benefit more from certain types of drug treatment than others, depending on the presence of other conditions (Table 27.3).

Thiazide diuretics

Thiazide diuretics remain the cornerstone of antihypertensive therapy. They are inexpensive and have been used to treat hypertension for almost 40 years. More importantly, they have been the pivotal agents in most large therapeutic outcome studies, including recent studies in the elderly, where positive benefits have been demonstrated for cardiovascular and cerebrovascular disease. For maximum benefit, these drugs should be prescribed at the lowest effective dose or in combination with potassium sparing agents.

Adverse effects. These are discussed in Chapter 35. Most disadvantages of diuretics relate to their adverse biochemical effects. Those that have caused concern include hypokalaemia, hypomagnesaemia, hyperuricaemia, hyperlipidaemia and glucose intolerance.

Table 27.3

Associated condition	Diuretic	β blocker	ACE inhibitor	Calcium antagonist	α blocker
Diabetes	Problems with higher doses	Prolonged hypoglycaemia with non-selective agents	Yes	Yes	Yes
Gout	No	Yes	Yes	Yes	Yes
Dyslipidaemia	Controversial	Controversial	Yes	Yes	Yes
Ischaemic heart disease	Yes	Yes	Yes	Yes	Yes
Heart failure	Yes	No	Yes	Problems with verapamil and some dihydropyridines	Yes
Asthma	Yes	No	Yes	Yes	Yes
Peripheral vascular disease	Yes	No	Care needed	Yes	Yes
Renal artery stenosis	Yes	Yes	No	Yes	Yes

Loop diuretics

Loop diuretics have no clear advantages over thiazide diuretics, when used as monotherapy, in terms of efficacy or adverse effects. Their major role is in patients with renal insufficiency or in combination with vasodilator drugs in resistant hypertension. In general they cause fewer metabolic problems than longer acting thiazide diuretics and related compounds. The risk of eighth nerve damage most commonly occurs with ethacrynic acid, and least commonly with bumetanide, and is seen mainly in patients with renal impairment who received large doses.

Potassium sparing diuretics

Potassium sparing diuretics are mainly used in combination with thiazide diuretics in the treatment of hypertension and may have some advantages over larger doses of thiazide diuretics in terms of preventing hypokalaemia, arrhythmias and sudden death. The main adverse effects are hyperkalaemia and hyponatraemia. Hyperkalaemia is most likely to occur in patients with poor renal function, and in those receiving ACE inhibitors and/or potassium supplements. Triamterene and amiloride are generally preferred to spironolactone. Although spironolactone is a more effective antihypertensive agent than other potassium sparing diuretics and is useful in primary and secondary aldosteronism, its role in the treatment of hypertension is severely limited because of the high incidence of impotence and gynaecomastia in men.

β-Adrenoceptor antagonists

Most clinicians now use β_1 selective adrenoceptor antagonists in the management of hypertension because of the lower incidence of adverse effects resulting from blockade of the β_2 receptor. Examples include atenolol, metoprolol and celiprolol. β-Adrenoceptor antagonists have additional effects which make them suitable for use in certain groups of hypertensive patients. They are particularly useful in patients with anxiety and related symptoms, angina pectoris and certain arrhythmias. The value of β blockers in reducing stroke and cardiovascular disease compared with diuretics is difficult to assess from the large intervention studies. In general the two groups are equally effective in reducing blood pressure but there may be a slight advantage in favour of diuretics in preventing stroke.

Adverse effects. The majority of the adverse effects of β blockers relate to blockade of the cardiac, vascular and bronchial smooth muscle receptors, and reduced myocardial reserve, asthma, peripheral vascular insufficiency and prolonged hypoglycaemia following insulin therapy have all been described in susceptible individuals. A withdrawal syndrome characterised by nervousness, tachycardia, worsening angina and increased blood pressure has been described and is probably related to 'upregulation' or supersensitivity of the β adrenoceptors. Other adverse effects include: nightmares, depression and insomnia with lipid soluble drugs, such as propranolol; tremor and tachycardia with drugs that have partial agonist activity, such as pindolol; and postural hypotension with drugs that have additional α-blocking effects, such as labetalol.

Calcium channel antagonists

All members of this group lower blood pressure by dilating the peripheral resistance arterioles. An increase in sympathetic tone occurs as a result of increased baroreceptor activity, particularly with the dihydropyridine group, which includes nifedipine, nicardipine, amlodipine, isradipine and felodipine. Calcium channel antagonists are effective antihypertensive drugs which combine well with most other agents. However, diltiazem and verapamil have significant depressant effects on cardiac muscle and conduction and therefore are likely to cause problems when combined with β-adrenoceptor antagonists. The dihydropyridine calcium antagonists are more selective as vasodilators and have less cardiac depressant effects than verapamil and diltiazem. Reflex sympathetic activation also helps to maintain cardiac output.

Adverse effects. The most important adverse effects are direct extensions of their therapeutic action. Excessive inhibition of calcium influx can cause serious cardiac depression, including cardiac arrest, bradycardia, atrioventricular block and congestive heart failure. Minor toxicity, which usually does not result in drug withdrawal, includes flushing, oedema, dizziness, gingival hyperplasia, nausea and constipation. Doubts have recently been expressed about the long term safety of short acting dihydrophyridines.

Angiotensin converting enzyme inhibitors

All currently available ACE inhibitors reduce blood pressure in patients with essential and renal hypertension. Patients with high plasma renin activity show the greatest decreases in blood pressure but reductions also occur in those with low plasma renin activity and in anephric subjects. ACE inhibitors offer an important option in the treatment of hypertension, either as first line treatment in diabetic patients or when other established drugs are contraindicated, ineffective or poorly tolerated.

Adverse effects. When captopril was first introduced it was considered to have such serious adverse effects that it was only recommended in hypertension resistant to other forms of therapy. Neutropenia, serious renal damage with proteinuria, skin rashes, loss of taste and angio-oedema were identified. Most of these effects were related to the high doses employed and are rarely seen at currently recommended doses. The most common adverse effect of ACE inhibitors is cough, which has been reported to occur in 3–22% of patients receiving the drug. The cough is non-productive and occurs more commonly in women and non-smokers, and is probably dose related. Changing the medication may be required and losartan, a new angiotensin II receptor antagonist, at present appears to be a useful alternative which does not cause cough. Although severe hypotension is relatively common when these drugs are used to treat congestive cardiac failure, severe hypotension can also occur in hypertensive patients whose renin–angiotensin system is activated as a result of renovascular disease or intensive diuretic therapy. It is most likely to occur after the first dose but can occur after the second and third doses. Acute renal insufficiency has also been described in patients with bilateral renal artery stenosis or unilateral renal artery stenosis in a single kidney. To maintain glomerular filtration in this condition, marked efferent glomerular arteriolar tone is achieved by high levels of angiotensin II. ACE inhibition removes this tone and decreases the glomerular filtration rate. ACE inhibitors inhibit the release of aldosterone from the adrenal cortex by reducing angiotensin II levels and hence increase serum potassium concentrations. This is usually mild but can cause problems in patients with renal impairment and in those receiving potassium and/or potassium sparing diuretics. Other uncommon effects, mostly seen with high dose captopril therapy, include angio-oedema, neutropenia, proteinuria and taste disturbances.

α-Adrenoceptor antagonists

Doxazosin is now the preferred antihypertensive agent in this group of compounds. It is selective for the α_1 receptor, it can be given once a day and has a lower incidence of adverse effects, particularly first dose hypotension.

Adverse effects. Most adverse effects of α-adrenoceptor antagonists are due to extension of their pharmacological properties. Hypotension, dizziness, headache, reflex tachycardia, nasal congestion and impaired ejaculation have all been reported, especially with non-selective drugs. First dose syncope seems to be related to venodilatation and is most likely to occur in patients on large doses of loop diuretics and/or organic nitrates.

Other antihypertensive agents — centrally acting

Centrally acting drugs methyldopa and clonidine are now rarely used in the management of hypertension, mainly because of their central sedative and depressive properties. They are sometimes combined with other agents in the management of resistant hypertension and are generally effective in renovascular hypertension.

Adverse effects. Sudden cessation of therapy (especially clonidine) can result in rebound hypertension. Methyldopa causes a number of hypersensitivity reactions: haemolytic anaemia, pancreatitis, myocarditis, hepatitis, a lupus-type syndrome and allergic rashes. Parkinsonism has rarely been reported.

Other antihypertensive agents — direct acting

Direct acting vasodilators minoxidil, hydralazine and diazoxide are also rarely used in patients with hypertension owing to a high incidence of adverse effects. They are now considered to be fourth line drugs as adjunctive therapy in patients with uraemia and severe resistant hypertension. Nitroprusside is used principally for rapid reduction of blood pressure in hypertensive crises and to maintain hypotensive anaesthesia. It is particularly beneficial in patients with cardiac failure due to hypertension.

Adverse effects. The most common adverse effect relate to their potent vasodilator activity. Headache, palpitations, sweating, flushing and peripheral oedema have been widely reported. In patients with ischaemic heart disease, reflex tachycardia and sympathetic nerve stimulation can result in angina and cardiac arrhythmias. Specific adverse effects include hyperglycaemia with diazoxide, a lupus-type syndrome and peripheral neuropathy with hydralazine, hypertrichosis with minoxidil, and cyanide and/or thiocyanate poisoning with prolonged administration of sodium nitroprusside.

Rationale for drug combinations of antihypertensive therapy

Most antihypertensive agents have additive effects on blood pressure when used in combination and in some instances can reduce adverse effects. Diuretics usefully combine with vasodilators which cause salt and water retention and β-adrenoceptor antagonists can be used to prevent the reflex sympathetic activity caused by these drugs. ACE inhibitors and potassium sparing diuretics potentiate the antihypertensive effects of thiazide and loop diuretics and help prevent some of the adverse metabolic effects. The combination of diuretics and ACE inhibitors is particularly useful in patients with associated heart failure, and the dihydropyridine calcium antagonists combined with β blockers are of major benefit in patients who also have angina.

Management of severe hypertension

There is usually no justification for rapidly reducing blood pressure in the majority of patients unless major complicating factors such as encephalopathy, pulmonary oedema or dissecting aneurysm are present. In the absence of these factors oral regimens should be used which are similar to those recommended for non-malignant hypertension, although these should be initiated in hospital. For urgent therapy of acute severe hypertension, sublingual nifedipine is now relatively standard therapy in this country. It consistently reduces systolic and diastolic blood pressure by about 20% within 20–30 minutes and seems to be relatively safe, even in the presence of cerebral symptoms. Intravenous nitroprusside has no clear advantages over nifedipine in conscious patients, except possibly when severe heart failure is present. Labetalol by mouth is also effective and produces smooth reductions in blood pressure without associated tachycardia.

Preoperative management of hypertension

In the past there was a reluctance to control hypertension before operation for fear of inducing hypotension which was refractory to treatment during anaesthesia. In general the dangers of continuing antihypertensive medication during surgery are less than the dangers of stopping the drugs. For some drugs, notably the thiazide diuretics, β-adrenoceptor antagonists and ACE inhibitors, the drugs would have to be discontinued at least 1 week before surgery to ensure significant loss of antihypertensive activity. There is evidence that β-adrenoceptor antagonists may protect against marked swings in blood pressure during tracheal intubation and that they should not be stopped before surgery. However, patients treated with labetalol, an α- and β-blocking drug, are reported to be very sensitive to halothane. As a general rule anti-hypertensive drugs should not be stopped before anaesthesia unless they are causing hypotension.

DRUGS USED IN CONTROLLED HYPOTENSION

The controlled reduction of arterial blood pressure during surgery has proved surprisingly free from complications. Fundamentally, arterial blood pressure, as an indication of cardiovascular integrity, is easy to measure but is of limited physiological significance. Well-being is more dependent on tissue perfusion, usually assessed clinically from indicators such as electrocardiograph, electroencephalograph, urinary output or acid–base status. This has certain implications for the conduct of anaesthesia and the selection of drugs. The main hypotensive effect should result from peripheral vasodilatation rather than cardiac depression and should be easily controllable, either because the main agent has a rapid onset and short duration of action or because it interacts with a short acting adjuvant such as halothane or isoflurane. Conversely, the chosen drug should be capable of providing stable conditions when the desired level of hypotension is attained. Ideally, the hypotensive agents used should not interfere with blood pressure autoregulation, but if they do so it is important that marked swings be avoided.

Hypotensive anaesthesia may be employed during surgery for aneurysm, middle ear, spinal, radical cancer and plastic procedures. Each of these needs slightly different conditions and even these may vary during the course of the operation. It is improbable that a single hypotensive drug ideal for all situations will be found. The anaesthetist can only become familiar with the available agents and select the most appropriate in the prevailing circumstances.

Sodium nitroprusside (Nipride)

Sodium nitroprusside was introduced into clinical practice in 1929 and was suggested as a suitable agent for intraoperative induced hypotension in 1962.

Pharmacology

The primary action of sodium nitroprusside is to produce relaxation of smooth muscle. This effect is common to all smooth muscle and is not vasculospecific. It is the result of intracellular release of nitric oxide, which activates guanylate cyclase, resulting in accumulation of cyclic guanosine monophosphate (cGMP). The release of nitric oxide from sodium nitroprusside probably takes place after it has undergone reduction and lost cyanide.

Cardiovascular system
Cardiac function. Cardiac output is usually maintained or even increased. Heart rate usually rises to a degree comparable with that occurring with nitroglycerin. Tachycardia, which may be an early sign of nitroprusside toxicity, may be controlled by use of β-adrenergic blocking agents such as labetalol. Neither the cardiac conducting system nor myocardial contractility is affected.

Coronary artery blood flow tends to increase but myocardial oxygenation may be reduced by cyanide-induced cytochrome oxidase inhibition, reduction in coronary perfusion pressure or failure of autoregulation. Sodium nitroprusside, by causing preferential dilatation of muscularised channels, may divert blood flow from functionally more important nutritive capillary channels, which, being without muscle, are undilated. Its use may also, however, be accompanied by reduction in oxygen demand, and lactate accumulation is uncommon.

In summary, it could be said that hypotension produced by sodium nitroprusside is accompanied by myocardial haemodynamic changes, the overall effect of which is equivocal, but that electrocardiographic abnormalities suggest that adverse effects tend to outweigh favourable factors.

Non-cardiac function. Total peripheral resistance decreases, often by as much as 60%, despite compensatory increases in plasma concentrations of adrenaline, noradrenaline and renin. Central venous pressure is consistently reduced. Pulmonary artery pressure also decreases but may show a rebound increase after nitroprusside is withdrawn. Systemic blood pressure is reduced by sodium nitroprusside but control values are rapidly regained when it is withdrawn. Withdrawal may be followed by rebound hypertension, probably resulting from raised plasma renin concentrations. The mechanism of renin release is of interest in that it suggests several points of pharmacological attack in dealing with rebound hypertension. Hypotension reflexly stimulates renal sympathetic nerves to produce the proteolytic enzyme, renin. Renin, in turn, gives rise to the decapeptide, angiotensin I, which is cleaved by the converting enzyme to the octapeptide, angiotensin II. Both angiotensins I and II act as vasoconstrictors and stimulate the release of catecholamines from the adrenal glands and central nervous system, thereby initiating the synthesis of further renin. This cycle can be interrupted by β-adrenergic blocking agents, clonidine and ACE inhibitors.

Tissue hypoxia may occur, resulting in part from precapillary dilatation with reduction in resistance, without concomitant venular dilatation. This reduces the arteriolar–venular pressure gradient and functional capillary density.

Moderate haemorrhage occurring during sodium nitroprusside-induced hypotension appears to have no adverse effect on cardiac output, mean arterial pressure, left cardiac work or blood flow to cerebral, coronary, renal or hepatic circulations.

Platelet function. Platelet aggregation may be reduced in a dose dependent manner, with increase in bleeding time.

Respiratory system. Several mechanisms, including increased dead space to tidal volume ratio, increased intrapulmonary shunting and inhibition of compensatory vasoconstriction in under-perfused lung tissue, may produce hypoxaemia.

Central nervous system. Cerebrovascular resistance usually decreases, the effect on cerebral blood flow probably being the resultant of this factor and changes in arterial blood pressure. Mean arterial blood pressures of 50–55 mmHg are not usually associated with significant reduction in cerebral blood flow.

Intracranial pressure tends to parallel cerebral blood flow when compliance is low. If, however, capacitance vessels are dilated in preference to resistance vessels, intracranial pressure may rise without increase in cerebral blood flow, especially where the initial pressure is high or when the drug is given as a bolus. It may be reduced, but not eliminated, by hyperventilation. In neurosurgical practice nitroprusside should probably be withheld until the skull has been opened. Autoregulation of cerebral blood flow may be inhibited and exaggerated swings in systemic blood pressure should be avoided. The absence of cycloplegia may be an asset.

Spinal cord blood flow decreases initially but returns to normotensive values within 30–40 minutes, suggesting an autoregulatory mechanism.

Renal system. Sodium nitroprusside does not appear to cause significant specific renal damage; however, toxic metabolites, thiocyanate and cyanide, have a low renal clearance and dosage should be minimised in the presence of renal insufficiency.

Hepatic system. There is evidence to suggest that the liver has an important role in the metabolism of sodium nitroprusside and dosage should be minimised in the presence of hepatic dysfunction.

Nitroprusside toxicity. At least two metabolites of nitroprusside, cyanide and thiocyanate, may cause toxicity. It has also been suggested that hydrogen peroxide may be a toxic product, possibly by facilitating the release of cyanide from sodium nitroprusside.

Thiocyanate. Whereas conversion of cyanide to thiocyanate is slow, renal excretion is even slower (half-life up to 7 days). Toxicity is significantly increased in the presence of renal impairment. Concentrations greater than $110 \mu g \, ml^{-1}$ produce drowsiness, lethargy, nausea and vomiting. High concentrations may affect thyroid function.

Cyanide. Fatalities have usually been attributed to overdosage. Cyanide rapidly enters the red blood cell and may affect oxygen transport or tissue oxygenation processes by blocking the actions of cytochrome oxidase and probably other enzymes. Pyruvate metabolism is interrupted and lactate produced. Toxicity is usually associated with concentrations of free cyanide in excess of $8 \mu g \, 100^{-1}$. Warning signs include resistance to hypotensive action, tachycardia, development of metabolic acidosis and elevation of venous oxygen tension. During prolonged exposure biochemical monitoring is recommended. Monitoring of lactate, or more conveniently of bicarbonate, is probably preferable to direct estimation of cyanide in expired air or blood or of serum thiocyanate. Risk factors may include hypoalbuminaemia or cardiopulmonary procedures.

Management of sodium nitroprusside toxicity. Suggested remedies involve attempts to facilitate the inactivation of cyanide or to potentiate the hypotensive effect of sodium nitroprusside, thus reducing dosage. An example of the former approach is administration of sodium thiosulphate, which is required by the enzyme rhodanase to form thiocyanate. This is probably the drug of choice. Dicobalt edetate is an alternative. High dose hydroxycobalamin (vitamin B_{12a}) combines with cyanide to form cyanocobalamin and is also a useful cyanide antagonist.

The alternative approach, namely potentiation of sodium nitroprusside with reduction in dosage, has included combinations with trimetaphan, β-adrenergic blockers, ACE inhibitors and calcium channel blockers. It has been suggested that 'closed loop' control of blood pressure might reduce dosage and the risk of toxicity. This approach has not, however, shown consistent superiority over manual control by an experienced anaesthetist.

Sodium nitroprusside in pregnancy. Sodium nitroprusside has been used successfully during pregnancy, for example in neurosurgical emergencies. Animal studies have, however, resulted in fatal concentrations of cyanide in the fetus.

Special contraindications. These include Leber's optic atrophy, tobacco amblyopia, liver dysfunction and neurological deficits arising from vitamin B_{12} deficiency, and patients with disturbance of cerebral blood flow or hypothyroidism should also be treated with caution.

Dosage and administration. The ampoule containing 50 mg is diluted initially in 2 ml 5% dextrose. The resulting solution may be diluted in 250–1000 ml of 5% dextrose, 0.9% sodium chloride or sodium lactate solution. The solution should be protected from light to prevent decom-

position, and used within 24 hours of preparation. The maximum dose should not exceed 1.5 mg kg^{-1} min^{-1} and a method capable of very accurate delivery should be used. Recommended doses have tended to become lower as experience has been gained. Sudden withdrawal increases the risk of rebound hypertension.

Drug interactions. The response to sodium nitroprusside may be increased in patients taking antihypertensive medication and by anaesthetic agents such as halothane or isoflurane. Prolongation of non-depolarising muscle block has been reported in animals but not confirmed in man.

Glyceryl trinitrate (Tridil)

Glyceryl trinitrate has been used in the treatment of angina pectoris for more than 100 years, and intraoperatively for over 20 years.

Pharmacology

The fundamental action of glyceryl trinitrate, like other nitrates, is to produce direct dilatation of smooth muscle. Intracellular release of nitric oxide activates guanylate cyclase, which in turn results in accumulation of cGMP.

Cardiovascular system. Glyceryl trinitrate acts on the vasculature and on the heart. Relaxation of both arterial and, predominantly, venous smooth muscle occurs. Venodilatation is most marked at lower infusion rates (up to 50 µg ml^{-1}). Pulmonary venous tone is reduced. Peripheral and pulmonary vascular resistance also decrease. Systemic arterial pressure decreases, systolic more than diastolic, which may assist coronary perfusion. General tissue perfusion appears to be well maintained.

Cardiac effects. Heart rate is usually unaltered. Left ventricular pressure, end-diastolic pressure, heart volume and myocardial oxygen demand are all reduced. Cardiac output tends to decrease, but seldom to a marked degree. Excessive reduction can be restored by low dose dopamine without abolishing the beneficial effects of glyceryl trinitrate on myocardial function. Coronary vascular resistance is reduced, especially in the presence of coronary artery disease. Glyceryl trinitrate may dilate large coronary conductance vessels, thereby enhancing collateral blood flow and redistributing blood to subendocardial ischaemic areas.

Sudden withdrawal of glyceryl trinitrate, unlike sodium nitroprusside, is not followed by rebound hypertension, although plasma adrenaline and noradrenaline concentrations are higher with glyceryl trinitrate.

Central nervous system. Intracranial pressure usually rises in normal subjects, often producing headache. If intracranial pressure is already raised there is often a further increase, related to the initial value. When systemic hypotension is profound, intracranial pressure may be lowered but show rebound increase when arterial pressure is restored. Overall, it appears that cerebral blood flow is quite well maintained and autoregulation unaltered.

Fate in the body. Nitroglycerin undergoes biotransformation in the liver by reductive hydrolysis catalysed by the enzyme glutathione organic nitrate reductase. Metabolites are inactive and the brief duration of action appears to be correlated with plasma concentrations of nitroglycerin.

Dose and administration. Glyceryl trinitrate should be diluted to a final concentration of $400\,\mu g\,ml^{-1}$ or less in 5% dextrose in water or 0.9% sodium chloride. Recommended dose range is $10–200\,\mu g\,min^{-1}$, although up to $400\,\mu g\,min^{-1}$ may be required. Suggested initial dose is $25\,\mu g\,min^{-1}$, increasing by $25\,\mu g\,min^{-1}$ at 5 minute intervals until the required level of hypotension is obtained. An accurate method of administration must be used.

Side-effects, precautions and contraindications. Hypersensitivity to nitrates, severe anaemia, hypovolaemia, pre-existing hypotension, intracranial trauma or haemorrhage are contraindications to the use of glyceryl trinitrate. Caution is advised in the presence of hypothyroidism, hypothermia, malnutrition, liver or renal disease. With long term use methaemoglobinaemia may be sufficient to impair oxygen delivery. Glass or rigid polyethylene infusion devices should be used. Contact with polyvinylchloride may reduce activity by 40%.

Trimetaphan (Arfonad)

Trimetaphan is a thiothanium derivative. It is unstable and is available as the camphorsulphonate.

Pharmacology

Cardiovascular system. Trimetaphan is classified primarily as a ganglion blocking drug. It blocks both sympathetic and parasympathetic ganglia competitively by occupying receptor sites and prevents stimulation of postsynaptic membranes by acetylcholine released from presynaptic nerve endings. It may also lower blood pressure by at least two other mechanisms, namely a direct dilator effect on peripheral vessels and the release of histamine from mast cells. Neither of these additional mechanisms may be of importance under ordinary circumstances but could explain, for example, the hypotension found in sympathectomised subjects. Both preload and afterload are reduced secondary to diminished venular and arteriolar tone. Hypotension tends to be greater in hypertensive patients. The onset of action is rapid, usually within 3 minutes, and hypotension continues for 15–30 minutes. Heart rate usually increases, both as a compensatory mechanism and possibly also as result of parasympathetic blockade. Tachycardia may be controlled by β-adrenoreceptor blockers, although this is likely to reduce cardiac output. Although it has a negative inotropic effect, cardiac output also tends to decrease because of decreased venous return. Coronary blood flow is reduced. Trimetaphan may sensitise the myocardium to sympathomimetic drugs.

Respiratory system. Oxygen saturation decreases, possibly as a result of drug induced suppression of hypoxic pulmonary vasoconstriction.

Central nervous system. Cerebral blood flow usually decreases, although this is seldom significant if mean arterial blood pressure remains over 50 mmHg. Epidural blood flow is reduced. Raised intracranial pressure may be aggravated, particularly if hypotension is induced rapidly.

Renal system. Renal blood flow and glomerular filtration rate are reduced; renal vascular resistance increases.

Indications and clinical usage. Trimetaphan has been widely used to produce intraoperative controlled hypotension. It has also been employed to improve perfusion during and after cardiac surgery, to control hypertensive crises of various origins and to attenuate the cardiovascular response to tracheal intubation. It has been used to control cerebral blood flow and intracranial pressure in pre-eclampsia. During aortic cross-clamping it controls the increases in cardiac output and cardiac work more effectively than some other agents.

Dosage and administration. The ampoule containing 250 mg is usually diluted to a concentration of 0.1% with normal saline or dextrose–saline. Solutions of 0.05% (elderly patients) or 0.25% (when fluid intake is restricted) are also used. The 0.1% solution is usually started at a rate of about 60 drops (3 or 4 mg) per minute and adjusted to maintain the required blood pressure. The undiluted solution has also been used by intermittent bolus injection, usually starting with a dose of 50 mg followed by smaller increments, as required, at about 10 minute intervals. Trimetaphan should not be mixed with other substances but combined infusions of trimetaphan and sodium nitroprusside appear to offer some advantages. Initially, a 1:10 ratio of sodium nitroprusside to trimetaphan was suggested but it is possible that ratios of 1:2.5 or 1:5 may provide more stable conditions.

Drug interactions. Trimetaphan may potentiate and prolong the effects of non-depolarising muscle relaxants and, being partly metabolised by pseudocholinesterase, may also increase the duration of action of succinylcholine. It should not be used in the presence of any abnormality of plasma cholinesterase, whether of genetic, drug induced or hepatic origin. Insertion of acrylic cement monomer produces a further decrease in both stroke volume and cardiac output. Local infiltration at the operation site with adrenaline, noradrenaline or ephedrine may antagonise the effects of trimetaphan.

Use during pregnancy. Trimetaphan is best avoided in pregnancy because of the risk of inducing ileus in the newborn.

Side-effects, precautions and contraindications.

Fluctuations in arterial blood pressure may occur rapidly, especially when marked release of histamine occurs. Tachyphylaxis may be a problem. Severe arteriosclerosis, cardiac disease or pyloric stenosis are regarded as contraindications. Caution is advised when using this, or any drug, to induce hypotension in the elderly. Similarly, the risk of adverse responses is increased in patients with diabetes mellitus or hepatic, renal or adrenal insufficiency, or those on steroid medication. Hypoglycaemia and hypokalaemia have been reported.

α-Adrenoceptor blocking drugs

These include phentolamine, phenoxybenzamine, chlorpromazine, droperidol and volatile anaesthetic agents. They exert their hypotensive effect by blocking postganglionic sympathetic fibres. Only phentolamine and the volatile agents have a sufficiently short duration of action for intraoperative use (<1 hour) but phentolamine is unsuitable because of its cardiac stimulant effect. Both halothane and isoflurane have been used successfully.

β-Adrenoceptor blocking drugs

These are widely employed as part of a hypotensive technique but only those without an intrinsic sympathomimetic effect are suitable. Using β blockers, bleeding can be minimised by control of the heart rate and cardiac output without the need for a profound reduction in arterial blood pressure. Propranolol 40 mg t.i.d. may be prescribed before operation or given intravenously (1–2 mg) during anaesthesia. Apart from its hypotensive properties it blocks the tachycardia induced by directly acting vasodilator agents or ganglion blocking drugs. Labetalol is widely employed to induce hypotension and with its combined α- and β-blocking actions may be preferred to other drugs. Its duration of effect (α 30 minutes; β 90 minutes) makes it sufficiently flexible for intraoperative blood pressure control.

VASOPRESSORS

These drugs are widely used in anaesthetic

Table 27.4 Actions of some non-catecholamine vasopressor drugs on sympathetic adrenergic receptors

	Direct	Indirect	α_1 effects	β effects
Ephedrine	+	+	+	β_1 and β_2
Methoxamine	+	+	++	–
Metaraminol	++	+	++	–
Phenylephrine	++	+	++	–

practice to compensate for sympathetic blockade induced by spinal or epidural local anaesthetic block. Catecholamines whose primary action is on the heart are considered elsewhere (Chapter 25). In addition to their use during regional block, vasopressors may also be used to support the peripheral circulation during the removal of phaeochromocytoma or when hypotension occurs during anaesthesia with volatile drugs, particularly isoflurane. These drugs are not recommended for use in patients who are in 'shock'.

Vasopressors act on tissues innervated by sympathetic fibres whose postganglionic endings release noradrenaline. Some of these drugs exert their effects by direct action on the receptor but others act indirectly by stimulating the release of noradrenaline. Noradrenaline, adrenaline and phenylephrine are purely directly acting, whereas ephedrine, methoxamine and metaraminol have both direct and indirect activity (Table 27.4).

Ephedrine

This drug is widely used to maintain systemic arterial blood pressure during regional block with local anaesthetics. It has inotropic and chronotropic actions on the heart and increases peripheral resistance. It is preferable to either fluid loading or methoxamine for maintaining blood pressure in elderly patients during spinal anaesthesia. It is also less likely to reduce placental blood flow in obstetric patients than drugs with more pronounced α_1-agonist activity. It crosses both the placenta and the blood–brain barrier readily and has been used in the treatment of narcolepsy. Ephedrine is sometimes used as a bronchodilator because of its β_2-stimulant effects and it is effective when taken by mouth.

Tachyphylaxis may occur due to depletion of noradrenaline stores. The usual intravenous bolus dose is 3–6 mg, which can be repeated as necessary up to 30 mg. For a more sustained effect the drug can be given by intramuscular injection (15–30 mg). Alternatively, it may be diluted in normal saline and given as a slow intravenous infusion, although care must be taken to avoid inducing tachyarrhythmias.

Methoxamine

This drug is devoid of β effects and does not cross the blood–brain barrier. It has very pronounced α_1 properties and is sometimes used during spinal or epidural block. It causes a reflex sinus bradycardia (due to its effect on blood pressure) which responds to atropine. In large doses methoxamine can block β receptors. It has a longer duration of action (30–60 minutes) than ephedrine. It is usually given intravenously in a dose of 2–5 mg.

Metaraminol

This is similar to methoxamine with prominent direct α_1 effects on vascular smooth muscle. The dose is 0.5–5 mg by slow intravenous bolus injection or 15–100 mg in 500 ml normal saline by infusion. Metaraminol has a longer duration of action than noradrenaline and has the potential to induce a prolonged increase in blood pressure.

Phenylephrine

This drug has a short duration of action (5–10 minutes) when given intravenously. It is a selective α_1 agonist and is used to increase peripheral resistance when cardiac output is preserved. It is also used as a nasal decongestant and as a mydriatic. It can be given as a bolus intravenously in a dose of 40–100 µg or by infusion at 10–20 µg min^{-1}.

PHAEOCHROMOCYTOMA

None of the endocrine causes for hypertension is more fascinating and challenging for the clinician than phaeochromocytoma. Its protean manifestations can make diagnosis difficult, yet its sinister prognostic implications demand prompt recognition and expert management. Diagnosis depends upon clinical suspicion, demonstration of high levels of free catecholamines in plasma or urine, or localisation by appropriate imaging techniques.

The dominant secretory products, and those largely responsible for the clinical symptomatology, are noradrenaline, adrenaline and, to a lesser extent, dopamine, However, these chromaffin tumours belong to the amine precursor uptake decarboxylase (APUD) series of cells and can elaborate other peptide hormones including L-dopa, vasoactive intestinal peptide, somatostatin, renin, parathormone, enkephalins and endothelins.

Diagnosis may be made by estimation of plasma catecholamine concentrations, urinary excretion of hydroxymethyl mandelic acid, computed tomography and magnetic resonance imaging.

Surgical extirpation of the tumour is the only curative therapy but should only be performed as an elective procedure after careful pharmacological preparation. α-Methyl-p-tyrosine (AMPT) inhibits tyrosine hydroxylase and blocks the rate limiting conversion of tyrosine to dopa in the catecholamine synthesis pathway. AMPT is particularly useful in patients with malignant phaeochromocytomas or in those for whom surgery is contraindicated. However, a tumour partially suppressed by AMPT may still cause major pressor responses during surgery; the addition of an α-adrenoceptor antagonist is essential and phenoxybenzamine remains the drug of choice. Phenoxybenzamine is a mixed α_1/α_2 non-competitive adrenergic antagonist. It blocks α receptors, mainly α_1, irreversibly, but also has effects at the α_2 receptor when given in large doses. The therapeutic dose should start at 10 mg 12-hourly, increasing to 10 mg 6-hourly. As a consequence of prolonged catecholamine stimulation, these patients often suffer from intravascular volume depletion, and postural hypotension requiring fluid replacement is a frequent complication in the perioperative period. The usefulness of phenoxybenzamine can be limited by side-effects such as nausea, sedation, weakness and dependent oedema.

When α blockade is established, unopposed, β-adrenergic stimulation, in the form of tachycardia and other arrhythmias, may become apparent, particularly if the tumour secretes adrenaline in addition to noradrenaline. Concomitant β-adrenergic blockade, usually with propranolol, is recommended.

Phentolamine is an α-adrenergic antagonist, equipotent at both α_1 and α_2 receptors, which has a short duration of action. It can be used as an intravenous infusion (0.1–2.0 mg min^{-1}) for the rapid control of paroxysmal hypertension associated with phaeochromocytoma.

The pure α-blocking drug, prazosin, is not recommended because it is a competitive antagonist which can therefore be displaced from its receptor by increases in plasma catecholamine concentrations. Theoretically, the mixed competitive α- and β-adrenoceptor antagonist, labetalol, might be useful in the pharmacological management of phaeochromocytoma. However, both its α- and β-antagonist actions are weak and it interferes indirectly with estimation of both plasma and urinary adrenaline.

Two days before surgery, the dose of phenoxybenzamine is increased to 0.5 mg kg^{-1} 4-hourly to ensure that as many α receptors as possible are irreversibly blocked. This regimen, first described by Ross in 1967, has proved safe and effective in attenuating potentially disastrous pressor crises during induction of anaesthesia and surgical manipulation. Even so, given the wide range of vasoconstrictor peptides that can be released, it is not surprising that the pressor episodes cannot be fully blocked by adrenoceptor blockade alone. Intraoperative hypertension should be controlled with rapid onset, short acting agents such as sodium nitroprusside (< 4 µg kg min^{-1}) and tachycardia or arrhythmias with esmolol (20–300 µg kg min^{-1}).

Cyclophosphamide, vincristine and dacarbazine have been administered in combination with α-adrenoceptor blockade to produce tumour shrinkage and enhanced biochemical response in patients with malignant phaeochromocytoma.

Other drugs that may be associated with pressor crises unrelated to phaeochromocytoma are:

- Glucagon
- Metoclopramide
- Droperidol
- Adrenocorticotrophin
- Suxamethonium
- Histamine
- Phenothiazines
- Naloxone
- Tricyclic antidepressants.

Anaesthetic management

It is important that the patient arrives in the anaesthetic room in a tranquil state. Benzodiazepines such as temazepam and diazepam are suitable for premedication and should be given in sufficient dosage. A barbiturate may be used but droperidol and the phenothiazine group of drugs, which may provoke pressor crises, should be avoided. Morphine should be avoided because of its potential to release histamine, and atropine because of its vagolytic effect.

The pressor response to tracheal intubation can be effectively suppressed by high doses of fentanyl or alfentanil, and judicious doses of thiopentone. Sodium nitroprusside and esmolol may also be used for this purpose, either singly or in combination.

Although there are insufficient data to recommend the use of propofol for induction of anaesthesia in these patients, its haemodynamic effects — direct and indirect myocardial depression, inhibition of central sympathetic discharge and resetting of the baroreceptor response — may be advantageous.

Vecuronium is a suitable muscle relaxant as it is devoid of autonomic effects and does not provoke catecholamine release through histamine liberation. A high dose intravenous opioid technique can be effectively supplemented with propofol, benzodiazepines or a volatile agent. Enflurane and isoflurane are less commonly associated with the sensitising effects of catecholamines on the heart than halothane.

FURTHER READING

Induced hypotension
Chaudhri S, Colvin J R, Todd J G, Kenny G N 1992 Evaluation of closed loop control of arterial pressure during hypotensive anaesthesia for local resection of intraocular melanoma. British Journal of Anaesthesia 69: 607–610
Johnson C C 1929 The actions and toxicity of nitroprusside. Archives of International Pharmacodynamics and Therapeutics 35: 480–496
Kaplan J A, Dunbar R W, Jones E L 1976 Nitroglycerine infusion during coronary artery surgery. Anesthesiology 45: 14–21
Magill I W, Scurr C F, Wyman J B 1953 Controlled hypotension by a thiophanium derivative. Lancet i: 219–220
Moraca P P, Bitte E M, Hale D E, Wasmuth C E, Poutasse E F 1962 Clinical evaluation of sodium nitroprusside as a hypotensive agent. Anesthesiology 23: 193–204
Murrell W 1879 Nitroglycerin as a remedy for angina pectoris. Lancet 1: 80
Randall L O, Peterson W G, Lehman G 1949 The ganglionic blocking action of thiothanium derivatives. Journal of Pharmacology and Experimental Therapeutics 97: 48–57
Rindone J P, Sloane E P 1992 Cyanide toxicity from sodium nitroprusside: risks and management. Annals of Pharmacotherapy 26: 515–519

Vasopressors
Wright P M C, Fee J P H 1992 Cardiovascular support during combined epidural and general anaesthesia. British Journal of Anaesthesia 68: 585–589

Management of phaeochromocytoma
Fonseca V, Bouloux P-M 1993 Phaeochromocytoma and paraganglioma. Baillière's Clinical Endocrinology and Metabolism 7(2): 509–541
Lewis I H, Yousif D, Mullis S L, Homma S, Gabrielson G V, Jebara V A 1994 Management of a cardiac phaeochromocytoma in two patients. Journal of Cardiothoracic and Vascular Anaesthesia 8: 223–230
Platts J K, Drew P J T, Harvey J N 1995 Death from phaeochromocytoma: lessons from a post-mortem survey. Journal of the Royal College of Physicians of London 29: 299-306
Ross E J, Prichard B N, Kaufman L, Robertson A I, Harries B J 1967 Preoperative and operative management of patients with phaeochromocytoma. British Medical Journal 28: 191–198

Blood

SECTION CONTENTS

28

Blood

S. D. Nelson
W. F. M. Wallace

The composition of blood is extremely complex and the physical, chemical and cellular constitution of the blood can significantly change within a few seconds in response to stressful stimuli. The commonly used blood profiles, blood cell count, coagulation screen, electrolytes, etc. provide only a 'freeze frame' picture of a rapidly changeable status; however, these investigations are helpful in indicating the direction and degree of deviation from the normal at the time of sampling. This chapter examines the production, regulation and function of the blood cells, red and white, platelets and coagulation factors.

CELLULAR ELEMENTS OF THE BLOOD

In the adult the red cells, white cells and platelets are, under normal circumstances, produced almost entirely in the bone marrow (in the fetus they are also formed in the liver and spleen). Bone marrow contains a pool of stem cells capable of multiplication and differentiation to fully functional mature cells of the various lines. These pluripotent stem cells (haemocytoblasts) are small mononuclear cells, morphologically indistinguishable from lymphocytes. In addition, it is clear that stem cells also constitute a proportion of the circulating leucocyte population, presumably having migrated from the bone marrow, as the transfusion of an appropriate number of peripheral blood mononuclear cells can reconstitute haemopoietic function in a patient whose marrow has been ablated by cytotoxic agents or radiotherapy.

The processes leading to stem cell commitment to a particular line are outside the scope of this chapter. However, once committed, cell multiplication and differentiation are under tight control, so that the marrow produces and releases exactly the number of cells required to maintain normal haematological values in the healthy individual. Some of the biological growth factors (cytokines) that stimulate red and white cell production — erythropoietin, G-CSF (granulocyte colony stimulating factor), GM-CSF (granulocyte-monocyte-CSF), etc. — have been identified, and through recombinant DNA engineering technology are now available commercially. Research reports indicate that thrombopoietin will quickly follow, permitting selective stimulation of the marrow as required.

Red blood cells

The blood in a healthy adult contains approximately 4.5×10^{12} red cells per litre in women (normal haemoglobin (Hb) 12.5–15 g dl^{-1}) and 5×10^{12} in men (normal Hb 13.5–17 g dl^{-1}).

Erythrocyte characteristics

The red cells are biconcave discs approximately 7 μm in diameter and 2 μm thick; they have no nucleus. The stroma of the red cell is mainly phospholipid; its membrane consists of a lipid bilayer that is high in unesterified cholesterol, and there is an integrated glycoprotein content that influences the viscoelastic properties of the red cell so that it is readily deformable. This enables the red cell to pass along capillaries, which may be considerably less than 7 μm in diameter. The energy required for maintenance of the red cell's advantageous shape and intracellular ionic content is produced by glucose metabolism. Supported by the phospholipid framework is the red cell's content of haemoglobin (mean corpuscular haemoglobin (MCH) 32–35 pg). Exposed to a high oxygen partial pressure, the molecular configuration of haemoglobin is subtly altered to become oxyhaemoglobin. In the tissues, at low oxygen tension, the carried oxygen is released, oxyhaemoglobin now becoming deoxygenated. The conformational change of giving up oxygen

makes haemoglobin accept hydrogen ions more readily, facilitating the generation of bicarbonate ions from carbon dioxide. The red cells thus ferry oxygen to the tissues from the lungs and aid transport of carbon dioxide from the tissues to the lungs.

Erythrocyte formation (erythropoiesis)

In the marrow the most primitive cell which can be recognised as committed to red cell production is the proerythroblast. This cell is capable of mitotic activity without maturation, so that the pool of red cell precursors is capable of great expansion when needed. In Romanowsky stained smears, the proerythroblast has opaque basophilic cytoplasm with minimal signs of cytoplasmic haemoglobin formation. Where the essentials for cell maturation and haemoglobin production are present, the proerythroblasts mature in an orderly fashion within the marrow, passing through morphologically identifiable stages of early, intermediate and late normoblasts. Both nuclear maturation and cytoplasmic maturation occur; the basophilia of the cytoplasm gradually reduces, being replaced by the oxyphilic staining characteristics of haemoglobin, while with progressing maturation the cell shrinks, the nuclear chromatin condenses and finally the nuclear remnant is lost, probably by fragmentation or possibly by extrusion. At this stage the red cell is ready for release into the general circulation, where it circulates as a reticulocyte for a day or two before becoming a fully mature 'normocyte'.

The process described above is controlled by the circulating hormone *erythropoietin*, which is secreted mainly by the kidneys. Erythropoietin is the stimulus to maturation by committed stem cells into erythrocytes. The process is controlled by a feedback loop, being inhibited by a rise in circulating red cell numbers, and stimulated by anaemia and also by hypoxia. The latter effect is important in acclimatisation to altitude. The common factor stimulating erythropoietin synthesis is a reduced oxygen content of the blood, detected by the renal tubular cells, which have a high energy requirement for their active reabsorption of sodium ions. Satisfactory erythropoiesis depends on the availability of the building materials for haemoglobin (iron, globin, haem, etc.); at the same time nuclear maturation must proceed synchronously with haemoglobinisation.

Nuclear maturation is dependent on the presence of adequate amounts of vitamin B_{12} and folic acid. Deficiencies of these factors slow the maturation of nuclei relative to cytoplasmic development and the red cells become *megaloblastic*. The chromatin condensation and shrinkage which is characteristic of nuclear maturity takes place only slowly, while haemoglobin production proceeds apace. The erythroblasts remain large; their mature cytoplasm now contains a greater than normal amount of haemoglobin and, even at the latest megaloblast stages, nuclear structure is still visible (and therefore nuclear function presumably remains). In any event, many of the red cells are not suitable for 'general release' but remain within the marrow. A proportion cannot sustain their integrity and are destroyed within the marrow (ineffective erythropoiesis); the retention of erythroblasts within the marrow for longer than normal increases the proportion of these cells present and produces the microscopic appearance of megaloblastic hyperplasia.

Haemoglobin

The other major element in the maturation of red cells is, of course, the production within the cell of haemoglobin. The haemoglobin molecule is a roughly spherical complex comprised of two pairs of polypeptide (protein) chains which loosely envelop a haem subunit. Haem is a porphyrin derivative and contains an atom of iron in the ferric Fe^{3+} state. In normal adult haemoglobin (Hb A) the globin molecules are referred to as α and β chains. Fetal haemoglobin (Hb F), although also having two α-globin chains, differs from Hb A in having differently configured subsidiary globin molecules, referred to as γ chains. In normal adult blood there is also a third minor haemoglobin component Hb A_2, which has two α and two γ chains.

Abnormal haemoglobins. Abnormalities of globin production may be quantitative or qualitative (or both). Quantitative globin deficiencies (the *thalassaemia* syndromes) arise when there is failure to produce the normal quantity of a particular globin chain, frequently because of loss or mutation of one of the genetic loci controlling globin synthesis. When the deficiency involves β chains there is a resulting deficiency of Hb A. In an attempt to correct this defect, excess γ and δ chains are produced. In the heterozygous condition, beta thalassaemia minor, the blood picture is that of a mild hypochromic anaemia and there are above-normal levels of Hb A_2 and Hb F. This condition is most often asymptomatic. It is now clear that synthesis of β chains or any of the other globins is regulated at several genetic loci. In the heterozygous state described above the abnormality is clinically mild. However, when a β-thalassaemia abnormality is inherited from both parents, the resulting clinical picture may be that of a congenital anaemia severe enough to necessitate repeated transfusion (thalassaemia major). Quite frequently, however, the patient inherits two different molecular defects and the clinical condition falls between the major and minor thalassaemias and is recognised as thalassaemia intermedia. In this condition there may be a need for transfusion at relatively frequent intervals. When the thalassaemia abnormality involves α-chain synthesis, not only is Hb A production effected but Hb F and Hb A_2 are also reduced. Even in the heterozygous state α-thalassaemia is a significant anaemia that can cause intrauterine fetal loss. Homozygosity or compound heterozygosity will usually result in fetal loss.

Qualitative abnormalities of the globin chains are equally important. If any of the globin molecular chains have an abnormal spatial configuration, their resulting haemoglobin molecules may fail to bind haem; or they may have reduced or increased oxygen affinity; or they may have abnormal physical characteristics. One obvious example is Hb S (sickle cell haemoglobin). Hb S homozygotes suffer from *sickle cell disease*. Oxygenated Hb S is quite a flexible molecule, but reduced Hb S loses solubility and tends to precipitate into rigid elongated crystals so that the erythrocyte forms an inflexible sickle shape and cannot pass through the capillaries. Sickle cell disease is therefore mainly a circulatory/thrombotic problem. The management of homozygous Hb S disease is outside the scope of this book; but even the heterozygote with sickle cell trait is at some risk, particularly if he or she undergoes significant hypoxia. The abnormal haemoglobin gives an advantage in some populations as the gene confers resistance to one type of malaria. The Hb S gene is present in people of Afro-Caribbean descent and a small number of Hb S sufferers are also found in some Arabic areas in the Middle East. The sickle cell trait occurs in 40% of the population in West Africa and in 10% of the black American population. If there is any reason to suspect the presence of Hb S, a simple and cheap laboratory test is readily available.

Finally, anaemia may be due to deficiencies of haem production. Haem synthesis involves the synthesis of protoporphyrin IX plus availability of iron. Abnormalities of porphyrin synthesis, while not uncommon, are of course overshadowed by the contribution of iron deficiency in causing anaemia.

Apart from foodstuffs that have been fortified with added iron, the major source of iron in our diet is nutrients of animal origin, in particular foods that contain haemoglobin, myoglobin or ferritin, which is an intracellular storage protein for iron reserves. Apart from females in the reproductive period, iron homeostasis is remarkably complete, although small amounts are excreted in the faeces.

Dietary iron is absorbed into the mucosal cells of the duodenum and jejunum, where it is oxidised to the ferric (Fe^{3+}) state and temporarily stored as ferritin. Elsewhere in the body, iron is available from the metabolism and recycling of the elements of haemoglobin. When iron is required, Fe^{3+} is released from the intestinal mucosal cells; it attaches to the serum transport protein, transferrin, and is transported as ferric transferrin. Iron is thus available for synthesis of haemoglobin, myoglobin, cytochrome enzymes and indeed ferritin within the liver, etc. Developing red cell precursors can bind ferric transferrin, thus delivering a package of iron for haemoglobin synthesis. Unused ferritin stores in the mucosal cells are lost in the faeces as the cells are shed, thus avoiding the dangers of excess iron in the body.

Once delivered, ferric iron is reduced to the ferrous state and inserted into the centre of the protoporphyrin IX molecule to form haem. α- and β-globin chain dimers bind two haem molecules and quickly polymerise to the α_2-β_2 tetramers of the haemoglobin molecule.

Most frequently, the metabolic processes limiting haem production are dictated by the availability of iron. Where haem production is deficient, it follows that the mature red cell membrane (rather like a sack) is not full to capacity and the mean corpuscular haemoglobin is less than normal; the red cells are smaller than normal (microcytic). Women through their menses and pregnancies can deplete their body stores of iron, and a good mixed diet provides only just enough iron to preserve their haemoglobin synthesis. People who undertake extremely strenuous training in connection with sports may develop iron deficiency as a result of myoglobin excretion in the urine. However, in general any man who becomes iron deficient in the absence of a very grossly iron deficient diet should be considered to have bled.

Erythrocyte breakdown

When released into the circulation, mature, non-nucleated red blood cells are subject to physical and biochemical stresses of friction, shear stresses and toxic insults that ultimately exhaust the ability of the cell to maintain its flexible biconcave shape. At this time the red cell is effete and ripe for removal from the circulation. Cells that cannot maintain their flexibility and shape are trapped mainly in the spleen, some also in the liver, and are phagocytosed and destroyed. When the red cells are broken down the globin chains are digested and their amino acids become available for reuse. Iron-containing haem is converted to biliverdin, and in the human to bilirubin, which is excreted in the bile, while the iron is reused for haemoglobin synthesis. Under normal circumstances approximately 1% of red cells are destroyed (and replaced) daily. The average survival of a red cell in the circulation is 120 days. Red cells that have been damaged by burn injuries, etc. are destroyed more rapidly, and quite frequently red blood cells that have become chemically complexed to drugs such as α-methyldopa, penicillins, cephalosporins, etc. can excite an immune response in which an antibody destroys the red cell which carries the drug. Some red blood cells may be more fragile than normal. Red cells like other cells swell in solutions with lower osmotic pressure than normal plasma (hypotonic solutions), losing their discoid shape and becoming spherical, and this may lead to their rupture and destruction (haemolysis). Hereditary spherocytosis causes exactly this abnormal fragility and spherocytes haemolyse much more easily than normal biconcave erythrocytes. Deficiency of the enzyme glucose 6-phosphate dehydrogenase (G6PD) leads to an increased susceptibility to lysis by drugs and infection. This relatively common genetic deficiency also inhibits the killing and phagocytic activity of neutrophils. Excess erythrocyte breakdown is usually manifest by falling haemoglobin and rising bilirubin and serum lactate dehydrogenase. Serum haptoglobin estimation is often helpful in pinpointing haemolytic problems — haptoglobin binds free haemoglobin released into the circulation, and where there is intravascular haemolysis haptoglobin levels are markedly reduced.

Blood groups

The red cell membrane is not simply a packaging structure for carrying haemoglobin. It has, of course, another important characteristic — among the membrane proteins are those that carry and express the antigens known as agglutinogens, which determine the blood groups. Landsteiner's identification of the ABO blood group system nearly 100 years ago has stood the test of time; and the identification of the rhesus (Rh) groups in the late 1930s brought blood transfusion from an experimental procedure to a recognised therapeutic modality. The science of blood transfusion serology, and the provision of blood products for human use, is now a medical specialty in its own right. There are many agglutinogens on the surface of human red cells. A total of 28 blood group systems permutate to

give over 500 000 000 000 possible human blood group phenotypes.

The substances defining our red cell ABO groups are glycoproteins, and these are found not only on the exposed surfaces of the red cell membrane but also in many other tissues — kidney, liver, lung, etc. A and B blood group antigens are inherited as mendelian dominants: a person who inherits group A from one (or both) parents will have group A red cells. In the absence of B group substance, the individual will develop an antibody to group B (anti-B agglutinin) in the serum, presumably stimulated by contact with bacterial antigens from the bowel (the A and B antigens are structurally similar to antigens found on the cell walls of many intestinal micro-organisms). Similarly, a group B patient will have anti-A, and a group O individual will have anti-A and anti-B. The A and B antigens are expressed also on tissue cells, and the A and B group glycoproteins are present in the body fluids. In blood transfusion practice it is highly desirable to give blood of the correct ABO group, but in an emergency blood of group O may be given to patients of group A or B. By the same token, blood for transfusion should be matched with the recipient's rhesus (D) group. For logistical reasons blood grouping tests on donor blood do not usually include identification of its full rhesus phenotype. There are 47 distinct antigens within the rhesus system. However, a significant number of patients requiring transfusion are found to have antibodies to non-D rhesus antigens. They may have been immunised by a previous blood transfusion or, if female, by a pregnancy. To date some 28 human blood group systems have been identified; they include MNSS, Kell, Duffy, Kidd and Lewis.

Cross-matching

Serological testing before transfusion is now quite sophisticated and all good blood bank laboratories can reliably identify serological incompatibilities. The major transfusion risk to a patient remains the clerical error — blood given for one reason or other to the wrong patient. In the conscious patient the administration of incompatible blood manifests with prostration, pain in the renal angle and pyrexia; subsequently, if more than 100 ml of incompatible blood have been given, renal failure and rapidly developing jaundice result. In the anaesthetised patient, the main indication that incompatible blood has been used is the development of otherwise unexplained hypotension. The offending transfusion should of course be stopped at once and further measures should be directed to maintaining renal perfusion and function. Further information is obtained from serological investigation, spectroscopic examination of the serum for free haemoglobin, and urine for casts, haemoglobin, etc.

Anaemia

Anaemia (and hence deficient oxygen carrying capacity) is usually defined as a reduction in the total haemoglobin below 10 g dl^{-1}, although some haemoglobinopathies may give rise to deficient oxygen carriage even in the presence of a normal haemoglobin level. However, in view of the dangers of viral contamination of blood for transfusion and the beneficial effects of the decreased blood viscosity and increased blood flow that accompany reduced haemoglobin levels, circulating levels of haemoglobin significantly less than 10 g dl^{-1} are quite acceptable for many procedures requiring general anaesthesia.

In the patient who is mildly or moderately anaemic the anaesthetist should, however, attempt to consider diagnoses. A simple classification of anaemia is based on the mean red cell volume (MCV) and haemoglobin content (MCH). A very high proportion of anaemias can be diagnosed and treatment instituted on the basis of the tabulated findings below (RDW = red cell distribution width, i.e. range of cell diameters).

Normal MCV Normal MCH	Low MCV Low MCH	High MCV (Normal/high MCH)
Uraemia (Urea⩾15.0)	Haemoglobinopathy (Normal RDW)	Vitamin B_{12}/ folate deficiency
Haemolysis	Iron deficiency (Increased RDW)	Marrow replacement
Recent blood loss	Chronic blood loss	
Hypothyroidism		

If time is available, the anaesthetist should correct anaemia, where possible, by the appropriate haematinics rather than by blood transfusion, which may cloud the diagnosis. Frequently, however, clinical pressures will dictate management, and urgent major surgery may mean that it is necessary to transfuse first and then make the diagnosis.

White blood cells

The blood normally contains 4–11×10^9 white cells per litre. They are lymphocytes, granulocytes and monocytes, of which the granulocytes (polymorphonuclear leucocytes) are the most numerous (Fig. 28.1).

Lymphocytes

Current evidence is that lymphocyte formation starts with the lymphopoietic stem cell in the marrow. Differentiation to form lymphocytes may take place in situ in bone marrow, or the precursor cell may enter the circulation and migrate to, and undergo further differentiation in, the thymus and the spleen or other secondary lymphoid tissues.

Lymphocytes entering the circulation before differentiation are believed to have extensive potential in terms of their life span and ability to develop in a variety of directions. Cells processed in the thymus are referred to as T cells and are responsible for cellular immunity. Cells processed elsewhere (spleen, lymph nodes, etc.) are referred to as B cells, and they are responsible for humoral immunity. This terminology (T and B cells) is derived from experimental work in chickens, in which it has been found that removal of the bursa of Fabricius, a gut-associated lymphoid organ, produces inability to make antibodies. In mammals which do not have a bursa, the transformation from precursor to B cells probably takes place in fetal liver, and perhaps spleen.

Further differentiation, often in response to antigenic or other stimulation, produces populations of lymphocytes whose functions are aimed at removing noxious stimuli from the body.

PLURIPOTENT STEM CELL

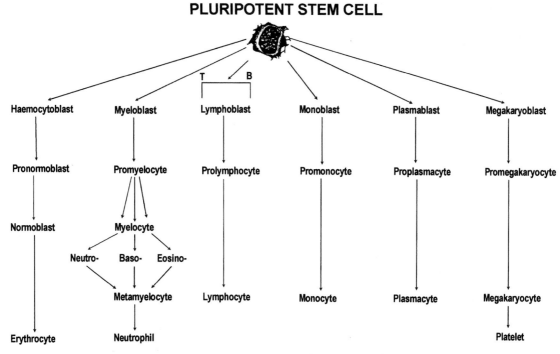

Figure 28.1   Differentiation of blood cells from a common bone marrow precursor.

B cells differentiate into activated B cells and further to plasma cells. T cells differentiate into four types: helper/inducer T cells and suppressor T cells, which both regulate B-cell production of antibodies; killer T cells (also known as effector or cytotoxic T cells); and memory T cells. The subsets of lymphocytes with differing functions can be identified by means of mouse monoclonal antibodies which pick out surface antigen structures peculiar to the functional group of lymphocytes.

Granulocytes

The granulocytes (neutrophils, eosinophils, basophils) all contain cytoplasmic granules, which in turn contain enzymes and other biologically active substances that are involved in inflammatory and allergic reactions. By comparison with the lymphocytes the development of granulocytes and their functions are relatively simple. Pluripotential stem cells (again in the marrow) differentiate into myeloblasts, then to promyelocytes. These cells are capable of mitotic activity.

Specific cytoplasmic granule formation identifies the myelocyte stage; mitosis is still possible but now the cells are identifiable by means of their granulation as being neutrophils, eosinophils or basophils. At the myelocyte stage, cytoplasmic differentiation is virtually complete; nuclear maturation proceeds. The nucleus, from being spherical, becomes kidney shaped, then elongated (band form) and finally segments in the multilobed polymorph, which is released into the peripheral blood.

The overall function of the neutrophil granulocytes is to rid the body of bacteria and other unwelcome substances by a phagocytic activity which is called into action in the inflammatory reaction or in the presence of necrotic tissue. Their function depends on their motility, ability to recognise a noxious stimulus (chemotaxis), and when at the scene, to degranulate, releasing lytic enzymes that deal with the offending agent; or they may kill and phagocytose bacteria and other particles.

Those granulocytes with specific granules (the eosinophils and basophils) probably have some phagocytic activity, although their main function takes a slightly different direction. Eosinophils are attracted to the site of local antigen–antibody complexes, and they are also found in relation to sites in which mast cells and basophils have been collected. They are particularly involved in the defence of the body against the larvae of parasitic helminths such as *Schistosoma* species, and they are frequently involved in other reactive processes where the antigenic stimulus is less well defined. The basophil granulocytes have only a minor phagocytic activity. Their involvement is mainly with immediate hypersensitivity reactions. Basophils and mast cells have receptors for immunoglobulin (IgE), and are degranulated in the presence of the appropriate antigen. Histamine is released by them (under the influence of antigen stimulated T lymphocytes) and is responsible for the vascular and other manifestations of immediate hypersensitivity.

Monocytes

The cells that develop into circulating monocytes probably originate in the marrow as monoblasts. These, in a Romanowsky preparation from the marrow, are morphologically indistinguishable from myeloblasts. In some leukaemias monoblasts are recognisable by virtue of the fact that the peripheral blood contains a high proportion of monocytes, both primitive and mature. The maturation process from monoblast through the promonocyte to mature monocyte is analogous to granulocytic maturation. Promonocytes are capable of mitosis and are identified by their content of mature monocytic cytoplasm. As the promonocyte develops, its nucleus becomes indented and often partly lobulated. At this stage monocytes become able to migrate from the marrow, probably via the peripheral blood to the tissues where they remain dormant or may become active as tissue macrophages. Their production is regulated mainly by a cytokine, GM-CSF. Their function is not simply that of phagocytosis: they appear to be able to process antigens and enable the activation of locally attracted T lymphocytes. They also have a role in the activation of the coagulation sequence.

HAEMOSTASIS

The processes leading to a halt in bleeding following injury to a blood vessel are extremely complex. Blood in circulation remains fluid because of a balance between factors that initiate and promote coagulation and other factors that inhibit coagulation and promote fibrinolysis. A further factor in achieving haemostasis lies in the constriction of arterioles particularly in close relation to the site of injury. Sympathetic nervous activity may play a part in vasoconstriction, but for arterioles in the immediate vicinity of an injury constriction is stimulated by the local concentration of serotonin, which appears to be passively ferried to the site by blood platelets. Once platelets are activated to initiate clotting, they also release prostaglandin PGI_2, which produces further vasoconstriction (see below).

Platelets

The physiological initiators of coagulation are the circulating platelets in the blood. These cytoplasmic fragments of bone marrow megakaryocytes have an intrinsic tendency not only to adhere to non-endothelial surfaces (platelet adherence) but to each other as well, this latter function being referred to as platelet aggregation. As long as the vascular endothelium remains intact (and inert vis-à-vis platelet function), platelets in the circulation undergo attrition quite slowly. In the event of damage to the vascular endothelium, whether in artery, arteriole, capillary or venule, platelet activity is dramatically altered. Damaged endothelial and tissue cells release tissue platelet activators into the surrounding plasma; collagen fibres in the supporting tissues are exposed; and all these factors induce platelet adherence to the damaged area. New platelets aggregate to the initial platelet plugs and the resultant platelet aggregates undergo a permanent change (viscous metamorphosis) with release of clotting activators and vasoconstrictors. The platelet plug becomes the site of deposition of a fibrin overlay which seals the vascular gap and arrests haemorrhage. The platelet aggregates release activators of the coagulation process, which starts an

INTRINSIC SYSTEM

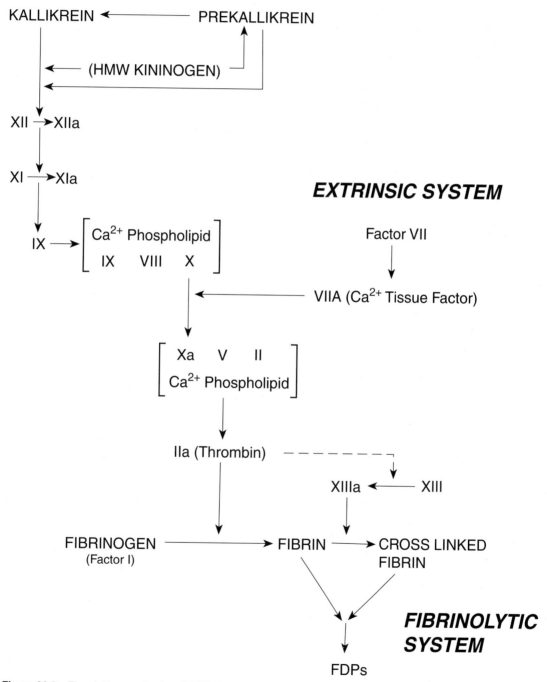

Figure 28.2 The clotting mechanism (HMW high molecular weight, FDP fibrin degradation products).

extremely complex series of reactions in the coagulation proteins of the plasma. Clotting activity is also induced by contact between the plasma and tissue cells outside the intact vascular endothelium; this phase of coagulation is referred to as the extrinsic phase, i.e. peripheral to the circulating coagulation protein.

Blood coagulation

Plasma-borne intrinsic clotting system

The intrinsic phase of coagulation is extremely complex and detailed consideration of it is outside the scope of this book; however, an abbreviated description of the intrinsic phase of coagulation is helpful. The proteins involved in coagulation can circulate in an inactive form until the milieu intérieur is disturbed. The coagulation sequence may be activated at various points, the end-point being the cleavage of fibrinogen to form fibrin. An abbreviated illustration of the coagulation system is shown in Figure 28.2.

Fibrinolytic system

In parallel with the complex coagulative system, a balancing fibrinolytic system exists. The fact that the blood in circulation remains fluid is testimony to the equilibrium between activation of coagulation on the one hand, and the influence of the fibrinolytic system on the other. The fibrinolytic system centres on plasminogen, which can be activated to plasmin, a serine protease, by several activators, including urokinase, streptokinase, kallikrein and extrinsic activators which are released from the damaged vessel wall. Plasminogen activation is thus initiated at the same instant as coagulative activity, and the fact that clotting does occur demonstrates that coagulation is activated more quickly than fibrinolysis. It is in the interests of homeostasis and restoration of the intact circulation that fibrinolysis be permitted to occur as an orderly process, when haemostasis has been reliably secured. Resolution/resorption of an established thrombus is not solely the province of the fibrinolytic system, particularly as plasmin can not readily gain access to the deeper portions of a clot. Recanalisation of established thrombi undoubtedly occurs but is often a slow process, involving the digestive and absorptive enzymatic processes of acute and chronic inflammation.

FURTHER READING

Appelbaum F R 1995 Allogenic marrow transplantation and the use of haematopoietic growth factors (review). Stem Cells 13: 344–350

Colon-Otero G, Menke D, Hook C C 1992 A practical approach to the differential diagnosis and evaluation of the adult patient with macrocytic anemia. Medical Clinics of North America 76: 581–597

Ellis M H, Avraham H, Groopman J E 1995 The regulation of megakaryocytopoiesis (review). Blood Reviews 9(1): 1–6

Faruqi R M, Di Corleto P E 1993 Mechanisms of monocytic recruitment and accumulation (review). British Heart Journal 69 (suppl 1): S19–29

Heriberg S M, Galan P 1992 Nutritional anaemias (review). Baillière's Clinical Haematology 5: 143–168

King M J 1994 Blood group antigens or human erythrocyte: distribution, structure and possible functions. Biochimica et Biophysica Acta 197(1): 15–44

Lee J H, Kiein H G 1995 Collection and use of circulating hematopoietic progenitor cells (review). Hematology/Oncology Clinics of North America 9: 1–22

Massey A C 1992 Microcytic anemia. Differential diagnosis and management of iron deficiency anemia (review). Medical Clinics of North America 76: 549–566

Quesenberry P J 1995 Hemopoietic stem cells, progenitor cells and cytokines. In: Beutler E G, Lichtman M A, Coller B S, Kipps T J (eds) Williams haematology, 5th edn, pp 211–228. McGraw-Hill, New York

Rizza C R, Jones P 1987 Management of patients with inherited blood coagulation defects. In: Bloom A L, Thomas D P (eds) Haemostasis and thrombosis, 2nd edn, pp 465–493. Churchill Livingstone, Edinburgh

Shapiro Linda H, Look T A 1995 Transcriptional regulation in myeloid cell differentiation. Current Opinion in Haematology 2: 3–11

Weatherall D J 1995 The thalassemias. In: Beutler E G, Lichtman M A, Coller B S, Kipps T J (eds) Williams haematology, 5th edn, pp 581–615. McGraw-Hill, New York

29

Drugs used in haematology

S. D. Nelson

BLOOD AND BLOOD FRACTIONS

In modern transfusion practice in Western countries, the use of whole blood has virtually ceased. This change is based on the fact that whole blood can readily be fractionated, and that the use of whole blood is not necessarily the optimum therapy for any particular patient in the clinical situation.

Fresh whole blood contains red blood cells, white blood cells, platelets, albumin, clotting factors and a wide variety of globulins with antibody activity. Instinctively one might argue that after significant haemorrhage the patient has bled whole blood and should therefore have whole blood replaced. However, a less superficial analysis will reveal that the patient's most significant loss is blood volume, and perhaps oxygen carrying capacity, while platelets, leucocytes, albumin, clotting factors and immunoglobulins remain in or close to the normal range. Transfusion of a synthetic plasma expander and an appropriate volume of packed red cells will remedy the major deficit, and other fractions need to be used only when they are specifically indicated. In addition, whole blood and its fractions may transport infective agents, in spite of the most broadly based screening procedures presently available, and there is increasing concern about agents that have yet to be identified. This latter fact emphasises the need to use blood and its fractions sparingly, and only for the strictest of indications. Donors are at present screened for syphilis, hepatitis B and C and for the human retroviruses — HIV-1 and -2. Any transfusion must be justified, and alternative therapies considered.

Collection and storage of blood, storage lesion

Blood for transfusion is collected by national and regional blood transfusion services and, after processing, packs of concentrated red cells, fresh frozen plasma, etc. are produced. Blood and concentrated red cells are preserved in a citrate–phosphate–dextrose anticoagulant, with adenine added to maintain levels of adenosine triphosphate (ATP), and can be stored for up to 35 days at a temperature of 2–4°C. During storage, red cell metabolism slows, there is a fall in intracellular 2,3-diphosphoglycerate, pH falls, and gradually the intracellular and extracellular electrolyte concentrations equilibrate. Thus there is an increase in the K^+ content of the plasma component of the stored blood — this may rise to over 30 mmol l^{-1} by the end of shelf life, although the actual amount of K^+ in the pack is small, only 2–3 mmol for red cell concentrate. The red cells tend to become nearly spherical, and as a result survive less well in the circulation when transfused.

BLOOD TRANSFUSION

A number of different preparations are available that can be used to supplement the oxygen carrying capacity of the circulating blood.

Whole blood

As detailed above, whole blood transfusion is now an increasingly rare option. Blood transfusion services are (wisely) more and more reluctant to release fresh whole blood before the completion of tests for transmissible diseases, and platelet function and factor VIII activity rapidly decay with storage. In the past, fresh whole blood has been considered suitable for use when massive transfusions are required, to avoid dilutional reductions of platelet and factor VIII availability. In practice, however, we are now increasingly forced to use platelet and coagulation factor concentrates as necessary, under the haematologist's guidance.

Red cell concentrate

This is the usual preparation when transfusion is required to correct anaemia or in acute haemorrhage.

Red cell concentrate (leucocyte depleted)

This may be indicated in patients who have developed antibodies to white cells, or to reduce the risk of this in patients receiving multiple transfusions.

All these are unsterilised and carry some risk of transmission of infection.

Synthetic substitutes for haemoglobin

Both shortage of blood for transfusion and increasing worry over undetected infective agents in donated blood make the concept of a synthetic substitute attractive. Two approaches are being followed: wholly or partly synthetic haemoglobin, or totally unrelated compounds, the perfluorocarbons. Either haemoglobin or a perfluorocarbon can form the base to transport oxygen, but these 'blood substitutes' obviously do not perform the metabolic, regulatory and protective functions of blood. None has been developed sufficiently to be used widely in clinical practice.

Haemoglobin preparations

Haemoglobin can be released from lysed human red cells, and stroma-free haemoglobin has been extensively studied. Several problems occur when the molecule is not within the protective environment of the cell. In particular, the oxygen dissociation curve is shifted to the left. In addition, the haemoglobin molecule dissociates from a tetramer into a dimer and this is rapidly cleared by the kidneys. Modifications of the molecule by chemical cross-linking to increase stability or to create macromolecules have helped to normalise the p_{50} and extend the life in the circulation, and the possibility of encapsulating haemoglobin within a liposomal envelope is being studied, but problems remain.

Haemoglobin can now be made by genetic modification of, for example, *Escherichia coli*, by recombinant DNA techniques to produce 'recombinant haemoglobin', which is undergoing clinical trials at the time of writing. When perfected, this should be an inexpensive raw material for a red blood cell substitute, free from infectious agents. Recombinant expression, combined with site directed mutagenesis, is also a technique that can facilitate modification of the functional properties of haemoglobin.

Perfluorocarbons

Perfluorocarbons are liquids whose molecules contain 8–10 carbon atoms combined with fluorine. They dissolve oxygen in simple physical solution, thus obeying Henry's law. The liquids are insoluble in water, and thus are administered as aqueous emulsions consisting of small droplets of fluorocarbon of 0.1–0.2 μm in diameter. As with the lipid emulsions used for parenteral nutrition, egg yolk phospholipid and poloyxamers are commonly used as emulsifiers. In general, perfluorocarbon molecules are biologically inert and therefore do not pose toxicological risk from metabolic degradation. Intravenous perfluorocarbon emulsions are cleared from the blood by phagocytosis of emulsion particles by reticuloendothelial macrophages, and ultimately by elimination through the lung in expired air. Newer 'second generation' perfluorocarbons can also be removed by plasmapheresis.

Platelets

The normal blood platelet count is 150–400 × 10^9 l^{-1}. The presence of a normal number of functional platelets is essential to adequate haemostasis; in general, a platelet count greater than 90–100 × 10^9 l^{-1} is compatible with adequate haemostasis in the absence of (surgical) injury.

Platelet concentrates may be prepared from routine whole blood donations (most commonly), or from single donors using cell separator procedures (plateletpheresis). From a single unit donation, after processing, a platelet concentrate provides about 50 × 10^9 platelets in 50 ml of plasma/anticoagulant. Plateletpheresis donations yield about 300 × 10^9 platelets per donation. Platelet concentrates are now stored for up to 5 days at 20–24°C with continual gentle mixing, although storage longer than 48 hours causes damage and gradual loss of haemostatic function for the stored platelets (storage lesion). Nevertheless, 5-day-old platelet concentrates still retain significant clinical activity.

Platelet usage

Thrombocytopenia associated with overt bleeding is the classic indication for platelet transfusion. Dosage has, in general, been calculated empirically, once a need for platelets is identified. The custom is to use 6–10 units (sometimes 12) of pooled donor platelets. The expected platelet count increment can easily be calculated, but the biological variability in numbers and function of transfused platelets renders this a sterile academic exercise. An empirical and perfectly adequate estimate of the platelet increment in a 70 kg patient is that one unit of platelet concentrate raises the platelet count by 5 × 10^9 l^{-1}.

It is clear that patients with grossly reduced platelet counts (< 5–10 × 10^9 l^{-1}) are at risk of potentially fatal internal haemorrhage; few would disagree with a policy of giving prophylactic platelet transfusions to a patient whose count is less than 5 × 10^9 l^{-1}. (Some years ago, the figure would have been 10 × 10^9 l^{-1}.) For thrombocytopenic patients whose platelets are in the region of 10–25 × 10^9 l^{-1}, many haematologists would delay platelet transfusion until there is evidence of haemorrhage from two sites — skin purpura counting as one, and overt epistaxis, haematuria, etc. counting as a second.

Perioperative platelet transfusion

Inevitably some thrombocytopenic patients will present for urgent surgical intervention. Some knowledge of the cause of each patient's blood problem is relevant to management because where the platelet deficit results from an auto-immune process, the response to unsupported platelet transfusion may be suboptimal and short lived. Firm data are lacking concerning the value of giving intravenous immunoglobin (as for idiopathic thrombocytopenic purpura) or fresh frozen plasma before giving platelets, but these modalities of therapy are certainly worthy of inclusion in a formal trial. Despite these theoretical reservations, in the acute situation the anaesthetist should aim at restoring and maintaining a peripheral blood platelet count of the order of 60–$80 \times 10^9 \, l^{-1}$. With adequate arterial haemostasis and in the absence of local (wound) infection, this level of platelet population will usually prevent significant haemorrhage.

Management of platelet dysfunctional states

There are numerous hereditary and acquired conditions characterised by platelet dysfunction that result in bleeding tendencies of varying severity — for example, some variants of Von Willebrand's disease may require not only plasma replacement but also platelet transfusion. The platelet defect associated with aspirin administration may also be so severe as to justify platelet transfusion, and active bleeding can occur even with a platelet count of greater than $100 \times 10^9 \, l^{-1}$. Platelet transfusions are immediately indicated where the bleeding is either retinal or intracranial, and also where it follows cardiopulmonary bypass procedures or where massive transfusion has been necessary (massive being defined as more than one complete blood volume transfusion in 24 hours).

Leucocyte concentrates

The development of cell separating machines has enabled the preparation not only of granulocyte concentrates but also of mononuclear cell enriched preparations. The latter contain a sufficient proportion of cells with stem cell potential and are used to reconstitute the marrow activity in patients with certain haematological and epithelial malignancies who are undergoing highly toxic anticancer chemotherapy.

Granulocyte concentrates have been used in a few centres since 1977 in the treatment of life threatening infections. They are thought *not* to be of value in the patient with septicaemia who maintains an adequate peripheral blood neutrophil count. However, in some cases of severe bacterial infection, severe leucopenia may occur either as a result of 'toxaemia' or sometimes as a side-effect of antibiotics prescribed. In these cases granulocyte concentrates may be of great value in the acute emergency. It is, however, important to remember that they are likely to induce immunity to HLA antigens, and may lead to difficulties with red cell and/or platelet transfusions at later dates. The provision of HLA-matched granulocytes, while in theory practicable and desirable, is in practice not possible for logistical reasons.

Outside the intensive care unit, patients with profound granulocytopenia, mainly in haematology units, are at risk of severe, life threatening bacterial, and more particularly disseminated fungal infections or fungal abscesses. In these patients, treatment with recombinant human granulocyte-monocyte colony stimulating factor (GM-CSF) can shorten the period of neutropenia. There is some evidence that granulocyte concentrates can be life saving, although in an 'odds against' situation.

Finally, a rare dysfunctional granulocyte disorder, chronic granulomatous disease, may justify granulocyte transfusion in an emergency. These cases are unlikely to be seen in anaesthetic practice.

Peripheral blood mononuclear cell concentrates are now routinely prepared for autoreconstitution of the marrow in patients undergoing chemotherapy for acute leukaemia and high grade non-Hodgkin's lymphoma. Usually these peripheral blood stem cell (PBSC) preparations are prepared when the patients are in remission from their primary disease, and are preserved in liquid nitrogen until the treatment schedule dictates their use. At this time trials of PBSC rescue in the management of carcinoma of the breast are under way, and further trials in the management of other carcinomas can be foreseen.

PLASMA AND PLASMA FRACTIONS

Plasma protein fraction (PPF, HPPF)

This product is prepared from pooled plasma that has not been snap frozen to preserve coagulation factors. Accordingly it provides effectively no coagulation activity. In order to avoid transmission of viruses (hepatitis, etc.) plasma protein fraction is always treated either by pasteurisation or with a virucidal detergent solution. It is of particular value in replacing plasma protein loss, and thus maintaining blood volume and plasma oncotic pressure in, for example, severe burns, peritonitis, etc.

Fresh frozen plasma

This is prepared from donor blood as part of the process of preparing platelet concentrates and packed cells. The plasma from which platelets have been removed is frozen in single donor packs to below −20°C within 6 hours of collection; for storage, refrigeration at −40°C is preferable. Fresh frozen plasma contains virtually all of the procoagulant activity of normal plasma, but it should be emphasised that the clotting factors are not concentrated above normal circulating levels. Fresh frozen plasma should be ABO compatible with the recipient. It should not be used prophylactically but only when there is clear evidence of a bleeding tendency. The dosage should be guided by coagulation tests but, in the adult, significant correction toward normality may require the administration of up to four packs. If there is a need to raise the patient's coagulation factor levels by more than 20%, this can be done with fresh frozen plasma only at the risk of circulatory overload.

Albumin

Salt-free concentrates of human albumin are available in various strengths up to 20% from the National Blood Transfusion Service and also from commercial sources. Their use is indicated to ameliorate the osmotic effects of severe protein deficiency. However, in conditions such as adult respiratory distress syndrome, increased capillary permeability makes attempts to reduce oedema by increasing plasma oncotic pressure relatively ineffective.

Coagulation factors

Fibrinogen cannot be prepared free of hepatitis virus and is no longer available as a separate concentrate.

Cryoprecipitate

This is prepared by collecting the precipitate formed as the plasma from a single donation is frozen and slowly thawed. It contains about 50% of the fibrinogen, fibronectin and factor VIII of the donation, in a volume of about 20 ml.

Factor VIII concentrate

This is highly purified factor VIII, used in the treatment of haemophilia A. It is treated chemically and by heat to inactivate viral contaminants (though non-A, non-B hepatitis virus may persist despite treatment). A synthetic factor VIII derived from human recombinant DNA (rfVIII) has been developed, but is still very expensive and may have added antigenicity problems.

Artificial plasma expanders

Several colloidal solutions are employed at present as substitutes for human plasma proteins, or for other properties that they possess. They are substituting largely for albumin, which has a molecular weight of 65 000. They fall into three groups: dextrans, gelatins and hydroxyethylated starches. These preparations do not have any oxygen carrying capacity.

Dextrans

Dextrans are polysaccharides made by fermentation of sucrose by a strain of *Leuconostoc mesenteroides* and subjected to subsequent hydrolysis and fractionation to obtain compounds of differing average molecular weight:

1. Dextran 70 intravenous infusion is a 5.5–6.5% solution of average mol. wt. 70 000.

2. Dextran 40 intravenous infusion is a 10% solution of average mol. wt. 40 000
3. Other preparations, e.g. 60 000, 110 000 and 150 000, are also available in some countries, but they are less popular than formerly because they cause tight rouleaux formation of the red cells and hence laboratory difficulties in reading blood cross-matching tests.

Dextran 70 has similar colloid osmotic pressure to plasma, and is therefore effective as a plasma expander. Because of its lower molecular weight, and because it is supplied in a slightly more concentrated form, Dextran 40 is more osmotically active. It will therefore temporarily attract extravascular fluid into the circulation and give an initially greater effect than higher molecular weight preparations. However, this apparent benefit is transitory and is more than offset by the greater incidence of renal complications with Dextran 40.

About half of an infused dose of Dextran 70 is excreted within 24 hours, while 5–10% remains in the circulation at 7 days. Some undergoes metabolism, mainly in the liver, to carbon dioxide and water. Dextran 40 is eliminated more rapidly, 60% being excreted in the urine within 6 hours. As well as expanding the circulating volume, dextran has other effects, which may limit the quantities infused.

Dextran has an antithrombotic effect due to a combination of several factors. Platelet adhesiveness is reduced, this effect being maximal 1–2 hours after dextran infusion, and factor VIII activity is also reduced. However, there is no observable effect on primary haemostasis with Dextran 40 or Dextran 70 in the doses normally used clinically (up to 1 g kg^{-1}) (Bergqvist 1982). Studies of operative blood loss in dextran treated patients have not been entirely conclusive, but there is no important increase and dextran can be given in doses of up to 1–1.5 g kg^{-1} to normal patients. However, caution should be exercised in any patient with a congenital or acquired haematological deficit, or who is receiving heparin.

Dextran 70 has been used in varying doses in the prophylaxis of postoperative deep venous thrombosis. A typical regimen would be 500–1000 ml per day initially, reducing after 3 days to 500 ml on alternate days for 10 days. A reduction in infusion rate is required because of gradual accumulation of higher molecular weight fractions with their slower rate of elimination, and consequent danger of circulatory overload. The effectiveness of dextran has not been proven in all trials but most reports have been encouraging.

In the management of microcirculatory insufficiency, dextran 40 has been used more than dextran 70, although there is probably little difference in their effectiveness, and dextran 40 may be more likely to lead to renal or circulatory overload problems.

Severe hypersensitivity reactions to dextrans have been reported, although the incidence is low — only about 1 in 10 000 for life threatening reactions. Ljungstrom et al (1984) have suggested that these reactions can be dramatically reduced in frequency by 'hapten inhibition', i.e. prior injection of a very low molecular weight dextran — dextran 1, mol. wt. 1000 (not available in the UK at present).

Dextrans, particularly those of lower molecular weight (<70 000), can cause renal problems because they are excreted intact by the kidneys and can cause intrarenal obstructive uropathy. This is more likely when renal perfusion is already reduced, as in the shocked patient. These difficulties can be eliminated by careful attention to the renal function of patients receiving dextran:

1. Do not give more than 1 litre day^{-1}.
2. Do not give if urine output is less than 1500 ml day^{-1}.
3. Stop if urine specific gravity rises above 1045.
4. Do not give if blood urea is above 10 mmol l^{-1}.

Gelatin solutions

These belong to three groups: oxypolygelatins, modified fluid gelatin and urea-linked gelatin (polygeline, Haemaccel). They are of average mol. wt. 30 000–35 000, so that they remain in the circulation for a much shorter time than the dextrans. Side-effects and effects other than those due to volume loading and dilution appear to be minimal. They have the advantage that there is little if any interference with platelet function. Anaphylactoid reactions are thought to be more common than with dextrans, but the incidence with polygeline, which is cross-linked with hexamethylene di-isocyanate, has been reduced markedly from that in early studies with the removal of this substance in manufacture.

Hydroxyethylated starch (HES)

This is prepared from amylopectin, a polymer of starch, which is resistant to the action of α-amylase. A preparation with a molecular weight of about 450 000 (hetastarch) is the most commonly available; pentastarch has a molecular weight of about 250 000. Hydroxyethyl starch is broken down by α-amylase in the blood, and the resulting smaller molecules are excreted by the kidneys. The half-life of hetastarch is initially (in the first 48 hours) 1.5–3.8 days, and the terminal half-life as much as a month, so that multiple dosing may lead to accumulation (Klotz and Kroemer 1987). In general, the uses and effects of hetastarch are similar to those of dextran, but it has little effect on coagulation. There is, however, a reduction in factor VIII that is greater than that due simply to dilution. This effect is less with pentastarch. Like the other plasma expanders, there is a low but definite incidence of anaphylaxis.

DRUGS AFFECTING HAEMOSTASIS

Haemostasis is a complex interplay between processes that promote clotting and other reactions that inhibit it. The anaesthetist may wish to promote one or other side of the haemostatic equilibrium, and the drugs available can affect a number of the constituent factors in the coagulation/fibrinolysis process.

Blood vessels

The intact vessel wall has a significant role in maintaining the fluid state of the blood and promoting its flow. Endothelial cells are a source of some of the plasma coagulant factor VIII. They also secrete a platelet inhibitor and a vasodilator prostacyclin (PGI_2). Damage to a blood vessel exposes tissue (collagen) fibres and a tissue coagulant factor, 'thromboplastin', is released. Prostacyclin activity is antagonised, permitting vasoconstriction, and the haemostatic equilibrium moves towards coagulation.

There are no drugs that can cause haemorrhage primarily by an effect on the vessel wall; however, desmopressin can increase the plasma factor VIII level in patients with mild haemophilia, and ethamsylate is said to reduce capillary oozing and blood loss after tonsillectomy.

Desmopressin

This substance, which is [1-deamino,8-D-arginine] vasopressin, or DDAVP, is a synthetic analogue of vasopressin and is of value in the diagnosis and treatment of diabetes insipidus. Its secondary value as a haemostatic promoter lies in the rise in factor VIII which follows its administration. For this use, it is given in a dose of 0.4 µg kg^{-1} at the time of surgery and 6-hourly afterwards. In patients with mild haemophilia given DDAVP, factor VIII may achieve a haemostatic level for a sufficient time to cover minor surgical procedures or dental extractions. It can also be used in patients whose factor VIII levels have been reduced by large volume transfusions. The primary action of desmopressin should not be forgotten, and significant water retention regularly follows its use in the doses mentioned. Restriction of water intake during its use is usually the only measure required.

Ethamsylate (Dicynene)

This is used as a systemic haemostatic agent. It has been shown to selectively inhibit some prostaglandins, and probably has a weak constrictor effect on the smallest arterioles. Ethamsylate is claimed to reduce blood loss following procedures such as tonsillectomy (and probably endometrial resection). The evidence for any activity is inconclusive (see review by Verstraete 1977).

If the anaesthetist is convinced of its activity, ethamsylate 750–1000 mg is given by intramuscular injection with the premedication. Alternatively, 1000 mg may be given intravenously at induction of anaesthesia. After operation a further 750–1000 mg may be given, followed by 500 mg every 4–6 hours.

Adverse effects in the conscious patient include nausea, headache, skin rashes and sometimes hypotension.

Drugs affecting the function of platelets

The management of numerical platelet deficiency has already been mentioned. Drugs that interfere with the function of platelets produce an effect similar to thrombocytopenia. The most important of these are acetylsalicylic acid (aspirin), sulphinpyrazone and dextran. The non-steroidal anti-inflammatory drugs also diminish platelet function, but as (apart from aspirin) this is a relatively minor effect, these drugs will not be discussed in this chapter.

Acetylsalicylic acid

This widely used substance is effective as an analgesic, anti-inflammatory and antipyretic. It has also a very marked effect on platelet function both in vivo and in vitro. A dose of 300 mg aspirin can significantly prolong the bleeding time in healthy people. This effect occurs through acetylation (and inactivation) of platelet cyclo-oxygenase, with resulting failure of synthesis of endoperoxidases and thromboxane A_2. A fully 'aspirinised' platelet is rendered useless, and this effect lasts for the life of the platelet — 4–6 days. Administration of aspirin is of value in preventing myocardial infarction, and aspirin is more and more widely used in patients who are awaiting cardiac or vascular surgery. In the event of planned surgery, aspirin should be stopped 7–10 days before operation, and can be reinstated 6 hours afterwards.

Long continued aspirin administration may also reduce the synthesis of some of the plasma clotting factors, in particular II, VII, IX and X, although the concentrations of these factors are not usually brought below haemostatic levels. A significant proportion of patients given long term aspirin will become anaemic, usually due to gastrointestinal bleeding. Uncoated aspirin tablets can produce gastric erosions and on occasion quite serious bleeding. Enteric-coated aspirin preparations are available, although even this formulation is not entirely free of gastrointestinal irritation. With the above caveat, aspirin is an extremely safe drug. Hypersensitivity is rare but can manifest as severe bronchospasm or angio-oedema.

Dipyridamole (Persantin)

This drug has a marked vasodilator effect and was initially used in angina pectoris; it was, however, only of marginal value and has been abandoned as a primary treatment for angina. Studies show it to diminish platelet aggregation in vitro; in the living patient its administration is not associated with any significant tendency to bleed. It is now used in conjunction with warfarin to prevent embolism from cardiac and vascular implants, in a dose of 400 mg daily. In some patients its vasodilator activity can give rise to troublesome headaches, but in general side-effects are rare.

Epoprostenol (prostaglandin I_2, prostacyclin, PGI_2)

PGI_2 has a potent vasodilator effect and also inhibits platelet aggregation. Its vasodilator effect is short lived on cessation of administration, but the antiplatelet effect continues for up to 2 hours. PGI_2 is not widely used, although it has been tried in the prevention of platelet activation during haemodialysis and other procedures involving extracorporeal circulation.

Drugs affecting the coagulation proteins

Production of these proteins depends on good nutrition, liver function and the presence of vitamin K. The action of vitamin K is antagonised by two groups of compounds, the coumarins and the indanediones. A large number of commercially available anticoagulants are available based on the parent compounds but only one example of each will be discussed, namely, warfarin and phenindione. Both prevent the γ-carboxylation of glutamic acid, thus resulting in the synthesis of inactive forms of factor II, VII, IX and X, antigenically similar to the base molecule but with little coagulative activity. This phenomenon is referred to as the PIVKA effect (*p*rotein formed *i*n *v*itamin *K* *a*bsence). Coagulation may also be inhibited by heparin and related compounds, which primarily act to inhibit factor Xa but also in higher dosage diminish the action of thrombin, not only on fibrinogen but also in promoting platelet aggregation.

Warfarin sodium

Warfarin sodium is rapidly absorbed from the intestine and peak concentrations are reached 1–2 hours after ingestion; however, its maximum effect is not realised until 36–48 hours, as time is required for the decay of existing, normally active coagulation proteins. Warfarin is largely bound to plasma albumin and this significantly inhibits its diffusion into red cells, cerebrospinal fluid, urine and breast milk. Warfarin is used in the management of deep venous thrombosis and pulmonary embolism, and also in the prevention of embolism in atrial fibrillation and after arterial and open heart surgery. In deep venous thrombosis the usual treatment protocol is to administer 10 mg of warfarin on day 1 and again on day 2. Maintenance treatment, usually in the range 3–7 mg daily, is started on day 3. Dosage is controlled by the prothrombin clotting time, nowadays reported as the International Normalised Ratio (INR), the therapeutic range being 2.0–3.5.

The major risk of warfarin treatment is overdosage and resultant haemorrhage, although hypersensitivity reactions have been reported. Skin reactions, including epidermal necrosis, are sometimes seen. Drug interactions, in particular those involving displacement from protein binding sites and hepatic enzyme inhibition, are unfortunately frequent. It is particularly important to be wary of aspirin compounds, which strongly potentiate warfarin, in addition to interfering with platelet function, as also do the non-steroidal anti-inflammatory agents, metronidazole and trimethoprim-sulphamethoxazole. In spite of the risks, an increasing number of patients suffering from angina pectoris, but in whom bypass surgery or angioplasty are not contemplated, are being given warfarin with aspirin. In these patients, and especially in the elderly, the INR should be maintained close to the lower end of the therapeutic range. On the other hand, barbiturates and glutethimide inhibit the action of warfarin. Warfarin should be given with caution to patients suffering from hypertension and those with a history of peptic ulcer or diverticulitis. Haemorrhage associated with overdosage often gives rise to concern. In mild cases, stopping warfarin for 48 hours may suffice to arrest bleeding. In more severe cases, blood transfusion may be required or it may be adequate to restore coagulative activity with fresh frozen plasma. It is rarely necessary to use a concentrate, such as factor IX concentrate NBTS. The action of warfarin can be reversed in 24–36 hours by the administration of synthetic vitamin K, aceto-menaphthone in a dose of 5–10 mg. Larger doses render the patient refractory to warfarin for up to 3 weeks, so that if the indication for anticoagulant therapy continues, heparin or one of the low molecular weight heparinoids must be used instead.

Phenindione

The absorption, distribution, mode of action and indications are similar to those of warfarin. Phenindione is, unfortunately, more frequently associated with hypersensitivity reactions, which can be extremely severe. Nowadays phenindione is used only in patients who cannot tolerate warfarin. The usual dose is 200 mg in divided doses on the first day, 100 mg on the second and maintenance thereafter with 25–150 mg in divided doses at 12-hourly intervals, as indicated by the INR. Drug interactions are similar to those of warfarin.

Heparin

This is not a single substance but a complex of sulphated mucopolysaccharides prepared from either beef lung or porcine intestinal mucosa. Available heparins have a molecular weight in the range 5000–35 000 and are available as sodium, calcium or lithium salts. Dosage is expressed in international units. When injected intravenously heparin is active at once and interferes with coagulation mainly by potentiation the effect of antithrombin III on factor Xa and also by preventing the formation of thrombin from prothrombin, and fibrin from fibrinogen. In low doses its main activity is in the potentiation of antithrombin III. It is rapidly broken down and metabolised, having a half-life of 1–2 hours in the blood. The main application of heparin is in the treatment of venous thrombosis and pulmonary embolism, but it is also widely used as a prophylactic against these conditions and as the anticoagulant for procedures involving extracorporeal circulation. In established venous thrombosis the usual practice is to inject a loading dose of 7500–10 000 units, followed by a constant infusion for several days in a daily dose of 20 000–40 000 units, depending on the monitoring laboratory tests, in particular the activated partial thromboplastin time (APTT). Treatment is deemed adequate when the APTT is prolonged to 60–120 seconds. If the APTT becomes excessively prolonged (more than 180 seconds), this need not necessarily give rise to anxiety; it is usually sufficient to reduce the heparin dosage unless the patient is bleeding overtly. If necessary, circulating heparin can be antagonised within a few minutes by protamine sulphate 50 mg given intravenously. In the treatment of deep venous thrombosis or pulmonary embolism it is customary to change to oral anticoagulants after 3–4 days when the patient's condition is stable.

Heparin may also be used in small doses (Minihep) as a prophylaxis against thrombosis in patients undergoing surgery who are deemed to be at significant risk. The usual dose is 5000 units given subcutaneously, 2 hours before operation, and repeated every 8–12 hours until the patient is mobile. At this dosage level, laboratory control is not required. The complications of heparin therapy are mainly related to bleeding; however, alopecia, osteoporosis and thrombocytopenia also occur, although infrequently. It is thought that heparin related thrombocytopenia is due to activation of the coagulation process with consequent platelet consumption. As with the oral anticoagulants, drug interactions are important. Heparin has many significant pharmacological incompatibilities; the most important of these are the aminoglycoside antibiotics, erythromycin and many of the cephalosporins — they should not be mixed with heparin in infusion bags. In recent years research efforts aimed at isolating and purifying the active antithrombin binding region of heparin have proved successful and it has become possible to discard, as it were, the molecular fragments of heparin that are inactive. The resulting low molecular weight heparinoids are now available and are in widespread clinical use.

Low molecular weight heparins

Numerous low molecular weight (LMW) heparins are available from various manufacturing companies. Their quoted molecular weight varies between 3000 and 8000. All the LMW heparins contain the antithrombin III-specific pentasaccharide unit of unfractionated heparin and as a result they all inhibit factor Xa. Depending on molecular size, some may also directly inhibit the action of thrombin. LMW heparins are given by subcutaneous injection in a single fixed daily dose, which is obviously more convenient than the use of heparin, and many hospitals have now adopted a low molecular weight protocol for the prevention of deep venous thrombosis in the perioperative period. A regimen such as the following is entirely satisfactory, although dosage may vary according to the preparation chosen. For patients with a low to moderate risk of venous thrombosis enoxaparin 20 mg is given once daily by subcutaneous injection; treatment should be continued for 7–10 days or until the risk of thrombosis has diminished. The initial dose should be given approximately 2 hours preoperatively. In those patients with a higher risk of thrombosis the dose may be increased to 40 mg daily. In the event of haemorrhage occurring in a patient who has been given LMW heparin, the agent may be neutralised with protamine sulphate given by slow intravenous injection. The dose of protamine used should be sufficient to neutralise the amount of LMW heparin available. 100 antiheparin units of protamine (1 mg) will neutralise 100 units of LMW heparin (approximately 1 mg).

Cardiopulmonary bypass and extracorporeal circulation

Patients having cardiac surgery go on cardiopulmonary bypass, which requires high dose heparinisation of 3–4 units ml^{-1} to prevent intracirculatory coagulation. It should be noted that the introduction of the bypass pathway causes a decrease in both platelet number and function. There may also be a decrease in the concentration of plasma coagulation factors. During operation heparin must be infused so as to maintain adequate anticoagulation — as mentioned above the half life of heparin in the circulation is approximately 1–2 hours.

As an alternative to standard heparin some units are now using LMW heparins in approximately similar dosage, a single bolus being adequate for an operation lasting up to 4 hours. When bypass is to be discontinued, heparin and its fractions can be neutralised with protamine sulphate. A small proportion of patients, approximately 3–5%, suffer significant postoperative bleeding and, while possible defects in surgical haemostasis should not be overlooked, it appears the most common problem is one of platelet dysfunction. Therapy is based on this premise and an initial bolus of platelets from 10–12 platelet concentrates should be given. Laboratory assays may identify severe depletion of coagulation factors and in these circumstances fresh frozen plasma and/or cryoprecipitate are given when there is evidence of significant coagulation factor deficiency or hypofibrinogenaemia, respectively.

Drugs affecting protease inhibitors

The protease inhibitors as a group have an anticoagulant effect by interfering with the activation of various steps in the coagulation chain. The most important naturally occurring protease inhibitor is antithrombin III, which, as its name suggests, antagonises thrombin. It also has important inhibitory activity against factors IXa, Xa, XIa and XIIa, and a reduction in the amount of antithrombin III available almost certainly leads to a state of hypercoagulability; patients congenitally deficient in antithrombin III suffer from frequent thrombotic episodes. Since the action of heparin is mediated primarily through antithrombin III, it follows that very low circulating antithrombin III levels render heparin relatively ineffective and on occasions it may be necessary to administer antithrombin III concentrates, which are available from the National Blood Transfusion Service. A dose of 1.2–5.0 units kg^{-1} will raise the antithrombin III level to about 0.6 units ml^{-1}, which is sufficient to maintain antithrombin activity. The biological half-life is about 2 days, so that antithrombin III treatment must be given at intervals suitably calculated to maintain circulating antithrombin levels.

Drugs affecting the fibrinolytic system

Fibrinolysis is a complex chain of reactions leading ultimately to activation of the major factor, plasminogen, which is converted to plasmin by several activators, including urokinase, streptokinase, kallikrein and extrinsic activators which are found in the vessel wall. Inhibitors of the fibrinolytic system are also available for clinical use and include aminocaproic acid, tranexamic acid and aprotinin.

Fibrinolytic activators

Streptokinase. Activators of the fibrinolytic system include streptokinase, which is a partly purified extract from cultures of group C haemolytic streptococci. Many patients have a high titre of circulating antistreptococcal antibodies, which, in theory at least, can neutralise streptokinase, and this activity must be overcome if streptokinase is to be fully effective. Streptokinase now plays a major part in the early management of myocardial infarction and a typical regimen is as follows. A loading dose of 600 000 units is infused over a period of 30–60 minutes, if felt appropriate under cover of intravenous hydrocortisone to avoid allergic reactions. After the initial loading dose streptokinase 100 000 units h^{-1} is infused for 72 hours. If necessary, streptokinase may be continued for a further 3 days, after which the body's immune response to the streptococcal protein leads to significant difficulty. The major side-effects of streptokinase are haemorrhage and allergy. Haemorrhage may be controlled by administration of fresh frozen plasma and, if necessary, tranexamic acid or aprotinin. Allergic problems may be combatted with corticosteroids, particularly hydrocortisone. Streptokinase is contraindicated in patients with severe hypertension, coagulation defects, cerebral metastases or peptic ulcer, and its use should be avoided in patients who have undergone surgery within the previous 10 days.

Urokinase. This is an enzyme extracted from human urine or from cultures of human kidney cells. It acts by direct conversion of plasminogen to plasmin. It has been used in the treatment of pulmonary embolism but its major application has been in the treatment of hyphaema (haemorrhage into the anterior chamber of the eye), and it is also of value in unblocking arteriovenous shunts and intravenous cannula. For local use in hyphaema 5000 units dissolved in 2 ml saline may be introduced via a suitable irrigator into the anterior chamber through a small incision into the cornea just inside the temporal limbus. For clotted shunts and intravenous cannula 5000–25 000 units of urokinase dissolved in 5 ml of saline are instilled into the affected limb of the shunt, which is then clamped off for 2–4 hours. Although theoretically attractive in the treatment of, for example, pulmonary embolism, urokinase has not in fact been widely used. This is probably because it can exert its action only on the tip of the thrombus in a blood vessel that is completely occluded. Many workers believe that urokinase, and to a lesser extent streptokinase, have little advantage over more conventional anticoagulants, particularly heparin.

Recombinant tissue plasminogen activator

(alteplase). Alteplase is a glycoprotein that activates the conversion of plasminogen to plasmin directly. When administered intravenously alteplase binds to fibrin, for which it has high affinity, and is relatively specific for fibrin in established clots. Alteplase is cleared rapidly from the circulating blood: the level in plasma falls to 50% of the initial level within 5 minutes and to less than 10% after 20 minutes. Large scale trials in the use of alteplase in early myocardial infarction have shown that it has a beneficial effect similar to that of streptokinase. Alteplase has the advantage of being a human product and therefore non-immunogenic, but because of expense its role in the management of myocardial infarction appears to be limited to situations where streptokinase cannot be given or where the brevity of its half-life is of significant advantage.

Anistreplase. This is a thrombolytic enzyme complex of plasminogen-streptokinase activator temporarily blocked by an anisoyl group. After intravenous injection, this group is cleft from the complex and plasminogen becomes activated, with a half-life of approximately 90 minutes. Contraindications and adverse side-effects are similar to those of streptokinase and, as anistreplase is significantly more expensive than streptokinase, the latter would appear to be the thrombolytic agent of choice, both in early myocardial infarction and even where thrombolysis is required at extracardiac sites.

Fibrinolytic inhibitors

Aminocaproic acid. This is readily absorbed from the gastrointestinal tract and becomes widely distributed throughout the body fluids. Excretion is via the kidneys, most of a single dose being excreted unchanged within 12 hours. It acts by inhibiting plasminogen activation and also inhibits the activity of plasmin. It is indicated in severe haemorrhage associated with excessive fibrinolysis and can be of considerable value in haemorrhage following surgery to the lower urinary tract. It is given orally or by intravenous injection: if orally, the dose is 3–6 g 4 or 6 times a day; if intravenously, 4–5 g are given in the first hour, followed by 1 g every 8 hours until bleeding has been controlled. Aminocaproic acid should be used with caution in patients with renal impairment and is contraindicated in patients with disseminated intravascular coagulation and with predominant activation of the coagulation phase.

Tranexamic acid. This has the action of aminocaproic acid but is approximately 10 times more potent weight for weight. The indications are as for aminocaproic acid, the usual dose being 1–1.5 g orally, 2 or 3 times a day, or 0.5–1 g by slow intravenous injection, 2 or 3 times a day. The solution is pharmacologically incompatible with penicillin.

Aprotinin. This is a polypeptide proteinase inhibitor with a molecular weight of about 6500. Aprotinin acts as an inhibitor of proteolytic enzymes, which of course include plasmin and some plasminogen activators. It has been used in acute pancreatitis, when it is of doubtful value, and in hyperfibrinolytic states. For hyperfibrinolysis a dose of 500 000 units is given slowly intravenously, followed by a continuous infusion of up to 50 000 units hourly. Allergic reactions, including urticaria, bronchospasm and even anaphylaxis, have been reported. There are no absolute contraindications to its use, although it is pharmacologically incompatible with corticosteroids and with nutrient solutions containing amino acids or fat emulsions.

REFERENCES AND FURTHER READING

Bell K 1995 Blood transfusion in the critically ill (part 1). British Journal of Intensive Care 5: 329–339

Bell K 1996 Blood transfusion in the critically ill (part 2). British Journal of Intensive Care 6: 10–15

Bergqvist D 1982 Dextran and haemostasis: a review. Acta Chirurgica Scandinavica 148: 633–640

Beutler E, Masouredis S P 1995 Preservation and clinical use of erythrocytes and whole blood. In: Beutler E G, Lichtman M A, Coller B S, Kipps T J (eds) Williams haematology, 5th edn, pp 1622–1635. McGraw-Hill, New York

Blood Transfusion Task Force 1991 Product liability for the hospital blood bank. In: Waltar B (ed) Standard haematology practice, pp 217–230. Blackwell Scientific, Oxford

De Bono D P 1995 Thrombolytic therapy of acute myocardial infarction. Baillière's Clinical Haematology 8: 403–412

Kakkar V V 1987 Prevention of venous thromboembolism. In: Bloom A C, Thomas D (eds) Haemostasis and thrombosis, 2nd edn, pp 802–819. Churchill Livingstone, Edinburgh

Klotz U, Kroemer H 1987 Clinical pharmacokinetic considerations in the use of plasma expanders. Clinical Pharmacokinetics 12: 123–125

Ljungström K G et al 1983 Prevention of dextran-induced anaphylactic reactions by hapten inhibition. Acta Chir Scand 149: 341–343

McCullough J 1995 Blood procurement and screening. In: Beutler E G, Lichtman M A, Coller B S, Kipps T J (eds) Williams haematology, 5th edn, pp 1618–1622. McGraw-Hill, New York

Taylor J 1996 Guide to platelet transfusion. British Journal of Intensive Care 6: 54–56

Verstraete M 1977 In: Haemostatic drugs: a critical appraisal, pp 26–39. Martinus Nijhoff, The Hague

Verstraete M 1995 Thrombolytic therapy of non cardiac disorders. Baillière's Clinical Haematology 8: 413–424

Respiratory system

Respiratory system

J. P. Jamison

STRUCTURAL BASIS OF RESPIRATORY TRACT FUNCTION

Mouth, nose and pharynx

The mouth is normally closed in quiet breathing, but when there is heavy ventilatory demand such as in severe exercise, mouth breathing supervenes and provides a significant reduction in resistance to flow at the expense of some loss of air warming, which may contribute to exercise induced asthma. Swallowing requires closure of the lower airway and nasopharynx and opening of the crico-oesophageal sphincter. A key movement is elevation and forward displacement of the cricoid cartilage. Some authors emphasise the importance of posterior deflection of the epiglottis acting as a flap valve to close the lower airway. When swallowing liquids, the epiglottis does not usually bend backwards; its contribution to preventing entry into the lower airway may be largely by directing the flow to either side of the centrally placed larynx.

The nose provides very effective moistening and warming of the inhaled air. The mucosa is moist and vascular and thrown into folds, which increase its surface area. The lumen is thereby narrowed, thus increasing the nasal resistance to airflow. In health, upper airway resistance is greater than lower airway resistance. Patency of the nasopharynx is dependent on muscular tone, which is diminished during sleep. Very severe obstruction to airflow can occur in this region. In common with the larynx and extrathoracic trachea, negative intraluminal pressure during inspiration is not balanced by corresponding negative extraluminal pressure. These airways therefore tend to collapse and increase their resistance during inspiration. When combined with decreased muscular tone during sleep, obstructive sleep apnoea may result, leading to periods of arterial desaturation.

Larynx

This provides one of the non-respiratory functions of the respiratory system — phonation. Its respiratory functions are to help prevent ingress of foreign material and to assist in the removal of sputum by its role in coughing. Laryngeal oedema may produce life threatening airway obstruction.

Tracheobronchial tree

The walls comprise a mucosa, connective tissue, smooth muscle, nerves, glands and cartilage. The outer aspects of the intrathoracic airways are tethered by the alveolar walls, which, being under tension from their elasticity, help to dilate the airways. The alveoli also exert a negative pressure outside the intrathoracic airways during inspiration that helps to dilate them, in contrast to the collapse that tends to occur in the extra-thoracic airways during this phase of respiration. The intrathoracic airways tend to collapse during expiration as a result of the positive pressure in the alveoli, as well as the reduction of traction from their elastic walls.

Mucus is secreted in part from intraepithelial goblet cells and in part from ducted serous and mucous glands. Mucous plaques form, floating on a serous layer. The tips of cilia from the pseudostratified columnar epithelium are engaged in the mucous plaques and waft them upwards towards the glottis. Further down the bronchial tree the ducted glands disappear and the pseudostratified columnar epithelium loses its goblet cells. At a lower level the epithelium loses its cilia and becomes cuboidal. The presence of cilia at a lower level than mucous secretion ensures that secretions are effectively cleared. Cilia are absent in the larynx and final expectoration of sputum requires coughing.

There are about 15 generations of branching in the bronchial tree. The increase in number of airways at each dichotomous branching causes a progressive decrease in airflow resistance with each generation after the segmental bronchi, despite the reduction in airway diameter (Fig. 30.1). This low resistance offered by healthy bronchioles contrasts markedly with the high resistance offered by arterioles in the control of blood flow.

Cartilage provides rigidity to larger airways and therefore prevents collapse when the airways are subject to compressive transmural pressures, such as occur during forced expiration. The tracheal cartilages are U-shaped, closed anteriorly; in the bronchi, these become irregular plates; cartilage is absent in the bronchioles.

The smooth muscle of the airways forms a sheet between the open ends of the cartilage plates in the trachea; in the bronchi and bronchioles the smooth muscle forms a gentle spiral or circular layer. The muscle is single-unit in type. Innervation from the vagus provides parasympathetic cholinergic and non-cholinergic non-adrenergic efferents to the smooth muscle and glands and afferents from pulmonary receptors. The upper airways receive a sparse sympathetic nerve supply, but most of the bronchial smooth muscle receives no sympathetic innervation, sympathetic innervation of the lung being limited to its vascular supply.

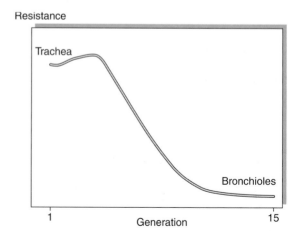

Figure 30.1 Most of the resistance to flow in the lower respiratory tract is in the large airways.

Arterial supply to the bronchi carries oxygenated blood from the aorta. Venous drainage delivers deoxygenated blood partly to the systemic veins and partly to the pulmonary veins.

The airways have no gas exchange function until the level of the respiratory bronchioles, which have alveoli opening off their walls. The respiratory bronchioles therefore have the dual functions of conducting airflow and gas exchange.

Inflammatory cells, mast cells and immune competent cells are present to provide their contribution to cellular and humoral immunity. Immunoglobulin A (IgA) is secreted into the lumen. IgE is prevalent in hypersensitive individuals.

Alveoli

The structure of the alveoli is adapted to their gas exchange function by providing a very large surface area (about $70\,m^2$) of thin alveolo-capillary membrane (about $0.5\,\mu m$). The type 1 pneumocytes which form the greater part of the alveolar epithelium are flattened cells connected to each other by tight junctions. The basement membranes of the epithelium and endothelium are fused in places. Type 2 pneumocytes are more rounded, with bulging cytoplasm containing the surface active agent, surfactant, in lamellated inclusion bodies.

There are occasional scavenger cells in the alveolar spaces — called alveolar macrophages. These move across the capillaries by diapedesis. Having phagocytosed foreign material, they may either re-enter the interstitial spaces of the alveolar walls and hence travel to the lymphatic system of the lung or they may move along the airway surfaces until they reach the mucociliary escalator and become expectorated.

The connective tissue of the alveolar walls contains an extensive network of elastin fibres synthesised by fibroblasts. These provide an elastic skeletal structure for the alveoli.

Lymphatic system

There are no lymphatic capillaries in the inter-alveolar septa, but they are present in adjacent septa and vascular sheaths. There is an extensive network in the walls of the bronchioles and larger conducting airways. The pleural lymphatics form a separate but interconnecting system. Lymph nodes abound in the hilar regions and drain into the venous system in the right and left neck veins.

MECHANICS OF VENTILATION

Movements of breathing

During inspiration the thoracic cavity increases its anteroposterior, vertical and to a lesser extent its transverse dimensions. Increase in the vertical dimension is achieved by descent of the hemidiaphragms. At rest the ribs run obliquely downward and forward from their costovertebral joints to their costochondral junctions. Thus elevation of the anterior ends of the ribs during inspiration increases the anteroposterior dimension of the thoracic cavity. This movement is achieved by contraction of the external intercostal muscles, the fibres of which run obliquely downwards and forwards. This elevation of the anterior ends of the ribs is known as the 'pump handle' movement. At rest, the middle of the ribs lies inferior to a plane joining the anterior and posterior ends of the ribs. Thus elevation of the ribs also increases the transverse dimension of the thoracic cavity. This movement is known as the 'bucket handle' movement.

In addition to the muscular force acting on the thoracic cage there are also elastic forces. Elastic forces from within the chest wall arise principally from the elastic cartilages. Elastic forces within the lung arise from the alveolar walls — elastin connective tissue fibres and surface tension at the air–fluid interface contribute about equally to this elastic force. If the muscles of respiration are relaxed, the chest takes up the position where the elastic recoil from the lungs, which tends to collapse the lungs, is exactly balanced by the elastic recoil from the chest wall, which tends to expand the lungs. The lungs and chest wall exert their force on each other through the pressure in the small quantity of lubricating pleural fluid in the pleural cavity. The expansile elastic force of the chest wall pulling against lung elastic recoil creates a pressure in the pleural cavity which is negative with respect to atmospheric pressure. The pressure is maintained because the pleural fluid is inexpandable and the cavity is normally sealed against the entry of fluid or air. The volume of air in the lungs at the end of a quiet expiration is the *functional residual capacity* (FRC). This is the position taken up by the respiratory system when the muscles relax. In health there is often a short pause at this phase of the respiratory cycle. This is an efficient position to rest because no muscular effort is required. Because inflation decreases the outward springiness of the chest wall and increases the elastic recoil of the lungs, the latter will exceed the thoracic cage elastic forces at volumes greater than the FRC. Consequently the lungs will deflate under their elastic recoil if not opposed by the contraction of the inspiratory muscles. This is the normal mechanism of quiet expiration. The elastic energy stored in the lungs by inflation is used to provide a passive force for expiration. Thus it is only necessary for the intercostal muscles and hemidiaphragms to relax to allow quiet expiration.

More powerful expiratory movements require additional muscular effort. The hemidiaphragms may be forced upward by the increased abdominal pressure generated by contraction of the abdominal muscles. Depression of the ribs may be achieved by contraction of the internal intercostal muscles, the fibres of which run downwards and backwards to the rib below. Other muscles arising from the spine or shoulder girdle and attached to the ribs can be used as accessory muscles of respiration to increase the force on the rib cage when necessary, e.g. during exercise or in the presence of respiratory disease which increases the airway resistance or decreases lung or chest wall compliance.

Coughing

Stimulation of irritant receptors in the respiratory tract or mechanical receptors in the larynx and trachea may give rise to coughing. This consists of an inspiration, then a forced expiratory effort against a closed glottis. The glottis is opened when the air pressure is high, allowing a sudden release of air through narrowed and vibrating airways, expectorating mucus and foreign material.

STATIC LUNG MECHANICS

This term refers to experimental measurements of ventilatory function made when there is no air flow. The consequence of absence of airflow is that the contribution normally made by airway resistance is eliminated, allowing elastic recoil to be analysed more fully using static pressure/volume curves. The slope of these plots ($\Delta V / \Delta P$) is the *lung compliance* and its reciprocal ($\Delta P / \Delta V$) is the lung elastance. Compliance is the term that is more commonly used and it represents the distensibility of the lung. The normal value is 0.2 l per cmH_2O in adults. Values higher than the upper limit of normal indicate larger volume increases per unit pressure resulting from loss of elastic recoil, e.g. after the destruction of elastin fibres in emphysema. Lower values indicate stiff lungs, such as result from the replacement of elastin fibres with collagen or in the presence of surfactant deficiency which leads to high surface tension forces in the alveoli. Maximum compliance generally occurs at volumes near to the FRC. At higher lung volumes the alveoli approach the limit of distensibility of the elastin network. At lower lung volumes, the small size of the alveoli favours collapse, by the law of Laplace. This law states that:

$$P = 2T/r,$$

where P is the excess pressure inside a spherical surface (such as an alveolus) required to maintain stability, T is the tension in the wall and r is its radius of curvature. At any particular volume, a higher transpulmonary pressure is required during lung inflation than during deflation (Fig. 30.2). This is referred to as *hysteresis*. It has been shown that a film of lung extract spread on saline has a lower surface tension than saline. This is due to *surfactant*, produced by type 2 pneumocytes, which is a combination of various surface active materials such as dipalmitoyl lecithin, other lipids and proteins. Surfactant

Volume

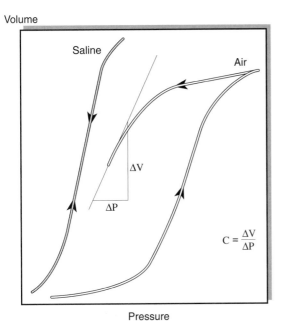

Pressure

Figure 30.2 Static transpulmonary pressure–lung volume curves in isolated lung inflated with air and saline. Lung compliance (slope $\Delta V/\Delta P$) is shown at its maximum (about FRC). Inflation of the lung with air from low volumes requires high pressures; lower pressures are sufficient to maintain volumes after inflation. This hysteresis is abolished and compliance increased when the lung is inflated with saline, which abolishes surface tension forces.

lowers surface tension of all alveoli but its effect is greater on small than on distended alveoli, an important property that assists in stabilising small alveoli. This property is also demonstrable in isolated surfactant films on saline. Reducing the surface area over which a given quantity of surfactant is spread reduces the surface tension. It is probable that reducing the surface area increases the surface concentration of the surfactant molecules, allowing a greater surface tension-reducing effect. Furthermore, the hysteresis described for lung inflation/deflation is also present for an isolated surfactant film on saline when the surface area is expanded and contracted at respiratory frequencies. The surface tension is higher when the surface is being expanded. It has been suggested that surfactant goes into solution when the film is concentrated by reducing the surface area. This makes less surfactant available during subsequent expansion. These surface active properties are abol-

ished by inflating isolated lung with saline instead of air. The saline inflated lung has a much higher compliance and does not show hysteresis in its static pressure/volume curve.

The reduction of surface tension by surfactant increases the interstitial fluid pressure in the alveolar walls. This reduces the distending transmural pressure across pulmonary capillary walls and reduces the fluid filtration pressure. In surfactant deficiency there is capillary congestion and fluid accumulation in the interstitial spaces and eventually in the alveolar spaces. Modification of the chemical constitution of the intra-alveolar exudate leads to the formation of a hyaline membrane, which is a characteristic pathological feature of respiratory distress syndrome. Surfactant may be administered intra-bronchially, from where its surface coating properties help it spread throughout the alveolar system. It is a very effective therapy for the respiratory distress syndrome of pre-term birth.

Gravity has an effect on the regional distribution of lung compliance. In the upright posture the weight of the lung deflates the bases and distends the apices. In quiet respiration the bases are at an optimal volume for high compliance, whereas the apices are stretched to volumes where their compliance is reduced. Thus inhaled tidal air goes preferentially to the bases. At residual volume the bases are collapsed to volumes where their compliance is reduced, whereas the apices have been brought into a volume range where their compliance is more nearly optimal. At residual volume inhaled air therefore goes first to the apices. A smaller range of volume increase is available at the apices because gravity limits the deflation of the apices at residual volume. With expiration, the first air out tends to come from the bases because they are on a steeper part of the compliance curve, and the last air out tends to come from the apices. At low lung volumes some airways close off completely so that air flow from that region ceases. This is the basis of the measurement of *closing volume*. In this technique, nitrogen levels are measured during exhalation after a breath of oxygen. The first air expired comes from the conducting airways where no mixing occurred between the inhaled oxygen and the nitrogen-containing air previously in the lungs. This air therefore contains no nitrogen. Anatomically it corresponds to the air in the spaces where no gas exchange can take place. It would not include dysfunctional alveoli where no gas exchange occurs but where mixing can occur. This volume is therefore the anatomical dead space. At the end of exhalation there is a rise of the nitrogen concentration. This is thought to occur when high nitrogen-containing areas (low ventilation regions) are emptying without dilution from low nitrogen-containing regions (highly ventilated regions). This can occur when the airways from the latter regions close. The volume above residual volume at which this occurs is called the closing volume. The sum of the closing volume and the residual volume is known as the closing capacity.

In health, the closing capacity should be well below the FRC. Increase of the closing capacity occurs in conditions where the airways become narrowed. This is often coupled with an increase of the FRC, but in anaesthesia the FRC is decreased by loss of end-expiratory diaphragmatic muscle tone. There is then a greater risk that airway closure will occur, leading to atelectasis behind the airway closure and consequent ventilation/perfusion mismatching and hypoxia.

STATIC LUNG VOLUMES

A spirometer is a device that collects and records the volumes of inhaled or exhaled air (Fig. 30.3). This may be used to measure *tidal volume*, which is the volume inhaled or exhaled during breathing. Typically this is about 0.5 l at rest. This volume can be increased during exercise by using reserves in both inspiration (*inspiratory reserve volume*) and expiration (*expiratory reserve volume*). The maximal volume which can be inhaled or exhaled is the sum of the resting tidal volume, the inspiratory reserve volume and the expiratory reserve volume. This is called the *vital capacity* and is typically about 10 times the resting tidal

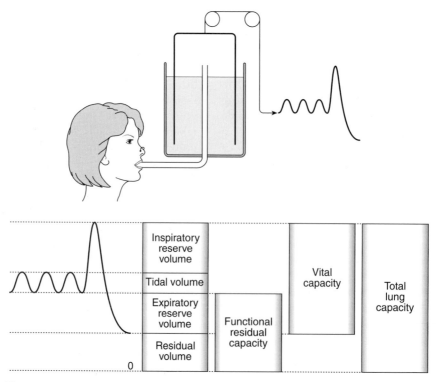

Figure 30.3 Measurement of lung volumes using a water filled spirometer.

volume. The respiratory frequency at rest is typically 12–14 breaths per minute. The volume of air ventilating the lungs per minute (*minute volume*) is calculated by multiplying the tidal volume (volume of air in one breath) by the respiratory frequency (number of breaths per minute). Thus the minute volume is about $6 \, l \, min^{-1}$ at rest and can increase some 25-fold to about $150 \, l \, min^{-1}$ in severe exercise. Somewhat larger increases can be achieved voluntarily (*maximum breathing capacity*). At the end of a full expiration, limitation of chest wall excursion prevents complete collapse of the lungs. The volume of air then left in the lungs is called the residual volume. As it cannot be breathed out, its size cannot be measured by simple spirometry. Instead the dilution principle is used. A marker gas, usually helium, is added to the spirometer. The subject inhales the helium-containing gas mixture. The helium is diluted by the helium-free air previously in the lungs, and the degree of dilution reflects this volume. In practice the volume of air in the lungs at the end of a quiet expiration, the functional residual capacity (FRC), is measured by switching the subject to rebreathe from a helium containing spirometer at the end of a quiet expiration, and allowing several minutes of normal breathing for the helium to mix thoroughly between the spirometer and the lungs. The residual volume and other lung capacities can then be obtained by addition or subtraction of the named volumes measured by spirometry. The *total lung capacity*, for example, can be obtained by adding the residual volume, inspiratory and expiratory reserve volumes and the tidal volume. Note that the term 'capacity' is used for sums of named 'volumes'. The FRC is important because it is the volume of air in the lungs most of the time. Its function is to provide a large volume of air from which oxygen can be taken up and into which carbon dioxide can be added without changing the fractional concentrations very much, thereby helping to maintain constancy of the arterial partial pressures of the respiratory gases.

DYNAMIC LUNG MECHANICS

When air flows into or out of the lung, pressure gradients are required along the conducting airways to overcome their resistance to flow. Airway resistance is an entity that reflects the frictional opposition to flow and is calculated as the pressure gradient per unit air flow rate. Poiseuille showed that resistance is a constant that is independent of pressure and rate of flow, provided the flow is laminar and the coefficient of viscosity, length and radius of the tube are constant. The radius of the tube is the most critical factor, being raised to the fourth power. Flow is laminar in the airways only at low flow rates, less than $1 \, l \, s^{-1}$, such as occur in quiet breathing. In this range, flow rate increases proportionately with pressure. With onset of turbulent flow, the relationship between flow rate and pressure becomes curved and less steep, i.e. the resistance is apparently increased. Turbulence is likely to occur when Reynolds number is exceeded. This number is higher, and turbulence more likely, with high velocity of flow, large diameter, high density and low viscosity.

Measurement of *airway resistance* is difficult. Flow rate is relatively easily measured. The rate of change of volume measured by a high frequency response spirometer can be used, or a pneumotachograph which measures flow rate from the pressure drop across a resistive wire grid. Alveolar pressure is more difficult to measure. There are several methods available but the most accurate is whole body constant volume plethysmography. In this technique, the subject is seated in a sealed cabin breathing the cabin air. Pressure changes in the cabin air are then proportional to alveolar pressure changes. Simultaneous recording of alveolus–mouth pressure gradients and rate of flow enable airway resistance to be calculated. The technique is difficult and expensive, therefore simpler inexpensive tests are more usually deployed to assess airway calibre indirectly. The problem with these tests is that their interpretation is more difficult because they do not separate airway resistance from other factors. The simplest is the *peak expiratory flow rate*. The subject inhales deeply and then blows with a maximal effort into a peak flow meter. This instrument records the highest flow rate that has been exceeded for more than a fraction of a second. This measurement is useful for frequent monitoring of airway obstruction and can be done by the patient at home. It is also useful in emergencies. A more informative and less effort dependent technique is to record a full *forced expiratory manoeuvre*. The forced expiratory manoeuvre consists of inhaling to total lung capacity, exhaling as fast as possible and maintaining the maximal exhalation down to residual volume. The usual graph produced is a plot of volume exhaled against time (Fig. 30.4). The maximal volume expired is known as the *forced vital capacity* (FVC). The volume expired at the first second is known as the one *second forced expiratory volume* (FEV_1). The rate at which volumes of air can be exhaled is affected by numerous factors: the voluntary effort, the muscular strength, the freedom of movement of the thoracic cage and abdomen, freedom from pain or discomfort, the elastic recoil of the lungs and thoracic cage, and the resistance offered by the airways. Despite the complexity of these factors, the simplicity of the measurement makes this test the single most useful lung function test. Two abnormal patterns may be observed: *obstructive ventilatory defect* and *restrictive ventilatory*

defect. The former is characterised by a greater reduction in the FEV_1 than in the FVC, so that the FEV_1:FVC ratio is reduced below the lower limit of normal, which is about 70%. In the restrictive ventilatory defect, the FEV_1 and FVC are reduced in parallel and the FEV_1:FVC ratio is preserved or even increased. The principal pathophysiological significance of the obstructive ventilatory defect is that the resistance of the airways is increased. This interpretation is valid provided the force applied to drive the airflow is normal. The principal pathophysiological significance of the restrictive ventilatory defect is loss of lung compliance leading to loss of lung volume. Again this is valid only if the applied ventilatory force is normal. Since compliance reflects distension of the alveoli, this ventilatory defect locates the pathological process to the alveolar walls.

A useful alternative method of recording the forced expiratory manoeuvre is to plot the flow rate against volume (Fig. 30.5). The inspiratory

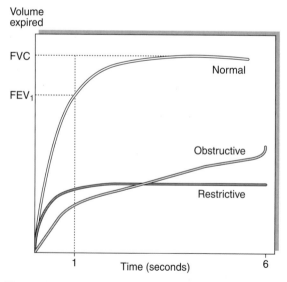

Figure 30.4 Volume–time records of the forced expiratory manoeuvre in a normal subject, a patient with an obstructive ventilatory defect and a patient with a restrictive ventilatory defect.

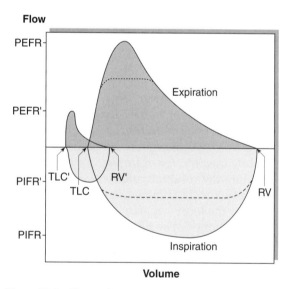

Figure 30.5 Flow–volume records of the forced expiratory–inspiratory manoeuvre. PEFR, PEFR′/PIFR, PIFR′: peak expiratory/inspiratory flow rate in a normal subject and a patient with an obstructive ventilatory defect. The marked concave expiratory phase is a feature of small airway compression due to loss of elastic tissue in emphysema. TLC, TLC′/RV, RV′: total lung capacity/residual volume. ...., Compressible intrathoracic large airway obstruction. - - - - -, compressible extrathoracic large airway obstruction.

phase may be included to complete a *flow–volume loop*. The highest flow rate during expiration is the peak expiratory flow rate (PEFR), as may be recorded directly using a peak flow meter. The flow rates at low lung volumes are less effort dependent and also reflect small airway function better than other indices of airway obstruction. Since many diseases affect the small airways first, this may be a more sensitive measurement in early disease. This advantage is, however, offset by the greater variability of these flow measurements.

The obstructive ventilatory defect is often associated with other abnormalities of lung function. The PEFR will be reduced. There is airway closure at higher lung volumes than normal. This contributes to the reduction in the FVC and leads to an increase in residual volume. The functional residual capacity is also increased. Much of this increase can be explained by increased inspiratory muscle activity, although there is also an increase in lung compliance that is poorly understood. The hyperinflation helps to distend the airways and reduce airway resistance. Some of the additional work of breathing caused by the airway obstruction is thus transferred from frictional flow resistance to increased distension against lung elastic recoil. Consequently, many asthmatic patients find it more difficult to breathe in than to breathe out, despite the greater airway resistance during expiration, although this change in lung volume does decrease the total work of breathing. The greater impairment of the inspiratory phase of the flow–volume loop in extrathoracic airway obstruction and the converse in intrathoracic airway obstruction may be demonstrated by flow–volume loops, thereby providing helpful non-invasive information to determine the site of airway obstruction.

Reversibility of airway obstruction and its variability are important features of the airway narrowing that occurs in asthma. Reversibility may be tested by administering a β_2-selective agonist such as salbutamol by aerosol and measuring airway function 10 minutes later. Variability may be tested by recording PEFR three times a day for 2 weeks.

CONTROL OF AIRWAY CALIBRE

Airway calibre may be affected by many factors acting at various sites — in the lumen, in the airway wall itself or outside the airway. In the lumen, an increased rate of secretion or depressed removal mechanisms may lead to sputum retention and airway obstruction; in the wall, increased tension in the smooth muscle or increased wall thickness by inflammatory infiltration may lead to airway narrowing; outside, an increased pressure or loss of support from the elastic tissue in the alveolar walls may lead to airway narrowing that is particularly marked during forced expiration. The smooth muscle tone is under parasympathetic nervous control from the vagus nerve, acetylcholine being the neurotransmitter substance. Parasympathetic tone is maximal in the early morning at about 4 a.m. This contributes to diurnal variation in airway calibre, a pattern that is exaggerated in asthma, leading to nocturnal wakening with cough or wheeze. Although there is little or no sympathetic innervation of bronchial smooth muscle, there are β_2-adrenergic receptors. These respond to circulating adrenaline from the adrenal medulla, increasing the intracellular levels of cyclic 3,5-adenosine monophosphate (cAMP), relaxing the smooth muscle and dilating the bronchi. Phosphodiesterase breaks down the cAMP. This mechanism is amenable to enhancement by therapeutic intervention using exogenous β_2-selective stimulants or phosphodiesterase inhibiting drugs such as the theophyllines. Non-cholinergic, non-adrenergic (NANC) nerves are present. Convincing evidence has been found to suggest that vasoactive intestinal polypeptide (VIP) is released as a neurotransmitter effecting bronchodilatation. Other neurotransmitter substances have been proposed as non-cholinergic bronchoconstrictor neurotransmitters, including substance P and other neuropeptides. Prostaglandins have various effects on the airways. For example, most studies have found $PGF_{2\alpha}$ to raise bronchomotor tone and PGE_2 to lower it. Histamine is a bronchoconstrictor. Leukotrienes, which include slow reacting substance of anaphylaxis, give prolonged bronchoconstriction. Platelet activating factor is also a potent bronchoconstrictor agent. Many of these substances are present in mast cells and other inflammatory cells. Their complex interactions and role in asthma are currently under investigation.

CONTROL OF BREATHING

It is conventional to consider this topic in two parts: nervous aspects and chemical aspects. Nervous aspects of the control of breathing are concerned with controlling the pattern of breathing and may provide substantial stimulation of respiration during exercise. Chemical aspects are concerned with regulation of the overall rate of ventilation of the lungs to maintain constancy of the arterial blood gases and hydrogen ion concentration. Both aspects are fully integrated and interdependent.

Nervous aspects

The *respiratory centre* in the medulla oblongata has its own inherent rhythm which will spontaneously maintain the required alternating motor nerve outflow to maintain respiration (Fig. 30.6). The respiratory centre receives multiple inputs which modify this inherent rhythm. Concerned with the pattern of breathing, there are external influences on those neurones in the respiratory centre which fire during inspiration. The *pneumotaxic centre* in the upper pons and the pulmonary stretch receptors acting through vagal afferent nerves inhibit the inspiratory neurones of the respiratory centre, while the *apneustic centre* in the lower pons facilitates the inspiratory neurones. If the inhibitory influence of either the pneumotaxic centre or the vagus is removed, the respiratory centre will produce deeper breaths, but the respiratory frequency will also be reduced so that the minute volume does not change. If both the pneumotaxic centre and the stretch receptor influences are removed, then there will be grossly exaggerated and prolonged inspiratory efforts, interrupted by short gasps of expiration. This pattern is called apneustic breathing and is maintained by the apneustic

centre in the lower pons. Apneustic breathing may be prevented by electrical stimulation of the afferents from the pulmonary stretch receptors as they travel in the vagus. Rhythmic activity, maximal at end-inspiration, may be recorded in these vagal afferents. The inhibition of inspiration by pulmonary stretch is called the Hering–Breuer reflex. In bronchoconstriction this reflex is activated at larger lung volumes because the airway narrowing decreases the stretch of the receptors, perhaps contributing to the increase in lung volumes that occurs in airway obstruction. It is not known whether these mechanisms have much importance in humans. The stretch receptors are slowly adapting. There are also rapidly adapting receptors which influence respiration. These receptors have been more difficult to study. Their effects include inhibition of expiration, induction of deep inspirations, bronchoconstriction and coughing. They are stimulated by deflation, leading to shortening of expiration and a rapid shallow pattern of breathing. Periodically they have the apparently opposite effect of causing deep augmented breaths which prevent the slow collapse of small airways. They are located just below the bronchial epithelium and are stimulated by inhaled irritants. In response, they cause bronchoconstriction and mucosal secretion. Stimulation of irritant receptors in the larynx and upper trachea leads to bronchoconstriction and coughing. The hypothalamus has influence on the medullary respiratory centre for temperature regulation and emotional changes in the pattern of breathing. The motor area of the cerebral cortex may be the site of an exercise centre which stimulates the respiratory centre to increase ventilation in exercise. Apart from this influence, the nervous aspects of ventilatory control are principally concerned with adjusting the pattern of the rate and depth of breathing so that the work of breathing is kept to a minimum. At higher tidal volumes than optimal, the same minute volume and alveolar and arterial gas tensions can be achieved by decreasing the rate of breathing. The work of breathing is, however, greater because of the increased work against lung elastic recoil. At higher respiratory frequencies the work of breathing is increased because of increased work being done to overcome airway resistance.

Chemical aspects

The principal function of the respiratory system is to maintain constancy of the arterial partial pressures of oxygen and carbon dioxide (Pa_{O_2}, Pa_{CO_2}) and pH. Their levels are monitored by the peripheral and central chemoreceptors. While the nervous networks described above determine the pattern of breathing, the level of activity is normally set by the chemoreceptors. Oxygen lack, hypercapnia and acidosis are the drives to ventilation which are integrated in the respiratory centre to produce the appropriate negative feedback control of ventilatory minute volume. There are differences in sensitivity to changes in levels of the respiratory gases, oxygen and carbon dioxide (see Fig. 30.7). The ventilatory response to hypercapnia is principally due to the central chemoreceptors, with a contribution from the peripheral chemoreceptors. The increase in ventilation in response to hypoxic hypoxia is mediated by the peripheral chemoreceptors. The central chemoreceptors are actually depressed by hypoxia. Both the peripheral and central chemoreceptors respond to acid pH but there are differences in their sensitivity and speed of response.

The *central* or *medullary chemoreceptors* lie in the brainstem close to the respiratory centre (Fig. 30.6). They are located in the ventral part of the medulla, and, being close to the surface, are exposed to cerebrospinal fluid. The central chemoreceptors respond to changes in hydrogen ion concentration. As carbon dioxide readily crosses the blood–brain barrier into cerebrospinal fluid and into the interstitial fluid of the brain, the local [H⁺] (and thus the pH) in the brain closely follows the arterial P_{CO_2}, i.e. carbon dioxide acts through its effect on pH. This system operates to maintain the arterial P_{CO_2} at 40 mmHg (5.3 kPa), and an increase in Pa_{CO_2} will lead to an increase in minute ventilation in order to blow off the excess carbon dioxide and return the Pa_{CO_2} and thus the [H⁺] at the receptors to normal. There is an almost linear relationship

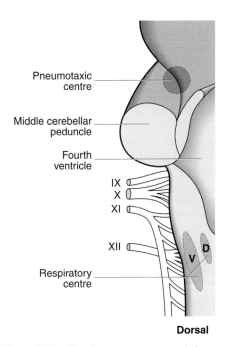
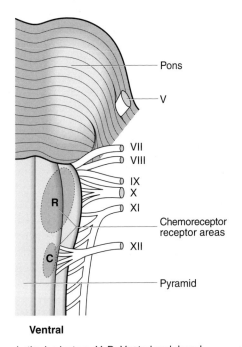

Figure 30.6 Respiratory neurones and chemoreceptor areas in the brainstem. V, D, Ventral and dorsal groups of respiratory neurones; R, C, rostral and caudal chemosensitive areas.

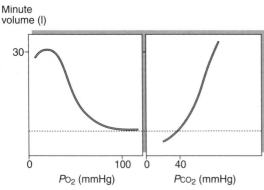

Minute volume (l)

P_{O_2} (mmHg) P_{CO_2} (mmHg)

Figure 30.7 Ventilatory response to hypoxia without hypercapnia (left panel) and to hypercapnia without hypoxia (right panel).

between Pa_{CO_2} increased by breathing a carbon dioxide-containing gas mixture and minute ventilation (Fig. 30.7). The slope of such a 'carbon dioxide response curve' is a measure of the sensitivity of the respiratory centre to carbon dioxide, and it is often depressed in chronic carbon dioxide retention.

The *peripheral chemoreceptors* are discrete bodies, a few millimetres in diameter, which lie close to the aorta and carotid arteries (aortic and carotid bodies, respectively). They have a very high rate of blood flow for their size — some 40 times relatively higher than that to the brain. This flow rate is important because it provides for the metabolic needs of the chemoreceptors themselves without having a significant effect on the partial pressures of the gases in the tissue fluid bathing the chemosensitive cells. While this high flow rate is maintained, the chemoreceptors are sensitive only to arterial blood chemistry. They do not respond to anaemia, which reduces the arterial blood oxygen content but does not change the Pa_{O_2}. Their blood flow is reduced by sympathetic vasoconstrictor nerves activated in hypotension. There is therefore effective stimulation of the chemoreceptors by severe life threatening haemorrhage.

Acid–base changes affect ventilation mainly through the peripheral chemoreceptors. H^+ does not readily cross the blood–brain barrier, so the effects of changes in blood pH on the central chemoreceptors are slower in timescale than those due to H^+ derived from carbon dioxide. In metabolic acidosis, for example in diabetic ketoacidosis, increased $[H^+]$ stimulates breathing, reducing Pa_{CO_2} and thus tending to reduce $[H^+]$. This results in the picture of metabolic acidosis with respiratory compensation.

PULMONARY CIRCULATION

The pulmonary arteries, distributing arteries and arterioles supply blood flow to the pulmonary capillaries in the alveolar walls at low pressure. A pulmonary artery flotation (Swan–Ganz) catheter may be used to monitor these pressures (Table 30.1). Perfusion pressure (mean arterial pressure – mean venous or atrial pressure) is thus only a fraction of that in the systemic circulation, while the rate of blood flow is essentially the same. Thus the resistance to blood flow offered by the pulmonary circulation is much less than that of the systemic circulation. In health, pulmonary vascular resistance does not regulate total pulmonary blood flow (cardiac output) but has marked influence on the regional distribution of blood flow within the lung and the matching of perfusion to ventilation. There are sympathetic noradrenergic vasoconstrictor nerves but their contribution is not clear. In the upright posture, the hydrostatic pressure due to gravity dilates the vessels at the lung bases, while allowing alveolar pressure to collapse the vessels at the apex during diastole. In the midzones, flow is maintained throughout the cardiac cycle but the resistance to flow is dependent on alveolar pressure, which is sufficient to collapse the pulmonary

Table 30.1 Average normal pressures above midthoracic level in recumbent subjects

	Pressure (mmHg)
Right ventricle	
systole	25
diastole	10
mean	15
Capillary wedge	8
Right atrium	
maximum	13
minimum	3
mean	7

capillaries at the point downstream where the intracapillary pressure falls below the external compression pressure from the alveoli. Oxygen lack has a marked vasoconstrictor effect on pulmonary arterioles. Physiologically the advantage of this response is that blood flow is directed away from those regions of the lungs that are underventilated and therefore hypoxic. When the whole lung is hypoxic, however, the increase in total resistance to flow leads to pulmonary hypertension.

The pulmonary vascular endothelium is an important tissue. It is the largest surface area of endothelium of any organ in the body. Receiving the entire cardiac output, it is well placed to process the blood. The pulmonary endothelium produces or modifies various vasoactive agents, including noradrenaline, adrenaline, endothelium derived relaxing factor, endothelin and prostaglandins. Nitric oxide is an endothelium derived relaxing factor that is a vasodilator in the pulmonary circulation, as it is in the systemic circulation. Nitric oxide modifies the reaction of vascular smooth muscle to oxygen and further research in this area may explain the opposite effects of oxygen on pulmonary and systemic arterioles.

CARRIAGE OF GASES BY BLOOD

Oxygen is carried by blood in two ways: in simple physical solution and in loose association with haemoglobin. The amount in simple solution is small — 3 ml l^{-1} blood. Although small in quantity, the dissolved oxygen is important because it represents the concentration that interfaces between the blood and the tissue fluid. The partial pressure of oxygen required in the gaseous phase to equilibrate with the blood is proportional to the concentration in physical solution (Henry's law). Thus partial pressures of the gases in solution are a useful guide to concentration gradients for diffusion. In a typical normal subject, Pa_{O_2} is 95 mmHg (12.7 kPa) and mixed venous partial pressure of oxygen ($P\bar{v}_{O_2}$) is 40 mmHg (5.3 kPa). The quantity of oxygen carried by haemoglobin is 1.34 ml g^{-1} Hg or 200 ml/l^{-1} blood for normal blood. Each haemo-

globin molecule is composed of a haem component, which is derived from porphyrin rings and contains iron in the ferrous state, and a globin component, which is protein (see also Ch. 28). There are four such units in each molecule. Most normal adult haemoglobin has two α globin chains and two β. Fetal haemoglobin contains two α and two γ chains. Disease states may affect the globin chains and upset the stability of the haemoglobin or its oxygen carriage. While the globin part of the molecule does not actually carry any oxygen, it does affect the affinity of the binding sites with the iron in the haem moiety. The affinity of the sites is also affected by the presence of other oxygen molecules and various substances found in the red blood cell. The relationship between P_{O_2} and oxygen content is a sigmoid curve (Fig. 30.8). The foot of the curve is caused by an increase in the affinity of haemoglobin for oxygen after some oxygen molecules have combined. The plateau of the dissociation curve is caused by the saturation of the binding sites with oxygen. It provides a reserve for oxygen carriage by blood when the P_{O_2} is reduced, e.g. at high elevations above sea level. The steep part of the curve is positioned for optimum loading and unloading of oxygen. This position is shifted to the right (Bohr shift) by high temperature, increased P_{CO_2}, increased hydrogen ion concentration and increased 2,3-diphosphoglycerate concentrations. Each of these occurs as a consequence of increased metabolism or in hypoxia. The shift of the dissociation curve to the right under these conditions favours the release of oxygen when most required. The steep part of the curve is located by the partial pressure of oxygen which produces 50% saturation of the haemoglobin (P_{50}). The P_{50} is 26 mmHg in arterial blood and shifts to 29 mmHg in mixed venous blood (Fig. 30.9).

Carbon dioxide is carried by blood in three ways: in simple physical solution, as carbamino compounds and as bicarbonate ions. The amount in solution is 10 times that of oxygen, even though the partial pressure of carbon dioxide is less than half that of oxygen in arterial blood — typically 40 mmHg (5.3 kPa); carbon dioxide is over 20 times as soluble as oxygen in blood. The

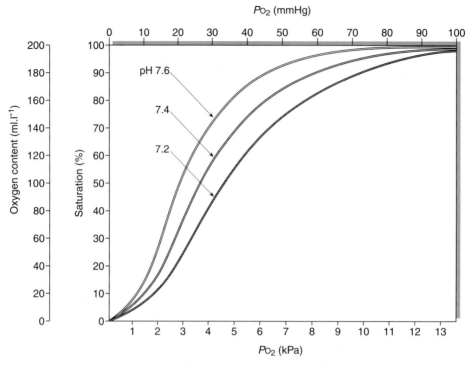

Figure 30.8 Oxygen–haemoglobin dissociation curve. Normal curve and displacement to right and left with pH change (see text for other factors causing displacement). Oxygen content values are for a haemoglobin level of 15 g dl^{-1}.

carbamino compounds are formed by reaction of carbon dioxide with amino groups in proteins. The globin moiety of haemoglobin is the most significant protein in blood to form carbamino compounds. The amount of carbon dioxide carried in this way is only one tenth of the total and its importance for the exchangeable carbon dioxide is reduced by the slowness of the reaction. Eight-tenths of the carbon dioxide in blood has reacted with water to produce hydrogen ions and bicarbonate ions. This reaction is slow in the plasma but fast inside red blood cells, where the reaction is catalysed by carbonic anhydrase. Bicarbonate ions produced in the red cells diffuse into the plasma in exchange for chloride ions to preserve electrical neutrality. The hydrogen ions are buffered by the haemoglobin. Reduced haemoglobin has a higher affinity for hydrogen ions than oxyhaemoglobin. This contributes to a shift of the relationship between carbon dioxide and P_{CO_2} to the left in venous blood (Haldane effect) (Fig. 30.9). The Haldane effect enables

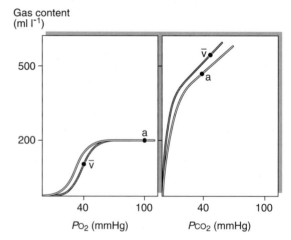

Figure 30.9 Blood gas content when equilibrated at various partial pressures of oxygen (left panel) and carbon dioxide (right panel). a, Arterial blood; v̄, mixed venous blood.

venous blood to carry more carbon dioxide with a lesser increase in partial pressure. Quantitatively this effect is greater than the Bohr shift of the oxygen dissociation curve. There is a much steeper relationship between content and partial pressure for carbon dioxide than for oxygen in blood. Thus an increase of only 6 mmHg (1 kPa) is required to add 45 ml carbon dioxide per litre of blood, 10 times lower than the 60 mmHg (8 kPa) required to extract 50 ml oxygen per litre of blood. A further difference between carbon dioxide and oxygen is that there is no saturation level for carbon dioxide carriage. This is because there is an effectively unlimited number of water molecules for reaction with carbon dioxide. This difference between the gases has an important significance for gas transfer.

GAS TRANSFER IN THE LUNG

The movement of gases between the alveoli and the blood is by diffusion down partial pressure gradients and by reaction with the blood. An essential requisite of normal gas transfer is that regional blood flow is matched to regional ventilation. This is described by the ventilation:perfusion ratio (V/Q), which is the rate of alveolar ventilation to a region divided by the rate of blood flow to that region.

The rate of diffusion of the gases is enhanced by the favourable dimensions of the alveolo-capillary membrane, which provides short diffusion distances over a large surface area. Carbon dioxide is the more freely diffusible because of its higher solubility than oxygen in the aqueous components of the membrane. The total partial pressure gradient is approximately equally divided between the gradient required to drive diffusion and the gradient required to drive the reaction with the blood. The partial pressure of oxygen in mixed venous blood is typically 40 mmHg (5.3 kPa) at rest, which is 60 mmHg lower than the partial pressure of oxygen in the alveoli (100 mmHg or 13.3 kPa). The corresponding pressures for carbon dioxide are 46 mmHg in mixed venous blood and 40 mmHg in the alveoli — a gradient one-tenth that for oxygen. This difference reflects the greater diffusibility of carbon dioxide. Both gases equilibrate fully with the blood perfusing normal alveoli. Despite its less favourable partial pressure gradient, carbon dioxide equilibrates more

quickly than oxygen. Oxygen equilibrates in about half a second, by which time the blood has traversed about three-quarters of the full distance across the pulmonary capillary bed at rest. There is thus some reserve diffusion time available.

Matching perfusion to ventilation is imperfect even in healthy lungs. Regions of the lung that are ventilated but not perfused with blood that is capable of gas exchange comprise the dead space of the respiratory tract. Air in the conducting airways accounts for the anatomical dead space, typically 150 ml. Physiological dead space includes alveoli in which no gas exchange can occur. In health, physiological dead space is not measurably larger than anatomical dead space. Ventilation of dead space is an unavoidable waste of muscular effort but does not directly impair the blood gases. Impairment of blood gases does result from perfusion of regions of the lung in which no effective gas exchanging ventilation occurs. The conducting airways are perfused by the bronchial circulation supplied by systemic arteries. The bronchial circulation provides nourishment to the conducting airway walls and does not take part in gas exchange. The venules therefore carry deoxygenated blood. Some of the venous drainage from the bronchial circulation joins with venules from the pulmonary capillaries (venous admixture) and reduces the partial pressure of oxygen of blood returning from the lungs to the left heart from the 100 mmHg after full equilibration with alveolar air to 95 mmHg. There is thus a normal alveolo-arterial partial pressure difference for oxygen. Shunts and mismatch of regional ventilation:perfusion ratio have similar effects on the arterial blood gases — the arterial oxygen is reduced but the arterial carbon dioxide is not increased and may even decrease. This is because of the plateau on the oxygen dissociation curve that is not on the carbon dioxide curve. Blood draining well ventilated regions of the lung can compensate for poorly ventilated regions for carbon dioxide but not for oxygen because the oxygen content cannot be increased above the normal plateau (except to a very limited extent by dissolved oxygen). The response to high oxygen inhalation can be used to distinguish between true shunts, in which there is no available gas exchange, and $\dot{V}/\dot{Q}$ mismatch, where there is a variation in $\dot{V}/\dot{Q}$ ratios but there is some gas exchange in even the poorly ventilated regions. Increased fractional concentration of inhaled oxygen (F_iO_2), by supplying a higher concentration of oxygen to underventilated alveoli, can compensate for the underventilation in $\dot{V}/\dot{Q}$ mismatch, but improvement in the presence of a true shunt is limited to the slightly increased dissolved oxygen in the ventilated regions of the lung.

The alveolar gas equation is often used to determine the alveolar partial pressure of oxygen as direct precise measurement is difficult. A simplified version of the alveolar gas equation is:

$$P_AO_2 = P_IO_2 - P_ACO_2/R,$$

where R is the respiratory exchange ratio ($\dot{V}CO_2/\dot{V}O_2$).

It is usual to assume full equilibration for carbon dioxide and therefore to take the arterial P_aCO_2 for alveolar P_ACO_2. If there is a steady state, this equation provides a rapid bedside check for venous admixture which causes an increase in the alveolar–arterial P_O_2 difference. Note that the alveolar P_{CO_2} divided by the difference between inhaled and alveolar P_{O_2} gives the respiratory exchange ratio, which is 0.8–0.9 on a typical diet. Calculated values outside this range in a steady state may suggest a laboratory error in blood gases. In unsteady states more complex versions of the equation are available.

THE RESPIRATORY SYSTEM UNDER STRESS

Exercise

During exercise there is an increase in minute volume proportionate to the rate of work, up to the anaerobic threshold when the steepness of the response increases. The maximal minute volume can be $150 \, l \, min^{-1}$ in a healthy adult. No mechanism has been described that links metabolic demand to ventilation and accounts for this magnitude of response. There are marked changes in muscle and mixed venous blood chemistry in exercise. The chemoreceptors are, however, on the arterial side of the circulation.

After passage through the lungs the arterial blood chemistry has been largely restored to resting levels. Above the anaerobic threshold the metabolic acidosis due to overspill of lactate is only partly corrected by the lungs, and the partial correction lowers the P_aCO_2 below resting levels. Muscle and joint movement, and possibly muscle chemical receptors, are stimulated during exercise and may reflexly stimulate ventilation. There is no simple relationship between stimulation of these receptors, V_{O_2} and the ventilatory response. An exercise centre in the brain that stimulates the respiratory centre in the medulla has been proposed. Stimulation of the cortex can simultaneously cause somatic movement and increase in ventilation. The increase in ventilation occurs even if movement is prevented by peripheral nerve block. An integrative theory that fits much of the experimental data is that the exercise centre provides the principal drive to ventilation during exercise, while the chemoreceptors maintain constancy of the arterial blood gas partial pressures, much as they do at rest. In severe exercise there is probably further ventilatory drive from chemoreceptor stimulation by a falling P_aO_2 and pH. Muscle and joint receptors may also provide some additional drive.

Oxygen uptake increases from $0.25 \, l \, min^{-1}$ at rest to $3 \, l \, min^{-1}$ or more in very fit subjects. Transfer of the increased volumes across the alveolocapillary membrane is achieved by the increased partial pressure gradients, by using the reserve transfer capacity and by increasing the transfer capacity itself. Dilatation of capillaries and opening of closed capillaries contribute to this enhancement.

Hypoxia

All steps in the delivery of oxygen to the tissues are subject to disease. This leads to four types of hypoxia: hypoxic hypoxia, where there is failure of the respiratory system to maintain a normal P_aO_2; anaemic hypoxia, where the reduction in the haemoglobin concentration of the blood leads to a fall in the oxygen content even though the P_aO_2 is normal; stagnant hypoxia, where the circulatory system fails to provide an adequate rate of blood flow; and histoxic hypoxia, where the cells themselves fail to utilise the oxygen normally.

Respiratory failure

When respiratory disease progresses until the lungs are no longer able to carry out their primary function to maintain constancy of the Pa_{O_2} with or without a rise in Pa_{CO_2}, then respiratory failure has developed. It has been suggested that, for subjects at sea level while resting, levels of Pa_{O_2} below 60 mmHg (8 kPa) and Pa_{CO_2} above 49 mmHg (6.5 kPa) should be used to define a level of loss of respiratory function sufficient to use the term respiratory failure. Since the exchange of oxygen is more difficult than the exchange of carbon dioxide both in their diffusibility and in their carriage by blood that renders oxygen susceptible to $\dot{V}/\dot{Q}$ mismatch, respiratory failure commonly leads to hypoxic hypoxia alone but never to hypercapnia alone. Hypoxic hypoxia without hypercapnia is referred to as type 1 respiratory failure. Hypoxic hypoxia with hypercapnia is referred to as type 2 respiratory failure. Hypoxic pulmonary vasoconstriction, so useful regionally to help preserve homogeneity of $\dot{V}/\dot{Q}$ ratios, leads to pulmonary hypertension when global. Eventually the right ventricle fails under the increased afterload (cor pulmonale).

Effects of high altitude

Hypoxia stimulates an increase in ventilation of the lungs through the peripheral chemoreceptors. This hyperventilation reduces the Pa_{CO_2}, which in turn acts as a brake on the ventilatory response to hypoxia and therefore limits the preservation of a normal P_{O_2}. After 1 or 2 days at high altitude, the cerebral tissue fluid alkalosis is corrected by ion pumping across the blood–brain barrier. This reduces the braking effect from the central chemoreceptors. After 1 or 2 weeks, renal compensatory excretion of bicarbonate ions and reduced excretion of hydrogen ions restores the pH of the blood, further reducing the braking effect from the hypocapnia and thus allowing an enhanced ventilatory response. The Pa_{O_2} therefore increases with acclimatisation to altitude. Other acclimatisation events include an increase in the haemoglobin concentration as a result of erythropoietin release from the kidney, improved oxygen release by a shift of the dissociation curve to the right as 2,3-diphosphoglycerate concentration in the red blood cells increases and improved tolerance by the tissues to low P_{O_2}.

Diving

There is a steep increase in the pressure with depth below sea level. The depth of submersion is very limited if surface pressure breathing through a snorkel tube is employed because the excess pressure that can be generated to inflate the lungs is limited to about 50 cmH$_2$O. At greater depths the pressure of gas inhaled usually corresponds to that of the surrounding water. The partial pressure of oxygen increases, while the difference between the inspired and alveolar levels is maintained. Similarly the alveolar partial pressure of carbon dioxide is maintained fairly steady or allowed to rise slightly. This means that the inspired/alveolar percentage concentration differences for both gases decrease markedly, while the actual volumes remain unchanged when measured under the usual standard conditions. During exercise under these conditions, alveolar ventilation tends to be impaired, leading to raised P_{CO_2} levels.

Toxicity from high P_{O_2} depends on the level and duration of exposure. A pressure six times that at sea level may be tolerated for several hours before toxic effects occur. Nitrogen has anaesthetic effects beyond 4 atmospheres and is substituted with helium at higher pressures. Another problem with nitrogen is decompression sickness, caused by the formation of gas bubbles as the dissolved nitrogen comes out of solution if decompression occurs too rapidly. Helium confers protection because of its lower solubility in body tissues.

A further problem with nitrogen is its high density at high pressure. This produces much higher resistance to airflow. The lower density of helium substantially reduces the work of breathing during diving.

Drowning

The larynx is initially closed and may prevent aspiration of water, but more usually there is aspiration after the break point of breath-holding. The break point depends on the central nervous system, lung volume, metabolic rate and initial PO_2 and PCO_2. Previous hyperventilation allows a lower PaO_2 to develop because the reduced $PaCO_2$ decreases the drive to the respiratory centre. The amount of available oxygen stored in the lung at total lung capacity is usually under 1 litre, which is unlikely to last more than 30 seconds in a drowning subject. Similarly, the quantity available in the blood is very limited. Stores of carbon dioxide are greater and the steeper dissociation curve for this gas means that the rate of rise of $PaCO_2$ is much lower than the rate of fall of PaO_2. The acute hypoxia will produce loss of consciousness probably at 30–45 mmHg. Residual cerebral damage and death depend on the duration and severity of the hypoxia and the temperature. Aspiration of water leads to further damage. If the drowning occurs in fresh water, most is absorbed into the circulation, where haemodilution, hyponatraemia and haemolysis may occur if large volumes have been inhaled, especially in children. Airway resistance is increased by reflex bronchospasm and compliance decreases because of dysfunction of pulmonary surfactant. Ventilation:perfusion mismatch and pulmonary oedema may develop.

Sea water, being hypertonic, is not initially absorbed but draws fluid from the circulation into the alveoli. This flooding of the alveoli leads to marked ventilation:perfusion imbalance. Theoretically the loss of fluid from the circulation will lead to haemoconcentration and hypernatraemia, but significant changes are unusual.

NON-RESPIRATORY FUNCTIONS OF THE LUNG

Voluntary control of movements of the chest and respiratory tract provides the apparatus for speaking, laughing, bracing the trunk for skeletal movements and carrying out the Valsalva manoevre.

The pulmonary circulation is the only circulation to receive the entire cardiac output. It is therefore well placed to process the blood rapidly. It performs important filtering functions, removing any foreign material larger than capillaries before the blood circulates to the brain.

There are many metabolic functions fulfilled by the lungs. The lung synthesises many chemicals, notably surfactant and proteolytic enzymes, which, if not opposed by α_1-antitrypsin as a result of a congenital deficiency, will destroy the elastin fibres in the lung, leading to severe emphysema. Cigarette smoking is especially liable to disrupt the delicate balance between the activity of proteolytic and antiproteolytic activities in lung tissue in α_1-antitrypsin deficiency. Some chemicals pass through the lung without being metabolised. They are therefore enabled to act as hormones with systemic effect. Others are actively metabolised, which enables the chemical's action to be terminated and remain local. Noradrenaline, being a neurotransmitter substance with local effects, is metabolised in the pulmonary circulation, reducing its spillover into the systemic blood; whereas adrenaline, being a hormone with generalised systemic effects, is not removed by metabolism as it passes through the pulmonary circulation. The lung endothelium provides angiotensin converting enzyme which catalyses the conversion of angiotensin I to angiotensin II. This metabolism produces a useful product. Angiotensin converting enzyme also contributes to the metabolism of bradykinin, which is inactivated by this enzyme. The lungs are an important site for the inactivation of prostaglandins, e.g. PGE_1 and $PGF_{2\alpha}$. Blood-borne histamine is not metabolised, even though the necessary enzymes are in the lung tissue. Unlike histamine, 5-hydroxytryptamine is taken up and metabolised by pulmonary capillary endothelial cells.

FURTHER READING

Bates D V 1989 Respiratory function in disease. Saunders, Philadelphia

Comroe J H 1974 Physiology of respiration, 2nd edn. Year Book Medical, Chicago

Cotes J E 1993 Lung function, assessment and application in medicine, 5th edn. Blackwell Scientific, Oxford

Jamison J P, McKinley R K 1993 Validity of peak expiratory flow variability for the diagnosis of asthma. Clinical Science 85: 367–371

Nunn J F 1993 Applied respiratory physiology, 4th edn. Butterworth, London

West J B 1990 Ventilation/blood flow and gas exchange, 5th edn. Blackwell Scientific, Oxford.

Widdicombe J, Davies A 1991 Respiratory physiology, 2nd edn. Edward Arnold, London.

31

Drugs acting on the respiratory system

G. G. Lavery

The respiratory system consists of a central control system (the respiratory centre in the brainstem), a bellows (the diaphragm and other muscles of respiration), a gas conduction system (the tracheobronchial tree) and a gas exchanger (the respiratory bronchioles, alveolar sacs and pulmonary circulation). Drugs may act on any one (or several) of these subunits.

GENERAL THERAPEUTIC MEASURES

Oxygen therapy

Oxygen is the most important 'drug' that can be applied to the respiratory system. The purpose of oxygen supplementation is to achieve satisfactory arterial oxygen saturation in patients who cannot achieve this while inspiring ambient air (21% oxygen). The factors involved in oxygen supplementation are: inspired concentration (F_iO_2), flow rate, delivery device (mask or nasal specula) and the presence or absence of 'hypoxic drive'.

The rate and depth of breathing are controlled by the respiratory centre situated in the medulla oblongata. Normally this structure is stimulated by the H^+ concentration in the cerebrospinal fluid. This is indirectly controlled by the arterial P_{CO_2}, as summarised by the following relationship:

$$CO_2 + H_2O \rightleftharpoons H_2CO_3 \rightleftharpoons H^+ + HCO_3^-.$$

Thus if P_{CO_2} increases, more H^+ ions are generated and stimulation of the respiratory centre is increased. A secondary stimulus to breathing is severe hypoxia (i.e. very low arterial P_{O_2}) but this is of less importance in most individuals. A small number of patients with significant chronic obstructive pulmonary disease (COPD) exhibit chronically increased arterial P_{CO_2}, to which the respiratory centre becomes insensitive. In this situation, only a relatively low arterial P_{O_2} maintains normal respiratory drive. In such patients, the use of high F_iO_2 may be unwise, as potentially it may cause significant increases in P_{O_2} and thus remove respiratory drive, leading to a life threatening rise in P_{CO_2} and profound respiratory acidosis.

The above situation is uncommon and yet fear of abolishing hypoxic drive has dictated that many patients suffering from COPD receive insufficient (24–35%) oxygen supplementation. Many patients remain grossly hypoxaemic to avoid a problem which in most does not exist! Unless there is current evidence to support the existence of hypoxic drive in an individual patient (or it has been documented during a previous clinical episode) all patients should receive the F_iO_2 that ensures an adequate arterial P_{O_2}.

High F_iO_2 (>60%) can only be delivered using a high flow of oxygen, 10–15 l min^{-1}, via a close fitting mask which has a reservoir bag. Masks without reservoir bags and masks which work on the venturi principle (to cause dilution of 100% oxygen with room air) are rarely capable of delivering more than 50% oxygen to the patient, even if the wall control is set at 100%. Nasal specula are similarly inefficient, are particularly ineffective in patients who are mouth breathing, and do not allow humidification of inspired gases.

Humidification and inhaled drugs

The upper respiratory tract normally warms and humidifies ambient air before it reaches the lower airways. In patients with respiratory insufficiency this mechanism fails because of increased respiratory rate and mouth breathing. Medical gases have zero humidity and are very cool at the point of delivery. Long term inhalation of cold, dry oxygen will result in (1) thick inspissated secretions that are impossible to expectorate, and (2) paralysis of the mucous membrane transport system which utilises a carpet of mucus and beating cilia to help remove foreign and unwanted material. Thus it is imperative that gases be humidified and warmed before being inspired by the patient. Oxygen can be humidified by being bubbled through a simple water bath. This becomes more efficient if a thermostatically controlled heated water bath is used.

The epithelium of the respiratory tract has a large surface area and an excellent blood supply. This allows administration of drugs by inhalation or (in the case of drugs used in cardiopulmonary resuscitation) direct injection into the airways. Inhaled drugs are administered either as nebulised particles or from pressurised inhalers. 8% of the dose is deposited in the large airways and only 4% reaches the alveoli. The remainder (almost 90%) reaches only the phaynx, larynx and trachea. Much is subsequently swallowed and then absorbed via the gastrointestinal tract, and a proportion is absorbed through the respiratory tract epithelium. Differences in the particle size of the aerosol makes only marginal differences to this pattern of drug distribution.

Antibiotic prescribing

Antibiotic therapy should be guided by the sensitivities of the pathogenic organisms cultured from the respiratory tract. Distinguishing normal flora and colonising organisms from pathogens may be difficult, as sputum samples are notoriously insensitive. In life threatening infections, bronchoalveolar lavage or bronchoscopic brush specimens may be used to make a diagnosis. A second influence on the choice of antibiotic(s) is tissue penetration. Some antibiotics penetrate well into lung tissue, while others do not (e.g. aminoglycosides).

Removal of secretions, eradication of infection and re-expansion of collapsed segments of lung can also be hastened by the use of aggressive regular chest physiotherapy. This may require multiple treatment sessions and should also be available at night when many patients tend to experience respiratory difficulties.

Mechanical ventilation

The 'ultimate' in respiratory support, mechanical ventilation, should be instituted in patients who have a potentially reversible underlying cause for their respiratory insufficiency. It should be initiated when clinical indicators suggest that overt respiratory failure is unavoidable and not when respiratory arrest has already occurred.

CONTROL OF AIRWAY CALIBRE

Respiratory function may be significantly influenced by changes in the calibre of the larger airways, as this influences gas flow to the more distal areas where gas exchange takes place. This affects tidal volume, respiratory rate and the ability to cough and expectorate. Reduction in airway calibre may also increase the work (and therefore oxygen cost) of breathing.

Like many other organ systems, airway calibre is controlled by two opposing systems, as summarised in Table 31.1. Increase in cyclic 3,5-adenosine monophosphate (cAMP) leads to sequestration of intracellular calcium, bronchial smooth muscle relaxation and bronchodilatation. Reduction in cAMP causes bronchoconstriction. In constrast, increase in cyclic 3,5-guanosine monophosphate (cGMP) causes bronchoconstriction, while reduction in intracellular cGMP is associated with bronchodilatation. The other factors involved are the presence or absence of mast cell-derived histamine and other mediators which may promote bronchoconstriction.

INFLUENCING AIRWAY CALIBRE: BRONCHODILATORS

Reversal of bronchoconstriction is a common

therapeutic goal for which there are three main classes of drug: β-adrenoreceptor agonists, methylxanthines and anticholinergic agents. These may be administered by a variety of routes and may be used in combination if required.

β_2-Adrenergic receptor agonists

Many sympathomimetics, e.g. adrenaline, isoprenaline, ephedrine and orciprenaline, have been used as bronchodilators; however, the cardiovascular effects (see below) mediated by these β_1-adrenoreceptor agonists limit their use. In addition, such agents are potentially dangerous when administered frequently during acute bronchoconstriction because high plasma levels, when associated with hypoxaemia, are known to sensitise the myocardium to their arrhythmogenic side-effects. Thus β_2-adrenergic receptor agonists are preferred as bronchodilatators because they are relatively selective for bronchial smooth muscle. It should be noted, however, that selectivity is only relative, and β_2-adrenergic receptor agonists may, at high dose, produce side-effects typical of β_1-agonists: tremor, anxiety, nausea and vomiting, headaches, dizziness, hypertension, tachycardia, tachyarrhythmias and the metabolic effects of adrenaline, i.e. hyperglycaemia, increased plasma insulin and increased release of free fatty acids.

Salbutamol

This is a selective β_2 agonist usually administered by inhalation from either a pressurised aerosol, which delivers $100\,\mu g$ per puff (usual dose 1–2 puffs), or a powder insufflator (metered dose $500\,\mu g$). The therapeutic effect lasts for 4–6 hours. In hospitalised patients who are unable to use a pressurised aerosol, 2.5 ml of a $1\,mg\,ml^{-1}$ aqueous solution may be administered as nebulised drug in a stream of oxygen using a special

Table 31.1 Factors controlling airway calibre

Bronchodilatation	Bronchoconstriction
Steroids	Mast cell degranulation
Sodium cromoglycate	Inflammatory mediators
Sympathetic stimulation	Parasympathetic stimulation
β_2 Agonists	Sympathetic blockade
Methylxanthines	
Anticholinergics	
Ca^{2+} antagonists?	

facemask (e.g. Hudson inhaler). The same solution can be nebulised and introduced into the inspiratory gas flow of patients receiving mechanical ventilation. The drug may also be administered parenterally, usually as an intravenous infusion at $3–20\ \mu g\ min^{-1}$, the dose being titrated to therapeutic effect. Side-effects are rare with the pressurised aerosol or powder insufflator because they deliver a small dose near to the site of action with little systemic absorption. The use of the nebulised solution (larger dose) or parenteral administration increases the frequency and severity of side-effects. Metabolism involves hepatic conjugation and the metabolites are excreted in the urine and faeces. Unchanged drug is also excreted in the urine.

Other actions of salbutamol include the inhibition of uterine contractions and it may be administered by intravenous infusion in an attempt to prevent premature labour. Recent work also suggests that administration of salbutamol may prevent tissue damage mediated by oxygen free radicals and that this is a function of its activity at β_2-adrenergic receptors.

Terbutaline is the other frequently used agent in this group; it is very similar to salbutamol and is supplied as a pressurized aerosol ($250\ \mu g$/puff) Some patients who experience sympathomimetic side-effects to salbutamol tolerate terbutaline better (and vice versa). Other agents include *fenoterol, reproterol* and *rimiterol*, which are available as aerosols. Rimiterol is the shortest acting of the group, having an effective duration of action of only 2 hours.

Methylxanthines

This group of substances are plant alkaloids and include theophylline and its derivates, theobromine and caffeine. Theophylline is the parent compound for a group of bronchodilators. Aminophylline (80% theophylline) is the ethylene diamine salt, which is more water soluble than theophylline. Other derivatives, e.g. diprophylline and proxyphylline, are of little therapeutic value, being either poorly absorbed or too short acting.

Caffeine

Theophylline

Theobromine

The methylxanthines have effects on several organ systems (see below); many of these effects mimic those of β agonists. The proposed mode of action is as follows:

- phosphodiesterase inhibition, which increases the levels of cAMP by reducing breakdown
- potentiation of the effect of other drugs that stimulate cAMP production, e.g. sympathomimetics
- release of calcium from sarcoplasmic reticulum, causing an increase in cytoplasmic calcium and an augmentation of muscular contraction
- inhibition at adenosine receptors, which modulate the effects of cAMP and influence calcium ion influx.

Therapeutic effects

Respiratory system. Theophylline and aminophylline are administered primarily for their bronchodilating effects. Respiration may also be helped by stimulation of respiratory drive and an increase in diaphragmatic and intercostal muscle strength. Bronchodilatation reduces the work of breathing and therefore the 'oxygen cost of breathing', which, in severe respiratory distress, may result in 20% of cardiac output being diverted to the respiratory muscles. Mucociliary clearance may be improved by methylxanthines.

Central nervous system. Central stimulation occurs, increasing minute ventilation. With increasing dose, this leads to restlessness, agitation, insomnia, tremor, nausea, and grand mal seizures. These effects may occur within or only slightly above accepted therapeutic concentrations.

Cardiovascular system. There is both a positive chronotropic and inotropic effect, vaso- and venodilatation, causing reduced systemic and pulmonary vascular resistance, venous pooling and reduced left ventricular end-diastolic pressure. These haemodynamic effects benefit patients in left ventricular failure and/or with pulmonary oedema. With increasing dose, tachycardia and tachyarrhythmias become frequent.

Other systems. Increased urinary output is common after administration of methylxanthines. This is partly due to the increase in cardiac output but also reflects a direct effect on renal tubular function. A more sinister effect is an increase in the secretion of both gastric acid and pepsin.

Clinical use

The role of theophylline and its derivates have been questioned in asthma and COPD and they do have significant side-effects. Nevertheless they are commonly employed, especially after failure to respond to nebuliser treatment. The intravenous loading dose of aminophylline is 5–6 mg kg^{-1} over 10–20 minutes. Toxic effects will be precipitated by rapid administration. Therapy may continue with an infusion of 0.5 mg kg^{-1} h^{-1}. Because of altered pharmacokinetics this infusion rate must be modified in smokers ($\times 1.6$), those receiving drugs such as cimetidine, erythromycin ($\times 0.5$) and severe cirrhosis or congestive cardiac failure ($\times 0.3$). The target plasma level is 10–20 mg l^{-1}. Plasma levels must be monitored if undertreatment or toxicity are to be avoided. Aminophylline must never be administered intramuscularly or subcutaneously because it has a pH of 9.4.

Theophylline is rapidly and consistently absorbed after oral administration but rapid elimination causes unpredictable plasma levels. Unfortunately absorption of rectal or sustained release formulations is even less predictable.

Theophylline is 40% protein bound and 90% is metabolised in the liver by the cytochrome P-450 system. The remainder is excreted unchanged in the urine. The half-life is 7–9 hours in non-smokers, 4–5 hours in smokers, 3–6 hours in children and 20–30 hours in those with liver cirrhosis.

Ingestion of theophylline in overdose is relatively common. Signs and symptoms are as described above, to which should be added hypokalaemia. This is severe and difficult to correct and, in these cases, many deaths are due to cardiac arrhythmias or arrest secondary to gross hypokalaemia. Management (see Ch. 51) involves urgent potassium replacement, symptomatic treatment and possibly haemoperfusion.

Anticholinergic drugs

Within the bronchial tree, parasympathetic stimulation increases guanylate cyclase activity and thus cGMP levels, which causes bronchoconstriction. Thus any agent that reduces cholinergic stimulation may act as a bronchodilator. In the seventeenth century anticholinergics (e.g. inhaled smoke from *stramonium* leaves) were known to alleviate asthma-like symptoms. Ipratropium bromide is the only anticholinergic bronchodilator in clinical use today.

Ipratropium bromide

Ipratropium produces modest bronchodilatation by competitively inhibiting cholinergic receptors on bronchial smooth muscle and (perhaps) by stabilising mast cells. It has a synergy with the more potent β_2 agonists and is used in both acute asthma and COPD. An additional desirable property is the lack of atropine-like effects. Despite being an anticholinergic, ipratropium preserves mucociliary clearance. Ipratropium is administered as a pressurised aerosol (1–2 puffs, 3–4 times a day, 20 µg per puff), as aerocaps — a gelatin capsule containing 40 µg of ipratropium bromide powder for inhalation, or as a liquid (250 µg ml^{-1}), which may be nebulised. Maximal effect occurs approximately 2 hours after aerosol inhalation and lasts 4–6 hours. Systemic absorption is minimal.

MEMBRANE STABILISERS

Disodium cromoglycate

This is a non-steroid membrane stabiliser which has a prophylactic role in conditions triggered by allergic and/or atopic mechanisms. It is used in bronchial asthma and also allergic rhinitis and conjunctivitis. In asthma it reduces the frequency of acute bronchoconstriction by stabilising mast cells. This is probably achieved by closing calcium channels and thus preventing entry of calcium ions, which is the trigger to mast cell degranulation. Since it has a preventative action only, disodium cromoglycate must be taken regularly (normally 3–4 times per 24 hours), even when the patient is asymptomatic.

For use in the respiratory tract it is supplied as an inhaled powder (Spincaps), as a pressurised aerosol (approximately 50 µg per puff) and as a solution for nebulisation (20 mg in 2 ml). Duration of effect is 3–6 hours. Occasionally pharyngeal discomfort may be produced but otherwise it is free of worrying side-effects and is safe if taken in overdose.

STEROIDS

Steroid therapy is indicated in acute severe asthma and in some patients with COPD. In asthma, short-term intravenous steroid therapy significantly reduces the frequency of hospital admission rates. The effect is due to the glucocorticoid action of steroids and several modes of action have been suggested:

- inhibition of inflammatory response
- inhibition of arachidonic acid metabolites (e.g. bronchoconstrictor prostaglandins)
- inhibition of platelet activating factor (which has bronchoconstrictor and proinflammatory actions)
- prevention of mast cell degranulation (membrane stabilisation)
- synergism with catecholamines (endogenous or therapeutically administered).

The lipid soluble steroid molecules enter cells and bind to intracellular receptors. As a result specific genes are activated, leading to changes in ribonucleic acid (RNA) production and protein synthesis. The synergism with β agonists occurs due to increased availability of cell membrane β-agonist receptor sites, increased binding affinity of such sites and increased adenyl cyclase activation. Peak response to steroids is 6–12 hours after intravenous administration and therefore the decision regarding their use should be made as early as possible.

Steroid therapy may be administered by inhalation or intravenously. The former route is unreliable in acute attacks and is therefore used only for 'prophylaxis' in order to reduce the frequency of acute attacks and/or reduce the dose of other bronchodilators (see below). Dosage for intravenous steroids is controversial. Hydrocortisone 0.5 mg kg^{-1} h^{-1} or 4 mg kg^{-1} i.v. every 4 hours is commonly advocated, although methylprednisolone 1 g 6-hourly has been suggested. The duration of therapy is usually several days, although at any appropriate point the intravenous regimen may be replaced by oral prednisolone in a reducing dose starting with 40–60 mg day^{-1}.

Improvement after steroid therapy does not occur in all patients with COPD and, in those who do respond, the benefit is less convincing than in acute asthma. Nevertheless in COPD with persistent wheeze unresponsive to bronchodilator therapy, steroids can be of benefit. The dose is similar to that employed in acute asthma.

Beclomethasone propionate

This steroid is administered by pressurised aerosol (200 µg per puff) given 3–4 times a day as a prophylactic measure. It is usually prescribed in association with an inhaled selective β$_2$ agonist. There is little systemic absorption and few side-effects if given in normal doses.

RESPIRATORY STIMULANTS

Respiratory stimulants are agents that have a direct effect on respiratory drive (analeptics). Many analeptics are of no clinical relevance today — for example, strychnine, which blocks central inhibitory pathways. There is no common structural pattern to this group of drugs — for example, acetazolamide and methylprogesterone are structurally unalike, yet both increase respiratory drive. In addition, respiratory stimulation may be achieved by other agents which antagonise the depressant effect of previously administered drugs on the respiratory centre.

Analeptics

Clinically useful agents in this group include doxapram and nikethamide, which act by stimulating central excitatory pathways. Although useful in a number of clinical situations, it must be stressed that ventilatory support is often the best (and safest) treatment for respiratory depression. Analeptics may be used to reverse opioid induced respiratory depression without diminishing the analgesic effect. They may also help avoid or postpone respiratory failure in patients with an acute exacerbation of long standing COPD. It should be noted, however, that many of these patients do not have a problem with respiratory drive but with the ability to breathe effectively. In addition, if analeptics are used, the underlying cause for the acute decompensation must be addressed, as there is an upper limit to the total dose of analeptic that can be administered. Other respiratory effects include increased cough and sneezing.

As might be expected from agents causing central excitation, the side-effects are restlessness, agitation, confusion and headache. These symptoms may be difficult to identify in a patient who is already distressed and in respiratory difficulty. If toxicity increases, grand mal epileptiform attacks may occur. Increased heart rate and arrhythmias are common (these are frequently associated with hypoxaemia and hypercarbia in any case). Hypotension may occur, although doxapram alone tends to cause an increase in arterial pressure.

Doxapram

This is the most frequently used analeptic because it stimulates the respiratory centre preferentially and has relatively less effect on cortical and spinal sites. This gives doxapram, a pyrrolidinone compound, a higher therapeutic index than the other agents in the group. It is unusual in that it also acts on carotid sinus chemoreceptors. Although not standard practice, its use has been advocated (1) to stimulate deep breathing in the perioperative period and thus reduce the incidence of chest infection, (2) to cause hyperventilation in order to facilitate blind nasal intubation, and (3) to reduce the incidence of apnoeic attacks in premature infants.

In its main role, doxapram should be administered as a slow bolus of 0.5 mg kg^{-1}, which will normally cause respiratory stimulation for 5–10 minutes. An infusion of 1–2 mg min^{-1} may be used to provide further respiratory stimulation, although this is not an answer to chronic hypoventilation.

Nikethamide

Nikethamide and its derivative, *ethamivan*, are acid amines that stimulate the respiratory centre. There is relatively greater excitation of the cerebral cortex than with doxapram and so the therapeutic index is decreased. There is little evidence that either agent has any action on carotid chemoreceptors. Nikethamide is usually administered intravenously. A dose of 0.5–1.0 g will be effective for up to 30 minutes. It is metabolised to nicotinamide and, after methylation, is excreted in the urine. The equivalent dose of ethamivan is 100 mg.

Naloxone

Naloxone, a derivative of oxymorphone, is an opioid antagonist which is devoid of agonist activity (see Ch. 17). It is used clinically to reverse respiratory depression, analgesia, sedation and the other effects of opiates and opioid drugs. It does not reliably antagonise the effects of buprenorphine and has no effect on respiratory depression due to other drugs or conditions.

Naloxone hydrochloride is available for clinical use as a colourless solution supplied in 1 ml ampoules containing 0.4 mg (400 µg), or in 2 ml ampoules containing 0.02 mg (20 µg) ml^{-1}, i.e. a 20-fold reduction in concentration. The latter formulation is for use in neonates and infants. Naloxone may be administered intramuscularly as well as intravenously, acts within 2 minutes and has a clinical effect for 30–60 minutes, depending on route of administration, dose and the duration of action of the opioid being antagonised. A continuous infusion may be indicated if the opioid agonist effect is expected to outlast the duration of effect of a single dose of naloxone, e.g. antagonism of dextropropoxyphene, dihydrocodeine or codeine.

Dosage in adults is 400–2000 µg intravenously, which may be repeated. If there is no apparent improvement after large doses, then the existence of opioid induced respiratory depression (or other opioid effects) should be questioned. Naloxone can be diluted in dextrose or saline for continuous infusion. The concentration and rate of infusion will be dictated by the clinical situation. Such dilute solutions are stable for up to 12 hours. In children, 10 µg kg^{-1} is the usual initial intravenous dose, although occasionally a total dose of 100 µg kg^{-1} may be required. In neonates, 10 µg kg^{-1} should be administered intravenously, intramuscularly or subcutaneously and repeated as indicated.

Flumazenil

This is an imidazobenzodiazepine which has no effect on the central nervous system but binds competitively to benzodiazepine receptors. It is effective for pure agonists, e.g. diazepam, mida-zolam, partial agonists, inverse agonists and partial inverse antagonists. Administration results in reversal of benzodiazepine effects — reduction in anaesthesia or sedation, including reversal of drug induced respiratory depression.

It is a water soluble compound available in 5 ml ampoules containing 100 µg ml^{-1}. Clinically it is administered intravenously as a 0.2 mg bolus followed by 0.1 mg increments until the appropriate reversal of sedation and other effects. The duration, after a single intravenous bolus, is variable (15–140 minutes) and dose dependent. Maximum dose is 1 mg, although larger amounts may be employed with monitoring and observation in the intensive care unit. Due to the relatively short and unpredictable duration of effect, resedation is a major danger, particularly when long acting benzodiazepines have been used. In such circumstances flumazenil may be diluted in dextrose or saline and administered as a continuous infusion at a rate of 0.1–1.0 mg h^{-1}.

Flumazenil is metabolised almost totally by the liver, where it undergoes carboxylation to an inactive form. Dosage must therefore be reduced in liver dysfunction. No adjustment is necessary in renal failure. Since flumazenil has no significant effects in the body (except its competitive displacement of benzodiazepine molecules), it appears to be safe even when massive doses (100 mg as an intravenous bolus) have been administered. Use in patients suffering from epilepsy is not recommended because the rapid withdrawal of benzodiazepine effect may precipitate seizures.

SURFACTANT

This is a lipid–protein complex that lines the alveolar surface of the lung and is produced by type II alveolar cells in normal mature lungs. It reduces surface tension at fluid–gas interfaces. Loss of this effect has two results: (1) an increase in surface forces and therefore a decrease in lung compliance, and (2) an increase in the pressure gradient between pulmonary capillaries and the pulmonary interstitial space, thus encouraging interstitial oedema even at relatively normal microvascular pressures. Loss of surfactant activity can occur as a consequence either of lack of production of normal surfactant or of inactivation of surfactant by the presence of plasma proteins or other substances (e.g. sea water) in the alveolar spaces. Clinically such conditions occur in neonatal respiratory distress syndrome (RDS), due to lack of surfactant production in the immature lungs of premature infants, or in adult respiratory distress syndrome (ARDS), when both lack of production and inactivation are thought to occur.

The main constituent of natural surfactant is dipalmitoylphosphatidylcholine (DPPC). The protein components are responsible for the spreading effect of surfactant on the alveolar surface. The use of surfactant as a therapeutic agent is well established in RDS and has been shown to significantly reduce morbidity and mortality. To date porcine, bovine and synthetic surfactant has been used in neonates. The normal procedure is to instil liquid surfactant into the large airways and distribute the drug by rotating, tilting and positioning the neonate.

Beractant

This is a bovine lung extract, suspended in 0.9% saline, composed of lipids, phospholipids, fatty acids and proteins enriched with DPPC, palmitic acid and tripalmitin. Each millilitre of this off-white liquid contains 25 mg of phospholipid. It is indicated for the treatment of RDS in premature neonates weighing more than 700 g and receiving mechanical ventilation. Warmed beractant (Survanta) should be introduced by intratracheal instillation just above the tracheal bifurcation. To optimise distribution of the agent, the dose is divided into 2–4 aliquots, each administered with the neonate in a different position. After each aliquot, the neonate should be ventilated for 30–60 seconds before changing position. The drug is usually given within 8 hours of birth to neonates who exhibit signs of serious RDS and may be repeated up to 6-hourly for up to four doses.

In ARDS, however, surfactant dysfunction is a secondary problem and there are many practical problems in the administration of exogenous surfactant in adults not found in neonates. Its use in ARDS is still only on a trial basis and there is no convincing evidence of benefit at present. Again, both animal and synthetic forms of surfactant have been used.

Exosurf

In 1992–1993 a large multicentre trial evaluated a synthetic surfactant, Exosurf, in ARDS. Exosurf is a mixture of DPPC, hexadecanol and tyloxapol. In ARDS, positioning the patients to ensure even and widespread distribution of the agent is not feasible. Thus Exosurf (100 mg) was administered into the inspiratory limb of the ventilator circuit, from a specially heated and pressurised nebuliser, as an aerosol. However, the trial was terminated prematurely when it became clear that, at best, the Exosurf treated group had the same 30 day mortality as the control group.

PULMONARY VASODILATORS

The use of pulmonary vasodilators has been advocated in the treatment of severe acute lung injury associated with ARDS. ARDS is typified by arterial hypoxaemia, bilateral patchy opacification on chest radiograph, pulmonary hypertension with increased pulmonary vascular resistance and decreased lung compliance. There are several mechanisms behind the development of pulmonary hypertension with increased pulmonary vascular resistance, including pulmonary hypoxic vasoconstriction, aggregation of white cells and platelets in the pulmonary capillary bed, release of vasoactive substances by leucocytes, and cytokine release. The problem may be exacerbated by therapeutic manoeuvres such as mechanical ventilation with high levels of positive end-expiratory pressure, which increase mean intrathoracic pressure and thus contribute to increased pulmonary vascular resistance. The use of either intravenous or inhaled agents that vasodilate the pulmonary vascular bed may reduce pulmonary vascular resistance, pulmonary hypertension and the resultant right ventricular dilatation or failure.

Intravenous prostaglandins

The problem with using a systemic vasodilator to dilate the pulmonary circulation is that it will exacerbate the hypotension which is usual in patients with ARDS. Since prostaglandins are metabolised in the lungs, it was reasoned that intravenous infusion of a suitable vasodilator prostaglandin into the central veins would produce vasodilatation in the pulmonary vascular bed. Subsequent breakdown within the pulmonary circulation might be expected to prevent systemic spillover and the resultant arterial vasodilatation and hypotension. Both prostaglandin E_1 and prostacyclin were evaluated in this role and, although effective, it was found that the doses required to reduce pulmonary vascular resistance were frequently so great that pulmonary metabolism could not prevent spillover of the agents into the arterial circulation. In addition, the entire pulmonary circulation is influenced by such intravenous agents, including those vessels supplying non-ventilated areas of lung tissue. This results in an increased right-to-left shunt and a deterioration of arterial oxygen saturation.

Nitric oxide

Nitric oxide (NO) is a gas which is generated in minute amounts within the body, where it acts as a second messenger to activate guanylate cyclase, increase cGMP levels and thus produce relaxation of vascular smooth muscle (it was also termed endothelial derived relaxing factor). It also decreases platelet adhesion and aggregation. Abnormalities of nitric oxide production are thought to occur in many clinical conditions — systemic sepsis, atherosclerosis, essential hypertension and diabetic angiopathy.

Inhaled nitric oxide results in pulmonary vasodilatation, or reversal of induced pulmonary vasoconstriction, but only in the ventilated areas of the lung. This limit to the scope of vasodilatation prevents an increase in the right-to-left shunt through non-functional areas of lung and a resultant worsening in arterial hypoxaemia.

NO is supplied in a concentration of 1000 p.p.m. in nitrogen and, when used clinically, is diluted in an air–oxygen mixture to produce concentrations of 20–80 p.p.m. delivered via a mechanical ventilator. It has an effective half-life within the body of less than 0.5 seconds before it combines with haemoglobin to form NOHb (nitrosyl-haemoglobin) and also methaemoglobin and nitrate. NOHb subsequently generates nitrites and nitrates which are excreted over the subsequent 48 hours. The former is converted to nitrogen gas, while the latter is excreted in urine or converted to ammonia (NH_3), reabsorbed and converted to urea. Thus the vasodilating effect of nitric oxide is confined to the lung, with no spillover into the systemic circulation.

Inhaled nitric oxide (80 p.p.m.) causes a minor degree of bronchodilatation and an increase in bronchial mucosal blood flow. Other effects are:

- prolonged bleeding time
- mutagenicity — has been reported in rat primary lung cells
- rebound pulmonary vasoconstriction on cessation of treatment.

The place of nitric oxide in the treatment of ARDS is still uncertain and there is an ongoing multicentre trial. As a result of its targeted effect on the lung, it would appear to have several advantages over intravenous vasodilators.

FURTHER READING

Barnes P J 1991 Nerves, neurotransmitters and asthma. In: Seymour C A, Summerfield J A (eds) Horizons in medicine, vol 3, pp 14–29. Transmedica Europe,

Berggren P, Lachmann B, Cursedt T, Grossman G, Robertson B 1986 Gas exchange and lung morphology after surfactant replacement in experimental adult respiratory distress syndrome induced by repeated lung lavage. Acta

Anaesthesiologica Scandinavica 30: 321–328

Fredholm B B 1985 On the mechanism of action of theophylline and caffeine. Acta Medica Scandinavica 217: 149–153

Goldstein G, Luce J M 1990 Pharmacologic treatment of the adult respiratory distress syndrome. Clinics in Chest Medicine 11(4): 773–788

King E, Garner 1984 Respiratory failure in the critically ill. In: Sibbald W J (ed) Synopsis of critical care, 2nd edn, pp 51–66. Williams & Wilkins, Baltimore

Lachmann B 1987 The role of pulmonary surfactant in the pathogenesis and therapy of ARDS. In: Vincent J L (ed) Update on intensive care and emergency medicine, vol 3, pp 123–134. Springer, Berlin

Moncada S et al 1991 Nitric oxide: physiology, pathophysiology and pharmacology. Pharmacological Reviews 43: 109–142

Newman S P, Killip M, Pavia D, Moren F, Clarke S W 1983 Do particle size and airway obstruction affect the deposition of pressurized inhalation aerosols? Thorax 38: 233

Popa V 1986 Beta-adrenergic drugs. Clinics in Chest Medicine 7(3): 313–330

Rossaint R, Falke K J, Lopez F, Slama K, Pison U, Zapol W M 1993 Inhaled nitric oxide for the adult respiratory distress syndrome. New England Journal of Medicine 328: 399–405

Shannon D C, Bunnell J B 1976 Dipalmitoyl lecithin in RDS. Pediatric Research 10: 467

Silver M R, Bone R C 1988 Acute respiratory failure and chronic obstructive pulmonary disease. In: Ledingham I McA (ed) Recent advances in critical care medicine (3), pp 31–52. Churchill Livingstone, Edinburgh

Tuxen D V, Oh T E 1990 Acute severe asthma. In: Oh T E (ed) Intensive care manual, 3rd edn, pp 192–201. Butterworth, London

Wong S C, Ward J W 1977 Analeptics. Pharmacology and Therapeutics 3: 123–165

Ziment I 1986 Steroids. Clinics in Chest Medicine 7(3): 341–354

32

Oxygen flux and delivery

J. P. H. Fee
W. F. M. Wallace

Local or general lack of oxygen (hypoxia) is probably the most common cause of acute and chronic morbidity and death. In the resuscitation of the seriously injured, during anaesthesia and intensive care, hypoxia is a central challenge capable of causing not only avoidable death but also severe and tragic permanent brain damage. In this chapter we describe the delivery of oxygen to the metabolising tissues (oxygen flux) at rest and during exercise, and how this is frustrated by the major classical varieties of hypoxia: stagnant, anaemic and hypoxic. (The fourth variety sometimes quoted — histotoxic — is a failure to utilise the oxygen provided, rather than a failure of oxygen flux.)

OXYGEN FLUX AT REST

This depends on three body systems: firstly, the respiratory system; secondly the haemopoietic system; and, thirdly, the circulatory system. The role of the respiratory system is to saturate the blood with oxygen in the lungs; the role of the haemopoietic system is to provide an adequate circulating level of haemoglobin; and the role of the circulatory system is to deliver the arterial blood in appropriate amounts throughout the body. Failure of the first system leads to hypoxic hypoxia; failure of the second leads to anaemic hypoxia, and failure of the third at a local or general level leads to stagnant hypoxia. The role of these various systems can be quantified in terms of total available oxygen.

Total available oxygen

This refers to the total amount of oxygen that leaves the left ventricle in the arterial blood each minute. It is thus available for uptake by the body tissues. It can be calculated from the equation:

Total available oxygen = [cardiac output].[haemoglobin concentration × ml O_2 g^{-1} Hb].[saturation] + dissolved oxygen.

Dissolved oxygen is proportional to the partial pressure of oxygen and is usually very small in relation to the combined oxygen and will be ignored at this stage. In an average person total available oxygen then equals:

$[5 \, l \, min^{-1}].[150 \times 1.34 = 200 \, ml \, O_2 \, l^{-1}].[100/100]$
$= 1 \, l \, O_2 \, min^{-1}.$

Thus in the average person around 1 litre of oxygen is available to the tissues each minute under resting conditions. It may at first seem strange that the resting oxygen consumption of about 250 ml min^{-1} is only a quarter of that available. This can be explained by the fact that about half the resting circulation goes to 'high oxygen extractors', tissues that extract a high proportion of the available oxygen, and the other half goes to 'low oxygen extractors', tissues that extract little of the available oxygen. The high extractors include the brain, the heart and the liver. These tissues extract around two-thirds to three-quarters of the available oxygen, and the venous blood draining them is only about 40% saturated and hence a dark bluish colour — this is true of the blood in the jugular vein, the coronary sinus and the hepatic veins.

The low extractors include mainly the skin and the kidneys. Under average circumstances there is a considerable skin blood flow, which is determined by the temperature regulating needs of the body and is greatly in excess of metabolic needs. Thus blood returns to the heart still highly saturated, e.g. 80–90%. The kidneys usually receive a quarter of the entire resting cardiac output. Although they are active metabolically (ionic pumps consume considerable amounts of oxygen), the blood flow is vastly in excess of the requirements of these small organs (under 0.5%

body weight) and so the blood in the renal veins is bright red and still almost fully saturated. Thus a mixture of all the venous blood returning to the heart (mixed venous blood is best sampled from the pulmonary artery) is around 70% saturated. As will be seen, this situation changes markedly during strenuous exercise.

OXYGEN FLUX AND DELIVERY DURING EXERCISE

Exercise constitutes the greatest challenge to oxygen delivery, and is most accurately assessed in terms of oxygen consumption. In an athlete, this assessment of cardiorespiratory fitness is achieved by measuring the greatest oxygen uptake that can be sustained. Some relevant figures are given in Table 32.1. It will be seen that exercise intensity is described in METs, where 1 MET is the resting metabolic rate (somewhat higher than the basal metabolic rate, which is recorded after a prolonged period of complete rest, ideally overnight, with a similar period of starvation, in a thermoneutral environment and with the subject in a relaxed state). For convenience 1 MET is taken to correspond to an oxygen consumption of 3.5 ml kg^{-1} min^{-1} (American College of Sports Medicine). For a 70 kg man this would be 245 ml min^{-1}.

The maximal METs achieved by an individual varies with age, and particularly with cardiorespiratory fitness. A minimum of around 2 METs is needed to walk at a minimal pace. Moderately brisk walking on the level would constitute

Table 32.1 Examples of oxygen consumption at rest and during three levels of exercise. Exercise at 10 METs (10 times the resting oxygen consumption) would indicate a good level of fitness in a middle aged man; 15 METs would be a high level of fitness in a young person and 20 METs would represent a good competition standard in an aerobic activity

Oxygen consumption		Total available oxygen (ml min^{-1})	Extraction (%)
METs	ml min^{-1}		
1	250	1000	25
10	2500	4000	67.5
15	3750	5000	75
20	5000	6000	83.3

about 5 METs, and 10 METs would be the maximum for many adults. Younger people, and particularly fit athletic individuals, can reach 15 METs, and world champions in sports associated with very high levels of energy expenditure, such as cross-country skiing, would reach about 20 METs.

Assuming a haemoglobin level of 150 g l^{-1} (15 g dl^{-1}), it is possible to work out approximately the cardiovascular performance necessary for the above achievements (Table 32.2). The examples given would apply to 20-year-old individuals with a maximal heart rate (fit or unfit) of 220 − age (years) = 200, and a body mass requiring a cardiac output of about 5 l min^{-1} at rest. Note that the fitter the individual, the lower the resting heart rate and the higher the stroke volume at rest and exercise. Combining Tables 32.1 and 32.2, it can be seen that at increasing levels of activity with an increasing proportion of the cardiac output going to exercising muscle, the overall extraction percentage increases. The very fit individual has a relatively large and powerful heart and so is capable of high stroke volumes at rest (leading to increased vagal tone and a lower resting heart rate) and even higher stroke volumes during exercise.

For the vast majority of people there is adequate ventilatory reserve, so maximal cardiac output determines maximal exercising ability. Exceptionally fit individuals may have a circulation that can return deoxygenated blood to the lungs at a rate which exceeds the lung's ability to maintain a normal alveolar oxygen level, and so a degree of desaturation would result. As will be seen, this occurs regularly at high altitudes.

ASSESSMENT OF FITNESS FROM OXYGEN FLUX AND UPTAKE

The gold standard or reference method of assessing physical fitness from an overall cardiorespiratory point of view is to measure maximal oxygen uptake. By definition, this is the maximal amount of oxygen that an individual can take up and use per minute. It may be expressed in litres per minute, or, to allow for body size, in millilitres per kilogram per minute. In order to assess maximal oxygen uptake the subject exercises at increasing rates until the oxygen uptake has levelled off.

In practice the subject will usually start at a level of exercise appropriate to the estimated level of fitness. Thus an athlete may start by jogging on a treadmill at 10 km h^{-1}, while an older or unfit person would walk initially at, say, $2-3 \text{ km h}^{-1}$. The effort is increased, usually every 3 minutes, by increasing the speed, and in some cases slope, of the treadmill, until the subject cannot increase or maintain the effort. Apart from the definitive levelling off of oxygen consumption, other indications that the subject is likely to have made a maximal effort include a respiratory exchange ratio (carbon dioxide production: oxygen consumption) greater than unity, indi-

Table 32.2   Heart rate, stroke volume (SV) and cardiac output (CO) to give the total available oxygen shown in Table 32.1, assuming full saturation, haemoglobin 150 g l^{-1} and maximal heart rate of 200 beats per minute (b.p.m.; normal for age 20). The average person exercises at 10 METs, the fit at 15 METs and the very fit at 20 METs. Exercising cardiac outputs correspond to the exercise total available oxygen levels in Table 32.1, as 5 litres of arterial blood with the above properties contain 1 litre of oxygen

Fitness	Resting			Maximal exercise		
	Heart rate (b.p.m.)	SV (ml)	CO (ml)	Heart rate (b.p.m.)	SV (ml)	CO (ml)
Average	72	70	5040	200	100	20 000
Fit	60	85	5100	200	125	25 000
Very fit	50	100	5000	200	150	30 000

cating the hyperventilation brought on by the production of lactic acid as metabolism becomes increasingly anaerobic, a heart rate around the predicted maximum and a lactate level in the blood (often sampled by ear lobe puncture) 5–10 times the resting level of around 1 mmol l^{-1}.

As indicated in Tables 32.1 and 32.2, a person of average fitness will have a maximal oxygen consumption of around 2.5 l min^{-1} and a champion endurance athlete will reach around twice that amount. Expressed in millilitres per kilogram per minute the values will range from around 30–40 in the average individual to twice that in the extremely fit.

OXYGEN FLUX AT HIGH ALTITUDES

With decreasing barometric pressure but a maintained percentage of oxygen, at high altitudes the problem for oxygen flux is a decreasing partial pressure of oxygen in the ambient atmosphere. This is reflected in the alveolar oxygen pressure to which blood in the pulmonary capillaries is exposed. Thus blood in these capillaries is exposed to a falling partial pressure of oxygen, so that the reserve indicated by the plateau of the blood oxygen dissociation curve is eroded and the steep portion of the curve is reached, at which point blood leaves the lungs appreciably desaturated. In fact, the x axis of the dissociation curve can be labelled from right to left with altitude, corresponding to the alveolar oxygen pressure found at that height.

Two points should now be noted. Firstly, the partial pressure of oxygen in the alveoli declines more quickly than would be predicted from the decline in total barometric pressure. This is because the water vapour pressure depends on temperature and not altitude, so that, with the lungs at core temperature, it has a similar value to the normal carbon dioxide pressure and this is maintained irrespective of the altitude because humidifying mechanisms in the upper airways prevent the lungs from drying out. Secondly, as hypoxia reaches a point indicated by the start of the steep descent of the dissociation curve, the carotid and aortic body chemoreceptors stimulate ventilation and so the alveolar oxygen level

is raised (and the carbon dioxide level is lowered by the increased alveolar ventilation).

Owing to the plateau of the blood oxygen dissociation curve, there is little if any evidence of hypoxia until around 2000 metres. This corresponds to the pressure maintained in commercial aircraft cabins to minimise the transmural pressure gradient between the inside and outside of the craft while avoiding hypoxic effects for healthy passengers, although patients with respiratory failure and an already low arterial oxygen pressure would be made worse in these conditions unless given supplementary oxygen. Above 2000 metres increasing hypoxia develops and, particularly when there has not been previous acclimatisation, there is a risk of the unpleasant effects of high altitude or mountain sickness.

High altitude sickness

This consists of a variety of effects, including headache, nausea and vomiting, general malaise, and, in extreme cases, fatal pulmonary or cerebral oedema. The effects are attributable to two main causes: hypoxia, which impairs the function of all body tissues; and the fall in the body level of carbon dioxide, due to hyperventilation, which leads to a respiratory alkalosis, contraction of cerebral resistance vessels, cerebral ischaemia and exacerbation of the effects of hypoxia on the brain.

Compensation in the days and weeks after first exposure to a high altitude includes decreased renal excretion of hydrogen ions and consequent decreased addition of bicarbonate ions to the renal circulation, together with an elevated erythropoietin level, leading to secondary polycythaemia. The fall in circulating bicarbonate level allows pH to return towards normal. Since [H$^+$] is proportional to $P\text{CO}_2/[\text{HCO}_3^-]$, the ratio can be normal with numerator and denominator correspondingly reduced. Return of the hydrogen ion level towards normal allows a further increase in ventilation, and the hypoxia is further alleviated by the increased oxygen carrying power of the blood as the secondary polycythaemia develops. However, compensation at altitudes above 5000 metres is barely adequate for even moderate activity, and in the longer term hypoxia leads to contraction of pulmonary resistance vessels, pulmonary hypertension and the risk of eventual right ventricular failure as in the cor pulmonale of respiratory failure.

In the short term, supplementary oxygen can reverse this vicious circle. If atmospheric pressure is half normal, then breathing oxygen at twice the normal percentage should give a normal partial pressure of oxygen and reverse the adverse effects. An alternative short term treatment for severe mountain sickness is to place the sufferer in an airtight plastic container and inflate the pressure towards sea level pressure. Again, this deals with the problem by correcting the alveolar oxygen pressure, but neither supplementary oxygen nor maintenance in a capsule at sea level pressure is practicable for long term activity.

Studies by John B. West of conditions at or simulating those at the summit of Mount Everest suggest that the maximal oxygen consumption there is around 1 litre (4 METs), achieved by severe hyperventilation (alveolar carbon dioxide around 7.5 mmHg (1 kPa)) and a greater than normal shift of the oxygen dissociation curve between lungs and tissues. Thus in the lungs the curve moves markedly to the left, owing to the low carbon dioxide level and high pH. In addition, the severe hyperventilation with very cold air may lower alveolar temperature, thus moving the curve further to the left and at the same time slightly lowering saturated water vapour pressure. All this facilitates oxygen loading. Then, in the tissues with a high rate of carbon dioxide production and a normal core temperature, the curve would swing markedly to the left, optimising oxygen unloading.

OXYGEN FLUX IN RESPIRATORY FAILURE

Respiratory failure provides another example of hypoxic hypoxia. In this case the alveolar oxygen content is depressed by inadequate ventilation rather than by inadequate oxygen in the inspired air at high altitudes. However, unlike the situation at high altitudes, respiratory failure is often associated with a high carbon dioxide level in the alveoli, again due to the inadequate ventilation. Thus, instead of a respiratory alkalosis, a respiratory acidosis is often present and this is compensated for in the kidneys by increased secretion of hydrogen ion into the tubules and increased generation of bicarbonate, so that the blood level rises. Instead of a reduction in cerebral blood flow, this tends to increase; however, the effect is again unfavourable because the increased flow raises cerebral capillary blood pressure and favours cerebral oedema with consequent headaches. In severe cases the combination of hypoxia, a high carbon dioxide level (hypercapnia) and cerebral oedema lead to a depressed level of consciousness.

As with the hypoxic hypoxia of high altitudes, respiratory failure also induces increased formation of erythropoietin and secondary polycythaemia. As at high altitudes, the combination of tissue hypoxia, raised pulmonary vascular resistance, due to hypoxia, and increased viscosity of blood lead to heart failure (cor pulmonale).

Oxygen treatment of respiratory failure

As with the hypoxic hypoxia of high altitudes, the logical and the effective treatment is by breathing oxygen-enriched air; however, when carbon dioxide retention is present, this carries considerable risks. The patient with hypoxia and hypercapnia clearly exhibits a depressed response by the chemoreceptor reflex to gas pressures that would cause marked hyperventilation in normal people. The activity of the medullary respiratory centre is subnormal, and complete removal of the hypoxic drive mediated through the peripheral chemoreceptor response to hypoxia tends to suppress ventilation severely, so that carbon dioxide builds up and a fatal acute respiratory acidosis may occur.

In this situation, a modest rise in the inspired oxygen can relieve potentially fatal hypoxia without so depressing ventilation that a potentially fatal respiratory acidosis develops. In practice, around 24–28% oxygen is often effective. Regular monitoring of the arterial blood gases is essential while the appropriate level of oxygen is decided.

In the longer term, treatment with mildly oxygen enriched air for considerable periods of the day has been shown to reduce pulmonary hypertension and improve the heart failure.

OXYGEN FLUX IN ANAEMIA

Since total available oxygen is directly proportional to the blood haemoglobin concentration (neglecting the very small amount of dissolved oxygen), it follows that anaemic hypoxia reduces this total in proportion to the severity of the anaemia. Thus, for any given cardiac output, and assuming full saturation, the available oxygen will be reduced by 50% if the haemoglobin is half normal and by 75% if it is one-quarter normal. This is particularly important during exercise, when most of the available oxygen is used. At maximal exercise, cardiac output cannot be further increased and arterial blood oxygen saturation is about 100%, so it follows that someone who, when healthy, could exercise at 10 METs (Table 32.1) by using 2500 ml min^{-1} of the 4000 ml min^{-1} available, would, with 50% of normal haemoglobin, now have only 2000 ml min^{-1} of oxygen available. There are then two consequences: first, maximal exercising ability is impaired, with less total oxygen available than was previously extracted; and second, in order to maximise oxygen consumption, the extraction ratio must rise. This can be accomplished partly by an increased level of 2,3-diphosphoglycerate which increases in red cells during anaemia. Thus the percentage of extraction can rise to reduce the deficit in the maximal oxygen consumption. Nevertheless, someone of moderate fitness can be reduced from normal activity to inability to walk at a normal rate when moderate to severe anaemia is present. The anaemic hypoxia leads to early fatigue during exercise, and in someone who depends on moderate exertion to earn a living this can be severely disabling.

Thus the main compensation for anaemic hypoxia is an increased cardiac output at all levels of exertion and, once maximal cardiac output has been reached, exertion cannot be further increased.

One favourable factor in this situation is that anaemia reduces the work of the heart at a given cardiac output by reducing blood viscosity. Viscosity in major blood vessels depends heavily on the haematocrit. Thus with mild to moderate anaemia, a relatively sedentary lifestyle can be maintained with few symptoms because oxygen flux is maintained by an increased cardiac output without much increase in cardiac work.

OXYGEN FLUX IN GENERAL AND LOCAL CIRCULATORY FAILURE

Both these conditions constitute stagnant hypoxia. General circulatory failure may be due to cardiac disease (central circulatory failure) or to an imbalance between vascular volume and vascular capacity (peripheral circulatory failure or shock). Peripheral circulatory failure is commonly a consequence of reduced blood volume due to haemorrhage or loss of extracellular fluid, as in intestinal obstruction, or there may be hypotension due to peripheral vasodilatation, as in septic shock. In such conditions the circulation generally is inadequate and stagnant hypoxia is present throughout the body, whereas in local circulatory failure the problem is confined to one region. Thus there may be narrowing of the coronary, cerebral and leg arteries, giving rise to conditions such as angina pectoris or myocardial infarction, transient ischaemic attacks or cerebral infarction, and intermittent claudication or gangrene of the distal leg, respectively.

Stagnant hypoxia in heart failure

In heart failure the circulation is impaired by a reduced perfusion pressure. At rest and increasingly with exercise the cardiac output is lower than that required. At rest this leads to vasoconstriction in less essential areas, such as the skin and splanchnic area, to maintain the vital cerebral and coronary circulations. Thus these areas have a reduced pressure at the arterial end of the capillary bed. In addition, the lower part of the body has an increased venous pressure due to a raised central venous pressure. These effects lead to cold peripheries, in some cases blue with peripheral cyanosis and features of mild hepatic and renal failure due to inadequate perfusion (prehepatic and prerenal forms of the organ failure).

With exercise the cardiac output and oxygen flux fall progressively below those required. Exercise is limited, depending on the severity of the condition, and is maintained by a very high extraction ratio of oxygen from the blood, so that mixed venous oxygen saturation falls to very low levels. Provided the circulating haemoglobin level is normal and oxygen saturation in the arteries close to 100%, the only effective treatment is that which improves cardiac output. In most cases this will consist of drugs; in cases where cardiac output is limited by bradycardia a pacemaker may be helpful; in severe cases, cardiac transplant is the only effective treatment.

Local stagnant hypoxia

This can affect any tissue but common major problems involve the coronary, cerebral and leg circulations. In all these cases the situation is similar — when oxygen delivery is borderline, symptoms of malfunction appear intermittently, and when delivery is seriously impaired (often suddenly) there is inadequate oxygen to maintain the tissues and necrosis occurs. Borderline inadequacy of the circulation to the heart and leg muscles gives rise to stagnant hypoxia when the rate of work exceeds a threshold level, giving rise to the pain of ischaemic muscle due to stimulation of pain fibres by the metabolic products of muscle that is exercising at a level which cannot be sustained by the available blood supply. In the heart this is experienced as angina pectoris and in the leg as intermittent claudication. Since the brain is devoid of pain fibres, ischaemia produces no pain, but there is temporary loss of function with ischaemic hypoxia, often leading to attacks of loss of vision or sudden falling (drop attacks) when posterior aspects of the brain are affected.

Temporary ischaemia and reperfusion

This occurs in situations where the circulation

is occluded for a period and then resumes. Examples of such situations are removal of an embolus (embolectomy), e.g. to a leg or pulmonary artery, recanalisation of a coronary artery by thrombolytic agents which activate plasminogen to plasmin so that fibrinogen is broken down, and deliberate arrest of the circulation to provide a relatively bloodless field for surgical operations such as knee joint replacement and hand surgery. The effects of such ischaemia can be local and general and depend on the bulk of the ischaemic tissue and the duration of ischaemia.

The effects of ischaemia can be studied on the conscious human subject by applying a cuff to the wrist or upper arm at a pressure above systolic. During a period of circulatory arrest to the hand, little will be felt in the first 15–30 minutes, but the accumulation of metabolic 'products', such as accumulation of carbon dioxide and hydrogen ions, and depletion of oxygen (hypoxia) can be seen when the occlusion is ended and is followed by the pink flush of reactive hyperaemia, precisely located to the ischaemic segment. If the cuff is maintained for longer periods, or if the ischaemic forearm muscles are exercised, a dull ache will appear and gradually become worse, indicating that a considerable build-up of metabolites is necessary to produce pain.

At the other extreme, a limb that has suffered prolonged arrest of the circulation, for example due to crushing for a period of 12–24 hours, is likely to show evidence of serious damage in the form of progressive swelling and will release products of tissue damage which may have serious general effects, including cardiac arrhythmias due to release of excessive potassium from the damaged muscle cells.

In between these extremes the limbs can be deprived of circulation for 1–2 hours without evidence of injury, and cardiac muscle can survive for several hours. The limit for thrombolytic therapy to the heart is around 6 hours after occlusion, although towards the end of this period there is likely to be considerable damage which can lead to problems during reperfusion, and recovery of the damaged but viable tissue may take months.

OXYGEN FLUX DURING HYPERBARIC CONDITIONS

Hyperbaric conditions are commonly encountered during scuba and deep sea diving (where the person is exposed to the ambient pressure and breathes air or other gases at that pressure — each 10 metres of depth adding about 1 atmosphere to the pressure) and are also produced in hyperbaric chambers for medical treatment. In both cases the total alveolar pressure must equal the ambient pressure, e.g. 2–3 atmospheres in the usual hyperbaric chamber or 10 or more atmospheres with diving.

There are two main consequences of a raised alveolar gas pressure: local effects on the lungs and general direct effects on the body tissues, including effects that follow dissolution of gases widely throughout the body, which takes a considerable time to complete.

Firstly, the local effects on the lung tissues. Here oxygen is the main danger. If, for example, air is breathed at 10 atmospheres, then the partial pressure of oxygen will be approximately 10 times normal, i.e. over 1000 mmHg (133 kPa). This level of oxygen is highly toxic, probably due to oxidation and production in tissues of highly reactive oxygen radicals which produce progressive damage with time. The solution for divers is to adjust the oxygen percentage breathed so that a normal alveolar oxygen is maintained. Thus 2% oxygen at 10 atmospheres will give a partial pressure of oxygen much the same as 20% at 1 atmosphere. The reason that the oxygen level is higher than that predicted from the atmospheric pressure is that water vapour pressure in the alveoli is governed by temperature and is unchanged at high pressures so that the other gases constitute a slightly higher percentage of the total pressure.

The second effect of the high alveolar pressure is that more gas will be dissolved in the blood and in the tissues, the amount dissolved being directly proportional to the pressure (Henry's law). This is taken advantage of in the treatment of carbon monoxide poisoning by the administration of a high (even hyperbaric) level of oxygen. If alveolar oxygen pressure rises fivefold, then the dissolved oxygen in the blood rises from 3 to 15 ml l^{-1}. Thus as well as displacing carbon monoxide from haemoglobin, the increased dissolved oxygen can contribute to oxygen flux to the tissues. With an atmosphere of pure oxygen at 2 atmospheres the alveolar oxygen pressure can rise almost 15-fold. This raises the dissolved oxygen in the blood to about 45 ml l^{-1}, which is a significant proportion of the normal total arterial oxygen content of 200 ml l^{-1} of blood.

With deep sea diving, the increased partial pressure of nitrogen, generally regarded as an inert gas, can have a noticeable effect on cerebral function. Initially there may be feelings of panic, or possibly elation, and with increasing nitrogen pressures dangerous disorientation and confusion occur (nitrogen narcosis, rapture of the deep). For this reason, an even more inert gas, usually helium, is required to dilute the low concentration of oxygen appropriate at high pressures.

Another widely known problem of high pressure nitrogen develops on return to breathing at 1 atmosphere — the 'bends'. This problem results from the formation of nitrogen bubbles as the dissolved nitrogen comes rapidly out of solution when the individual is rapidly decompressed. The bends are painful joints due to nitrogen bubbles within them, but the same problem can occur in the lungs (the chokes) and in the brain, leading to scattered areas of damage or even strokes. The amount dissolved depends on the amount of increased pressure and the duration of exposure. Thus a brief exposure to a high pressure (bounce diving) leads to less solution of gas (and less risk of decompression sickness) than prolonged exposure (saturation diving) when the dissolved gas has time to come into equilibrium with the increased gas pressure in the body fluids. Data have been accumulated so that by following a known profile of the extent and duration of increased pressure a safe programme of gradual decompression can be prescribed. When problems of decompression arise (because the prescribed programme has not been followed, or possibly as a result of individual susceptibility) the individual requires rapid recompression, which redissolves the gas bubbles; compression chambers are available at strategic points for this purpose.

HISTOTOXIC HYPOXIA

This is the fourth variety of hypoxia in the classical description. The term refers to hypoxia of tissues because the enzymes which use the oxygen have been poisoned, typically by cyanide. In this situation oxygen flux is normal and the patient's colour is normal, but at high levels of cyanide death occurs rapidly because the vital oxidative source of energy is suddenly cut off and all cellular activity ceases. All forms of hypoxia tend towards this end-point of cellular hypoxia, dysfunction and death.

A rather similar problem impairs oxygen flux when the oxygen dissociation curve for blood is shifted markedly to the left, as in hypothermic tissues (e.g. in trench foot), or when someone receives massive transfusion with stored blood which has been depleted of 2,3-diphosphoglycerate; here also the oxygen flux to the microcirculation is not followed by delivery to the surrounding tissues.

MONITORING OXYGEN FLUX AND DELIVERY

Since normal oxygen flux depends on a normal level of circulating haemoglobin, full saturation of arterial blood with oxygen and normal perfusion of tissues, these three factors are monitored. In addition, evidence of local hypoxic cellular dysfunction can be sought.

In practice, all of these four factors must be continuously reviewed in conjunction with the general clinical situation in all patients under general anaesthesia and in patients subject to intensive care. Measurement of the partial pressure of oxygen in arterial blood adds further to the picture and is an important measurement in its own right, as described below.

Monitoring the haemoglobin level

Haemoglobin levels are assessed preoperatively in patients to be anaesthetised for elective surgery and are measured regularly in those liable to further blood loss or extensive haemodilution.

In certain circumstances it may be necessary to test for abnormalities of haemoglobin which interfere with the carriage of oxygen. Some of these produce a blue discoloration, which is literally cyanosis (blue colour) but does not in such circumstances indicate desaturation of the remaining normal haemoglobin.

Monitoring saturation

Saturation is assessed in a number of ways. Clinical observation of the presence and severity of cyanosis is fundamental. Central cyanosis is an indicator of arterial desaturation, either from hypoxic hypoxia or from an extensive right-to-left shunt. Its presence indicates a significant amount of desaturated haemoglobin in the tissues observed. The blood is present in superficial small vessels in the mouth or conjunctiva and it is generally accepted that 5 g dl^{-1} (50 g l^{-1}, or a third of the normal total haemoglobin) must be desaturated to produce the definite blue colour that denotes cyanosis. Thus it would be impossible to detect cyanosis in someone with less than 5 g dl^{-1} total haemoglobin; conversely, it is relatively easy to detect in someone with polycythaemia, and in this case does not necessarily imply a serious fall in saturation.

Assessing arterial desaturation from the appearance of cyanosis assumes that circulation to the part is normal, as decreased perfusion would cause stagnant hypoxia and peripheral cyanosis. Thus blue discoloration of cold peripheries (ears, fingers) suggests peripheral rather than central cyanosis and indicates local stagnant hypoxia rather than general hypoxic hypoxia. On the other hand, cyanosis of a well perfused, and hence warm, extremity does suggest central cyanosis and this is the basis of monitoring by oximetry (see below).

Saturation is not easily measured directly in arterial blood because procedure is complicated, involving measuring oxygen content and relating it to oxygen capacity using the time honoured Van Slyke method. In practice it can be inferred from measurements of the oxygen pressure in arterial blood and estimated indirectly from blood colour by pulse oximetry.

Pressure of oxygen in arterial blood

This is a valuable measure in itself and the saturation of blood can normally be inferred from it. A sample is taken from any artery (most commonly the radial artery) under conditions that avoid contamination by air and with rapid analysis to avoid changes due to metabolism by the cellular elements in the blood. The normal arterial oxygen pressure (PO_2) varies between about 80 and 120 mmHg (about 10–16 kPa) and at this level saturation can be assumed to lie between 95 and 100%. In older people without obvious pulmonary disease, oxygen pressure may fall to about 70 mmHg (about 9 kPa) corresponding to a saturation between 90 and 95%. Below this level the plateau of the blood oxygen saturation curve merges into the steep descent. Thus at an oxygen pressure of 60 mmHg (8 kPa) saturation is just below 90%, and by 50 mmHg (6.6 kPa) saturation is little over 80% and falling rapidly. Thus it is logical that the carotid bodies normally stimulate ventilation at around 60 mmHg (8 kPa), and below 50 mmHg (6.6 kPa) is regarded clinically as dangerously hypoxic.

Pulse oximetry

This method is now widely used in the assessment of blood oxygen saturation. It depends on the different colours of oxygenated haemoglobin (red) and deoxygenated haemoglobin (blue). The tissues are transilluminated by two frequencies of light so that the proportion of oxygenated haemoglobin can be measured. By relating the results to arterial pulsation in the part (finger or ear) it is possible to eliminate effects due to other factors influencing tissue colour. It is thus a very accurate method of measuring oxygen saturation of the blood. Since arterial oxygen pressure can change widely at normal to high values without much change in saturation, the method is not an accurate measure of oxygen pressure in this range.

As poor tissue perfusion causes local desaturation (peripheral cyanosis), the saturation measured (accurately) by a pulse oximeter is not an accurate indicator of arterial oxygen saturation when perfusion is impaired. Equally, when the patient is breathing a high concentration of oxygen, arterial oxygen saturation may be normal, while the arterial carbon dioxide level is increased due to hypoventilation. Thus the instrument should be regarded as an accurate indicator of local blood saturation but its limitations should be borne in mind. A low reading could indicate poor local perfusion rather than general arterial desaturation; a normal reading does not necessarily indicate adequate pulmonary ventilation.

Monitoring of intramucosal pH in the gut

This is an emerging method of assessment that could be a valuable early indicator of developing splanchnic hypoxia. The principle is that vasoconstriction in the splanchnic area occurs early in the response to developing circulatory failure and hence generalised stagnant hypoxia. Vasoconstriction in the splanchnic area leads to stagnant hypoxia there and this can be detected by a change in the intracellular pH of the mucosal cells, e.g. in the stomach. The method is to measure the local carbon dioxide pressure by a tube passed into the stomach and to combine this assessment of tissue carbon dioxide pressure with the arterial bicarbonate level to calculate intracellular pH using the Henderson–Hasselbalch relationship.

With this method the intracellular pH (normally around 7.3, slightly lower than blood pH) can be shown to fall in ischaemic, and hence hypoxic, mucosal cells. The method should give early warning of gut ischaemia in patients with circulatory difficulties, and is potentially valuable because it could also give early and precise warning of the changes in the ischaemic gut which allow endotoxins and organisms to cross the damaged wall and lead to development of the potentially lethal complication of septic shock.

FURTHER READING

Fiddian-Green R G 1995 Gastric intramucosal pH, tissue oxygenation and acid–base balance. British Journal of Anaesthesia 74: 591–606

Hanning C D, Alexander-Williams J M 1995 Pulse oximetry: a practical review. British Medical Journal 311: 367–370

Hutton P, Clutton-Brock T 1993 The benefits and pitfalls of pulse oximetry. British Medical Journal 307: 457–458

Kindwall E P 1993 Hyperbaric oxygen — more indications than many doctors realise. British Medical Journal 307: 515–516

Nunn J F 1993 Applied respiratory physiology 4th ed. Butterworth, London

Oh T E 1996 Gastric tonometry to monitor tissue oxygenation: more than a gut feeling? British Journal of Anaesthesia 76: 604–605

Sykes J J W 1994 Medical aspects of scuba diving. British Medical Journal 308: 1483–1488

Renal system

SECTION CONTENTS

33

Renal physiology

P. McNamee

RENAL PHYSIOLOGY

The practising anaesthetist frequently encounters critically ill patients suffering multiple organ failure, including renal failure. On a day to day basis, he or she administers drugs which may directly affect renal function, which are metabolised or excreted by the kidney or which may have potentially adverse effects upon renal function. The population in general is ageing, bringing more patients with comorbid illnesses including renal impairment into anaesthetic practice. An understanding of basic renal physiology and the role of the kidney in the regulation of the internal environment is essential to safe practice.

This chapter will review the elements of renal function, the mechanisms controlling renal function and the effects of a variety of drugs and clinical situations upon renal function.

RENAL ANATOMY

The kidney consists on a macroscopic level of a number of elements: the cortex, which surrounds a central region — the medulla; and the renal pelvis, which connects the kidney to the ureter, which in turn conducts urine formed within the kidney to the urinary bladder. The medulla of the kidney may be subdivided into outer and inner regions.

Roughly 20% of resting cardiac output is directed to the kidneys, making renal blood flow in terms of volume per weight of tissue amongst the richest of all organs. Renal blood flow in the adult is therefore approximately 1250 ml min^{-1}, with a corresponding plasma flow of 700 ml min^{-1} and glomerular filtrate formation of 120 ml min^{-1} or 170 litres in 24 hours. Blood enters the kidney via the renal artery, which runs alongside the ureter through the hilum of the kidney. Within the kidney the renal artery branches, progressively forming the interlobular, arcuate and cortical radial arteries. These arteries branch to form the afferent arterioles, which give rise to the glomerular capillary beds. The venous system is similar to the arterial system in terms of divisions.

Renal blood flow is unique in that it traverses two capillary networks in series: the glomerular capillary network arising from the afferent arteriole, and a peritubular capillary network arising from the efferent arteriole (Fig. 33.1). The glomerular capillary network is embedded within Bowman's capsule, forming the renal corpuscle. The peritubular capillary network surrounds the renal tubules within the medulla of the kidney.

The nephron

The functional unit of the kidney is the nephron. The nephron is composed of the glomerular capillary network, the proximal tubule, the loop of Henle, the distal tubule and the collecting duct. There are roughly one million nephrons in each adult kidney. This provides a great reserve and ensures effective homeostasis even when up to 70% of nephrons have been lost.

Functionally there are two types of nephron: cortical or superficial nephrons, arising within the cortex of kidney, and juxtamedullary nephrons, arising from around the corticomedullary junction. The majority of nephrons are cortical — in a proportion of roughly 8 to 1. They have short loops. Juxtamedullary nephrons, on the other hand, arise close to the corticomedullary junction and have long loops that penetrate deeply into the medulla. The blood supply of the tubules descending deep into the medulla is derived from the efferent arteriole, which gives rise to the vasa recta — long straight capillaries with a

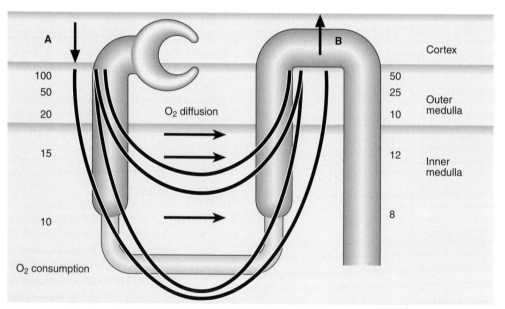

Figure 33.1 Figure 33.1 shows blood flow to the nephron. Blood supply to the interstitium of the kidney is via the vasa recta. Blood enters the vasa recta at point A and exists at point B. The afferent and efferent vessels are closely apposed. Oxygen is consumed as a result of active solute absorption by the tubular cells reducing the oxygen content of blood leaving the vasa recta. As a result, diffusion of oxygen from the afferent to the efferent vessels occurs, leaving the interstitium of the kidney critically hypoxic. The numbers indicate tissue pO$_2$ mmHg. (Adapted with permission from M Brezis, S Rosen, P Silvan and F H Epstein. 1984 Kidney Int 226: 375)

hairpin shape similar to the loops of Henle. Blood returning from the peritubular capillaries is carried to the cortex by the ascending vasa recta. In terms of function the juxtamedullary nephrons are more effective in the production of concentrated urine and conservation of sodium and water, making them of particular importance at times of physiological stress. The cells of the kidney that consume most energy are those involved in the active reabsorption of filtered sodium, i.e. tubular cells. The blood supply to the cells of the juxtamedullary nephrons, while ideal for the preservation of a hypertonic medulla, means that these cells are always relatively hypoxic, which has significant clinical consequences.

Juxtaglomerular apparatus (JGA)

This structure comprises the cells of the macula densa (found within the thick ascending limb of the loop of Henle), lacis cells and specialised cells at the vascular pole where the afferent and efferent arterioles enter and leave the glomerulus. The JGA secretes renin, which is ultimately responsible for the activation of angiotensin II and the release of aldosterone. The JGA also plays a role in the regulation of glomerular filtration.

Urine formation

Glomerular filtration

The process that eventually results in urine formation begins with plasma ultrafiltration across the glomerular capillary wall. The process is similar to that in any capillary and is governed by Starling's forces, being proportional to membrane permeability and the balance between hydraulic and oncotic pressure gradients.

Blood enters the glomerular capillary network via the afferent arteriole. The filtration barrier comprises the endothelial cells of the glomerular capillary, the basement membrane and the epithelial cells of Bowman's capsule, which are attached to the basement membrane by means of podocytes. The most important element of the filtration barrier is the basement membrane, which is both size and charge selective. The glomerular filtration barrier permits the free filtration of water and water soluble substances into Bowman's space. The passage of colloid — cells and proteins — is largely prevented, resulting in a protein-free filtrate. The normal glomerular filtration rate in man is around 125 ml min^{-1}. Total daily filtrate is therefore around 180 litres. The flux of filtrate or glomerular filtration rate (GFR) is given by the equation:

$$\text{GFR} = K_f \text{ (hydraulic pressure gradient}$$
$$- \text{oncotic pressure gradient)},$$

which can be expanded to

$$J_v = K_f \left[(P_{GC} - P_{BS}) - (P_P - P_{BS}) \right],$$

where J_v is the flux across the glomerular capillary (GFR), K_f is the filtration coefficient, P_{GC} is the hydrostatic pressure within the glomerular capillary, P_{BS} is the hydrostatic pressure within Bowman's space, P_P is the oncotic pressure within the glomerular capillary and P_{BS} is the oncotic pressure within Bowman's space (Fig. 33.2A).

Control of glomerular filtration rate

The oncotic pressure gradient increases progressively throughout the length of the glomerular capillary because it is determined by plasma protein concentration. As filtration of water and contained solute across the glomerular capillary occurs, the concentration of protein remaining within the capillary rises and may become sufficiently large to prevent filtration. This situation, however, is probably of importance only when renal blood flow is low. The role of capillary permeability in regulation of the GFR is incompletely understood and under normal circumstances is probably not of major importance. The situation of the glomerular capillaries, interposed between the afferent and efferent arterioles, permits rapid regulation of the GFR by alteration of afferent and efferent arteriolar tone.

Glomerular hydraulic pressure is affected by changes in both afferent and efferent arteriolar tone. Increased afferent arteriolar tone reduces systemic pressure transmission to the glomerular capillary. Dilatation of the afferent arteriole

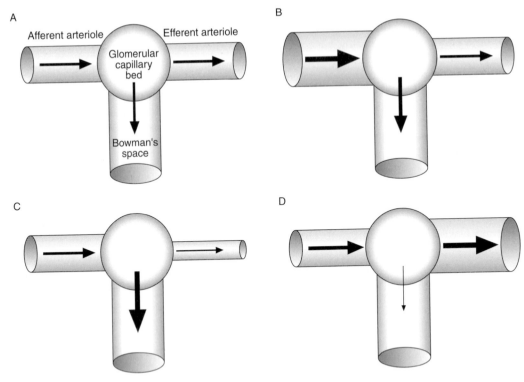

Figure 33.2 (See text for explanation).

increases transmission of systemic pressure to the glomerular capillary, increasing hydraulic pressure (Fig. 33.2B). On the other hand, increased efferent arteriole tone increases intraglomerular pressure, while efferent arteriole dilatation reduces glomerular capillary hydraulic pressure (Figs 33.2C, D). Renal plasma flow is a function of the total pressure differential across the kidney (arterial pressure – venous pressure) and the total renal resistance (which is a function of both afferent and efferent arteriolar tone):

$$\text{renal plasma flow} = \frac{\text{pressure gradient}}{\text{total renal resistance}}$$

It can be seen that increased afferent or efferent arteriolar tone will decrease renal plasma flow. Increased afferent arteriolar tone will tend to decrease both renal plasma flow and GFR, but increased efferent arteriolar tone, although decreasing renal plasma flow, will tend to increase GFR.

Regulation of glomerular filtration rate and renal plasma flow

Blood pressure varies widely within the physiological range; however, despite this, renal blood flow and GFR remain fairly constant. This is achieved mostly by alterations in renal arteriolar resistance. Two principal intrarenal mechanisms responsible for regulation of GFR and renal plasma flow are autoregulation and tubuloglomerular feedback.

Autoregulation

When the blood pressure increases within the physiological range, renal blood flow remains relatively constant. Similarly when systemic blood pressure falls, renal blood flow is also maintained relatively constant. From the equation above it is apparent that maintenance of renal blood flow, despite variation in perfusion pressure, can be achieved only by alteration of renal vascular resistance. Most of the alteration in renal resistance responsible for maintenance of renal blood flow occurs within the afferent arterioles. The mechanisms responsible for this autoregulation of renal blood flow within the physiological pressure range are incompletely understood. At its simplest level it is believed that alteration of tone in myogenic stretch receptors within the wall of the afferent arteriole is responsible, i.e. increased pressure stretches the vessel walls, activating stretch receptors which increase smooth muscle tone, thus increasing resistance and decreasing renal blood flow. The process also operates in reverse — decreased systemic pressure leading to reduced afferent arterial resistance and maintenance of renal blood flow. The afferent arteriole is maximally dilated at a mean arterial pressure of 70–80 mmHg and consequently a decrease in pressure below this level leads to decreased renal plasma flow and also decreased GFR.

Tubuloglomerular feedback

This is the mechanism whereby tubular fluid flow may affect the glomerular filtration rate. It results from a feedback loop from the macula densa to its parent glomerulus. The macula densa is capable of sensing alterations in tubular fluid flow. Precisely what is sensed by the cells of the macula densa is unclear — it may be the concentration of NaCl, Na^+ or Cl^-. When an alteration occurs, the macula densa signals to its parent glomerulus, altering the GFR. Alteration in the GFR may be achieved by variation of the afferent or efferent arteriolar tone or glomerular permeability as a result of altered mesangial cell tone. The mode of signal mediation is uncertain and may involve local angiotensin II production or prostanoids.

Clinical relevance

The concepts of both autoregulation and tubuloglomerular feedback are both of clinical importance. A fall in systemic blood pressure normally leads to alteration in both afferent and efferent

arteriolar tone which preserves both renal blood flow and GFR. When hypotension occurs in the presence of renal artery stenosis, however, although renal resistance may be reduced by afferent or efferent arteriolar dilatation, increased renal blood flow is limited by the presence of the stenosis, leading to decreased renal perfusion and decreased GFR. This is a particular problem in patients taking angiotensin converting enzyme (ACE) inhibiting drugs. Under normal circumstances ACE inhibitors induce efferent arteriolar dilatation and decreased filtration pressure; however, efferent arteriolar dilatation also decreases total renal resistance, thus increasing renal blood flow. There may also be some afferent arteriolar dilatation and, overall, both renal plasma flow and GFR are preserved. In the patient with renal artery stenosis, however, while efferent arteriolar dilatation may be induced, increased renal blood flow is prevented by the presence of stenosis leading to decreased GFR (Fig. 33.3). This is of particular importance in patients with a single functioning kidney with renal artery stenosis where the introduction of an ACE inhibitor may induce acute renal failure.

Tubuloglomerular feedback is relevant to the development of acute tubular necrosis. When renal perfusion is decreased, glomerular filtration continues because the hydraulic pressure needed to maintain filtration is relatively modest. Decreased interstitial blood flow, however, leads to tissue hypoxia. Hypoxia inhibits Na^+,K^+-ATPase activity, decreasing filtrate reabsorption. Failure of reabsorption results in increased loss of filtered sodium. If this continued for any length

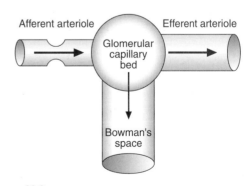

Figure 33.3

of time it would lead to volume depletion and worsened renal perfusion. Failure of sodium chloride reabsorption is sensed at the macula densa, however, and the JGA signals to its parent glomerulus, decreasing glomerular filtration. Decreased glomerular filtration reduces the amount of sodium that must be reabsorbed, consequently reducing sodium loss.

Under normal circumstances autoregulation and tubuloglomerular feedback ensure that renal plasma flow and GFR remain constant. In situations of stress, e.g. hypovolaemia, other factors are of increased importance in the regulation of both renal plasma flow and GFR. Hypotension increases sympathetic activity and the renin–angiotensin system is activated. These effects lead to systemic vasoconstriction; however, at a local level within the kidney, vasodilating prostanoids such as prostaglandin E_2 (PGE_2) are released, leading to local vasodilatation and preservation of renal blood flow. In addition PGE_2 tends to inhibit Na^+ movement across the luminal border, this reduces renal tubular Na^+ reabsorption and reduces renal oxygen consumption as a result of decreased Na^+,K^+-ATPase activity. In this way cellular energy consumption is reduced and energy conserved is available for the maintenance of cellular integrity. It should be apparent that non-steroidal anti-inflammatory drugs (NSAIDs), by inhibiting the release of prostaglandins, can have adverse effects upon both renal blood flow and GFR. Under normal circumstances, the renin–angiotensin system is not activated and prostaglandins do not play a major role in the regulation of renal plasma flow or GFR. However, if prostaglandin production is inhibited at a time of physiological stress, the effect may be to induce acute renal failure. The combined effects of both ACE inhibitors and NSAIDs in patients suffering coincident stress are now probably the most common cause of acute renal failure.

Measurement of glomerular filtration rate

Measurement of GFR is an essential part of the evaluation of renal function. GFR reflects the sum of filtration rates of all functioning nephrons and is therefore an index of total renal function. Measurement of GFR allows the assessment of the severity of renal disease and is also helpful in determining the correct dosage of drugs excreted by the kidney.

CFR may be measured using the polysaccharide inulin. This substance is freely filtered but is neither secreted nor reabsorbed by the tubular cells. Urinary inulin therefore reflects GFR:

urinary inulin = urine volume × urine inulin concentration;

filtered inulin = Plasma inulin concentration × GFR.

Since all filtered inulin must enter the urine,

$$GFR = \frac{U_V \times U_I}{P_I},$$

where U_V is the urine volume, U_I is the urine inulin concentration and P_I is the plasma inulin concentration.

In practice inulin is rarely used as an indicator of GFR. It requires an infusion of inulin, steady-state conditions and measurement of inulin concentration, which is technically difficult. Creatinine clearance is used as an alternative in clinical practice and is reasonably accurate. Creatinine is secreted by the cells of the distal nephron and consequently creatinine clearance overestimates GFR by roughly 10%:

$$creatinine\ clearance = \frac{U_C \times U_V}{P_C},$$

where U_C is the urinary creatinine concentration, U_V is the urinary volume and P_C is the plasma creatinine concentration. Creatinine clearance is usually estimated using a 24 hour collection of urine. The figure $U_C \times U_V$ represents the total amount of creatinine excreted in a 24 hour period. In the steady state, this represents daily creatinine generation. Creatinine generation reflects muscle mass and is relatively constant, certainly on a day to day basis. Hence once creatinine generation has been accurately determined, plasma creatinine may be used to deduce creatinine clearance — assuming that muscle mass and hence creatinine generation remain stable. A drawback of the use of creatinine concentration as a reflection of GFR is that, as GFR declines, the initial rise in creatinine concentration is relatively small.

A number of drugs in common clinical practice interfere with the secretion of creatinine, including trimethoprim and cimetidine. Administration of these drugs inhibits creatinine secretion, the consequence is decreased urinary creatinine excretion, a rise in the serum creatinine level and an apparent fall in creatinine clearance.

Renal tubular function

The glomerular filtration rate is roughly 125 ml min^{-1} or 180 l day^{-1}. The normal urinary output, however, is roughly 1 litre, implying that more than 99% of glomerular filtrate is reabsorbed by the renal tubules. The renal tubule is not a homogenous structure. It can be divided into a number of functional regions.

An understanding of the mechanisms of solute handling within the tubule is of importance in appreciating the actions of many drugs, both physiological and toxic upon renal function. It is also of importance in appreciating the renal mechanisms that come into play in acid–base disturbances, electrolyte disturbances and in patients suffering from acute renal failure.

The tubule may be divided into functional areas:

- the proximal tubule
- the loop of Henle
- the distal tubule
- the collecting duct.

The areas may be further subdivided according to function; this chapter will provide only a broad outline of the more clinically relevant parts.

Almost all of the energy consumed by the cells of the kidney is used in the process of active reabsorption of filtered solute. Although the solute reabsorbed by tubular cells may differ along the length of the nephron, the process of reabsorption is similar. Reabsorption of solute by tubular cells is driven by the activity of the cell membrane enzyme Na$^+$,K$^+$-ATPase. This enzyme, although responsible for reabsorption, is not located on the luminal border of the cell membrane but rather on the basolateral border. Solute enters the tubular cell via channels or transporter proteins on the luminal border (Fig. 33.4A). The solute is then driven from the cell by the activity of Na$^+$,K$^+$-ATPase on the basolateral border. The activity of Na$^+$,K$^+$-ATPase creates an electrochemical gradient that facilitates the movement of solute from the tubular lumen into the tubular cell. The channels and transport proteins on the luminal side of the cell vary, permitting variation of the substances reabsorbed. Na$^+$, being the most abundant ion in the filtrate, is of greatest importance. The mechanism of Na$^+$ entry into the tubular cell varies, depending on the nature of the transport protein or channel on the luminal border. Na$^+$ may be reabsorbed as a result of antiporter proteins, which exchange Na$^+$ for positively charged ions such as K$^+$ and H$^+$; Na$^+$ is also reabsorbed via cotransporters which facilitate recovery of filtered amino acids and glucose. Water reabsorption occurs passively through the tight junctions between tubular cells. Although itself a passive process it occurs as a result of active solute reabsorption. The reabsorption of Na$^+$ and water raises the relative concentration of other filtered ions, such as K$^+$, creating a concentration gradient which promotes their reabsorption.

The proximal tubule

Within the proximal tubule, 50–55% of the glomerular filtrate is reabsorbed. The luminal transport and exchange proteins vary in their density and abundance throughout the length of the proximal tubule, resulting in selective differences in reabsorption along the proximal tubule.

Within the earliest part of the proximal tubule, the principal solute reabsorbed is NaHCO$_3$. The mechanism of reabsorption is illustrated in Figure 33.4B. H$^+$ ion is exchanged for Na$^+$ ion by an antiporter on the luminal membrane of the proximal tubular cell. The H$^+$ ion secreted associates with HCO$_3^-$ in the filtrate forming H$_2$CO$_3$, which, in the presence of carbonic anhydrase — found in high concentration within the vesicles of

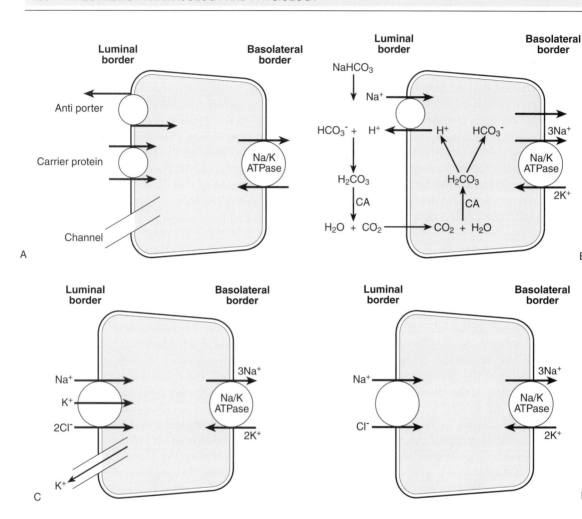

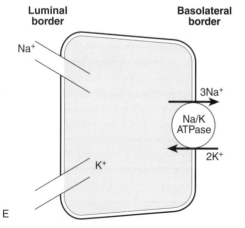

Figure 33.4 Transport mechanisms in the kidney. A: Proximal tubular reabsorption of solute. B: Proximal tubular reabsorption of bicarbonate. C: Sodium reabsorption in loop of Henle. D: Distal tubule reabsorption of sodium and chloride. E: H+ secretion and potassium reabsorption in collecting duct.

the brush border of the proximal tubular cells — dissociates to form water and carbon dioxide. Carbon dioxide diffuses freely across the tubular cell membrane where, in the presence of intracellular carbonic anhydrase it forms H_2CO_3, which in turn dissociates to form H^+ ion — which feeds the H^+,Na^+-antiporter. Na^+ is pumped from the cell by the action of Na^+,K^+-ATPase, and HCO_3^- follows, maintaining electrical neutrality. Thus in the early part of the proximal tubule $NaHCO_3$ reabsorption is achieved as a result of the action of Na^+,K^+-ATPase on the basolateral border of the tubular cell. As $NaHCO_3$ is reabsorbed, water reabsorption occurs passively via the tight junctions. The early proximal tubule has a high reflective coefficient for Cl^-. As $NaHCO_3$ and associated water are reabsorbed, the concentration of Cl^- within the filtrate rises, so that in the more distal part of the proximal tubule, where the reflection coefficient for Cl^- is lower, Cl^- moves down a concentration gradient, Na^+ accompanies the Cl^-, maintaining electrical neutrality, and water follows through the intercellular space as a result of osmotic shift. Thus the reabsorption of NaCl in the proximal tubule occurs partially as a result of a concentration gradient created by the selective active reabsorption of $NaHCO_3$ in the first part of the proximal tubule. It has been estimated that at least 30% of proximal tubular NaCl reabsorption occurs passively as a result of $NaHCO_3$ reabsorption.

Within the earliest part of the proximal tubule the reabsorption of Na^+ is facilitated by the presence of an antiporter on the luminal membrane. In the more distal parts of the proximal tubule the movement of Na^+ into the cell is facilitated by the presence of cotransporter proteins on the luminal membrane, which permit the entry of Na^+ combined with other solutes, including glucose and amino acids. The movement of Na^+ from the cell into the interstitium is as a result of the action of Na^+,K^+-ATPase on the basolateral cell border.

Clinical relevance

The proximal tubule is the site in which almost all filtered bicarbonate is reabsorbed. A failure of reabsorption of $NaHCO_3$ leads to bicarbonaturia and the development of metabolic acidosis (proximal or type II renal tubular acidosis). Carbonic anhydrase inhibitors inhibit the reabsorption of $NaHCO_3$, leading to diuresis. Such drugs induce metabolic acidosis and bicarbonaturia. Theoretically carbonic anhydrase inhibitors should act as effective diuretics because they are capable of inhibiting the reabsorption of large amounts of Na^+ in the proximal tubule. The effects of carbonic anhydrase inhibitors are blunted, however, because the reabsorption of Na^+ throughout the rest of the nephron can be greatly increased in response to hormonal signals.

The loop of Henle

This may be subdivided into three main functional areas: the thin descending limb, the thin ascending limb and the thick ascending limb. Although the thin parts of the limb are of importance in establishing a concentration gradient within the interstitium of the kidney, they are metabolically relatively inactive, having low levels of Na^+,K^+-ATPase. The thin descending limb is largely impermeable to water. However Na^+ diffuses from the interstitium, where it is in high concentration, into the lumen, and this is the basis of the countercurrent multiplier system that is responsible for the creation of a high osmotic gradient within the interstitium of the kidney.

The thick ascending limb is metabolically very active: 35–40% of filtered Na^+ is reabsorbed in this limb. Within the thick ascending limb reabsorption of Na^+ is also dependent on the activity of Na^+,K^+-ATPase located on the basolateral cell border. The receptor on the luminal border permits the entry of 1 Na^+, 1 K^+ and 2 Cl^- ions (Fig. 33.4C). Na^+ is pumped from the basolateral cell membrane by Na^+,K^+-ATPase and Cl^- follows, maintaining electrical neutrality. The intercellular tight junctions of the thick ascending limb are very tight and almost impervious to water, preventing water from following solute into the interstitium. The consequence is that the concentration of the filtrate within the tubular lumen decreases progressively along the length of the thick ascending limb. On the other hand, the concentration of Na^+ within the interstitium increases and, as mentioned above, some of this diffuses down the concentration gradient into the lumen of the thin descending limb. A large proportion of the K^+ which is reabsorbed diffuses back into the lumen of the thick ascending limb. Back diffusion of K^+ ensures that the lumen of the thick ascending limb is positively charged. This positive charge promotes the reabsorption of Ca^{2+}, which also occurs within the thick ascending limb.

Clinical relevance

The $Na^+,K^+,2Cl^-$ receptor of the thick ascending limb is the site of action of the loop diuretics. It is believed that the commonly used loop diuretics, frusemide and bumetanide, both act by occupying the binding site of Cl^-. The presence of these diuretics inhibits the movement of Na^+ into the cell, leading to diuresis. Further effects include a reduction in the positive charge normally found on the thick ascending limb, which in turn leads to reduced Ca^{2+} and Mg^{2+} reabsorption and consequently increased calcium and magnesium loss within the urine. The loop diuretics may be associated with the development of hypomagnesaemia. They may also be used to promote urinary calcium loss in the management of hypercalcaemia.

As mentioned above, the tight junctions of the thick ascending limb are largely impervious to water so that the filtrate becomes progressively more dilute throughout its length. Inhibition of Na^+ reabsorption in the thick ascending limb makes the production of a very dilute urine impossible. The thick ascending limb is also responsible for the creation of the concentration gradient found within the interstitium of the kidney as a result of the countercurrent multiplier. Na^+ reabsorbed by the thick ascending limb is in high concentration within the interstitium of the kidney, from where it diffuses into the thin descending limb, providing increased tubular Na^+, which is reabsorbed in the thick ascending limb. Inhibition of Na^+ reabsorption within the thick ascending limb significantly reduces the concentration gradient within the interstitium, which in turn makes the production of a highly

concentrated urine impossible, as will be seen when the collecting duct is considered later.

The distal tubule

Within the distal tubule 5–8% of filtered Na^+ is reabsorbed. The energy necessary for reabsorption of Na^+ within the distal nephron is supplied by the activity of Na^+,K^+-ATPase on the basolateral border of the tubular cell. The luminal border within the distal tubule contains a cotransporter for Na^+ and Cl^- (Fig. 33.4D). It is within the distal tubule that the filtrate is reduced to its most dilute state.

Clinical relevance

The cells of the distal nephron are responsive to a number of drugs in common usage. Thiazide diuretics act by inhibiting the NaCl cotransporter. As a consequence, natriuresis results, leading to increased Na^+ delivery to the collecting duct. Thiazide diuretics inhibit the production of a maximally dilute urine. Thiazide diuretics also have the effect of promoting increased calcium reabsorption within the distal nephron by mechanisms that are unclear. In contrast to the loop diuretics, diuretics acting on the distal nephron do not significantly affect the ability of the kidney to produce a concentrated urine. This is of particular relevance with regard to thiazide diuretics with a prolonged half-life. Since they may induce volume contraction and induce the release of antidiuretic hormone (ADH), hyponatraemia is a more likely consequence of the use of these thiazide diuretics than of loop diuretics (see below).

The collecting duct

Within the collecting duct 2–3% of filtered Na^+ is reabsorbed. As with the other tubular segments it is possible to divide the collecting duct into a number of subdivisions: the cortical collecting duct, the outer and inner medullary collecting ducts and the common collecting duct, each of which has slightly different functions — these will not be described in detail. However, the cortical collecting duct has two cell types of importance: principal cells, which reabsorb Na^+ and secrete K^+, and intercalated cells, which are involved in H^+ secretion and K^+ absorption (Fig. 33.4E). The cells of the cortical collecting duct are aldosterone responsive, and reabsorption of Na^+ and secretion of K^+ and H^+ are increased in response to increased aldosterone levels. The mechanism of secretion of K^+ and H^+ depends upon the insertion of an appropriate channel on the tubular border. The expression of these channels is promoted by the presence of aldosterone.

Within the collecting duct the final adjustment of urinary concentration is made. The cells of the medullary collecting duct are ADH responsive. Activation of ADH receptors on the basolateral membrane of collecting duct cells promotes the insertion of water channels, called aquaporins, within the collecting duct cells, permitting water movement from the lumen to the interstitium; this allows the collecting duct to equilibrate with the interstitium, producing a maximally concentrated urine of 1200 mosmol kg^{-1}. The osmotic gradient found within the kidney is dependent upon the activity of the thick ascending limb. When the thick ascending limb is maximally active, an osmotic concentration of up to 1200 mosmol kg^{-1} can be established within the renal interstitium. In the absence of ADH, a maximally dilute urine corresponding to the concentration of the filtrate leaving the distal tubule is produced — 50 mosmol kg^{-1}.

The collecting ducts and more distal parts of the distal convoluted tubule are hormone responsive. The proximal tubule and thick ascending limb are responsible for the reabsorption of up to 95% of filtered Na^+; however, this process of reabsorption is largely independent of hormonal control. Within the more distal nephron Na^+ reabsorption is to a large extent under the control of hormones such as aldosterone and atrial natriuretic peptide. The presence of aldosterone increases expression on the luminal membrane of Na^+ channels, permitting the entry of Na^+ into the cells. In the absence of aldosterone, 3–4% of filtered Na^+ may be lost in the urine. When

aldosterone is maximally present and renal function is normal, urinary Na^+ loss may be reduced to as little as 1 mmol l^{-1}.

Clinical relevance

The potassium sparing diuretics, spironolactone, amiloride and triamterene, have their effects on the collecting duct. Spironolactone is a direct aldosterone antagonist and is effective only in hyperaldosteronaemic states. Amiloride and triamterene inhibit the transtubular transport of NaCl by blocking luminal channels.

The final osmolality of the urine is determined within the collecting duct. Volume contraction occurs in patients taking diuretics, which stimulates ADH release. In such patients the presence of ADH leads to water abstraction from the collecting duct and the production of a concentrated urine. Abstracted water is reabsorbed into the peritubular capillaries, leading to dilution of plasma Na^+. Since thiazide diuretics do not affect the thick ascending limb, the interstitial concentration gradient is unaffected by their use and consequently thiazides, although less potent than loop diuretics, may cause hyponatraemia, due not to Na^+ deficiency but to excessive water retention. The efficient operation of the thick ascending limb is essential to the establishment of an osmotic gradient within the interstitium of the kidney. If such a gradient is not established ADH will have decreased effect upon the reabsorption of water. Thick ascending limb activity is inhibited by the loop diuretics. The effect is that, while increased ADH production may be induced by loop diuretics, water abstraction from the collecting duct is reduced. Hyponatraemia is therefore less likely to occur with loop diuretic use than with the use of thiazides. Hyponatraemia is particularly likely with the use of thiazides with long half-lives.

Patients with impaired renal function due to decreased nephron reserve may not be able to establish an effective concentration gradient within the interstitium. In the absence of such a gradient, ADH is ineffective and a state of nephrogenic diabetes insipidus results.

Renal blood flow and oxygen consumption

Glomerular filtration is not an oxygen intensive process. Most oxygen utilised by the kidney is required for the activity of Na^+,K^+-ATPase. Since tubular cells facilitate the movement of Na^+ across the tubular border, Na^+,K^+-ATPase activity, and hence oxygen consumption, is directly proportional to the amount of filtrate reabsorbed and, as described above, reabsorption is a tubular function.

The tubular capillary network is supplied from the efferent arteriole via the vasa recta. Because of the close apposition of incoming, highly oxygenated vasa recta and outflowing, less well oxygenated vasa recta, it is believed that oxygen diffuses from the incoming to the outgoing vasa recta, leaving the interstitium of the kidney hypoxic.

Clinical relevance

In situations of physiological stress, e.g. hypoxia, hypotension, locally active prostanoids, particularly PGE_2, produce local vasodilatation, increasing interstitial blood flow. They also inhibit the transport of Na^+ across the luminal membrane, reducing the activity of Na^+,K^+-ATPase and hence reducing oxygen consumption. NSAIDs in times of stress may significantly increase interstitial hypoxia and cell damage by reducing interstitial blood flow and increasing transtubular Na^+ transport. Drugs such as amphotericin promote increased Na^+ movement across cell membranes and therefore induce increased oxygen consumption as a result of increased Na^+,K^+-ATPase activity. Under situations of stress, these drugs, by increasing oxygen consumption, may induce hypoxic cellular injury, leading to acute tubular necrosis.

CONTROL OF RENAL FUNCTION
Sodium

As described above, the reabsorption of filtered Na^+ is the most energy intensive process performed by the kidney. Na^+ is the principal extracellular cation; it is the main determinant of extracellular volume, and consequently intravascular volume, and it is also a major contributor to extracellular osmolality. Maintenance of extracellular volume, and hence total body sodium and sodium concentration, is essential to the regulation of the internal environment and the kidney plays a key role in this. Although the kidney functions to maintain total body sodium and sodium concentration, it does so only in response to signals from a variety of sensors.

Total body sodium

The principal determinant of extracellular volume is total body sodium. The daily intake of sodium is 100–300 mmol day^{-1}. The plasma Na^+ concentration is 140 mmol l^{-1} and, as the normal glomerular filtration rate is 180 l day^{-1}, the total amount of Na^+ filtered each day is 25 000 mmol. To maintain total body sodium the amount excreted by the kidneys each day must be equal to the amount taken in, i.e. of the 25 000 mmol Na^+ filtered each day only 150 mmol or 0.5% is lost in the urine. Should more than this be lost extracellular volume depletion and hypotension will result. Should more than this be reabsorbed, extracellular volume expansion will occur, leading ultimately to the development of pulmonary oedema. Total body sodium is not monitored by the body but, as extracellular volume is determined by total body sodium, indicators of extracellular volume act as signals of total body sodium to the kidney. These are blood pressure, renal perfusion and atrial stretch. Increased atrial stretch leads to the release of atrial natriuretic peptide, which promotes increased glomerular filtration and decreased Na^+ reabsorption by the renal tubules. Similarly, increased intravascular volume increases cardiac output and blood pressure. This leads to inhibition of sympathetic activity, which induces increased renal Na^+ loss. Increased renal perfusion, as a result of increased blood pressure, inhibits the release of renin and consequently reduces aldosterone production, leading to increased

Na^+ loss by the kidney. Conversely, decreased intravascular volume leads to increased sympathetic tone, increased aldosterone production and inhibition of release of atrial natriuretic peptide.

Plasma sodium concentration

The normal intake of water each day is roughly $30 \, ml \, kg^{-1}$ or approx $2 \, l \, day^{-1}$. Plasma sodium concentration is a reflection of both total body sodium and total body water. Of the 2 litres of water taken in each day, roughly 500 ml is lost insensibly. The remainder is excreted by the kidneys. If more water is taken in each day than is lost, hyponatraemia will result; on the other hand, excessive water loss results in hypernatraemia.

A fall in extracellular osmolality leads to a fall in intracellular osmolality. This can only be achieved, in the short term at any rate, by movement of water from the extracellular to the intracellular space. Similarly, increased extracellular osmolality is followed in the short term by the movement of water from the intracellular to the extracellular space.

Plasma osmolality is tightly regulated between 275 and 290 $mosmol \, kg^{-1}$. Increased osmolality stimulates the release of ADH from the posterior pituitary. Stimulation of collecting duct ADH receptors results in increased water movement from the lumen to the interstitium via aquaporins, leading to a concentrated, lower volume urine. Simultaneously, the thirst centre is stimulated, leading to increased water intake. When plasma osmolality falls, ADH release is inhibited, thirst is reduced and a dilute urine is produced because water abstraction cannot occur in the absence of water channels.

Clinical relevance

Plasma sodium concentration is a function of both total body sodium and total body water. Hyponatraemia is commonly encountered in hospital practice. It may be due to decreased total body sodium or increased total body water. If due to sodium depletion it should be treated with sodium repletion; if due to excess water it should be treated by water restriction. It is important to be able to distinguish between the two situations because management of each condition is quite different.

Total body sodium is the principal determinant of extracellular volume. In the hyponatraemic patient, if there is evidence of volume contraction (hypotension, postural hypotension, decreased skin turgor, etc.) then total body sodium is probably decreased and the patient should be treated with Na^+-containing fluids. On the other hand, if the patient appears euvolaemic or there is evidence of volume expansion (oedema, hypertension, pulmonary congestion), then, even in the presence of hyponatraemia, total body sodium is not decreased and the administration of Na^+-containing fluids is inappropriate. The management is water restriction rather than Na^+ administration. While in the oedematous patient it is possible clinically to recognise that total body sodium is increased, the situation in the non-oedematous patient is more difficult, and although clinical parameters such as blood pressure may be helpful, accurate determination of the state of hydration may necessitate the insertion of a central line and measurement of central venous pressure.

Hypernatraemia is much less frequently encountered clinically than hyponatraemia because it is a hyperosmolar state that induces thirst in a conscious patient, which in turn leads to increased water intake and correction of $[Na^+]$. Hypernatraemia may arise as a result of water depletion or excess total body sodium. As in hyponatraemic states, distinction between the two requires clinical assessment. Increased total body sodium leads to increased extracellular volume, increased blood pressure and the development of oedema. In the absence of signs of volume expansion, water deficiency is more likely to be the cause. Treatment of hypernatraemia due to water deficiency involves the administration of water, while hypernatraemia due to increased total body sodium necessitates salt restriction.

Potassium

Potassium is the most abundant intracellular ion, being found in a concentration of approx. 150 mmol l^{-1}. Only 2% of total body K$^+$ is found in the extracellular space, the concentration being in the range 3.5–5 mmol l^{-1}. Na$^+$,K$^+$-ATPase is the enzyme responsible for establishing the gradient between the intracellular and extracellular compartments. The maintenance of the low extracellular [K$^+$] is essential to normal neuromuscular function and even small changes in extracellular [K$^+$] may lead to serious complications, such as arrhythmias and muscular paralysis.

As is the case with Na$^+$, both total body K$^+$ and extracellular [K$^+$] are regulated. The kidney is principally concerned with the regulation of total body K$^+$ and, although this has an effect upon extracellular [K$^+$], the regulation of the ratio of intracellular to extracellular [K$^+$] is a function of Na$^+$,K$^+$-ATPase and is affected by multiple factors, including [H$^+$], hormones, such as insulin and catecholamines, and the availability of oxygen.

Total body potassium

Total body K$^+$ is a function of the balance between daily intake and output. Daily intake of K$^+$ is roughly 1 mmol kg^{-1} or 70 mmol day^{-1}. Of this, almost all is excreted by the kidney. Some is lost through the gastrointestinal tract and in sweat but this is not under physiological control. Within the proximal tubule, thick ascending limb and early distal nephron, almost all filtered K$^+$ is reabsorbed. The excretion of K$^+$ is a function of secretion by the principal cells of the collecting duct. The hormone promoting K$^+$ secretion, as has been mentioned above, is aldosterone.

Aldosterone release from the adrenal is stimulated by angiotensin II. States of volume contraction that lead to decreased renal perfusion and activation of the renin–angiotensin system are associated with hyperaldosteronism and increased K$^+$ secretion.

Aldosterone production is also induced by increased plasma [K$^+$]. Thus a rise in plasma [K$^+$] will itself induce hyperaldosteronism, and conse-quently increased secretion of K$^+$ by the principal cells. Hyperaldosteronism increases the expression of Na$^+$ and K$^+$ channels on the luminal border of the principal cells, leading to increased K$^+$ secretion and Na$^+$ reabsorption. Increased K$^+$ secretion may also be induced also by increased distal urine flow.

Renal failure or a failure of aldosterone production both lead to reduced K$^+$ excretion and increased total body K$^+$.

Extracellular potassium concentration

The extracellular [K$^+$] is closely regulated. The kidney is involved in regulation of plasma [K$^+$], in so far as alteration of total body K$^+$ will affect it. However, the precise regulation of [K$^+$] is a function of multiple factors, particularly Na$^+$,K$^+$-ATPase activity, which is influenced by several factors, including extracellular pH, insulin, catecholamines and [K$^+$] itself.

Extracellular pH

Extracellular pH is controlled within a narrow physiological range. Alteration in [H$^+$] is prevented in large measure by buffering. Much of the body's buffering capacity is provided by the movement of H$^+$ from the extracellular to the intracellular compartment. Electrical neutrality across the cell membrane is maintained by the movement of K$^+$ from the intracellular to the extracellular space in exchange for H$^+$. States of metabolic acidosis are therefore usually associated with the development of hyperkalaemia, as a consequence not of increased total body potassium but of movement of K$^+$ from the intracellular to the extracellular compartment.

Catecholamines and insulin

β$_2$ agonists, such as adrenaline, promote the movement of K$^+$ from the extracellular to the intracellular compartment. Similarly insulin promotes the movement of K$^+$ from the extracellular to the intracellular space.

Clinical relevance

Renal failure leads to a failure of K$^+$ excretion

and the development of hyperkalaemia because of increased total body K^+. Hyperkalaemia also occurs in states of hypoaldosteronism. In both of these cases, total body K^+ is increased. The only effective long term treatment is to promote K^+ loss from the body — in the case of hypoaldosteronism by the administration of mineralocorticoid and in the case of renal failure by promoting improved renal function or by dialysis therapy.

Hypokalaemia may also be life threatening and may arise as a result of depletion of total body K^+ or as a result of alteration of the ratio of intracellular to extracellular K^+. Depletion of total body K^+ occurs when gastrointestinal losses are excessive, as in severe diarrhoeal and vomiting states. K^+ depletion may also occur as a result of hyperaldosteronism. Normally extracellular $[K^+]$ is within the range 3.5–5 mmol l^{-1}. Patients with $[K^+]$ less than 3 mmol l^{-1} are in considerable K^+ deficit and require repletion. The maximal rate of K^+ repletion is roughly 10 mmol h^{-1}.

Hyperkalaemia may occur by shift of K^+ from the intracellular to the extracellular space without a change in total body K^+. This situation arises in insulin deficient patients, those taking non-cardioselective β blockers and in situations of metabolic acidosis. It may also occur in hypoxic patients where oxygen intake is insufficient to meet the demands of Na^+,K^+-ATPase, allowing K^+ to diffuse from the intracellular to the extracellular compartment. Under these circumstances, hyperkalaemia should be treated by correction of the underlying problem.

Life threatening hyperkalaemia occurring as a result of increased total body K^+ may also be treated, in the short term, by promoting the movement of K^+ from the extracellular to the intracellular space — by the administration of insulin, catecholamines and by the correction of metabolic acidosis. While these measures may be helpful in preventing fatal arrhythmias, in the longer term management must be aimed at the reduction of total body K^+. Calcium gluconate should also be administered as a membrane stabilising agent.

Hydrogen ion

The normal plasma $[H^+]$ is 40 nmol l^{-1}. Although several orders of magnitude lower in concentration than other ions, such as Na^+ and K^+, even small alterations in $[H^+]$ lead to significant changes in pH. The kidney contributes to H^+ homeostasis by regulation of HCO_3^- concentration. This is achieved by two mechanisms: firstly, by reabsorption of almost all filtered bicarbonate, and, secondly, by the regeneration of HCO_3^-, a process that involves the secretion of H^+.

The normal daily load of H^+ is approximately 1 mmol kg^{-1} day^{-1} or 70 mmol day^{-1}. H^+ is initially buffered within the plasma, limiting alteration of pH. The principal physiological buffer is HCO_3^-. In the process of accepting H^+ ions, HCO_3^- is consumed. In the proximal tubule, as described above, HCO_3^- is reabsorbed but is not regenerated by this process. The process of HCO_3^- regeneration occurs in the collecting duct and is a function of the intercalated cells. These cells secrete H^+ and in the process HCO_3^- is generated within the cells. This HCO_3^- is transported from the basolateral border of the cell in association with Na^+. H^+ secreted by the intercalated cells is lost in the urine, either as NH_4^+ or as titratable acid. Quantitatively, NH_4^+ is of much greater importance.

Although of central importance in the regulation of $[HCO_3^-]$, acid–base disturbances arising from disordered renal function are much less common than metabolic disturbances, such as ketoacidosis or lactic acidosis (described elsewhere). Respiratory disturbances also lead to acid–base disturbance (also dealt with elsewhere).

Conclusion

The kidney is of central importance in the regulation of electrolyte, acid–base and water balance. It is the site of action of many commonly administered drugs. An understanding of renal physiology helps in the management of many clinical disturbances of fluid and electrolytes. It may prevent the inappropriate administration of drugs that may induce nephrotoxicity.

34

Drugs in renal disease

J. P. Alexander

The annual incidence of acute renal failure in the UK is about 180 per million. Substantial renal impairment may occur in up to 5% of patients undergoing major surgery, and the mortality is high (20–80%). Prevention is therefore important, particularly as modern methods of treatment do not appear to have led to improvements in survival.

Tubular function

The proximal renal tubules receive the brunt of drug induced injury. There is progressive concentration of toxic drugs and metabolites as water is absorbed during passage down the nephron. Proximal tubular damage is common, although mild injury may not be obvious. Some drugs concentrate in cells during repeated administration (e.g. gentamicin), while ischaemia and vasoconstriction may lead to extensive damage and acute renal failure. The medullary thick ascending limb of the loop of Henle has a high oxygen demand and low oxygen supply from the medullary countercurrent exchange and is thus particularly vulnerable to relatively mild hypoxic insults.

Influence of renal disease on pharmacokinetics

Drugs are cleared by passive glomerular filtration and by active tubular excretion and may return to the circulation by passive reabsorption from the renal tubule. Drug clearance is the sum of renal and non-renal clearance and may be estimated from the former. As renal function deteriorates, the concentration of endogenous substances in urine increases. Blood urea is a poor index of renal drug elimination, being influenced by protein uptake, metabolism, hepatic function, heart failure, gastrointestinal haemorrhage and urine output. Plasma creatinine depends on age, sex and muscle mass but is easily determined, and is usually an adequate measure of renal function.

Inulin clearance is the marker of choice for quantifying glomerular function, but is impractical for routine clinical work. Clearance of endogenous creatinine gives a reasonable indication of glomerular filtration, the normal value for a 70 kg person being 100–130 ml min^{-1}. Creatinine clearance is calculated from the equation:

$$\frac{UV}{P} = C,$$

where U is the creatinine concentration in urine, V is the volume of urine (ml min^{-1}), P is the creatinine concentration in plasma and C is the creatinine clearance (ml min^{-1}) and approximates to the glomerular filtration rate. However, endogenous creatinine is not an ideal marker either, as it is also eliminated by tubular secretion and non-renal mechanisms. As renal function declines, creatinine clearance progressively overestimates glomerular filtration rate to a peak ratio of approximately 1.7, as clearance as determined by inulin declines to 30 ml min^{-1}.

Bioavailability

Bioavailability and absorption can in theory be altered by multiple factors. In renal failure, gastrointestinal upsets are common and gastric pH may be increased due to urea conversion to ammonia by urease and by the use of antacids. Absorption of ketoconazole, iron salts and tetracycline is pH dependent. Delayed gastric emptying is common, although apparently normal, in patients receiving chronic dialysis. Gastric emptying may be delayed in patients receiving chronic ambulatory peritoneal dialysis during

the treatment phases. In contrast the plasma concentrations of propranolol and other β blockers, dihydrocodeine, encainide and propoxyphene are increased after oral dosage secondary to a decreased first pass metabolism through the liver or gastrointestinal tract.

Drug distribution

Little is known about changes in metabolism in uraemia, but there is a great deal of evidence that drug distribution changes. Apparent volume of distribution (V_D) depends on plasma protein binding, tissue binding and total body water. The catabolism of severe illness will result in decreases in binding proteins. Many drugs are bound to some extent to either albumin (acidic drugs) or α_1-acid glycoprotein (AAG) (basic drugs). Uraemic patients exhibit serum levels of AAG up to three times those seen in normal serum. Clindamycin, lignocaine and disopyramide are all bound to AAG, although free (active) concentrations of lignocaine remain unchanged. On the other hand, binding of acidic drugs to albumin is usually decreased in patients in renal failure. Phenytoin is the classic example, but because the unbound and active fraction may be normal, loading doses should not be altered and maintenance dosage should be closely monitored.

There may be concentration in the central compartment at the expense of the peripheral compartment — the apparent V_D of digoxin is said to decrease by 30–45% secondary to displacement from tissue binding sites by endogenous uraemic substances. Loading and maintenance doses should probably be reduced by one-half to two-thirds of normal.

Conversely, increased apparent distribution volumes have been found for many drugs, including phenytoin, diazoxide, penicillin G and some cephalosporins. These changes in distribution are associated with decreased plasma protein binding, which will increase the apparent V_D and decrease the plasma levels of the drug. A relative hypoalbuminaemia in renal failure allows more unbound or free drug to exist. Highly bound drugs are most likely to demonstrate overdose effects because a relatively small change in binding will lead to a large increase in unbound drug. Cardiac glycosides, benzodiazepines, anticonvulsants, hypoglycaemic agents and neuromuscular blocking drugs all demonstrate this effect. When protein binding is decreased, more free drug is available to distribute to sites of action. Because distribution is increased, plasma levels are lower, yet more drug has passed to receptor sites, where a greater response may be observed than the lower serum level would suggest. Thus low serum levels may not indicate subtherapeutic amounts. Lower protein binding will make more drug available for elimination; in renal failure this will have to be by the hepatic route unless the molecular size allows removal by dialysis. Metabolic acidosis also affects protein binding. Endogenous organic acids accumulate in uraemia, and bind to plasma proteins, thus displacing protein bound drugs. The precise nature of the changes in protein binding in uraemic patients is not understood. The defective binding is not corrected by dialysis but is corrected by successful renal transplantation. It would appear more likely that altered albumin synthesis and structure are involved. Protein binding of some drugs (quinidine, trimethoprim, chloramphenicol) is unchanged in renal failure.

Drug metabolism

Renal failure may have a significant effect on both renal and non-renal mechanisms of drug metabolism. In particular, many drugs undergo hepatic biotransformation to water soluble metabolites before renal excretion, although there are considerable difficulties in investigating the effects of renal failure on the liver. Uraemic inhibitory factors may compete for binding sites within the liver, but changes in protein binding, liver blood flow or changes within the kidney, which contains many of the same metabolic enzymes that are found in the liver, all tend to confuse the picture. The non-renal clearance of imipenem differs in patients with acute versus chronic renal failure. Some metabolites are pharmacologically active; acetylation metabo-

lites of sulphonamides may retain the toxic properties of the parent compound. Norpethidine, the N-demethylated metabolite of pethidine, accumulates in renal failure and can cause central nervous system excitation. Metabolites of cefotaxime and morphine are active, as is N-acetylprocainamide, the main metabolite of procainamide. The minor metabolite of morphine, morphine-6-glucuronide, is pharmacologically active, much more potent than morphine, and accumulates in renal failure.

Dialysis

The normal kidney has both excretory and metabolic functions and is involved in the active production of various substances including renin, erythropoietin and calcitriol (1,25-dihydroxy-vitamin D_3). With progressive loss of renal function, creatinine and urea start to accumulate as the glomerular filtration rate approaches 50% of normal, which is the functional equivalent of loss of one kidney. When creatinine clearance falls to less than 30 ml min^{-1}, patients may become symptomatic, with complaints of fatigue, lack of energy and anorexia. Metabolic disturbances such as hyperphosphataemia, hypocalcaemia, hyperkalaemia, metabolic acidosis and anaemia are common. When end-stage renal disease is reached (creatinine clearance of approximately 10 ml min^{-1}), patients are ill, with malaise, dyspnoea, nausea, vomiting and confusion. At this stage dialysis is indicated to correct the electrolyte and fluid disturbances.

The choice of the dialysis method for the individual patient will depend on the clinical situation and the technical expertise available.

Haemodialysis

Haemodialysis involves the diffusion of small and medium-sized molecules, including uraemic toxins, into a dialysate solution across a semipermeable membrane. Haemofiltration is a form of high permeability treat-ment in which fluid and solutes up to high molecular weight (10 000) are removed without the need for any dialysis fluid. Considerable amounts of infused replacement fluid must be given to the patient to compensate for the transmembrane losses.

Peritoneal dialysis

Although haemodialysis is 10–20 times more efficient than peritoneal dialysis, critically ill patients may react unfavourably to intermittent haemodialysis, with large fluid and electrolyte shifts leading to cardiovascular instability and life threatening arrhythmias. Peritoneal dialysis is a relatively cheap option and can be used where haemodialysis is not available, vascular access fails or the patient is haemodynamically unstable. Continuous ambulatory peritoneal dialysis (CAPD) has been the most successful form of peritoneal dialysis, and here dialysate exchanges are performed by the patient.

Continuous therapies

Continuous slow removal of fluids or solutes by either continuous haemofiltration or by continuous haemodialysis techniques may be tolerated better in some patients with cardiovascular instability, respiratory failure, acute renal failure and multiple organ failure. Techniques include either continuous arteriovenous haemofiltration or continuous arteriovenous haemodialysis. Venovenous techniques (continuous venovenous haemofiltration or haemodialysis) require the use of a blood pump.

Effects of dialysis

Standard dialysis membranes typically remove small molecules of molecular weight less than 500. Drugs of higher molecular weight (e.g. vancomycin) or highly protein bound (phenytoin) or widely distributed in body tissues (digoxin, tricyclic antidepressants) are not effectively removed by dialysis. However high-flux dialyser membranes remove molecules of up to a molecular weight of 10 000 and will therefore remove vancomycin (mol. wt. 1486). A rebound in plasma drug concentrations may occur when drug is removed from the blood more rapidly than it redistributes from tissue compartments. This

phenomenon has been noticed particularly with aminoglycosides and vancomycin, and post-dialysis plasma levels should be measured 2 hours and 6–12 hours after treatments, respectively. In general, the clearance of most drugs by peritoneal dialysis is quite low, although the peritoneal membrane will allow passage of large molecules such as albumin. Drugs that have the potential to be removed in significant amounts include aminoglycosides, vancomycin, amoxycillin, ampicillin, ticarcillin, many cephalosporins, amantadine, 5-fluorocytosine, phenobarbitone, atenolol, sotalol and lithium. If peritoneal dialysis is intermittent, doses of drugs should be administered when the procedure is finished, and routine monitoring of plasma levels performed where appropriate to ensure efficiency and safety. Many antibiotics have been given into the peritoneal cavity and in general the bioavailability and ability to be absorbed into blood exceeds 50%. However, intravenous administration is usually preferred in the treatment of CAPD peritonitis. Amphotericin B is very irritating to the peritoneal membrane. While continuous renal replacement techniques are becoming more popular, drug removal via continuous haemofiltration and haemodialysis is relatively inefficient compared with intermittent haemodialysis, because blood flow rates are quite low. It is impossible to predict in any individual exactly how one procedure may affect drug clearance and therefore plasma drug concentrations should be monitored when possible.

MODIFICATION OF DRUG THERAPY IN RENAL DISEASE AND DIALYSIS

When the glomerular filtration rate is greater than 30 ml min^{-1} it is seldom necessary to modify usual doses, except perhaps for certain antibiotics and cardiovascular drugs. Usually the initial or loading dose is essentially unaltered for patients with renal dysfunction. Maintenance doses are adjusted by either lengthening the interval between doses or by reducing the size of individual doses. In practice a combination of both methods is used. Serum levels are only of value if the time from administration of the last dose and the elimination half-life is known. For best estimate of peak concentration, blood samples should be taken 1–2 hours after an oral dose and 0.5–1 hour after an intravenous or intramuscular dose. It should be remembered that dosing recommendations are usually derived from pharmacokinetic studies performed in patients with stable renal failure and not in patients with acute renal dysfunction.

Diuretic therapy

Loop or high ceiling diuretics, such as frusemide or bumetanide, are the agents of choice, as thiazide diuretics tend to lose their efficacy when creatinine clearance falls to 30 ml min^{-1}. Addition of metolazone may be indicated if the patient is resistant, but this requires careful monitoring (see also Ch. 35).

DRUG NEPHROTOXICITY

Drugs can injure the kidney through dose related toxic effects on the renal vasculature or on tubular epithelial cells, or through non-dose related immunological mechanisms. Among the drugs most commonly incriminated have been the penicillins, thiazides, sulphonamides, paracetamol, frusemide, co-trimoxazole, phenobarbitone, phenylbutazone and rifampicin. Acute risk factors such as volume depletion, aminoglycoside use, exposure to radiographic contrast media, use of non-steroidal anti-inflammatory drugs, septic shock and pigmenturia augment the risk of acute renal failure in the face of drug exposure. A special form of active tubular absorption is pinocytosis, which occurs with drugs of the aminoglycoside group. The drug binds to the luminal brush border of the proximal tubular cell, and a pinocytic vesicle forms which fuses with the lysosomes and then is broken down, causing acute tubular acidosis. Sudden deterioration of renal function is seen when plasma creatinine concentrations reach 200–300 μmol l^{-1} (2.2–3.3 mg dl^{-1}). Table 34.1 lists the non-anaesthetic drugs most commonly associated with deterioration of renal function, although the list is not exhaustive.

Non-steroidal anti-inflammatory drugs

Phenacetin has long been recognised as a cause of papillary necrosis and obstructive uropathy, but the active metabolite paracetamol (acetaminophen *USP*) is widely available. Metabolites of paracetamol, especially *p*-aminophenol, are concentrated in the renal papillae. Oxidised metabolites of *p*-aminophenol bind to sulphydryl-containing tissue macromolecules and deplete stores of reduced glutathione, and cause cell necrosis. However, the most common renal complication of non-steroidal anti-inflammatory drug use is acute prerenal failure due to decreased activity of prostaglandins. Prostaglandins are synthesised in the kidney, and the principal ones PGE$_2$, PGD$_2$ and PGI$_2$ (prostacyclin) are powerful vasodilators. In normal conditions these do not play a big part in the maintenance of the renal circulation, and drugs such as indomethacin have little effect on the kidney. In a patient with increased amounts of vasoconstrictor substances, such as angiotensin II, noradrenaline or antidiuretic hormone, however, vasodilatory prostaglandins become important in maintaining renal blood flow. Clinical conditions such as congestive cardiac failure, cirrhosis of the liver with ascites, diuretic induced volume depletion, salt restriction and the nephrotic syndrome will cause the release of vasoconstrictor substances to maintain blood pressure. In these circumstances inhibition of prostaglandin synthesis (cyclo-oxygenase inhibition) by non-steroidal anti-inflammatory drugs may cause unopposed renal arteriolar constriction, leading to acute renal insufficiency or renal tubular necrosis.

Another form of renal toxicity that may be induced by these drugs is hyperkalaemia. Prostaglandins directly stimulate the release of renin, and the resulting inhibition of cyclo-oxygenase leads to a hyporeninaemic hypoaldosteronism with subsequent hyperkalaemia. Stopping the drug quickly reverses the hyperkalaemia, but serum potassium may need monitoring in patients having potassium supplements or potassium sparing diuretics. Acute interstitial nephritis and the nephrotic syndrome have also been

Table 34.1 Drugs considered to have occasional nephrotoxicity

Group	Drug	Comments
Antibiotics		
Sulphonamides		Crystal formation with earlier members, sulphadimide in normal dosage
	Acetazolamide	Worsens acidosis
	Co-trimoxazole	Deterioration in renal function; trimethoprim preferred; occasional interstitial nephritis
Penicillins		Injectable preparations contain Na^+ or K^+ — reduce dosage in renal failure
Cephalosporins	Second and third generation	Reduce dosage — loading dose unchanged
Aminoglycosides		All toxic; tobramycin and netilmicin preferred to gentamicin: monitor levels
Tetracyclines	Tetracycline,	Toxic, antianabolic effect may produce fatal uraemia
	Oxytetracycline	Toxic, antianabolic effect may produce fatal uraemia
	Doxycycline	Safe — can be used in normal dosage
Antifungal	Amphotericin B	Distal tubular dysfunction
Antituberculous	Rifampicin	Occasional nephropathy — may colour urine red
Analgesics	Phenacetin	Should never be prescribed
	Aspirin	Can cause nephropathy
	NSAID	Isolated reports of renal damage; cyclo-oxygenase inhibition
	Pencillamine, gold	Nephropathy
Sedatives, hypnotics	Barbiturates	Acidosis increases tubular reabsorption
	Phenytoin	Toxic effects and drug interactions common — monitor plasma levels
Cardiovascular	Digoxin	Increased sensitivity with electrolyte disturbances
	β blockers	Reduce dosage
	Antihypertensive	Adjust dosage according to therapeutic response
Diuretics	Thiazides	Not effective if GFR <20 ml min^{-1}
	Frusemide	Effective when GFR <20 ml min^{-1} but occasional nephropathy or dehydration
Cytotoxic, uricosuric	Sulphinpyrazone	Urate crystals deposited in urinary tract
	Allopurinol	Preferred in renal failure
	Cisplatin	Nephrotoxic in one-third of treated patients
Other	Radiological contrast	Occasional deterioration, probably undeserved reputation but may be dose related or associated with volume depletion
	Cimetidine	Accumulates in renal failure, affects metabolism of other drugs
	K^+ deficiency	Leads to nephropathy

GFR, glomerular filtration rate.

described. Any clinical situation in which elevated circulating levels of angiotensin II and catecholamines exist must be considered a high risk setting for the development of non-steroidal anti-inflammatory drug-induced renal failure. Since an activated renin–angiotensin system characterises the anaesthetised state, the implications for anaesthetists are obvious. These drugs are widely used and require careful monitoring.

DRUG USE IN ANAESTHESIA IN THE RENAL FAILURE OR ANEPHRIC PATIENT

The importance of overhydration and underhydration, electrolyte shifts and acid–base distur-bances on the pharmacokinetics of drug action have already been discussed. Drugs that act mainly on the central nervous system must be fat soluble and hence are normally reabsorbed during passage through the kidneys. The duration of action of such agents therefore depends on redistribution, metabolism or excretion via the lungs, and not on renal function. This applies to the intravenous induction agents, opioid anal-gesics and inhalational agents, but not to the water soluble non-depolarising relaxants which are highly ionised at body pH.

Preoperative medication

Virtually all the standard premedicant drugs

have been used, although dosage schedules may need to be modified in view of the increased sensitivity to the undesirable effects of medication that is seen in renal failure patients. Plasma protein binding of both diazepam and midazolam is decreased in end-stage renal failure, and although one active metabolite of diazepam, desmethyldiazepam, is said not to accumulate after repeated dosing, the parent drug certainly will, while the renal clearance of the active metabolite of midazolam, 1-hydroxymidazolam, is decreased.

Induction agents

There is no requirement to reduce the induction dose of thiopentone, but the rate of administration should be decreased to minimise the effects of any relative overdosage of free drug to the heart and circulation. The disposition of etomidate and propofol are unaltered in renal failure, although the latter may produce profound circulatory changes in ill patients. The dose of other hypnotic and sedative drugs may need to be reduced, while the response to neuroleptics is unpredictable.

Choice of muscle relaxant

Acidosis slows down the metabolic degradation of non-depolarising relaxants. Gallamine, tubocurarine and alcuronium have all been used in patients in renal failure and reports of prolonged curarisation recorded. Although pancuronium has generally been satisfactory in clinical practice, as an alternative excretory pathway exists via the liver and biliary systems, there have been isolated reports of prolonged curarisation after its use in renal failure. Since only 15–20% of a dose of vecuronium is excreted by the kidney, and atracurium does not require either renal or hepatic routes for elimination, either should be suitable for the patient with little or no renal function. In critically ill patients receiving vecuronium infusions, the active metabolite 3-desacetylvecuronium may accumulate and give rise to prolonged neuromuscular block lasting several days. Atracurium is probably the best drug available at present. Laudanosine, a major

metabolite of atracurium, has central nervous system stimulant properties in animals. Higher plasma concentrations of laudanosine have been found in patients in renal failure but not in sufficient amounts to produce toxic effects, and it is thought that even prolonged infusions of atracurium in renal failure do not produce levels of laudanosine that are likely to be epileptogenic. New relaxants that require consideration are mivacurium, rocuronium and ORG 9487. The dose of mivacurium required to give good intubating conditions is 0.2 mg kg^{-1}, which leads to significant histamine release that may prove to be unsafe in ill patients. Rocuronium has been used successfully in renal failure patients, although the duration of neuromuscular block was longer than that in normal patients. ORG 9487, an analogue of vecuronium, has a very rapid onset, comparable with that of suxamethonium, and a short duration of action. Renal failure prolongs the duration of action of the anticholinesterase agents neostigmine, pyridostigmine and edrophonium by at least 100%, as they are excreted mainly by the kidney. Patients with chronic renal failure have normal serum cholinesterase unless there is atypical cholinesterase inheritance, so that there is no contraindication to the use of suxamethonium, provided serum potassium levels are not greater than 5.5 mmol l^{-1}.

Inhalation agents

Methoxyflurane is no longer available in the UK. Almost 50% of the drug is metabolised in man and prolonged anaesthesia is likely to produce nephrotoxic concentrations of fluoride ion (50 μmol l^{-1}); oxalate crystals have been found in transplanted kidneys after methoxyflurane anaesthesia. There have been isolated reports of acute renal failure after enflurane anaesthesia in patients with pre-existing renal disease. Although peak inorganic fluoride levels in blood do not produce clinically significant postoperative impairment of renal function in normal patients, there may be a transient impairment after enflurane anaesthesia (serum fluoride levels of 15 μmol l^{-1}). This is evident where the duration of anaesthesia exceeds 2–4 MAC (minimum alveolar concentration) hours. Anaesthesia with all inhalational agents temporarily depresses renal blood flow, glomerular filtration rate and urine production, but there are usually no lasting effects. Halothane in low concentration has been widely used in renal failure and transplant patients. Patients given isoflurane demonstrate no renal impairment after anaesthesia. Either drug can be recommended. These volatile agents have the additional advantage of potentiating the neuromuscular blocking action of many non-depolarising muscle relaxants, especially vecuronium and atracurium, so that dosage of the latter can be reduced. This effect is particularly noticeable with isoflurane. It is too early to speculate as to whether the newest agents, sevoflurane and desflurane, have a place in renal failure patients. Both drugs are expensive. Sevoflurane is less stable than halothane and exposure for 1 MAC hour produced a mean inorganic fluoride level of 22.1 μmol l^{-1}. As yet, there has been no evidence of gross renal damage in man or animals. Desflurane, although less subject to biotransformation than any other agent, is unlikely to replace isoflurane for these patients.

Analgesic drugs

Nearly all the major analgesic drugs cause a fall in urine production and a rise in circulatory antidiuretic hormone levels. Fentanyl or derivatives may be the analgesics of choice in renal failure, although respiratory failure due to unexpected high levels of sufentanil has been described. Although these drugs are rapidly metabolised in the liver, the elimination half-life of fentanyl is prolonged by 45% in renal failure, and the possibility of respiratory depression after continuous infusions into the epidural space should not be dismissed. Norpethidine, the metabolite of pethidine, accumulates in renal failure and has an excitatory effect on the nervous system. Prolonged effects of opioid analgesics in anuric patients have been described, and accumulation of the opioid or its metabolites or enterohepatic recirculation postulated. Evidence that the kidney has an important role in the elimination of opioid narcotics is accumulating. The pharmacokinetics of a single oral dose of

dihydrocodeine is altered in patients in renal failure. Uraemic patients appear to be exceptionally susceptible to the effects of intrathecal opioids. Although the kinetics of morphine are unchanged in patients in renal failure, increased plasma concentrations of morphine-3- and -6-glucuronides and perhaps normorphine are found. Morphine-6-glucuronide is an active metabolite that relies on renal excretion for elimination.

Immunosuppression

Patients undergoing renal transplant require long term immunosuppression with azathioprine, which inhibits purine synthesis. A dose of 5 mg kg^{-1} is given intravenously during the operation, together with a loading dose of hydrocortisone (3 mg kg^{-1}), and both are continued in reduced dosage orally postoperatively. If there is a high risk of rejection, cyclosporin A is given orally in the postoperative period.

Local and regional anaesthesia

The local anaesthetic esters procaine, 2-chloroprocaine and tetracaine undergo enzymatic hydrolysis with plasma cholinesterase. The toxicity of these agents is inversely proportional to their rate of degradation. The metabolism of the amide-type drugs (bupivacaine, etidocaine, lignocaine, mepivacaine, prilocaine and ropivacaine) is more complex. Inactive metabolites formed in the liver are normally excreted by the kidney. Accumulation of metabolites is minimised by the use of the longer acting bupivacaine and etidocaine, which are both highly bound to protein when in the bloodstream. A case of bupivacaine cardiotoxicity in a renal failure patient has been reported. Although renal failure will delay excretion of the metabolites of lignocaine, problems are unlikely to arise unless significant hepatic dysfunction is also present.

Colloid plasma substitutes

When patients with terminal renal failure are infused with hydroxyethyl starch, dextran 40 or gelatine, increases in plasma volumes are greater as compared with normal patients, and last twice as long. Although low molecular weight dextrans do not appear to be nephrotoxic if given in recommended doses to patients with normal hydration and normal renal function, acute renal failure may be precipitated if shock or hypovolaemia is present. The renal tubular cells become grossly swollen with vacuoles containing dextran. With current knowledge of the fate of these substances in the body, their use in patients with poor renal function or those receiving a kidney transplant should be treated with caution. However, some European transplant units use liberal quantities of dextran to maintain adequate plasma volume and a high central venous pressure (1 g kg^{-1} of dextran 40, 60 or 70).

FURTHER READING

Aronson S 1993 Monitoring renal function. In: Miller R D (ed) Anesthesia, 4th edn, pp 1293–1317. Churchill Livingstone, New York

Aronson S 1995 Controversies: should anesthesiologists worry about the kidney? IARS 1995 Review Course Lectures: 68–73

Brezis M, Rosen S 1995 Mechanisms of disease: hypoxia of the renal medulla — its implications for disease. New England Journal of Medicine 332: 647–655

Gillum D M, Brennan S 1992 Acute renal failure. In: Hall J B, Schmidt G A, Wood L D H (eds) Principles of critical care, pp 1899–1912. McGraw-Hill, New York

Grand round 1994 Nephrotoxicity of non-steroidal anti-inflammatory drugs. Lancet 344: 515–518

Hakin R M, Wingard R L, Parker R A 1994 Effect of the dialysis membrane in the treatment of patients with acute renal failure. New England Journal of Medicine 331: 1338–1342

Hunter J M 1994 Muscle relaxants in renal disease. Acta Anaesthesiologica Scandinavica 38(suppl 102): 2–5

Lederer E D, Gillum D M 1992 Dialysis in the critical care patient. In: Hall J B, Schmidt G A, Wood L D H (eds) Principles of critical care, pp 1920–1929. McGaw-Hill, New York

McGeown MG 1992 Clinical management of renal transplantation. Kluwer, Dordrecht

Mazze R I 1990 Anesthesia and the renal and genitourinary systems. In: Miller R D (ed) Anesthesia, 3rd edn, pp 1791–1808. Churchill Livingstone, New York

Mini-symposium: kidney 1992 Current Anaesthesia and Critical Care 3124–3161

Muther R S 1992 Acute renal failure; acute azotemia in the critically ill. In: Civetta J M, Taylor R W, Kirby R R (eds) Critical care, 2nd edn, pp 1583–1597. Lippincott, Philadelphia

Perneger T V, Whelton P K, Klag M J 1994 Risk of kidney failure associated with the use of acetaminophen, aspirin and nonsteroidal anti-inflammatory drugs. New England Journal of Medicine 331: 1675–1679

Ronco P M, Flahault A 1994 Drug induced end-stage renal disease. New England Journal of Medicine 331: 1711–1712

St Peter W L, Halstenson C E 1994 Pharmacologic approach in patients with renal failure. In: Chernow B (ed) The pharmacologic approach to the critically ill patient, 3rd edn, pp 41–79. Williams & Wilkins, Baltimore

Suthanthiran M, Strom T B 1994 Medical progress: renal transplantation. New England Journal of Medicine 331: 365–376

Sweny P 1995 Management of acute renal failure in the intensive care unit. Current Anaesthesia and Critical Care 6: 625–628

Turney J H 1994 Acute renal failure — some progress? New England Journal of Medicine 331: 1372–1374

35

Diuretics

C. C. Doherty

Diuretics are used in a diversity of disorders but their principal application remains that of conditions associated with excessive extracellular fluid, where the object of treatment is to produce a decrease in oedema without compromising the circulating blood volume. The proper use of diuretics requires knowledge of their pharmacology and understanding of the fundamental role which the kidney plays in body salt and water homeostasis.

GENERAL CONSIDERATIONS

Actions on the kidney

The clinical efficacy of a diuretic is related to a variety of factors, including site and duration of action, rate of excretion, dietary sodium intake, the activity of counterregulatory mechanisms (renin–angiotensin and sympathetic systems) and diuretic dose. Diuretics are almost all highly protein bound and enter the urine primarily by the organic anion or cation secretory pathways in the proximal tubule. Spironolactone does not require access to the tubular lumen because it diffuses into the collecting tubule across the basolateral membrane and then binds to the cytosolic aldosterone receptor. Once within the lumen, the ability of loop and thiazide diuretics to inhibit sodium reabsorption is partly dose dependent, being determined by the rate at which the diuretic is delivered to its luminal site of action (Rose 1991). The most powerful natriuretic agents are frusemide and ethacrynic acid, the thiazides are of moderate strength, while acetazolamide, amiloride, triamterene and spironolactone are weak diuretics.

The currently available compounds can be divided into five groups on the basis of their preferential effects on different segments of the nephron involved in tubular reabsorption of sodium chloride and water (Lant 1985):

1. Loop diuretics — a heterogeneous group of agents that act on the thick ascending limb of Henle's loop and have a powerful short lived diuretic effect, complete within 4–6 hours.
2. The benzothiadiazines and related variants, which localise their effects to the early portion of the distal tubule.
3. The potassium sparing diuretics, which act exclusively on the sodium–potassium hydrogen exchange mechanism in the late distal tubule and cortical collecting duct. The action of drugs in groups 2 and 3 is prolonged to between 12 and 24 hours.
4. Diuretics chemically related to ethacrynic

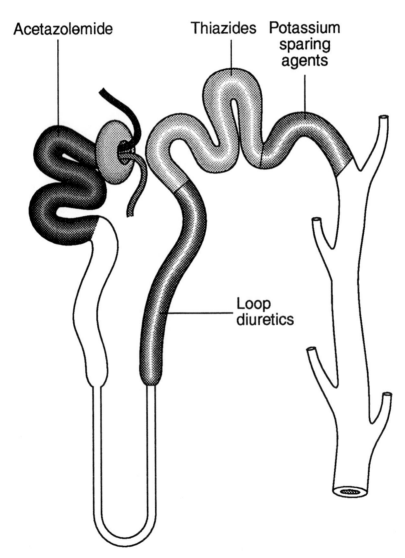

Figure 35.1 Nephron sites of action of individual groups of diuretics.

acid, but with the unusual property of combining within the same molecule the property of saluresis and uricosuria. These compounds have actions to different individual extents in the proximal tubule, thick ascending limb and early distal tubule and are known as polyvalent diuretics.

5. A mixed group of weak or adjunctive diuretics, which includes the vasodilator xanthines such as aminophylline, and the osmotically active compounds such as mannitol (Fig. 35.1).

Diuretics may also be classified according to mechanism rather than site of action.

Thus some diuretics may be classified as transport inhibitors, as they inhibit ionic transport processes for sodium, chloride and bicarbonate ions in the renal tubule; they are the most important group in clinical usage. The mechanisms of inhibition involved vary: thiazides interfere with the Na^+,Cl^- cotransporter in the distal tubule, acetazolamide affects the rate limiting step of the carbonic anhydrase catalysed conversion of carbonic acid to carbon dioxide, and loop diuretics decrease sodium reabsorption by competing for the chloride site on the $Na^+,K^+,2Cl^-$ cotransporter. Spironolactone competitively inhibits aldosterone binding to its cell receptor, resulting in an increase in the number of open sodium channels.

Various salts and crystalloids, e.g. urea and mannitol, are non-absorbable and act as osmotic agents. Such agents may induce a diuresis despite the maximal operation of pituitary antidiuretic hormone (ADH), and will therefore prevent the usual postoperative oliguria that occurs due to release of this hormone. Osmotic diuretics act via their effects on tubular fluid composition and renal perfusion and not by interaction with specific transporters.

Lithium carbonate and demeclocycline are not true diuretics but are known to block the effect of ADH on the collecting duct, thus promoting loss of water without significant loss of solute, an effect utilised to treat states of inappropriate ADH release. Such agents have been termed aquaretics, and other small peptide antagonists of vasopressin with aquaretic activity may be clinically available in the near future.

Endogenous natriuretic peptides stored in the heart and vascular endothelial cells have been shown to cause natriuresis, vasodilatation and suppression of the renin–angiotensin system. Diagnostic uses may be defined in the future for plasma measurements of these peptides, while therapeutic roles may be found for neutral endopeptidase inhibitors which decrease their metabolic breakdown (Struthers 1994).

In addition to the effects of diuretics on monovalent ion excretion by the kidney, there are also important effects on divalent ion excretion (calcium, phosphate, magnesium), acid–base balance and uric acid excretion.

Clinical use of diuretics

The following discussion on clinical use of diuretics is centred on disorders that are common in anaesthetic practice; other conditions in which diuretic therapy is of value (nephrolithiasis, hypercalcaemia, etc.) are not considered here (Table 35.1).

Cardiac failure

Diuretics are an essential component of the treatment of both acute and chronic left heart failure; they reduce the main symptoms of heart failure (oedema, fatigue and shortness of breath) by increasing renal sodium excretion, so reducing circulating blood volume and oedema. In acute left heart failure, their venodilator effect offers a useful additional property.

Table 35.1 Indications for diuretics

Oedematous disorders	Non-oedematous disorders
Cardiac failure	Hypertension
Liver disease	Recurrent nephrolithiasis
Renal disease	Nephrogenic diabetes insipidus
	Acute dilutional hyponatraemia
	Acid–base disorders
	Forced diuresis in poisoning
	Glaucoma
	Mountain sickness

The pathophysiological response of the kidneys to heart failure closely resembles the physiological response to hypovolaemia. In both states, baroreceptors sense a fall in pressure which results in release of ADH, an increase in sympathetic nervous tone and activation of the renin–angiotensin system. In hypovolaemia the resulting salt and water retention ceases when venous volume is restored. By contrast, in heart failure, salt and water retention may continue, despite adequate filling of the venous system, so long as the cardiac output remains inadequate. The extent to which increasing venous return can increase stroke volume (via the Frank–Starling mechanism) is limited, however, and knowledge of the configuration of the Frank–Starling curve is an important consideration before diuretics are administered for preload reduction. If the heart is on the flat portion of the Frank–Starling curve, relatively little change in stroke volume will occur as left ventricular end-diastolic pressure (LVEDP) falls; conversely, on the ascending limb of the Frank–Starling curve, large changes in cardiac index may accompany small decreases in preload (Fig. 35.2). The filling pressure at which the Frank–Starling curve flattens is influenced by ventricular compliance; thus in the stiff failing ventricle, a fall in LVEDP results in a much greater decrease in stroke volume than a similar fall in LVEDP in the failing ventricle with normal compliance. In conditions of left ventricular hypertrophy, such as hyper-

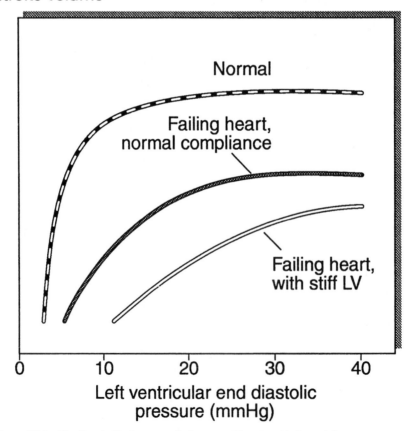

Figure 35.2 The Frank–Starling curve in the normal heart and in heart failure.

tension, aortic stenosis and hypertrophic cardiomyopathy, the heart is operating at end-diastolic dimensions on the steep segment of the Frank–Starling curve, and attempts to reduce elevated filling pressures in these situations may result in important decreases in cardiac index. In this setting, afterload reduction (hydralazine, nitroprusside) and inotropes take precedence over diuretics.

Most of the available data on the acute haemodynamic response to intravenous frusemide are based on studies of patients with acute pulmonary oedema following myocardial infarction. In these patients frusemide administration led to a 'morphine-like' effect, accompanied by a rise in venous capacitance and a fall in pulmonary capillary wedge pressure before any significant fluid loss. The initial fall in preload in such patients following intravenous frusemide is therefore due to venodilatation rather than diuresis. In chronic heart failure or hepatic cirrhosis, diuretics commonly induce an opposite effect — systemic vasoconstriction — occurring before the diuresis and lasting as long as 2 hours.

Diuretics should not be given to patients with acute right heart failure (e.g. due to a large pulmonary embolism or right ventricular infarction), as they may cause a precipitious drop in cardiac filling pressures, hypotension and shock.

The optimal left atrial pressure for any given patient with heart failure depends in part on the underlying aetiology of the heart disease. Vigorous diuretic therapy is recommended in cases of dilated cardiomyopathy to reduce heart size and prevent further dilation. Such patients are likely to have flat Frank–Starling curves and therefore tolerate diuresis without a large fall in cardiac index. Diuretics should be used with caution, if at all, in heart failure associated with abnormalities in diastolic filling, such as in constrictive pericarditis, hypertrophic cardiomyopathy or aortic stenosis.

Diuretics remain the first line treatment for the congestive symptoms of heart failure, with thiazides the initial choice for mild heart failure, while for severe heart failure loop diuretics are indicated. Spironolactone may be a useful additional drug in patients refractory to loop diuretic

therapy. Diuretics can interact adversely with other drugs commonly used in heart failure, especially digitalis, as diuretic-induced hypokalaemia and hypomagnesaemia potentiate digoxin toxicity and cardiac arrhythmias. The initiation of therapy with an angiotensin converting enzyme (ACE) inhibitor drug (captopril, enalapril) in patients taking diuretics may precipitate severe hypotension, and for this reason diuretics should be withheld for several days before starting an ACE inhibitor for congestive heart failure.

Acute renal failure

The term acute renal failure encompasses a number of clinical conditions associated with an abrupt deterioration in glomerular filtration rate (GFR). These conditions include acute tubular necrosis, severe prerenal azotaemia, acute urinary tract obstruction, acute interstitial nephritis and acute glomerulonephritis. In acute glomerulonephritis which is characterised by sodium retention, oedema and hypertension, diuretics may be of considerable value in control of hypertension and pulmonary congestion when present. The use of diuretics in acute tubular necrosis is more controversial.

The reduction in GFR that occurs in acute tubular necrosis may result from a variety of pathophysiological events, including renal vasoconstriction, back-leak of filtrate across damaged tubular epithelia or obstruction of tubular flow by intraluminal precipitation of tubular debris. The relationship between these tubular events and renal haemodynamics is incompletely understood. However, the ability of diuretics such as frusemide and mannitol to induce renal vasodilatation and increase tubular flow rate has led investigators to attempt prevention or alteration of the course of acute tubular necrosis by intervention with diuretics. Despite many studies, the therapeutic efficacy of diuretics in established acute renal failure is unproven; in particular there is no evidence that conversion of oliguric to non-oliguric acute renal failure with use of high dose frusemide has any influence on the mortality of this syndrome (Lameire 1995). The uncritical use of intravenous frusemide when oliguria develops in diverse clinical situations is to be deprecated; if such patients are concurrently receiving aminoglycoside or cephalosporin antibiotics, diuretics may potentiate nephrotoxicity and ototoxicity.

A different issue is the prophylactic use of diuretics in patients at high risk of acute renal failure (patients undergoing open heart surgery, with extracorporeal perfusion, biliary surgery in jaundiced patients, abdominal aortic aneurysm repair, trauma, especially with rhabdomyolysis, and exposure to known nephrotoxins). Prophylactic mannitol given before abdominal surgery in jaundiced patients, or to patients with severe crush injuries, appears to lessen the severity of renal failure in these two settings only. The evidence of a beneficial effect is less compelling in the other disorders mentioned (Reineck 1986). Where incipient acute renal failure is due to hypovolaemia, and volume repletion with central venous pressure measurement has failed to restore a normal urine flow rate, a trial of intravenous mannitol (50–100 ml of a 25% solution) is reasonable. In other instances where a disorder which can cause acute tubular necrosis is known to be present (e.g. acute intravascular haemolysis with haemoglobinuria due to incompatible blood transfusion, rhabdomyolysis with myoglobinuria), prophylactic administration of mannitol is reasonable if acute oliguria develops. This is, however, only effective if given in the early phase and caution is necessary if fluid overload is present, as pulmonary oedema may be precipitated.

Other medical conditions

Liver disease. Despite anatomical normality, the kidney exhibits a wide spectrum of functional derangements in patients with liver disease, including decreased GFR and impaired renal sodium handling.

Treatment of ascites in cirrhotic patients is associated with a high incidence of diuretic-induced complications, including azotaemia, hyponatraemia, hypokalaemia, hyperuricaemia, metabolic acidosis and metabolic alkalosis. Initial therapy must include rigid dietary sodium restriction (10–20 mmol day^{-1}) and fluid restriction to avoid dilutional hyponatraemia. A distal potassium sparing agent, e.g. spironolactone 100 mg b.d., is the drug of first choice, and if no natriuresis occurs with maximum dosage of spironolactone, frusemide 40–80 mg daily should be added. Diuretic combinations in cirrhotic patients are particularly likely to produce a wide array of complications, including massive fluid and electrolyte losses, profound circulatory collapse, hepatorenal syndrome, acute renal failure and hepatic encephalopathy. Patients with liver disease and severe hypoalbuminaemia (less than 2 g dl^{-1}) in whom there is evidence of marked intravascular volume depletion (orthostatic hypotension) may benefit from intravenous administration of albumin concentrate (20% salt-poor, 100–200 ml daily) as part of the treatment regimen. In patients with massive ascites where intravenous diuretic therapy is considered necessary for rapid diuresis, the administration of intravenous albumin before the intravenous diuretic may enhance its efficacy and prevent circulatory complications.

Renal disease.

- *Nephrotic syndrome.* The ideal diuresis is a slow one resulting in a gradual loss of oedema of about 0.5–1.0 kg day^{-1} in an adult patient. Only in certain circumstances is rapid diuresis with intravenous frusemide or bumetamide, usually in association with infusion of volume expanders, indicated.

- *Chronic renal failure.* In the presence of renal insufficiency, diuretic access to the tubular lumen is limited by the decrease in GFR and, probably more importantly, by impaired tubular secretion. It is appropriate to consider separately the indications, benefits and risks of diuretic therapy in patients with chronic renal failure and those with acute renal failure (see above).

The common indications for diuretics in patients with chronic renal failure are hypertension, cardiac failure and nephrotic oedema. The benzothiadiazide diuretics may be effective until the GFR falls below 20 ml min^{-1}. Below this level of GFR, or in the event of unresponsiveness, loop diuretics are necessary, and in some instances high doses of frusemide may be required (40–200 mg daily). Neurosensory hearing loss is a well recognised complication of the potent loop-acting diuretics and is particularly likely to occur in patients with severely impaired renal function, usually in conjunction with high doses. If diuretic therapy causes sufficient depletion of total body sodium, intravascular volume falls; as a result, renal blood flow and GFR may fall, causing exacerbation of renal failure. In the volume contracted state, urea clearance by the kidney is impaired to a greater degree than that of creatinine, and changes in the latter are a more reliable index of adverse diuretic effect on renal function. In view of the risks of potentially lethal metabolic acidosis and hyperkalaemia, potassium sparing drugs should be avoided in patients with chronic renal failure.

Hypertension. The precise mechanism by which diuretics lower blood pressure remains uncertain. Contraction of the plasma and extracellular fluid (ECF) volume appears to play an important role in the initial lowering of blood pressure, but there is also a long term action associated with a lowering of peripheral vascular resistance. A liberal salt intake can overcome the antihypertensive effect of thiazide therapy. The effect of thiazides on the metabolic profile (hyperlipidaemia, hyperglycaemia, hyperuricaemia) is a cause of concern with respect to their long term usage in hypertension.

Although loop diuretics are more potent in terms of natriuresis than the thiazides, their antihypertensive effects are inferior to the former. Loop diuretics are indicated in hypertensive patients in the following clinical situations: (1) hypertension that is primarily volume dependent (e.g. patients with chronic renal failure); (2) hypertensive crises; (3) in combination with antihypertensive drugs that cause fluid retention, e.g. minoxidil, hydralazine.

Failure to respond

The response to a short acting diuretic such as frusemide is that sodium excretion increases above baseline for the 6 hour period that the diuretic is acting, but then falls to low levels for the rest of the day, because the ensuing volume depletion activates compensatory sodium retaining mechanisms. A patient who does not respond to 40 mg of frusemide in the morning should therefore receive an increased single dose of 60 or 80 mg, rather than being given 40 mg twice a day.

Some oedematous patients are, however, resistant to conventional doses of a loop diuretic and this can arise from two general mechanisms, each of which is treated differently. First, the rate of diuretic excretion in cardiac failure, cirrhosis and renal failure can be diminished from renal hypoperfusion or severe hypoalbuminaemia. In this situation increasing the single dose will increase the plasma levels and increase the rate of drug delivery to the kidney. In advanced chronic renal failure (GFR <15 ml min^{-1}) the effective dose can be as high as 200 mg of intravenous frusemide. The second mechanism of diuretic resistance may operate despite adequate levels of drug excretion if there is (1) an increase in angiotensin II, aldosterone and noradrenaline levels in cardiac failure and hepatic cirrhosis, (2) flow dependent distal nephron hypertrophy, and/or (3) a reduction in the number of functioning nephrons in chronic renal failure. In this setting, effective fluid removal sometimes requires administration of the diuretic two or three times a day.

In patients who remain resistant to high dose intravenous loop diuretic therapy given several times a day: (1) 24 hour sodium excretion should be estimated, and if over 100 mmol day^{-1}, adequate diuresis is occurring and the reason for persistent oedema is excess sodium intake; (2) combination therapy with a loop and a thiazide-type diuretic may be tried, or improvment in renal function and therefore diuretic responsiveness may be sought through changes in posture. Patients with cardiac failure and hepatic cirrhosis have renal vasoconstriction that is exacerbated by standing. In this situation supine posture enhances venous return, cardiac output and creatinine clearance. Thus diuretic therapy may be most effective if given in the early afternoon or evening when the patient can remain supine.

Cardiac oedema may require a combination of

diuretic agents that act at different parts of the renal tubule, e.g. use of a loop diuretic with a distal tubule aldosterone antagonist. In resistant heart failure it is rational to combine diuretics with a low dose of an ACE inhibitor (e.g. enalapril 2.5 mg) to block synthesis of angiotensin II and break the vicious cycle of increasing vascular resistance and falling cardiac output. In severe cases of nephrotic syndrome, failure to respond to oral diuretic therapy may occur, and dramatic improvement may follow a change to intravenous administration.

Intravascular volume depletion may exist in some instances of oedematous disorders associated with hypoalbuminaemia (cirrhosis, nephrotic syndrome) — such hypovolaemia causes a decrease in GFR, and the consequent increase in proximal tubular reabsorption reduces the amount of sodium delivered downstream to the site of diuretic action; increased aldosterone secretion may also contribute to the blunting of natriuretic effect. In this situation, infusion of 100 ml of 20% salt-poor albumin before diuretic administration may restore diuretic responsiveness. In chronic renal failure, when the GFR falls below 25 ml min^{-1}, thiazide diuretics are ineffective and loop diuretics are required. The uraemic patient may, however, require dosages exceeding those used in patients with normal renal function, thus in chronic uraemia 250–500 mg frusemide may be necessary to induce diuresis.

Complications of diuretic therapy

Some complications may occur even when diuretics are correctly used, others occur due to injudicious use. Diuretics are the most common cause of adverse drug reactions in old age, which is not surprising as around one-fifth of people over 65 take diuretics. Some complications are common to all diuretics, while others may be encountered with one diuretic but not with others (Table 35.2).

Extracellular fluid volume depletion

Diuretics invariably result in some degree of ECF reduction, which will initiate a sequence of compensatory haemodynamic and hormonal alterations. The haemodynamic changes result in reduced stroke volume and a fall in arterial blood pressure, which causes an increase in heart rate. If cardiac output is not maintained, orthostatic hypotension, dizziness and syncope will be the presenting complaints. The compensatory hormonal changes that occur are an increase in the circulating levels of aldosterone and ADH. The primary purpose of the compensatory changes is to correct the compromised ECF volume by enhancing renal salt and water retention, they will also, however, aggravate several other side-effects of diuretics by reducing the excretion of urea, uric acid, calcium and free water, while increasing the excretion of potassium.

Table 35.2 Complications of diuretics

Thiazides	Loop diuretics	Potassium sparing diuretics	Carbonic anhydrase inhibitors
Hyperlipidaemia	Urinary retention	Hyperkalaemia	Metabolic acidosis
Hypercalcaemia	Ototoxicity	Gastrointestinal upset	Nephrolithiasis
Impotence		Nephrolithiasis	
		Metabolic acidosis	
(Common to both)			
Hypovolaemia, hypotension, uraemia			
Hypokalaemia			
Hyponatraemia, hypernatraemia			
Metabolic alkalosis			
Hyperuricaemia			
Hyperglycaemia			
Induction of hepatic encephalopathy			
Hypersensitivity reactions			

Hypokalaemia

Three main factors regulate distal potassium secretion: the intracellular potassium content, the intratubular fluid volume and rate of flow, and the intraluminal negativity that develops consequent to the reabsorption of sodium. By affecting these three mechanisms, diuretics augment the urinary excretion of potassium. Two additional side-effects of diuretic therapy which also promote distal potassium wasting are diuretic-induced volume depletion (resulting in secondary hyperaldosteronism) and metabolic alkalosis (increases intracellular potassium). The frequency with which hypokalaemia will develop, and its severity, depend on several factors, namely: the dosage and duration of action of the diuretic agent, dietary potassium and salt intake, the age of the patient and the level of circulating mineralocorticoid activity.

The major symptoms of potassium depletion are fatigue, muscular weakness and ultimately paralytic ileus. Serious side-effects of hypokalaemia result from the myocardial irritability that develops, predisposing to ventricular arrhythmias, especially in the setting of acute myocardial infarction or concurrent digitalis therapy. However, diuretics do not usually cause important reduction in total body potassium and available evidence suggests that hypokalaemia requires correction only when the plasma potassium falls below 3 mmol l^{-1} (Morgan & Davidson 1980). Contrary to universal belief, loop diuretics are less likely than the thiazides to cause important hypokalaemia.

Potassium sparing agents, such as amiloride, triamterene or spironolactone, reduce potassium loss by their action on the distal tubule, and may induce dangerous hyperkalaemia when given to: (1) patients with reduced GFR (less than 30 ml min^{-1}), (2) diabetic patients who may have hyporeninism, (3) patients taking potassium supplements or potassium-containing salt substitutes, and (4) elderly patients with age related reduction in GFR.

Azotaemia and renal failure

Diuretic administration can result in decreased renal function. Initially, the rise in blood urea is consequent to the tubular compensatory mechanisms mediated by ECF volume depletion (increased tubular reabsorption of salt and water is accompanied by increased absorption of urea). The subsequent reduction in the rate of urine flow further reduces the excretion of urea, as the clearance of urea is a function of urine flow rate. This results in a rise in blood urea at a time when the GFR is still close to normal; hence the clearance of creatinine, which depends on filtration, remains normal. Consequently, the ratio of urea concentration to that of creatinine rises disproportionately, giving the classical findings of prerenal azotaemia.

Hyponatraemia

This is a common complication of diuretic therapy which may develop acutely in oedematous states, especially if a loop diuretic is used, or insidiously when a thiazide is used. In general, the degree of hyponatraemia is modest and the patient is asymptomatic. Severe hyponatraemia (Na$^+$ below 120 mmol l^{-1}) is rare, and may produce symptoms ranging from muscle cramps, apathy and altered mental status to coma. The principal mechanism by which diuretics cause hyponatraemia is impairment of the ability to dilute the urine appropriately. The loop diuretics interfere with sodium reabsorption in the ascending limb of Henle's loop, and thus limit the amount of solute-free water that the kidneys can generate. The thiazides act in the distal convoluted tubule and also impair urinary dilution but not concentration (which is primarily a medullary function).

Treatment of diuretic-induced hyponatraemia depends on the aetiology and severity of the disorder. Mild asymptomatic hyponatraemia will usually respond to a reduction in, or discontinuation of, diuretic therapy combined with fluid restriction. Severe symptomatic hyponatraemia, on the other hand, is a medical emergency with significant risk of death or neurological morbidity. Acute symptomatic, severe hyponatraemia of any aetiology should be corrected to mildly hyponatraemic levels (125–130 mmol l^{-1}) within

24 hours, using hypertonic saline. It is important to avoid rapid overcorrection to eunatraemic levels as this may result in a specific central nervous system lesion of pontine myelinolysis (Laureno & Karp 1988). Paradoxically, the loop diuretics, specifically frusemide, are used in therapy of acute severe hyponatraemia of dilutional type (e.g. the TURP syndrome). In this situation frusemide is administered in conjunction with intravenous hypertonic saline.

Hypernatraemia

The urine produced by all diuretic agents is relatively hypotonic to plasma, at least until the compensatory mechanisms result in the preservation of free water and production of a concentrated urine. As such, the initial response is one of increased free-water clearance as urine flow rates increase, an event that is particularly evident with osmotic diuretics such as mannitol. If, at this stage of diuresis, the ability of the patient to drink or express thirst is impaired, as in stroke victims, then hypernatraemia will ensue. If undetected and uncorrected this may progress to hyperosmolar coma, and such coma may erroneously be attributed to the cerebrovascular accident rather than the electrolyte disorder.

Metabolic alkalosis

This is a common complication of diuretic therapy. Three main mechanisms are involved in the generation and maintenance of diuretic-induced metabolic alkalosis: volume depletion, mineralocorticoid excess and potassium depletion. A rise in circulating aldosterone levels may result in increased exchange of sodium for hydrogen ion and increased bicarbonate reabsorption by the distal nephron. Potassium depletion can result in intracellular acidosis, thus stimulating secretion of hydrogen ion by the renal tubule and therefore the absolute amount of bicarbonate reabsorption. Correction of diuretic-induced metabolic alkalosis requires normalisation of ECF volume with isotonic saline solutions and correction of potassium depletion.

Metabolic acidosis

This acid–base disorder will invariably develop with the use of carbonic anhydrase inhibitors and often, although to a lesser degree, with potassium sparing diuretics. The most common use of carbonic anhydrase inhibitors (e.g. acetazolamide) is in the treatment of chronic glaucoma, and the observation of unexplained metabolic acidosis in elderly patients should always prompt a query for ophthalmic medications. The potassium sparing diuretics, by blocking distal sodium reabsorption, will interfere with the ability of the distal tubule to secrete hydrogen, thus reducing the ability of the kidney to generate bicarbonate. Spironolactone is particularly prone to induce acidosis because of its specific antialdosterone effect.

Miscellaneous complications

Hypersensitivity reactions that have been reported with diuretics include skin rash, acute pancreatitis, acute interstitial nephritis, vasculitis, pulmonary oedema and haematological disorders. Deafness, occasionally irreversible, has been reported with frusemide and ethacrynic acid given in large doses. Muscle pain and cramps may occur with loop diuretics given in high doses. Gastrointestinal disturbances may occur with any of the diuretic agents, but are especially common with spironolactone. Urinary retention may be precipitated by vigorous diuresis in elderly male patients with partial prostatic obstruction. Triamterene may induce nephrolithiasis, with stones that contain triamterene. Chronic spironolactone administration has been associated with a variety of endocrine disorders, including impotence and gynaecomastia in males, and breast soreness and irregular menstruation in females. This is most likely the result of the antiandrogenic effect of spironolactone at receptor sites. Triamterene blocks dehydrofolate reductase and may cause megaloblastic anaemia and pancytopenia. This appears to occur exclusively in patients with alcoholic cirrhosis who take high doses of the drug.

Volume depletion induced by diuretics has

been associated with an increased incidence of venous thrombosis and pulmonary embolism, particularly in the paediatric age group and in patients with severe nephrotic syndrome.

Important drug interactions

The combination of frusemide and first generation cephalosporins is nephrotoxic, and in the past was one of the most common causes of drug induced acute renal failure. Thiazides, because they decrease sodium reabsorption in the proximal tubules, indirectly may increase reabsorption of lithium and induce lithium toxicity in those with mania receiving long term treatment with lithium. The hypokalaemia which may result in combination with steroids and carbenoxolone has already been referred to. Non-steroidal anti-inflammatory drugs (NSAIDs) such as indomethacin may inhibit the diuretic response to frusemide, this may occur because prostaglandins have an effect on salt transport at the site of action of frusemide. In elderly patients the combination of diuretic therapy with NSAIDs or ACE inhibitor drugs is a common cause of acute renal failure. The loop diuretics displace warfarin from its binding site to albumin, resulting in the acute availability of the free anticoagulant to exert its effect, hence the intermittent tendency to increase the prothrombin time when these agents are used together.

INDIVIDUAL DIURETIC DRUGS

Benzothiadiazines (thiazides and hydrothiazides)

Pharmacology

All benzothiadiazines possess a chlorine or pseudohalogen group at position 6 and a sulphamoyl group at position 7. They are highly protein bound and, like the loop diuretics, are thought to gain access to their renal locus of action via the probenecid-sensitive organic acid secretion pathway. They depress sodium chloride transport in the distal tubule just proximal to the site of potassium exchange and cause moderate natriuresis equivalent to 5–10% of the filtered sodium. The major difference between the various benzothiadiazines lies in the time course of their biological activity: whereas, for example, bendrofluazide has an elimination half-life of only 3 hours, the half-life of hydroflumethiazide is 17 hours, and that of polythiazide is approximately 26 hours. These differences reflect variations in lipid solubility, volumes of distribution and renal clearances.

Chlorthalidone and clorexolone are members of the pthalimidine group and both possess prolonged biological activity with elimination half-life of approximately 40–50 hours. The quinazolinones, in particular metolazone, have been the subject of much study, as it appears they have some distinctive features not shared with conventional benzothiadiazines. In particular, metolazone is able to retain its natriuretic potency in advanced renal insufficiency, resembling in this respect the loop diuretics.

The chlorobenzamides — clopamide, indapamide and xipamide — may be considered together. Clopamide and indapamide have been introduced as diuretics, but indapamide is unusual in being marketed as a fixed dose, single drug therapy specifically for the treatment of hypertension. At low dosage it exerts negligible saluretic effects, yet effectively lowers blood pressure by reducing vascular smooth muscle tone. At higher doses indapamide shares with the other two compounds the classic renal locus of action of the benzothiadiazines — the cortical diluting site. The elimination half-life of clopamide is about 6 hours, that of xipamide is about 14 hours and that of indapamide is about 15–20 hours.

Indications

Benzothiadiazines are used mainly to relieve oedema due to moderate heart failure when the patient is not desperately ill and severe pulmonary oedema is not present. They are also used in small doses to lower blood pressure, either alone or in combination with other antihypertensive drugs, and their hypotensive effect is probably due to reduction of plasma volume combined with reduced peripheral vascular resistance.

Side-effects

Benzothiadiazines have a number of adverse effects and, in addition to those listed in Table 35.2, they have been reported to cause neonatal thrombocytopenia when given in late pregnancy. Mild hypokalaemia occurs commonly, but only certain patients are at sufficient risk to require measures to correct this. Prevention of hypokalaemia in such patients may be achieved by addition of potassium supplements (e.g. Slow-K or Sando-K tablets, which contain 8 and 12 mmol of potassium, respectively), or a potassium sparing diuretic, to maintain the plasma potassium at 3.5 mmol l^{-1} or above.

Dosage

The thiazides differ in potency on a weight-for-weight basis and are usually given as an oral daily dosage, e.g. cyclopenthiazide (Navidrex) 0.5–1.0 mg or chlorthalidone 50–100 mg. It has been shown that cyclopenthiazide 0.125 mg (one-quarter of the conventional dose) produces a similar hypotensive effect to 0.5 mg of the drug without adversely affecting the biochemical profile (McVeigh et al 1988).

LOOP DIURETICS
Frusemide (furosemide *USP*)

Frusemide is a sulphonamide derivative of anthranilic acid but differs chemically and pharmacologically from the thiazides. Frusemide has both haemodynamic and renal tubular effects; the haemodynamic response involves: (1) increased renal blood flow with redistribution of flow from outer to midcortical zones, and (2) reduction in systemic venous capacitance. These effects are probably mediated via the renin–angiotensin system and vasodilatory prostaglandins. Frusemide-induced renal vasodilatation is thought to play only a minor role in the natriuretic response. Frusemide gains access to its site of action by being transported through non-specific secretory pathways for organic acids in the proximal tubule; it subsequently acts to inhibit the active transport of sodium in the thick ascending limb of Henle's loop, and as a direct result the passive absorption of calcium and magnesium are also inhibited. Inhibition of solute absorption in the thick ascending limb markedly inhibits both renal diluting and concentrating ability. The urine tends to be isotonic with plasma or slightly dilute, bicarbonate excretion is increased and urinary pH rises. Potassium loss occurs to a lesser extent than with the thiazides, as the duration of action is shorter and the ion exchange mechanism in the distal tubule is not directly affected. The mechanism of increased potassium excretion in the urine with loop diuretics involves both the indirect effects of increased flow rate and the inhibition of the common transport system for sodium, chloride and potassium in the luminal cell membrane. The natriuresis amounts to 30% of filtered sodium.

Frusemide has a very steep dose–response relationship, which has led to the label 'high ceiling diuretic'. It has a pK_a of 3.80, possesses low lipid solubility and is extensively bound to plasma protein. The onset of action with oral therapy produces a peak diuresis within 20–30 minutes and the major effect of the drug is complete in 3–4 hours. Bioavailability of oral frusemide is approximately 50–60% and the kinetic disposition of the drug fits most closely an open two-compartment model with an elimination half-life ranging from 19 to 100 minutes. The response to intravenous administration occurs within 2–3 minutes. The drug is chiefly excreted in the urine and faeces; only a little is metabolised.

Indications

Frusemide is used in patients with pulmonary oedema and is of particular value by intravenous injection in the emergency situation; it not only induces a vigorous diuresis but also reduces the preload on the heart. Oral therapy is used in patients with long standing cardiac, renal or hepatic oedema who no longer respond to thiazide diuretics. Frusemide can be used with blood transfusion in severe anaemia where cardiac failure is imminent; it allows transfusion without increasing blood volume which would precipitate heart failure.

Dosage

In oedematous disorders the initial dose is usually 40–80 mg and this may be increased to 160 mg daily; in treatment of heart failure, if patients require more than 40–80 mg a day of frusemide, it may be appropriate to add a converting enzyme inhibitor (e.g. captopril 12.5 mg or enalapril 2.5 mg) rather than further increase diuretic dosage. In patients with advanced renal failure, very large doses may have to be given (250–500 mg daily) but deafness is an attendant risk.

Side-effects

The response to loop diuretics may be torrential (e.g. 10 litres in 24 hours) and care must be taken to avoid hypotension and vascular collapse. Other side-effects are as listed in Table 35.2.

Ethacrynic acid

Ethacrynic acid is an aryloxacetic acid derivative and its pharmacological actions closely resemble those of frusemide. The peak diuretic response usually occurs within 15–20 minutes and results in excretion of 15–25% of the filtered load of salt. Intravenous ethacrynic acid can cause acute uricosuria. It has a pK_a of 3.50, possesses good lipid solubility and is extensively bound to plasma protein. Metabolism of the drug involves degradation in both the liver and proximal tubular cells of the nephron. The renal site of action of ethacrynic acid is the thick ascending limb of Henle's loop, where microperfusion studies have shown that it acts by inhibiting active chloride transport. As with other loop diuretics, it is not clear how much of the diuretic response is due solely to direct interference with transport systems at specific membrane sites, and how much to secondary effects resulting from a release of intrarenal mediators and the associated redistribution of blood flow within different zones of the kidney. The conventional oral dosage of ethacrynic acid is 50–200 mg daily or 50 mg by intravenous injection in emergencies.

During studies of ethacrynic acid analogues, compounds were discovered which surprisingly displayed combined saluretic and uricosuric properties (uricosuric saluretics or polyvalent diuretics). Indacrinone is a loop diuretic possessing these dual activities, and this is thought to reflect different renal activities of the constituent enantiomers. Tienilic acid has similar properties.

Bumetanide

Systematic alteration of the basic sulphamoyl benzoic acid structure led to the development of bumetanide in 1975. This powerful loop diuretic is similar to frusemide with the exception of a phenoxy group in position 4 for the pseudohalogen CF_3 normally situated there, and a butylamino substitution at position 3. Bumetanide has a pK_a of 3.60, is highly bound to plasma protein and is rapidly and completely absorbed from the gastrointestinal tract. The elimination half-life is between 60 and 90 minutes. The main renal site of action is the thick ascending limb of Henle's loop, where it inhibits sodium chloride absorption, and the alterations in renal haemodynamics evoked are also similar to those of frusemide. It differs from frusemide in its milligram potency, 1 mg having the equivalent effect to 40 mg of frusemide.

POTASSIUM SPARING DIURETICS

There are four commercially available potassium sparing diuretics. All act on the distal nephron to cause a modest natriuresis (less than 5% of the filtered sodium load), while conserving potassium. Two are steroidal compounds, spironolactone and potassium canrenoate, and their action is to abolish the aldosterone dependent portion of distal sodium reabsorption. The other two agents, triamterene and amiloride, are non-steroidal in structure and they act on luminal transepithelial sodium reabsorption independently of the presence of mineralocorticoids. The major role of these drugs is as potassium sparers in combination with other diuretics in congestive heart failure and hepatic cirrhosis with ascites.

Spironolactone

Pharmacology

Aldosterone enters cells of target organs by diffusion across the plasma membrane, following which it combines with a cytoplasmic receptor protein, and is then translocated as a steroid–receptor complex into the nucleus. This causes enhanced transcription of the messenger ribonucleic acid (mRNA), which is then translated into new proteins within the cytoplasm and also the plasma membranes. The manner in which these mineralocorticoid-induced proteins activate transepithelial sodium transport remains uncertain, but induction of mitochondrial tricarboxylic acid cycle enzymes has been implicated. Spironolactone is a synthetic steroid lactone with structural resemblances to the natural hormone aldosterone, resulting in competition with the mineralocorticoid for binding to its receptor protein in the distal nephron, thereby preventing reabsorption of sodium chloride and increasing potassium reabsorption. It is relatively ineffective when given alone, and is usually given with a thiazide or loop diuretic to obtain added diuretic effect or prevent hypokalaemia.

Indications

Spironolactone is most useful in states where excessive secretion of aldosterone contributes to oedema formation, e.g. cirrhosis. It may also help in oedema of cardiac failure which is resistant to therapy. In Conn's syndrome of hypertension due to an aldosterone secreting adrenal tumour, spironolactone may be useful in both treatment and diagnosis.

Dosage

Spironolactone is readily absorbed from the intestinal tract and is given in tablet form, 25 mg four times a day. Maximum diuresis is delayed up to 4 days, and if the response is inadequate 200 mg total daily dosage may be given.

Side-effects

As spironolactone reduces renal potassium loss, there is a risk of dangerous hyperkalaemia, especially if given to patients with diabetes mellitus, impaired renal function or those treated concomitantly with potassium supplements, ACE inhibitors or cyclosporin. An important point to remember in this context is that commercial salt substitutes, e.g. Selora, consist of potassium chloride. Drowsiness, mental confusion and gynaecomastia are other adverse effects in addition to those listed in Table 35.2.

Potassium canrenoate

This is the potassium salt of one of the important metabolites of spironolactone, and as it is freely water soluble it is available for intravenous use. It has a relative potency, compared with spironolactone, of about 0.30:1.

Triamterene

Triamterene is a pteridine derivative and is not chemically related to other diuretics. It has a pK_a of 6.20, is bound approximately 50% to plasma protein and the elimination half-life is between 2 and 4 hours. It acts on the distal tubule to depress cell membrane permeability to sodium and indirectly decrease potassium loss. It also increases uric acid excretion (thiazides reduce it). It is not a very effective diuretic (maximal natriuresis 2–3% of filtered sodium) and is normally used in combination with other diuretics which inhibit sodium reabsorption in the proximal tubule of loop of Henle. It is well absorbed after oral administration and is excreted partly unchanged and partly in metabolite form. Its effect lasts up to 24 hours.

Indications

Triamterene may be used in cardiac failure, cirrhosis and nephrotic syndrome.

Dosage

The oral dose is 50 mg twice daily but up to 300 mg may be required.

Amiloride

This is a pyrazine carboxamide derivative with a pK_a of 8.70, oral bioavailability of about 50% and elimination half-life of about 6–9 hours. There is no evidence that it undergoes metabolic degradation in humans. Stop flow, micropuncture, microperfusion and microelectrode studies have localised the action of amiloride to the distal nephron, and in particular the cortical collecting duct. It causes modest saluresis with decreased excretion of potassium and a rise in urine pH. It is used in oedematous states and for potassium conservation with thiazide or loop diuretics. The oral dosage is 5–20 mg daily.

Side-effects

All potassium sparing diuretics may cause hyponatraemia, and older patients, especially women, are particularly at risk. Co-amilozide, identified as the proprietary drug Moduretic, accounts for 38% of reports. Hyponatraemia is characterised by failure of ADH suppression despite low plasma osmolality and high fluid intake. The serum sodium can fall as low as 105 mmol l^{-1} without total body salt depletion.

OSMOTIC DIURETICS

Mannitol

Mannitol is a polyhydric alcohol which is filtered across the glomerulus but not reabsorbed to any significant extent in the tubules, and is therefore excreted with its isosmotic equivalent of water. If given orally it will cause osmotic diarrhoea. Because transport processes in the thick ascending limb and more distal nephron remain intact, however, the major diuresis is water and, to a considerably lesser extent, salt.

Indications

Mannitol is most commonly used in cerebral oedema to reduce brain volume and lower intracranial pressure by shrinkage of brain cells. A further application is based on the observation that infusion of hypertonic mannitol causes intravascular volume expansion and dilation of the afferent renal arteriole with increased renal plasma flow and intratubular pressure. These properties have led to its use in preventing acute renal failure in conditions that predispose to development of acute tubular necrosis, e.g. aortic aneurysm surgery or jaundiced patients undergoing surgery. Mannitol has also been advocated in the early stages of acute oliguria following trauma, major surgery or other circulatory insult, the intention of such treatment being to 'open up' the kidney and thereby prevent acute renal failure or convert it from the oliguric to the non-oliguric form. Patients with decreased renal function, however, have diminished ability to eliminate mannitol, with potentially disastrous consequences. Retained mannitol draws water into the intravascular space by osmosis, resulting in hyponatraemia and sudden increase in intravascular volume, which may precipitate pulmonary oedema (Borges et al 1982).

Dosage

Mannitol is given by intravenous infusion of 10 or 20% solution, 50–200 g over 24 hours, preceded by a test dose of 200 mg kg^{-1} by slow intravenous injection.

Side-effects

Chills, fever and thrombophlebitis may occur. Tissue necrosis has resulted from extravasation. The acute expansion of blood volume that occurs with mannitol may precipitate pulmonary oedema. Hyperkalaemia may be worsened in renal failure, as movement of water out of the intracellular compartment creates a chemical gradient favouring potassium exit from cells.

Urea

This is also an effective osmotic diuretic but has side-effects that render it inferior to mannitol. These include arrhythmias, haemolysis and a bleeding tendency.

CARBONIC ANHYDRASE INHIBITORS (acetazolamide, dichlorphenamide)

Acetazolamide

Pharmacology

Acetazolamide acts in the proximal tubule to inhibit the action of carbonic anhydrase. This enzyme facilitates the formation of carbonic acid in the tubular cells, which in turn dissociates to produce hydrogen and bicarbonate ions. The hydrogen ions are exchanged for sodium in the glomerular filtrate so that body sodium is conserved. This reabsorption of sodium in exchange for hydrogen ions requires a supply of hydrogen ions, and this depends on the action of carbonic anhydrase. Inhibition of the enzyme reduces the supply of hydrogen ions, with the result that sodium and bicarbonate remain in the lumen of the tubule. Thus, an alkaline urine with a high sodium bicarbonate content results and the increase in sodium excretion leads to a diuresis.

Potassium excretion is also increased because it normally competes with hydrogen ions in the exchange with sodium, and when hydrogen ion excretion is reduced more potassium will be lost. The excretion of persistently alkaline urine produces a metabolic acidosis, resulting in respiratory compensation by the elimination of carbon dioxide and a reduction in plasma bicarbonate. This in turn inhibits the diuretic effect by reducing the amount of sodium bicarbonate presented to the renal tubules, and drug tolerance develops.

Indications

Acetazolamide and dichlorphenamide are only weak diuretics and have their main application in treatment of glaucoma (they inhibit the formation of aqueous humour and therefore lower intraocular pressure). Acetazolamide has also been used to increase bicarbonate excretion in patients with severe alkalosis (e.g. gastric alkalosis, posthypercapnic alkalosis) and to alkalinise the urine in order to solubilise certain compounds (e.g. uric acid in myeloproliferative disorders). Acetazolamide may prevent mountain sickness by causing metabolic acidosis, which stimulates respiration and therefore minimises hypoxaemia.

Dosage

Acetazolamide is usually given orally, 250 mg–1 g per 24 hours, and the duration of action is about 12 hours.

Side-effects

Hyperchloraemic metabolic acidosis may occur and rarely may be associated with nephrocalcinosis and formation of renal calculi in patients on long term therapy.

COMBINED DIURETICS

The widespread use of fixed combinations of thiazide or loop diuretics with potassium sparing diuretics is illogical, as in most patients long term diuretic therapy has little effect on potassium balance. Potassium sparing diuretics are necessary in only a small minority of patients who develop clinically significant hypokalaemia during use of thiazide or loop diuretics alone, or in whom hypokalaemia is particularly risky, e.g. in patients taking cardiac glycosides or drugs that prolong the QT interval, including sotalol and some other antiarrythmic agents, imipramine and phenothiazines. The debate on preventing potassium depletion has yet to be resolved. Combined diuretic preparations have a tendency to cause hyponatraemia and uraemia in elderly patients with impaired renal function. The use of combined diuretics does not eliminate the need to check serum electrolyte concentration. Some patients go on to develop hyperkalaemia, which is more likely to cause cardiac arrhythmias and sudden death than is potassium depletion.

REFERENCES

Borges H F, Hocks J, Kjellstrand C M 1982 Mannitol intoxication in patients with renal failure. Archives of Internal Medicine 142: 63–66

Lameire N, Verbeke M, Vanholder R 1995 Prevention of clinical acute tubular necrosis with drug therapy. Nephrol Dial Transplant 10: 1992–2000

Lant A 1985 Diuretics; clinical pharmacology and therapeutic use (part II). Drugs 19: 162–168

Laureno R, Karp B I 1988 Pontine and extrapontine myelinolysis following rapid correction of hyponatraemia. Lancet i: 1439–1440

McVeigh G, Galloway D, Johnston D 1988 The case for low dose diuretics in hypertension: comparison of low and conventional doses of cyclopenthiazide. British Medical Journal 297: 95–98

Morgan D B, Davidson C 1980 Hypokalaemia and diuretics: an analysis of publications. British Medical Journal 281: 905–908

Reineck H J 1986 Diuretic use in renal failure. In: Eknoyan G, Martinez-Maldonado M (eds) The physiological basis of diuretic therapy in clinical medicine, pp 277–291. Grune & Stratton, New York

Rose B D 1991 Diuretics. Kidney International 39: 336–352

Struthers A D 1994 Ten years of natriuretic peptide research: a new dawn for their diagnostic and therapeutic use? British Medical Journal 308: 1615–1619

Metabolism and energy balance

SECTION CONTENTS

36

Metabolism and temperature regulation

R. S. J. Clarke

METABOLISM

Metabolism, respiratory quotient and respiratory exchange ratio

The body consumes fuel and produces energy for all the processes of maintaining life. These include the activity of vital organs, such as the heart, liver, brain and secretory glands, the activity of muscle at rest and during exercise and the maintenance of a constant body temperature. Ionic pumps consume about half the resting energy requirement. The energy output is expressed in kcal or kjoules. Metabolism involves the consumption of oxygen and the production of carbon dioxide and the ratio of these and the overall oxygen consumption depend on the nature of the fuel.

When carbohydrate is burned in a bomb calorimeter the chemical reaction is

$$C_6H_{12}O_6 + 6O_2 = 6CO_2 + H_2O$$

That is, the number of CO_2 molecules produced is the same as the number of O_2 molecules consumed. This ratio is known as the respiratory quotient (RQ) and for carbohydrate is 1.0. When carbohydrate is burned in 1 litre of oxygen, $4\,kcal.g^{-1}$ of energy is released.

The corresponding formula for fat is

$$C_{17}H_{35}COOH + 26O_2 = 18CO_2 + 18H_2O$$

and the RQ = 26/18 or approximately 0.7. When fat is burned in 1 litre of oxygen, the energy output is $9\,kcal.g^{-1}$.

The equations for proteins are more complex

and combustion in the body is rarely complete but in a calorimeter the RQ is approximately 0.8 and the energy produced is around 4 kcal.g^{-1}.

In the living organism metabolism is not completed in one process but passes through intermediary stages. However, the end-result is the same and over a long period the RQ represents the diet consumed. Over a short period carbohydrate may be converted into fat with consumption of oxygen but no output of carbon dioxide. Conversely, in violent exercise lactic acid is formed and on entering the blood is buffered by HCO_3^- to yield H_2CO_3 and liberate CO_2. This gives an RQ that exceeds 1.0. Production of lactic acid is by anaerobic glycolysis and builds up an oxygen debt. On recovery from the exercise, oxygen is consumed in excess of the carbon dioxide output and the RQ falls to a low value.

Acidaemia or alkalaemia from metabolic causes can unbalance the output of carbon dioxide with no effect on the oxygen consumption. Purely respiratory changes can also influence the ratio: for instance voluntary hyperventilation can wash out excessive quantities of carbon dioxide with minimal increase in oxygen consumption. In this case CO_2 output from the body does not represent CO_2 production. The CO_2 output:O_2 uptake is termed the respiratory exchange ratio and in stable conditions this equals the body respiratory quotient.

Basal metabolic rate

The term basal metabolic rate (BMR) is given to the energy output of an individual under conditions of complete rest, both physical and mental, in a postabsorptive state and at a comfortable temperature. It is usually expressed in relation to surface area and the BMR of an adult male of 50 years of age is approximately 37 kcal m^{-2} h^{-1}.

Measurement of caloric output is very difficult in man and the figure is usually derived from the oxygen consumption if the RQ is known or assumed. Oxygen consumption is relatively easy to measure by having the patient breathe in and out of a Benedict–Roth bell spirometer filled with oxygen and with a carbon dioxide absorber. The rate of decline of the volume of the spirometer

represents the oxygen consumption. Carbon dioxide production is more difficult to measure and involves collection and analysis of expired gas; hence, this measurement is often omitted and the RQ is assumed in a fasting state to be 0.75. For clinical purposes the BMR is often not expressed absolutely: for instance +50 is used for 50% above the appropriate values for the patient.

Factors influencing the metabolic rate include:

- *Surface area*, which is well correlated with the BMR in healthy individuals; the value quoted is usually per square metre.
- *Age and sex*. The BMR per square metre declines with age from 57 kcal m^{-2} h^{-1} at the age of 2 years to 35.5 kcal m^{-2} h^{-1} at 60 years. At all ages it is higher in males than females (related in part to the lower percentage of fat and hence higher percentage of lean body mass that produces energy in males).
- *Undernutrition*, which reduces the metabolic rate and is a protective mechanism during prolonged starvation.
- *Body temperature*. For every 0.5°C rise in body temperature, the basal metabolism rises by 8%. This is a consequence of the effect of temperature on all chemical reactions. It leads to an increase in oxygen consumption, carbon dioxide production and pulmonary ventilation and these consequences are often a reason for controlling pyrexia in patients.
- *External temperature*. Exposure to a cold environment leads to increased metabolism (e.g. increased muscle tone, shivering) in order to maintain normal body temperature. Exposure to a hot environment also raises metabolic rate by increased cardiac action, sweating and a rise in overall body temperature.
- *Thyroid function*, which has a major influence on metabolic rate, with an increase in thyrotoxicosis of up to +100 and a decrease in myxoedema to as low as –40.
- *Adrenaline*, whether exogenous or endogenous, which increases metabolism for a few hours by stimulating cardiac action and tremor as well as by stimulating catabolism generally.
- *Food*, which generally stimulates metabolism, an effect most marked with proteins and least

with carbohydrates. The effects of a protein meal are more marked 3–5 hours after ingestion, declining slowly thereafter. This effect is known as the specific dynamic action of protein and averages about 20% over 4–6 hours. The mechanism of this (and of fat in the diet) is attributed to a stimulating action on metabolism of fatty acid residues which are left after the —NH_2 groupings have been removed from the amino acids. The small increase in metabolism with carbohydrate ingestion is probably due to energy stored as glycogen rather than glucose and does not represent energy expenditure. Overall, the effect of a mixed diet is to increase metabolism by 50–150 kcal daily.

- *Exercise*, which has the most profound effect on metabolism, with a rise in oxygen consumption from a resting value of 250 ml to as much as 4 litres or more in extremely fit athletes.

Biochemistry of metabolism

The process of total breakdown of foodstuffs into carbon dioxide, water and nitrogenous compounds is known as catabolism. It may conveniently be divided into three phases. The first (digestion) takes place in the gut, in which polysaccharides, fats and proteins are broken down into monosaccharides, fatty acids and glycerol and amino acids. In the second phase these substances are transported to the liver where they are further reduced to acetic acid, α-ketoglutaric acid, oxaloacetic acid and some final residues of CO_2, H_2O and NH_3. During this phase about one-third of the energy available from complete catabolism is released. Finally, in the third phase the above three acids are broken down in various cycles, resulting in further production of CO_2 and H_2O and the release of their residual energy.

All chemical reactions involve energy exchanges and most catabolic processes are exothermic or give out energy. The most important chemical stores of this energy are the phosphate components such as the high-energy adenosine triphosphate (ATP), adenosine diphosphate (ADP), creatine phosphate and others. Low energy phosphates include adenosine monophosphate (AMP), glucose 1-phosphate, glucose 6-phosphate and others of the Embden–Meyerhof pathway.

The other important high-energy store is in acetyl coenzyme A (acetyl CoA). This has the general formula R—CO—S—R_1, the bond between the acid R—CO group and the thio group involving high energy storage. It can be used, for instance, in storing the energy released when pyruvic acid, $CH_3.CO.COOH$ is oxidised to acetic acid, $CH_3.COOH$. Later, when the bond is broken and the acetyl portion split off from the mercaptan, the energy can in turn convert ADP to ATP.

Many forms of tissue oxygenation consist more precisely of addition of water followed by dehydrogenation. This is a form of anaerobic oxidation but requires a hydrogen acceptor; the most common is the coenzyne nicotinamide adenine dinucleotide (NAD). This is converted in the process to NAD.2H, which in the presence of oxygen can be restored to NAD. It is an essential part of the metabolic production of energy to be discussed, although the hydrogenation of NAD itself is not an energy transferring reaction.

Carbohydrate metabolism

The process of digestion (see Ch. 38) results in the breakdown of polysaccharides (e.g. starch) and disaccharides (e.g. sucrose and lactose) to monosaccharides (e.g. glucose and fructose), in which form they can be absorbed into the bloodstream. Once absorbed they circulate as free sugars, to be converted in the liver or muscle to glycogen or be broken down by a complicated chain of reactions to carbon dioxide and water.

Glycogen is the form in which glucose is stored in the body and there are about 60 g in the liver and about 150 g in the muscle. Other tissues store much less glycogen, and the brain in particular depends on a continuous supply of glucose for its metabolic activity, otherwise irreversible damage will follow. Glycogen is a polysaccharide which is insoluble, exerting no osmotic pressure, but is still reactively broken down to glucose when required. However, the glycogen in the muscle can only be used to fuel muscle activity and cannot easily re-enter the blood, even when there is hypoglycaemia. The steps involved in glycogen formation are:

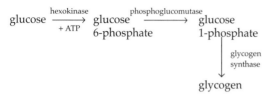

Although glucose is the main source of glycogen, other sugars, together with fatty acids, glycerol and amino acids after deamination, can be stored in this form and all these anabolic reactions are promoted by insulin.

Glycogenolysis or the breakdown of glycogen to glucose occurs through the same intermediaries but different enzymes. The first step involves adenyl cyclase in removing phosphate groups from ATP, leaving cyclic AMP, and transferring the phosphate to active phosphorylase, which in turn catalyses the formation of glucose 1-phosphate. This is converted by phosphoglucomutase to glucose 6-phosphate and in the liver (but not the muscle) glucose 6-phosphatase removes phosphate from the latter to provide free glucose. The whole process is initiated by the presence of adrenaline and glucagon, which stimulate the adenyl cyclase.

Glycolysis or the breakdown of glucose 6-phosphate to pyruvic acid occurs through many intermediaries (Embden–Meyerhof pathway). These are as follows :

glucose 6-phosphate $\longrightarrow$ fructose   (1)
6-phosphate
(fructose and mannose enter the metabolic pathway here)
fructose 6-phosphate + ATP $\longrightarrow$ fructose   (2)
1,6-diphosphate + ADP
fructose 1,6-diphosphate $\longrightarrow 2 \times$ (3)
3-phosphoglyceraldehyde
3-phosphoglyceraldehyde + ADP $\longrightarrow$ (4)
3-phosphoglyceric acid + ATP
3 phosphoglyceric acid $\longrightarrow$ phosphoenol   (5)
pyruvic acid
phosphoenol pyruvic acid + ADP $\longrightarrow$ (6)
pyruvic acid + ATP

The net energy yield from these reactions is conversion of three molecules of ADP to ATP for each molecule of glucose 6-phosphate. In addition, two NAD.2H molecules are produced, which on oxidation yield a further six ATP molecules.

The final phase in the breakdown of glucose to CO_2 and H_2O takes place through the Krebs citric acid cycle with the production of acetyl CoA as the energy transfer mechanism. The chain is:

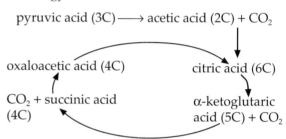

In the breakdown of 1 glucose molecule, 2 pyruvate molecules are formed, yielding, as described above, 8 ATP molecules. However, the dissimilation of the 2 pyruvate molecules to 2 acetyl CoA molecules and the dissimilation of the acetyl CoA to CO_2 and H_2O yields a further 30 ATP molecules.

This whole process is largely dependent on oxygen to regenerate the NAD and fuel the citric acid cycle. In the absence of oxygen (anaerobic metabolism) the Embden–Meyerhof pathway yields only 2 rather than 8 molecules of ATP and pyruvate is converted to lactic acid rather than undergoing complete dissimilation. In addition, the pyruvic acid acts as a hydrogen store by being converted to lactic acid, thus freeing more NAD:

NAD.2H + $\longrightarrow$ NAD +
$CH_3.CO.COOH$ $CH_3.CHOH.COOH$
(pyruvic acid)   (lactic acid)

This reaction is reversible and is not to be regarded as a metabolic pathway but as a temporary expedient until oxygen becomes available for the aerobic dissimilation of pyruvic acid.

Factors regulating blood glucose

The fasting blood glucose level is 4.5–5.5 mmol l^{-1}, with a peak after meals to approximately

7.5 mmol l^{-1} and a fasting trough of 3.5 mmol l^{-1}. The regulation of the blood glucose takes place in the liver and it is there that excess of glucose and other sugars, glycerol, fatty acids and deaminated amino acids are converted into glycogen. The hepatic cells are freely permeable to glucose and the liver is normally pouring out glucose to maintain a steady blood level while other tissues consume it. This process is controlled partly by the balance of glucose itself, the whole variety of intermediates and energy stores such as ATP, NAD and acetyl CoA. However, the hormones adrenaline, glucagon, cortisol and growth hormone tend to raise blood glucose by glycogenolysis and gluconeogenesis from fat and protein residues. The actual glycogen stores in the liver are limited and in starvation last only 24 hours at most, so the importance of gluconeogenesis must be stressed. Muscle tissue can metabolise fatty acids and ketone bodies but the brain can metabolise only glucose and requires a constant supply.

When the blood glucose level rises, insulin, secreted by the β cells of the islets of the pancreas, comes into play. It firstly promotes the entry of glucose from extracellular fluid into cells and then activates enzymes which oxidise it, convert it into glycogen and bring about its conversion to fat and amino acids. In addition insulin antagonises the reverse reactions, glycogenolysis, and gluconeogenesis, and all those hormones that have a catabolic action.

Fat metabolism

The term 'fat' embraces, firstly, triglycerides, which are formed from one molecule of glycerol and three molecules of a fatty acid such as palmitic (with 16 C atoms), stearic (with 18 C atoms) and oleic (with 18 C atoms and unsaturated). Secondly, there are the phospholipids (e.g. lecithin), sphingomyelins and cerebrosides. Thirdly, there are soaps and fat soluble substances such as steroid hormones, cholesterol and certain vitamins that are closely associated with fats.

The digestive phase of the metabolism of neutral fats results in their breakdown into glycerol or monoglycerides and fatty acids and in this form they are taken into the intestinal cells. From this position the longer chain fatty acids (>14 C atoms) with glycerol are reformed into neutral fat and this passes on to the lymphatics as chylomicrons. The remaining fatty acids pass directly to the bloodstream. All these forms of fat and fat derivatives circulate combined with plasma protein as lipoprotein.

The fate of these lipoproteins can be divided into:

1. Storage as neutral fat in fat depots under hormonal control. The stores of fat in the body are large — about 7 kg in an adult, representing more than a month's total food energy, compared with the carbohydrate stores of only 0.5 kg.
2. Oxidation in the liver to produce energy. The first phase is breakdown of fat by hepatic lipase into glycerol and fatty acids. The glycerol then passes through the carbohydrate pathways and the fatty acids are broken up into acetyl CoA units containing 2 C each (β-oxidation). These fragments in turn are completely oxidised to CO_2, H_2O and energy through the citric acid cycle, provided there is sufficient oxaloacetic acid available from carbohydrate metabolism. Once it is used up, this oxaloacetic acid cannot be reformed from acetyl CoA.
3. Fat is built up into the structure of all tissues in the form of lecithins and cholesterol derivatives.

Ketone bodies and ketosis

The 2-C fragments produced by β-oxidation, as described above, have an alternative pathway:

$$\text{fatty acids} \xrightarrow{\text{liver}} \text{2-C fragments} \xrightarrow{\text{liver}} CO_2 + H_2O + \text{energy}$$

$$\downarrow \text{liver}$$

$$CH_3.CO.CH_3 \underset{\text{kidneys}}{\overset{\text{lungs}}{\longleftarrow}} CH_3CO.CH_2.COOH \underset{\text{tissues}}{\overset{\text{other}}{\longrightarrow}} CO_2 + H_2O + \text{energy}$$

acetoacetic acid

$$\updownarrow$$

$$CH_3.CHOH.CH_2.COOH$$
β-hydroxybutyruc acid

The other pathway consists of condensation of 2-C units to form the 4-C molecule acetoacetic acid. This passes out of the liver, circulates at a low level and is metabolised by most tissues in the body as an alternative to glucose. However, if normal oxidation of acetyl CoA in the citric acid cycle slows down, more fatty acids are converted to acetoacetic acid and, as its metabolism is strictly limited, the plasma level rises. Acetoacetic acid can freely convert by dehydrogenation to form β-hydroxybutyric acid, a reversible reaction. It also passes into lungs and urine and by the loss of CO_2 can form acetone. These three products derived from fatty acids are collectively known as ketone bodies.

A low level of circulating keto acids is normal but even brief periods of starvation (e.g. 2–3 days) and insulin deficiency can cause a sharp rise. This leads to a metabolic acidosis and increased excretion of H^+ (buffered by ammonia to NH_4^+) in the urine. As the proportion of fat in the diet increases, ketosis becomes more likely, but there are marked racial differences in ability to tolerate fat. The peoples of northern Canada and Alaska normally have high fat diets that would cause gross ketosis in those used to typical European diets.

Protein metabolism

Proteins are complex molecules consisting of amino acids linked together in chains, and smaller groups of amino acids are known as polypeptides. When foreign protein is ingested, it is broken down in the gastrointestinal tract to its constituent amino acids and only these are absorbed. Free amino acids then circulate in the blood in small quantities until utilised for some particular process. Foreign protein does not normally reach the bloodstream intact and, if it does, dangerous reactions may occur.

Amino acids in the plasma are in dynamic equilibrium with those in the tissues and constitute the 'amino acid pool'. This is purely a functional concept for all body proteins and is constantly in a state of change. Approximately 80–100 g of tissue protein is broken down and resynthesised daily and this is also the approximate daily protein requirement to maintain equilibrium.

Amino acids are lost from the pool by:

1. deamination with excretion of the nitrogenous residues and metabolism of the remainder
2. loss in the urine, which is not reabsorbed
3. Loss in hair, skin and nail formation.

Amino acids enter the pool by:

1. reamination of non-nitrogenous residues in circulation which might come from carbohydrate or fat sources
2. transamination resulting essentially in formation of a new amino acid from amino acid and other residues
3. being absorbed after the breakdown of ingested protein.

Essential and non-essential amino acids

There are about 21 important amino acids, ranging from the simplest, glycine and alanine, to the more complex molecules containing sulphur, iodine, a benzine or other ring or various organic acids. Most of these can be synthesised and transaminated but a few (eight is the current figure) must be taken in as such in adequate amounts for normal growth and development.

The essential amino acids are:

1. Valine.
2. Leucine.
3. Isoleucine.
4. Threonine.
5. Methionine, which can be converted to cysteine — both are important sources of sulphur for such substances as taurine. Methionine is also a source of methyl groups, which are essential for such reactions as conversion of noradrenaline to adrenaline.
6. Phenylalanine — which can be converted to tyrosine, thyroxine and the catecholamines.
7. Tryptophan — which is essential for the formation of 5-hydroxytryptamine or serotonin.
8. Lysine.

In addition, two other amino acids that are required for healthy growth are:

9. Histidine — which is the precursor of histamine
10. Arginine — which forms part of the cycle of urea formation and also takes part in creatine formation.

Metabolism of the amino acids

Amino acids that are not required either undergo transamination to form other amino acids or deamination, both occurring in the liver. Deamination results in the production of ammonia, which is highly toxic and is rapidly converted in the liver cells into urea. However, this process is not a simple combination of NH_3 (2 molecules) + CO_2 (1 molecule) to form $CO(NH_2)_2$ with the elimination of water. Instead the Krebs urea cycle catalyses the process through several intermediaries:

$$\text{ornithine} \xrightarrow{+NH_3+CO_2} \text{citrulline} \xrightarrow{+NH_3} \text{arginine} \rightarrow \text{ornithine} + \text{urea}$$

The resulting urea is almost non-toxic until very high concentrations are reached, and is normally eliminated steadily by the kidney.

The non-nitrogenous residues of amino acids enter the common metabolic pool and may be broadly classified into glucogenic and ketogenic. The former break down to pyruvic acid and enter the citric acid cycle. The latter break down to acetyl CoA, requiring adequate oxaloacetic acid for full metabolism.

It is apparent from the concept of an amino acid pool that the urinary urea cannot be said to come solely from ingested protein and amino acids. However, it is largely exogenous in origin and on a protein-poor diet only a minimum of urea is produced (and for this reason the urine volume falls greatly). Most of the sulphur, and hence of the acidity of the urine, is also derived from ingested sulphur-containing amino acids (in meat).

The creatinine in the urine is largely derived from endogenous metabolism and is unaffected by diet. It is formed from surplus creatine phosphate in the muscles and, although more is lost during muscular work, the 24 hour output is remarkably constant.

Metabolic acidosis

This is also referred to as non-respiratory acidosis and is characterised by a low plasma bicarbonate or base deficit, which is accompanied by a lowered blood pH, although this may be partly compensated for by a fall in the arterial P_{CO_2}. The principal causes are:

1. Anaerobic metabolism, as described above, which results in the production of lactic acid from glucose, instead of full breakdown to carbon dioxide and water, with the much greater energy yield. It is a normal accompaniment of exercise but also occurs when the blood supply of the tissues is inadequate for their metabolic needs, due to such causes as cardiac failure, peripheral vascular disease or hypovolaemic shock.

2. Ketoacidosis, where fat metabolism ends with acetoacetic acid and β-hydroxybutyric acid rather than complete catabolism. This happens when there is inadequate insulin for breakdown of acetyl CoA, as in diabetes, or inadequate acetoacetic acid in the citric acid cycle, as in starvation.

3. Renal failure, leading to inability to conserve bicarbonate and selectively secrete hydrogen ions. As a result, a diet rich in protein with its sulphate and phosphate residues will result in metabolic acidosis.

4. Excessive loss of bicarbonate from the digestive tract. This occurs in all forms of severe diarrhoea, such as infantile gastroenteritis, cholera and dysentery. Specific surgical causes include small bowel fistula and ileostomy, with loss of large volumes of alkaline secretions.

Obesity

The topic of obesity is included here for convenience, but it must be stressed that it is a nutritional rather than a metabolic disorder. It results essentially from an intake of food in excess of the energy expenditure. Causes include overfeeding in early childhood, an environment predisposing to excessive intake of food or alcohol, loss of interest in one's appearance and a sedentary lifestyle.

The general effects are entirely harmful, the obese being prone to hypertension and atheroma of the main vascular beds and to diabetes. Excessive weight also causes strain and wear on the joints of the back and lower limbs. There are many added risks in subjecting obese patients to anaesthesia but, in particular, the condition predisposes to reductive metabolism of halothane.

TEMPERATURE REGULATION

Purpose of temperature regulation

The internal temperature in man is normally maintained at a relatively constant level (36.5–37.5°C) in spite of wide changes in environmental temperature. This constancy of the internal environment, known as homeothermia, is not a feature of all animal species and is exhibited only by birds and mammals. The reason for the constancy must be, as Claude Bernard put it, 'La fixité du milieu intérieur est la condition de la vie libre'. More precisely, it can be said that by providing a uniform temperature at which enzymes can act, their efficiency is improved, and the higher animals gain an advantage over simpler forms. However, it must not be thought that the temperature of the whole body remains constantly within the above range. There is minor physiological cycling with time and there are gross anatomical variations from one part to another.

Variation in temperature between different regions of the body must be considered first because, only after defining what is meant by body temperature, is there any meaning in its regulation. The temperature of the 'core' of the body varies little but within the core the liver is the hottest part and therefore probably the main source of heat production. The temperature in the blood of the heart and great vessels is about 0.25°C lower than that of the liver. The rectal temperature is almost the same as the latter but may rise above it and this can only mean that the faeces are a source of heat production. Even if this source of confusion is not clinically important, the faeces do insulate a thermometer in the rectum from rapidly-occurring changes else-where. The best indication of core temperature is probably the aortic blood and the nearest point for measuring this is the middle of the oesophagus. This is therefore the best site for detecting rapid changes, although mouth or rectum are more convenient and quite adequate for detecting diurnal changes.

While the temperature of the core may be relatively constant, its extent is not. That is to say, in warm conditions the core embraces all but the surface of head, thorax and abdomen and extends into the upper arms and legs. Under cold conditions, not only the skin but all the muscles of the body wall and limbs are allowed to cool so that the temperature of vital tissues is maintained.

The muscle temperature at rest is probably 30–35°C, according to the distance from the heart, but during exercise it rises rapidly above that of the core. Skin temperature varies more widely still, from an axillary temperature very close to that of the aorta and a hand temperature under comfortable conditions similar to that of muscle, to finger temperatures of 5°C under cold conditions. In extreme conditions this may lead to freezing of extremities (frostbite). As in the heart and brain, function in peripheral tissues depends on temperature. Muscles and joints move more slowly when cold, and tactile acuity falls off. While the possible temperature range in skin and muscle is greater than in the central tissues, the optimum for complicated functions is probably not greatly different.

Normal variations in body temperature

Diurnal variation is the natural cycling of temperature from a low point at about 4 a.m. to a peak around 8 p.m. The range is about 36.0–37.3°C and is probably mainly due to the rise during the working phase of the day and a falling off in the resting phase. The cycle is reversed during regular night work.

Menstrual variation. The morning temperature is at its lowest during menstruation, rising slowly thereafter but exhibiting a further sharp rise during ovulation and remaining higher during the second half of the cycle. The mechanism appears to be the thermogenic action of progesterone and its metabolic products.

Age. Infants and old people have less efficient temperature regulating mechanisms. Marked rises occur in babies with crying and minor illnesses and undue stress cannot be placed on such peaks of temperature. However, equally important is the inability to maintain temperature when anaesthetised or debilitated, in part due to deficient regulation but also to the high ratio of body surface area to mass. Any vasodilatation during anaesthesia therefore leads to a rapid loss of heat unless temperature is monitored and maintained artificially. Old people also can become hypothermic due to low metabolic rate in the presence of debility, alcoholic intoxication or minor degrees of myxoedema.

Control of body temperature

Body temperature is usually raised by internal heating, but heat can be taken up via the skin or digestive tract. Cooling, on the other hand, is usually due to a fall in environmental temperature. The temperature regulating mechanisms are therefore regulated to continuous loss of heat and, since man's environment is nearly always colder than 37°C, the extent of the loss must be regulated. This regulation is not equally efficient under all circumstances and man combats heat or cold more effectively if he has been previously exposed to them, i.e. if he is acclimatised.

Central temperature receptors. The concept of a central area for detecting temperature changes and correcting them has given way, as in the control of respiration, to the concept of a central coordinating area with both central and peripheral temperature receptors. Experiments at the beginning of the twentieth century showed that destruction of an area in the anterior hypothalamus abolished the ability to regulate body temperature. Furthermore, receptors sensitive to heating have been stimulated in animals, both electrically and by heat, and sweating and vasodilatation obtained. Discharge from single neurones has even been correlated with local hypothalamic temperature. It has been harder to demonstrate the existence of cells sensitive to cold but there is some evidence for it. However, there must also be a mechanism for altering the 'setting' of the central regulation. The diurnal and menstrual rhythms and the situation during fever suggest that these influence the temperature regulating centre to maintain temperature constant at a different level. In man it can be shown that, at any one time, the receptors are sensitive to changes of ±0.2°C.

The existence of these central receptors can be simply demonstrated by the experiment of immersing a leg, with the circulation occluded, in hot water for 1 hour. Although the limb becomes very uncomfortable, there is no generalised sweating or vasodilatation until the tourniquet is released and warm blood flows centrally. A different mechanism may be demonstrated by exposing the leg to radiant heat. Within 25 seconds there is vasodilatation in the hand and a rise in heart rate, which occurs whether the circulation from the irradiated area is free or occluded. A rapid, nervously-mediated response to cold can be also shown, so there are clearly central and peripheral thermal receptors that play a synergistic role in response to temperature change, the cutaneous receptors being rapid in action and able to prevent any central change rather than waiting for it to occur.

Heat production

This may be divided into:

1. Basal heat production (BMR), occurring throughout all the tissues of the body but particularly in the liver, which is the centre of most of the metabolic processes (see above). This amounts to about 40 kcal m^{-2} h^{-1} or about 1700 kcal day^{-1}.
2. Additional heat production as a result of work that takes place in all the working muscles and in the cardiac muscle. This increases the basal heat production by 1000–1300 kcal day^{-1} but in heavy work 1000 kcal h^{-1} is possible.
3. Additional heat production due to the specific dynamic action of protein metabolism and of food generally (see above).

4. Additional heat production to maintain temperature when cold. This includes purely behavioural responses such as voluntary muscular effort, thermal muscle tone, which is an irregular discharge of nerve impulses at different frequencies, and true shivering. Shivering involves rhythmic discharge of nerve impulses and is mediated in the central nervous system by the rubrospinal rather than the pyramidal tracts. Initiation of shivering is normally by impulses from the skin and it is a common experience that non-specific impulses can evoke a shiver if the body is cold. However, it has been shown that cold blood flowing up the internal carotid arteries to the hypothalamus can also be responsible for shivering and this mechanism probably governs the severity of shivering under normal circumstances.

Heat loss

This is almost entirely from the skin in man and is brought about by the four standard physical mechanisms of radiation, connection, conduction and evaporation. Small amounts of heat are also lost in the expired air, urine and faeces.

Radiation means transfer of heat from a warmer body to a cooler one without direct contact. It can occur through air or a vacuum and depends on surface area and the temperature difference between the surfaces. It occurs from exposed surfaces and to some extent from clothes (which in turn are heated by conduction), and in temperate climates accounts for about 60% of heat loss. However, because the skin temperature changes little from resting to hot conditions it is not a flexible source of heat loss. Alternatively, heat may be taken up by radiation, as from an electric heater or the direct rays of the sun.

Conduction is the transfer of heat within one material or between two substances that are in contact. Again the extent of heat transfer depends on temperature differences but also on the conducting properties of the materials. For instance, air and water are bad conductors of heat, as are wood, paper, fat, clothing and the various synthetic insulations, but metals are good conductors. It follows therefore that within the body conduction is not an important method of heat transfer, the outward flow of warm blood being the only significant factor. Because of the small area of tissue in contact with solid objects there is little heat loss by this means, but rapid conduction does explain the danger of touching metals at temperatures below zero.

Convection consists of the warming of the air next to the skin. This air rises, to be replaced by cooler air, and the greater the flow of air, the greater the heat loss. The same phenomenon also occurs in water but the rate of flow of the water is too slow for it to be important. In both air and water, convection can be greatly aided by movement, so that the fluid next to the skin is carried away more rapidly, to be replaced by cold air and water. The same mechanism applies in reverse when exposed to a hot wind or hot water, although the former, if dry, will facilitate evaporation.

Evaporation means the conversion of molecules of water in the liquid phase to the gaseous phase; the process is accompanied by the uptake of heat from the surroundings. In quantitative terms, when 1 g of water is converted into water vapour, 0.58 kcal of heat is taken up from the skin, or 580 kcal l^{-1} of sweat. This amount is huge compared with the 100 kcal required to raise the temperature of 1 litre from 0 to 100°C. This is the most important means of heat loss when the body temperature is rising and is facilitated by dryness and movement of the surrounding air. It is the only means available when the air temperature rises above that of the body. In addition, about 300 ml of water are lost with the expired air per day, giving a heat loss of about 200 kcal. This is uncontrolled in man but plays an important part in the dog.

Control of cutaneous blood flow. All the above methods of heat loss depend upon transfer of heat from the deep tissues to the surface. Transfer by conduction is inefficient and slow, so the main route is via the bloodstream. Heat loss by radiation, convection and conduction is governed by the skin temperature, which depends on both capillary vasodilatation and blood flow. The main areas of heat elimination are the palmar surfaces of the distal phalanges, with diminishing activity in the more proximal phalanges and the hands. This gradation is proportional to the number of arteriovenous anastomoses in these areas and experiments with nerve blockade have shown that the control is largely by the degree of sympathetic vasoconstrictor tone.

The efficiency of the skin of body and proximal parts of the limbs as areas of heat loss is reduced by a covering of hair or clothing. It must be emphasised, therefore, that the peripheral arteriovenous anastomoses provide the most rapidly acting and complete degree of vasodilatation in the body. There is also evidence for the release of a vasodilator polypeptide, bradykinin, in the sweat glands, which, spreading through the skin, dilates the vessels surrounding the gland. A secondary factor in heat loss within the limbs is the countercurrent arrangement of an artery surrounded by two venae comitantes. As the blood travels down the vessel it gives up heat to the blood returning centrally, thus protecting the core from the extreme degrees of venous cooling. In cold conditions nearly all the venous return in the limbs is by these deep veins.

Sweating

Water comes to the skin surface by two mechanisms: insensible perspiration and sweating.

Insensible perspiration is due to simple diffusion through the epidermis and is almost continuous and uncontrolled. It amounts to 600–800 ml day^{-1}.

Sweating occurs through two types of gland, eccrine and apocrine. The eccrine glands are responsible for temperature regulation and occur all over the body, particularly on the palms, soles and head. They are under the control of sympathetic nerves but in this instance the transmitter is acetylcholine, atropine having an inhibitory effect. The sweat secreted contains sodium, potassium, chloride, urea and lactic acid. The sodium chloride concentration varies from 0.1 to 0.4% and one of the adaptations of acclimatisation to tropical environments is a reduction in the salt content of sweat, due possibly to increased adrenocortical activity. Heavy sweating results

in losses as high as 1.5 litres in an hour, which can continue throughout the day. Replacement of the water loss is instinctive but excessive sodium loss can result in cramps and other signs of extracellular dehydration, unless sodium chloride is given as well. Acclimatisation results not only in the production of a more dilute sweat but sweating also occurs at a lower skin temperature. In heat-adapted people the ability to sweat is increased and a given level of physical work can be carried out with less rise in core temperature.

The apocrine glands are mainly associated with the hair follicles and are in the axilla and round the genitalia. They are stimulated by adrenaline and are responsible for the sweating of fear, excitement or nausea.

Control of thermal sweat secretion, like the skin blood flow, is by both central and peripheral mechanisms. The central control can be demonstrated more easily by the inhibition of sweating when the hands are suddenly cooled. Sweating ceases after 1–2 minutes but only if the circulation to the hands is free. However, more recent experiments have also shown a very good correlation between 'deep' skin temperature and the rate of sweating.

Hyperthermia

Fever

This means a raised central temperature due to excess of heat production over heat loss and can result from:

- infections due to a wide variety of organisms
- destruction of tissue, as in many non-infective diseases, neoplasms, rheumatic fever, etc.
- damage to part of the basal ganglia or hypothalamus resulting in loss of control.

The term pyrogen is applied to substances that produce fever, most commonly products of bacterial and leucocyte breakdown. They are lipopolysaccharides and were often found as contaminants of intravenous infusions before disposable materials became universal. They are not destroyed by boiling or autoclaving but only by dry heat at 160°C. Since as little as 0.1 µg injected intravenously in man can produce fever, adequate removal has proved very difficult.

It seems that the bacterial pyrogen reacts with a substance in the plasma to produce endogenous pyrogen. It, in turn, acts on the temperature regulating centre to 'set' the mechanism at a higher level. The effect of this is an intense vasoconstriction accompanied by shivering, which persists until the 'desired' temperature is reached.

Heatstroke

This is rare in temperate climates but occurs in older people exposed to hot conditions in cities, as well as in troops and others in deserts without adequate water. The temperature may rise to 44°C, the patient is comatose with a dry skin and often incontinent. Recovery is possible with rapid surface cooling. The cause has nothing to do with action of the sun's rays on the back of the neck, as was once thought, but is rather a failure of sweating due to dehydration. It is also likely in temperatures around 40°C with around 100% humidity because sweating can only cool the body when the sweat evaporates freely.

Hypothermia

The physiology of lowered body temperature is the same whatever the cause, but the emphasis below is on controlled hypothermia for surgical procedures or therapeutic hypothermia, while special problems of accidental hypothermia will be described later. Hypothermia is present when the core temperature falls by 5°C or more. The term 'moderate' hypothermia is usually applied to body temperatures of 25–30°C, and 'profound' hypothermia to 5–10°C.

Metabolism

Reduction of the oxygen *requirement* of the specialised tissues (brain, liver, heart, etc.) is the main purpose of controlled hypothermia and, although it is only possible to measure oxygen *consumption*, all the evidence is that they are in fact the same:

- The oxygen consumption during rewarming is no greater than during cooling for the same temperature.
- There is no increase in blood lactate during rewarming unless there has been circulatory arrest.
- There is no damage to vital organs after moderate hypothermia unless there has been gross venous congestion. Damage to the brain after profound hypothermia is rare and is probably due to excessively rapid cooling with development of temperature gradients.

V'ant Hoff in 1884 showed that the rate of a chemical reaction fell exponentially with temperature and this has been shown to be true of oxygen consumption. Experimentally the Q_{10}, or ratio of oxygen consumption at 37°C to oxygen consumption at 27°C is about 2.1 and this ratio continues to apply as the temperature is lowered (5% per degree centigrade). It is, however, difficult to achieve the same temperature throughout the body, therefore only an approximation to the ratio can be arrived at. Carbon dioxide production also falls in a similar manner.

Cardiovascular system

The heart rate slows linearly with temperature due to a direct effect on the sinoatrial node. When this depression reaches a critical point impulses from the atrioventricular node may excite the ventricle and ventricular ectopic beats are more likely. Atrial fibrillation may occur. The effect of further cooling of the heart varies with age, oxygenation, etc. If it is young and healthy, and particularly if the coronary circulation is maintained by total body or coronary perfusion, the rate slows until asystole occurs at about 20°C. However, certain factors predispose to the progression of ventricular ectopic beats, ventricular tachycardia and ventricular fibrillation and this last may occur as high as 32°C. These factors appear to be:

- rapid changes in K, Ca, H or CO_2 tension
- hyperkalaemia
- respiratory acidosis

- myocardial hypoxia from poor coronary perfusion or a paroxysmal tachycardia
- lack of analgesia/sympathetic stimulation
- mechanical irritation.

Systole lengthens much more than in vagal slowing and the QRS complex is spread out. The QT interval is also prolonged and there may be ST elevation. During moderate hypothermia there is also often an additional upward deflection or Osborn wave on the downstroke of the R wave.

In general, cardiac output, coronary blood flow and oxygen consumption fall with temperature. The decline in cardiac output, however, is mainly due to bradycardia, as the stroke output changes little. Efficiency is probably unimpaired during moderate hypothermia but does fall off with more severe cooling. Coronary blood flow falls slightly but a greater proportion of the cardiac output goes to the coronary arteries because of the prolongation of diastole. Oxygen uptake falls less than that of non-working muscle and there is no evidence of any failure of the myocardium to extract oxygen.

The arterial blood pressure falls, but not markedly, until the temperature reaches about 25°C, but the peripheral resistance is maintained by increased viscosity of the blood rather than by vasoconstriction. Below this temperature, however, there is a fall in peripheral resistance due to the direct effect of cold on the blood vessels. Vasomotor reflexes are maintained in moderate hypothermia, although they are slower to develop — for example, compensation for rapid blood loss is not as rapid as in normothermia.

Respiration

In general this is depressed both in rate and depth, partly by an effect on the medulla and partly by depression of stretch receptors and nerve conduction. Spontaneous respiration usually ceases about 25°C. The natural effect of this is accumulation of carbon dioxide and this is further aided by dilatation of the bronchioles, increasing the anatomical dead space (+75%).

On the other hand, carbon dioxide production decreases and a patient's spontaneous respiration at 26°C may be quite sufficient to sustain life in spite of some rise in P_{CO_2}.

With regard to transport of respiratory gases, a decline in blood temperature increases the solubility. The volume of oxygen dissolved in arterial blood in a normothermic individual breathing air is 0.3 ml dl^{-1} blood, and when the blood temperature is lowered to 10°C the figure rises to 3.2 ml dl^{-1} blood. Under these conditions dissolved oxygen forms a significant part of the tissue oxygen requirement.

The other way in which hypothermia influences oxygen transport is by the Bohr effect — that is, by shifting the oxygen dissociation curve for haemoglobin to the left. As a result the blood takes up slightly more oxygen at the high P_{O_2} of the pulmonary capillaries but only gives it up at a lower P_{O_2} within the tissues. If the P_{CO_2} is also low from overventilation the two effects are additive and it is desirable to ensure that the P_{CO_2} does not fall. Although this effect could lead to a degree of tissue hypoxia, it is offset by the larger amount of oxygen carried per unit volume of blood. In the last resort, tissue oxygenation often depends more on blood flow through that tissue than on minor differences in oxygen transport.

Haematological changes

The process of coagulation slows as temperature falls as a consequence of inhibition of enzymatic action and slowing of chemical reactions. In addition, the platelets become sequestrated from the circulation. It is therefore possible in venovenous cooling to avoid heparinisation even though blood is exposed to passage along tubes. Other changes include haemoconcentration due to loss of plasma into tissue spaces, and sequestration of leucocytes. Haemoconcentration is a factor in the phenomenon of 'sludging', which may lead to intravascular coagulation. However, it is difficult to explain the rarity of serious consequences when haemoconcentration is so common; other factors must be involved in the rare cases of localised circulatory obstruction.

Acid–base balance

The effect of hypothermia on blood pH and bicarbonate in vivo is the resultant of many factors, some physical, some physiological and some pathological. In the patient it is not easy to predict the metabolic state accurately, and beyond moderate hypothermia with uninterrupted cardiac action, it is desirable to measure pH and related variables. However, there are certain principles governing disturbances during hypothermia.

1. In vitro change in pH. Blood cooled in a syringe has a rise in pH of 0.0147 units per degree centigrade. This is because cooling slows the dissociation of H_2CO_3 to H^+ and HCO_3^-.

2. Reduction in buffering power of blood. This is because the dissociation of protein and haemoglobin buffers is reduced. These are normally the main buffers of the blood because their pK is near the pH of blood but, with cooling, the emphasis shifts to the less efficient bicarbonate system. This effect means that a rise in P_{CO_2} from 40 to 50 mmHg (5.3–6.6 kPa):

at 37°C results in a fall in pH of 0.06
at 27°C results in a fall in pH of 0.15.

There is a similar reduction in ability to neutralise a metabolic acidosis.

3. Carbon dioxide becomes more soluble. Solubility of all gases rises as temperature falls, and in the case of carbon dioxide this leads to an increase in carbonic acid. In practice this effect approximately balances the reduction in dissociation of carbonic acid mentioned above and the pH changes little in vivo.

4. Carbon dioxide production falls. This has been discussed earlier and means that unless there is a reduction in alveolar ventilation the arterial P_{CO_2} falls, with cerebral vasoconstriction and other circulatory effects resulting from this.

5. Metabolic acidosis. It was stated above that hypothermia per se does not lead to accumulation of acid metabolites. However, certain factors in clinical hypothermia do frequently have this effect:

a. Total circulatory (cardiac) arrest and occlusion of the circulation to certain tissues (e.g. in aortic surgery) are the main causes of metabolic acidosis. Even if the cardiac output or total pump output is adequate for the total oxygen requirements, certain tissues may be underperfused and they will produce lactic acid. This is more likely when there are extreme gradients, as in rapid core cooling compared with slower surface cooling.

b. Production of lactic acid is accentuated by shivering and by hypoxia. Even imperceptible shivering in the absence of complete muscle paralysis increases blood lactic acid. This factor applies particularly to the re-warming rather than to the period of cooling.

c. The liver is less able to metabolise lactate and citrate at low temperatures.

d. The renal tubule cells are almost inactive at low temperatures so the renal mechanisms for retention of base are impaired.

e. Stored blood has a pH of 6.3–7.0 and massive transfusion leads to a temporary metabolic acidosis. After rewarming, when the citrate is metabolised bicarbonate is formed and a metabolic alkalosis results.

Hepatic function

When body temperature falls to 30°C glucose metabolism in the liver virtually ceases and the blood sugar rises to a high level if glucose solutions are infused. One effect of a high blood glucose level is an osmotic haemodilution as water is drawn from cells into vascular and extravascular compartments. With rewarming the blood glucose returns rapidly to normal.

Cold also impairs the ability to metabolise citrate. For instance, in the dog at 28°C, citrate metabolism is reduced by 40% from that at 37°C. At 37°C 500 ml of stored blood can probably be infused over 5 minutes without a rise in citrate, whereas at 28°C 500 ml must be spread over 10 minutes. The effect of the citrate is to bind the serum calcium, reducing the effective concentration. This leads to cardiac irregularities, hypotension that is resistant to pressor agents and muscle weakness.

Renal function

As the body temperature and cardiac output

fall, so renal plasma flow is reduced. In fact the latter is reduced more than the former, indicating a selective renal vasoconstriction. The result is a reduction in the glomerular filtrate. The cold also depresses tubular reabsorption of fluid so that the final volume of urine may be almost unaffected. However, the ability to absorb or reject certain ions is reduced and the urine tends to resemble a filtrate of plasma. Below 20°C renal function is suppressed almost completely.

Central nervous system

The cerebral oxygen consumption falls to about one-third at 25°C and cerebral blood flow falls similarly. Furthermore, the cerebral vascular resistance can still compensate for alterations in blood pressure down to 25°C. The cerebrospinal fluid pressure and brain volume fall (unless shivering occurs) and the brain becomes firmer, which facilitates neurosurgery. The electroencephalograph (ECG) develops large δ waves at 25–27°C. Approximate safe periods for cerebral ischaemia are 3 minutes at 37°C, 10 minutes at 30°C, 15 minutes at 25°C and 60 minutes at 15°C.

The spinal cord is somewhat less sensitive to ischaemia than the brain but can also be damaged by circulatory occlusion unless the temperature is lowered or circulation is maintained artificially.

Accidental hypothermia

Hypothermia can occur in healthy people who are immersed in the sea after shipwreck or exposed on mountains with inadequate protective clothing. It is particularly likely in elderly people living in inadequately heated rooms, because of their lowered metabolic rate and reduced ability to increase heat production by exercise. The risk in general is increased by alcohol, which causes peripheral vasodilatation, and sedation, which reduces general activity. Chlorpromazine is particularly effective in lowering body temperature by (1) peripheral vasodilatation, (2) depression of the temperature regulating centre, (3) reduction in muscle tone, and (4) inhibition of shivering. The term 'moderate' applies to core temperatures of 30–34°C and 'severe' to temperatures below 30°C.

Treatment on site consists in removing wet clothing and preventing further heat loss. The patient should be kept horizontal with a minimum of muscular activity, which could return a bolus of cold blood to the heart. The ECG should be monitored as soon as possible. In hospital, external rewarming is effective if the patient is breathing and heart beating, but if the temperature is below 30°C cardiopulmonary resuscitation may be required, followed by internal rewarming, ideally by extracorporeal means. Simultaneous management of other problems, such as drowning, may also be necessary.

FURTHER READING

Carli F, MacDonald I A 1996 Perioperative inadvertent hypothermia: what do we need to prevent? British Journal of Anaesthesia 76: 601–603

Hensel M 1981 Thermoreception and temperature regulation. Academic Press, London

Holdcroft A 1980 Body temperature control in anaesthesia, surgery and intensive care. London, Baillière Tindall

Weinberg A D 1993 Hypothermia (review). Annals of Emergency Medicine 22: 370–377

37

Body fluid balance and nutrition

C. McAllister

MAJOR BODY FLUID COMPARTMENTS

The adult body is 45–60% water by weight, the actual percentage depending on age, sex and amount of fat. Most body tissues are 70–80% water except for bone (20%) and fat (10%). Individuals with a higher fat or lower muscle mass will have less water as a percentage of their weight. Consequently women have a relatively lower total body water, and in both sexes the percentage falls with age (Table 37. 1).

Total body water is divided into two main functional compartments: the intracellular fluid and the extracellular fluid. Extracellular fluid can be further subdivided into interstitial fluid and the intravascular fluid component or plasma. For clinical purposes the intracellular fluid volume is considered to be 30–40% of body weight, depending on age and sex, or about two-thirds of body water, and the extracellular fluid 20% of body weight, or about one-third of body water (Fig. 37.1). Plasma is about 3.75–4.5% of body weight (7.5% of body water).

Table 37.1   Approximate water content as a percentage of total body weight

Age (years	Male (%)	Female (%)
1–5	65	65
10–16	60	60
17–39	60	50
40–59	55	47
60+	50	45

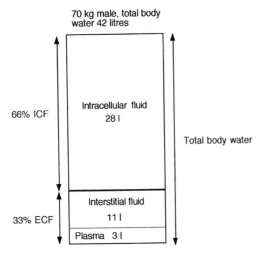

Figure 37.1 Approximate body fluid compartment volumes of a 70 kg young adult male.

Solute composition

Units of measurement

The SI unit of concentration is moles per litre (mol l^{-1}). One mole of any substance is its molecular weight in grams and contains 6.02×10^{23} molecules of that substance (Avogadro's number). A millimole is one thousandth of a mole, or the molecular weight in milligrams (mg). The molarity of a solution is the number of moles of solute per litre of solvent, and the molality of a solution is the number of moles of solute per *kilogram* of solvent. In clinical practice concentrations are expressed as millimoles per litre (mmol l^{-1}) (Fig. 37.2).

Solutes dissolved in water cause a reduction in the number of water molecules compared with an equal volume of pure water. Osmosis is the diffusion of water molecules from an area of high water concentration to a lower one across a membrane that is permeable to water but not solute. The pressure required to stop this movement is the osmotic pressure of the solute solution.

Osmotic pressure exerted by particles in a solution is determined only by the *number* of particles of whatever size per unit weight of solution. The unit of osmotic pressure is the *osmole* and one osmole is equal to a mole of undissociated solute. Thus for non-electrolytes, 1 mosmol = 1 mmol, but if the solute dissociates then there will be an increased number of osmotically active particles. So, in an ideal solution, 154 mmoles of NaCl in 1 kg of water (0.9% saline) would produce twice as many osmotically active particles — 308 mosmol kg^{-1}. In fact solutions are not

Plasma			Interstitial fluid		Intracellular fluid	
Cations	mmol l^{-1}	mmol l^{-1} water	Cations	mmol l^{-1}	Cations	mmol l^{-1}
Na+	142	153	Na+	145	Na+	10
K+	4	4.3	K+	4.1	K+	150
Ca++	2.5	2.7	Ca++	2.4	Ca++	< 0.1
Mg++	0.7	0.8	Mg++	0.8	Mg++	20
Anions			Anions		Anions	
Cl-	104	112	Cl-	117	Cl-	3
HCO$_3$-	24	26	HCO$_3$-	27.1	HCO$_3$-	7
Phosphate	1.1	1.2	Phosphate	1.1	Phosphate	100
					Protein	

Figure 37.2 Approximate solute concentrations of body fluid compartments.

ideal and ionic interaction reduces this number. In the case of 1 kg of 0.9% saline this reduces the osmolality by a factor 0.93 (the osmotic coefficient) to 286.4 mosmol kg^{-1}.

The *osmolality* is the number of particles present in a given weight of solvent, so 1 mosmol dissolved in 1 kg of water has an osmolality of 1 mosmol kg^{-1}. *Osmolarity* is the number of particles present in 1 litre of solvent. Although in dilute solutions, such as body fluids, the quantitative difference between the two is minimal (less than 1%), it is in fact the number of osmols per kilogram of water and not per litre of solute that determines the osmotic pressure. Also, it is osmolality that is measured in practice, by the depression of the freezing point of water. Each osmol of any solute added to 1 kg of water depress the freezing point by 1.86°C. Plasma has a freezing point of about –0.521°C, giving an osmolality of 0.280 osmol kg^{-1} or 280 mosmol kg^{-1}.

Extracellular fluid

The interstitial and intravascular fluid compartments are separated only by a capillary membrane freely permeable to all plasma solutes, except protein and lipids. Consequently, since they differ significantly only in protein content (20 g l^{-1} in interstitial fluid, 70 g l^{-1} in plasma), they are considered equivalent for clinical purposes. The dominant ion in the extracellular fluid is Na$^+$ and this, together with the anions Cl$^-$ and HCO$_3^-$, accounts for over 90% of the osmolality of the extracellular fluid. Thus sodium balance regulates extracellular fluid volume.

The fact that the electrolyte concentrations in the plasma and interstitial fluids are not exactly the same is due to the effect of the negative charges of the different protein concentrations, the Gibbs–Donnan effect. Briefly: the presence of a non-diffusible anion (protein) on one side of a membrane (plasma) increases the concentration of diffusible cations (Na$^+$ and K$^+$) and decreases the concentration of diffusible anions (Cl$^-$ and HCO$_3^-$).

Intracellular fluid

The extracellular and intracellular fluid compartments are separated by the cell membrane, a selective barrier that is freely permeable to water but not sodium. Since any transcompartmental osmotic differentials will result in the diffusion of water to the compartment with the higher osmolality, at equilibrium there are no osmolal gradients between compartments. There are, of course, specialised areas of the body where there are dramatic osmolal gradients maintained by active, energy dependent processes, for example in the kidney.

Intracellular fluid osmolality determines the intracellular fluid volume. This is controlled by the membrane Na$^+$,K$^+$ pump which exchanges two intracellular Na$^+$ ions for three extracellular K$^+$ ions. Consequently, in contrast to the extracellular fluid, the predominant intracellular fluid ion is K$^+$. The dominant intracellular fluid cations are phosphate and protein.

WATER BALANCE

Normal plasma osmolality is maintained by regulation of water output and intake. Hypothalamic osmoreceptors maintain plasma osmolality within the range 275–290 mosmol kg^{-1}, primarily by the action of antidiuretic hormone (ADH) control of renal water excretion and, secondarily, by thirst. Thirst is not perceived until after the urine is maximally concentrated. Volume status is regulated by vascular stretch receptors (baroreceptors), which also influence ADH secretion and thirst. Significant changes in ADH secretion are produced by a 1% change in plasma osmolality but require a 10% change in volume, i.e. osmoreceptors are more sensitive than baroreceptors. However, volume status overrides osmolality. Hence the infusion of a litre of 0.9% saline produces a diuresis, or the loss of a litre of iso-osmotic fluid (e.g. in haemorrhage) results in thirst and ADH secretion.

Maximum and minimum urine osmolality in response to ADH are 1400 and 30 mosmol kg^{-1}, respectively. Since 650 mosmol of solute products must be excreted per day, the minimum or obligatory urine output is 500 ml day^{-1}, although the usual is around 1000 ml day^{-1}. Maximum urine output is about 20 l day^{-1}. Renal impairment causes a progressive decline in the ability to produce concentrated urine. Other sources of obligatory water loss are the respiratory tract (400 ml), skin (500 ml) and faeces (200 ml). Thus the minimum water loss per day is 1600 ml. Obviously losses from these sites will vary depending on intake, activity, ambient temperature and humidity, and bowel function. Losses must be at least matched by water ingested, water content of food (about 700 ml) and the water of oxidation of carbohydrate (about 350 ml). Fasting stable patients require about 35 ml kg^{-1} day^{-1} of water.

MINERALS

Sodium

Sodium balance

Total exchangeable body sodium is about 40 mmol kg^{-1} (i.e. 2800 mmol in a 70 kg individual), of which over 90% is extracellular. There are no mechanisms for regulating intake, which varies widely but is around 150 mmol day^{-1} in a Western diet. Non-urine sodium losses are trivial in health (around 20 mol day^{-1} in sweat and faeces) and balance depends on renal excretion, which can vary from less than 10 to over 400 mmol day^{-1}. The sodium requirement of hospitalised patients is around 85 mmol day^{-1}; however, patients with abnormal losses (e.g. bowel fistula diarrhoea) may require at least two or three times this.

Potassium

Function and balance

Potassium is the major determinant of intracellular osmolality (and hence volume) and is intimately involved in neuromuscular function. Total exchangeable body potassium is about 50 mmol kg^{-1} for men and 40 mmol kg^{-1} for women. All but 2% is intracellular, i.e. of the total body potassium of around 3000 mmol only 60 mmol is in the extracellular fluid. Like sodium there are no mechanisms for regulating potassium intake, which is 50–150 mmol day^{-1} in a Western diet. Losses in sweat are less than

5 mmol day^{-1} and in faeces usually under 20 mmol day^{-1}. Potassium balance is maintained by the kidney, normal urinary potassium ranging from about 30 to over 150 mmol day^{-1}.

Potassium requirements of hospitalised patients must be individualised but are usually between 50 and 100 mmol day^{-1}. It is usually omitted in the first 24 hours after surgery because the stress response raises plasma potassium.

Hypokalaemia

Hypokalaemia results from increased urinary and gastrointestinal losses or from redistribution from extracellular to intracellular fluids. Causes of the latter include alkalosis, insulin and β_2 agonists. Plasma potassium concentration is low (3.1–4.2 mmol l^{-1}) and represents a tiny fraction of the total body potassium; however, it is the ratio of extracellular to intercellular potassium concentration that is the major determinant of the resting membrane potential across excitable cell membranes; hence, severe plasma hyperkalaemia (>6.5 mmol l^{-1}) or hypokalaemia (<2.5 mmol l^{-1}) can lead to potentially fatal cardiac arrhythmias and skeletal muscle weakness.

In the absence of transcellular shifts, each 1 mmol decrease in plasma potassium can represent a total body deficit of at least 150 mmol. Intravenous replacement potassium should never be faster than 0.5 mmol kg^{-1} h^{-1} and usually not more than 10–20 mmol h^{-1}, to allow time for intracellular redistribution.

Hyperkalaemia

Hyperkalaemia results from decreased renal excretion or from redistribution from intracellular to extracellular fluid. Causes of transcellular shift include acidosis, insulin deficiency rhabdomyolysis and drugs. Factitious hyperkalaemia results from mishandling of specimens.

Phosphorus

Distribution and function

Total adult body phosphate is about 23 000 mmol or 10 g kg^{-1}, of which 85% is in bone. Over 99% of the non-bone phosphate is intracellular, mostly as organic phosphates; it is the dominant intracellular anion. The intracellular:extracellular concentration ratios are of the order of 100:1, and plasma levels are between 0.8 and 1.5 mmol l^{-1}. Cellular phosphate is required for cell wall structure (phospholipids), nucleic acid generation, glucose metabolism, high energy bonds (adenosine triphosphate (ATP), phosphocreatine), oxygen transport (2,3-diphosphoglycerate) and as a buffer.

Phosphate balance

Daily intake is around 30–40 mmol, with a minimum requirement of about 20 mmol day^{-1}. Balance is maintained by the kidney, hence renal failure leads to hyperphosphataemia and renal losses cause hypophosphataemia. The most common causes of hypophosphataemia result, however, from redistribution of phosphate from extracellular to intracellular fluid due to alkalosis, insulin, glucose and β$_2$ agonists (the same causes as intracellular potassium redistribution). Consequently hypophosphataemia can be a complication of parenteral nutrition, particularly high glucose loads with added insulin, in malnourished patients ('refeeding hypophosphataemia') and of the treatment of diabetic ketoacidosis. In starved patients with depletion of total body phosphate, the refeeding hypophosphataemia can be severe (less than 0.32 mmol l^{-1}) and phosphate is routinely provided in total parenteral nutrition at about 10 mmol 1000 kcal^{-1}. More may be required.

Some important clinical consequences of severe hypophosphataemia are listed in Table 37.2. Treatment is by oral or intravenous phosphate, up to about 60 mmol day^{-1}, titrated to achieve a plasma level greater than 0.8 mmol l^{-1}. Various potassium or sodium phosphate salts are available for intravenous use — for example, Addiphos (Pharmacia), which contains 2 mmol ml^{-1} phosphate and 1.5 mmol ml^{-1} potassium.

Hyperphosphataemia up to three times normal is well tolerated in the short term. However, if the concentrations of calcium and phosphate (mmol) multiplied together is greater than 6, ectopic cal-

Table 37.2 Complications of severe, persistent hypophosphataemia

- ↓ ATP in red blood cells, white cells and platelets → haemolysis, ↓ neutrophil function and ↓ platelet aggregation
- ↑ red blood cell oxygen affinity due to in ↓ 2,3 diphosphoglycerate (2,3 DPG) → ↓ Oxygen delivery
- Hypotension
- Heart failure
- Paraesthesia, confusion, convulsions, coma
- Weakness
- Hypoventilation, difficulty in weaning from ventilator

cification results; consequently dialysis dependent patients are routinely given antacids, which act as phosphate binders.

Calcium

Over 99% of total body calcium is in the skeleton. Plasma calcium is about 50% ionised, 40% is plasma protein bound and about 10% is complexed with anions such as citrate, phosphate and bicarbonate. The normal total calcium level in plasma is 2.2–2.64 mmol l^{-1}, and of ionised calcium 1.14–1.3 mmol l^{-1}. It is the concentration of *ionised* calcium that affects physiological processes such as neuromuscular function. Most laboratories report *total* calcium concentration and an allowance must be made for plasma protein concentration. One such is to correct the reported plasma calcium by 0.025 mmol l^{-1} for each g l^{-1} the albumin deviates from 40. Instruments that report free or ionised calcium overcome this problem.

Calcium deficiency

In anaesthetic practice this is most often seen in conditions such as acute pancreatitis, after parathyroidectomy and with massive transfusion of citrated blood. As symptoms are related to ionised rather than total calcium concentrations, they may also occur with a normal total calcium level, if the ionised fraction decreases. This may be caused by alkalosis, particularly respiratory alkalosis due to hysterical overbreathing. The classical symptoms of hypocalcaemia are increased neuromuscular excitability, tetany, laryngospasm and muscle cramps.

The normal daily intake of calcium is about 20 mmol, of which 40% is absorbed. Minimum daily requirement is at least 5 mmol a day, which may be added to total parenteral nutrition, although precipitation may occur if large amounts of calcium and phosphate are administered together.

Calcium chloride BP, USP: $CaCl_2.H_2O$

The usual 10% solution contains 0.68 mmol ml^{-1} calcium. It should be injected slowly intravenously.

Calcium gluconate BP, USP: $[CH_2OH(CHOH)_2—COO]_2Ca.H_2O$

Calcium gluconate 10% contains 0.22 mmol ml^{-1} calcium. It is the preparation of choice for treatment of hypocalcaemic tetany. It may also be used in place of chloride, as contrary to past opinion it is equally effective in raising the plasma ionised calcium concentration and is less toxic to local tissues should extravasation occur.

Magnesium

Magnesium is the fourth most abundant cation in the body and the second most abundant within the cells, i.e. it is primarily an intracellular ion, where it is a component of several enzyme systems, especially those involved in transfer of high energy phosphate radicals to ATP, and is important in neuronal transmission and muscle contractility. Normal plasma magnesium concentration is 0.7–1.2 mmol l^{-1}, of which about 35% is protein bound, while within cells there is a concentration of about 20 mmol l^{-1}, varying between tissues.

Magnesium deficiency

Magnesium depletion can occur in malnourished patients, those with prolonged diarrhoea or fistulas, or with diuretic therapy.

Clinical symptoms of deficiency may develop with plasma concentrations below 0.5 mmol l^{-1}. The picture is similar to that of calcium deficiency characterised by hyperexcitability or tetany, as well as cardiac arrhythmias and electrocardiographic changes similar to those of potassium

deficiency. Hypomagnesaemia may often be associated with hypokalaemia and digitalis toxicity.

The daily requirement of magnesium is about 0.17–0.25 mmol kg^{-1} in well-nourished patients, but may be several times higher in those with chronic depletion.

Magnesium sulphate BP, USP: $MgSO_4.7H_2O$

This salt is available in several concentrations. The usual concentration, a 50% solution, contains 2.03 mmol ml^{-1}, and 5–10 ml can be used for the acute treatment of hypomagnesaemia, with supplemental doses as required.

PARENTERAL NUTRITION

Patients are not starved to health. The best form of nutrition is an adequate well balanced diet. If this is not possible then supplements or total artificial enteral feeds are the next best option. The indication for total parenteral nutrition (TPN) is the inability to deliver adequate nutrition via the gastrointestinal tract for more than 7–10 days, for whatever reason, e.g. prolonged ileus, obstruction, pseudo-obstruction, intestinal fistula, malabsorption and pancreatitis. The threshold for commencing TPN will obviously be lower in patients who are malnourished on presentation. Feeding should be converted to enteral nutrition at the earliest opportunity as, apart from being expensive, there is a higher complication rate with TPN.

Constituents of TPN

Patients receiving TPN require an energy source, protein, essential fatty acids, minerals and essential organic and inorganic micronutrients.

Carbohydrate

Glucose is the standard carbohydrate used in TPN today. Others such as sorbitol, fructose and ethanol have been used, but are now of historical interest only. It is physiological, can be metabolised by all body tissues and is essential for some (e.g. brain). It stimulates the secretion of insulin (an anabolic hormone) and blood levels can be easily and rapidly measured. Glucose would appear then to be the perfect source of all the body's energy requirements. Unfortunately there is a limit to the body's ability to oxidise glucose.

Up to an infusion rate of $3–5 \text{ g kg}^{-1} \text{ day}^{-1}$ in healthy volunteers there is a progressive increase in glucose oxidation. Beyond this an increasing percentage of glucose is converted to glycogen or fat, an energy and oxygen consuming process, and by $8 \text{ g kg}^{-1} \text{ day}^{-1}$ about 50% is stored. The ability of the stressed patient to oxidise glucose is if anything decreased (insulin resistance), so the maximum amount of glucose that can be usefully handled by patients is probably around $4 \text{ g kg}^{-1} \text{ day}^{-1}$ or 280 g for a 70 kg man, which is about half of the energy requirement of the vast majority of patients. Infusion of glucose at a rate much in excess of this leads to hyperglycaemia, associated with an increase in the overall infection rate, hypophosphataemia, liver dysfunction and increased metabolic stress associated with the storage of glucose as fat. The energy shortfall of 40–50% should be provided in the form of lipid.

Lipid

Lipid emulsions are isotonic, rich in essential fatty acids, calorie-dense and pH neutral. The essential fatty acid, linoleic acid, is converted in vivo to arachidonic acid, a semi-essential fatty acid. Deficiency leads to an essential fatty acid deficiency syndrome, characterised by dermatitis, alopecia, delayed wound healing and increased susceptibility to infection. Linolenic acid is considered essential in the infant, for eye and brain development. Biochemical evidence of a deficiency syndrome can be seen in patients receiving fat-free parenteral nutrition after about a month. Clinical evidence may take twice as long.

All preparations available in the UK at present are soya bean oil emulsions. The fat particles in Intralipid (Pharmacia), emulsified by egg yolk phospholipid, are of the same order of size as chylomicrons and are similarly hydrolysed by lipoprotein lipase. Intralipid is available as 10%, 20% and 30% solutions. A litre of 20% Intralipid contains 200 g fat and 22 g glycerol, providing 1800 kcal and 200 kcal, respectively. Intralipid fatty acids (50% of which are linoleic acid, 8% α-linolenic acid) are composed entirely of long chain triglycerides. Mixtures of medium and long chain triglycerides are available (Lipofundin MCT/LCT, Braun) and are popular in continental Europe. Despite theoretical advantages of more complete oxidation and more rapid clearance from the blood they have not been shown to be superior to standard lipid emulsions in clinical practice.

The minimum requirement of soya bean fat to prevent essential fatty acid syndrome is about 15 g day^{-1}, which corresponds to 500 ml of 10% Intralipid twice a week or 7.5% of the daily energy requirement. In practice 30–50% (1.0–$1.5 \text{ g kg}^{-1} \text{ day}^{-1}$) of the energy requirements are provided as fat. More than this can lead to hyperlipidaemia, especially in the critically ill patient in whom fat should not exceed $1.0 \text{ g kg}^{-1} \text{ day}^{-1}$.

Protein

In health, minimum high quality protein requirements are of the order of $0.75 \text{ g kg}^{-1} \text{ day}^{-1}$. Dietary protein is absorbed as amino acids and provided as such in TPN. The amino acid content of TPN is described in terms of grams of nitrogen per day (1 g nitrogen = 6.25 g protein). TPN nitrogen requirements vary, being lower in the elderly, frail and female and higher in the young, male and muscular. Daily requirements are about $0.15–0.25 \text{ g kg}^{-1} \text{ day}^{-1}$, which is equivalent to 0.9–$1.5 \text{ g kg}^{-1} \text{ day}^{-1}$ of protein. Stable patients with bowel failure are at the lower end of this range, while acutely ill patients with trauma or sepsis are at the upper.

Body proteins are composed of 20 amino acids. Eight can not be synthesised by healthy adults in amounts sufficient to maintain nitrogen balance — the essential or non-dispensable amino acids. However, young children and adults with certain conditions are unable to synthesise adequate amounts of some 'non-essential' amino acids — the conditionally essential amino acids (Table 37.3).

Table 37.3 Essential, non-essential, conditionally essential amino acids and some conditions causing their essentiality

Essential	Non-essential	Conditionally essential		Conditions causing essentiality
Isoleucine	Alanine	Histidine	⟶	Infants, uraemia
Leucine	Asparagine	Arginine	⟶	Critically ill
Lysine	Aspartate	Cyst(e)ine	⟶	Neonates, liver disease
Methionine	Glutamate	Glutamine	⟶	Acutely ill
Phenylalanine	Glycine	Tyrosine	⟶	Phenylketonuria, premature babies,
Threonine	Proline			liver disease
Tryptophan	Serine			
Valine				

Current commercial amino acid preparations are solutions of laevo isomers of synthetic crystalline amino acids (except glycine, which has no isomers), the dextro isomers being non-utilisable for protein synthesis by man (except for small amounts of D-methionine and D-phenylalanine). Ideally amino acid solutions should contain all the essential and conditionally essential amino acids as well as a broad mix of the non-essential amino acids in proportions comparable with those found in high quality protein. Standard solution composition varies but none contain all the amino acids because of difficulties in formulation as a consequence of the physicochemical properties of certain amino acids. Thus, although currently available solutions contain all of the essential amino acids, none contain glutamine, except Glamin (Pharmacia), which has recently become available. Interestingly, glutamine and tyrosine are in the form of dipeptides in Glamin, thus overcoming some of the stability problems.

Branched chain amino acids (leucine, isoleucine and valine) bypass the liver and are metabolised by skeletal muscle and heart, and so probably should be more generously provided in amino acid solutions compared with the other essential amino acids. Despite theoretical advantages the infusion of branched chain amino acids in liver failure has not been shown to be beneficial.

Amino acid solutions are supplied in differing concentrations e.g. Vamin 9, 14 and 18 (Pharmacia). The number refers to the grams of nitrogen in each litre. Thus Vamin 18 contains 18 g nitrogen per litre, which is equivalent to 112 g protein.

Amino acids are traditionally not included in calculations of energy supplied, and to prevent their utilisation as an energy substrate non-protein energy sources are normally provided in the ratio of 100–150 kcal to 1 g nitrogen.

ENTERAL NUTRITION

Enteral nutrition includes oral supplementation, drink feeding and tube feeding. Oral supplements are just that — supplements — i.e. they are not designed to be nutritionally complete. Depending on the patient the emphasis may be on protein ($12 \, g \, l^{-1}$, $1.0 \, kcal \, ml^{-1}$) or caloric supplementation ($1.5 \, kcal \, ml^{-1}$, protein $7.2 \, g \, l^{-1}$). Either way they should contain 100% RDA (recommended daily allowance, USA) of essential micronutrients, trace elements and vitamins per litre.

Drink feeds, on the other hand, provide a complete source of nutrition, in a liquid form and in a reasonable volume (1.5–2.0 l), for patients who are unable to eat solids but who can drink — for example, those with upper intestinal obstruction. The particular drink feed chosen is unimportant but it should be palatable. There is increasing evidence of the beneficial effects of oral supplementation and drink feeding in surgical patients, especially the elderly and malnourished. Most enteral feeding in hospitals is in the form of tube feeding and the rest of this discussion confines itself to this form.

Advantages of enteral nutrition

For many years TPN was the major means of artificial nutrition in surgical patients. However, the benefits of enteral feeding are increasingly appreciated and, where possible, this is now the route of choice. Some of the reasons for this are:

- Cost — currently less than one-fifth that of TPN.
- It is physiological — polymeric feeding solutions provide a mixture of all nutrients that is similar to that encountered in a normal diet.
- Maintenance of gut mucosal integrity and digestive function, probably secondary to stimulation of trophic intestinal hormones, and perhaps improved intestinal immunity and gut barrier function.
- Reduction in hyperglycaemia and cholestasis.
- Enteral nutrient solutions contain many substances that may have beneficial effects, such as fibre, small peptides, medium chain triglycerides and increased amounts of immuno-modulatory amino acids (e.g. glutamine and arginine). (Immunomodulatory = the favourable effect of substances on the host's defence systems against potential pathogens and injury.
- Reduction in overall infection rates.

Disadvantages of enteral nutrition

- Tube complications: malposition, unplanned extubation, ulceration
- Gastric dilatation/aspiration
- Diarrhoea
- Metabolic: hyper/hypokalaemia, hypo/hypernatraemia, hyperglycemia, hypo/hyperphosphataemia.

Enteral nutrition solutions

Polymeric feeds

Polymeric solutions are the most commonly used feeds in clinical practice. They contain a mixture of nutrients similar to that found in a normal diet and are therefore balanced, but are iso-osmolar (glucose is replaced by non-lactose glucose polymers) and low residue. Although the addition of fibre to polymeric formulations may have beneficial effects on gut barrier function, this has not

been shown to prevent constipation in patients on long term polymeric feeding. Most commercially available polymeric feeds are fibre-, lactose- and gluten-free and contain 1 kcal ml^{-1}. Energy dense feeds with 1.5 kcal ml^{-1} or more are available, the extra calories provided mostly as fat (e.g. Pulmocare).

Semi-elemental and elemental feeds

In patients with malabsorption syndromes, e.g. Crohn's disease and short-bowel syndrome, elemental or semi-elemental feeds may be used. These feeds are composed of amino acids or short polypeptides, respectively, glucose polymers, medium and long chain triglycerides, as well as 100% RDA of trace elements and vitamins. Elemental and semi-elemental formulations provide nutrients in a more absorbable form. They have also been used in patients with bowel fistulae as they have minimal residue. Patients with malabsorption secondary to pancreatic insufficiency are best treated with pancreatic supplements.

Feeds for special conditions

Respiratory disease. Patients with carbon dioxide retention are frequently undernourished; however, feeding promotes further carbon dioxide production and consequently enteral diets with a high fat to carbohydrate ratio are available (e.g. Pulmocare). Fat has a lower respiratory quotient than carbohydrate (0.7 and 1.0, respectively), thus less carbon dioxide is produced for an equivalent amount of oxygen consumption. Unfortunately, despite this theoretical advantage they have not been shown to facilitate ventilator weaning. These feeds also have a high energy:volume ratio (1.5 kcal ml^{-1}) and have been used where volume is restricted.

Liver disease. The characteristic plasma amino acid profile of patients with hepatic encephalopathy is an increase in the aromatic amino acids (phenylalanine, tyrosine, methionine, and tryptophan) in conjunction with a decrease in the branched chain amino acids (valine, leucine and isoleucine). The clinical features include fluid

556 ANAESTHETIC PHARMACOLOGY AND PHYSIOLOGY

overload and sodium retention. These patients also tolerate long chain triglycerides poorly.

The optimum feed will therefore have a high proportion of branched chain amino acids, low fat content (predominantly as medium chain triglycerides), low sodium content and 100% of the RDA of vitamins and trace elements (e.g. Hepatic-Aid). Feeds used in liver disease are supplements and are complete feeds. For patients with chronic but stable liver disease who are not encephalopathic, standard polymeric feeds, if required, are tolerated.

Vitamins

The vitamins are 13 organic micronutrients that are essential for health. In general the fat soluble vitamins (A, D, E and K) have membrane and structural functions, whereas the water soluble vitamins B_1 (thiamine), B_2 (riboflavin), B_5 (pantothenic acid), B_6 (pyridoxine), B_{12} (cyanocobalamin), niacin, folate, C (ascorbic acid) and biotin are involved in enzymatic reactions. All the available enteral feeds contain vitamins in excess of that recommended for healthy adults (Table 37.4), but supplements may be required in patients with pre-existing deficiencies or who have excess requirements.

Although stores of the fat soluble vitamins A,

D and E in the liver are usually substantial, stores of the water soluble vitamins and vitamin K are low, even in health. Vitamins should be given in at least the recommended amounts to all patients receiving parenteral nutrition. It is not practical that these should be added individually and there are various multivitamin preparations available, fat soluble (Vitlipid N), water soluble (Solvito N) and combined (Cernevit). Vitamin recommendations for parenteral use differ from the oral but are designed to be appropriate for the vast majority of patients receiving TPN (Table 37.4). The reasons for the different recommendations are:

1. The oral recommendations are for healthy adults. An increased allowance is provided in enteral formulations as these are used in patients, whose requirements are higher.
2. Patients requiring TPN are considered more likely to have a further increase in requirements.
3. Bioavailability of the fat soluble vitamins is variable (especially A).
4. Relatively high doses of the water soluble vitamins are well tolerated as there is a wide margin of safety. Hypervitaminosis syndromes are almost unknown for the water soluble vitamins, except in cases of mega-vitamin abuse.
5. Hypervitaminosis syndromes can rarely occur

Table 37.4 United Kingdom (UK) reference nutrient intake (RNI), American Medical Association (AMA) recommended daily allowance (RDA) for oral vitamins, AMA intravenous (i.v.) multivitamin recommendations and available multivitamin preparations (UK)

Vitamin	UK RNI (oral)	AMA RDA (oral)	AMA (i.v.)	Cernevit (Clintec)	Vitlipid N (Pharmacia)	Solvito N	Multibionta (Merck)
A (iu)	2000–2300	4000–5000	3300	3500	3300	NP	10 000
D (iu)	0 (if > 65 yrs 400)	400	200	220	200	NP	NP
E (iu)	>3 mg	12–15	10	10.2	10	NP	5
K (mg)	0.001 kg^{-1}	2–4 weekly	NR	0	0.15	NP	NP
B_1 (thiamine) (mg)	0.8–1.1	1–1.5	3	3.51	NP	3.2	50
B_2 (riboflavin) (mg)	1.1–1.3	1.1–1.8	3.6	4.14	NP	3.6	10
B_5 (mg)	3–7	5–10	15	17.25	NP	15	25
B_6 (pyridoxine) (mg)	1.2–1.5	1.6–2.0	4.0	4.5	NP	4.0	15
Niacin (mg)	12–17	12–20	40	46	NP	40	100
B_{12} (µg)	1.5	3	5	6	NP	5	NP
Folate (µg)	200	400	400	414	NP	400	NP
C (mg)	40	45	100	125	NP	100	500
Biotin (µg)	10–200	150–300	60	69	NP	60	NP

NP, not present; NR, not recommended.

with vitamins A (mucocutaneous desquamation, liver disease and intracranial hypertension in children) and D (hypercalcaemia).

6. The American Medical Association (AMA) do not recommend vitamin K in multivitamin preparations in case of interference with warfarin therapy.

Trace elements

The essential trace elements (chromium, cobalt, copper, iodine, iron, manganese, molybdenum, selenium and zinc) are inorganic micronutrients that play an important role in basic cellular function. They act as cofactors in enzymatic reactions (copper, manganese, molybdenum, selenium and zinc) and as antioxidants. With the exception of iron and zinc, there are substantial body stores of trace elements and deficiency states have usually been described only after prolonged deprivation.

Zinc losses are increased in patients with diarrhoea, gut fistula, burns and hypercatabolic states, leading to deficiency within a few weeks.

Iron body stores are often critical, especially in females and the elderly.

Cobalt is to the vitamin B_{12} molecule (cyano-*cobal*amine) as iron is to the haemoglobin molecule, except that the cobalt atom is surrounded by four substituted pyrrole rings. Deficiency syndromes are those of B_{12} deficiency and cobalt is provided as vitamin B_{12}.

With the exception of iron and zinc, body levels of trace elements are rarely measured. Replacement is usually empirical, using the additive Additrace (Pharmacia), which contains nine trace elements, including fluoride. This contains the recommended daily intravenous allowance, based on probable requirements for most patients requiring intravenous artificial nutrition, while leaving a margin of safety for those elements that have a higher risk of toxicity (selenium, zinc and iron). In patients with increased losses, additional zinc supplementation may be required. Table 37.5 lists the trace elements, some of their functions and the estimated daily requirements of patients receiving TPN.

Table 37.5 Essential trace elements, functions, deficiency states, daily intravenous requirements and the contents of one ampoule of Additrace (Pharmacia)

Trace element	Physiological function	Deficiency effects	Estimated daily i.v. requirements	Additrace
Chromium	Glucose metabolism Peripheral insulin activity Fat metabolism	Glucose intolerance Weight loss Peripheral neuropathy	0.2–0.4 µmol 0.01–0.02 mg	0.2 µmol
Cobalt	Part of the corrin ring in vitamin B_{12}	B_{12} deficiency	Given as B_{12}	Not present
Copper	Synthesis of haemoglobin Immune system	Anaemia Neutropenia	5–20 µmol 0.3–1.3 mg	20 µmol
Iodine	Synthesis of thyroid hormones	Goitre Hypothyroidism	1 µmol 0.131 mg	1 µmol
Iron	Component of haemoglobin, myoglobin and cytochrome system	Anaemia	20 µmol 1.2 mg	20 µmol
Manganese	Energy and fat metabolism	Lipid abnormalities Dermatitis	5 µmol 0.3 mg	5 µmol
Molybdenum	Xanthine oxidase (DNA metabolism). Sulphite oxidase (sulphur amino acid metabolism)	Intolerance to sulphur amino acid metabolism — irritability, coma, tachycardia	0.2 µmol 0.02 mg	0.2 µmol
Selenium	Glutathione peroxidase — protects membrane lipids from oxidation	Myopathy; myalgia; cardiomyopathy (Keshan disease); macrocytosis	0.4–0.8 µmol 0.03–0.06 mg	0.4 µmol
Zinc	Growth and reproduction Promotes wound healing and humoral immunity	Diarrhoea; dermatitis; alopecia; immune deficiency	50–100 µmol 2.5–6.4 mg	100 µmol

FURTHER READING

Payne-James J, Grimble G, Silk D (eds) 1995 Artificial nutrition support in clinical practice. Edward Arnold, London

Rose B D 1994 Clinical physiology of acid–base and electrolyte disorders. McGraw-Hill, New York

Worthley L I G 1994 Synopsis of intensive care medicine. Churchill Livingstone, Edinburgh

38

Gastrointestinal physiology

I. C. Roddie

MOUTH AND SALIVARY SECRETIONS

Mastication

Mastication aids the swallowing and digestion of food by breaking it into smaller pieces, moistening it and lubricating it with salivary mucus. Food is prepared into moist, soft boli of suitable size for swallowing. People unable to masticate because of tooth or mouth problems can not manage hard, dry or large items of food; they require it to be suitably prepared before ingestion.

Saliva

Saliva is secreted by three pairs of salivary glands into the buccal cavity. The parotid glands are serous glands which secrete a watery fluid containing ptyalin. The sublingual glands are mucous glands secreting mucins. The submandibular glands are mixed and secrete both. Normally 1.5 litres of saliva are secreted per day.

Composition

When secreted into the salivary ducts, saliva has a salt concentration similar to that in plasma. As it traverses the salivary ducts it gradually becomes hypotonic as sodium chloride is reabsorbed and potassium and bicarbonate are secreted. When it enters the mouth it is hypotonic and alkaline.

It contains digestive enzymes, an amylase called ptyalin, which can break down starch into smaller polysaccharides, and a lipase, derived from glands on the dorsum of the tongue. It also contains mucus, which lubricates the food for swallowing. Saliva contains agents that combat mouth infections. These include lysozyme and the immune antibody IgA.

Control of secretion

The flow of saliva is controlled reflexly. The main efferent nerves for the reflexes are the parasympathetic cholinergic fibres supplying the glands. Stimulation of these nerves produces a copious salivary flow accompanied by strong vasodilatation. The vasodilatation has been attributed to vasoactive polypeptides, such as vasoactive intestinal polypeptide (VIP) and bradykinin, formed or released when the glands are activated. When sympathetic nerves are stimulated, the glands secrete a scanty juice, rich in organic constituents, and their blood vessels constrict.

The reflex centres for salivation are in the medulla but the reflexes are strongly influenced by higher centres, which can facilitate or inhibit them. Salivary reflexes are both unconditioned and conditioned. Stimulation of sensory nerve endings in the mouth by food, manipulation of teeth or anaesthetic/surgical interventions in the mouth elicit salivary flow though unconditioned reflexes. However, conditioned reflexes are also effective, as Pavlov showed in his dogs. Thinking about food (or the dentist's drill!) can make the mouth water.

Functions

Saliva has a small role in digestion. Although it contains an amylase and a lipase, food spends so little time in the mouth that little digestion occurs before it enters the stomach, where the pH is not optimal for its enzymes. These enzymes could have a cleansing role by digesting food debris that would otherwise accumulate around the teeth and other oral structures.

By moistening and lubricating the food, it helps the mouth mould food into boli of suitable size and consistency for swallowing. Chemical agents must be in aqueous solution to stimulate taste receptors. Saliva facilitates taste by dissolving these agents.

Salivary secretion is important in preventing infection in the mouth. The flow of saliva continually flushes away food particles and cell debris from the mouth so that bacterial colonisation is discouraged. In addition, saliva contains lysozyme and IgA, which are hostile to invading microorganisms.

When salivary secretion is reduced, the resulting dry mouth makes mastication, swallowing and speech difficult. Nervous orators need to keep sipping drinks to keep their mouths wet. Taste is impaired because the molecules that stimulate taste buds do not go into solution. The loss of saliva's cleansing power leads to mouth infections, ulceration of the mucous membranes and damage to tooth enamel. However, no problem arises from lack of digestive enzymes because their role can be assumed by others further down the digestive tract.

Swallowing

Swallowing (deglutition) is the act that shifts food boli from the mouth to the stomach via the oesophagus. It is customary to divide the act into three stages. The first or *oral* phase is a voluntary one whereby the tongue pushes or throws a bolus of food backwards on to the posterior pharyngeal walls. The second or *pharyngeal* phase is an unconditioned reflex. The reflex has the usual afferent and efferent limbs and a reflex centre to coordinate the response. The swallowing centre lies in the medulla oblongata. The afferent limb is triggered by food impacting against the pharyngeal walls. This sets up impulses which travel to the swallowing centre via the vagus, trigeminal and glossopharyngeal nerves. The reflex response is effected through the facial, hypoglossal and trigeminal nerves. It consists of a complex sequence of events including: (1) a wave of contraction in the pharyngeal muscles, which carries the food past the opening to the larynx to the upper oesophageal sphincter; (2) inhibition of breathing and closure of the glottis associated with raising of the larynx; (3) opening of the upper oesophageal sphincter; and (4) delivery of the bolus to the lumen of the upper oesophagus. It should be noted that stimulation of the receptors in the posterior pharynx does not invariably trigger a swallowing reflex. Stimulation of the posterior pharyngeal walls with a spatula or intubation device may trigger retching rather than swallowing. In the third or *oesophageal* phase of swallowing, a peristaltic wave of contraction passes down the oesophagus, driving the bolus in front of it. Peristaltic waves consist of a wave of contraction preceded by a wave of relaxation. Before the contraction wave reaches the lower oesophagus, the lower oesophageal sphincter relaxes to allow passage of the bolus into the stomach.

The upper and lower oesophageal sphincters are normally closed so that the intraoesophageal pressure is negative, approximating to intrathoracic pressure. Swallowing occurs several hundred times per day, even during sleep, and is associated with swallowing small amounts of saliva. Air may be swallowed with the saliva and, when excessive, gas builds up in the digestive tract. Some gas is absorbed but the rest is expelled via the mouth (belch) or via the rectum (flatus).

Problems with swallowing

Swallowing is a complex reflex and precise timing of the sequence of the events is important. Factors such as anaesthesia, alcoholic stupor, motor neurone disease, etc., which compromise the effectiveness of the neural control, can impair it. Material destined for the stomach may be passed to the lungs via the larynx, causing aspiration pneumonia.

Problems with the lower oesophageal sphincter can also cause dysphagia. Occasionally the VIP secreting nerve cells controlling relaxation of this sphincter are defective. This causes achalasia, where a failure of the sphincter to relax during swallowing allows food to accumulate at the bottom of the oesophagus. The oesophagus can become enormously dilated.

The sphincter is normally kept closed and this is important in preventing reflux of acid gastric contents into the lower oesophagus. Incompetence of the sphincter allows such reflux. The resulting irritation of the lower oesophageal mucosa causes pain (heart burn).

THE STOMACH AND GASTRIC SECRETION

The stomach is a large distensible sac in which food can be stored and partially digested before being released at suitable rates into the small intestine. Its glands secrete about two litres of gastric juice per day.

Gastric juice

Composition

The main constituents of gastric juice include the *pepsinogens*, proteolytic proenzymes secreted by the chief (peptic) cells, *hydrochloric acid* and *intrinsic factor* secreted by the oxyntic (parietal) cells, and *mucin* secreted by the mucous cells in the gastric mucosa.

Pepsinogens have no proteolytic effect until they reach the cavity of the stomach, where they are converted to pepsin by hydrochloric acid. Pepsin hydrolyses the bonds between certain amino acids in protein, splitting it up into polypeptide chains. Its pH optimum is about 1–2, so it is active only as long as it remains in the stomach.

Hydrochloric acid is secreted by the oxyntic cells and can be produced at a pH of about 1. Secretion of hydrochloric acid is stimulated by (1) histamine acting on H_2 receptors on mucosal cells, (2) acetylcholine acting on M_1 muscarinic receptors and (3) by gastrin acting on gastrin receptors on the walls of oxyntic cells. Histamine has a vital role because H_2-receptor blocking drugs abolish acid secretion almost completely, despite vagal and gastrin activity.

The cells secrete hydrogen using a hydrogen–potassium pump with energy derived from ATP. The acid reaches the surface of the cells through small canaliculi in their cytoplasm. The hydrogen is generated from the dissociation of H_2CO_3 catalysed by carbonic anhydrase, which has a high concentration in these cells. The bicarbonate generated in the dissociation passes back into the blood, accounting for the 'alkaline tide' seen after a meal. A pH of 1 implies a hydrogen ion concentration of 100 mmol l^{-1}, so at this stage, hydrogen ions are the most common cations in the fluid. With an internal cellular pH of just over 7, the proton pump overcomes a million-fold gradient.

Control of secretion of gastric juice

Gastric juice secretion is controlled by nerves and hormones. The secretory process for gastric juice takes place in three phases. The first phase (*vagal phase*) is a reflex response to the thought of food or the act of chewing food and is mediated through the vagus nerve. The vagal phase is responsible for the secretion of about half the juice in response to a meal. It is affected by emotional stimuli: fear and anxiety can inhibit gastric secretion; conversely, anger and rage can augment acid secretion. The centres responsible for this are thought to be in the hypothalamus. This phase anticipates and limits the buffering action of food on gastric pH. Gastrin release is also stimulated by a rise in gastric pH, an example of negative feedback.

The second phase is the *gastric phase*, in which food and food products in the stomach stretch its wall and excite receptors which cause release of the hormone gastrin.

The final phase is the *intestinal phase*, in which food products in the small intestine inhibit gastric secretion of acid and pepsinogen through nervous and hormonal mechanisms.

Functions of gastric juice

Gastric juice plays a significant, but not critical, role in protein digestion through its proteolytic enzyme pepsin. In its absence, protein breakdown is effected by pancreatic proteases, trypsin and chymotrypsin.

The hydrochloric acid is useful in killing harmful bacteria ingested with food. It activates pepsinogen by converting it to pepsin. It also reduces the valency of iron in ingested food from the trivalent ferric form to the divalent ferrous form in which it is absorbed.

Mucous secretion is important in providing a protective coating for the gastric mucosal cells. Although pepsin digests ingested protein, it does not normally attack the walls of the stomach because they are protected by this flexible mucous coat. In addition, bicarbonate is secreted into this mucous layer and buffers the relatively small number of hydrogen ions that penetrate it. If the protection provided by the mucous layer fails, ulceration of the mucosa may result. The mucous coat may be disrupted by excessive acid secretion, aspirin, non-steroidal anti-inflammatory drugs (NSAIDs), and infections in the stomach with the *Helicobacter pylori* bacterium. The disruption can lead to peptic ulceration. Prostaglandins normally promote mucous secretion, and NSAIDs and aspirin act by inhibiting prostaglandin synthesis in the stomach mucosa. Another factor protecting against ulceration is the rapid rate of regeneration of gastric mucosal cells: the mucous membranes of the gut are constantly renewing themselves.

Finally, intrinsic factor is needed for absorption of vitamin B_{12} in the terminal ileum and thus for normal erythropoiesis. Chronic gastritis can lead to atrophy of the gastric mucous membrane. A problem for such patients is anaemia, due in part to poor absorption of iron due to lack of hydrochloric acid and in part to poor absorption of vitamin B_{12} due to lack of intrinsic factor.

Gastric motility

The stomach acts as a hopper to store ingested food and deliver it at an appropriate rate to the small intestine for further digestion and absorption. A major inconvenience after surgical removal of the stomach is inability to take large meals; small frequent meals are required. The stomach, like the urinary bladder, shows 'receptive relaxation' — an ability to increase its volume with little increase in internal pressure.

The smooth muscle in the stomach wall is usually active even when the stomach is empty. When it is filled, regular waves of peristaltic contraction run down the body of the stomach from below the fundus to the pylorus about three times a minute. They mix and propel the contents. Mixing waves stop short of the pylorus so that food is churned back and forth by a recip-rocating action. As each propulsive wave reaches the pylorus, a squirt of gastric juice passes through the pyloric sphincter into the duode-num. Fluids can leave the stomach almost imme-diately. For example, oral glucose in solution given to a patient with hypoglycaemia can be ab-sorbed in a few minutes. The peristaltic activity in the stomach is coordinated through its vagal innervation. After vagotomy, gastric motility is reduced and less coordinated. The emptying time of the stomach is lengthened. The smooth muscle still contracts because these are local pacemakers in the stomach wall but the contractions are less effective in propelling gastric contents.

BILE AND THE GALLBLADDER

Bile is produced in the liver, stored and concen-trated in the gallbladder and discharged periodi-cally into the second part of the duodenum, where it assists in the digestion and absorption of fat. Its formation is a continuous process and about 500 ml day^{-1} is produced. Production takes place in the liver cells, and the bile, when formed, collects in small canaliculi in the liver lobules. The canaliculi collect into bile ducts, which come together outside the liver to form the common hepatic duct. The cystic duct from the gallbladder joins the common hepatic duct to form the common bile duct, whose opening into the duodenum is guarded by the sphincter of Oddi.

Composition of bile

Bile is 97% water, an alkaline fluid with inorganic salt concentrations similar to those in pancreatic juice. Its brown/green colour is due to the bile pigments, bilirubin and biliverdin, derived from haem after erythrocyte breakdown. Its most im-portant functional constituents are the bile salts, the sodium salts of taurocholic and glycocholic acid. In addition it contains lipid material, such as cholesterol, lecithin and fatty acids.

Control of bile secretion

Although bile secretion is a continuous process, the rate of secretion is increased by vagal nerve stimulation, the hormone secretin and by bile salts. Substances that increase flow are called choleretics.

Bile is not released into the alimentary tract immediately it is formed. When the sphincter of Oddi is closed the bile passes back up the cystic duct to the gallbladder, where it is stored and concentrated. Water is reabsorbed and the solid content of the bile rises from about 3 to 10% . The pH falls towards neutrality and the bile salt concentration rises 5–10-fold.

The gallbladder contracts and empties its con-tents after a meal is taken, when acid, fatty acids and amino acids enter the duodenum. These agents stimulate release of the hormone chole-cystokinin (CCK) from the intestinal mucosa. CCK contracts the smooth muscle in the gallbladder wall and relaxes the muscle in the sphincter of Oddi to drive the contained bile into the duo-denum. Vagal parasympathetic nerves are motor to the gallbladder muscle but their importance in regulating gallbladder function, relative to that of CCK and other gut hormones, is unclear.

Functions of bile

Bile pigments

Bile is the vehicle that excretes blood pigments. When old erythrocytes are removed from the circulation by the reticuloendothelial system, the contained haemoglobin is broken down. The iron is removed for storage in the liver and the globin is returned to the amino acid pool. The haem pigment is converted to bilirubin, which is carried to the liver. Bilirubin is not very soluble in water and is held in solution by binding to albu-min as it travels to the liver. Here the albumin is removed and the bilirubin is conjugated with glucuronic acid by the enzyme glucuronyl trans-ferase. Bilirubin glucuronide is more water soluble than bilirubin. In this form it is trans-ported into the bile canaliculi and excreted with the bile. The bile pigments have no digestive function in the intestine.

Bile salts

The bile salts are important in fat digestion and

absorption. They are steroid substances manufactured in the liver. They aid fat emulsification by reducing surface tension. Emulsification breaks fat into smaller particles, which provide a greater surface area to interact with lipase.

Bile salts have hydrophilic and lipophilic ends. They form complexes (micelles), with the hydrophilic ends on the outside and lipophilic ends facing the centre. Lipids which are poorly soluble in water collect on the inside (the hydrophobic part) of these complexes. Micelles thus confer water solubility on lipids and aid their transport across the mucosal wall for absorption. In the absence of bile salts, fat digestion and absorption is impaired and most ingested fat is passed as neutral fat in the faeces. There is also failure to absorb fat soluble vitamins. Failure to absorb vitamin K can lead to a bleeding tendency. Bile salts and lecithin also form micelles with cholesterol in the gallbladder, helping to prevent formation of cholesterol gallstones.

Bile salts are reabsorbed in their passage down the intestine, mainly by an active process in the terminal ilium. They return to the liver in the portal vein, where they stimulate bile formation and are re-excreted. This recirculation of the bile salts is called the enterohepatic circulation.

PANCREATIC EXOCRINE SECRETION

The pancreas secretes 1–2 litres of juice into the second part of the duodenum each day and plays an important part in the digestion of fat, protein and carbohydrate.

Composition

Pancreatic juice is alkaline because of its bicarbonate content, which is about five times that of plasma. Its pH, of about 8, helps to neutralise the acid gastric contents when they move into the small intestine.

Its proteolytic enzymes include *trypsin* and *chymotrypsin*, secreted as the proenzymes trypsinogen and chymotrypsinogen. When in the duodenum, trypsinogen is converted to trypsin by the enzyme, *enterokinase*, secreted from the mucosal cells of the small intestine. When formed, trypsin activates many of the other proenzymes, including trypsinogen and chymotrypsinogen. The ensuing catalytic chain reaction ensures a rapid rise in active enzyme concentration. Pancreatic juice also contains peptidases and enzymes that break down elastin, deoxyribonucleic acid (DNA) and ribonucleic acid (RNA).

For lipolysis, the principal enzyme is *pancreatic lipase*, which splits triglycerides into glycerol and fatty acids. Its action is assisted by a coenzyme, colipase. There are also enzymes that act on phospholipids and cholesterol esters.

For carbohydrate digestion, *pancreatic amylase* digests starch, breaking it down into dextrins and smaller polysaccharides and eventually disaccharides. Normally little of this enzyme leaks into the blood; however, in acute pancreatitis it leaks into the blood more freely and a high blood level is a marker for the disease.

Control of pancreatic juice secretion

Vagal juice

The pancreas has a vagal innervation and stimulation of the vagus results in the production of a small volume of juice, rich in enzymes. The flow of vagal juice is reflexly stimulated by the act of chewing food or by mental anticipation of a meal. This allows the digestive enzymes to be secreted into the pancreatic ducts well before the food reaches the duodenum. When the nerves are active, the zymogen granules in the acinar cells are mobilised and released by exocytosis into the pancreatic ducts. The proteolytic enzymes are secreted in an inactive form so that they do not damage the gland tissues. They become active only after they reach the small intestine.

Secretin juice

When food products enter the small intestine, they induce release of the hormone secretin from the intestinal mucosal cells. This hormone circulates in the blood and stimulates the pancreatic ducts to produce a copious watery juice rich in bicarbonate but poor in enzymes. It flushes the enzymes, secreted in response to vagal nerve activity, into the duodenum.

Pancreozymin/CCK juice

Subsequently, another hormone, pancreozymin/cholecystokinin is released from the mucosal cells which, like vagal nerve activity, stimulates the acinar cells in the pancreas to secrete an enzyme-rich juice.

Functions of pancreatic juice

The bicarbonate in pancreatic juice is important for neutralising the acid gastric contents entering the small intestine. Raising the pH to around neutrality protects the intestinal mucosa and provides an optimal pH for the many enzymes that act in the intestinal lumen. Because of its many digestive enzymes, which act on most varieties of foodstuff, adequate secretion of juice is essential for normal digestion. If pancreatic secretion is impaired, there is incomplete digestion of fats, carbohydrates and protein and incompletely digested food appears in the faeces. The stools are bulky from undigested food residues, buoyant due to the high fat content and foul-smelling due to the action of bacteria on the undigested food.

THE SMALL INTESTINE

The small intestine is about 300 cm long. It commences as the duodenum, the second part of which receives the common bile and pancreatic ducts. The duodenum continues into the jejunum and then the ileum, which opens into the caecum. Entry to the system is controlled by the pyloric sphincter, and exit by the ileocaecal valve. Most of the food in a meal leaves the stomach within 4–6 hours, depending on its size and content, especially fat content, and the small intestine within 10 hours of ingestion.

Mucous membrane

Surface area

The small intestine is concerned chiefly with absorption of digested food products and provides a large surface area for this purpose. The large surface area results from several anatomical factors. The mucosa of the small intestine is thrown into folds which look like valves and are called *valvulae conniventes*. The mucosal surface has finger-like projections (*villi*), about 0.5 mm long, which project into the lumen with a density of about 40 mm^{-2}. In addition to this the luminal surface of the mucosal cells (enterocytes) has *microvilli* which form their brush borders.

Mucosal regeneration

The mucous membrane has a high rate of turnover of mucosal cells. Cells at the top of the glandular crypts are constantly being sloughed off into the lumen and new cells are constantly being generated at a similar rate at the base of the crypts to replace them. The mucosal cells are thought to be completely replaced in a few days in humans and in a few hours in some small animals.

Lymphoid tissue

The mucosa contains much lymphoid tissue. In the upper part it consists of solitary nodules but the nodules are aggregated in the lower small intestine into larger masses called Peyer's patches. Each villus has a central lymphatic, the contents of which eventually drain into afferent lymphatics. These carry the lymph to lymph nodes in the mesentery. Efferent lymphatics, including the thoracic duct, carry the lymph from the nodes back to the great veins.

Secretory activity

Between 1 and 2 litres of intestinal juice are secreted per day. It is alkaline and contains a number of digestive enzymes. The enzymes are not secreted by exocytosis but are derived from the enzyme-containing mucosal cells shed from the mucosal surface. The enzymes complete the digestive splitting of foodstuff into products suitable for absorption. *Aminopeptidases* and *dipeptidases* break down polypeptides to amino acids. *Maltase*, *sucrase* and *lactase* split the respective disaccharides into monosaccharides. *Nuclease* splits nucleic acid into pentose sugars and purine and pyrimidine bases.

There are many mucus secreting cells in the mucous membrane and their secretions form a gel layer that covers and protects the mucosa. Vagal stimulation increases mucus secretion, as does irritation or inflammation of the intestinal wall. In addition to protecting the mucosa the mucus helps to lubricate the food in its passage along the gut.

Absorptive activity

Water and salts

Water. Each day about 10 litres of water are presented to the small intestine; 1.5 litres of this is derived from drinks or food and the remainder, about 8.5 litres, is derived from digestive secretions. The small intestine absorbs most (about 8.5 litres) of this water load, leaving only 1.5 litres or so to proceed to the large intestine. Absorption of water is passive. It depends on the active reabsorption of sodium and the end-products of digestion. Water follows these substances to maintain osmotic equilibrium between the intestinal contents and the blood.

Sodium. Sodium is absorbed by the enterocytes using an active sodium pump mechanism which facilitates the absorption of glucose and amino acids by carrier mechanisms. Chloride follows the sodium ions to maintain electrical equilibrium between the luminal fluid and the blood. Potassium absorption results mainly from its movement down its electrochemical gradient. Linkage of salt and glucose absorption by a symport mechanism is the basis of oral rehydration therapy (see Ch. 40, p. 592). Using this therapy for patients with gastroenteritis, an approximately isotonic and equimolecular solution of salt and glucose (some potassium may be added) is absorbed almost as rapidly as an intravenous infusion. Proximal tubular cells in the nephron have a similar symport system.

Calcium. Calcium absorption is adjusted to meet the body needs for calcium and this is effected through the vitamin D mechanism. Normally only a fraction (about 50%) of ingested calcium is absorbed. A metabolite of vitamin D — 1,25-dihydroxycholecalciferol — is produced in amounts related to the serum calcium level. When the calcium level falls, the level of 1,25-dihydroxycholecalciferol rises. In the gut it increases the amount of calcium binding protein in the mucosal cells, which facilitates calcium absorption. Certain substances, such as oxylates and phosphates, interfere with calcium absorption by forming insoluble calcium salts in the gut.

Iron. The percentage of dietary iron absorbed is normally even smaller (less than 10%) than that of calcium. It is absorbed in amounts that replace the amount of iron lost from the body. This tends to be higher in women than men because of menstrual loss of blood. The body must limit iron uptake because it has no effective mechanism for excreting that in excess of body needs. Excessive deposits of iron are toxic to tissues, especially those of the liver and pancreas.

Iron is absorbed in the upper part of the small intestine by an active process involving a transcellular carrier. It is absorbed in the ferrous (divalent) rather than the ferric (trivalent) form. The hydrochloric acid in gastric juice converts the ferric form of iron common in the food into the ferric form, which can be absorbed.

In the cells there is a substance called apoferritin which combines with iron to form ferritin. The polypeptide iron carrier in plasma is called transferrin. When this carrier becomes desaturated, it takes up iron from the ferritin and the resulting apoferritin can take up more iron from the gut. When mucosal cells are discarded and pass into the faeces, their iron stored as apoferritin is lost with them.

End-products of digestion

Carbohydrates. In the small intestine, maltose is split into two glucose molecules by maltase, lactose into glucose and galactose by lactase, and sucrose into fructose and glucose by sucrase. These molecules can be absorbed rapidly by the gut. Glucose and galactose are absorbed by an active process that is facilitated by sodium and inhibited by phlorhizin. Fructose is absorbed by an independent mechanism involving facilitated diffusion. The absorbed monosaccharides are carried by the portal blood to the liver.

Proteins. The protein presented to the small intestine is derived from ingested protein (50%), the enzymes in the digestive juices (25%) and the cellular debris cast off by the mucosa (25%). Protein substances are absorbed into the portal blood as amino acids. Some of these are produced by enzymes in the lumen of the gut but others are produced in the mucosal walls by the dipeptidases and aminopeptidases in the brush border of the mucosal cells.

The individual amino acids are absorbed by a variety of active processes using different carriers. Laevo isomers of amino acids are absorbed more rapidly than the dextro isomers, which are thought to be absorbed by passive diffusion. As with glucose absorption, sodium can facilitate the transport of amino acids. Certain congenital diseases can affect the absorption of particular amino acids.

In infants, some protein can be absorbed as undigested protein. This is accomplished by pinocytosis and accounts for the absorption of antibodies in maternal milk. The ability of proteins to cross the mucosal wall is lost in adults. If it persists, absorption of foreign proteins can set up immune reactions in the gut wall, which can cause allergic reactions to food. Food allergies are more common in children than in adults.

Antigens from foreign organisms are taken up by lymphoid tissue in the gut wall and stimulate the immune system to produce antibodies. IgA produced as a result of this returns to the mucosal cells where it provides defence against further exposure to the foreign organisms.

Fats. After fat has been emulsified in the lumen of the gut, it is acted on by pancreatic lipase and colipase to form glycerol and fatty acids. Fatty acids and other lipids are taken up by micelles which make the relatively water insoluble compounds soluble and facilitate their transport into the mucosal cells. The glycerol can move into the cells by diffusion. In the cells, the short chain fatty acids are absorbed directly into the blood, where they are carried as free fatty acids. The long chain fatty acids are re-esterified with glycerol to form triglycerides inside the mucosal cells. With the addition of cholesterol, phospholipid and protein, the triglycerides are formed

into chylomicrons. These are extruded from the cells by exocytosis and taken up by the lacteals in the mucosal villi. They are returned to the circulation via the lymph and are responsible for the milky colour of intestinal lymph after a fatty meal. Levels of lipoprotein in the blood influence the development of arterial disease and vascular occlusion and so contribute to the genesis of myocardial infarction.

Intestinal motility

The smooth muscle of the small intestine causes movements which propel its contents by peristalsis or mix its contents by segmentation contractions. The muscle is provoked to contractile activity by stretch of the intestinal wall by incoming food. Although this activity is modulated by extrinsic autonomic nerves, it can occur in the absence of extrinsic innervation through local pacemaker activity in the myenteric plexus of the gut wall. An isolated segment of gut in an organ bath shows regular spontaneous contractions about 10 times per minute. The rate and force of the contractions is increased by parasympathetic nerve stimulation and by acetylcholine. Sympathetic nerve stimulation, adrenaline and noradrenaline slow and weaken the contractions.

After abdominal surgery, motility in the intestines is often reduced and may cease (*paralytic ileus*). This is due to several factors, including trauma to the muscle from handling the intestines, sympathetic nerve activity in response to shock and disturbance of electrolyte balance. It causes intestinal obstruction because gut contents will not move forward without contractions of the gut wall. Usually the condition is temporary and movements begin again spontaneously within hours or days of the surgery. Return of peristaltic activity can be inferred from bowel sounds heard by auscultating the abdomen.

THE LARGE INTESTINE

Each day 1–2 litres of material is presented to the colon through the ileocaecal valve. In the metre or so of colon traversed, water and some salts are absorbed and about 250 ml of semisolid material is presented to the rectum for defecation. Faecal bulk and intestinal transit time are strongly influenced by the fibre content, especially bran, of the diet. A high fibre diet may give a transit time of 1 day with a faecal weight around 400 g day^{-1}. With a low fibre diet, transit time is 3–4 days and faecal weight under 100 g day^{-1}.

Secretory activity

The dominant cells in the colonic mucosa are mucus secreting cells and mucins secreted by them form a protective layer over the mucosa. They also act as a lubricant to facilitate movement of faeces. There is net secretion of potassium and bicarbonate into the colon so that prolonged diarrhoea may cause hypokalaemia and a non-respiratory (metabolic) acidosis.

Absorptive activity

Active sodium absorption, similar to that seen in the small intestine, occurs in the colon. The negatively charged chloride ions follow the positively charged sodium ions. To maintain osmotic equilibrium between the colonic contents and the blood, water passively follows the sodium chloride. Thus, most of the water presented to the colon from the small intestine is reabsorbed before the colonic contents reach the rectum.

Motor activity

The ileocaecal valve is normally closed but opens each time a peristaltic wave reaches the terminal ileum and allows a squirt of ileal contents to enter the caecum. The ileocaecal valve also prevents reflux of caecal contents into the ileum. The colon exhibits the same segmentation and peristaltic movements seen in the small intestine. Another type of movement, not seen in the small intestine, is the mass action contraction. In this movement there is simultaneous contraction over a wide length of colon which moves faeces from one part of the colon to another.

Isolated colon strips show rhythmic contractile activity similar to, but slower than, that seen in the small intestine. This activity is coordinated through local nerve plexuses in the bowel wall. In the intact animal, the activity is modulated by autonomic nerve activity. Parasympathetic activity causes an increase, and sympathetic nerve activity a decrease, in the rate and strength of the contractions. Psychological states can modify large bowel activity to cause either diarrhoea or constipation. These effects are presumably mediated via extrinsic nerves.

Distension of the colonic wall is a powerful stimulus to contraction and colonic movements are more apparent when the bulk of the faecal material it contains is increased. Dietary fibre, which increases faecal bulk, promotes colonic movements. It has been suggested that high levels of fibre intake diminish the incidence of diverticulitis and colonic cancer by lowering intraluminal pressure and reducing transit time, during which bacteria could generate carcinogens.

Intestinal flora

The small intestine contains relatively few bacteria because of the digestive action of its enzymes and the relatively rapid transit through the system. However, the colonic contents have a rich bacterial flora which accounts for about 25 % of faecal weight. Some of these bacteria are beneficial, in that they manufacture vitamins such as vitamin K for the body. Others are probably harmful, as young animals treated with antibiotics have greater growth rates than untreated ones. The flora is also responsible for the production of some of the gases found in the colon and some of the amines produced by degradation of amino acids.

Protection against harmful bacteria is afforded by lymphoid tissue in the wall, which can be activated by the antigens of pathological bacteria and other micro-organisms. The antibodies so formed are taken up by the mucosal cells and provide some immunity against further infection with those organisms.

Defecation

The large intestine acts as a hopper to store

faeces for evacuation at convenient intervals. In some ways, its function is analogous to that of the stomach. The stomach's capacity to store food eliminates the need for continuous feeding and the storage capacity of the large intestine eliminates the need for continuous defecation. A problem for patients who have undergone colectomy is having to wear an ileostomy bag over the stoma to collect and store the relatively fluid faecal material being presented to it continually by the small intestine. A proximal colostomy in the right iliac fossa presents similar problems. On the other hand, a distal colostomy in the left iliac fossa transmits a more formed faeces at less frequent intervals, illustrating the storage and water absorbing functions of the colon.

Defecation is a spinal reflex with its reflex centres in the sacral segments of the cord. The afferent limb consists of sensory fibres from stretch receptors in the wall of the rectum. Stretch of these receptors, when of sufficient strength, triggers the wish to defecate. The efferent limb involves parasympathetic cholinergic activation of rectal smooth muscle and inhibition of the anal sphincters. The reflex can be voluntarily inhibited by keeping the voluntary anal sphincter closed. It can also be facilitated by voluntary relaxation of the anal sphincter together with voluntary contraction of the diaphragm and then the abdominal muscles to raise intra-abdominal pressure. This drives colonic contents into the rectum and reinforces the involuntary spinal reflex.

FURTHER READING

Allen A, Flemstrom G, Garner A, Kivilaakso E 1993 Gastroduodenal mucosal protection. Physiological Reviews 73: 823–857

Davison J S 1989 Gastrointestinal secretion. Wright, London

Johnson L R (ed) 1994 Physiology of the gastrointestinal tract, 3rd edn. Raven Press, New York

Lewis J H (ed) 1994 A pharmacological approach to gastrointestinal disorders. Williams & Wilkins, Baltimore

39

Physiology and control of nausea and vomiting

L. D. Paxton

Nausea and vomiting have from prehistoric times been important concerns to man, and even before his understanding of other major organ systems, gut symptomatology played an important part in both cultural activities and medical remedies. (*Nausea* and *nautical* have a common linguistic origin, indicating the familiarity of the ancients with seasickness.) Physiologically, vomiting is a primitive reflex providing a protective function to the animal, and is found not only in mammals but in other vertebrate and invertebrate animals. Vomiting mechanisms have evolved to detect and expel from the body toxic substances that have been ingested. Detection involves both peripheral and central elements, with connecting pathways and integrative mechanisms, leading to activation and coordination of expulsive muscle contractions.

Definitions

Nausea is a subjective sensation and is the desire to vomit without any expulsive muscular actions. Severe nausea may be further associated with hypersalivation and vasomotor disturbances. Nausea may be brief or prolonged, or come in waves, and may either precede vomiting or occur in isolation. Vomiting may alleviate the symptom.

Retching is the laboured rhythmic activity of the respiratory musculature that usually precedes or accompanies vomiting. Vomiting is neither synonymous with retching nor an invariable consequence of it.

Vomiting (emesis) is the production from the mouth of gastric contents by expulsive reflex somatic muscular contraction. Passive regurgitation results from loss of sphincter tone in the pharynx and oesophagus without strong contraction of the abdominal muscles.

PHYSIOLOGY

The physiology of vomiting involves both central and peripheral structures; although these are interconnected they will be discussed separately.

Central structures

The concept of well defined anatomical areas within the brainstem which control homeostatic functions has given way to more broadly spread functional zones. These areas have connections to the other control zones (respiratory and cardio-vascular) in the medulla and pathways to higher and lower parts of the central nervous system. The *chemoreceptor trigger zone* (CTZ) is located in the area postrema, one of the four circumventricular organs, which lie outside the blood–brain barrier. The CTZ is U-shaped, about 4 mm long in man and is in close proximity to the fourth ventricle. The absence of the blood–brain barrier here allows the transfer of both non-polarised and polarised chemicals (endogenous and exogenous) directly into the CTZ from the cerebrospinal fluid (CSF).

A large number of neurotransmitters are found in the CTZ (Fig. 39.1). Serotonin, dopamine and acetylcholine may be the dominant transmitters involved in transmission of the information to the vomiting centre from the CTZ. The *nucleus of the tractus solitarius* (NTS) and the *vagal nuclei* receive afferent input from the vagus nerve and are interconnected with the CTZ. The afferent inputs are modulated in these areas and then

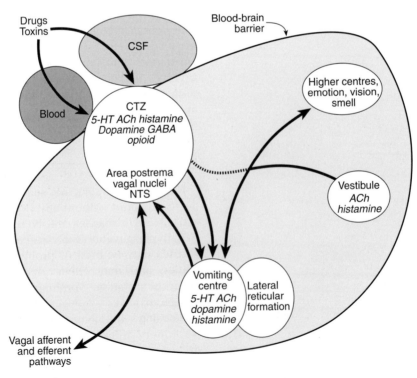

Figure 39.1

impulses pass to the 'vomiting centre' where, if appropriate, the emetic reflex is initiated.

Vomiting centre

The *vomiting centre* is located in the dorsolateral reticular formation of the brainstem, the Bötzinger complex. This area coordinates all the events in the emetic reflex, from the prodromal symptoms to the profound changes in respiratory musculature and upper gastrointestinal system motility that precede emesis. In the vomiting centre the predominant transmitters (and receptor types) appear to be serotonin (5-HT$_3$), dopamine (D$_2$) and acetylcholine (muscarinic M$_3$).

The emetic reflex is a highly integrated physiological and protective reflex involving precise temporal coordination between autonomic and somatic motor components. Irrespective of the mode of stimulation of the vomiting centre, the motor component is the same. The efferent stimuli pass down the vagus nerve to the upper gastrointestinal tract, the phrenic nerve to the diaphragm and the intercostal nerves to the abdominal and intercostal muscles.

Peripheral structures

These include both afferent (80%) and efferent (20%) pathways in the vagus nerve from the upper gastrointestinal tract. There are both cholinergic and non-cholinergic nerve fibres in the vagus; the non-cholinergic neurones may have serotonin as transmitter. Two types of vagal afferent receptors are involved in the emetic response:

1. *Mechanoreceptors*, located in the muscular wall of the distal stomach and proximal duodenum, which are activated by distension or contraction of the gut wall.
2. *Chemoreceptors*, located in the gut mucosa of the upper small bowel, which monitor the intraluminal contents. They are activated by acid, alkali, hypertonic solutions and irritants (classically copper sulphate). Serotonin may play an important part in the transmission from these chemoreceptors. Evidence for this includes a high concentration in the upper

gastrointestinal tract of enterochromaffin cells which are rich in serotonin. When these are stimulated they release serotonin into the surrounding tissues and so activate the afferent vagal pathways. These cells may also act as a reservoir of serotonin.

After a meal, a large number of gut hormones are released, including gastrin and motilin. These hormones may induce emesis if injected directly into the CSF around the area postrema and their role may possibly be to sensitise the area postrema in the event of poisoning. Vagotomy (subdiaphragmatic) abolishes both the mechano- and chemoreceptor responses.

Although not strictly 'peripheral', there are also inputs to the vomiting centre from other sense organs from cranial nerves and descending pathways from the cortex and hypothalamus. Visual and olfactory responses may act as a first line of defence, dissuading the person or animal from eating a potentially toxic substance in the first place. Stimulation of the vestibular system by rhythmical motion (motion sickness) or head / position disorientation (space sickness) leads to emesis. The evolutionary significance of these is uncertain, but it is a cause of discomfort for those who suffer motion related sickness. Sudden movement of the head leads to labyrinthine stimulation, which may potentiate opioid related and postoperative nausea and so should be avoided as far as possible following surgery. The cholinergic (M$_3$) receptor is probably dominant in this form of emesis.

Behavioural and psychological inputs may further modulate the emetic response, either to suppress it or to activate it without pathophysiological stimulation. Learned responses can be important — a patient who has experienced severe nausea or vomiting with, for example, chemotherapy may become nauseated even by such a tenuously related experience as driving past the hospital where treatment was given. Severe pain may also be a cause of nausea and perhaps vomiting.

Although different stimuli appear to cause vomiting by different mechanisms, there is often summation of effects; for example, opioids (acting on the CTZ) are more likely to cause sickness in the ambulant patient (labyrinthine upset) and sickness is more likely to follow an emetic stimulus if the patient can hear and see another patient who is actually vomiting.

Emetic reflex

This is the motor response to a perceived poisoning and involves both inhibitory and excitatory phenomena. Nausea may be the initial symptom, which may lead rapidly or slowly to emesis. The emetic reflex could potentially cause severe damage to the upper gastrointestinal tract if it was not coordinated. Immediately before retching and vomiting there is inhibition of the peristaltic and propulsive waves of the upper gastrointestinal tract, mediated through non-cholinergic and non-adrenergic neurones and thought to involve vasoactive intestinal peptide or possibly nitric oxide. There is a corresponding central inhibition of respiration due to inhibition of inspiratory neurones in the ventrorespiratory group in the medulla. This inhibitory signal appears to be the first event in the emetic reflex and there is no retching without this inhibition having preceded it. It is protective for the animal, as there could be disastrous consequences if vomiting and inspiration occurred together. This is then followed by rhythmical, coordinated contraction of the diaphragm and abdominal muscles. There is a large retrograde contraction of the upper small intestine which moves gastric and small bowel contents into the upper stomach and lower oesophagus; this is probably mediated by cholecystokinin and substance P. Simultaneously there is a relaxation of the hiatal diaphragmatic fibres and the lower oesophageal sphincter, with the protrusion into the lower thoracic cavity of the proximal stomach, thus removing the acute angle of the lower oesophageal and gastric junction and forming a funnel into which the gastric contents flow. The complex functional nature of the lower oesophageal sphincter has to be changed to allow the retrograde movement of gastric contents and this is achieved by this change in the position of the stomach relative to oesophagus and diaphragm.

All these phenomena occur with retching and may be repeated until there is vomiting. Vomiting (emesis) involves an additional coordinated relaxation of both the upper oesophagus (the upper oesophageal sphincter is opened with the contraction of the geniohyoid muscle) and the pharyngeal muscles, allowing expulsion of gastric contents. There are other associated postural changes so that the relative efficiencies of the muscle groups can be enhanced — for example, holding on to fixed objects, bending over, etc. After expulsion of gastric contents there is a pause in retching to allow for respiration, which up till this point has been inhibited, to continue.

Receptors involved in emesis

Because emesis involves activity at several discrete locations in the body, it is more difficult to ascribe emetic effects, or the antiemetic effect of a drug to action at one particular type of receptor. Four different receptor types have been the main focus of interest. These are *muscarinic cholinergic*, *histamine H_1*, *dopamine D_2* (different from the vascular dopamine receptor) and *serotonin 5-HT_3*. Dopamine D_2 receptors are found in high concentration in the area postrema, which contains the CTZ. Histamine H_1 receptors are concentrated in the nucleus tractus solitarius, which processes sensory information relating to emesis, and in the dorsal motor nucleus of the vagus. This nucleus and the nucleus ambiguus also contain muscarinic cholinergic receptors, and these initiate the motor components of vomiting. Serotonin has more recently been identified as an important mediator of emesis, and is dealt with in more detail below.

In addition to these receptors, it has been suggested that enkephalins are involved in some parts of this process. Enkephalins or opioids may cause release of dopamine in the CTZ, with stimulation of dopaminergic receptors, and cytotoxic drugs, by inhibiting the enzymes that break down enkephalin, may allow them to build up, causing nausea.

In contrast, there may be an enkephalin-mediated antiemetic 'tone', expressed at the vomiting centre, not the CTZ, and probably an effect on synaptic transmission there. These effects may be mediated by µ and δ receptors respectively.

Acupuncture, which is known to influence enkephalin concentrations, has been shown to have an antiemetic action.

Serotonin (5-hydroxytryptamine, 5-HT)

A precise functional role or roles for 5-HT has yet to be fully established; however, 5-HT is involved in a number of diverse activities including sleep, mood, behaviour, possibly memory, cardiovascular control (Bezold–Jarisch reflex), smooth muscle contraction and relaxation, modulation of pain at the spinal cord level and platelet activation, and as described above it has an important role in emesis.

5-HT is synthesised from L-tryptophan (an essential amino acid) in a two step pathway. There is active uptake of L-tryptophan in the tissues involved in the synthesis of 5-HT, e.g. nerve terminals, which may be a further limiting factor in its synthesis. Following release into the synaptic cleft the activity of 5-HT is terminated by active reuptake into the presynaptic nerve terminal. To date, four main subtypes of 5-HT receptor have been discovered, each receptor subtype having specific roles.

The 5-HT$_3$ receptor is different to the other 5-HT receptors in that it forms a ligand gated ion channel similar to the muscarinic acetylcholine receptor, whereas the 5-HT$_1$, 5-HT$_2$ and 5-HT$_4$ receptors are G-protein coupled. Activation of the 5-HT$_3$ receptor leads to a rapid depolarisation of the cell membrane and the influx of sodium and calcium into and potassium out of the cell. The 5-HT$_3$ receptor is found only on neurones, both in the central and peripheral nervous systems, and is located pre- and postsynaptically. Peripherally the receptors are found in the upper gastrointestinal tract, and in the central nervous system they are found in a number of areas, including high concentrations in the area postrema, the hippocampus, the trigeminal and vagal nuclei and in the spinal cord. In the spinal cord the receptors are found in the substantia gelatinosa where they are involved in the perception and processing of pain signals.

Postoperative nausea and vomiting and preanaesthetic fasting

Many events in the perianaesthetic period may have an influence on the associated postoperative morbidity and wellbeing for the patient undergoing anaesthesia. Many of the anaesthetic drugs used in modern anaesthetic practice have an effect on the CTZ and vomiting centre, either directly or indirectly — for example, stimulation of the CTZ by opioid agonist drugs, inhibition of 5-HT by indirect effects of propofol, stimulation of the vestibular apparatus. Nitrous oxide may cause gut distension and also increase middle ear pressure, leading to stimulation of the vestibular apparatus. Gastric stasis due to a number of factors, and pain as a result of the surgical procedure, may also contribute to postoperative nausea and vomiting. The prevention and treatment of postoperative nausea and vomiting has assumed a more important role in perianaesthetic management of patients as the overall morbidity from anaesthesia has improved. In the majority of cases postoperative nausea and vomiting has no significant morbidity except for the discomfort experienced by the patient; however, there may be serious consequences, including aspiration of gastric contents, rupture of the oesophagus, wound dehiscence and disturbance of surgical reconstruction, especially in head and neck surgery and ophthalmic procedures, if the retching or vomiting are severe and prolonged. Nausea, retching and vomiting may occur after regional as well as general anaesthesia. The overall incidence of postoperative nausea and vomiting in the past 5–10 years has decreased from that reported in the 'ether era' 30–40 years ago. This in part is due to changes in drugs used and improvements in surgical and anaesthetic techniques. However, there are still subgroups of patients with a relatively high incidence, for example patients undergoing gynaecological, ear, nose and throat and ophthalmic procedures.

Pulmonary aspiration of gastric contents at the induction of anaesthesia is potentially life threatening and certainly one of the main reasons for patients to fast before elective procedures. A volume of gastric contents greater than 25 ml and a pH less than 2.5 have been cited as 'at risk' levels for the development of the acid pneumonitis syndrome. In fact these figures have arisen mainly from the need for an arbitrary target for comparison between studies of antacid regimens, and there is very little scientific data supporting these particular levels as the threshold for risk. Most information is extrapolated from animal work. Traditionally the fasting period has been a length of time ranging from 6 to 12 hours. This is probably due more to organisational restrictions with operating schedules than any physiological constraints. The supposed rationale of this period of fasting is to allow adequate time for the stomach to empty. Solids need to be liquefied before passage into the duodenum and so may have a gastric transit time of up to 8 hours, although usually not more than 4–6 hours. Gastric emptying for fluids is rapid, with 95% of ingested liquids emptied within 1 hour. The production of gastric secretions (50 ml h^{-1} — baseline) and saliva (1 ml kg^{-1} h^{-1}) is dependent on the ingestion of solids and liquids. There may indeed be a higher residual gastric volume in patients with a prolonged fast than in those who have taken clear fluids in the previous 2 hours, due to an accumulation of gastric secretions in the stomach. It thus seems to be that the duration of the fast for solids should be maintained but that for fluids be redefined for patients without any underlying pathology prolonging gastric emptying. Suggested guidelines include the following:

- no solid food on the day of surgery
- unrestricted clear fluids until 2 hours before surgery
- oral medications 1–2 hours before surgery, with up to 150 ml of water
- for those patients specially at risk, an H_2 receptor antagonist.

PHARMACOLOGY OF ANTIEMETIC DRUGS

Antiemetic drugs are used for symptomatic relief of nausea and vomiting and also in the prevention of these unpleasant symptoms in predictable situations, for example postoperatively or following chemotherapy and radiotherapy. The aetiology of radio- and chemotherapy induced nausea and vomiting is related to the amount of cellular damage in organs with a high cell turnover, particularly in the gut, where there is liberation both locally and systemically of hormones and transmitters. Serotonin is released in high quantities from the gut and, with the advent of specific antiserotonin agents, the prevention and treatment of emesis is more predictable in these situations. The nausea and emesis seen following anaesthesia seems to be more multifactorial, as seen from the complex input and number of receptors within the emetic mechanisms of the brainstem. There are therefore a large number of differing drug groups and classes that have antiemetic effects along with other class related side-effects, for example extrapyramidal symptoms and signs with phenothiazine drugs. The development of more specific antiemetics, of which the serotonin (5-HT_3) antagonists are the first example, has reduced the side-effects of these drugs.

There are many different antiemetic drugs available and the large number of studies in the literature show that the response to these drugs may be influenced by a wide number of variables which are very difficult to control, and so the reported efficacy of certain drugs may vary widely. Therefore, without clear guidance being available from studies, antiemetic usage may often be based on personal preference and experience and possibly on institutional protocols.

Table 39.1 shows the broad classes of drugs with antiemetic properties.

Anticholinergic drugs

Atropine; hyoscine (scopolamine)

The use of these drugs for their antiemetic effects has been in decline in recent anaesthetic practice, particularly as benzodiazepines are now used more frequently for premedication. *Hyoscine* crosses the blood–brain barrier more than atropine and so some of the side-effects are more pronounced with hyoscine. These include drowsiness, blurred vision, dizziness, dry mouth and difficulty with micturition, while confusion may

Table 39.1 Receptor affinity of antiemetic drugs.

Pharmacological group	Dopamine (D$_2$)	Cholinergic muscarinic	Histamine (H$_1$)	Serotonin (5-HT$_3$)
Anticholinergics				
Hyoscine	−	++++	+	−
Phenothiazines				
Chlorpromazine	++++	++	++++	+
Prochlorperazine	++++			
Fluphenazine	++++	+	++	−
Butyrophenones				
Droperidol	++++	−	+	+
Domperidone	++++			
Antihistamines				
Promethazine	++	++	++++	−
Diphenhydramine	+	++	++++	−
Benzamides				
Metocolopramide	+++	−	+	++
Serotonin antagonists				
Ondansetron	−	−	−	++++
Granisetron	−	−	−	++++

Modified from Hamik & Peroutka (1989) and Peroutka & Snyder (1982).

occur in the elderly. Hyoscine is a traditional anti-emetic, usually given in premedication (0.4 mg), and is combined with papaveretum in the preparation 'omnopon and scopolamine', which was an extremely popular premedicant in the past, now largely superseded by benzodiazepines. Its main side-effects are drowsiness and dryness of the mouth.

Hyoscine is a well proven remedy for motion sickness, and an effect on the vestibular apparatus may contribute to its action. Here it is given in the form of the hydrobromide (scopolamine), 1 mg of which contains 0.7 mg of the *laevo*-hyoscine base. Commercially available seasickness tablets usually contain 0.3 mg and one or two are recommended for protection for short journeys. Side-effects preclude the long term use of hyoscine for travel sickness.

A transdermal preparation has become available. This patch, containing 0.5 mg, is effective for up to 72 hours, but absorption is slow, reaching a steady-state plasma level only after 5 hours, so that the patch needs to be applied early, i.e. 5–6 hours before travel and similarly before operation. Studies have again shown only moderate efficacy in postoperative nausea and vomiting, but side-effects are slight.

Phenothiazines

This group of drugs has a number of widely differing therapeutic indications. Only the phenothiazines with significant antiemetic actions will be discussed in this section. Phenothiazine compounds share a common basic structure (Fig. 39.2), and in general have similar actions and side-effects. All have sedative effects and may cause extrapyramidal effects, which might range from restlessness to an oculogyric crisis. The pattern of side-effects will depend on the arrangement of side-chains attached to the parent molecule — for example, extrapyramidal manifestations may be greater in drugs with a piperazine ring structure. The symptoms abate with dose reduction or drug withdrawal. Occasionally tardive dyskinesia may occur with prolonged use. Other side-effects include blurred vision, urinary retention, cholestatic jaundice, blood dyscrasias, hypothermia, postural hypotension and neuroleptic malignant syndrome.

A. Diethyl aminophenothiazines

Chlorpromazine (Largactil)

Dose: oral, intramuscular and intravenous.

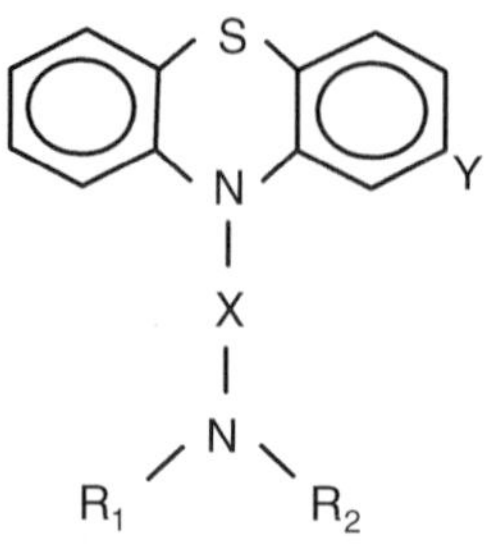

	Y	X	R_1	R_2
Chlorpromazine	Cl	$-(CH_2)_3-$	CH_3	CH_3
Promethazine	H	$-CH_2-CH-$ $\quad\quad CH_3$	CH_3	CH_3
Fluphenazine	CF_3	$-(CH_2)_3-$	N◯N$-CH_2-CH_2-OH$	
Prochlorperazine	Cl	$-(CH_2)_3-$	N◯N$-CH_3$	
Perphenazine	Cl	$-(CH_2)_3-$	N◯N$-CH_2-CH_2-OH$	
Trifluperazine	CF_3	$-(CH_2)_3-$	N◯N$-CH_3$	

Figure 39.2 General structure of phenothiazines.

There is a large dose range. For antiemetic/premedication the dose is 12.5–25 mg, either orally or intramuscularly.

Chlorpromazine has direct effects on the CTZ and may also depress temperature control and prevent shivering. The effects are due to inhibition of dopamine centrally. When initially developed, this drug was used as an adjunct to anaesthesia, before its introduction into the treatment of psychiatric illness. It may potentiate the effects of hypnotics, sedatives and anaesthetic agents.

Promethazine (Phenergan)

Dose: oral 10–25 mg, intramuscular or intravenous 25–50 mg.

Promethazine was first developed for its antihistamine effects but is more commonly used for its sedative/anticholinergic, antiemetic actions and prevention of motion related sickness. The sedative actions are quite marked and last longer than the antiemetic effects.

B. Phenothiazines with a piperazine ring

Perphenazine (Fentazin)

Dose: only oral formulation is now available; 2–4 mg, 1–2 hours preoperatively.

This phenothiazine is used less and less in anaesthetic practice and is usually given with premedication. The antiemetic effects are well recognised but there may be marked sedation. It has a role in anxiety states and in the management of psychiatric cases.

Prochlorperazine (Stemetil, Buccastem)

Dose: intramuscular, oral or sublingual; 12.5–

25 mg intramuscularly, 5–10 mg orally and 5 mg sublingually

Prochlorperazine has less potentiating effects on hypnotics than chlorpromazine and does not produce lethargy and hypotension. It may be used in the treatment of migraine, Ménière's syndrome and other labyrinthine disturbances.

Trifluoperazine (Stelazine)

Dose: 2–4 mg day^{-1}; sustained release preparation — 6 mg maximum daily dose.

Trifluoperazine has potent antiemetic effects but also causes marked sedation and extrapyramidal effects and is not used commonly as an antiemetic.

Butyrophenones

Droperidol (Droleptan)

Droperidol is the only member of this group used in anaesthesia. It is a moderately effective antiemetic, and is used in the dose range 0.25–1.25 mg. Some studies have suggested that the lower dose is at least as effective as the higher. In the past it was used in higher doses as part of a neuroleptic anaesthetic technique. After intravenous administration it is rapidly distributed, and eliminated mainly by hepatic metabolism, with a plasma half-life of approximately 2 hours. Side-effects include sedation or prolongation of recovery from anaesthesia; others are similar to those of phenothiazines. Dysphoria can occur, with restlessness and apprehension, but extrapyramidal effects are rare. A slight α-blocking effect may cause hypotension in some patients. It has no effect against motion sickness. Haloperidol has similar actions but a longer onset and duration of action.

Domperidone (Motilium)

Dose: oral 10–20 mg 6-hourly; rectally 20–60 mg 4–8-hourly.

This drug is structurally related to droperidol. It does not cross the blood–brain barrier to the same extent as droperidol so has fewer sedative side-effects. Domperidone has an affect both on the CTZ and by a peripheral action on the stomach by increasing gastric emptying. Timing of the dose of drug is important with domperidone to get maximal efficacy.

Antihistamines

There are a number of antihistamine drugs that also have antiemetic properties. They are useful in the suppression of motion related sickness and also in emesis following labyrinthine disturbances, including surgery. The mechanism of action for these effects is by an action on the CTZ. Most antihistamine drugs should be avoided in patients with porphyria, although cyclizine and chlorpheniramine are thought to be safe.

Cyclizine

Dose: oral, intramuscular, intravenous; 50 mg up to 3 times a day.

Cyclizine is a piperazine derivative, with both antihistaminic and antimuscarinic effects; the latter may be responsible for most of its antiemetic effect. Before the advent of the serotonin antagonist drugs it was part of the mainstay of antiemetic treatment after anaesthesia. The main side-effect appears to be drowsiness and therefore it has less indication in motion sickness, although it is available as an over-the-counter remedy. Its antimuscarinic actions may cause a dry mouth and tachycardia. Although it is an old drug, several recent studies have suggested that its moderate efficacy and low incidence of significant side-effects justify a resurgence in popularity.

It is also prepared in combination with morphine (Cyclimorph 10 = morphine 10 mg + cyclizine 50 mg) for ease of administration for the treatment of acute pain after surgery or trauma; however, there may be some risk in combining morphine with this agent — cyclizine has a longer half-life than morphine and tends to cumulate on repeated 6-hourly dosing. The combination has been criticised and implicated as a cause of pronounced sedation and perhaps respiratory depression. It is interesting to note that use of Cyclimorph has declined in the UK for this reason.

Cinnarizine (Stugeron)

Dose: oral 30 mg 2 hours before travel, then 15 mg 8-hourly for motion sickness.

This drug is available only in oral formulation. It is useful in preventing motion sickness and reducing the symptoms from labyrinthine disorders, including tinnitus and vertigo.

Dimenhydrinate (Dramamine)

Dose: oral 50–100 mg 2–3 times a day

This drug has similar indications to cyclizine.

Chlorpheniramine (Piriton)

Dose: oral, intravenous; 4 mg oral, up to 10 mg intravenously.

This antihistamine is effective in reducing pruritus from opioid drugs and may have synergistic activity with other antiemetic drugs, although it is not primarily used as an antiemetic.

Benzamides

Metoclopramide (Maxolon)

Dose: oral, intravenous; 10–20 mg up to 3 times a day.

Metoclopramide is structurally related to orthoclopramide, a procaine derivative. However, its side-effects are similar to those seen with phenothiazine derivatives. In high doses a range of extrapyramidal symptoms may develop. The antiemetic effects of metoclopramide are due to two main actions: centrally it blocks dopamine in the CTZ; and peripherally it hastens gastric emptying, abolishes irregular intestinal contractions and increases the tone of the lower oesophageal sphincter. Morphine sparing effects of metoclopramide have been described. The dura-

tion of antiemetic action is short so timing of the dose may be important and repeat doses may have to be given. A high dose regimen in patients receiving chemotherapy and radiotherapy is described but this is associated with a high incidence of side-effects, in particular those due to dopamine antagonism. At this high dose the effects of metoclopramide are probably due to 5-HT$_3$ antagonism, which was the early stimulus to look at these drugs in emesis.

Serotonin antagonists

The development of specific serotonin antagonist drugs has added an important arm to the treatment of nausea and vomiting, whether from radiation and chemotherapy or postoperatively due to the effects of anaesthetic and analgesic drugs. Among a large number of putative transmitters acting at the CTZ, serotonin appears to have a dominant role and therefore the drugs blocking its action will be effective antiemetics. Serotonin can be blocked peripherally in the gut and at the CTZ by these 5-HT$_3$ receptor antagonists. The first clinically available serotonin antagonist is ondansetron, and a number of other drugs with similar activity are being developed or have already been released into clinical use. These drugs have similar actions and side-effects but different pharmacodynamic profiles. Granisetron has a half-life longer than that of ondansetron but shorter than that of tropisetron, which makes dosing schedules for each drug different. Currently, ondansetron is the only drug in the group to have a licence for postoperative nausea and vomiting. Dolisetron is another serotonin antagonist undergoing trials. It has a moderate duration of action but is metabolised in the liver by a different pathway to the rest, which may be an advantage. The common side-effects for this group of drugs include constipation, dizziness, fatigue, headache and transiently elevated liver enzymes. Cardiac arrhythmias have been reported but the causal relationship has yet been established. This group of drugs has no sedative actions and does not cause extrapyramidal symptoms, in contrast to the other antiemetics discussed above.

Ondansetron (Zofran)

Dose: oral, intramuscular, intravenous; the dose is dependent on the indication; intravenous injection should be slow:

- For chemotherapy: *moderately emetogenic* — 8 mg orally 1–2 hours before or 8 mg i.v. just before starting and then 8 mg 12-hourly for 5 days; *highly emetogenic* — 8 mg i.v. before then 8 mg 2–4 hours later, then 8 mg 12-hourly for 5 days. Alternatively 32 mg before treatment then 8 mg 12-hourly for 5 days after this.
- For children: the dose is 5 mg m^{-2}.
- For postoperative nausea and vomiting: either 8 mg orally or 4 mg i.v. before induction. The dose for postoperative nausea and vomiting for some patients may be insufficient and higher and more frequent doses may be needed.

The drug is well tolerated by patients but may be less effective if vomiting is established or if the emesis is due to opioid analgesia. A number of studies comparing ondansetron with other antiemetics have appeared in the literature: ondansetron appears to be more effective than some of these drugs. The multimodal causality of postoperative nausea and vomiting makes it difficult to control all patient groups in these studies, so many more results will be needed.

Granisetron (Kytril)

Dose: oral, intravenous; 1 mg orally before chemotherapy / radiotherapy, then a further 2 mg if required; 3 mg by intravenous infusion.

The indications for this drug at the time of writing are only for chemotherapy or radiotherapy induced sickness.

Tropisetron (Navoban)

Dose: oral, intravenous; 5 mg before therapy and then daily for 5 days.

The indications are the same as for granisetron.

Cannabinoids

The cannabinoids have previously been noted to have antiemetic properties and nabilone has been available for the treatment of emesis due to chemotherapy for some years. Recently there have been reports of its use in preventing postoperative nausea and vomiting in gynaecological patients, with some limited success.

Nabilone (Cesamet)

Dose: oral; 2 mg.

This is used for control of nausea and vomiting in cancer therapy, but as yet has no licence for use in postoperative nausea and vomiting.

Other substances

Zingiber officinale (common ginger root)

Powdered ginger root has been used in traditional remedies for gastrointestinal complaints and is an excellent calmative. It has recently been studied in anesthesia for day surgery, and initial reports have indicated a significant antiemetic effect in comparison with placebo. The mechanism of action is as yet unknown, as is the active ingredient, but it appears to have effects in both motion related and postoperative sickness.

Non-pharmacological techniques

Non-pharmacological techniques for the prevention and treatment of emesis includes acupuncture and hypnosis. Acupuncture at the P6 or Neiguan point has been used with variable results in prevention and treatment of postoperative nausea and vomiting and hyperemesis gravidarum. Acupressure with either digital pressure or an elastic band with a plastic stud (Sea Band) applied at the same point seemed to have a limited effect. The use of hypnosis in patients with a previous history of severe postoperative nausea and vomiting has shown some effect but is not practical, owing to the large amount of time needed for each case, for mainstream practice.

FURTHER READING

Biebuyck J F, Watcha M F, White P F 1992 Postoperative nausea and vomiting. Anesthesiology 77: 162–184

Borison H L, Wang S C 1953 Physiology and pharmacology of vomiting. Pharmacological Reviews 5: 193–230

Hamik A, Peroutka S J 1989 Differential interactions of traditional and novel antiemetics with D_2 and 5-hydroxytryptamine-3-receptors. Cancer Chemotherapy and Pharmacology 24: 307–310

Palazzo M G A, Strunin L 1984 Anaesthesia and emesis 1. Etiology. Canadian Anaesthetists' Society Journal 31: 178–187

Palazzo M G A, Strunin L 1984 Anaesthesia and emesis 2. Prevention and management. Canadian Anaesthetists' Society Journal 31: 407–415

Peroutka S J, Snyder S H 1982 Antiemetics: neuroreceptor binding predicts therapeutic action. Lancet i: 658–659

40

Drugs acting on the gastrointestinal tract

W. McCaughey

ANTACID THERAPY

The stomach secretes acid and peptic enzymes in response to neural and humoral influences. Peptic ulceration has traditionally been managed by antacid therapy — drugs which raise the pH of stomach contents by directly neutralising acid, or by blocking acid production. Emphasis is now shifting toward mucosal protection, but this is hampered by poor understanding of the factors involved in the resistance of the gastric mucosa to acid damage. In anaesthetic practice, pulmonary aspiration of gastric acid can cause a severe pneumonitis, and various drugs are used to reduce the acid content of the stomach.

Gastric acid secretion is regulated by a number of mechanisms (Fig. 40.1):

- Neural: vagal stimulation releases acetylcholine, which acts on muscarinic M_3 receptors, leading to increased cytosolic Ca^{2+}.
- Hormonal: gastrin secreted by the G cells of the gastric antrum stimulates the parietal calls directly through gastrin receptors (increased Ca^{2+} as second messenger), and probably also indirectly by acting on enterochromaffin-like (ECL) cells to release histamine.
- Paracrine:
  —histamine acts via H_2 receptors to activate adenylate cyclase and increase cyclic adenosine monophosphate (cAMP)
  —there also are H_3 receptors which reduce acid secretion
  —somatostatin acts via G-protein coupled receptors to *inhibit* adenylate cyclase. (Acetyl-

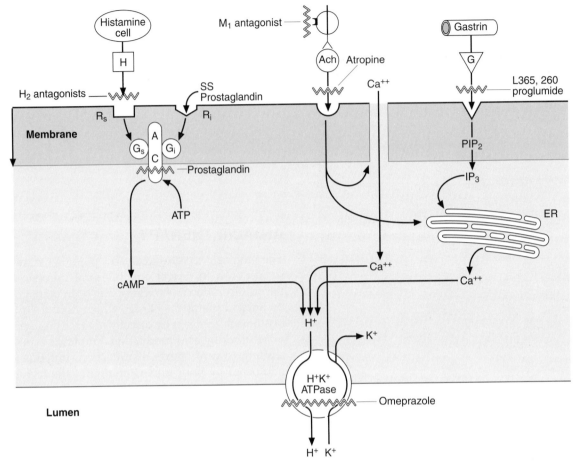

Figure 40.1 Model of gastric acid secretion and inhibition. Receptors for histamine (H), acetylcholine (Ach) and gastrin (G) are present on the parietal cell. Histamine stimulates adenyl cyclase (AC) via a stimulatory G protein (GS); somatostatin (SS) and prostaglandin oppose this. Acetylcholine and gastrin act through pathways involving inositol triphosphate (IP₃) and calcium. The two pathways converge on H⁺,K⁺ ATPase, the 'proton pump' of the parietal cell. (Reproduced with permission from Shamburek and Schubert 1993.)
(Rs, Ri, stimulatory and inhibitory receptors; PIP2, phosphatidyl inositol biophosphate; ER, endoplasmic reticulum)

choline and gastrin may act in part through histamine release.)

All these pathways converge to modulate the activity of the enzyme H⁺,K⁺-ATPase, the proton pump of the parietal cell (Shamburek & Schubert 1993). This is a membrane spanning protein, an adenosine triphosphate (ATP) dependent ion pump, exchanging K⁺ and H⁺ ions. This H⁺,K⁺-ATPase is closely related in structure to Na⁺,K⁺-ATPase.

Alkalis

Alkali antacids neutralise acid directly. *Sodium bicarbonate* and *sodium citrate* act rapidly, but have little buffering capacity. They are absorbed systemically, and repeated dosing may lead to metabolic alkalosis — the 'milk–alkali' syndrome characterised by hypercalcaemic alkalosis can result from chronic intake of sodium bicarbonate along with calcium carbonate or milk. However, this is not a problem with single or a few doses given before anaesthesia. Sodium citrate is normally used as a 0.3 molar solution, in a dose of 15–20 ml. Sodium bicarbonate is very rapidly effective, but has the disadvantage that a considerable volume of carbon dioxide is produced, possibly increasing the chances of regurgitation.

Aluminium and magnesium salts, such as *aluminium hydroxide, magnesium hydroxide* or *trisilicate*, possess greater buffering capacity and may be more appropriate for management of peptic ulcer symptoms. They are relatively unabsorbed (although absorption of aluminium increases by a factor of 10 if taken concurrently with orange juice or citric acid). These are particulate, in contrast to sodium bicarbonate and citrate which are clear solutions, and aspiration into the lungs of particulate antacids can lead to damage comparable with that caused by acid gastric contents (see below).

There is evidence that antacids (particularly those containing aluminium hydroxide) have a protective effect on the gastroduodenal mucosa (see below).

Aluminium- and magnesium-containing antacids frequently affect absorption of other drugs, but most interactions can be avoided by giving the drug at least 2 hours before or after the antacid. These interactions may be due to reduction (Al) or increase (Mg) in gastric or intestinal motility, to adsorption of drugs to antacid molecules, or to alkalinisation of urine — so the resulting picture is complex. Bioavailability of cimetidine or ranitidine is reduced when given with antacids. Magnesium is associated with diarrhoea; aluminium with constipation.

Histamine H$_2$-receptor antagonists

There is a diversity of histamine receptors. The H$_2$, H$_3$ and H$_4$ receptors are of interest in gastrointestinal pharmacology. H$_2$ receptors are G-protein receptors which act by increasing intracellular cAMP to stimulate gastric acid production, and blockade reduces acid secretion.

Chemistry. The H$_2$-blocking drugs resemble histamine in structure (Fig. 40.2).

Pharmacokinetics. H$_2$-blocking drugs are well absorbed orally, although concurrent antacid

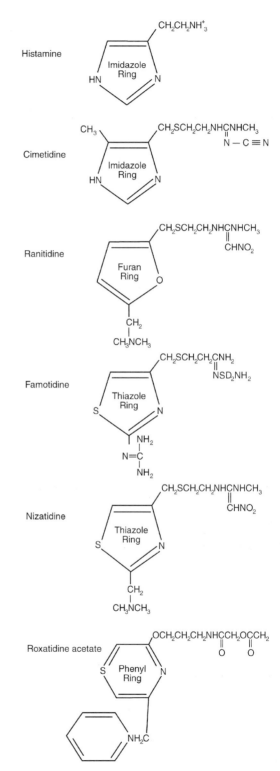

Figure 40.2 Structure of histamine H$_2$-blocking drugs.

Table 40.1 Pharmacokinetic values for H_2 blocking drugs

	Cimetidine	Ranitidine	Famotidine	Nizatidine
Absorption				
Bioavailability (%)	60	50	45	95
Time to C_{max} (h)	1–2	1–3	1–3.5	1–3
Distribution				
V_D (l kg^{-1})	0.8–2.1	1.0–1.9	1.1–1.3	1.2–1.6
Protein binding (%)	20	15	16	30
Elimination				
Plasma $t_{1/2}$ (h)	1.5–2.5	1.6–3.1	2.5–4	1.1–2.0
Relative potency	1	4–10	20–50	4–10

Modified with permission from Shamburek & Schubert (1993).

therapy may reduce availability by up to 30%. They are widely distributed in the body; they cross the blood–brain barrier and the placenta. Cimetidine, ranitidine and famotidine are extensively metabolised in the liver, and about one-third excreted unchanged in urine, while only one-third of nizatidine is metabolised. Elimination half-life is increased up to 10-fold in renal failure, and doses must be adjusted. Cimetidine and other H_2-receptor antagonists may also have an action at histamine receptors in other sites.

CNS. Side-effects such as headache, dizziness, sleepiness and even confusion and delirium have occurred. These are rare, but most likely to occur with cimetidine, which achieves highest cerebrospinal fluid levels.

Cardiovascular effects. Histamine causes increased cardiac inotropic action and increased atrial automaticity acting through H_2 receptors in the atria. The most common side-effect of H_2 blockade, although still uncommon, is development of bradyarrhythmias following intravenous bolus or infusion of cimetidine, or less commonly another antagonist. In contrast, a slight inotropic effect of ranitidine has been described, perhaps due to action at H_2-presynaptic receptors at the sympathetic myocardial junction resulting in an increase in noradrenaline levels. An exaggerated effect of dobutamine can occur with cimetidine as a result of reduced dobutamine metabolism.

Immune system. Suppressor T lymphocytes possess H_2 receptors and contribute significantly to the function of the immune system. Experimentally, cimetidine has been shown to enhance a variety of immunological functions both in vivo and in vitro because of its inhibitory effects on suppressor cell function. This may include a degree of antitumour activity. Conversely, H_2 blockade may be deleterious in patients with organ transplant and autoimmune disorders.

Drug interaction. Cimetidine binds to cytochrome P-450 hepatic mixed-function oxidase enzymes. This leads to enzyme inhibition and reduced metabolism of other drugs, for example benzodiazepines, theophylline, dobutamine, lignocaine, etc. This can be of clinical significance with drugs that have a narrow therapeutic margin and in particular if there is concurrent therapy with another enzyme inhibitor such as ciprofloxacin. The affinity of cimetidine for different P-450 isoenzymes, and thus its effects on different drugs, differs widely. Ranitidine has a 5–10-fold lesser effect, not likely to be of importance, and famotidine and nizatidine seem not to interact significantly.

Renal clearance of creatinine, and of cationic drugs which undergo active proximal tubular excretion, is reduced by cimetidine and to a lesser extent by ranitidine. For example, cimetidine therapy given to older male patients taking procainamide can cause steady-state concentrations of procainamide to rise to toxic levels.

H^+,K^+-ATPase inhibitors

The membrane bound H^+,K^+-ATPase enzyme exchanges H^+ and K^+ ions, resulting in a four million-fold gradient in [H^+], between a cytosolic pH of 7.3 and an intraluminal pH of 0.8. Benzimidazole inhibitors, such as omeprazole, lansoprazole and pantoprazole, bind covalently and irreversibly with the enzyme. There is also a group of inhibitors which competitively block potassium stimulation of the enzyme.

Omeprazole

This is a substituted benzimidazole, a lipophilic weak base (pK_a 4), which crosses cell membranes easily at physiological pH. It is a prodrug, which at the acidic intracellular pH in the gastric parietal cell converts to the active sulfenamide form, and also is trapped within the cell as it becomes lipophobic. After absorption, it is distributed to extracellular water (volume of distribution $0.31 \, l \, kg^{-1}$) but is preferentially concentrated in the parietal cells by acid trapping It is highly protein bound. Hepatic metabolism is rapid, with a plasma half-life of 0.5 –1.5 hours, but because of covalent binding to the H^+,K^+-ATPase, duration of action exceeds 24 hours.

Because of its pH dependent structure, orally administered omeprazole would be prematurely converted by gastric acid and poorly absorbed, and it is therefore formulated in enteric-coated granules, and is absorbed where the pH is above 6.

As the H^+,K^+-ATPase enzyme or 'proton pump' in parietal cells is responsible for the final step in the process of acid secretion, omeprazole blocks acid secretion in response to all stimuli. Single doses produce dose dependent inhibition, with increasing effect over the first few days, reaching a maximum after about 5 days. Doses of omeprazole 20 mg daily or greater are able virtually to abolish intragastric acidity in most individuals, although lower doses have a much more variable effect. It has also been shown to be highly effective in healing ulcers that have failed to respond to H_2-receptor antagonists, and has been extremely valuable in treating patients with Zollinger–Ellison syndrome. Omeprazole has produced short term healing rates superior to the histamine H_2-receptor antagonists in duodenal ulcer, gastric ulcer and reflux oesophagitis.

Side-effects are few, probably because of its selective concentration. Long term use can result in hypergastrinaemia, which in animal studies has led to ECL (enterochromaffin-like) cell carcinoidosis, but there is growing evidence that this is of little, if any, clinical significance in patients receiving proton pump inhibitors.

Omeprazole has the potential to partly inhibit the metabolism of drugs metabolised to a great extent by the cytochrome P-450 enzyme subfamily IIC (diazepam, phenytoin), but not of those metabolised by subfamilies IA (caffeine, theophylline), IID (metoprolol, propranolol) and IIIA (cyclosporin, lidocaine, quinidine). Since relatively few drugs are metabolised mainly by IIC compared with IID and IIIA, the potential for omeprazole to interfere with the metabolism of other drugs appears to be limited, but the half-lives of diazepam and phenytoin are prolonged as much as by cimetidine.

Lansoprazole and pantoprazole

These are 'second generation' proton pump inhibitors. Their mode of action is similar to that of omeprazole. Structural differences give more rapid absorption and greater bioavailability of lansoprazole. Lansoprazole has less effect on P-450 enzymes, while interaction with pantoprazole is insignificant. Lansoprazole has significant antibacterial effect on *Helicobacter pylori*.

Mendelson's syndrome

Prevention of pulmonary acid aspiration syndrome (Mendelson's syndrome) requires a combination of approaches, and only the pharmacological details will be dealt with here.

The main aim is to reduce both the volume and acidity of stomach contents. Many studies have used a volume of 25 ml and a pH of 2.5 as the 'danger level', but this is more a matter of statistical convenience than clinically proven. Vagal blockade using anticholinergics such as glycopyrrolate are effective in raising pH but reduce the tone of the lower oesophageal sphincter, thus potentially increasing the risk of regurgitation. They also cause discomfort by drying up salivary secretion and are thus not suitable in practice.

Alkali antacids are very effective at neutralising acid rapidly but, as described above, particulate antacids — especially aluminium salts — can cause pulmonary inflammation and are no longer widely used. Non-particulate antacids, sodium citrate or bicarbonate, have not been shown to cause damage, and are used in conjunction with H_2 blockers. They will neutralise acid already in the stomach, although 'pocketing' of the stomach contents may prevent mixing with and neutralisation of all the contents. Bicarbonate has the theoretical disadvantage of reacting to produce gaseous carbon dioxide in the stomach.

Histamine H_2-receptor blockers are the mainstay of prevention of Mendelson's syndrome at present. Probably the best protection is afforded by a combination of H_2-receptor blockade by ranitidine and a single oral dose of sodium citrate or bicarbonate. Because of its longer duration of action, and relative lack of enzyme inhibition, ranitidine is preferred to cimetidine for this purpose, although there is a latent period of 1–2 hours before it takes effect. Other blockers, famotidine and nizatidine, are probably equally effective in blocking acid secretion.

Omeprazole is more effective than H_2 blockers in producing achlorhydria when repeated doses are used in treating peptic ulceration or reflux oesophagitis. However, it is less effective than these in reducing volume and acidity of stomach contents when given as a single preoperative dose, and has no advantage over H_2 blockade in this situation.

Metoclopramide is frequently used in combination with antacid therapy. It increases the tone of the lower oesophageal sphincter and increases stomach emptying, and because of this may speed absorption of drugs from the small intestine.

CYTOPROTECTANTS/MUCOSAL PROTECTIVE DRUGS

Sucralfate

Aluminium-containing antacids exhibit cytoprotective activity or enhancement of natural mucosal defense mechanisms.

Sucralfate is a basic aluminum salt of sucrose, a complex of sucrose octasulphate and aluminium hydroxide. It has little or no antacid activity but, more importantly, has a major cytoprotective action, both protecting the mucosa from damaging influences and also causing accelerated healing. The molecular basis of these actions is not known and different actions may be related to its chemistry as an aluminium salt and to the sucrose octasulphate component. At acid pH (<4), it forms a very sticky gel polymer which adheres to epithelial cells and the base of ulcer craters. It appears to work through a number of relatively poorly understood mechanisms, enhancing several gastric and duodenal protective mechanisms:

- Interaction with local tissues. Sucralfate appears to augment the protective function of the mucus-bicarbonate barrier. This is partly due to increased bicarbonate and mucus secretion, and partly to an interaction with the unstirred layer overlying gastric epithelium, as well as by making the mucus gel more hydrophobic. It binds bile acids and pepsin and adheres to both ulcerated and non-ulcerated mucosa.
- Increase in mucosal blood flow, with improved cell viability.
- Stimulation of endogenous mediators of tissue injury and repair. Sucralfate stimulates endogenous synthesis and release by the gastric mucosa of prostaglandin E_2, inhibits thromboxane release, and increases production of endogenous sulphydryl compounds. Sucralfate also increases binding of epidermal growth factor to ulcerated areas and stimulates macrophage activity and epithelial cell proliferation and repair.

Clinical use. Sucralfate is used in the management of peptic ulceration and reflux oesophagitis and its cytoprotective effects may be of benefit in radiation induced mucosal damage elsewhere in the gastrointestinal tract.

Prophylaxis of stress ulceration in the intensive care unit is the major interest to the anaesthetist. Here it is given in a dose of 1 g every 6 hours via nasogastric tube. Several studies have shown sucralfate to be comparable in efficacy to H_2 blockers in preventing this complication. It has been claimed to result in a reduction in morbidity and mortality from nosocomial pneumonias in comparison with H_2 blockers, which, by raising gastric pH, eliminate the acid barrier to colonisation of the gut by pathogens, which sucralfate does not do. However, the results of comparative studies of the incidence of nosocomial pneumonia are conflicting.

Toxicity. Like other aluminium salts, pulmonary aspiration of sucralfate can lead to acute lung injury. There is some systemic absorption of aluminium, which is probably significant only in patients with renal impairment. Administration can be associated with a degree of hypophosphataemia, and there is also interference with absorption of some other drugs — for example, quinolone antibacterials, digoxin, quinidine and warfarin.

Misoprostol

Misoprostol is a synthetic prostaglandin E_1 analogue that has a mild gastric acid antisecretory action, as well as increasing acid and mucus production. It promotes ulcer healing, and has a protective effect on the gastric and duodenal mucosa, reducing the incidence of erosions induced by non-steroidal anti-inflammatory drugs (NSAIDs). It is given orally, 400–800 mg daily in divided doses, and is also marketed in combined preparations with NSAIDs, such as diclofenac. Studies of its effects on renal function are not consistent, but it probably does not reliably protect against the renal effects of NSAIDs.

Misoprostol is rapidly absorbed, and de-esterified to its acid form, which is equipotent to misoprostol. It is 85% protein bound; 65% is excreted renally, with a half-life of 1.5 hours.

Side-effects are relatively unimportant, mainly diarrhoea; however, prostaglandins do stimulate uterine contractions and misoprostol has been widely used as an abortifacient by women in Brazil, where abortion is legal only in cases of rape or incest, or to save the woman's life. Used in Brazil in cases of unwanted pregnancy, it is inefficient, and this use has led to fetal malformations — yet overall complications from illegal abortions may have been reduced by this use.

Bismuth compounds

These are frequently used along with antibiotics as part of 'triple therapy' aimed at the eradication of *Helicobacter pylori* in peptic ulcer disease.

Liquorice/carbenoxolone

Liquorice has an ulcer-healing property; *carbenoxolone* is a synthetic derivative of glycyrrhizinic acid, which is a constituent of liquorice. Their protective effect on gastric mucosa may be due to both increased prostaglandin levels and effects on the nitric oxide system.

The main side-effects of liquorice and carbenoxolone are hypokalaemia with salt and water retention, which predisposes to hypertension. This is thought to be due to inhibition of the enzyme 11β-hydroxysteroid dehydrogenase, which inactivates cortisol and corticosterone, leading to increased activation of renal mineralocorticoid receptors by cortisol. There may also be a central effect.

PROKINETIC DRUGS

The myenteric plexus (plexus of Auerbach) may be regarded as a third division of the autonomic nervous system. Gut motility depends on its function. Prokinetic drugs probably act mainly through cholinergic mechanisms, enhancing release of acetylcholine from cholinergic nerves in the myenteric plexus. This prokinetic action of metoclopramide and cisapride *may* be mediated through action at 5-HT$_4$ receptors in the gut wall. They have a partial agonist action at the 5-HT$_4$ receptors and at high dose also act as 5-HT$_3$ antagonists. Metoclopramide is also a potent dopamine D_2 antagonist both centrally and in the gut.

Metoclopramide

This is used principally as an antiemetic (see Ch. 29), but also for its prokinetic properties. It is a dopamine D_2 antagonist, but this is probably not important for its prokinetic action. It increases the tone of the lower oesophageal sphincter and hastens emptying of the stomach. Its main disadvantage is a significant incidence of dysphoric or parkinsonian reactions due to its antidopaminergic action.

Domperidone

Also a potent D_2 antagonist, this has similar antiemetic and prokinetic properties to metoclopramide, although probably with less efficacy than either, but does not readily cross the blood–brain barrier and thus has fewer central side effects.

Cisapride

This is an orally administered prokinetic agent that facilitates or restores motility throughout the length of the gastrointestinal tract. It is a substituted piperidinyl benzamide, chemically related to metoclopramide, but unlike metoclopramide and domperidone, cisapride is largely devoid of central depressant or antidopaminergic effects. It therefore has neither their central antiemetic action nor the side-effects related to dopamine blockade.

It increases lower oesophageal sphincter tone, increases the rate of gastric emptying, and reverses the morphine-induced delay in gastric emptying more effectively than metoclopramide. It is used in various disorders of motility, including oesophageal reflux, and has also been shown to be of use in some cases of intestinal pseudo-obstruction or ileus.

Oral bioavailability is 40–50%; it is highly protein bound, and it is metabolised in the liver with a half-life of about 10 hours.

Drug interactions. Increased motility may lead to increased absorption of drugs such as morphine, diazepam, etc., although the picture may be more complicated. Ranitidine reaches peak plasma concentration more rapidly, but bioavailability is reduced when given with cisapride.

Anticholinergics

Atropine and related drugs act at muscarinic cholinergic receptors. (At least five muscarinic receptor genes have been cloned and expressed.

Muscarinic receptors act via activation of G proteins: M_1, M_3 and M_5 muscarinic receptors couple to stimulate phospholipase C, while M_2 and M_4 muscarinic receptors inhibit adenylyl cyclase.) Cholinergic blockade can reduce gastric acid secretion by 40–50%. It is also used to reduce intestinal spasm, both therapeutically and to aid endoscopic procedures. Unselective drugs such as atropine and scopolamine (hyoscine) are of limited use because of side-effects such as dry mouth and tachycardia.

Pirenzepine

This is a tricyclic antimuscarine drug with an antisecretory effect on gastric secretion and inhibitory effect on oesophageal peristalsis. The cholinergic receptor on postganglionic intramural neurones of the submucosal plexus has recently been identified as an M_1 subtype, and that on the parietal cell as an M_3 subtype; pirenzipine is selective for the M_1 receptor. Selective M_1 blockade is as effective as atropine in reducing gastric secretion, and avoids side-effects.

Although anticholinergic drugs such as pirenzipine are becoming more widely used in management of peptic ulcer disease, they are not appropriate in anaesthetic practice because lower oesophageal sphincter tone is reduced (as with atropine), thus reducing the barrier to regurgitation.

Several atropine-like drugs are used as antispasmodics. These include:

- homatropine
- hyoscine
- hyoscine-*n*-butylbromide (Buscopan)
- propantheline (probanthine).

Some care should be exercised in their use in children and the elderly, as relative overdosage leading to signs of hyoscine poisoning has been reported.

LAXATIVES (with special reference to patients receiving terminal care)

The treatment of constipation and questions of use and abuse of laxatives are not normally of major interest to the anaesthetist; however, constipation is a particular problem in terminal care patients, especially where they are receiving opioid drugs for pain relief, and its prevention and management must be an integral part of their treatment.

A large number of other drugs may contribute to constipation:

- opioids
- prostaglandin inhibiting analgesics
- anticholinergics — phenothiazines, antiparkinsonian drugs, H_1 blockers, tricyclic antidepressants (anticholinergic side-effect)
- ganglion blockers
- monoamine oxidase inhibitors
- verapamil
- antacids containing calcium carbonate or aluminium hydroxide
- antidiarrhoeals
- laxatives used chronically.

Laxative drugs may be classified as:

- bulking agents
- faecal softeners
- osmotic laxatives
- stimulant laxatives.

Two terms are often used: laxatives and cathartics. Cathartics produce prompt fluid evacuation, while laxatives produce soft formed stools over a protracted period. Mechanisms of action vary, but the net overall effect is fluid accumulation within the bowel lumen by a hydrophilic action, an osmotic action and/or a direct action on mucosal cells to decrease absorption or to enhance secretion of water and electrolytes. Changes in Na^+,K^+-ATPase, adenylyl cyclase and prostaglandins may be involved in these actions.

Bulking agents

These are mostly unrefined substances of plant origin (bran, etc.). These preparations increase the bulk of stool and soften its consistency, largely by absorbing and holding water. They may diminish absorption of some minerals and drugs, but this is not usually clinically significant.

Faecal softeners

Liquid paraffin is contraindicated if there is any risk of aspiration. Interference with the absorption of fat soluble vitamins would not appear to be clinically significant.

Docusate sodium is an emulsifying and wetting agent. It has minimal laxative properties, but penetrates and softens the stool.

Saline and osmotic laxatives

Magnesium salts, e.g. magnesium sulphate (Epsom salt), sodium phosphates and polyethylene glycol–electrolyte solutions produce largely fluid stools and are useful in preoperative preparation of the bowel.

Lactulose is a semisynthetic disaccharide which is not absorbed from the gastrointestinal tract. It produces an osmotic diarrhoea of low pH and discourages the proliferation of ammonia-producing bacteria. It is therefore useful in the treatment of hepatic encephalopathy.

Osmotic laxatives like lactulose, sorbitol and lactilol rarely cause significant adverse effects.

Glycerol suppositories are useful in softening and lubricating passage of inspissated faeces.

Stimulant laxatives

These are among the most powerful, but prolonged use can aggravate constipation. Mechanisms of action are multiple and not well studied. They include increased permeability of the mucosa, leading to accumulation of water in the lumen; inhibition of intestinal Na^+,K^+-ATPase; increased synthesis of prostaglandins and cAMP.

Stimulant laxatives include diphenylmethane and anthraquinone derivatives.

Diphenylmethane derivatives (phenolphthalein, bisacodyl) are effective but potential toxicity should lead to dosage being limited to 10 days. Bisacodyl is used for bowel evacuation prior to diagnostic procedures.

Danthron (1,8-dihydroxyanthraquinone) derivatives occur in senna, cascara and rhubarb. They are highly effective; the main side-effect is excessive laxative effect and abdominal pain.

Danthron preparations should only be used in older patients and the terminally ill because of the risk of hepatotoxicity with this drug.

Unlike the bulk forming laxatives, which are unabsorbed, the diphenylmethane and anthraquinone drugs are absorbed in considerable amounts and excreted in bile, urine and breast milk.

ANTIDIARRHOEALS

Diarrhoea is often of infective origin but management is generally non-specific. It is also common following antibiotic therapy, which disturbs normal bowel flora, and replacement therapy using electrolyte solutions may be needed, and can be life saving in severe diarrhoea, especially in children. Oral rehydration is preferred, although parenteral fluids may be required. The standard oral rehydration solution promoted by the World Health Organization is simply made up from basic constituents:

- sodium chloride 3.5 g
- potassium chloride 1.5 g
- sodium citrate 2.9 g
- anhydrous glucose 20 g

- water to make 1 litre (in addition, drinks of water are allowed to those with mild to moderate dehydration).

Other treatment is aimed mainly at decreasing discomfort. Bulking agents such as methylcellulose, bran, etc. may be of use, but the mainstay of treatment of diarrhoea is opioid derivatives. These act mainly by an action at μ receptors, slowing transit time and thus allowing more time for absorption of fluids. There may also have an effect directly on the epithelial cells of the bowel, reducing secretion and / or increasing reabsorption.

Opium derivatives such as morphine and codeine phosphate have been used for a long time, but the piperidine derivatives *loperamide* (Imodium) and *diphenoxylate* (Lomotil) are now preferred. Both are μ receptor agonists, largely devoid of central opiate-like effects, and relatively insoluble in water, so that parenteral use and abuse are almost impossible.

A number of other classes of drug have shown potential in management of diarrhoea. These include gut specific α-adrenergic agonists, intestinal Cl⁻ channel blockers, somatostatin analogues and calmodulin inhibitors.

REFERENCES AND FURTHER READING

McCarthy D M 1991 Sucralfate (review). New England Journal of Medicine 325: 1017–1025

Newell S 1990 Cisapride: its use in children. British Journal of Hospital Medicine 44: 408–409

Rowbotham D J 1989 Cisapride and anaesthesia (editorial). British Journal of Anaesthesia 62: 121–123

Shamburek R D, Schubert M L 1993 Pharmacology of gastric acid inhibition (review). Baillière's Clinical Gastroenterology 7(1): 23–54

Thompson E M, Loughran P G, McAuley D M, Wilson C M, Moore J 1984 Combined treatment with ranitidine and saline antacids prior to obstetric anaesthesia. Anaesthesia 39: 1086–1090

41

The liver

J. M. Murray

ANATOMY

The liver is the largest organ in the body, weighing up to 1500 g. It is situated in the right upper quadrant of the abdomen and is shaped like a pyramid, the apex of which reaches the xiphisternum. The upper border lies approximately at the level of the nipples. There are two lobes, the right being approximately six times the size of the left in adults.

Lobular architecture

The minute structure of the liver comprises a mass of neatly arranged lobules within which blood flows along sinusoids past hepatic cells (Fig. 41.1). Blood is supplied by the hepatic artery and portal vein and flow is from the periphery inwards towards the central vein. The sinusoids are lined by endothelial cells and Kupffer cells, the latter forming part of the reticuloendothelial system. The centrilobular veins unite to form venules, the larger branches of which end in the inferior vena cava.

Blood flows from the periphery of the lobule to the central vein because the portal venous pressure is higher than that in the central vein. The hepatocytes at the periphery of a lobule therefore have a more abundant supply of oxygen and nutrients and cells nearest the centre of a lobule are most prone to oxygen lack due either to hypoxia or hypotension (centrilobular necrosis). The linear arrangement of hepatocytes along the sinusoids creates concentration gradients in the

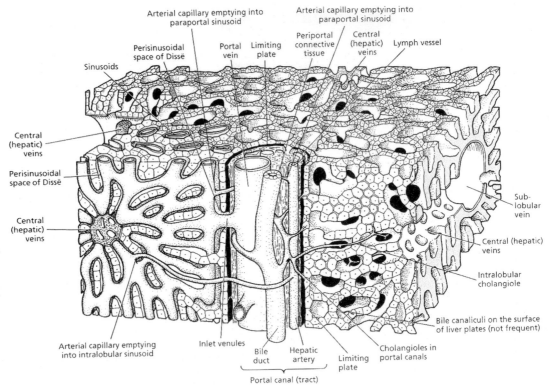

Figure 41.1 Liver lobule. (Reproduced with permission from Sherlock S, Dooley J (eds) 1993 Diseases of the liver and biliary system, 9th edn. Blackwell Scientific, Oxford.)

plasma and parenchyma for many of the substances extracted or released by hepatocytes. In the adult liver, 60–65% of cells are hepatocytes and 35-40% are non-parenchymal cells. Kupffer cells represent a third of non-parenchymal cells.

Every liver cell is associated with several bile canaliculi which drain into a ductal system culminating, in the liver, in the left and right hepatic ducts. Outside the liver these join to form the common hepatic duct. The cystic duct drains the gallbladder, and the common hepatic duct unites with it to form the common bile duct. This enters the duodenum, usually after receiving the pancreatic duct, at the sphincter of Oddi.

Functional architecture

The basic liver unit, the lobule, is an anatomical entity which does not adequately describe the functioning of the liver. It is considered that

the functional unit is the *acinus*, of which there are estimated to be 100 000 in a human liver (Fig. 41.2). Each acinus carries terminal branches of portal vein, hepatic artery and bile duct and with its neighbours forms a grape-like cluster of units. In contrast to the lobules, blood flow is from the centre of the unit outwards along the sinusoids to peripheral hepatic venules. The cells nearest the centre of the acinus are well oxygenated (zone 1) and are believed to be mainly involved in protein anabolism and catabolism. They contain the greatest concentrations of the aminotransferase enzymes. The oxygen supply deteriorates progressively towards the periphery (zones 2 and 3) and it is these cells that are most vulnerable to injury, whether it be viral, toxic or hypoxic in origin. Regions that are closer to the afferent vessels and bile ducts are less susceptible to such insults and may provide the base for possible regeneration. Cells in zone 3 have high

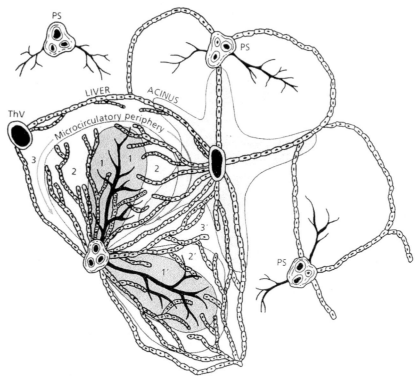

Figure 41.2 Liver acinus. PS, portal stalk containing portal vein, terminal bile ducts, hepatic arteriole; ThV, terminal hepatic vein. (Reproduced with permission from Sherlock S, Dooley J (eds) 1993 Diseases of the liver and biliary system, 9th edn. Blackwell Scientific, Oxford.)

levels of cytochrome P-450 and this is the area where phase I drug biotransformation takes place.

Cellular function

The hepatocyte

Electron microscopy shows that the hepatocytes contain all the organelles, such as mitochondria, endoplasmic reticulum and Golgi apparatus, found in other metabolically active cells.

The *mitochondria* have double membranes, the inner being folded to form grooves or cristae. Mitochondria are involved with the production of energy, particularly that involving oxidative phosphorylation. They have a high phospholipid content and contain many enzymes capable of oxidizing substrate, including fatty acids and the intermediates of the Krebs (citric acid) cycle.

Energy generated by this process is converted into high energy phosphate bonds of adenosine triphosphate (ATP).

The *endoplasmic reticulum* within the cell consists of two distinct parts. The rough endoplasmic reticulum, which is characterised by the presence on the tubular membranes of small particles of ribonucleic acid (RNA). The rough endoplasmic reticulum is responsible for protein metabolism, particularly that of albumin and the factors used in blood coagulation and enzyme synthesis. Glucose-6-phosphatase is synthesised and triglycerides are elaborated from free fatty acids and complexed with protein to be secreted by exocytosis as lipoprotein. The rough endoplasmic reticulum may take part in glycogenesis.

The smooth endoplasmic reticulum does not contain granules and is the site of drug biotransformation, conjugation of bilirubin and the synthesis of steroids. These include cholesterol and the primary bile acids which are conjugated with the amino acids glycine and taurine. The proportion of smooth endoplasmic reticulum is increased by enzyme-inducing drugs such as phenobarbitone. Most of the functions of the liver cell take place within the endoplasmic reticulum.

Lysosomes are vesicles which are found within the cytoplasm and contain hydrolytic enzymes. They are probably intracellular scavengers and act as storage sites for ferritin, lipofuscin, copper and bile pigment. They may also be involved in disorders affecting lipid metabolism.

Microtubules and *microfilaments* provide a supporting cytoskeleton. They are contractile, and control subcellular motility, vesicle movements and cell shape. Canalicular motility and bile flow may depend on microfilament function.

The Kupffer cell

These cells form part of the reticuloendothelial system and line the sinusoids. Kupffer cells predominate in the periportal regions and represent 80–90% of all resident macrophages in the body. They phagocytose large particles and contain vacuoles and lysosomes. They actively take up foreign particulate matter from the blood. This applies particularly to bacteria that enter portal blood from the gastrointestinal tract. Kupffer cells also phagocytose old cells, tumour cells, yeasts, viruses and parasites.

Kupffer cells are activated by generalised infections or trauma. They specifically phagocytose endotoxin and, in response, secrete a series of factors such as tumour necrosis factor, interleukins, collagenase and lysosomal hydrolases.

The Kupffer cell has specific membrane receptors for insulin, glucagon and lipoproteins. These cells express class II major histocompatibility antigens (see Ch. 44) and play a major role in the initiation of immune responses and graft rejection. In the fetus the Kupffer cells have a role in haemopoiesis. This function usually disappears within a few weeks of birth but the potential for producing red cells is retained throughout life. In disease conditions that destroy the bone marrow, particularly myelofibrosis, some red cell production occurs in the Kupffer cells in the liver.

The space between the hepatocytes and the Kupffer cells is known as the space of Disse. Although optically empty, this space contains the major components of the extracellular matrix, i.e. collagens, glycosaminoglycans and glycoproteins. The development of hepatic fibrosis is associated with a marked increase in the amount of collagens and other components of the extracellular matrix deposited in the space of Disse.

Normally this space contains tissue fluid which flows outwards into lymphatics in the portal zones. When sinusoidal pressure rises, lymph production in the space of Disse increases and this contributes to ascites formation where there is hepatic outflow obstruction.

BLOOD SUPPLY

The liver has a dual blood supply. About two-thirds of the blood perfusing the liver is venous and is supplied by the portal vein coming from the splanchnic region. This includes the digestive tract below the diaphragm, the spleen and the pancreas. One-third of the blood perfusing the liver is arterial, from the hepatic artery, which in 90% of cases arises from the coeliac axis.

Knowledge of the physiology and pharmacology of the hepatic circulation has grown rapidly in recent years. Abnormalities of the hepatic macro- and microcirculations appear to be a major determinant in the pathophysiology of many liver diseases. Alteration in the hepatic microcirculation in disease states is as a result of collagenisation of the space of Disse and formation of a basal lamina beneath the endothelium. These processes contribute to: (1) deprivation of nutrients intended for the hepatocyte, (2) diminished diffusion of drugs to the hepatocyte, and (3) the development of portal hypertension.

Portal venous system

This is a unique system in that it starts and ends in capillaries. The portal vein is formed in front of the inferior vena cava and behind the neck of the pancreas by the union of the superior mesenteric and splenic veins. It passes into the liver at the porta hepatis and its branches end in the hepatic sinusoids.

The hepatic portal vascular bed is interposed between the capillary network of the splanchnic territory and the hepatic sinusoids. The structure of the portal vein differs markedly from other veins. Valves are absent and flow can reverse in many pathological conditions, e.g.cirrhosis. Unlike other venous systems, a longitudinal muscle layer showing rhythmic activity is present in the adventitia. This phenomenon accounts for the stretch dependent myogenic tone of the portal vein. The myogenic tone can affect the compliance of the portal vein and is therefore an important modulator of portal pressure in vivo.

Portal blood flow ranges from 1000–1200 ml min^{-1} in healthy adults and this may double after a meal.

Hepatic arterial buffer response

This is an autoregulatory mechanism designed to prevent large fluctuations in total liver blood flow. Portal venous pressure is about 10 mmHg in humans, and hepatic venous pressure about 5 mmHg. The mean hepatic arterial pressure is much greater, at 90 mmHg. In the absence of a very marked pressure drop in the sinusoids, hepatic arterial blood would perfuse the portal system in a retrograde direction. This pressure drop is achieved by the dilating action of peri-arteriolar adenosine stores on hepatic arterioles and this forms the basis upon which hepatic flow is adjusted. It is hypothesised that, as portal venous flow reduces, less adenosine is removed from periarteriolar tissues. As a result local adenosine concentrations increase and the hepatic arterioles dilate. Although hepatic arterial flow changes in order to buffer alterations in the total flow there is no reciprocity of flow relationship; portal blood flow is not altered by changes in arterial flow.

The buffer response protects against hypoxic liver injury induced by hypovolaemia, low flow states and drugs. It is of most value when there is a large decrease in portal blood flow because the liver normally receives much more oxygen than

Table 41.1 Factors affecting liver blood flow

Increase	Decrease
Acute hepatitis	Positive pressure ventilation
Supine posture	Abdominal surgery
Food	Hypercarbia
Enzyme inducing drugs	Hypoxia
	Ganglion blocking drugs
	H_2-receptor antagonists
	Vasopressin
	Volatile anaesthetics
	Intravenous anaesthetic drugs

it requires and can readily extract more oxygen from the blood to compensate for altered delivery. It is also thought that the buffer response provides a means of regulating hepatic blood volume.

In summary, many factors influence the control and regulation of total hepatic blood flow (Table 41.1).

PHYSIOLOGY

The liver serves a variety of important functions related to macromolecular synthesis, energy generation and storage, catabolism and disposal of toxic substances and waste products of intermediary metabolism. The main functions are:

- Formation of bile
- Storage and utilisation: carbohydrate, vitamins, iron
- Synthesis: plasma proteins, urea, 2,5-hydroxycholecalciferol
- Metabolism: fat, cholesterol, polypeptide hormones
- Detoxification: steroid hormones, drugs and toxins.

Bile formation

Bile consists of water (97%), bile salts, pigments (bilirubin and biliverdin), cholesterol, fatty acids and inorganic salts. The *bile salts* are sodium and potassium salts of bile acids conjugated to glycine or taurine. These acids are derived from cholesterol. The bile salts, by reducing surface tension, emulsify fat before digestion and absorption in the small intestine. The bile salt molecule is hydrophilic at one end and hydrophobic at the other. This favours the formation of *micelles* in which the molecules are arranged with their hydrophilic surfaces facing out. This configuration assists in the absorption of lipids from the brush border of the intestinal epithelium. There is extensive (95%) enterohepatic reabsorption of bile salts from the small intestine.

Bilirubin

The majority of bilirubin is formed in the tissues by the breakdown of haemoglobin. It is bound to albumin, although some of it dissociates in the liver. Free bilirubin enters liver cells, where it is conjugated with glucuronic acid in the presence of glucuronyl tranferase. Bilirubin glucuronide is more water soluble than free bilirubin and is actively transported into the bile canaliculi. Some escapes into the blood, where it is loosely attached to albumin and is excreted in the urine. Most of the conjugated bilirubin passes into the bile ducts and is excreted through the intestine. Bacterial action in the intestine results in the formation of urobilinogens and these may be absorbed through the intestinal wall into the portal circulation. Small amounts of urobilinogen enter the systemic circulation and are excreted by the kidney. Although conjugated bilirubin does not readily cross the intestinal mucosa, a little unconjugated bilirubin may be formed and is subject to enterohepatic recirculation.

When conjugated or unconjugated bilirubin accumulates in the tissues, the sclera, skin and mucous membranes become yellow (icteric) and the patient is said to have *jaundice*. A total plasma bilirubin concentration of >30 µmol l^{-1} is necessary for this to become apparent. High concentrations of free (unconjugated) bilirubin occur in the presence of increased production (haemolysis), decreased uptake into liver cells, or defective intracellular binding or conjugation. When there is impaired transfer of conjugated bilirubin into bile canaliculi or biliary tract obstruction (tumour, duct atresia), conjugated bilirubin predominates. High plasma concentrations of unconjugated bilirubin are usually well tolerated but may cause kernicterus in the newborn, in whom the blood–brain barrier is not fully developed. High circulating concentrations of conjugated bilirubin may be associated with acute renal failure — the hepatorenal syndrome.

Saturation of albumin binding sites can occur at very high bilirubin concentrations and there may be competition with non-steroidal anti-inflammatory drugs, diuretics, salicylates and sulphonamides.

METABOLISM

Amino acids

Through a variety of anabolic and catabolic processes, the liver is the major site of amino acid interconversion. Amino acids used for protein synthesis are derived from dietary protein, metabolic turnover of endogenous protein (primarily from muscle) and direct synthesis in the liver. Most of the amino acids entering the liver by the portal vein are catabolised to urea (except for the branched chain types — leucine, isoleucine and valine). Catabolism or degradation of amino acids in the liver involves two major reactions: transamination and oxidative deamination.

Transamination is the process by which the amino group of an amino acid is transferred to a keto acid. This reaction is catalysed by a specific group of enzymes, the aminotransferases. These enzymes are found in significant amounts in liver but are also present in kidney, heart, lung and brain. As a result of transamination reactions, amino acids can enter the citric acid cycle to function in the intermediary metabolism of carbohydrates and lipids. Aminotransferases can also catalyse the reverse reaction — namely, the synthesis of amino acids from certain keto acids.

Oxidative deamination is the process that results in the conversion of an amino acid to a keto acid (and ammonia) and is catalysed in the main by L-amino acid oxidases. If the liver is severely damaged (e.g. in massive hepatic necrosis), utilisation of amino acids is impaired, free amino acids in the bloodstream increase, and an 'overflow' type of amino aciduria may occur.

Changes in serum proteins in liver disease reflect a multifactorial reaction, which includes a response to foreign agents and the effects of decreased protein synthesis. A change in the synthesis of a plasma protein in the liver may reflect variations in the *regulation* of synthesis rather than a change in *capacity* for this function.

Many plasma proteins are synthesised by the liver and, of these, albumin is the most prominent. The major functions of albumin in the serum are the regulation of oncotic pressure and the binding and transport of certain hormones, fatty acids, bilirubin, trace metals and toxic products. Albumin is processed exclusively by the liver and, in the normal adult, daily production is about 120–220 mg kg^{-1} body weight. Under conditions of reduced albumin half-life from excessive losses from the body, synthesis can be increased two- to threefold. Clinically decreased albumin synthesis can also result from an inadequate amino acid supply, as in starvation, protein calorie malnutrition or malabsorption syndromes. Plasma albumin concentrations correlate well with prognosis in chronic liver disease but, because of its 20 day half-life, it is a poor marker of acute liver damage. Prealbumin has a shorter half-life (1.5 days) and may be useful in predicting the prognosis of acute liver disease.

Other proteins produced by the liver include many of the blood clotting factors: fibrinogen, prothrombin and factors V, VII, IX and X. Factors II, VII, IX and X are vitamin K responsive and thus are dependent on normal intestinal fat absorption. Because factor VII has a short half-life, it is a useful guide to hepatic synthetic function.

Intermediate metabolism

The liver plays a vital role in glucose homeostasis and is the main site of gluconeogenesis. Apart from a minor contribution from the kidney, the liver alone is responsible for meeting the demands of other tissues for glucose and it is of prime importance in disposing of ingested carbohydrate, in particular glucose and fructose. It has the capacity to store carbohydrate as glycogen (glycogenesis), to convert excess glucose into lipid, to convert glycogen back to glucose (glycogenolysis) and to convert precursors such as lactate, pyruvate, alanine, other glucogenic amino acids and glycerol into new glucose (gluconeogenesis).

Glucagon, growth hormone and adrenaline stimulate glycogenolysis, in contrast to insulin and corticosteroids which promote glycogenesis. The opposing actions of the pancreatic hormones, insulin and glucagon, on glycogenolysis, gluconeogenesis and glycogenesis provide an effective control system for glucose homeostasis and energy substrate consumption.

In the fasting state, the body can mobilise endogenous carbohydrate, fat and protein to cover short term energy requirements. Stored fat and protein (mainly from muscle) provide the bulk of calories, with limited amounts supplied from carbohydrate.

Carbohydrate, primarily in the form of liver and muscle glycogen, is essentially a reserve for acute anaerobic production of high energy phosphate by glycolysis to lactate. This small glycogen mass is fundamental for survival in the short term. After depletion of liver glycogen, further glucose requirements are met by gluconeogenesis.

Reductions in blood glucose and insulin concentrations created by starvation stimulate the breakdown of reserves in the form of muscle and plasma protein and adipose tissue triglyceride. This metabolic activity may be augmented by activation of the sympathetic nervous system.

Stimulation of lipolysis increases fatty acid flux to the liver. Under conditions of excess acetyl coenzyme, or a relative shortage of oxaloacetate, acetoacetate, β-hydroxybutyrate and acetone (ketone bodies) are formed. The β-hydroxybutyrate:acetoacetate ratio in the blood is usually 3–6:1. The formation of ketone bodies is dependent on several factors: fasting, starvation and insulin activity. Insulin reduces ketone body formation by inhibiting lipolysis and stimulating esterification of fatty acids. Although the liver cannot utilise ketone bodies as an energy source, under aerobic conditions they can be utilised by muscle, heart tissue, kidney, brain and intestinal cells. The ability of the brain to use ketone bodies produced in the liver is a fundamental adaptation during starvation. It has been demonstrated that ketone bodies play a significant role in providing alternative energy for cerebral respiration.

Anaesthesia and surgery activate a stress response, which is mediated by the sympathetic nervous system. This is manifest by the suppression of insulin release with a corresponding increase in blood glucose concentrations. Anaesthetised patients are unable to utilise this 'available' energy source and are often in the fasted state before surgery, relying on gluconeogenesis to fuel cerebral respiration. This adaptation is all the more important if anaesthesia and surgery are prolonged. Elegant work by Biebuyck and associates (1972) has shown that halothane can increase the rate of glycogenolysis in the isolated perfused rat liver. This increase in glycogenolysis resulted in a rise in lactate concentration. However, in the intact animal exposed to halothane, glycogenolysis caused an increase in blood glucose concentration. It was postulated that the different effects of halothane on the isolated organ, and on the liver in vivo, may be due to the effects of halothane on cyclic adenosine monophosphate (cAMP) and phosphofructokinase activity.

Starvation may have implications for the liver during anaesthesia. Increased drug metabolism (including that of volatile anaesthetics) may occur and may generate a rise in free radical production. Hepatic glutathione, an antioxidant, protects the liver from exogenous toxins and drugs such as paracetamol or carbon tetrachloride and it has been suggested that, in some circumstances, a reduction in glutathione below a critical level would allow intermediates to bind to liver microsomal protein and cause cellular necrosis and triglyceride accumulation. Although glutathione may be important in preventing liver damage due to certain drugs, studies in animals and man have failed to show that it has a role in halothane induced liver injury.

ENZYME TESTS OF LIVER FUNCTION

Hepatocellular injury leads to the leakage of cellular contents into the circulation. The majority of biochemical tests of hepatocellular damage are based on the measurement of enzyme activity in the serum or plasma.

There are four main variables that will affect the activity of an enzyme in the circulation: (1) intracellular localisation of the enzyme; (2) activity in the liver cell; (3) amount of leakage from the cell; and (4) rate of disappearance of the enzyme from the circulation. The site of the lesion in relation to the distribution of enzyme activity within the liver is an important consideration when reviewing the value of particular enzymes as indicators of cellular damage in different types of liver disease. More than 50 enzymes have been identified in the serum or plasma. However, Sherlock (1989) has documented that 'the multiple functions of the liver are only exceeded by the number of biochemical methods designed to test them'. The original goal of such tests was to provide answers to two questions. Is hepatic disease present in a patient, and if so, what is the nature and severity of the disease?

Liver function tests are often used in circumstances where there is no liver pathology — for example, during therapy with a drug known to be potentially hepatotoxic — and are a measure of dysfunction rather than function. They are notoriously difficult to interpret owing to lack of specificity and they offer little quantitative information. Despite their drawbacks, liver function tests remain the first line of investigation because of their simplicity, their observer independence and their role in monitoring therapy.

Measurement of serum liver enzyme activities is the most common method of assessing hepatic injury after general anaesthesia. These enzymes include the aminotransferases, alkaline phosphatase, γ-glutamyl transpeptidase, 5'-nucleotidase and ornithine carbamoyl transpeptidase.

Alkaline phosphatase

This is a group of enzymes that hydrolyse phosphate esters at alkaline pH. Alkaline phosphatase activity mainly comprises contributions from liver, bone, intestine and, during pregnancy, the placenta. Alkaline phosphatase activity characteristically increases in bile duct obstruction and may precede jaundice. It is a poor discriminator between different causes of obstruction and, because of its distribution in other tissues, can occasionally give misleading information.

Aminotransferases

Aspartate aminotransferase (AST) and alanine aminotransferase (ALT) are the most widely used tests of liver function. AST is a cytoplasmic and mitochondrial enzyme, different isoenzymes being found in each. ALT occurs only in the cytoplasm and is almost exclusively a liver enzyme. In contrast, AST is found in other tissues and is a less specific marker of hepatocellular damage. Aminotransferase activity is particularly increased in acute hepatocellular injury (e.g. pre-icteric phase of acute viral hepatitis, infectious mononucleosis, drug induced) and may also be increased in chronic liver disease. In acute liver illness, ALT is a more sensitive and specific test than AST.

Dehydrogenases

The aminotransferases have proved to be the most popular hepatocellular enzymes over the years, but there are other enzymes that offer a greater degree of organ specificity.

Lactate dehydrogenase (LD) consists of five major isoenzymes, of which LD-5 predominates in hepatic tissue. This isoenzyme is often increased in hepatitis and other conditions involving hepatocellular damage. Increases in LD-5 activity may also be seen in hepatic malignancy, but the isoenzyme pattern will depend on the activity of the malignant process. Measurement of the isoenzymes has not, however, proved useful when compared with the other more easily performed enzyme assays, as the presence of lactate dehydrogenase in the cytoplasm of cells of many organs of the body gives it poor diagnostic specificity.

Isocitrate dehydrogenase

This enzyme is present in the cytoplasm of the liver cell but is also present in significant amounts in heart, kidney and skeletal muscle. Despite this wide tissue distribution, increases in the activity of this enzyme in the serum are almost totally confined to patients with liver disease, particularly acute viral hepatitis, infectious mononucleosis and toxic hepatitis. In chronic liver disease, isocitrate dehydrogenase shows changes similar to those seen with the aminotransferases. In cases of hepatic malignancy, activities are increased in more than 50% of patients, but it is worth noting that increases have been observed in disseminated malignancy without any apparent hepatic involvement. Isocitrate dehydrogenase does not therefore appear to offer any singular diagnostic advantage and its determination is not common in routine laboratory practice.

Sorbitol dehydrogenase

This enzyme is found almost exclusively in the liver, with only small amounts present in the prostate and kidney. Very little activity is present in the serum of healthy individuals. Increased sorbitol dehydrogenase activity occurs in patients with hepatocellular damage and in patients with congestive cardiac failure when secondary liver damage occurs as a result of hypoxia. Changes appear to parallel those of alanine aminotransferase, and sorbitol dehydrogenase offers little diagnostic improvement.

Glutamate dehydrogenase

This enzyme differs from those previously mentioned in that it is solely a mitochondrial enzyme. It is found mainly in liver, heart, muscle and kidneys. Its intracellular location suggests that increases in glutamate dehydrogenase would parallel the changes seen with aspartate aminotransferase.

Other enzymes

γ-glutamyl transpeptidase (GGT). This is a microsomal enzyme that has been used to complement the measurement of alkaline phosphatase in the assessment of hepatobiliary disease. Increased activity of the enzyme is confined to diseases of the pancreas and hepatobiliary system and, to a lesser extent, the kidney. Increased activity of

GGT is also commonly found in the presence of hepatic malignancies and in cirrhosis, although in the terminal stages of the latter disease there is a tendency for GGT activity to reduce. The test is used to confirm that high alkaline phosphatase activity is of liver origin. GGT is the best available screen for alcohol abuse.

Glutathione S-transferase (GST). This enzyme may offer some advantage over the standard aminotransferases in the investigation of drug mediated hepatic injury. The poor sensitivity of aminotransferases in detecting damage in certain types of liver pathology may partly lie in their distribution within the liver. The periportal hepatocytes contain the highest concentrations of the aminotransferases but the centrilobular hepatocytes, which are relatively deficient in aminotransferases, are more susceptible to damage from hypoxia and toxins. The GSTs are a group of dimeric proteins that constitute about 5% of the total hepatic cytosolic protein and they are thought to play a major role in drug detoxification.

Recently, the measurement of hepatic GST has been advocated as a superior marker of hepatocellular damage due to volatile anaesthetics. Because of its physical and chemical properties, plasma GST estimations may provide a sensitive measure of liver function or dysfunction. When immunological techniques are used to measure individual GST isoenzymes, a high degree of organ specificity can be achieved.

CHRONIC LIVER DISEASE

Alterations in drug disposition

One of the principle functions of the liver is to detoxify drugs by converting lipid soluble compounds to more water soluble ones which may then be excreted in the urine or the bile. Microsomal enzymes within the endoplasmic reticulum of the hepatocyte are responsible for this metabolism. Most drugs undergo an initial step (oxidation or reduction) and then are conjugated with glucuronic and sulphuric acid. The microsomal enzyme system employs molecular oxygen and cytochromes and the system is often referred to as the mixed function oxidase enzyme system.

In chronic liver disease the total hepatocyte mass is decreased and so the potential amount of drug presented to each individual cell for metabolism is increased. This increases enzyme activity within the cell by a process called substrate enzyme induction. As a result, it is only in the presence of very severe disease that drug metabolism becomes impaired.

Centrally acting analgesic and sedative drugs may have prolonged actions in patients with liver disease. This may not be a reflection of altered metabolism but reflects the fact that brain metabolism is abnormal in such patients. This is particularly true in patients with fulminant hepatic failure, in whom analgesic and sedative drugs must be given very cautiously. Similarly, hypoalbuminaemia and hyperglobulinaemia can result in disordered drug binding. Fluid and sodium retention are features of chronic liver disease and sodium-containing drugs (e.g. carbenoxolone, phenylbutazone) should be avoided. In the presence of biliary obstruction, drugs that are usually excreted in the bile may either accumulate or cause toxicity. Known hepatotoxic drugs should be avoided. Where possible, drugs that are normally excreted unchanged in the urine are preferred. Those drugs affecting the central nervous system or the coagulation cascade should be administered with care, and if necessary should be commenced with a reduced dosage.

Avoidance of halothane is sensible in terms of its detrimental effects on total liver blood flow and the degree to which this drug is metabolised (20%). Recent evidence suggests that possible hepatoxic effects of halothane are exacerbated in patients with alcoholic liver disease. The wide availability of isoflurane, desflurane and sevoflurane make the use of halothane in liver disease unnecessary.

Finally, any patient with liver disease presenting for operation is at high risk. All normal precautions should be taken and any coagulation disorders corrected before surgery.

THE GALLBLADDER AND ITS FUNCTIONS

In health, bile flows into the gallbladder when the sphincter of Oddi is closed. In the gallbladder, the bile is concentrated by the absorption of water. Liver bile contains 97% water, whereas the average water content of bile in the gallblader is 89%.

The presence of food in the mouth causes a reflex decrease in the resistance of the sphincter of Oddi. Contraction of the gallbladder is caused by cholecystokinin, which is released in response to the presence of fatty acids in the duodenum. Acid, the products of protein digestion, and Ca^{2+} also stimulate cholecystokinin release. Stimulation of the vagus nerve and release of secretin both stimulate the production of bile and simultaneously increase its water and bicarbonate concentration. Bile salts are important stimulators of bile secretion.

FURTHER READING

Biebuyck J F, Linch P, Krebs H A 1972 The protective effect of oleate and metabolic changes produced by halothane in rat liver. Biochemical Journal 128: 721–723

Sherlock S 1989 Biochemical assessment of liver function. In: Diseases of liver and biliary system 8th Ed. Blackwell Scientific Publications, Oxford

Endocrine system

42

Endocrine pancreas

A. B. Atkinson
W. F. M. Wallace

This chapter and the next review the current state of knowledge of the main endocrine glands, with special reference to anaesthetic practice. The most common disorders are those of the endocrine pancreas and this gland is the subject of the present chapter. Chapter 43 deals with other endocrine glands and their disorders, and also contains a description of the response (including endocrine) to trauma.

INSULIN AND GLUCAGON

The endocrine functions of the pancreas were discovered by Banting and Best in 1921, when they demonstrated the hypoglycaemic properties of pancreatic extract. Pancreatic hormones come from the million or so islets of Langerhans. In the islets, α, or A cells constitute about 20% of the cell population and secrete glucagon; β or B cells are around 70% and secrete insulin; δ or D cells secrete somatostatin; and there are also F cells, which secrete pancreatic polypeptide. The precise role of these last two hormones is not clear.

Insulin is formed as proinsulin, a polypeptide consisting of insulin (51 amino acid units) and a smaller connecting (C) peptide. These are found in storage vesicles in the islet cells, secreting mainly insulin and C peptide. The daily output of insulin is about 40 units; surges of secretion during meals are superimposed on a resting secretion rate of about 1 unit per hour. Insulin secretion can be influenced by stimulatory parasympathetic and inhibitory β sympathetic innervation, but the main control is by the plasma level of nutrients, especially glucose, and by hormones released by the gut during digestion of a meal.

Glucagon is a smaller polypeptide formed not only in the α cells but also in the upper gastro-intestinal tract. As well as its hyperglycaemic action, glucagon has a wider role in the control of metabolism and the reaction to stress. Gluca-gon, cortisol, growth hormone and adrenaline all play a part in opposing excessive insulin action and in raising the blood glucose level when hypoglycaemia, physical activity, injury, illness or major surgery demand it. The main therapeutic use of glucagon is to counteract severe hypoglycaemia.

ROLE OF INSULIN

While many endocrine hormones have been identified in the pancreas, the only one generally replaced in clinical practice is insulin; its normal role will now be reviewed.

Adequate nutrition requires four main phases: ingestion, digestion, absorption and assimilation. Insulin is essential for the last of these — the entry of the main assimilated substances (mono-saccharides, amino acids, fat products and potas-sium ions) into cells. Without the action of insulin these products accumulate in the extracellular fluid and are to varying degrees lost in the urine, leading to serious malnutrition as a major contri-butor to morbidity. Insulin is required mainly during the absorptive phase following a meal. This begins shortly after the first part of the meal enters the stomach, and continues, depending on the size of the meal, for up to 4–6 hours. In someone taking a moderate-sized breakfast and lunch at 07.30 and 12.30 respectively, and a larger evening meal at 18.00, pulses of insulin will be secreted regularly throughout the waking hours. There is less secretion during the hours of sleep.

With this intimate relationship between pro-cessing of ingested food and the secretion of insulin it is not surprising that insulin secretion is controlled by the factors associated with this processing — the entry of glucose and other nu-trients into the circulation and extracellular fluid, and the release into the circulation of various gastrointestinal hormones associated with diges-tion. Additionally, just as vagal activity initiates the early, cephalic, phase of digestion, so vagal activity is another factor controlling secretion of insulin. This pattern of control is confirmed by the finding that much more insulin is released by ingestion of a glucose meal than by the intra-venous infusion of the same amount of glucose. In this way the secretion of insulin is optimally synchronised with requirement for its action. If secretion of insulin were to begin too early this would lead to hypoglycaemia, while late release would allow a period of hyperglycaemia and glycosuria. As with a number of other hormones, insulin action needs to be terminated fairly promptly, and its half-life of about 5 minutes means that its circulating level will fall to one-eighth within 15 minutes of cessation of secre-tion, thus avoiding serious hypoglycaemia when absorption from the gut ceases.

With this sophisticated control, intimately related to requirements, it is not surprising that the insulin regimen of diabetics often falls short of the basic, although demanding, requirements of avoiding serious hyperglycaemia during absorp-tion of a meal, and subsequently avoiding serious hypoglycaemia when absorption ceases. Clearly a single daily injection of insulin cannot fulfil these requirements and is not normally consid-ered appropriate. A single injection cannot gen-erate the peaks of insulin secretion produced endogenously in response to a meal. When the exogenous insulin level is below the ideal insulin level, hyperglycaemia and potential glycos-uria occur; when it is above the ideal level between meals, there is a risk of hypoglycaemia. Both have potential short term and long term hazards.

The body can compensate to some degree for the shortcomings of exogenous insulin administra-tion by the actions of other hormones, e.g. adre-naline and glucagon can limit hypoglycaemia. However, modern techniques of administration are moving closer to the normal physiological control. Two injections a day are frequently used. These often contain mixtures of short and intermediate duration action insulin in an attempt to 'cover' the main ingestions of food. Many patients are now controlled with multiple injection regimens consisting of short acting insulin injections before each meal combined with a long acting insulin injection given at bedtime, the latter preventing morning hyperglycaemia and providing the necessary steady background serum insulin concentration.

During anaesthesia, as in everyday life, it is important to avoid the twin pitfalls of inadequate insulin activity, tending towards ketoacidosis, and excessive insulin activity, tending towards hypoglycaemia. These twin dangers will now be considered.

INADEQUATE INSULIN ACTIVITY

From consideration of the normal role of insulin in the assimilation of absorbed nutrients, it is clear that inadequate insulin activity will lead to excessive accumulation of nutrients in the extracellular fluid, with inadequate entry into cells influenced by insulin, notably skeletal muscle and fat cells and with the notable exception of brain cells. Much of the problem is centred on the handling of glucose and this will be considered first. Other nutrients present somewhat similar problems and will be considered later. It is worth mentioning at this stage that inadequate insulin activity may result from a variety of causes, e.g. destruction of the islet cells by disease, surgical removal of the pancreas and pancreatitis, but the general patterns of effects are similar. In non-insulin dependent diabetes mellitus there is often both deficient insulin secretion and insulin resistance. When considering management during anaesthesia, both insulin dependent (type I) and non-insulin dependent diabetes (type II) require expert endocrine management and careful use of fluids, including dextrose and insulin (although not all type II diabetics require insulin in these circumstances).

Problems with glucose can be considered under two main headings: excess glucose in the extracellular fluid, and inadequate glucose in cells. This has often been referred to as 'starvation in the midst of plenty'.

Excess glucose in the extracellular fluid

This in turn poses two particular problems: firstly, extracellular hyperosmolality; and, secondly, glycosuria. Glucose normally contributes around 5 to the total osmolality of around 290 mosmol l^{-1}. As its level rises, so osmolality is increased in proportion; therefore a fourfold rise in blood/extracellular glucose contributes 20 to the total and an eightfold rise contributes 40, or an extra 35 to the total. Thus fluid tends to be drawn out of cells, to the detriment of their function, and in extreme cases this can affect brain function and cause hyperosmolar coma.

Glycosuria results when the renal threshold for glucose is exceeded, so that the load presented to the tubular cells exceeds their tubular maximum. This happens when blood glucose rises to around twice its normal fasting level. In uncontrolled diabetes mellitus the level rises to 5–10 times the normal level and increasing amounts of glucose are filtered and not absorbed. As in the blood, this glucose has a powerful osmotic effect, and the unabsorbed glucose carries with it the excessive amounts of water and electrolytes which cause the classical symptoms of polyuria and polydypsia. When the patient is vomiting or in coma (discussed below) the fluid deficit cannot be restored by mouth and there is a risk of rapid depletion of body water and electrolytes, leading to a fall in extracellular fluid volume, a concomitant fall in plasma, and hence blood, volume and eventually peripheral circulatory failure.

Inadequate glucose in the intracellular fluid

When this occurs, active tissues, such as skeletal and cardiac muscle, which normally metabolise a blend of glucose and lipid are deprived of glucose and produce energy by the relatively inefficient and potentially harmful pathway of unbalanced lipid breakdown. Not only does this produce inadequate energy, but toxic ketone bodies such as acetoacetic acid and acetone are produced. A major effect is a huge rise in the hydrogen ion level in the body. The build up of ketone bodies and the lowering of pH constitute ketoacidosis. The acidosis can quite rapidly reach severe levels, and blood pH levels below 7.0 can occur in the advanced condition. Even before such severe levels are reached the acidosis leads to increasing malfunction of tissues, particularly the brain, and vomiting is induced. The loss of gastric acid may provide slight compensation for the acidosis but its main effect is to contribute to the loss of body fluids, leading to peripheral circulatory failure, as mentioned earlier. It is this intracellular acidosis and dehydration, coupled with circulatory failure, that leads to coma and potentially to death. The metabolic acidosis is buffered by bicarbonate, which steadily falls as a consequence and is partially compensated for by respiratory alkalosis following hyperventilation (Kussmaul respiration).

Other assimilation problems

While most of the effects of inadequate insulin are related to the above disturbances in glucose handling, parallel problems occur with the other nutrients. Uptake of amino acids and potassium ions into cells is impaired. This impairs tissue synthesis, especially in skeletal muscle, and contributes to the malnutrition produced by insulin deficiency. This process emphasises the usual anabolic role of insulin. In ketoacidotic crisis the blood potassium level rises at the expense of the intracellular level, leading to intracellular potassium depletion. In the patient developing insulin dependent diabetes mellitus, malnutrition and loss of body weight are often seen and occur because of the failure of protein synthesis, inadequate fat deposition and increased fat breakdown.

EXCESSIVE INSULIN ACTIVITY

Although hypoglycaemia occurs rarely as a result of an insulin secreting tumour (insulinoma) or a variety of other medical conditions, it is most commonly seen as a result of temporary excess of insulin in a diabetic patient treated with insulin, or, less commonly, in a patient being treated with oral hypoglycaemic drugs.

Excessive insulin activity produces its main and potentially fatal effect on cerebral function. Normally the brain relies almost entirely on glucose for its constant and high level metabolic requirements. When the circulating glucose level falls to about half the normal fasting level, the brain cells falter in their function, and as the blood glucose continues to fall, coma can develop rapidly. Withdrawal of glucose in this way leads to progressive impairment of consciousness, very like that produced by other disturbances that impede brain metabolism, such as hypoxia, acidosis and hypothermia. Initially, thought processes of the highest order are impaired, so that the patient cannot concentrate and carry out difficult mental tasks, such as working out problems or driving a vehicle safely. Diabetic patients are educated to recognise and manage appropriately the earliest symptoms of hypoglycaemia in order to abort hypoglycaemic attacks. However, in some cases the cerebral disturbances impair judgement, with consequent loss of patient awareness. In others with longstanding type 1 diabetes and in those with frequent hypoglycaemic events, warning symptoms are blunted or lost. In such cases friends and family may have to learn to recognise and treat early features of hypoglycaemia.

The body has its own automatic compensatory mechanisms in hypoglycaemia. Firstly, at approximately 3.7 mmol l^{-1} increased release of glucagon in response to hypoglycaemia mobilises hepatic glycogen. Secondly, there is activation of the autonomic system. This includes both sympathetic and parasympathetic activation. Sympathetic activation also raises the blood glucose level through activation of β receptors. The associated sympathetic effects of tremor and a hyperdynamic circulation (β effects) and sweating (a cholinergic effect) are useful alerting signs. The parasympathetic effects involve vagal stimulation of the stomach. Gastric stimulation, with its associated increase in gastric acid secretion, is probably of value in promoting a sense of hunger and in aiding rapid absorption of any glucose or sucrose taken. Increased growth hormone and cortisol secretion also occur but are of lesser importance.

ANAESTHESIA AND THE DIABETIC PATIENT

The key to adequate management of the diabetic patient is matching nutrient intake to insulin action. The period of starvation — often of uncertain duration — associated with anaesthesia and surgery seriously interferes with the desirable routine of diet, activity and insulin. This period of starvation can be kept as short as possible by having the patient at the start of an operation list. During the period of starvation — before, during and after the anaesthetic — maintenance of a supply of glucose for intracellular use is provided by infusion of glucose and concomitant administration of insulin by its addition to the infusion. In preparation for operation, frequent measurements of plasma glucose should be made. If bedside devices are used these must be regularly calibrated and quality assured. In the perioperative period only short acting insulin should be used. Although infusion of 5% dextrose cannot provide for adequate daily nutrition (2 litres contain only 100 g dextrose, which would supply only about 20% of the daily requirements of a sedentary adult), it provides, under insulin's action, a limited supply of glucose to the tissues and can readily maintain normal circulating levels required by the brain, as 5% dextrose (50 g l^{-1}) represents more than 50 times the normal plasma level. Without the action of insulin, much of the infused dextrose would be lost as glycosuria.

APPENDIX

This appendix refers briefly to different types of insulin and oral hypoglycaemic drugs and then outlines the principles of perioperative management of patients with diabetes mellitus, including those normally treated with insulin, and those normally managed on diet or diet plus oral hypoglycaemics.

Insulin preparations

These consist of various formulations of human insulin and of bovine and porcine insulin, which closely resemble it.

Soluble insulin (Actrapid, Humulin S, Velosulin, Hypurin Neutral)

These are simple aqueous solutions with a half-life of several minutes when given intravenously. However, they are usually given subcutaneously, when the onset of action is in about 30 minutes, with maximal effect in 2–3 hours and a duration of 6–8 hours. Flexible control of diabetes can be achieved using two or three such injections per day, but depot preparations are widely used in addition. These make use of zinc and protamine to prolong duration of action.

Isophane insulin, NPH (Humulin I, Insulatard)

These are suspensions of insulin and protamine with a medium duration of action, with onset at 1–2 hours, maximal effect 3–8 hours and duration up to 16 hours.

Insulin zinc suspensions, IZS (Ultratard, Humulin Zn)

Zinc retards the release of injected insulin and such formulations have a duration of 12–24 hours, depending on particle size. Semilente is amorphous, ultralente is crystalline, while lente is a mixture of the two.

Protamine zinc insulin, PZI (Hypurin Protamine Zinc)

This contains both protamine and zinc and has a still longer duration of action of 24–40 hours.

Oral hypoglycaemic drugs

These drugs are effective only in the patient with some endogenous insulin secretion. There are two distinct groups: the sulphonylureas and the biguanides.

Sulphonylureas

These act by stimulating the β cells of the pancreas to produce insulin. *Tolbutamide* has a short half-life of 5 hours, so it may be given in divided doses. It is metabolised in the liver and caution is therefore required in patients with liver failure. However, it can be used in patients with renal impairment. *Chlorpropamide* has a longer half-life of 35 hours and is therefore given as a single morning dose. It should be avoided in the elderly because of the risk of prolonged hypoglycaemia. *Glibenclamide* has an intermediate duration of action and is usually given once or twice a day.

Newer, third generation sulphonylureas, e.g. *gliclazide*, are now being used widely. They have a biphasic duration and are metabolised by the liver. They can be used in renal failure.

Biguanides

Their action is probably multifactorial, including delayed absorption of glucose from the gut (like pancreatic polypeptide), increased peripheral use and decreased gluconeogenesis. *Metformin* is usually given in divided doses. It should not be used in patients with renal or hepatic failure because of the risk of lactic acidosis.

No oral agents should be used in pregnancy.

Diabetes and surgery

Diabetes mellitus is the most common endocrine disorder encountered in anaesthetic practice. Despite this, there is no consensus as to what constitutes good control of blood sugar in the perioperative period, and the literature contains a large number of different regimens for management. No one regimen has been shown to be of greater benefit to the patient than any other (Milaskiewicz & Hall 1992).

The scheme proposed by Alberti & Thomas (1979) has gained wide popularity for its relative simplicity. An intravenous infusion containing KCl 10 mmol, and insulin 10 units in glucose 10%, 500 ml given at a rate of 100 ml h^{-1} forms the basis of this. The rate and content are adjusted on the basis of blood glucose estimations; however, this has not been shown to give better control than other regimens.

A more comprehensive plan for management of diabetes is given below.

Perioperative management of insulin dependent diabetes

1. The diabetologist should be informed about these patients and should be involved routinely in their management. The patients are suitable for day case surgery only where this is relatively minor, and only in patients with good diabetic control and suitable home circumstances.

2. Check laboratory plasma glucose plus capillary blood glucose four times a day before meals. If premeal values of 4–12 mmol l^{-1} are found, no advice is required, but if they are outside this range the diabetologist should be contacted at once.

3. For elective morning surgery:
a. Give the usual dose of fast acting insulin on the evening before operation.
b. If the patient is on medium acting insulin, give two-thirds the usual dose.
c. If the patient is on a multiple injection regimen, give usual fast acting insulin and half very long acting insulin on the evening before operation (e.g. Ultratard).
d. Start hourly capillary blood glucose monitoring at 7.00 a.m.

If glucose is less than 2 mmol l^{-1}, commence 500 ml 5% dextrose over 2 hours with no insulin. If the patient has symptoms of hypoglycaemia give 50% dextrose (if fasting), 10–40 ml intravenously. Do not exceed this amount.

If glucose is 2–5 mmol l^{-1}, commence 500 ml 5% dextrose over 6 hours.

If glucose is 5–10 mmol l^{-1}, commence 500 ml 5% dextrose plus 6 units soluble insulin over 4 hours.

If glucose is 10–15 mmol l^{-1}, commence 500 ml 5% dextrose plus 10 units soluble insulin over 4 hours.

If glucose is 15–20 mmol l^{-1}, commence 500 ml 5% dextrose plus 14 units soluble insulin over 4 hours.

If glucose is greater than 20 mmol l^{-1}, contact diabetologist.

Check capillary glucose hourly, changing dextrose infusion if necessary.

Add 80 mmol potassium per day to drip and give saline as well if required. If intravenous fluids are required for more than 24 hours, contact the diabetologist urgently.

4. When the patient is eating again, intravenous fluids can be discontinued and subcutaneous fast acting insulin given, depending on:
a. glucose before meal
b. how much is to be eaten
c. the patient's usual insulin requirement at that time
d. the response to the previous doses of insulin.

Thus decisions must be made at the time of eating, when a glucose estimation is available, and should not be written up in advance.

As a rough guide, if glucose is 4–10 mmol l^{-1} before a meal, 60–100% of the usual insulin requirement is a reasonable initial dose, as long as the response to this is known before the next meal and insulin is again prescribed.

Patients usually return to their standard preoperative insulin requirements within 24–48 hours.

If the patient becomes ill, urgent help should be sought from the diabetes team. It is easier to sort out porblems early and quickly during working hours, when laboratories are available, than to 'sit' on problems.

The doctor on call should be responsible for checking that the regimen is working and should monitor this actively and obtain help as necessary. A daily visit from a member of the diabetes team is most helpful.

Perioperative management of diet and tablet controlled diabetes

1. Check capillary glucose profile and single laboratory plasma glucose on day before operation. If glucose is greater than 15 or less than 4 mmol l^{-1}, contact the diabetes team urgently. Fast overnight before surgery as usual.

2. Omit oral hypoglycaemic agents on the morning of surgery. Check laboratory glucose 1 hour before operation, and capillary glucose hourly during surgery.

If glucose is less than 3 mmol l^{-1}, give 500 ml 5% dextrose without insulin over 2 hours (plus 10–40 ml 50% dextrose but no more than this if the patient is symptomatic).

If glucose is 3–5 mmol l^{-1}, give 500 ml 5% dextrose intravenously without insulin over 6 hours.

If glucose is 5–12 mmol l^{-1}, no intravenous glucose or insulin is needed.

If glucose is greater than 12 mmol l^{-1}, ask for advice from the diabetes team.

3. When the patient is eating again, oral hypoglycaemic agents should be restarted, as before, and the capillary glucose monitored four times a day until full recovery from the operation. At that stage monitoring can be reduced to before breakfast only.

4. If the patient is to fast for more than 24 hours, the diabetes team should be consulted.

Perioperative management of diet controlled diabetes

1. Check capillary blood glucose profile on the day before operation and perform a single laboratory plasma glucose estimation.

If laboratory glucose exceeds 15 mmol l^{-1}, consult the diabetes team.

If laboratory glucose is less than 15 mmol l^{-1}, fast overnight before surgery as usual.

2. Check fasting laboratory glucose 1 hour before operation.

If less than 12 mmol l^{-1}, no drip is required for diabetes (although one may be required for other reasons).

3. Check laboratory glucose after surgery.

If less than 12 mmol l^{-1}, the patient can resume usual diet.

If more than 12 mmol l^{-1}, consult the diabetes team.

4. If intravenous fluids are required for a surgical indication, use normal saline and 5% dextrose as usual, initially monitoring capillary blood glucose 2-hourly.

If glucose exceeds 10 mmol l^{-1}, consult the diabetes team.

5. If glucose is satisfactory (4–12 mmol l^{-1} before meals) and the patient is well 24 hours after surgery, reduce monitoring to single capillary blood glucose before breakfast each day. All patients must be monitored four times a day and advice sought from the diabetes team.

REFERENCES AND FURTHER READING

Alberti K G M M 1990 Diabetes and surgery. In: Rifkin H, Porte D (eds) Ellenberg and Rifkins' diabetes mellitus: theory and practice, 4th edn, pp 626–633. Elsevier, London

Alberti K G M M, Thomas D J B 1979 The management of diabetes during surgery. British Journal of Anaesthesia 51: 693–710

De Fronzo R, Hendler R, Christensen N 1980 Stimulation of counterregulatory hormonal responses in diabetic man by a fall in glucose concentration. Diabetes 29: 125

Felig P 1974 Insulin therapy: rates and routes of delivery. New England Journal of Medicine 291: 1031.

Milaskiewicz R M, Hall G M 1992 Diabetes and anaesthesia: the past decade. British Journal of Anaesthesia 68: 198–206

The Diabetes Control and Complications Trial Research Group 1993 The effect of intensive treatment of diabetes on the development and progression of long-term complications in insulin-dependent diabetes mellitus. New England Journal of Medicine 329: 977

43

Other endocrine glands

A. B. Atkinson
W. F. M. Wallace

In understanding the endocrine system, it is worth noting two general points: firstly, the parallels between nervous and endocrine control; and, secondly, the reserve of function that endocrine glands have.

Parallels between nervous and endocrine control

The parallels include the action of a transmitter substance (neurotransmitter or hormone) on a target cell to produce a specific effect (more diffuse in the case of a hormone), negative feedback, and for many but not all endocrine glands (in the present state of knowledge) cerebral control (mainly via the hypothalamus and pituitary in the case of the endocrine system). The differences become blurred in some situations. Thus the posterior pituitary consists of nerve axons releasing chemicals, but these chemicals (neurotransmitters/hormones) act diffusely at a distance; this is sometimes described as a neuro-endocrine effect. Again in the sympathetic system, discharge of nerves (neurotransmission) is usually accompanied by complementary secretion of the adrenal medulla (endocrine), with both the neural effects and the endocrine effects converging at the end-organ. Thus both sympathetic nerves and circulating catecholamines stimulate cardiac β adrenoceptors to cause tachycardia and increased contractility in a variety of conditions, including response to haemorrhage and trauma, and in strenuous exercise.

Reserves of function

As with other organs, such as the liver, there is considerable reserve of function in the normal individual so that destruction of cells by disease or surgical removal do not result in permanent failure of function unless considerable amounts of the gland are affected.

PITUITARY

The pituitary gland has two separate lobes with separate development and hypothalamic control. These two lobes are in such close proximity in a confined space that lesions that affect one part often affect both parts.

The anterior lobe (adenohypophysis) is derived embryologically from the gut. It has no direct link with the brain but receives controlling hormones from the hypothalamus via portal vessels passing down the pituitary stalk. The hormones include corticotrophin releasing hormone (CRH) which governs release of adrenocorticotrophic hormone (ACTH). Growth hormone secretion is stimulated by a releasing hormone, somatotrophin, and inhibited by somatostatin. Thyrotrophin releasing hormone (TRH) governs release of thyroid stimulating hormone (TSH). Secretion of prolactin is inhibited by dopamine, and the gonadotrophins follicle stimulating hormone (FSH) and luteinising hormone (LH) are both controlled by gonadotrophin releasing hormone (GnRH).

The posterior lobe (neurohypophysis) is derived from the brain and contains axons from hypothalamic neurones. It releases vasopressin (or antidiuretic hormone, ADH) and oxytocin in response to hypothalamic integration of inputs from osmoreceptors and more peripheral sense organs, e.g. volume receptors.

Disorders of the pituitary are uncommon but tend to have severe effects. The pituitary, like other endocrine glands, has considerable reserve function, but when deficiency arises there are profound effects. Loss of the gonadotrophic hormones leads to amenorrhoea and infertility, loss of growth hormone in childhood leads to growth failure, loss of vasopressin from the posterior lobe leads to inability to conserve water, and hence polyuria, while loss of trophic hormones for thyroid and adrenal function leads to profound deficiency of the corresponding hormones. When the entire gland is destroyed, these effects summate. In particular, the combination of hypothyroidism and cortisol deficiency leads to even poorer tolerance of physical stress than either of the two alone.

Excessive pituitary function is usually selective for a particular hormone, causing such conditions as acromegaly (excessive growth hormone), ACTH dependent hypercortisolism and hyperprolactinaemia. Across any pituitary surgery hydrocortisone is given parenterally and careful attention must be paid to fluid balance. If polyuria ensues, vasopressin should be given and excessive use of dextrose infusions omitted to avoid the risk of precipitating hyperosmolar hyperglycaemic coma.

THYROID

Just as the crucial activity of the pancreatic islets is to produce insulin, so that of the thyroid is to produce thyroxine and related hormones; in addition, it produces thyrocalcitonin, the effects of which are unrelated. As with loss of pancreatic function, so loss of the thyroid requires replacement treatment, with thyroxine but not with calcitonin. Thyroxine is the major circulating hormone, although that part converted peripherally to tri-iodothyronine is more active. In discussing actions of thyroid hormones and the effects of deficient and excessive thyroid activity, the word thyroxine will be used, for convenience, to describe the gland's endocrine output.

Iodine and the thyroid hormones

Iodine is a vital ingredient of thyroid hormone and is obtained from sea fish (iodide deficiency and goitre was, and in some parts still is, common in people living far from the sea), iodised salt, and to a lesser extent from bread, milk and vegetables. The daily requirement is around 100–200 µg. The element is absorbed as iodide and the follicular cells of the thyroid gland actively take up and store 95% of total body iodide. Tyrosine attached to thyroglobulin within the follicle is iodinated to mono- and di-iodotyrosine and combined with a second tyrosine molecule to make tri-iodothyronine (T_3) and tetra-iodothyronine, or thyroxine (T_4). The latter hormones are stored (bound to thyroglobulin) in follicular colloid and are released under the influence of TSH. This leads to breakdown of thyroglobulin, making the hormones available for secretion.

In states of iodine deficiency the reduced output of thyroid hormones removes negative feedback inhibition of the pituitary and TSH level rises and stimulates thyroid growth, causing goitre. Replacement of the iodine leads to shrinkage of the goitre.

Actions of thyroxine

This hormone controls the basal and resting metabolic rate of the body by acting on the mitochondria to increase their generation of energy by oxidative phosphorylation. This has three major effects: increased consumption of oxygen and substrates, increased generation of heat and increased available energy to the body organs generally, including the heart and the neuromuscular system. In practice this allows elevation of the metabolic rate and increased energy availability in the tissues in situations of serious stress, such as trauma and surgery. The control of the thyroid via TSH from the pituitary, in turn controlled by TRH from the hypothalamus, provides a link between the brain and the thyroid.

Inadequate thyroxine activity

This condition presents two major problems: a fall in basal metabolism and an inability to increase metabolism when required.

Fall in basal metabolism

The basal metabolic rate is defined as the level of metabolism necessary to maintain normal function when major factors tending to increase metabolism are at a minimum. Thus the basal state implies absence of exertion (complete rest

for several hours), absence of digestion and assimilation of food (fasting for the length of time it takes to deal with the previous meal, typically at least 6 hours), absence of thermal challenge (referred to as thermoneutrality, described by the conscious individual as being neither too hot nor too cold), and absence of mental stress, which can increase metabolism by, for example, sympathetic activity. It is not surprising that when this basal metabolism is depressed, so that energy available to tissues such as the heart and the neuromuscular system is inadequate, the individual shows signs of malfunction. Thus the three effects of thyroxine referred to above (increased oxygen consumption, increased heat production and increased available energy) are impaired.

Decreased consumption of oxygen is one of the hallmarks of the condition, although chemical tests have long since replaced its measurement for routine diagnosis. Decreased consumption of substrate in the mitochondria is probably one of the reasons for the excess fat deposition that can occur. It probably contributes to decreased appetite, inactivity of the alimentary system and constipation.

Inadequate basal heat production is to some extent compensated for by reflex vasoconstriction and decreased heat loss. This leads to the typically cold extremities and, when vasoconstriction cannot compensate, the risk of a serious fall in core temperature (hypothermia). For the hypothyroid patient the thermoneutral temperature is several degrees higher than normal and in a normal environment the patients constantly feel uncomfortably cold.

The decreased energy available to the tissues generally leads to widespread problems, including decreased rate and force of cardiac contraction, decreased electrocardiographic voltage, increased reflex relaxation times and general slowing of thought, speech and actions.

Inability to increase metabolism

Everyday stresses (physical activity, a cold environment) require increased metabolism, and unusually severe stresses (trauma, surgery) require a greater and longer-maintained surge of increased metabolism. Thus the hypothyroid patient is physically inactive and has cold intolerance. More seriously, such patients cannot respond adequately to life threatening trauma, e.g. multiple or widespread burns, which in normothyroid patients increases resting metabolic rate by as much as 50% above normal. This increased metabolism is required for the widespread response (vasoconstriction, tachycardia, increased ionic pumping and chemical synthesis) required for survival. Untreated hypothyroid patients are prone to collapse and death in these circumstances and require especially careful management in intensive care and during anaesthesia. Tri-iodothyronine is sometimes given in such situations because of its more rapid onset of action, but it may precipitate angina or cardiac failure in patients with heart disease.

Excessive thyroxine activity

The problem in this case is fundamentally the reverse of that seen in hypothyroidism. The basal metabolic rate is abnormally high because of increased mitochondrial activity. Oxygen consumption and substrate utilisation increase, excessive cellular energy is made available and heat production increases. In the presence of excess thyroxine the hyperactivity of tissues, with increased heat production, tremor and increased alerting mechanisms, generally lead not to increasingly rapid and effective thought processes but to an irritable excited state that often militates against normal calm thought and evaluation.

The somatic effects of excessive thyroxine can be related to increases in oxygen and substrate utilisation, energy availability and heat production. Increased oxygen consumption (and a corresponding increase in carbon dioxide production) lead to increased ventilation and this may be recognised by the patient as abnormal and interpreted as breathlessness.

Greater substrate utilisation (day and night) leads to depletion of body stores of fat and the tendency to lose weight. A natural consequence is an increased appetite and increased activity in the alimentary tract with increased frequency of defecation.

Greater energy availability has widespread consequences, including increased rate of cardiac contraction, shortened reflex time and muscle tremor.

One of the more unpleasant effects of excess thyroxine activity is the constant production of excessive heat. This threatens to elevate core temperature, and in thyrotoxicosis may do so. However, core temperature is usually maintained at the upper limit of normal by the hypothalamic reflexes which increase peripheral blood flow and sweating. This has two effects. Firstly, at rest, the patients feel uncomfortably warm, as normally the environmental temperature indoors is maintained at a level that suits the normothyroid individual. The picture presented to the brain by the peripheral receptors is probably of great significance for our comfort. When our peripheries are vasodilated and sweating is occurring we feel uncomfortably warm. Secondly, the overall effect of the high metabolic rate and increased heat production is general exhaustion. A major contributor is probably heat exhaustion, as the individual with a high basal and resting metabolic rate is in a constant state of vasodilatation and sweating. The increased cardiac output of the resting state (with a risk of high output cardiac failure when cardiac function is impaired by concomitant disease) erodes the reserve available during exertion, and hence the ability to exercise is curtailed.

Because some of the most serious and unpleasant effects are related to increased stimulation of β-adrenergic receptors, β blockers can relieve such effects in the short term. Longer term treatment requires drugs, such as carbimazole, that block synthesis of thyroid hormones. Since iodine is taken up very selectively by the thyroid gland, overactivity can be treated in appropriate patients by radioiodine (^{131}I), a β emitter that penetrates only some 2 mm.

Physiological diagnosis of thyroxine abnormalities

The detailed biochemical diagnosis of such abnormalities is beyond the scope of this book, but the levels of TSH are of considerable interest.

Because of the negative feedback control loop operating through the pituitary, the level of the trophic hormone changes reciprocally with that of thyroxine, although this can be overridden if required by TRH from the hypothalamus, a local hormone carried in the pituitary portal network of capillaries.

When the thyroid gland itself is underactive, removal of negative feedback leads to a rise in the level of TSH and when this rise is detected by diagnostic tests it provides strong evidence for the diagnosis of hypothyroidism. If hypothyroidism is diagnosed without elevation in TSH, the overall pituitary structure and function must be investigated in detail as the abnormality is then pituitary in nature. In hyperthyroidism, the increased feedback from the overactive gland suppresses release of thyrotrophin as the vast majority of cases of hyperthyroidism are not of pituitary or hypothalamic origin.

Anaesthesia in thyroid disorders

Adequately treated hypothyroidism does not constitute a major anaesthetic risk. However, if the level of thyroid activity is deficient, the missing hormone should be supplied at the level judged equal to the body's normal requirements. Non-urgent surgery should be postponed until the situation is well controlled. This usually takes from 6 to 8 weeks, but in an urgent situation the more rapidly acting agent, tri-iodothyronine can be used. In all such situations careful overall assessment is required for optimal outcomes.

In uncontrolled hyperthyroidism the risk is one of inducing thyrotoxic crisis. Surgery should be postponed, if at all possible, until the thyroid has been brought under control. If emergency surgery is required then large doses of β-blocking drugs can be used.

ADRENAL CORTEX

In considering the functions of these glands and their steroid hormones, it is worth noting that so-called 'steroid' therapy, which is essentially synthetic glucocorticoid therapy, is by far the most common cause of disturbance of adrenal cortical function. Some general properties of steroid hormones will now be considered, followed by a review of the main adrenal cortical hormones — cortisol and aldosterone.

Steroid hormones

Adrenocortical hormones and the gonadal hormones are derivatives of cholesterol. This fat soluble compound, perhaps best known as a major coronary risk factor, is an essential hormone precursor and is synthesised in the body. Because of their cholesterol derived, four ringed basic structure, with the possibility of vast numbers of different side-chain combinations, steroid hormones constitute a large family of compounds with numerous interrelated effects. Many such compounds are synthesised in the adrenal cortex and many others have been synthesised as pharmacological agents. The structures of cholesterol, hydrocortisone (cortisol), aldosterone and testosterone are given in Figure 43.1.

Cortisol is classified as a glucocorticoid hormone because of its profound effects on glucose metabolism. In particular it mobilises glucose from stores and non-glucose sources and raises the circulating glucose level. However, it also closely mimics the actions of aldosterone, the major mineralocorticoid, increasing reabsorption of salt and water in the nephron, thus tending to raise extracellular volume. *In vivo*, cortisol has less marked mineralocorticoid actions than aldosterone, but when present in high concentration its effect is substantial. One reason for pharmaceutical synthesis of novel steroids has been the desire to dissociate mineralocorticoid from glucocorticoid actions (the latter having a protein suppressing effect that is useful in suppressing unwanted inflammation in such diverse conditions as asthma and rheumatoid arthritis, inflammation depending heavily on protein synthesis). Some dissociation has been achieved but some synthetic anti-inflammatory glucocorticoids retain a residual mineralocorticoid effect.

The overlapping effects of corticosteroids are seen in other systems; for example, the male and female sex hormones both favour an adolescent growth spurt, despite having differing effects on

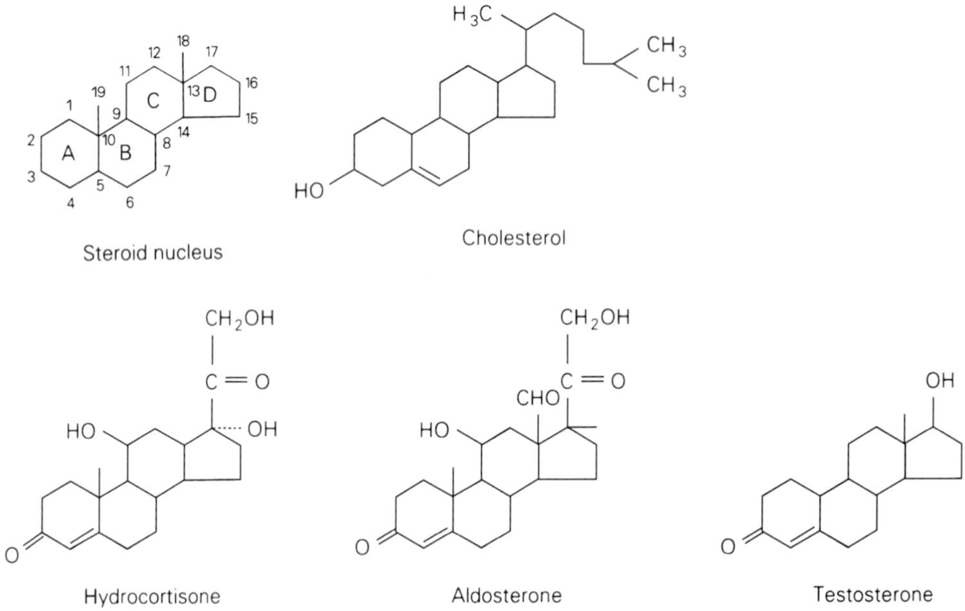

Figure 43.1 Structure of the steroid nucleus, cholesterol and three major steroid hormones.

secondary sexual characteristics. While most of the sex steroids are produced in the gonads, the adrenal glands also synthesise these hormones, mainly androgens. In both sexes these contribute to the development of axillary and pubic hair.

Cortisol

Before cortisone acetate therapy became available, adrenal failure led to death. The survival of patients after its introduction indicates that cortisol is the crucial adrenal hormone for maintenance of life. Therapy for loss of mineralocorticoid action is now usually given in addition.

As with thyroxine, cortisol secretion is controlled by a trophic pituitary hormone (ACTH) whose secretion is, in turn, regulated by feedback loops involving the adrenal gland (cortisol), the pituitary (ACTH) and the hypothalamus (CRH and vasopressin).

A point of crucial importance in medical practice is that long term therapy with high doses of glucocorticoid drugs such as prednisone leads not only to excessive cortisol-type effects (see later) but to negative feedback at pituitary level. This suppresses activity in the cells that produce

ACTH and the result is disuse atrophy of the adrenal cortical cells (inner layers — zonae fasciculata and reticularis), which produce cortisol. Should an emergency arise, the hypothalamic–pituitary–adrenal axis cannot respond in the usual fashion. This suppression is long lasting and steroid replacement therapy is the only effective treatment. Patients submitted to either emergency or elective surgery require parenteral hydrocortisone and careful attention to sodium balance in the perioperative period.

Circadian rhythm of cortisol

Secretion of cortisol in the normal person shows one of the clearest of the circadian (diurnal) rhythms, although within this framework secretion is episodic. The basic pattern is of a steep surge in the early morning, generally maintained high levels during the waking hours and a steady fall during sleep, with minimal levels between 12 midnight and 4 a.m.

This pattern has been shown to persist in people isolated from the outside world in deep caves or sound- and light-insulated laboratories without any indicators of time. On travel across time zones the pattern adapts to the new sleep/ waking, dark/light pattern. This indicates that it is a fundamental endogenous pattern embedded in the organism but linked with the sleep/activity rhythm. Clearly this requires the integrative activity of the brain, and experimental evidence points to a hypothalamic clock. In Cushing's syndrome of any type the circadian rhythm is frequently absent.

Since cortisol favours production of energy, including that produced from body protein, high levels produce a state of breakdown of body tissues (catabolism) and liberation of high levels of energy (high metabolic rate). In contrast, a low level of cortisol allows regeneration of body tissues and is compatible with the resting and sleeping state. The importance of the normal circadian rhythm becomes more apparent when we consider the problems of patients with, firstly, deficient cortisol secretion (with inadequate secretion during the day's activities and during stress), and, secondly, excessive secretion (which abolishes the normal fall in secretion during sleep).

Deficient cortisol activity

Those with virtually absent cortisol secretions (adrenal failure or suppression of cortisol secreting cells) have a profound inability to cope with the stress of everyday living. Loss of cortisol secretion leads to lethargy, nausea and postural hypotension so that even the upright posture cannot be maintained adequately and moderate exercise is impossible; major trauma is fatal. This suggests that the many and varied cellular actions of cortisol have the overall physiological effect of allowing people to deal with physical stress, and in particular of maintaining an adequate circulation and arterial blood pressure in the upright posture and following serious trauma. Through their varied effects, the production of steroids provides the necessary milieu for daily activity.

It has been found that injury leads to a surge of cortisol roughly proportional to the severity of the injury. Patients who cannot produce this cortisol surge are at serious risk of circulatory failure and death unless they are provided with exogenous cortisol to match the normal response. An early indication of unsuspected adrenal failure in such circumstances is a falling arterial blood pressure that fails to respond to the usual treatments, such as blood replacement and pressor agents. In the intensive therapy setting, it has recently become apparent that a number of critically ill patients without any history of previous steroid therapy are unable to produce an adequate pituitary–adrenal response. The increase in circulating cortisol in response to ACTH may be used to identify these patients and they may benefit from cortisol supplementation.

Excessive steroid production

Quite different problems arise with maintained high levels of cortisol, whether endogenous or exogenous. Excessive catabolic effects, maintained day and night, ensue. The provision of glucose for the production of energy is maintained at the expense of the body tissues, especially protein. Excess gluconeogenesis, the formation of glucose from protein, leads to depletion of protein in skeletal muscle (muscle wasting), protein depletion in skin (fragility and striae) and in bone (weakness due to destruction of the collagen fibres that make an important contribution to bone strength). Other effects, e.g. fat deposition, diabetes and hypertension, are also seen.

Aldosterone

As discussed earlier, cortisol has secondary mineralocorticoid actions and these contribute to its maintenance of the circulation by helping to regulate the extracellular, and hence blood, volume. However, the other major adrenal corticoid, aldosterone (produced in the outer layer or zona glomerulosa) is the main mineralocorticoid. It has negligible glucocorticoid action and its control is also different. While cortisol is controlled mainly by ACTH (with a dominant hypothalamic input) and is largely a stress hormone, aldosterone has a number of control mechanisms, the major one of which is the renin–angiotensin system. This system operates as a negative feedback loop to maintain extracellular volume and hence arterial blood pressure. It is probably triggered by a variety of monitors which measure blood volume and arterial blood pressure, but the role of the juxtaglomerular apparatus has been most clearly defined and seems to be dominant. The cells of this apparatus secrete renin when blood pressure falls in the afferent arteriole, as it will when systemic arterial pressure falls or when such a fall is prevented by the baroreflexes, which include renal vasoconstriction. Renin circulates and stimulates formation of angiotensin I, which in turn is converted into angiotensin II by angiotensin converting enzyme (ACE), an enzyme abundant in endothelial cells. One of the major actions of angiotensin II is to stimulate the release of aldosterone from the adrenal cortex. Aldosterone acts on the renal tubules to cause salt and water retention and hence conserves extracellular volume and in turn plasma volume and arterial blood pressure. The effects of deficient and excessive aldosterone action illustrate the above.

Deficient aldosterone action

As explained above, the effects of this are most marked in total adrenal failure when the mineralocorticoid action of cortisol is also lost. Extracellular volume and hence plasma volume become depleted and this contributes, along with cortisol deficiency, to the inability to maintain arterial blood pressure in day to day activity, especially when standing (postural hypotension) and failure to maintain arterial pressure, even in the supine position, after trauma or surgery. Conditions of isolated mineralocorticoid deficiency are also seen clinically.

Excessive aldosterone action

This produces a mirror image effect of increased retention of salt and water with consequent hypertension. Because aldosterone favours exchange of potassium and hydrogen ions for sodium ions in the tubules, there is excessive loss of potassium and hydrogen ions, leading to hypokalaemic alkalosis, which together with hypertension is characteristic of hyperaldosteronism of any type.

Therapeutic use of corticosteroids

Corticosteroids, particularly synthetic glucocorticoids, are widely used drugs with potent beneficial effects, e.g. in severe asthma, rheumatoid arthritis and in preventing rejection of transplanted organs. They also have potent adverse effects and, despite synthesis of many novel steroids, it has not been possible to divorce entirely these potentially serious side-effects from the beneficial effects.

Hydrocortisone

Hydrocortisone is rapidly absorbed orally, as are most other synthetic and natural steroids. It is carried in plasma, about 95% bound to a globulin, transcortin, some of the remainder being loosely bound to albumin. Its half-life is about 90 minutes, shorter than some of its synthetic analogues. Because of its indirect action, via nucleic acid, its effects (e.g. anti-inflammatory) last longer than the short half-life would suggest. Most inactivation of hydrocortisone is in the liver, by conjugation, etc., and the products and some unchanged hydrocortisone are excreted by the kidneys.

Synthetic steroids

The aim in synthesising new compounds is to dissociate mineralocorticoid from glucocorticoid effects. Apart from fludrocortisone, the common synthetic steroids are glucocorticoids. There is considerable variation in equipotent doses from an anti-inflammatory point of view. More importantly, there has been moderate but not complete dissociation of mineralocorticoid actions from glucocorticoid actions. However, many serious side-effects are glucocorticoid in nature (e.g. destruction of collagen leading to bone weakness and poor healing of tissues, impaired immune responses to infection) and so the glucocorticoid drugs can have side-effects that limit their use to conditions which seriously threaten life (severe asthma) or its quality (e.g. severe rheumatoid arthritis).

Prednisolone is widely used, both orally and parenterally, in the management of asthma, rheumatoid arthritis and other inflammatory conditions. Its 6 α-methyl derivative, methylprednisolone, has even less mineralocorticoid action and has been widely used in both soluble and depot form for local treatment of painful conditions. Dexamethasone has been used in the short term treatment of cerebral oedema.

Steroid therapy in relation to anaesthesia

Patients who have been on long term steroid therapy immediately before surgery, or within several months of it, are at risk of perioperative collapse, particularly circulatory collapse, due to inability to secrete the increased levels of cortisol needed in such circumstances. Such patients should be given supplementary hydrocortisone parenterally at the time of premedication, followed by further doses 6–8-hourly for 1 day for minor procedures and for 3 days or more for major surgery. High dosage steroid therapy has in the past been advocated for critically ill patients with septic shock, but this role has not been fully validated as initial improvement has been found to be followed by increased mortality

ADRENAL MEDULLA

As mentioned earlier, the sympathetic nervous system combines the two standard mechanisms of central physiological control: the nervous and the endocrine systems. The adrenal medulla augments the effects of sympathetic nervous activity. The time course of effects is quite different. Sympathetic nerves, like autonomic nerves in general, conduct at a velocity of around 1 m s^{-1}. With distances to heart and blood vessels, for example of the order of 0.5–1.5 metres, sympathetic nerves can produce their effects within a few seconds. However, catecholamines from the adrenal medulla must travel in the circulation to the heart and then through the lungs and to the peripheries to produce effects such as general vasoconstriction.

The sympathetic nervous system can usually compensate for loss of adrenal medullary hormones, e.g. after removal of the adrenal glands,

but dramatic effects can be produced by the rare tumour (phaeochromocytoma) which secretes adrenal medullary hormones. Adrenaline produces prominent β effects — tachycardia, hyperdynamic circulation, tremor and a raised metabolic rate (effects similar to thyrotoxicosis) — while noradrenaline produces peripheral vasoconstriction, a rise in total peripheral resistance and systemic hypertension. β- and α-receptor blockers, respectively, produce dramatic relief of these effects.

Anaesthesia in patients with phaeochromocytoma is extremely hazardous and patients with this diagnosis should be managed in centres with special expertise. The anaesthetic management is discussed fully in Chapter 27. If the diagnosis of phaeochromocytoma is suspected, cold surgery must be postponed until the diagnosis has been made (and appropriate management measures taken) or refuted.

PARATHYROIDS AND VITAMIN D

The four small parathyroid glands produce the hormone parathormone, which is essentially the guardian of the extracellular ionised calcium level. The major effect of this level is on the function of excitable tissues, especially the neuromuscular system, where ionised calcium levels determine the level of excitability, presumably by modifying the function of the channels that permit rapid entry of sodium ions and hence electrical activation of the tissues. A low level of extracellular calcium increases excitability and leads to tetany — muscle spasms that may vary from the minor discomfort of carpopedal spasm to life threatening laryngospasm in infants or general muscle spasms in adults. Sensory nerves are also affected, leading to tingling (paraesthesiae), while involvement of the central nervous system may cause epileptic attacks.

A high level of ionised calcium has the mirror image effect of reducing excitability, leading (centrally) to lethargy and depression and (peripherally) to muscle weakness and loss of tone.

Parathormone produces elevation of the extracellular ionised calcium level in three main ways. Firstly, it promotes osteoclastic activity in releasing calcium phosphate salts from the relatively huge calcium store in the bones of the skeleton. Secondly, it promotes urinary loss of phosphate ions by depressing phosphate reabsorption. Thirdly, it activates vitamin D by completing its hydroxylation in the kidney, and this in turn promotes increased absorption of calcium from the gut, thereby replenishing body stores.

ECTOPIC HORMONE PRODUCTION

Because tumour cells tend to assume more primitive characteristics, some acquire the ability to produce hormones that normal differentiation had abolished. Lung tumours are a well recognised example and the hormones produced include ACTH and vasopressin. The effects of these hormones are indistinguishable from excess production at the usual site or exogenous administration. Thus ACTH leads to cushingoid manifestations, especially body protein depletion, hyperglycaemia and hypokalaemia, while vasopressin leads to excessive water retention, with dilution of all the body fluid compartments, and hyponatraemia.

METABOLIC RESPONSE TO TRAUMA

This term is used to describe the widespread and profound changes in body metabolism which follow trauma in a characteristically predictable pattern. The response is produced by injury and major surgery and by any severe physical stress, e.g. severe infection or burns. Major features of the response are retention (or positive balance) of salt and water and depletion (or negative balance) of potassium and body protein (often referred to as negative nitrogen balance). The extent and duration of the disturbance are roughly proportional to the severity of the trauma.

While sympathetic nervous system responses, many hormones and other factors, such as the pro-inflammatory cytokine tumour necrosis factor (TNF), play a part in this response, many features are at least in part effects of sustained high levels of cortisol. This hormone, by its catabolic effects, leads to breakdown of body protein, especially skeletal muscle protein, and the consequent excretion of nitrogen (as urea) and potassium (from cells) in the urine. The mineralocorticoid action of high levels of cortisol leads to retention of salt and water and excretion of potassium. As mentioned earlier, secretion of high levels of cortisol with the requisite time course has been documented following trauma, and absence of such a response prevents both the metabolic changes and normal recovery of the patient.

There are two situations in which the metabolic response to trauma cannot occur adequately: firstly, in the patient who cannot secrete cortisol; and, secondly, in the patient who does not have the body substrates on which the cortisol acts, the latter applying to the severely malnourished patient who, in particular lacks skeletal muscle bulk. Both types of patient show a greatly increased mortality from trauma and major surgery. Malnourished patients have a reduced plasma albumin level and poor muscle strength, as exemplified by the handgrip test. Both these assessments have been shown to be effective predictors of mortality after major surgery.

ANAESTHESIA AND SURGERY IN THE PATIENT WITH ENDOCRINE ABNORMALITY

Having considered the vital role of the endocrine glands in maintaining normal body function, and in particular in responding to the high demands of surgery, it is not surprising that any endocrine disturbance must reduce the efficiency of this response — hypothyroidism and cortisol deficiency are notorious examples. Hence the aim must be to return the patient to as near normal as possible before surgery, by correcting deficiencies and excesses, and to help the patient to respond as normally as possible to stress, by maintaining levels of hormones as near as possible to the levels seen in the normal (optimal) stress response. Complications due to endocrine abnormality are much more difficult to manage once they have become established.

FURTHER READING

Arendt J 1996 Melatonin. British Medical Journal
312: 1242–1243

Bravo E L 1994 Evolving concepts in the pathophysiology,
diagnosis and treatment of phaeochromocytoma.
Endocrine Reviews 15: 356–368

Cooper D S 1991 Treatment of thyrotoxicosis. In: Braverman

L E, Utiger R D (eds) Werner and Ingbar's The thyroid: a
fundamental and clinical text, 6th edn, pp 887–916.
Lippincott, Philadelphia

Tyrell J B 1995 Glucocorticoid therapy. In: Felig P, Baxter J D,
Frohman L A (eds) Endocrinology and metabolism, 3rd
edn, pp 855–882. McGraw-Hill, New York

Responses to infection

44

Immunity

W. T. McBride
S. J. McBride

This chapter gives a brief introduction to the immune system, with more detailed consideration of the effects of anaesthesia and critical illness.

Many factors associated with the body's response to disease or altered status impinge on the immune system. These include infection, neoplasia, trauma, inflammation and pregnancy, together with environmental, psychological and iatrogenic factors. It follows that the immune system of many patients presenting for operation may be deranged and may be further affected by anaesthesia itself. The immunological effects of sepsis and trauma are of particular relevance in the intensive care unit.

Most diseases run their course without overt immunological sequelae but in some patients additional stresses, including surgery, drugs, infection, hypoxia and hypotension, may precipitate clinical manifestation of dysfunction. This may manifest as postoperative immunosuppression or imbalance between the pro- and anti-inflammatory response systems.

NORMAL RESPONSE OF THE BODY TO INFECTION

The natural immune response

The first line of defence against invading pathogens consists of the natural barriers to infection, which include the skin and the linings of the respiratory, gastrointestinal and genitourinary tracts. These have associated secretions that contain bactericidal and cleansing agents. The epithelial surfaces and their secretions function as a continuously renewed barrier to pathogenic penetration.

A second, non-specific, line of defence exists to protect against organisms that have successfully invaded the natural barriers. This includes granulocytes (neutrophils, eosinophils and basophils), natural killer cells (NK cells, a subgroup of lymphocytes) and enzyme systems, such as the complement cascade, which attempt to clear the system of infectious agents. NK cells are cytotoxic to various malignant and virally infected cells. They possess opioid receptors and their function may be modified by large doses of opioids. In contrast, catecholamines increase NK cell numbers and activity.

The adaptive immune response

Unlike the natural immune response, which does not specifically recognise antigen, adaptive immunity is highly specific for antigen, requires previous antigenic exposure and is enhanced after such exposure. This, in fact, constitutes a memory mechanism protecting the body against future encounters with antigen. Adaptive immunity encompasses both the humoral response, which leads to the production of antibodies by B lymphocytes, and the cell mediated immune response which depends on the T lymphocytes. It is highly complex and incompletely understood, but the key to understanding is the differentiation of white cells and their various functions, briefly introduced in Chapter 28.

As described there, precursor lymphocyte cells differentiate into two main lines, *B* and *T lymphocytes*. B cells further differentiate into activated B cells and *plasma cells*. T cells differentiate into four types: *helper/inducer T cells* (T_H or T_4 cells) and *suppressor T cells*, both of which regulate B-cell production of antibodies; *cytotoxic T cells* (also known as effector or killer T cells) and *memory T cells*. In the activation of an immune response, these cells interact in particular with a third line of cells, the antigen presenting cells (APCs) as described below.

Many types of cells involved in these processes

secrete hormone-like substances which act to communicate between them, and to mediate many of their effects; for example, activation of cells, triggering of their differentiation, and activation of specific genes. These are known as *cytokines* (or lymphokines if secreted by lymphocytes). Their nomenclature is somewhat confused, many having names that indicate the effect for which they were first described, e.g. tumour necrosis factor (TNF). The amino acid sequences of the cytokines are currently being elucidated and, once known, give rise to the prefix interleukin; for example, B-cell differentiation is stimulated by interleukin 4 (IL-4), formerly known as B-cell differentiating factor. The cytokines are discussed more fully below.

HUMORAL IMMUNITY

Humoral immunity is a specific response and involves the differentiation of B lymphocytes to plasma cells for the production of immunoglobulin, which is highly specific for each antigen. The beginning of this process is called the *induction phase*. This commences when T_H lymphocytes are activated by being exposed to antigen (see below and Figure 44.1). These activated T_H cells secrete cytokines, which in turn activate B cells, and this leads to clonal proliferation and results in a population of memory B cells and plasma cells with the capacity to recognise and respond to that antigen by antibody production. When memory B cells from this initial clonal expansion subsequently encounter the same antigen, a swift and greatly augmented response occurs. This is called the *effector phase*.

Immunoglobulins

The antibodies produced by plasma cells are large protein molecules, which are to be found in the globulin fraction of circulating plasma proteins. There are five types of these immunoglobulins, with different functions:

IgA — appears mainly in external secretions — tears, intestinal secretions, etc.

IgD — is involved in antigen recognition by B cells

IgE — histamine release from basophils and mast cells

IgG — complement fixation (crosses the placenta by active transport)

IgM — complement fixation.

They all have a common basic structure, consisting of two pairs of light and heavy polypeptide chains. Although similar, the immunoglobulins exhibit great diversity, so an enormous range of antigens can be recognised.

When an immunoglobulin binds to an antigen that it has recognised, there are several possible outcomes:

1. An inactive complex may be formed, which will be phagocytosed.
2. The antibody may act as an *opsonin*, attaching the antigen to a phagocyte and facilitating its phagocytosis, or it may coat parasite or virus cells making them susceptible to killer K cells, which kill them by direct contact;
3. The antibody may activate the complement system.

Complement is an important element in destruction of invading organisms. The complement pathway is a cascade of reactions involving plasma enzymes identified as C1–C9. The *classical* pathway for complement activation begins with the binding of C1 to immunoglobulins which have bound antigen. This results in the insertion of perforin molecules in the membrane of antibody sensitised cells, causing them to become leaky and to lyse. In addition C3 and C5 are activated, beginning a cascade which opsonises bacteria, attracts leucocytes, and by releasing histamine from granulocytes, mast cells and platelets causes local vasodilatation and hyperaemia. The cascade can also be activated by an *alternative* pathway, beginning with a circulating protein which recognises sugar residues in bacterial or viral coats and activates C3.

CELL MEDIATED IMMUNITY

This, likewise, is a specific response and depends on specific antigen presentation to T cells by specialised APCs. As with the clonal expansion of B cells, T cells undergo a similar induction phase, with production of memory T cells enabling a later effector response.

Antigen presentation

Should an antigen defeat the natural immune response, it is recognised by cells which form part of the adaptive immune response (Fig. 44.1).

B and T lymphocytes differ in their ability to recognise antigen. Both recognise it when it binds to membrane receptor proteins on the cell surface. B cells can react with antigen in its natural form, while T calls do not recognise antigen in solution, but only when it is presented at cell surfaces. Here it must be associated with histocompatibility (HLA) antigen of the cell. The difference may be because T cells can only recognise short peptide fragments of the antigenic protein.

Recognition is mainly carried out by the helper/inducer T lymphocyte (T_H cell). Antigen must be presented to the T_H cell on the membranes of APCs. These include macrophages which have phagocytosed the invading organism or foreign protein, and other cells strategically placed throughout the body in skin, mucosal surfaces, lymph nodes and the circulation. To do this, the APC first takes up the exogenous antigen, processes it and presents the relevant antigenic portion of the invading substance (the antigenic epitope) on its cell membrane. When an epitope is presented on the APC membrane within a specialised binding groove on the HLA class II molecule, antigen recognition can take place. (These may also be known as major histocompatibility class II (MHC class II) molecules, because they are coded for by a group of genes known as the major histocompatibility complex). The MHC molecules are membrane bound glycoproteins that are found on the surface of all nucleated cells. The antigen–MHC–T_H interaction leads to activation of the T_H cell. This may be considered as an inducing stimulus which leads to production of cytokines by both the APCs and the T_H cells and to the initiation of the cell mediated response, as well as antibody production through B lymphocytes.

Cytotoxic T cells may be activated by this process. They bind to infected cells and destroy

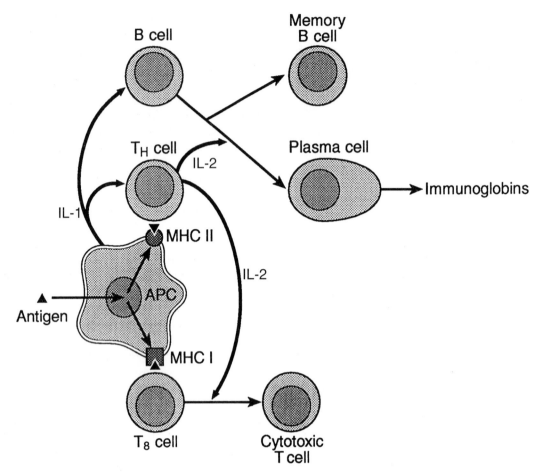

Figure 44.1 The adaptive immune response (see text for description).

them by releasing perforins, which punch holes in the cell membrane, as well as cytokines such as TNF, interferon, etc. This is important in defence against viral infection.

Other cells that are important in immunity include *enhancers* such as *mast cells*. These have receptors for the immunoglobulin IgE, which causes them to degranulate, releasing histamine, leukotrienes and kinins. This is also important in allergic and anaphylactoid reactions.

Influence of anaesthesia and surgery

This entire process may be influenced by anaesthetic and surgical procedures. A decrease in circulating monocyte numbers may impair antigen presentation. This occurs during cardiopul-monary bypass when monocytes adhere to the plastic tubing. A fall in relative T_H numbers may also impair antigen presentation. This occurs following thiopentone and vecuronium administration and is less marked in patients receiving dobutamine infusions. Downregulation of MHC class II expression on monocytes or lymphocytes may also lower immune responsiveness. Down-regulation of human MHC class II (HLA-DR) expression on lymphocytes and monocytes has been shown 10 minutes after high dose fentanyl anaesthesia at cardiac surgery. 2 hours after termination of cardiopulmonary bypass, there was a further downregulation of monocyte HLA-DR, with some recovery after 24 hours. Lymphocyte HLA-DR, in contrast, underwent downregulation 24 hours postoperatively. This indicates profound immunosuppression. This initial down-regulation in HLA-DR occurred before surgery commenced, suggesting a possible opioid effect. In vitro work has shown that IL-10, a product of the type 2 helper T cell (T$_{H2}$), causes selective downregulation of monocyte HLA-DR.

CYTOKINES

The cellular release of cytokines is central to the inflammatory reaction. These substances may be produced by lymphocytes, monocytes, granulo-cytes, eosinophils, endothelial cells and synovial cells. Cytokines are glycosylated and non-glycosylated polypeptides that act as the soluble messengers of the immune system. They are multifunctional and appear to work singly or synergistically with other cytokines to control both immune and non-immune cells such as endothelial cell. Cytokine production is under elaborate neurohumoral control. This is possible because leucocytes have opioid, adrenergic and cholin-ergic receptors.

It is helpful to consider cytokines as proinflam-matory and anti-inflammatory. Proinflammatory cytokines include TNF, IL-1, IL-6, IL-8, IL-12 and the interferons (IFN). Anti-inflammatory cyto-kines include IL-10, IL-1-receptor antagonist (IL-1ra), TNF binding proteins 1 and 2 (TNF-BP1 and TNF-BP2). These are also known as the soluble TNF receptors (TNFsrI and TNFsrII). In health the anti-inflammatory cytokines are found in plasma in appreciable quantities but the pro-inflammatory cytokines are present in very low concentrations or not at all.

The concept of cytokine balance

The proinflammatory cytokines have relatively short half-lives (less than 20 minutes). In order to avoid unwanted systemic effects, spillover into the systemic circulation is minimised by a system of membrane reservoirs. These consist of endo-thelial membrane-bound glycosaminoglycans which hold the cytokines close to the site of release. In addition, the anti-inflammatory cyto-kines form a fail-safe mechanism to prevent systemic upset by stray plasma proinflammatory

cytokines. In health there is a delicate equili-brium, termed the cytokine balance, between plasma pro- and anti-inflammatory cytokines. Although it is difficult to measure local concen-trations of cytokines in most tissues, broncho-alveolar lavage can be used to recover cytokines from the pulmonary tree. Lavage concentrations of TNF and IL-1, unlike plasma concentrations, correlate with the development of adult respira-tory distress syndrome (ARDS).

In health pro- and anti-inflammatory cytokines are in balance but this may be upset by trauma, sepsis and neoplasia. A good outcome correlates with a return to the balanced state, and thera-peutic interventions designed to bring this about are now emerging. The role of cytokine balance was well illustrated in Lyme arthritis, where clin-ical improvement correlated with an elevation in plasma concentrations of IL-1ra in relation to IL-1. In human meningococcal septicaemia, a linear relationship was found between concentra-tions of TNF soluble receptors and TNF concen-trations, up to TNF concentrations of 500 pg ml^{-1}. Where this linear relationship remained there was associated survival. However, in severe dis-ease, where plasma TNF was above 500 pg ml^{-1}, a corresponding increase in the TNF soluble recep-tors was not observed, and this 'imbalance' was associated with reduced survival.

So far, the use of human recombinant anti-inflammatory cytokine therapy in patients with multiple organ failure has been disappointing but a therapeutic role may emerge — for example, as prophylaxis before major surgery when there is a high risk of postoperative multiple organ failure.

The physiological function of cytokines in the inflammatory response

Background immunology

Leucocyte adhesion cascade. Leucocytes and vascular endothelial cells have adhesive molecules on their surfaces. Proinflammatory cytokines are known to upregulate a number of endothelial adhesive molecules. These form complementary ligands with leucocyte adhesive molecules, leading to rolling of the leucocyte along the vascular endothelium, followed by activation (triggering) and more intense adherence, degranulation or migration of the neutrophil. In addition, the cytokine cascade increases the prothrombotic potential of endothelium. The pathogenesis of this cytokine-induced inflammatory response will now be described.

The interaction between the leucocyte adhesive molecule L selectin and endothelial adhesive molecules P and E selectin leads to rolling of the leucocyte along the vascular endothelium. This is followed by more intense adherence mediated by the complementary binding of the integrin series of leucocyte adherence molecules (CD11b/CD18) with further endothelial adhesive molecules of the immunoglobulin superfamily (IgSF) series. It is important to realise that constitutive expression of integrins merely represents 'adherence potential'. It is thought that integrin-mediated adhesion requires prior activation of the leucocyte. This process is thought to be dependent on endothelial expression of bound macrophage inflammatory peptide (MIP-1β), IL-8, granulocyte-monocyte colony stimulating factor (GM-CSF), TNF, IL-1 and platelet activating factor (PAF). It is believed that activation involves phosphorylation of the cytoplasmic portion of the integrin protein. It is only after this has been accomplished that the leucocyte has realised its full adhesive potential. Even then, the cell must overcome the kinetic energy of the blood flow and the antiadherence effect of endothelium-bound highly negatively charged proteoglycans such as heparin sulphate.

Leucocyte activation in inflammation. Following the more intense adherence mediated by the integrin–IgSF interaction, diapedesis and/or degranulation can take place. Activated leucocytes adhering to endothelium release enzymes that degrade connective tissue elements such as endothelial basement membrane and endothelial cell junctions. They also secrete leucoattractant cytokines which recruit additional inflammatory cells into the subendothelial space. The barrier to plasma proteins entering the parenchymal intercellular spaces is thus breached and oedema occurs both by the osmotic action of the now extracellular proteins and the alteration of vasomotor control over the capillary vascular bed. This oedema is further exacerbated by the increased blood flow which follows breakdown of precapillary sphincter tone and relaxation of afferent arterioles. Endogenous neuropeptides and an increase in inducible nitric oxide synthase contribute to this vascular smooth muscle mediated response. This leads to the reduction in vascular resistance so familiar in the systemic inflammatory response syndrome. However, although overall flow through vascular beds is increased, because there is such a large opening up of hitherto redundant microvasculature, there is reduced flow at the level of individual capillaries. This relative stasis of flow in small vessels leads to sludging of red cells, in part caused by the obstructive effects of the large activated leucocytes blocking capillaries. The combination of activated endothelium, with its prothrombotic potential, and microvascular sludging leads to fibrin deposition with platelet activation.

Microvascular thrombotic events occur, firstly, because there is a reduction in the expression of endogenous anticoagulant, fibrinolytic and antiplatelet mechanisms and, secondly, due to an increase in concentrations of surface markers that have prothrombotic activity — for example, endothelial von Willebrand factor. In this situation red cells are damaged and a degree of intravascular haemolysis is common. Degradative enzymes released from activated leucocytes damage the intercellular matrix and parenchymal cells. The cells in this area now face an inadequate oxygen supply owing to impaired red cell flow, greater barriers to diffusion and competition from the highly metabolically demanding leucocytes. The extracellular milieu now becomes increasingly hostile, as there is a combination of reduced drainage of toxic metabolic waste products and large amounts of toxins from the inflammatory exudate cells. Chief among these are proteolytic enzymes and free radicals, which may kill cells outright or cause reversible loss of function. Because of oxygen starvation intracellular protective antioxidant supplies become depleted and cannot be regenerated while the inflammation proceeds. These are the processes which combine to provide the clinical picture of multiple organ failure, systemic inflammatory response syndrome and ARDS.

Predicting outcome in multiple organ failure. An increasing number of inflammatory mediators have been characterised and their role in the pathogenesis of multiple organ failure investigated. Predictive value in terms of clinical outcome has been assigned to some of them. It is now known that the development of ARDS in the intensive care patient may be predicted by elevated bronchoalveolar lavage IL-8, TNF and IL-1 and a fall in plasma concentrations of the soluble form of the adhesion molecule L selectin. This may be because generalised endothelial activation occurring early in ARDS leads to upregulation of endothelial ligands, which, in turn, bind the soluble L-selectin molecule, causing a marked decline in plasma concentrations. Possibly the resulting blockade of endothelial L-selectin ligands by soluble L selectin is a mechanism to avoid excessive neutrophil adhesion.

Pharmacological modulation of target cell (activated leucocyte) activity

Expression of adhesive molecules

Pentoxifylline has been reported to inhibit expression of granulocyte adhesive molecules, CD11a, CD11b, CD11c and CD18.

Rolling and tethering

This is less likely to occur in high flow states. Conversely, low flow states, such as aortic cross-clamping at cardiac surgery, will largely reduce the protective effect of flow. It is possible that intermittent positive pressure ventilation, by virtue of increasing pulmonary vascular resistance, will predispose to neutrophil lung infiltration, irrespective of whether or not a volatile or total intravenous technique is used. In adults anaesthetised and ventilated for 1 hour, there is a marked increase in neutrophil count (bronchoalveolar lavage) compared with a postinduction baseline value. This response is independent of whether anaesthesia is inhalational or intravenous, but is particularly prominent in smokers.

Triggering of adhesive molecules

This process involves protein phosphorylation in response to activation by endothelially expressed IL-1, IL-6, TNF, IFN, IL-8, monocyte inflammatory proteins and GM-CSF. It may be inhibited by increases in cyclic adenosine monophosphate (cAMP) and may be one mechanism by which adrenaline induces neutrophilia.

Adhesion

Adrenaline *in vitro* inhibits human monocyte spreading and adherences, an effect that can be blocked by propranolol and is thought to be cAMP-mediated, as cAMP analogues mimic the effect. In contrast, Met-enkephalin induces a dose dependent increase in macrophage spreading and adherence. This effect can be blocked by concurrent administration of adrenaline suggesting that both agents have conflicting effects on cAMP. The *in vitro* adherence of granulocytes to endothelium is inhibited by pentoxifylline. This has also been observed *in vivo*, where, in experimental administration of TNF to human and animal subjects, the resulting neutropenia caused by TNF-induced adherence is less pronounced if there is previous administration of pentoxifylline.

Adhesiveness of neutrophils to endothelium and other surfaces is enhanced by factors which decrease the negative charge that normally promotes cell separation through electrostatic repulsion. Cationic proteins such as lactoferrin are released by activated neutrophils and promote neutrophil adhesion. In contrast, large anionic molecules such as heparin inhibit neutrophil adhesion. Heparin, when added to in vitro systems, reduces adherence of activated neutrophils. This is particularly noted in TNF dependent adherence. Heparin also inhibits neutrophil carbohydrate ligands binding to P selectin (an adhesive molecule expressed on platelets and endothelial cells). The highest *in vivo* concentrations of heparin occur during cardiac surgery. This may be an important contributor to the lack of adverse clinical sequelae following cardiopulmonary bypass, a period during which there is upregulation of neutrophil adhesive molecules.

NEUTROPHIL FUNCTION

Basic immunology

In view of the important role of neutrophils in the development of multiple organ failure there has been much interest in the effects of anaesthetic agents on various measures of neutrophil function. Neutrophil adherence and degranulation are key steps in initiation of this process, which is the subject of recent reviews. The neutrophil activation process consists of polarisation and locomotion, adherence, phagocytosis and degranulation. Each of these aspects may be studied separately in vitro using specialised techniques.

Modulation by anaesthetic agents

Various in vitro studies have shown differing effects of anaesthetic agents on parameters of neutrophil function.

Neutrophil polarisation. There is some evidence that this is reduced by clinical concentrations of propofol and thiopentone but not by midazolam or Intralipid.

Neutrophil chemotaxis. This is reduced by propofol and Intralipid probably because of their lipid solubility. As far as volatile anaesthetic agents are concerned, lipid solubility correlates with reduced granulocyte migration. In some animal studies neutrophils show a naloxone-sensitive chemotactic response to endogenous opioids.

Neutrophil respiratory burst. This is inhibited by propofol and barbiturates in clinical concentrations. This effect is 10–100-fold greater for thiobarbiturates, such as thiopentone, compared with oxybarbiturates, such as methohexitone. It is thought that difference in activity depends on the presence of the sulphur atom. Neutrophils have opioid receptors and exposure to opioid peptides rapidly induces naloxone-reversible superoxide production in vitro at physiological concentrations.

LYMPHOCYTES

Proliferation

The proliferative response of lymphocytes is fundamental in the mounting of an effective immune response. This process may be studied in culture systems. Lectins such as phytohaemagglutinin, concanavalin A and pokeweed mitogen are often used selectively to induce B- and T-lymphocyte proliferation in vitro. β-Endorphin is a potent inhibitor of phytohaemagglutinin-induced human T-cell proliferation, an effect not blocked by naloxone. It has been suggested that endogenous opioids may contribute to the cell mediated immunosuppression seen after major stress and trauma.

The effects of propofol and Intralipid have been assessed in such a system. The drugs had no effect on cells obtained from normal healthy volunteers, but in surgical intensive care patients propofol caused a reduction in the proliferative response to pokeweed mitogen. This suggests that B-lymphocyte proliferation in critically ill patients may be inhibited by this drug.

Effects of anaesthesia on leucocyte subtypes in vivo

Following induction of anaesthesia with propofol or thiopentone aided by low dose fentanyl, a similar response in peripheral blood lymphocyte subpopulations has been reported. There was an increase in the numbers of total T lymphocytes, memory T lymphocytes and B lymphocytes for both drugs. NK cell numbers fell in both groups but there was one important difference. Propofol anaesthesia increased the number of helper T cells, whereas thiopentone had no effect.

Perioperative immunomodulation

There are several studies documenting a decline in intra- and postoperative IgM, IgG and IgA antibodies. The general picture is that, after regional or general anaesthesia, there is a similar slight decrease during the postinduction period, persisting briefly into the postoperative period. Such a dramatic decrease cannot be attributed to a sudden reduction in production, as IgG half-life is of the order of 3 weeks. The mechanism of this is unclear. The effect may be partly haemodilutional and partly due to the formation of immune antigen–antibody complexes, perhaps secondary to increased amounts of circulating endotoxin and other antigens which may arise as a consequence of hypotension or invasive procedures. The same mechanisms may explain the decrease in complement concentrations observed intra- and postoperatively. Furthermore, experimental in vitro and animal data have shown little effect of anaesthetic agents on T-cell dependent B-cell antibody production when used in therapeutic concentrations; however, prolonged exposure to toxic concentrations will inhibit antibody production.

In conclusion, many drugs used in anaesthesia and intensive care have immunomodulatory properties. The consequences of this will depend on the intrinsic immunosuppressive or pro- or anti-inflammatory properties of these drugs.

FURTHER READING

Adams D H, Shaw S 1994 Leucocyte-endothelial interactions and regulation of leucocyte migration. Lancet 343: 831–836

Allen J D, Herity N A 1996 Prospects for management of peripheral vascular failure in septic shock. British Journal of Anaesthesia 76: 177–178

Dale M M, Foreman J C, Fan T-P D (eds) 1994 Introduction to the immunology and pathology of host defence mechanisms. In: Textbook of immunopharmacology, pp 1–17. Blackwell Scientific, Oxford

Dinarello C A, Gelfand J A, Wolff S M 1993 Anticytokine strategies in the treatment of the systemic inflammatory response syndrome. Journal of the American Medical Association 269(14): 1829–1835

Girardin E, Roux-Lombard P, Grau G E, Suter P, Gallati H 1992 Imbalance between tumor necrosis factor alpha and soluble TNF receptor levels in severe meningococcemia. Immunology 76: 20–23

Miller L C, Lynch E A, Isa S, Logan J W, Dinarello C A, Steere A C 1993 Balance of synovial fluid IL-1 beta and IL-1 receptor antagonist and recovery from Lyme arthritis. Lancet 341: 146–148

Nomoto Y, Jhonokosi H, Karasawa S 1993 Natural killer cell activity and lymphocyte subpopulations during dobutamine infusion in man. British Journal of Anaesthesia 71: 218–221

Norenberg R G, Seth G K, Scott S M, Takaro T 1975 Opportunistic endocarditis following open heart surgery. Annals of Thoracic Surgery 10: 592–596

Shappel S B, Smith C W 1994 Acute inflammatory response. Granulocyte migration and activation. In: Wegner C D (ed) The handbook of immunopharmacology, pp 29–70. London: Academic Press

Shavit Y, Terman G W, Martin F C, Lewis J W, Liebeskind J C, Gale R P 1985 Stress, opioid peptides, the immune system and cancer. Journal of Immunology 135(2): 834s–837s

Strieter R M, Lukacs N W, Standiford T J, Kunkel S L 1993 Cytokines and lung inflammation: mechanisms of neutrophil recruitment to the lung. Thorax 48: 765–769

Zabel P, Wolter D T, Schonharting M M, Schade F U 1989 Oxypentifylline in endotoxaemia. Lancet 334: 1474–1477

45

Sepsis

K. G. Lowry

PATHOPHYSIOLOGY OF FULMINANT SEPSIS

Definitions

One of the greatest problems facing clinicians is sepsis. The recorded incidence has risen dramatically in recent years and current estimates are that between 15 and 20% of hospital inpatients will suffer a septic episode or complication. Unfortunately, but not surprisingly, more severely ill patients are at even greater risk.

The precise definitions of severe sepsis have varied with time and author, making comparison of clinical research difficult and hampering communication between clinicians. Further, it is well recognised that there is a group of patients who have all the pathophysiological changes of 'severe sepsis' but have no detectable infection. These inconsistencies have been addressed in a set of consensus definitions published jointly by the American College of Chest Physicians (ACCP) and the Society of Critical Care Medicine (SCCM). The definitions are set out below. Of particular note is the similarity between the systemic inflammatory response syndrome (SIRS) and severe sepsis, where the only difference is the triggering event. This addresses the clinical reality of the situation where, with the exception of antimicrobial therapy, treatment modalities are the same no matter what the primary cause.

Systemic inflammatory response syndrome

The systemic inflammatory response to a variety

of severe clinical insults. The response is manifested by two or more of the following conditions:

temperature >38°C or < 36°C
heart rate > 90 beats min^{-1}
respiratory rate > 20 breaths min^{-1} or
P_aCO_2 < 32 mmHg (<4.3 kPa)
white blood count >12 or < $4 \times 10^9 \, l^{-1}$.

Sepsis

The systemic response to infection. This systemic response is manifested by two or more of the following conditions as a result of infection:

temperature >38°C or < 36°C
heart rate > 90 beats min^{-1}
respiratory rate > 20 breaths min^{-1} or P_aCO_2
< 32 mmHg (<4.3 kPa)
white blood count > 12 or < $4 \times 10^9 \, l^{-1}$.

Severe sepsis

Sepsis associated with organ dysfunction, hypoperfusion or hypotension. Hypoperfusion and perfusion abnormalities may include, but are not limited to, lactic acidosis, oliguria or an acute alteration in mental status.

Septic shock

Sepsis with hypotension, despite adequate fluid resuscitation, together with the presence of perfusion abnormalities that may include, but are not limited to, lactic acidosis, oliguria or an acute alteration in mental status. Patients who are on inotropic or vasopressor agents may not be hypotensive at the time the perfusion abnormalities are measured.

Multiple organ dysfunction syndrome

The presence of altered organ function in an acutely ill patient such that homeostasis cannot be maintained without intervention.

Prognostic indicators

In fulminant sepsis certain features, at presentation, are predictive of a poor outcome:

- Hypothermia
- Hypotension
- Leucopaenia
- Previous antimicrobial therapy
- Inappropriate antibiotics
- Nosocomial infection
- Diabetes mellitus
- Congestive cardiac failure
- Lactic acidosis
- Decreased fibronectin
- Raised cyclo-oxygenase metabolites.

Some, such as cardiac failure, represent a host with poor physiological reserve, while others, such as lactic acidosis, represent severe disease with profound tissue hypoxia.

Mechanism of systemic inflammatory response

Regardless of the triggering event the mechanism of physiological derangement is the same. The simplest model proposes the activation of macrophages, by endotoxin in Gram-negative infections or by a variety of other insults, such as hypoxia, trauma, multiple transfusion, chemical injury or thermal burn. These macrophages subsequently release cytokines — tumour necrosis factor (TNF), interleukin 1 (IL-1), platelet activating factor (PAF) — that activate neutrophils, which then adhere to endothelial surfaces (Fig. 45.1). Degranulation of the activated neutrophils releases free radicals (e.g. hydrogen peroxide), which damage the endothelium. Circulating cytokines cause a reduction in cardiac contractility and vasodilatation and these, in conjunction with the endothelial damage, lead to organ dysfunction (see below).

Cardiovascular changes

In the cardiovascular system the earliest clinical sign of sepsis is tachycardia. This may be in response to pyrexia but is also thought to occur secondary to a reduction in myocardial contractility mediated by a substance, known previously as the myocardial depressant factor but whose real identity is probably TNF. In the systemic

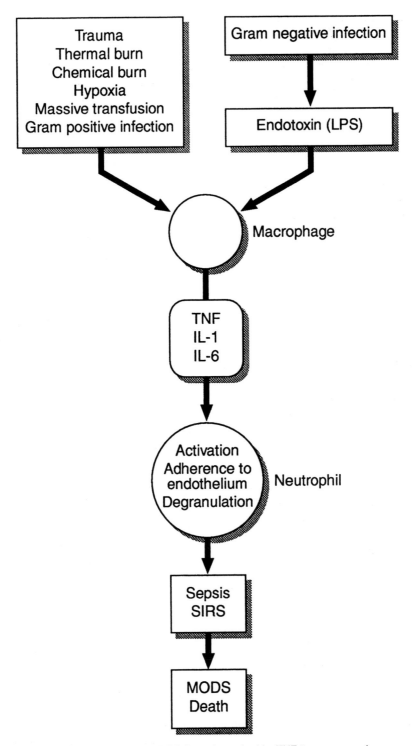

Figure 45.1   The sepsis cascade. LPS, lipopolysaccharide; TNF, tumour necrosis factor; IL-1, interleukin 1; IL-6, interleukin 6; SIRS, systemic inflammatory response syndrome; MODS, multiorgan dysfunction syndrome.

circulation vasodilatation is mediated by a substance released from damaged endothelium. This endothelium derived relaxant factor has a short half-life and only acts locally; it is probably locally synthesised nitric oxide. Despite the reduction in vascular resistance and the reduction in myocardial contractility, arterial blood pressure is initially maintained by an increase in cardiac output. With further reductions in systemic vascular resistance, mild hypotension ensues. As the syndrome develops, cardiac output starts to decrease, mediated in part by further reduction in contractility but also by reduced left ventricular filling secondary to pulmonary hypertension and right heart failure (see below). This, in the presence of an already very low systemic vascular resistance, leads to profound hypotension, hypoperfusion and tissue acidosis. The coronary circulation will also be hypoperfused by this stage, resulting in a marked deterioration of both cardiac output and arterial blood pressure.

Respiratory changes

In the respiratory system the first clinical sign is often tachypnoea, which may result in hypocapnia. Within the lung, changes in the distribution of blood cause an increase in ventilation/perfusion mismatch, with a resultant right to left shunt and hypoxaemia. Under the influence of platelet aggregating factor (PAF), platelet aggregates develop and behave like microemboli, blocking pulmonary capilliaries and increasing pulmonary vascular resistance. This occurs both directly and as a consequence of pulmonary vasoconstriction. Activated neutrophils adhere to pulmonary vascular endothelium and, by degranulating, cause its disruption. The combination of pulmonary hypertension and damaged, leaky endothelium predisposes to leakage of fluid into the pulmonary interstitium, even in the presence of normal pulmonary capillary wedge pressures. This non-cardiogenic pulmonary oedema is defined as adult respiratory distress syndrome (ARDS) and results in worsening hypoxaemia.

As outlined above, induced pulmonary hypertension may impair right ventricular output. This

is of particular importance given the myocardial depression seen in sepsis and the need for adequate filling of the left ventricle to maintain stroke volume and cardiac output.

Renal changes

The renal manifestations of sepsis are oliguria and uraemia. In the early phase of the syndrome the kidneys behave in a similar fashion to that in volume depletion. Glomerular filtration rate and renal blood flow are reduced. Later, endothelial damage occurs within the renal vasculature, and immune complexes (similar to those in glomerulonephritis) are deposited. The end-result is oliguria resulting from both renal and pre-renal causes.

Hepatic and coagulation changes

Coagulopathies are common is sepsis and are usually labelled as disseminated intravascular coagulopathy in type. The formation of microemboli and platelet aggregates and activation of the clotting cascade by damaged endothelium lead to consumption of clotting factors. In some Gram-negative infections, particularly meningococcal septicaemia, bleeding occurs into the tissues and presents as a non-blanching purpuric rash. In the liver, jaundice develops several days after a septic insult. Typically this is manifested by intrahepatic cholestasis with dilatation of biliary canaliculi. Further damage may be mediated through hepatic hypoxaemia as a result of imbalance between oxygen supply and demand. This may be exacerbated by the microstructure of the liver, where centrilobular hepatocytes are at a considerable diffusion distance from the perfusing capillaries.

Central nervous system changes

Often the earliest clinical sign of sepsis is confusion or obtunding of the affect. This occurs more frequently in the elderly and is thought of be related to relative cerebral hypoperfusion secondary to changes in systemic blood pressure and microvascular flow within the cerebral vessels. Intracerebral infection is not necessary for these changes to occur. Later, in severe sepsis, some patients develop a polyneuropathy with absence of deep tendon reflexes and muscle wasting.

THERAPY

The therapeutic interventions in sepsis can be conveniently considered under the following headings:

- prevention
- antimicrobial drugs
- organ support
- anti-inflammatory drugs
- immunotherapy
- others.

Prevention

Given the high overall mortality from severe sepsis, prevention must be of considerable importance. If sepsis occurs, early recognition and prompt treatment are essential. If septic shock develops, mortality increases from approximately 15% to more than 40%. General preventive measures include adequate nutrition, careful hand-washing etiquette, line care protocols and controlled antibiotic prescribing. Attempts to influence the rate and type of bacterial colonisation, and hence infection, by manipulating the microbial flora in the upper gastrointestinal tract by a regimen of selective digestive decontamination have been shown to significantly reduce the rate of nosocomial pneumonia but not to influence mortality.

Antimicrobials

In stressing that SIRS may not necessarily be caused by infection, it is imperative that a patient who fulfils the criteria for sepsis/SIRS is assumed to have an active infective process *until proven otherwise*. Antimicrobial therapy should, as in any other infective scenario, be targeted to the known or most likely organism or site. Inappropriate antibiotic prescribing is one prognostic indicator for a poor outcome in severe sepsis

because it simultaneously allows an infection to continue while selecting out resistant strains or organisms.

It is often the case, however, that a patient presents with sepsis/SIRS with no, or limited, information concerning a possible causal organism or site. In these circumstances antibiotic therapy must be broad spectrum and bactericidal. A good starting point is combined therapy using a β-lactam, an aminoglycoside and metronidazole given parenterally in large doses. This regimen should be adjusted to the most specific drugs when the organism and sensitivities have been established. If no organism can be identified, and there has been no clinical improvement after 48 hours, then antimicrobial therapy must be reviewed.

In patients who are immunocompromised, or who have been on a prolonged course of broad spectrum antibiotics (particularly third generation cephalosporins), the possibility of fungal infection must be borne in mind.

As in all prescribing, consideration must be given to the degree of renal or hepatic impairment in regard to the choice and dose of antibiotic.

Where the site of infection includes devitalised tissue or collections of fluid or pus, aggressive surgical debridement or drainage is necessary. Imaging techniques such as computed tomography or ultrasonography should be employed to search for potential septic foci.

Organ support

The mainstay of organ support is the maintenance of tissue perfusion and oxygen delivery. Oxygen delivery is the product of cardiac output and oxygen content, and in clinical practice it is manipulation of cardiac output that yields the greatest improvement in delivery.

As a consequence of systemic vasodilatation and the loss of circulating volume through leaky capillaries, these patients are both volume depleted and functionally hypovolaemic. Further, impaired myocardial contractility demands higher than normal filling pressures if cardiac output is to be maintained. *Volume replacement is a priority.* In mild hypotension the pressor response to volume replacement and urine output are useful guides to the adequacy of fluid replacement. In more severe cases, central venous pressure monitoring is a minimum requirement, with early consideration given to insertion of a pulmonary artery catheter to measure pulmonary capillary wedge pressure, cardiac output and vascular resistances.

The precise type of fluid, although receiving much attention in the literature, is not as important as ensuring that an adequate volume has been given, at least in adults. If the pressor response to volume loading is inadequate, or the hypotension is severe, then inotropic support should be initiated. The choice of drugs is more fully covered in Chapter 24, but this is less important than achieving an adequate perfusion pressure and cardiac index without severe side-effects such as arrhythmias.

Goal-directed therapy, advocated by Shoemaker and others, which seeks a cardiac index of greater than 4.5, oxygen delivery of more than 600 ml min^{-1} and oxygen consumption of more than 170 ml min^{-1}, is associated with improved survival, but this may be due as much to selecting patients with adequate physiological reserve as to its efficacy as a therapeutic modality in its own right.

Hypoxaemia should be corrected by oxygen administration in the first instance, with ventilatory support if required. In practice all the patients who fulfil the criteria for severe sepsis will require ventilation. The use of positive end-expiratory pressure (PEEP) is almost universal in an attempt to achieve satisfactory oxygenation while avoiding high inspired oxygen tensions. However, the negative effect of PEEP on cardiac output should be remembered, so that any improvement in oxygen saturation is not achieved at the expense of a greater relative reduction in cardiac output and thus oxygen delivery.

Anti-inflammatory drugs

Non-steroidal anti-inflammatory drugs

Given the inflammatory processes which are at the heart of sepsis/SIRS, the use of non-steroidal anti-inflammatory drugs (NSAIDs) has theoretical attractions. TNF and IL-1 produce inflammation by stimulation of arachidonic acid metabolism with the production of leucotrienes, thromboxane A$_2$ and prostaglandins. NSAIDs exert their therapeutic effects by inhibiting arachidonic acid metabolism and, theoretically, should prove beneficial in sepsis/SIRS. There are, however, potentially deleterious effects arising from the inhibition of prostaglandin synthesis, as these substances have beneficial effects on tissue blood flow and tend to reduce pulmonary arterial pressure. Ibuprofen has a more specific effect on thromboxane synthesis than on prostaglandin synthesis and has been more studied than other NSAIDs in sepsis. Human investigations show an improvement in haemodynamic and pulmonary function but not in mortality. Conversely, animal studies have reported increased survival. Not unexpectedly, some animal studies have shown a decrease in renal function after treatment with ibuprofen, presumably due to reduced renal blood flow.

Corticosteroids

These have considerable anti-inflammatory effects and help stabilise neutrophils and maintain endothelial integrity. Whereas many early studies reported an improvement in survival with corticosteroid treatment in sepsis, later, better controlled trials, although sometimes demonstrating an increase in shock reversal, failed to show an improvement in survival. There is also convincing evidence that the use of steroids leads to an increase in secondary infection. Current opinion is that pharmacological doses of corticosteroids are not indicated in sepsis/SIRS.

The only recognised use for steroids is as replacement therapy in adrenal failure and during the fibroproliferative phase of ARDS.

Immunotherapy

Apart from the potential role of endotoxin in initiating the sepsis cascade, it has long been recognised that exposure to endotoxin leads to the production of antibodies to it. These antibodies confer a degree of protection against further exposure to endotoxin originating from the same bacterial strain. Antibodies with reactivity to a broad range of endotoxin types were only able to be produced in the laboratory following the recognition of a mutant strain of *Escherichia coli* (J5), whose endotoxin consisted of only the lipid-A core. In the early 1980s Zeigler demonstrated that treatment with pooled human polyclonal antiserum to J5 could reduce mortality in Gram-negative sepsis. Such treatment, however, was impractical, firstly because of difficulties in obtaining supplies of the antibody and secondly because of the risk of transmission of infective agents which are potentially present with every pooled human blood product. The evolution of recombinant DNA technology solved both these problems and allowed the production of a variety of monoclonal antibodies to J5 endotoxin of either human or murine origin. Clinical trials with these agents produced conflicting results and, although the human antibody HA-1A received a product licence after the first phase III study demonstrated efficacy in Gram-negative sepsis, it was subsequently withdrawn when a second, larger study failed to demonstrate any beneficial effect.

Antibodies directed at endotoxin can only ever be of use in Gram-negative sepsis, whereas antibodies targeted at cytokines in the sepsis cascade could, theoretically, be effective irrespective of the triggering event. Recombinant technology allowed the production of antibodies to TNF of both murine and human origin. Unfortunately, despite promising results from animal trials, these too failed to produce the desired reduction in mortality in phase III trials. Indeed, there is some suspicion that in certain subgroups of treated patients mortality is increased, suggesting that TNF may have a protective role.

The antagonist to the IL-1 receptor was also produced by recombinant technology. This substance occurs naturally and, by preventing IL-1 reaching its receptor, downregulates the pro-inflammatory action of IL-1. Despite promising animal data, clinical trials in humans have been disappointing.

It would seem that the simplistic approach to controlling the sepsis cascade by blocking individual cytokines will not work. Rather, the system needs to be viewed as a dynamic whole, whose internal checks and balances usually generate an effective response to infection or injury. Further understanding of the balancing mechanisms between the proinflammatory and anti-inflammatory arms of the cascade are needed before effective strategies can be postulated.

Other therapy

A number of other therapeutic approaches have been tried in sepsis/SPRS but do not fall conveniently into any of the above groups:

- Inhibitors of neutrophil function
  pentoxyfylline
  adenosine
  aminophylline
  terbutaline
  caffeine
- Inhibitors of adhesion
  interleukin 4
  interleukin 8
  monoclonal antibodies to adhesion molecules
- Inhibitors of degranulation
  dapsone
- Antioxidants
  superoxide dismutase
  catalase
  glutathione
  vasoactive intestinal peptide (VIP)
  allopurinol
  oxypurinol
- Oxygen radical scavengers
  N-acetylcysteine
  mannitol
  ethanol
  vitamin E
  vitamin C
  dimethylurea
- Protease inhibitors
  soyabean tripsin inhibitor
  phenylmethylsulphonyl fluoride.

Of these, perhaps the most promising is pentoxyfylline, which reduces inflammation by blocking activation of neutrophils by endotoxin, TNF or IL-1. Further, it prevents neutrophil adherence to endothelium and may also inhibit neutrophil degranulation. Interestingly, some of the other agents that may inhibit neutrophil function also have vasodilating properties and thus may improve pulmonary function in sepsis. Neutrophil adherence is also reduced by IL-4 and IL-8, and degranulation inhibited by dapsone. The endothelial damage that occurs after adherence and degranulation is mediated by oxygen radicals and proteases. A variety of agents that scavenge oxygen radicals, or reduce concentrations of xanthine oxidase (the enzyme responsible for the production of superoxides) or inhibit proteases are also listed above. None of these has been shown to improve survival in man.

Lastly, physical methods of removing inflammatory compounds from the circulation have been tried. Ultrafiltration removes thromboxane and other leukotrienes from the circulation, as well as reducing the levels of TNF and PAF, and there have been recent reports of clinical improvement in severe sepsis following its use.

RECOMMENDED READING

American College of Chest Physicians / Society of Critical Care Medicine Consensus Conference 1992 Definitions for sepsis and organ failure and guidelines for the use of innovative therapies in sepsis. Critical Care Medicine 20: 864–874

Bone R C 1992 Phospholipids and their inhibitors: a critical evaluation of their role in the treatment of sepsis. Critical Care Medicine 20: 884–890

Bone R C 1992 Inhibitors of complement and neutrophils: a critical evaluation of their role in the treatment of sepsis. Critical Care Medicine 20: 891–898

Edwards J D 1991 Oxygen transport in cardiogenic and septic shock. Critical Care Medicine 19: 658–663

Eidelman L A, Sprung C L 1994 Why have new effective therapies for sepsis not been developed? Critical Care Medicine 22: 1330–1334

Lamy M, Thijs L G (eds) 1992 Mediators of sepsis. Springer, Berlin

Zeigler E J, McCutchan J A, Fierer J et al 1987 Treatment of Gram-negative bacteremia and shock with human antiserum to a mutant Escherichia coli. New England Journal of Medicine 307: 1225–1290

46

Antimicrobial drugs

N. N. Damani

The reported incidence of patients with infection in intensive care units varies widely, depending on the case mix and the type of intensive care, but in some cases is as high as 80%. Therefore anaesthetists working in intensive care require good knowledge of the commonly used antimicrobial drugs, including their spectrum of activity, pharmacokinetics, indications for use, interactions with other drugs and possible side-effects. This chapter gives a brief account of the modes of action of antimicrobials and mechanisms of bacterial resistance, followed by a description of individual drugs or groups of drugs. Drug dosage has been omitted because it depends greatly on the seriousness of the clinical infection and the organ function of the patient. Readers are therefore advised to consult the most recent edition of the *British National Formulary* (BNF) and *ABPI data compendium*. Antibiotics restricted to topical use or to specific indications that are of limited importance to anaesthetics have been excluded, as have antiviral, antiprotozoal and anthelmintic agents.

HISTORICAL BACKGROUND

The first therapeutically useful microbial agents were not antibiotics. It was the dream of the great German chemist Paul Ehrlich (1854–1915) to synthesise 'magic bullets' — organic chemicals capable of killing pathogenic organisms exclusively. In 1909, he discovered the effectiveness of arsenical compounds in the treatment of syphilis; before this, mercury had been used for treatment of syphilis since the sixteenth century, giving rise to the aphorism 'one night with Venus — a life time with Mercury'. Further progress did not occur until the production of sulphonamides in 1935, and then penicillin during the 1940s. The latter entered routine clinical use 10 years after discovery by Fleming and this was due to mass production of penicillin on a factory scale. One means of maintaining supply was extraction of penicillin from the patient's own urine and re-administration! The search for new and better antimicrobials has continued unabated since then, and currently more than 4000 antibiotics have been isolated from microbial sources and reported in the literature, and more than 30 000 semisynthetic substances have been identified, but only some 100 are used clinically, because of toxicity or of unsatisfactory pharmacokinetic properties.

EMERGENCE OF RESISTANCE

Recent reports on antibiotic resistance have caused alarm. The almost complete lack of oral anti-biotics with which to treat certain infections is cause for considerable concern, with conse-quences for increased hospitalisation for the treatment of multiresistant infections.

Emergence of methicillin resistant *Staphylococcus aureus* (MRSA), multiresistant coagulase-negative staphylococci, penicillin resistant pneumococci, vancomycin resistant strains of enterococcus (VRE) and multiresistant strains of Gram-negative organisms like *Pseudomonas aeruginosa*, *Burkholderia (Pseudomonas) cepacia*, *Enterobacter-iaceae* and *Acinetobacter* spp. have caused further concern. The emergence of multidrug resistant (MDR) *Mycobacterium tuberculosis* is of further concern because mortality in patients infected with MDR *M. tuberculosis* is reported as 40–60% in those who are immunocompetent and up to 80% in those who are immunocompromised.

There is more general evidence that mortality, hospitalisation, length of stay and cost of treat-ment is higher in patients who are infected with multiresistant organisms. Strict infection control measures in hospital are important to allow control and prevent cross-infection. These meas-ures are expensive and may be very difficult to achieve due to lack of isolation facilities. Out-breaks also lead to ward closures, with further implications for the delivery of an adequate health care service.

Control of antibiotic usage and avoidance of inappropriate use is therefore strongly advo-cated. Typically this requires the prescriber to be guided by locally agreed policies for antibiotic treatment and prophylaxis based on locally produced surveillance data. There is also a need for audit of antibiotic prescribing, and moni-toring of pathogen prevalence by type, ward or specialist unit on a regular basis so that tailor-made policies are made for individual units. This can only be achieved by close collaboration with the medical microbiologist. Control of antibiotic resistant microorganisms is a major challenge and the implications of failure to meet this chal-lenge means the eventual arrival of the post-antibiotic era, which many microbiologists predict will come about in the foreseeable future.

Most new antimicrobial agents emerge by a process of chemical modification of existing compounds, although a few novel substances continue to be described. Among new agents that are currently marketed, caution must be exercised because of toxic side-effects which will come to light only after extensive use. It is there-fore wise to husband our resources, and employ them in such a way as to preserve them.

MECHANISMS OF ACTION OF ANTIMICROBIAL DRUGS
Antibacterial mechanisms
Inhibition of cell wall synthesis

Unlike animal cells, bacteria possess a rigid outer cell wall surrounding the cell membrane, which protects the organism from its external environ-ment, particularly from osmotic effects. Cell wall damage or inhibition of cell wall synthesis usually leads to rupture and death of the cell. The penicillins and cephalosporins are the prime examples of antimicrobial drugs that act by inhi-biting cell wall synthesis; as mammalian cells do not have any comparable structure, these anti-

Table 46.1 Sites of action of antibacterial agents

Site	Agent	Principal target
Cell wall	Penicillins	Transpeptidase
	Cephalosporins	Transpeptidase
	Bacitracin	Isoprenylphosphate
	Glycopeptides	Acyl-D-alanyl-D-alanine
	Cycloserine	Alanine racemase/synthetase
	Fosfomycin	Pyruvyl transferase
Ribosome	Chloramphenicol	Peptidyl transferase
	Macrolides	Translocation
	Lincosamides	?Peptidyl transferase
	Fusidic acid	Elongation factor G
	Tetracyclines	Ribosomal A site
	Aminoglycosides	Initiation complex/translation
Nucleic acid	Quinolones	DNA gyrase (α subunit)
	Novobiocin	DNA gyrase (β subunit)
	Rifampicin	RNA polymerase
	5-nitroimidazoles	DNA strands
	Nitrofurans	DNA strands
Cell membrane	Polymyxins	Phospholipids
Folate synthesis	Sulphonamides	Pteroate synthetase
	Diaminopyrimidines	Dihydrofolate reductase

Reproduced with permission from Lambert H P, O'Grady F W 1992 Antibiotic and Chemotherapy, 6th edn, Churchill Livingstone, Edinburgh.

biotics are virtually non-toxic to mammalian tissues, except when hypersensitivity develops.

Inhibition of cell membrane function

In common with other living cells, bacteria possess a limiting cytoplasmic or cell membrane situated beneath the bacterial cell wall. This membrane acts as a selective permeability barrier and has active transport functions, thus controlling the internal composition of the cell. Agents such as polymyxin B and colistin (polymyxin E) which interfere with cell membrane function can cause leakage of internal constituents and cell death in many Gram-negative bacteria.

Inhibition of protein synthesis

Many antibiotics, such as the aminoglycosides, teracyclines, chloramphenicol and erythromycin, exert their antibacterial effect by inhibiting bacterial protein synthesis. The synthetic process is complex, the final stage involving ribosomal linkage of amino acids in a genetically determined sequence, and antibiotics can act at various points. Bacterial and mammalian ribosomes differ sufficiently to allow agents to interfere with bacterial protein production without significantly affecting mammalian cells.

Inhibition of nucleic acids

Some antimicrobial drugs, including the sulphonamides, trimethoprim, rifampicin and the quinolones, act by interfering with the synthesis or replication of nucleic acids, which are essential constituents of living cells. The discovery of the antibacterial activity of the first sulphonamides in the 1930s led to the elucidation of their mode of action. Bacterial cells require p-aminobenzoic acid (PABA) for synthesis of folic acid and ultimately deoxyribonucleic acid (DNA). Sulphonamides closely resemble PABA and by competitive inhibition they interfere with one stage of folic acid synthesis, while trimethoprim interrupts a later stage of this process. Combining them in preparations such as co-trimoxazole produces a synergistic antibacterial effect. Mammalian cells are generally unaffected by these drugs as they do not synthesise folic acid but must obtain it from external sources. The mode of action of rifampicin is by inhibition of bacterial ribonucleic acid (RNA) polymerase, while the quinolone drugs inhibit the enzyme DNA gyrase.

Antifungal mechanisms

There are still comparatively few effective antifungal drugs that are sufficiently non-toxic to allow their use in systemic therapy. Their modes of action are generally similar to those of the antibacterial agents. For example, the polyene antifungals nystatin and amphotericin B act on sterol groups in fungal cell membranes, while the imidazoles (miconazole, ketoconazole and itraconazole) interfere with synthesis of membrane sterols. Flucytosine and griseofulvin both inhibit nucleic acid synthesis, while fluconazole inhibits the formation of ergosterol, the principal sterol in the membrane of susceptible fungal cells.

MECHANISM OF RESISTANCE TO ANTIMICROBIAL AGENTS

There are several ways in which an organism may demonstrate resistance. *Intrinsic* resistance to an antimicrobial agent characterises resistance that is an inherent attribute of a particular species. Species vary widely in this respect and,

for example, a 'coliform' infection would not be treated with erythromycin or vancomycin, or a streptococcal infection with aminoglycosides, because these organisms are intrinsically resistant to these drugs.

Acquired resistance reflects a true change in the genetic composition of a bacterium, so that a drug that was once effective in vivo is no longer active. The major strategies that bacteria employ to avoid the actions of antimicrobial agents are outlined in Table 46.2.

Molecular genetics of antibiotic resistance

Bacteria can acquire resistance to antimicrobials either through chromosomal mutation or by plasmid transfer. Plasmids are extrachromosomal elements of bacterial DNA, which, like the chromosome, carry genetic information about antibiotic resistance. Plasmid-mediated resistance is generally of greater clinical importance than chromosomal, as bacteria that have undergone chromosomal mutation are usually metabolically impaired and less well able to multiply than non-mutant members of the population.

Plasmid-mediated resistance is usually based on the synthesis of proteins which either act as enzymes or change the cell wall in such a way

Table 46.2 General mechanisms of resistance to antimicrobial agents

Resistance mechanisms	Specific examples

Diminished intracellular drug concentration
  Increased efflux
 	
  Decreased outer membrane permeability
  Decreased cytoplasmic membrane transport
	Tetracyclines (e.g. tetA)
	Quinolones (e.g. norA)
	β–lactams (e.g. OmpF, OprD)
	Aminoglycosides (decreased energy)

Drug inactivation (reversible or irreversible)	β-lactams (β-lactamases) Aminoglycosides (modifying enzymes) Fosfomycin (glutathione binding) Chloramphenicol (inactivating enzymes)
Target modification	Quinolones (gyrase modifications) Rifampicin (DNA polymerase binding) β-lactams (penicillin binding protein) Macrolides (rRNA methylation)
Target bypass	Glycopeptides (vanA, vanB) Trimethoprim (thymine-deficient strains)

Reproduced with permission from Fraimow H S, Abrutyn E 1995 Pathogens resistant to antimicrobial agents. *Infectious Disease Clinics of North America* 9(3): 497–530.

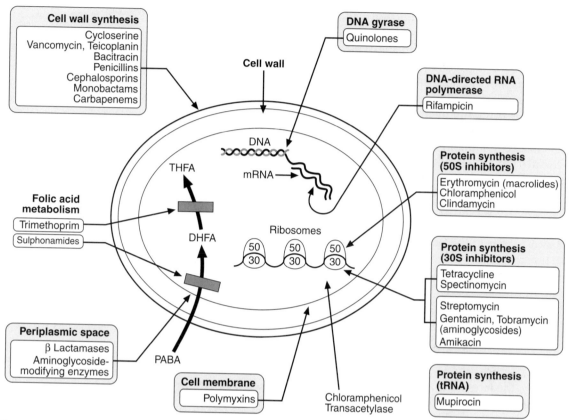

Figure 46.1 Sites of action of various antimicrobial agents. mRNA, messenger RNA; tRNA, transfer RNA; PABA, *p*-aminobenzoic acid; DHFA, dihydrofolic acid; THFA, tetrahydrofolic acid. (Reproduced with permission from Harold C Neu 1992 The crisis in antibiotic resistance, Science 257: 1064–1073.)

that the antibiotic can no longer penetrate. R (resistance) plasmids can be transferred from one bacterial cell to another by conjugation, transduction or transformation.

Another means of resistance transfer is by means of minute mobile elements of DNA (*transposons*), which are often found on plasmids and can move from plasmid to plasmid or to the chromosome. A transposon mediating single or multiple resistance can, after entering a bacterial cell, become incorporated in its plasmid or chromosome. Chromosomal and plasmid mediated resistance involve different mechanisms. It is not uncommon for more than one resistance mechanism to be present in a single bacterial strain.

Other mechanisms of antibiotic resistance

Enzymatic inhibition

Resistance to β-lactam antibiotics is due mainly to the production of β-lactamases, which are enzymes that inactivate these antibiotics by splitting the amide bond of the β-lactam ring. Among Gram-positive cocci, the only β-lactamase of major clinical significance is staphylococcal β-lactamase. Among Gram-negative bacilli the situation is more complex and enzymes are divided into various classes based upon their substrate profiles and their response to certain enzyme inhibitors.

Among aerobic bacteria, aminoglycoside resistance is most commonly due to aminoglycoside modifying enzymes that are capable of three general reactions: *N*-acetylation, *O*-nucleotidylation and *O*-phosphorylation. Resistance to chloramphenicol in Gram-positive and Gram-negative organisms is primarily mediated by an inactivating enzyme known as chloramphenicol acetyltransferase. This is an intracellular enzyme which inactivates the drug by 3-*O*-acetylation.

Membrane impermeability

Gram-negative bacteria have a lipid bilayer that acts as a barrier to the penetration of antibiotics into the cells. The outer portion of this layer consists of lipopolysaccharide, which is absent in Gram-positive bacteria. Lipopolysaccharide impedes entry of hydrophobic antibiotics, e.g. erythromycin, into the cell wall. The passage of hydrophilic antibiotics through the outer membrane protein is facilitated by the presence of porins which allow passage of antibiotics. Generally, the larger the antibiotic molecule, the more negative charge and the greater the degree of hydrophobicity, the less likely it is to penetrate through the outer membrane protein. Mutations resulting in the loss of specific porins can occur in clinical isolates and determine increased resistance to β-lactam antibiotics.

Promotion of antibiotic efflux

The major mechanism of resistance to tetracycline found in enteric Gram-negative organisms results from decreased uptake of tetracycline, due to an energy dependent active outward transport of antibiotic across the cell membrane.

Alteration of ribosomal target sites

Resistance to a wide variety of antimicrobial agents, including tetracycline, macrolides, lincosamides and the aminoglycosides, may result from alteration of ribosomal binding sites. Failure of the antibiotic to bind to its target site(s) on the ribosome disrupts its ability to inhibit protein synthesis and cell growth.

Alteration of target enzyme

β-Lactam antibiotics inhibit bacteria by binding covalently to penicillin binding proteins in the cytoplasmic membrane. These target proteins catalyse the synthesis of the peptidoglycan that forms the cell wall of the bacteria. Alteration of penicillin binding proteins can lead to β-lactam antibiotic resistance.

Overproduction of target enzyme

Sulphonamides compete with PABA to bind the enzyme dihydropteroate synthetase, thereby altering the generation of pteridines and nucleic acid. Sulphonamide resistance may be mediated by production of a dihydropteroate synthase that is resistant to binding by sulphonamides. The most common mechanism of transferable trimethoprim resistance occurs in a similar fashion, by making a drug resistant to dihydrofolate reductase.

PHARMACOKINETICS

Pharmacology must be taken into account when planning antibiotic treatment, particularly the choice of agent, route of administration and dosage. Antibiotics vary greatly in their absorption, blood concentrations, tissue diffusion, distribution in the body, metabolism, accumulation and excretion. Antibiotic pharmacokinetics also vary with the patient's age, disease and organ function.

The absorption rate after oral administration affects the blood concentration–time curve. Some antibiotics are well absorbed when taken by mouth, whereas others require parenteral administration. Tissue diffusion is very important in therapy, although the tissue concentration is difficult to determine. Antibiotic concentrations in well perfused tissue, such as lung and liver, are usually higher than in poorly perfused ones, such as eye or bone, and concentrations in body fluids are important in the treatment of certain infections.

Some antibiotics are metabolised in the liver but most are eliminated predominantly through the kidneys, by glomerular filtration and also, in some cases, by tubular secretion. Renal insufficiency leads to the accumulation of antibiotics whose primary route of elimination is through the kidneys, and this may cause toxic side-effects. Therefore the serum level of more toxic antibiotics must be monitored and the dose should be adjusted accordingly.

β-LACTAMS

The β-lactam family comprises a number of sub-families, i.e. penicillins, cephalosporins, monobactams and carbapenems. Each basic molecule has been widely modified to produce an extensive range of agents with varying antimicrobial and pharmacokinetic properties. The β-lactam agents are widely used and remain among the safest and most effective antibacterial agents available.

Penicillins

Narrow spectrum penicillins

Benzylpenicillin (penicillin G) is partially inactivated by gastric acid and is therefore given parenterally. It remains highly active against most streptococci, most *Neisseria* spp., *Treponema pallidum* and *Actinomyces israelii*. Many anaerobic micro-organisms are sensitive, with the exception of the *Bacteroides fragilis* group and *Clostridium difficile*. Benzylpenicillin is well tolerated

Table 46.3 Bacteriostatic and bactericidal agents

Bacteriostatic	Bactericidal
Erythromycin	Penicillins
Tetracyclines	Cephalosporins
Sulphonamides	Aminoglycosides
Trimethoprim	Vancomycin
Chloramphenicol	Fluoroquinolones
Clindamycin	Metronidazole
Ethambutol	Bacitracin
	Rifampicin
	Isoniazid
	Pyrazinamide

Note: Bactericidal agents are preferable to bacteriostatic agents when the phagocytic cells of the host either fail to penetrate to the site of infection (e.g. endocarditis) or are quantitatively or qualitatively impaired (e.g. in granulocytopenia).

and high doses are used in treatment of infective endocarditis, meningitis and actinomycosis. Following parenteral administration the drug diffuses readily into body tissues and fluids, although cerebrospinal fluid levels are low unless the meninges are inflamed. Excretion via the kidney is very rapid, giving a short serum half-life of about 20 minutes and negligible levels after 6 hours. Probenecid delays tubular excretion and prolongs serum half-life. Benzylpenicillin has few side-effects in normal dosage; however, administration at high dose is associated with nephritis and haemolytic anaemia. Penicillin hypersensitivity (allergy) varies from urticarial rash to fatal anaphylactic shock.

Phenoxymethylpenicillin (penicillin V) is acid stable and can be given orally in mild infections or for prophylaxis. Absorption may be unreliable, so it should not be used in serious infection. Procaine penicillin is a long acting penicillin that is given by intramuscular injection and gives therapeutic blood levels for up to 24 hours.

Antistaphylococcal penicillins

Flucloxacillin and cloxacillin are resistant to β-lactamase produced by staphylococci and their primary use is confined to the treatment of penicillin resistant staphylococcal infection. MRSA is unresponsive to treatment with these agents. Flucloxacillin and cloxacillin are available for both oral and parenteral use. Flucloxacillin is better absorbed from the gut than cloxacillin and has similar efficacy. Both drugs are mainly excreted via the kidney.

Broad spectrum penicillins

This group of penicillins have almost identical antibacterial activity but differ in their pharmacokinetics. They are active against certain Gram-positive and Gram-negative organisms but are inactivated by penicillinases produced by *Staph. aureus* and common Gram-negative bacilli.

Ampicillin can be given by mouth but less than half the dose is absorbed and absorption is further decreased by the presence of food in the gut. Higher plasma concentrations are obtained with the ampicillin esters bacampicillin and pivampicillin; their absorption is little affected by the presence of food. Ampicillin is well excreted in the bile and urine. Maculopapular rashes commonly occur with ampicillin (and amoxycillin), but are not usually related to true penicillin allergy. They almost always occur in patients with glandular fever; broad spectrum penicillin should not therefore be used for 'blind' treatment of a sore throat. Because of poor oral absorption diarrhoea is more common in patients receiving ampicillin.

Amoxycillin is a derivative of ampicillin that differs by only one hydroxyl group and has a similar antibacterial spectrum. It is better absorbed than ampicillin when given by mouth, producing higher plasma and tissue concentrations; unlike ampicillin, absorption is not affected by food in the stomach.

β-Lactamase-stable penicillin

Temocillin differs from other penicillins in its exceptional stability to β-lactamases and also in having a long serum life of 4.5 hours. It is active against Gram-negative organisms, with the exception of *Pseudomonas* and *Bacteroides* spp. It has no therapeutic activity against Gram-positive bacteria.

Antipseudomonal penicillin

Antipseudomonal penicillins, such as carboxypenicillin, carbenicillin and ticarcillin, are less active against Gram-positive cocci but are active against sensitive *Ps. aeruginosa*, which is their principal indication. They also have some activity against Gram-negative bacteria. Ticarcillin has now superseded carbenicillin by virtue of increased activity. The ureidopenicillins, e.g. mezlocillin, azlocillin and piperacillin, have an extremely broad spectrum of action that covers most Gram-negative bacteria including pseudomonas, streptococci, pencillin sensitive *Staph. aureus* and many anaerobes. They are often combined with one of the aminoglycosides for treatment of serious infection. The drugs are not acid stable and must therefore be given parenterally.

They diffuse readily into most tissue and are excreted mainly via kidney. Side-effects include sodium overload, hypokalaemia, dose related platelet dysfunction leading to prolonged bleeding time, and abnormalities of liver function tests. High doses may result in convulsions, especially in patients with impaired renal function.

Penicillin combined with β-lactamase inhibitors

The realisation that the β-lactam ring can be protected from destruction by β-lactamase inhibitors, such as clavulanic acid, sulbactam and tazobactam, has led to development of a number of penicillin + β-lactamase inhibitor combinations (Table 46.4). Although they lack antibacterial activity themselves, these inhibitors improve the spectrum of activity against resistant bacteria which produce β-lactamases. However, when bacterial resistance is due to reduced permeability of the cell wall, these agents are of no benefit.

Cephalosporins

Cephalosporins are the largest single class of antibiotics; they share many common features with the penicillins, including a similar chemical structure and mode of action. Substitutions of the side-chains on the original cephalosporin nucleus have produced a range of drugs with broader bacterial spectra, greater activity and improved pharmacokinetics. New cephalosporins continue to be developed and marketed, many having only minor differences from one another. Compounds developed before 1975 appear with -ph- and those later with -f-. They are usually divided into three generations. First generation cephalosporins are highly active against Gram-positive bacteria such as streptococci and staphylococci but are less active against Gram-negative bacteria because they are inactivated by several β-lactamases. Second generation cephalosporins are active against Gram-positive and Gram-negative bacteria (with the exception of *Ps. aeruginosa*) and are more stable against β-lactamases. Third generation cephalosporins are highly active against Gram-negative bacteria and some have

Table 46.4 A classification of the more complex antibiotic groups

1. β-lactam agents
   a. Penicillin group
      i. Narrow spectrum
         benzylpenicillin
         phenoxymethylpenicillin
         procaine penicillin
      ii. Antistaphylococcal
         flucloxacillin
         cloxacillin
         methicillin
         oxacillin
         dicloxacillin
         nafcillin
      iii. Broad spectrum
         ampicillin
         amoxicillin
         pivampicillin
         bacampicillin

      iv. β-lactamase stable penicillin
         temocillin
      v. Antipseudomonal
         azlocillin
         piperacillin
         carbenicillin
         ticarcillin
      vi. Penicillins combined with β-lactamase inhibitor
         ampicillin + clavulanic acid (Augmentin)
         ampicillin + salbactam (Unasyn)
         piperacillin + tazobactam (Tazocin)
         ticarcillin + clavulanic acid (Timentin)

   b. Cephalosporins

First generation	Second generation	Third generation	Third generation (with antipseudomonal activity)
cephazolin	cefamandole	cefotaxime	ceftazidime
cephalothin	cefuroxime	ceftriaxone	cefpirome
cefadroxil	cefaclor	cefoperazone	cefpiramide
cephalexin	cefotetan	ceftizoxime	cefepime
cephradine	cefoxitin	cefpodoxime	cefoperazone
cephapirin	cefonicid	cefibuten	
	cefmetazole	cefixime	
	cefprozil		

   c. Monobactam
      aztreonam
   d. Carbapenems
      imipenem
      meropenem

2. Aminoglycosides group

gentamicin	kanamycin
netilmicin	neomycin
tobramycin	sissomicin
amikacin	spectinomycin
streptomycin	

3. Quinolones group

Non-fluorinated	Fluorinated	
naladixic acid	ciprofloxacin	fleroxacin
cinoxacin	norfloxacin	temofloxacin
pipemidic acid	ofloxacin	sparfloxacin
piromidic acid	enoxacin	tosufloxacin
acrosoxacin	pefloxacin	clinafloxacin
oxolinic acid	amifloxacin	flumequin
	lomefloxacin	difloxacin

4. Macrolides, lincosamines and streptogramins group

Macrolides	Lincosamines	Streptogramins
erythromycin	lincomycin	pristinamycin
clarithromycin	clindamycin	virginamycin
azithromycin		
roxithromycin		
rosaramicin		
spiramycin		
josamycin		

5. Glycopeptides group
   vancomycin
   teicoplanin

antipseudomonal activity (Table 46.4). None of the cephalosporins has any activity against enterococci, *Listeria monocytogenes* or anaerobes, with the exception of cefoxitin (a cephamycin), which is active against many anaerobic bacteria, including *B. fragilis*.

Some cephalosporins can be given by mouth, while others require parenteral administration. Like the penicillins, most are well distributed throughout the body and achieve useful levels in bile, sputum and cerebrospinal fluid. They are mainly excreted via the kidney and therefore dosage of most cephalosporins must be reduced for patients with renal impairment to avoid drug accumulation. Haematological side-effects, such as thrombocytopenia and hypoprothrombin-aemia, are occasional complications. Cephalo-sporin hypersensitivity may develop in some patients, and up to 10% of penicillin-allergic patients will also react to cephalosporins and therefore use of these agents must be avoided.

Monobactam

Aztreonam is the first monobactam which is highly active against a wide range of aerobic Gram-negative bacteria and is stable to most β-lactamase enzymes produced by these organisms. Anaerobes and Gram-positive bacteria are resistant. The drug is poorly absorbed when taken by mouth and must be administered parenterally. It is widely distributed throughout the body and mainly excreted via kidney, with a serum half-life of about 2 hours.

Carbapenems

Imipenem

Carbapenems, of which imipenem was the first to be commercially available, are modified β-lactam antibiotics which are characterised by great stability to many of the newer extended spectrum β-lactamases and a very broad range of antibacterial activity.

Imipenem is active against most Gram-positive and Gram-negative species (including *Ps. aeruginosa*) and anaerobes. However, a few bacteria are resistant, including *Enterococcus* spp.

and MRSA. Imipenem is rapidly broken down to a toxic metabolite by human renal dihydropepti-dase-1 (DHP-1), so it has to be administered with cilastatin, an efficient inhibitor of DHP-1. Some metabolites of imipenem are neurotoxic, with effects such as tremor, seizure and confusional states. In two-thirds of the cases, seizures were associated with pre-existing central nervous system disorders or were the result of excessively high levels of imipenem metabolites in patients with renal failure.

Meropenem

Meropenem has similar activity to imipenem but the addition of a methyl group at C-1 on the carbapenem molecule gives meropenem greater stability to DHP-1, eliminating the need for cilastatin. Meropenem also appears to lack the seizure activity seen with imipenem. It penetrates well into tissues, including cerebrospinal fluid. Dosage reduction is required in patients with impaired renal function.

AMINOGLYCOSIDES

The aminoglycosides inhibit bacterial protein synthesis by interfering with ribosome function. They are active against some Gram-positive bacteria, particularly staphylococci, and many Gram-negative bacteria, including Pseudo-monas. Some aminoglycosides are also active against *M. tuberculosis*, but they have poor activity against streptococci and no activity against anaerobes.

The aminoglycosides are all poorly absorbed from the gut and therefore must be given parenterally in the treatment of systemic infections. After injection they are rapidly distributed through the body tissues, and excretion is mainly via the kidneys. Excretion may be delayed in the elderly and in patients with renal impairment.

There are now limited indications for clinical use of the earlier aminoglycosides. Streptomycin is almost restricted to the treatment of tuberculosis, while neomycin and framycetin are mainly used topically in skin, eye and ear infections. Of the newer agents, kanamycin is now

Table 46.5 Dialysability of antimicrobial agents

Antimicrobial	Haemodialysis	Peritoneal dialysis
Penicillin	+	−
Cloxacillin	−	−
Ampicillin	+	−
Piperacillin	+	+
Azlocillin	+	+
Cefamandole	+	−
Cefuroxime	+	+
Cefotaxime	+	?
Ceftriaxone	−	−
Ceftazidime	+	+
Imipenem	+	?
Co-Amoxical	+	+
"Timentin"	+	+
Aminoglycosides		
Gentamicin	+	+
Netilmicin	+	+
Amikacin	+	+
Tobramycin	+	+
Erythromycin	−	−
Clarithromycin	?	?
Azithromycin	?	?
Ofloxacin	−	−
Ciprofloxacin	−	−
Chloramphenicol	+	−
Clindamycin	−	−
Co-trimoxazole	+	−
Metronidazole	+	+
Vancomycin	−	?
Teicoplanin	−	?
Amphotericin B	−	−
Flucytosine	+	+
Keto/miconazole	−	−
Fluconazole	+	?

+, Dialysable; −, not dialysable; ?, no data available.

seldom prescribed, but gentamicin, tobramycin, netilmicin and amikacin are all extensively used in the treatment of serious infection, either alone or in conjunction with a β-lactam antibiotic where it shows bacterial synergy. Specific indications include severe Gram-negative infections, infections of unknown aetiology in neutropenic and other immunosuppressed patients, neonatal infections and endocarditis (in combination with penicillin or ampicillin).

The choice of aminoglycoside depends on a number of factors, including sensitivity of the infecting organism (if known), bacterial resistance, potential toxicity and cost. Tobramycin is usually the most active against *Ps. aeruginosa*; netilmicin is claimed to be the least toxic and may be preferred when prolonged treatment is required. Often there is little to choose between these four

agents and gentamicin should be prescribed for cost reasons, being by far the cheapest.

The principal side-effects of the aminoglycosides are ototoxicity, nephrotoxicity and neurotoxicity. Either vestibular or auditory nerve damage can occur, their relative frequency varying with different aminoglycosides. Neomycin, kanamycin and amikacin usually cause deafness, while streptomycin and the other aminoglycosides are more liable to cause vestibular damage. The frequency of ototoxic complications can be greatly reduced, if not entirely eliminated, by regular monitoring of serum levels and dosage adjustment, which must be done on all patients on aminoglycoside therapy but particularly in the elderly, in patients with renal impairment, and with prolonged therapy.

Nephrotoxicity occurs more frequently with gentamicin and tobramycin than with amikacin or netilmicin. The risk of nephrotoxicity increases if aminoglycosides are given concurrently with other potentially nephrotoxic drug(s) or with potent diuretics such as frusemide. Renal damage is usually reversible if treatment is stopped. Neuromuscular blockade with a curare-like effect can occur and may result in respiratory arrest, especially if muscle relaxants are also being used.

QUINOLONES

The currently available quinolones are chemical modifications of the basic nalidixic acid structure. They have antibacterial potencies 1000 times greater than that of nalidixic acid. Quinolones act by inhibiting bacterial DNA gyrase enzymes, which are crucial for DNA replication.

Fluoroquinolones are a new group of quinolones which are now widely used and include ciprofloxacin, ofloxacin, sparfloxacin, norfloxacin, etc. These agents are highly active against most common Gram-negative bacteria and gut pathogens, i.e. *Salmonella, Shigella* and *Campylobacter* spp. Ciprofloxacin is active against *Ps. aeruginosa*, although other pseudomonas such as *Burkholderia (Pseudomonas) cepacia* and *Stenotrophomonas (Xanthomonas) maltophilia* are often resistant. Activity against *Streptococcus pneumoniae* is only modest and it is not recommended for treatment of pneumococcal chest infection. Quinolones have no activity against anaerobic organisms and enterococci. Ciprofloxacin and ofloxacin are also active against chlamydia, mycoplasma and some mycobacteria. Although ciprofloxacin is effective against MRSA, development of high resistance against staphylococci has emerged recently and therefore its use should be restricted for the treatment of patients infected with MRSA and should be used with caution for staphylococcal infections in general.

The fluoroquinolones are well absorbed from the gut and there is wide distribution in the body, with preferential concentration in sites such as the lungs and prostate. Absorption is best in the fasting state and reduced when they are taken with preparations containing magnesium, aluminium, zinc or iron salts.

The major unwanted side-effects are gastrointestinal disturbances, skin rashes, photosensitivity and central nervous system toxicity. The central nervous system side-effects include headaches, dizziness, drowsiness, agitation, psychosis and convulsions. Crystalluria and nephrotoxicity can occur but are rare. They are not licensed for use in children and adolescents because of possible risk of arthropathy. Fluoroquinolones interact with warfarin (prolongation of prothrombin time), sucralfate (reduction of ciprofloxacin and norfloxacin serum levels). Ciprofloxacin and pefloxacin interfere with theophylline metabolism, so therapeutic drug monitoring of theophylline is advised.

MACROLIDES

The original macrolide, erythromycin, was discovered and first used in human infections in the early 1950s. Recently there has been a resurgence of interest in this class of antibiotics and two new macrolides have been introduced in the UK. Clarithromycin is a 6-O-methyl derivative of erythromycin, and azthromycin is the first of a new group of macrolides, called azalides. Macrolides inhibit microbial protein synthesis by binding to bacterial ribosomes. They may be bacteriostatic or bactericidal, depending on the organism and the antibiotic concentration.

Erythromycin

Erythromycin base is unstable at low pH and hence its gastrointestinal absorption is poor. Most erythromycin is inactivated by N-demethylation in the liver and excreted via the bile. Erythromycin is active against Gram-positive cocci, *Neisseria* spp., some Gram-positive rods (such as *Clostridium perfringens* and *Corynebacterium diphtheria*), *Bordetella pertussis*, *Campylobacter* spp., *Helicobacter pylori*, *Mycoplasma pneumoniae*, *Chlamydia* and *Legionella* spp. It has variable activity against *Haemophilus influenzae*.

The instability of erythromycin in the stomach, together with its dose related stimulant effect on gut motility, commonly produces nausea, abdominal pain and vomiting, particularly in adults. Diarrhoea is more likely to occur with high doses. Intravenous erythromycin lactobionate is irritant to veins and thrombophlebitis occurs in many patients. Cholestatic jaundice, associated with eosinophilia, occasionally occurs after 10–14 days of erythromycin administration; it can occur with any erythromycin ester, and is reversible on stopping therapy. Erythromycin can cause sensorineural hearing loss (usually reversible) when high dosages are given or in patients with renal and hepatic failure.

Clarithromycin

Clarithromycin has a similar antimicrobial spectrum to erythromycin but, together with an active 14-hydroxy metabolite, is more than twice as active against *H. influenzae*. It is more acid stable than erythromycin and is much better absorbed if given orally. Its serum half-life is three times that of erythromycin and its active metabolite persists in the blood for even longer — it need only be given twice a day, thus reducing the volume of fluid required for infusion. Other advantages over erythromycin include greater activity against most respiratory pathogens and less frequent gastrointestinal side-effects.

Azithromycin

The peak serum level of the drug is low but its serum half-life is long (60 hours). Levels in neutrophil and macrophage lysosomes are up to 40 times higher and the drug persists for long periods at high concentrations in the tissues. The antibacterial spectrum of azithromycin at the concentrations reached in tissue (but not plasma) includes a wide range of Gram-positive, Gram-negative and anaerobic organisms. It is twice as active against *H. influenzae* as clarithromycin or its metabolite, but is less potent in vitro than erythromycin against Gram-positive organisms. Erythromycin resistant streptococci and staphylococci are also considered resistant to azithromycin and clarithromycin.

LINCOSAMINES

Lincomycin was isolated in 1962 from the organism *Str. lincolnesis*. Its biological properties are similar to those of erythromycin, but it is chemically unrelated. Clindamycin is a semisynthetic derivative of lincomycin, is better absorbed and much more active. Since there are no therapeutic advantages for lincomycin over clindamycin, discussion will concentrate on the latter.

Clindamycin has good antistaphylococcal and antistreptococcal activity and greater activity than erythromycin against *B. fragilis*. However, it is not active against *Enterococcus* spp., *H. influenzae* and *N. meningitidis*. All the Enterobacteriaceae, *Acinetobacter* and *Pseudomonas* spp. are intrinsically resistant to clindamycin. Absorption of clindamycin is about 90% and is slightly delayed, but not decreased, by ingestion of food, whereas that of lincomycin is markedly decreased. The normal half-life of clindamycin is 2–4 hours. Most of the absorbed drug is metabolised, probably by the liver, to products with variable antibacterial activity. Appreciable dose modification should be made where there is concomitant severe renal and hepatic disease in the same patient.

Clindamycin has been successfully used in the treatment of staphylococcal infection, particularly in bone and joint infection, and used as a substitute in patients allergic to penicillin. It is effective for the prophylaxis and treatment of anaerobic infections and indicated where *B. fragilis* is suspected. It is often used in combination with other agents for treatment of intra-abdominal sepsis, infection of the female genitourinary tract and aspiration pneumonia and lung abscess.

Allergic reactions including rashes, fever and eosinophilia have been reported. Diarrhoea occurs in up to 10–30% of patients and is more common with oral administration. Occurrence of pseudomembranous colitis caused by *Cl. difficile* has been reported in 0.01–10% of treated patients.

GLYCOPEPTIDES

Vancomycin

This is widely used to treat serious staphylococcal, streptococcal and enterococcal infections, especially when other agents have failed or are contraindicated. It is used for treatment of infection associated with peritoneal dialysis, cerebrospinal fluid shunts and intravenous lines which is due to highly resistant coagulase-negative staphylococci. It is also used for treatment of infections caused by MRSA and prosthetic valvular endocarditis. Oral vancomycin 125 mg 6-hourly for 7–10 days is used to treat pseudomembranous colitis caused by *Cl. difficile*; metronidazole provides an alternative choice, is much cheaper and avoids development of VRE in the gastrointestinal tract and should be used as first line therapy.

Vancomycin should be infused slowly (i.e. 500 mg over at least 60 minutes or 1 g over at least 100 minutes) to avoid flushing of the upper body (red man syndrome) and hypertension caused by histamine release. Other side-effects include nausea, fever, chills, eosinophilia, anaphylaxis, rashes, renal failure and interstitial nephritis, ototoxicity (discontinue if tinnitus occurs); blood disorders include neutropenia and rarely agranulocytosis and thrombocytopenia. Serum level must be monitored. Combined treatment with vancomycin and aminoglycosides can cause synergistic nephrotoxicity and should be avoided if possible.

Teicoplanin

This is a naturally occurring mixture of several closely related compounds with a spectrum of activity similar to that of vancomycin, although some coagulase-negative staphylococci are less susceptible to teicoplanin. Unlike vancomycin, teicoplanin can be administered by intramuscular injection; it also has a much longer half-life than vancomycin and appears to have a reduced propensity to give rise to adverse reactions. It does not undergo extensive metabolism and is excreted almost entirely by the kidneys.

OTHER GROUPS

Tetracyclines

The tetracyclines are a group of closely related antibiotics very similar in their activity but with a difference in their pharmacokinetics. They are broad spectrum antibiotics and have activity against many Gram-positive and Gram-negative bacteria, as well as mycoplasma, rickettsiae and chlamydiae. Some bacterial species have now developed considerable resistance to these agents. Tetracyclines remain the treatment of choice in various chlamydial, mycoplasmal and rickettsial infections and also in brucellosis. Most of the tetracyclines are only available in oral preparations, but they can be obtained for parenteral use if required. Side-effects include minor gastrointestinal upsets, and these drugs should generally be avoided in renal failure.

Fucidic acid

This is used primarily as an antistaphylococcal agent. Drug resistant strains may emerge on treatment and therefore it is usually combined with other antistaphylococcal agents, i.e. flucloxacillin, erythromycin, etc. It is mainly used in the treatment of serious staphylococcal infection, osteomyelitis, septicaemia, endocarditis, pneumonia, cellulitis and wound infections.

Fucidic acid is well absorbed from the gastrointestinal tract. It may be given as an intravenous infusion whenever oral therapy is inappropriate. Fucidic acid has a unique ability for tissue penetration, has the advantage of providing high concentrations in soft tissue, sputum, bone tissue and sequestra, synovial fluid and intraocularly in the aqueous humour and in the vitreous body. It

is metabolised in the liver and excreted mainly through the bile — little or none being excreted through the urine; therefore, in a patient with hepatic or biliary dysfunction or when given with other drugs which have similar excretion pathways, regular monitoring of liver function is recommended. If fucidic acid is given intravenously it should be given into a large vein with good blood flow or through a central venous catheter to minimise the risk of venospasm and thrombophlebitis.

Sulphonamides

The first of these agents was introduced in 1935, and later modifications of the basic molecule produced a series of drugs with greater antibacterial activity and improved physical and pharmacological properties. Sulphonamides inhibit the enzyme dihydropteroate synthetase, thus interfering with the conversion of PABA as the first stage of folic acid synthesis.

They are 'broad spectrum' in their activity, being effective against a wide range of both Gram-positive and Gram-negative bacteria, as well as chlamydia and some protozoa. However, many groups of organisms that were previously sensitive have now developed sulphonamide resistance, including most strains of gonococci and many meningococci and *Enterobacteriaceae*. Increasing sulphonamide resistance and the availability of more effective and less toxic antibiotics have reduced the indications for sulphonamide therapy.

Minor gastrointestinal side-effects and skin rashes are not uncommon. Crystalluria and renal damage can occur with the less soluble sulphonamides. Stevens–Johnson syndrome (erythema multiforme) and blood dyscrasias such as agranulocytosis are rare but serious complications. Haemolytic anaemia may occur in patients with glucose 6-phosphate dehydrogenase deficiency.

Trimethoprim and trimethoprim–sulphonamide combinations

Trimethoprim was synthesised in 1956 and first marketed in 1969 as co-trimoxazole, a combination of trimethoprim and sulphamethoxazole. Trimethoprim inhibits the enzyme dihydrofolate reductase, preventing the conversion of folic acid to folinic acid and ultimately nucleic acid. It has a broad antibacterial spectrum but it is not active against *Pseudomonas* or *Neisseria* spp., or against most anaerobic bacteria.

Trimethoprim is well absorbed after oral administration and is widely distributed in most body fluids. The serum half-life is 8–12 hours and excretion is mainly via the kidneys, producing high urinary concentrations.

In co-trimoxazole (5 parts sulphamethoxazole to 1 part trimethoprim) the combined effects of trimethoprim and the sulphonamide on different stages of nucleic acid synthesis result in synergistic antibacterial activity, and the drug is bactericidal against a wide range of aerobic Gram-positive and Gram-negative organisms and some anaerobes.

In the past, co-trimoxazole has been used successfully in a wide variety of infections, particularly of the respiratory and urinary tracts. Since 1980 trimethoprim has been increasingly used alone for treating respiratory and urinary tract infections, being apparently equally effective and producing fewer side-affects. However, recently use of co-trimoxazole in the UK has been confined to treatment and prophylaxis of *Pneumocystis carinii* and toxoplasmosis and treatment of infection with *Nocardia* spp.

Minor gastrointestinal upsets and skin rashes can occur, more frequently with co-trimoxazole. Caution is necessary in elderly and potentially folate deficient patients, and folate supplement may be required during long term therapy. Serious blood dyscrasias occasionally follow co-trimoxazole therapy, probably associated with the sulphonamide component. Dosages should be reduced if renal function is impaired, and both trimethoprim and co-trimoxazole are best avoided in severe renal failure, during pregnancy and in neonates.

Chloramphenicol

Chloramphenicol is extremely active against a variety of organisms, including bacteria (Gram-positive and Gram-negative aerobic and anaerobic bacteria including *B. fragilis*), spirochaetes, rickettsia, chlamydia and mycoplasma. The three most common organisms of childhood meningitis, *N. meningitidis, H. influenzae* and *Str. pneumoniae*, are highly susceptible.

Chloramphenicol remains a useful antibiotic, but only as an alternative therapy in seriously ill patients who are allergic to penicillin. It can be used in typhoid fever or in areas where cost and availability make it the primary therapy. The third generation cephalosporins, e.g. cefotaxime and ceftriaxone, have superseded chloramphenicol for the treatment of bacterial meningitis.

Side-effects include dose-related but reversible bone marrow suppression with leucopenia and thrombocytopenia. Irreversible and fatal aplastic anaemia have been reported. A life threatening disorder (the 'grey baby syndrome') can occur, especially in preterm infants, with higher plasma concentration and therefore this antibiotic should be avoided.

Rifampicin

Rifampicin is highly active against many Gram-positive bacteria, some Gram-negative bacteria and other organisms such as mycobacteria and chlamydia. Its action is bactericidal and it readily penetrates leucocytes and kills intracellular organisms. Unfortunately, resistant mutants readily emerge, and rifampicin must therefore be given in conjunction with another antibiotic.

Rifampicin is well absorbed after oral administration, producing a high blood level which falls slowly. It is widely distributed throughout the body and intracellular penetration is particularly good. Excretion is partly biliary and partly in the urine.

Owing to its high activity against *M. tuberculosis*, rifampicin is now one of the first line antituberculous drugs, being used in conjunction with at least one other agent. It has been suggested that it should be reserved for this purpose to minimise the risk of the emergence of rifampicin resistant strains of mycobacteria. However, its use may be justified in other situations where there is no effective alternative therapy, such as severe infections due to antibiotic resistant staphylococci and chemoprophylaxis of invasive *H. influenzae* type b and meningococcal infection.

Rifampicin is generally well tolerated, although gastric disturbances and skin rashes can occur. Hepatotoxicity may develop on prolonged therapy, and especially if treatment is intermittent, an influenza-like syndrome is not uncommon. Rifampicin interferes with oral contraception (Family Planning Association advice for a 'missed' pill should be followed if rifampicin is prescribed to an oral contraceptive user). It also causes red coloration of urine, saliva and tears; soft contact lenses may be permanently stained.

Metronidazole and tinidazole

Metronidazole and tinidazole are closely related imidazole compounds with similar antibacterial and antiprotozoal activity. These agents are highly active against obligate anaerobic bacteria; aerobic bacteria are resistant. They are also effective against various species of protozoa, including *Trichomonas vaginalis*, *Giardia lamblia* and *Entamoeba histolytica*.

Metronidazole is well absorbed after oral or rectal administration; an intravenous preparation is available for use in seriously ill patients. The plasma half-life is about 8 hours. It diffuses well into most tissues and body fluids, including the cerebrospinal fluid. The drug is extensively metabolised in the liver, and unchanged drug and metabolites are mainly excreted via the kidneys.

Metronidazole is indicated in a wide variety of infections caused by anaerobic, or mixed aerobic and anaerobic organisms. These include postoperative surgical and gynaecological wound infections, intra-abdominal sepsis, cerebral and lung abscesses, and pseudomembranous colitis. It is also used prophylactically in abdominal and gynaecological surgery and in treatment of susceptible protozoal infections such as trichomonal vaginitis, amoebiasis and giardiasis.

Nausea, furred tongue and a metallic taste are fairly common side-effects. Peripheral neuropathy has occasionally been reported after prolonged treatment. Metronidazole may potentiate

the effect of some oral anticoagulant drugs, and alcohol should be avoided as disulfiram-like reactions may occur.

Nitrofurantoin

This is a synthetic nitrofuran compound that is active against most of the common urinary tract pathogens, except *Pseudomonas* and *Proteus* spp. It is well absorbed when given by mouth, and high levels are quickly obtained in the urine, but tissue concentrations remain low, and for this reason use is restricted for treatment and prophylaxis of urinary tract infection.

ANTIFUNGAL DRUGS

Relatively few effective antifungal agents are available for use in the treatment of systemic fungal infections. The more important of these are briefly considered in this section; drugs that are restricted to topical use in superficial fungal infections have been omitted.

Amphotericin B

Amphotericin B is a polyene antifungal antibiotic that is effective against a wide range of yeasts and other fungi, acting by interference with cell membrane function. The drug is insoluble in water and is not significantly absorbed when given by mouth. It can be given intravenously after conjugation with sodium deoxycholate. Tissue concentrations are low and very little of the drug enters the cerebrospinal fluid. Elimination from the circulation is slow, with a serum half-life of about 24 hours. Urinary excretion is minimal.

Amphotericin is the most useful drug for the treatment of systemic fungal infections. It is indicated in generalised candidiasis, cryptococcal meningitis, aspergillosis, and other deep seated mycoses. It is administered by slow intravenous infusion, dosage increasing from an initial $0.25 \text{ mg kg}^{-1} \text{ day}^{-1}$ to a maximum of $1.0–1.5 \text{ mg kg}^{-1} \text{ day}^{-1}$. Once full dosage is established, treatment on alternate days may be sufficient. Monitoring of serum concentration of amphotericin B is not indicated; however, the patient's renal function should be monitored frequently and the treatment interrupted or the dosage temporarily modified if renal function deteriorates. Plasma potassium concentration and haemoglobin should also be monitored. Amphotericin can also be given orally to treat gastrointestinal candidiasis, and topical preparations are available for local treatment of superficial infections.

Parenteral therapy with amphotericin is frequently accompanied by toxic effects, including local irritation and phlebitis, pyrexia, and nausea and vomiting. Anaemia, hypokalaemia and impairment of renal function also commonly occur, the last usually being reversible when dosage is reduced.

Three other amphotericin B formulations are available in the UK: amphotericin B colloidal dispersion (Amphocil), liposomal amphotericin B (AmBisome) and amphotericin B lipid complex (Abelcet). They are less nephrotoxic than amphotericin B deoxycholate, but sufficient comparative trials have not been done to determine whether any of these has superior efficacy to amphotericin B. The most logical current indication is that these can be used in patients with renal failure to limit toxicity, rather than where there is a failure to respond to conventional doses of amphotericin B. All new amphotericin B formulations are very expensive.

Flucytosine

This is a synthetic pyrimidine derivative that is active against certain yeast-like fungi, such as *Candida albicans* and *Cryptococcus neoformans*. It acts by interfering with nucleic acid synthesis. However, resistance in yeasts is not uncommon and can develop during treatment. Other fungi are resistant. The drug is well absorbed after oral administration, has a half-life of about 4 hours, and is largely excreted in the urine. It diffuses well throughout the body and into the cerebrospinal fluid.

In combination with amphotericin B, flucytosine is indicated in systemic fungal infections such as generalised candidiasis or cryptococcal meningitis, but sensitivity testing of the yeast is always advisable. To avoid resistance developing during therapy, flucytosine is seldom used on

its own in serious infections, but is prescribed in conjunction with another antifungal agent, usually amphotericin B. Its use as a single drug is restricted to candidiasis of the lower urinary tract and some forms of chromomycosis.

Toxic effects of flucytosine include nausea, vomiting, neutropenia and thrombocytopenia. Serum concentrations of flucytosine should be measured in all patients; this is essential when there is renal impairment, or when the drug is given in combination with amphotericin B, to ensure adequate therapeutic concentrations and to avoid excessive concentrations that can cause toxic effects.

Imidazole drugs

Imidazole compounds include miconazole, ketoconazole and itraconazole. These compounds have broad spectrum antifungal activity and are effective against the dermatophytes, yeasts and some other fungi. They can be used in the treatment of systemic fungal infection; miconazole and other imidazole derivatives are also available as topical applications. Miconazole is poorly absorbed after oral administration but can be given parenterally by intravenous infusion. It diffuses well into most body tissues but not into the cerebrospinal fluid. It is rapidly metabolised in the liver and there is little urinary excretion. Ketoconazole is well absorbed when given by mouth, although antacids and cimetidine inhibit absorption. Absorption of itraconazole from the gastrointestinal tract is incomplete, but is improved if the drug is given with food. Toxicity is generally low but changes in liver function are not uncommon with ketoconazole, and fatal hepatotoxicity has been reported.

These drugs have been successfully used in some fungal mycoses but their proper therapeutic role needs to be defined; in serious fungal infection amphotericin remains the drug of first choice.

Fluconazole

This is a triazole antifungal agent with some chemical similarity to imidazole. It is particularly active against *Candida* spp. The drug is well absorbed after oral administration, diffuses widely

Table 46.6 Recommendations for the chemoprophylaxis of endocarditis

1. *Dental extractions, scaling or periodontal surgery under local or no anaesthesia*
   a. For patients not allergic to penicillin and not given penicillin more than once in previous month:
   Amoxycillin
   Adults: 3 g single oral dose taken under supervision 1 hour before dental procedure
   Children 5–10 years: half adult dose
   Children under 5 years: quarter adult dose
   b. For patients allergic to penicillin:
   Clindamycin
   Adults: 600 mg single oral dose taken under supervision 1 hour before dental procedure
   Children 5–10 years: half adult dose
   Children under 5 years: quarter adult dose
   Under general anaesthesia
   c. For patients not allergic to penicillin and not given penicillin more than once in the previous month:
   Amoxycillin intravenously or intramuscularly
   Adults: 1 g intravenously or 1 g in 2.5 ml 1% lignocaine hydrochloride intramuscularly at the time of induction plus 500 mg by mouth 6 hours later
   Children 5–10 years: half adult dose
   Children under 5 years: quarter adult dose
   or
   Amoxycillin orally
   Adults: 3 g oral dose 4 hours before anaesthesia followed by a further 3 g by mouth as soon as possible after the operation
   Children 5–10 years: half adult dose.
   Children under 5 years: quarter adult dose
   or
   Amoxycillin and probenecid orally
   Adults: amoxycillin 3 g together with probenicid 1 g orally 4 hours before operation.
   Special risk patients who should be referred to hospital:
   i. Patients with prosthetic valves who are to have a general anaesthetic
   ii. Patients who are to have a general anaesthetic and who are allergic to penicillin or who have had penicillin more than once in the previous month
   iii. Patients who have had a previous attack of endocarditis
   Recommendations for these patients are:
   d. For patients not allergic to penicillin and who have not had penicillin more than once in the previous month:
   Adults: 1 g amoxycillin intravenously or 1 g amoxycillin in 2.5 ml 1% lignocaine hydrochloride intramuscularly plus 120 mg gentamicin intravenously or intramuscularly at the time of induction; then 500 mg amoxycillin orally 6 hours later
   Children 5–10 years: amoxycillin half adult dose; gentamicin 2 mg/kg body weight.
   Children under 5 years: amoxycillin quarter adult dose; gentamicin 2 mg/kg body weight
   e. For patients allergic to penicillin or who have had a penicillin more than once in the previous month:
   i. Adults: vancomycin 1 g by slow intravenous infusion over at least 100 minutes followed by gentamicin 120 mg intravenously at the time of induction or 15 minutes before the surgical procedure
   Children under 10 years: vancomycin 20 mg/kg by intravenous infusion followed by gentamicin 2 mg/kg intravenously
   or
   ii. Adults: teicoplanin 400 mg intravenously plus gentamicin 120 mg intravenously at the time of induction or 15 minutes before the surgical procedure
   Children under 14 years: teicoplanin 6 mg/kg intravenously plus gentamicin 2 mg/kg intravenously
   or
   iii. Adults: clindamycin 300 mg by intravenous infusion over at least 10 minutes at the time of induction or 15 minutes before the surgical procedure, followed by 150 mg orally or 150 mg by intravenous infusion over at least 10 minutes 6 hours later
   Children 5–10 years: half adult dose
   Children under 5 years: quarter adult dose

2. *Surgery or instrumentation of upper respiratory tract*
   Recommended cover is for 1(a)–1(e)(iii), but postoperative antibiotics may have to be given intramuscularly or intravenously if swallowing is painful

3. *Genitourinary surgery or instrumentation*
   For patients with sterile urine the suggested cover is directed against faecal streptococci and is as for 1(d), 1(e)(i) or 1(e)(ii) above.* If the urine is infected prophylaxis should also cover the pathogens involved

Table 46.6 (*contd*)

4. *Obstetric and gynaecological procedures*
   Cover is suggested for patients with prosthetic valves or patients who have had a previous attack of endocarditis and is as for 1(d), 1(e)(i) or 1(e)(ii) above because of the risk from faecal streptococci.*

5. *Gastrointestinal procedures*
   Cover is suggested for patients with prosthetic valves or patients who have had a previous attack of endocarditis and is as for 1(d), 1(e)(i) or 1(e)(ii) above because of the risk from faecal streptococci*

Clindamycin regimes are not suitable for this purpose.
Reproduced with permission from the Endocarditis Working Party of the British Society of Antimicrobial Chemotherapy, 1993.

throughout the body and is mainly excreted in the urine. It is effective in treating oropharyngeal and oesophageal candidiasis, particularly in immunocompromised patients and in treating urinary candidiasis. Side-effects include nausea, abdominal discomfort, diarrhoea and flatulence. Rash, angio-oedema, anaphylaxis and Stevens–Johnson syndrome have been reported.

ANTITUBERCULOUS DRUGS

In the UK, treatment of tuberculosis is according to the recommendations published by the Joint Tuberculosis Committee of the British Thoracic Society; variations occur in other countries. Tuberculosis is treated in two phases:

1. *Initial phase.* The concurrent use of at least three drugs during the initial phase is designed to reduce the population of viable bacteria as rapidly as possible and to prevent the emergence of drug resistant bacteria. Treatment of choice for the initial phase is the daily use of isoniazid, rifampicin and pyrazinamide; ethambutol is added if drug resistance is thought likely. Streptomycin is now rarely used in the UK but may be added if the organism is resistant to isoniazid. The initial phase drugs should be continued for 2 months.

2. *Continuation phase.* After the initial phase, treatment is continued for a further 4 months with isoniazid and rifampicin; longer treatment is necessary for non–pulmonary tuberculosis or for resistant organisms.

Rifampicin and streptomycin have already been discussed. Three other important drugs, isoniazid, pyrazinamide and ethambutol, are briefly described here.

Ethambutol

Ethambutol is active against *M. tuberculosis*. Resistance can emerge fairly rapidly if the drug is used alone and therefore it is combined with other antituberculous agents. The most important adverse effect is impairment of vision due to retrobulbar neuritis.

Isoniazid

Isoniazid was first synthesised in 1912, but its antituberculous effectiveness was not recognised until the 1950s. The drug is well absorbed after oral administration, and diffuses widely throughout the body, including the cerebrospinal fluid, and penetrates into macrophages, where it affects intracellular mycobacteria. It is inactivated by acetylation in the liver, and individuals fall into two distinct groups of fast and slow acetylators. Both the free and inactivated forms of the drug are excreted in the urine.

Isoniazid is used for the prophylaxis and treatment of tuberculosis. Prophylactically it may be given on its own to close contacts of the disease. Therapeutically it is prescribed in conjunction with other antituberculous drugs, such as isoniazid, rifampicin and pyrazinamide.

Toxicity is uncommon on normal dosage but occurs more frequently on high dose therapy, especially among slow acetylators. Toxic effects include psychotic symptoms, peripheral or optic neuritis and hepatitis.

Pyrazinamide

Pyrazinamide has moderate bactericidal activity against *Mycobacterium tuberculosis*. It can be given by mouth and diffuses particularly well into the cerebrospinal fluid.

ROLE OF SELECTIVE DECONTAMINATION

Selective decontamination of the digestive tract (SDD) is a measure intended to reinforce failing mucosal defences and to enhance the 'colonisation resistance' of the mucosae of the critical care patient. It was first described in the early 1980s by Stoutenbeek and van Saene, who used it in intensive care trauma patients. Their regimen involved the topical application of a non-absorbable mixture of amphotericin, polymyxin and tobramycin to the oropharynx and stomach, along with a short initial course of cefotaxime to treat any infection present or incubating on intensive care admission. This study, which used historical controls, demonstrated a dramatic reduction in nosocomially infected patients (81 versus 16%) and mortality (85 versus 0%). Since then many SDD trails have been conducted on both unselected and specialist intensive care patient populations. The results have been more encouraging in trauma, high risk surgical and liver transplant patients than in unselected inten-

sive care populations. Patients already infected on admission to intensive care and medical patients benefited least from SDD.

Gram-positive bacterial colonisation and emerging antibiotic resistance are legitimate concerns surrounding the use of SDD. Mucosal overgrowth with coagulase-negative staphylococci, enterococci and *Staph. aureus* has been widely experienced, in some cases involving multiresistant strains. Widespread multiresistant species have emerged in some centres. There is no consensus among SDD trialists as to the importance of these observations.

SDD remains a controversial treatment modality in the intensive care unit. The routine use of SDD in a general intensive care unit and in medical patients cannot be supported by the available evidence. Those most likely to benefit are patients with a good potential for recovery, who are not infected on admission, but are at high risk of nosocomial infection. These include major trauma, solid organ transplantation, upper gastrointestinal surgery and perhaps some neurology patients. Very rigorous prospective microbiological surveillance and traditional infection control will always be necessary.

FURTHER READING

British Society for Antimicrobial Chemotherapy Working Party 1991 Laboratory monitoring of antifungal chemotherapy. Lancet 337: 1577–1580

British Society for Antimicrobial Chemotherapy Working Party 1994 Management of deep candida infection in surgical and intensive care unit patients. Intensive Care Medicine 20: 522–528

Kucers A, Bennett N M 1987 The use of antibiotics, 4th edn. Heinemann, Oxford

Lambert P H, O'Grady F W 1992 Antibiotic and chemotherapy, 6th edn. Churchill Livingstone, London

Mandell G L, Douglas R G, Bennett J E 1993 Principles and practice of infectious diseases: handbook of

antimicrobial therapy. Churchill Livingstone, New York

Ormerod L P 1990 Chemotherapy and management of tuberculosis in the United Kingdom: recommendations of the Joint Tuberculosis Committee of the British Thoracic Society. Thorax 45: 403–408

Reese R E, Betts R F 1993 Handbook of antibiotics, 2nd edn. Little, Brown, Boston

Simmons N A. Recommendation for endocarditis prophylaxis 1993 Journal of Antimicrobial Chemotherapy 31: 437–438

Webb C H 1992 Selective bowel decontamination in intensive care — a critical appraisal. Reviews in Medical Microbiology 3: 202–210

Life cycle

SECTION CONTENTS

47

Conception and pregnancy

Neil McClure
W. Thompson

Chromosomal division

Each cell of the human body contains a copy of all the genetic information of the body, coded in strands of deoxyribonucleic acid (DNA) and contained in 48 chromosomes. During cell division by mitosis the chromosomes are duplicated, and each daughter cell acquires a full diploid number of chromosomes. Sexual reproduction, however, requires the offspring to inherit genes from both parents. Thus the germ cells in their final division undergo a reduction division, meiosis, in which half the chromosomes go to each daughter cell, to give a haploid number of chromosomes. When the sperm and ovum unite in fertilisation, the resulting cell, the zygote, therefore has a full diploid complement of chromosomes, half from the mother and half from the father. (Some mitochondrial nucleic acid is passed down purely from the mother.) The processes that lead to fertilisation of the ovum and development of the fetus are described in this chapter.

OVULATION

The ovulation cycle is divided into the pre-ovulatory ('follicular' or 'proliferative') phase and the postovulatory ('luteal' or 'secretory') phase. The terms 'proliferative' and 'secretory' refer to the endometrial response to the follicular hormones, while the terms 'follicular' and 'luteal' refer to the appearance of the follicle before and after ovulation. During any one menstrual cycle approximately 1000 oocytes begin to develop in response to hormonal stimulation, although only one, usually, achieves full maturation and is released. The control of follicular development is highly complex. Basically, the system consists of a series of feedback loops between the hypothalamus, anterior pituitary gland and ovary. At the beginning of the cycle serum oestrogen levels and therefore negative feedback by oestrogen on the hypothalamus have fallen to a low level. Thus the frequency and amplitude of the pulses of gonadotrophin releasing hormone (GnRH) from the hypothalamus increase and stimulate the production of follicle stimulating hormone (FSH) from the anterior pituitary. This, in turn, induces the granulosa cells surrounding the ovarian germ cells to grow, divide and secrete oestrogen. Oestrogen results in increased FSH receptor expression. FSH and oestrogen then induce luteinising hormone (LH) receptor expression. LH release from the pitu-

itary also increases and the follicle, now able to respond to the LH, undergoes final maturation, with separation of the oocyte and its surrounding granulosa cells and the spontaneous release of the follicular contents, known as ovulation. By this stage the follicle has reached its greatest diameter of approximately 20 mm. After ovulation the graafian follicle becomes the corpus luteum, so called because of its yellowish discoloration, which results from the cholesterol stores laid down for the intense luteal phase steroidogenesis.

Figure 47.1 illustrates the hypothalamic–pituitary–ovarian endocrine cycle.

ENDOMETRIUM AND MENSTRUATION

As the ovarian follicles grow and as oestrogen levels rise, regeneration of the endometrium is stimulated and a protective mucinous layer of

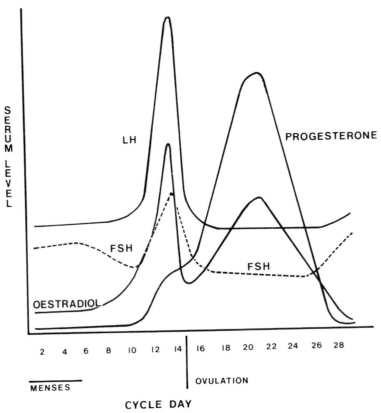

Figure 47.1 The hypothalamic–pituitary–ovarian endocrine cycle.

carbohydrate is produced from the glandular and stromal cells. The stroma increases in volume, the glands lengthen through it and the spiral arteries extend to the surface of the endometrium. In this proliferative phase the endometrium thickens from 0.5 to 5.0 mm. Before ovulation the changes in the endometrium may be thought of as regenerative or reparative. After ovulation the endometrium is stimulated not only by oestrogen but also by progesterone. In this phase its role is to receive and nurture the embryo during implantation. Oestrogen continues to induce growth in the glands and spiral arteries, which become more coiled and tortuous. Under the influence of progesterone, however, the secretions that were contained in vacuoles within the glandular cells are secreted into the glandular lumen and from there into the uterine cavity.

If implantation occurs, the embryonic cells secrete human chorionic gonadotrophin (hCG). This directly stimulates the corpus luteum, replacing the falling levels of LH and FSH. Thus progesterone production is maintained until the placenta produces sufficient levels for the corpus luteum to become redundant, usually between the 5th and 8th weeks of pregnancy.

If implantation has not occurred the whole cycle must recur so that a new oocyte can be released for fertilisation. Thus, the corpus luteum regresses, the hormone concentrations decrease, the endometrium is left without hormonal support and menstruation occurs. The spiral arteries undergo rhythmic vasoconstriction and vasodilatation, which leads to stasis and ischaemia within the endometrium. This is mediated, at least in part, by local changes in the relative balance of the vasoconstrictor and vasodilator prostaglandins. Red cells leak into the endometrial stroma, producing interstitial haemorrhages and ultimately worsening ischaemia. Eventually, the binding membrane of the endometrium is broached and blood leaks into the uterine cavity. Thereafter, a plane of separation develops between the spongiosum and basalis layers of the endometrium and the upper two-thirds are shed. Unless excessive, the menstrual flow normally fails to clot, as the endometrium is rich in plasminogen activators. As menstruation

occurs, follicles are already growing and developing in the ovary as part of the new cycle.

MENARCHE AND MENOPAUSE

These physiological events are the two ends of the female reproductive life. Menarche is part of puberty. Typically it is preceded, in sequence, by thelarche (the development of the breasts in response to increasing levels of oestrogen), adrenarche (the appearance of pubic and axillary hair in response to an increase in adrenal androgen secretion) and a linear growth spurt.

The early increases in serum oestrogen levels are in part responsible for the growth spurt, and they are also responsible for the development of adult female fat distribution and for uterine and vaginal growth. The oestrogen levels required to bring about these events are, however, considerably less than those required to stimulate endometrial growth and menstruation. Initially the menstrual cycles are anovulatory and the periods are relatively pain free; however, as the system matures and ovulation occurs so the cycles become regular, and primary, prostaglandin induced dysmenorrhoea develops.

Menopause, the cessation of menstruation, occurs during the climacteric. This is the period in a woman's life when she experiences the symptoms of, and has the endocrinological markers for, the menopause. After menopause, serum oestrogen levels are low. As a result bones begin to thin and osteoporosis develops. Similarly, in the absence of oestrogen the risk of ischaemic heart disease increases significantly. There is now good evidence that oestrogen replacement therapy helps to protect both against subsequent heart disease and fractures of the long bones or vertebrae. Of more immediate importance to the patient, however, is the decrease in hot flushes, bladder instability, vaginal dryness, loss of libido and moodiness, all symptoms associated with the menopause.

Hormone replacement therapy can be given orally, vaginally, transdermally or by subdermal implant. If the uterus is present, however, progestogens should be given for 12 days at least 3-monthly to protect the endometrium.

Unopposed oestrogen may lead to endometrial hyperplasia with the possibility of atypia and ultimately endometrial carcinoma. Recently the introduction of combined continuous oestrogen hormone replacement therapy (continuous low dose progestogen with continuous oestrogen) has provided hormone replacement without the inconvenience of withdrawal bleeds. Because of the apparent similarity between hormone replacement therapy and the combined oral contraceptive pill, it initially had a long list of contraindications. It is now apparent that, in particular, it is not associated with an increased risk of venous thrombosis.

CONCEPTION

Except for a few other primates, the human is the only species to maintain a regular monthly cycle of ovulation and menstruation; however, the human, as a species, has a low fertility rate of only 20% in any one ovulatory cycle.

Fertilisation occurs in the ampulla of the fallopian tube. The oocyte is probably collected by the cilia on the fimbriae of the fallopian tube, which have 'sticky' sites for oocytes. The fallopian tube also has a small negative internal pressure.

Sperm, however, must be transported from the external cervical os through the cervical mucus, the uterine cavity and the length of the fallopian tubes. To assist this, at ovulation the cervical mucus changes from a thick impenetrable substance to a stretchy, clear, watery substance easily permeable to sperm.

It is believed that human oocytes retain their potential to be fertilised for a maximum of 24 hours after ovulation. By contrast, sperm probably retain their ability to fertilise for at least 48 hours, although they can retain motility for up to 7 days. As the oocyte is released from the follicle it completes its first meiotic division. One set of chromosomes is therefore shed from the nucleus and forms the first polar body. The second meiotic division is completed at the moment the sperm penetrates the oocyte.

Treatment of infertility

In general this subject is beyond the scope of this book, but one aspect is mentioned because of its occasional relevance to the anaesthetist in the intensive therapy unit.

Ovulation may be stimulated by removing the negative feedback of oestrogen on the hypothalamus and pituitary. Clomiphene citrate, or less commonly tamoxifen, blocks the oestrogen receptors so that FSH levels rise. Alternatively, the ovary may be stimulated directly by a pump that injects tiny doses of GnRH either subdermally or intravenously, or by using human menopausal gonadotrophin. Excessive stimulation may, however, lead to the ovarian hyperstimulation syndrome in which gross oedema of the ovaries, pleural effusions and ascites lead to depletion of extracellular fluid volume with increased blood viscosity and a risk of renal failure.

In vitro fertilisation can now exceed the natural conception rate of about 20%, and, as a further technique for use when the numbers of sperm available are particularly low, the sperm may be injected directly into the oocyte cytoplasm.

EMBRYO DEVELOPMENT AND IMPLANTATION

After fertilisation the zygote divides to form, initially, a ball of cells (the morula). As the cells continue to divide they excrete fluid which collects to form a cyst within the morula, which now becomes the blastocyst. The cells that will form the embryo are concentrated at one end of this cyst (the embryonic pole), while the cells that line the sac are known as the trophoblast cells and will ultimately form the placenta. At the blastocyst stage the zona breaks down, probably in response to the uterine fluid, and the embryo hatches, ready for implantation. Transportation of the embryo to the uterus takes approximately 3 days. A further 3 days are spent in the uterus before implantation, which therefore occurs on about day 21 of the cycle.

At implantation the trophoblastic cells over the embryonic pole align with the epithelial cells of the endometrial surface. Their microvilli then interrelate and adhere. The trophoblast cells grow between the uterine epithelial cells and through their basement membrane. The entire embryo then follows and is eventually covered over by uterine epithelium. At the site of implantation there is a marked angiogenic response. The trophoblast divides into two layers: an inner cellular cytotrophoblast and an outer syncytiotrophoblast. Lacunae form in the syncytiotrophoblast and quickly fill with maternal blood as the capillaries are invaded. The syncytium then advances further into the endometrium to form primitive villi with a cytotrophoblast and an inner mesodermal lining. Fetal vessels form within the mesoderm and a placental circulation is established when the heart starts to beat approximately 21 days after fertilisation. The main portion of the placenta develops from the trophoblast over the embryonic pole. The remainder of the syncytium gradually regresses. Eventually the spiral arteries are invaded and their muscular walls destroyed to provide a low pressure circulation for maternal blood.

THE FETUS

Development

Growth of the fetus is traditionally divided into three phases: (1) fertilisation to implantation; (2) the period of organogenesis (implantation to the end of the 8th week (10th menstrual week)); and (3) the period of organ growth (from phase 2 until delivery). This has important implications for the potentially adverse effects of drugs.

Phase 1, blastogenesis, which is covered above, is the most vulnerable period. Drugs or other toxic agents encountered at this time have an 'all or none' effect — they may kill the embryo, but are unlikely to cause congenital malformations. If there is slight injury, the embryo may be able to survive without permanent damage, as the cells still retain their 'totipotency' and are able to replace injured cells by newly formed cells.

In phase 2, embryogenesis, the inner cell mass forms a second sac which grows within it to form the amniotic cavity. The inner cell mass then organises into two layers: the ectoderm, within which is the amniotic cavity, and the endoderm, which lines the blastocyst cavity. The two layers

fairly quickly become separated by a mesodermal layer. The primitive streak then appears as a ridge on the ectodermal plate, bulging into the amniotic cavity. There is considerable mesodermal growth under the streak, which becomes grooved, and a further concentration forms the head process. Over the next few days the embryonic plate lengthens and the coelomic cavities form. By now the embryo is 3 weeks old (5 weeks menstrual age). At this stage the primitive heart begins to pulsate, the neural tube closes and the pronephros appears. By 4 weeks the limb buds have formed and by 5 weeks the embryo is recognisably human. By 8 weeks organogenesis is almost complete. It is the rapid rate of cell division that renders the embryo so susceptible to the teratogenic properties of both drugs and infections at this time.

The teratogenic effects of drugs during this phase are likely to lead to major structural abnormalities. The type of abnormality produced depends both on the exact timing of exposure and on the nature of the drug or toxin. During development specific genes are expressed according to a precise sequence, and toxins may cause abnormal development either by inhibiting expression or by inducing it at an inappropriate time or to an excessive amount. The timing of exposure will obviously be critical in determining the effect, and specific combinations of abnormalities are likely to be associated with damage at particular stages of organogenesis. In addition some drugs and toxins tend to affect specific systems — for example, the drug thalidomide led to skeletal abnormalities but otherwise normal growth and normal intelligence.

During this second phase the bulk of the amniotic fluid is produced from the membranes and placenta. Later, however, it is increasingly made up of fetal urine. Thus it is that if the fetus is distressed the amniotic fluid volume falls as renal blood flow is compromised. Alternatively, if there is a blockage to the fetus's ability to swallow amniotic fluid, such as oesophageal atresia, polyhydramnios develops.

Phase 3, the fetal phase, begins at the end of the 8th week, when all the major systems have formed. The main events still to occur are complete closure of the palate, differentiation of the external genitalia and histogenesis of the nervous system. Ultrasonography at 18–24 weeks can detect some fetal abnormalities, such as neural tube defects, and an open neural tube is also suggested by raised levels of α-fetoprotein at amniocentesis. Drug toxicity at this stage will result in functional rather than major structural abnormalities, or in behavioural abnormalities as a consequence of interference in the final maturation and myelinisation of the nervous system.

Circulation

During phase 3 the placenta acts as fetal lung, kidney and liver. The fetal circulation is therefore adapted to allow the delivery of well oxygenated blood to the brain (Figure 47.2). The maternal blood entering the placenta in the uterine arteries has a saturation of around 98%, but the level in the maternal blood sinuses is lower. There is also an arteriovenous gradient across the

placenta, which is greater than that across the lung because tissues of the placenta are thicker and less permeable than those of the alveoli.

This unfavourable situation is compensated for by the leftward shift of the fetal blood oxygen dissociation curve relative to adult blood. The fetal haemoglobin (haemoglobin F) has a greater affinity for oxygen than does adult haemoglobin (haemoglobin A). This is because in fetal haemoglobin β chains found in adult haemoglobin are replaced by γ chains, which bind 2,3-diphosphoglycerate less efficiently, leading to greater affinity for oxygen. Adult haemoglobin begins to appear in the fetal circulation at around 20 weeks of gestation, and comprises 20% by the time of birth. This rises to 90% by the age of 4 months as fetal haemoglobin is not manufactured after birth.

Fetal blood leaving the placenta in the umbilical vein is about 80% saturated. As blood returns to the fetus through the umbilical vein it crosses the ductus venosus into the inferior vena cava to bypass the liver. It mixes with systemic

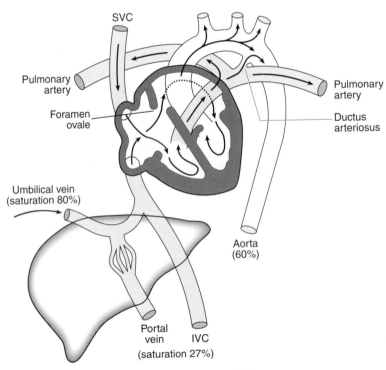

Figure 47.2 Fetal circulation (showing O_2 saturation).

and portal blood, and the resulting mixed blood in the inferior vena cava has a saturation of approximately 67%. At the heart, the angle of entry is such that blood is directed to the foramen ovale in the atrial septum. Oxygenated blood from the inferior vena cava therefore escapes the right ventricle and lungs and moves, instead, straight into the left ventricle and from there to the aortic arch and the cerebral circulation. By contrast, relatively deoxygenated blood from the superior vena cava passes into the right ventricle and the pulmonary artery. There, however, pressures are relatively high, and blood is forced through the ductus arteriosus into the lower pressure of the descending aorta and back to the placenta by the umbilical arteries.

Changes in circulation and respiration at birth

At birth, the neonate has to undergo a major change from the fetal situation, in which gas exchange is carried out by the placenta, to an air-breathing state. The changes are summarised in Figure 47.3.

In the fetus the left and right hearts pump in parallel, whereas they pump in series in the adult. The peripheral resistance is relatively low in the fetus and pressures in the left ventricle are thus less than in the right, allowing blood to pass through the foramen ovale. However, the lungs are collapsed, so that pulmonary resistance is high, and pulmonary artery pressure is higher than aortic pressure, so that blood from the pulmonary artery is diverted through the ductus arteriosus to the aorta.

At birth, the placenta is suddenly removed from the circulation, so peripheral resistance rises and aortic pressure rises to exceed pulmonary artery pressure. The infant responds to the asphyxia that follows the cutting off of oxygena-

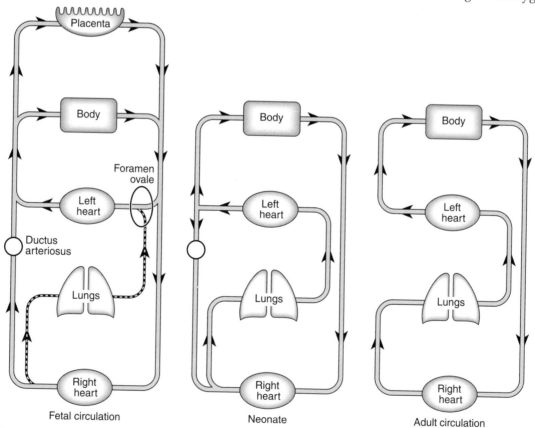

Figure 47.3   Changes in fetal circulation at birth.

tion by the placenta by gasping several times, which leads to expansion of the lungs. Following expansion of the lungs, pulmonary vascular resistance falls to less than one-fifth of the in utero value and pulmonary blood flow increases. The foramen ovale is closed by the increase in left atrial pressure caused by the increased flow of blood returning from the lungs. The ductus arteriosus constricts immediately after birth and normally closes completely over a period of around 24–48 hours. Closure of the ductus is probably mediated by the rise in P_{aO_2} after birth, together with changes in humoral factors. Prostaglandins seem to maintain patency, as in cases of failure to close, or incomplete closure of the ductus, administration of a prostaglandin synthase inhibitor, such as indomethacin, may induce closure.

MATERNAL PHYSIOLOGICAL ADAPTATIONS IN PREGNANCY

The changes imposed on the mother both by the endocrinology of the fetoplacental unit and by the sheer physical presence of the pregnancy within the abdominal cavity are considerable. The fetus is a parasite: all of its energy is derived from the mother and all of its waste is returned to the mother.

Placental endocrinology

Initially the placenta produces hCG in exponentially increasing amounts. After the 6th week of pregnancy the rate of increase slows and values peak by the 13th week. The levels then diminish to a plateau. HCG is necessary to prevent the regression of the corpus luteum and to ensure its continued production of oestrogen and progesterone and the preservation of the endometrium. However, by the 7th week of pregnancy the placental production of these hormones far exceeds that of the corpus luteum.

Other placental products include relaxin, placental thyrotrophin and placental lactogen. Relaxin, together with progesterone, allows the stretching of muscle fibres and the softening of ligaments. This is primarily to decrease the rigidity of the pelvis and thereby increase its diameters for childbirth; however, in effect it leads to pelvic arthropathy and sore backs for many. Placental thyrotrophin and hCG both increase the maternal thyroid function slightly. Placental lactogen is a growth hormone-like substance and thus antagonises the action of insulin.

Systemic physiological changes

Cardiovascular system

During pregnancy, considerable extra demands are made of the cardiovascular system. The uterine blood flow increases from 70 ml min^{-1} to 700 ml min^{-1}. Oxygen consumption at rest increases by 10–15%, much of this being utilised by the fetus. To help satisfy this, the red cell mass increases by 18–25%, but as there is a relatively greater increase in plasma volume, the haemoglobin level tends to fall. Plasma volume increases progressively, from around 2600 ml before pregnancy, to reach a plateau value of approximately 3800 ml by 32–34 weeks. The normal haemoglobin level in a healthy pregnant woman at term is 12.5 g dl^{-1}; values below 11 g dl^{-1} are likely to indicate iron deficiency. The increased red cell mass is due to increased erythropoietin levels. The overall increase in blood volume not only allows for the increase in vascular space and the increased oxygen needs but also helps compensate for the average blood loss of 500 ml at delivery.

Cardiac output increases throughout the first trimester, at the end of which it is 40% higher than before pregnancy, but there is little rise after that. This is accompanied by a rise in heart rate of 10–15 beats per minute, and an increase in stroke volume of 10%. In addition, especially in multiple pregnancies, increased fractional shortening of ventricular diameters contributes to the overall inotropic effect. However, all these changes also mean that the cardiac reserves are diminished in pregnancy. The increase in cardiac output is proportionally greater than the increase in oxygen demand, partly because hormone-induced (oestrogen, progesterone and relaxin) peripheral vasodilatation leads to a fall in peripheral resistance and thus contributes to the development of a hyperdynamic circulation.

Pressure on the inferior vena cava from the uterus and induced peripheral vasodilatation result in a decreased venous return. Thus, in later pregnancy, it has been shown that moving from a left lateral to a supine position leads to an increase in femoral vein pressure from 8 to 24 mmHg as the vena cava is obstructed, with a 22% fall in cardiac output. An alternative return pathway exists via the paravertebral and azygos veins, which may explain why all women do not overtly suffer the *supine hypotensive syndrome*.

While the systolic blood pressure is largely unchanged in pregnancy, the diastolic pressure decreases in the first two trimesters, returning to its initial value by term. It is not until near term that the reduction in the arteriovenous oxygen gradient is lost.

Anatomical changes (see below) mean that the apex of the heart is displaced upward and to the left. This is not functionally significant but the heart appears enlarged on radiographs and the electrocardiographic pattern is altered.

Respiratory system

As pregnancy progresses and the uterus grows, the diaphragm rises, the subcostal angle widens, and the transverse diameter of the chest increases by 2 cm. There is a 20% fall in the residual volume of the lung; however, diaphragmatic movement is not 'splinted' and in fact tidal volume and minute volume both increase by up to 40%, while respiratory rate is unchanged.

These changes are mediated by a 'resetting' of the sensitivity of the respiratory centre, i.e. a reduction in its threshold P_{CO_2}. Functionally, this results in a reduction in Pa_{CO_2} to 4 kPa and this facilitates the transfer of carbon dioxide from the fetus, whose Pa_{CO_2} is 6 kPa. Reduced Pa_{CO_2} is accompanied by a respiratory alkalaemia (pH 7.44), with reduced circulating bicarbonate and, as there is no change in renal handling of bicarbonate, there is less reserve to cope with conditions causing acidosis. The increased sensitivity of the respiratory centre also means that there is an exaggerated response to exercise, which can easily lead to a reduction in Pa_{CO_2} by 2 kPa, with resulting dyspnoea and cerebrovascular vasoconstriction and dizziness.

Gastrointestinal system

Gastrointestinal motility is decreased, as is the tone in the lower oesophageal sphincter. This is again primarily due to progesterone and relaxin and can lead to reflux oesophagitis and constipation. Reduced competence of the lower oesophageal sphincter is especially important in anaesthetic practice because, in combination with an increase in intragastric and fall in intra-oesophageal pressures, it leads to increased risk of regurgitation of stomach contents and potentially to pulmonary aspiration. Although transit times are generally increased, gastric emptying in pregnancy and in labour is essentially normal — but is markedly delayed by opioid drugs given for the pain of labour.

Secretion of gastric enzymes and acid is decreased but saliva production is unaltered. Dental caries are increased and the gums can become oedematous and bleed easily.

Renal function

This is significantly altered in pregnancy. The increased circulating volume results in an increase in renal blood flow with a concomitant increase in glomerular filtration. The filtered load of some substances can therefore exceed the tubular reabsorptive capacity, leading, for example, to glycosuria. The increased filtration of sodium is also balanced by increased reabsorption controlled by the increases in aldosterone (secondary to increases in renin and angiotensin I and II) and in deoxycorticosterone from the placenta. Overall, the plasma osmolality is reduced in pregnancy, although the antidiuretic hormone (vasopressin) levels are normal. The maternal osmoreceptors, therefore, appear to be reset. In total there is a cumulative water retention in pregnancy of 7.5 litres accompanied by 900 mmol sodium.

PARTURITION

The stimulus for parturition remains unidentified. From animal studies it would appear that high levels of progesterone during pregnancy inhibit uterine smooth muscle contractions. Immediately before the onset of labour oestrogen output increases and progesterone output decreases. The change in the ratio rather than the amounts of these hormones probably results in the myometrial production of prostaglandins. These, in turn, sensitise the myometrium to oxytocin from the maternal posterior pituitary gland. In the clinical situation the obstetrician can induce labour by the vaginal administration of prostaglandins, by rupturing the amniotic membranes to release cervical prostaglandins and/or by the administration of intravenous oxytocin.

In established labour, uterine contractions are rhythmical and regular, occurring at least once in 10 minutes, and of increasing frequency and amplitude. From the onset of labour to full dilatation of the cervix is the first stage of labour; the time from full dilatation to expulsion of the fetus is the second stage; the third stage is from the birth of the baby until the delivery of the placenta. The third stage is usually managed actively with an intramuscular injection of an oxytocic, but some units manage the third stage 'naturally' by encouraging the mother to put the baby to the breast to induce release of oxytocin from the pituitary gland. This not only lets down milk but also contracts the uterus.

Preterm labour

In the UK preterm labour is defined as labour before 37 completed weeks of pregnancy and after 24 weeks. Since the mid-1970s major advances in neonatology have resulted in dramatically improved survival rates for these babies, but fetal morbidity and mortality rates remain high for the very immature baby and for those under 750 g at birth. Such babies typically have significant difficulties with breathing, temperature regulation, feeding and combating infection. Respiratory problems associated with immaturity are due to the inability of the immature fetal lungs to secrete surfactant, which typically is not properly produced before 32 weeks. Surfactant reduces surface tension and prevents the alveoli from collapsing at the end of each exhalation and thus improves lung compliance. In utero its production is stimulated by chronic fetal stress or by the exogenous weekly administration of corticosteroids to the mother; however, in combination with β_2 mimetics, given to arrest preterm labour, corticosteroids have been reported to cause pulmonary oedema. The efficacy of the β_2 mimetics is questionable and they rarely prevent labour for more than 48 hours — this may be long enough to allow the steroids to work.

48

Drugs in pregnancy

D. M. McAuley

Increasing public awareness of the potential harm to the developing fetus has greatly influenced drug (including alcohol and nicotine) consumption during pregnancy. However, treatment is sometimes required for medical conditions in the mother and even, to some extent, the baby, while anaesthesia may be indicated for surgical conditions or caesarean section. All new drugs must be carefully evaluated before use in pregnancy and an understanding of the extensive maternal physiological alterations and of the placental transfer of drugs is required to minimise adverse effects in both mother and baby.

DRUG DISPOSITION IN PREGNANCY

Uptake

While nausea, heartburn and fear of fetal drug effects may lead to reduced drug intake, pregnancy per se has little effect on gastric emptying or the absorption of drugs from the gastrointestinal tract. Established labour may cause an unpredictable delay in gastric emptying, which is also markedly slowed by systemic opioids and, to a lesser extent, by epidural opioids. Absorption from the small intestine may therefore be delayed in labour, with the possibility of increased plasma drug concentrations post partum. Increase in minute ventilation (30% by the 7th week and 50% at term) and reduction in functional residual capacity (20% at term) results in more rapid uptake of inhalational agents.

Distribution

Total body water may increase by 6–8 litres during pregnancy. Plasma volume increases by 20% at mid-gestation and by 50% at term, while rises in extravascular water may be around 5 litres with generalised oedema. Thus, the apparent volume of distribution, particularly for polar drugs, is increased. The increase in body fat of 3–4 kg acts as a depot for fat soluble drugs.

Albumin is a major binding protein for drugs, e.g. anticonvulsants, benzodiazepines, fentanyl. The decrease in plasma concentration from 35 to 25 g l^{-1} results in fewer binding sites, leading to an increase in the free drug fraction. This is exacerbated by the increase in late pregnancy of non-esterified fatty acids which compete for albumin binding sites. Basic drugs, including local anaesthetics, most opioids and β-blockers, are bound to α_1-acid glycoprotein (AAG). Plasma concentrations of this protein are more variable, with no consistent trend in pregnancy.

Elimination

Liver

Liver blood flow does not change significantly during pregnancy. Induction of hepatic enzymes by progesterone enhances drug metabolism, whereas oestrogen has the opposite effect; the net effect depends on the oestrogen:progesterone ratio. Smoking and alcohol also cause enzyme induction. This will influence the clearance of drugs such as phenytoin and diazepam.

Serum cholinesterase activity decreases by 24% at term, with a further reduction post partum, causing slower metabolism of suxamethonium, although this is rarely clinically important.

Placenta and fetus

Some drug metabolism may occur in the placenta, which contains multiple forms of the cytochromes P-450. The human fetal liver has the adult complement of enzymes but, at term, activity is only about half that of the adult. Glucuronidation is poorly developed but sulphation activity in the term fetus is similar to that of adults.

Renal

Renal blood flow and glomerular filtration rate increase by about 50% from early pregnancy. Drugs, usually polar and water soluble, that have substantial renal excretion are therefore cleared more rapidly.

Placental transfer of drugs

Anatomy

Maternal blood is carried to the placenta by the uterine arteries, which divide into spiral arteries in the basal plate. Blood is spurted from these into the intervillous spaces. Fetal blood arrives via the two umbilical arteries which ultimately form capillaries in the tips of the fetal villi. Exchange occurs with maternal blood in the intervillous space.

The human placenta is haemomonochorial, i.e. a single layer of trophoblast separates maternal blood from the fetal capillaries. At term it unites with the endothelium overlying fetal capillaries to form the vasculosyncytial membrane. Transcellular aqueous pathways exist within this lipid membrane but the area of these channels relative to total placental surface is very small (approximately 10^{-5}:1). Thus, lipid soluble substances diffuse rapidly, while diffusion of polar molecules and ions is very restricted. Maternal placental blood flow is double that of umbilical blood flow. However, flow within various areas of the placenta is not uniform and considerable shunting occurs.

Mechanisms of exchange

The rate of transfer across the placenta depends not only on the chemical properties and concentration of free drug, but on uteroplacental blood flow, placental surface area, and the diffusion distance across the placental membrane. Factors such as aortocaval compression, uterine tone and maternal disease are therefore important.

Most drugs used for anaesthesia and analgesia are transferred by passive diffusion, which depends on the concentration gradient present. The speed of transfer also depends on molecular size, spatial configuration, degree of ionisation (if an electrolyte) and lipid solubility. Substances of low molecular weight diffuse readily but as size increases the lipid solubility becomes more important. Thus, water soluble molecules up to 100 daltons cross rapidly, but lipid soluble drugs transfer easily at molecular weights up to approximately 1000 daltons. For most drugs, lipid solubility is the major determinant of membrane transfer. Transfer rate for drugs of moderate to high solubility is dependent on blood flow rate on either side of the placenta.

Polar drugs undergo partial ionisation at body pH. Membrane permeability to the unionised form of a weak electrolyte is much greater than to the ionised moiety, transfer of which is very slow. The transfer of drugs which are highly protein bound to plasma proteins is small compared with free drugs. Other mechanisms of placental transfer include facilitated diffusion (glucose, lactate), active transport (amino acids, water soluble vitamins, some ions), pinocytosis (immunoglobulins) and bulk flow (water and some solutes.)

Breaks in the villi may result in fetal material entering the maternal circulation and vice versa. In this way rhesus isoimmunisation may occur.

Fetal factors

While maternal plasma albumin concentrations decrease throughout pregnancy, the opposite is true for the fetus, so that, at term, the fetal albumin concentration exceeds maternal. This increases the maternal to fetal transfer rate and the fetal:maternal (F:M) ratio of drugs such as diazepam may exceed unity at delivery. The fetal plasma concentration of AAG always remains below maternal.

Fetal plasma pH is approximately 0.1 unit below maternal. This results in greater ionisation of basic drugs, e.g. lignocaine, in fetal plasma compared with maternal; the converse is true for acidic drugs. Equilibration across the placental membrane depends on the concentration of non-ionised drug. Hence, for basic compounds, the plasma concentration of free drug tends to be greater in the fetus — so-called 'ion-trapping'. This effect is more marked in the acidotic fetus.

Measurement of placental transfer

Study of placental transfer in humans is limited to drugs given for therapeutic reasons and measurement of their concentrations in the mother and umbilical cord at delivery. The umbilical vein (UV) concentration is a measure of placental transfer rate on first exposure but does not give any indication of the drug content of the infant. The umbilical artery (UA) concentration gives a better indication of the amount of drug present in the fetus after equilibration with fetal tissues. The UA:UV ratio is an index of the extent of fetal tissue equilibration and direction of transfer.

Information is also available from animal studies, including the chronically cannulated ewe. This allows serial sampling of maternal and fetal blood and other fluids. Direct extrapolation of data to the human may, however, be misleading. Considerable research has also been carried out using the isolated perfused human placenta. Effects of differing flow rates and perfusate composition can be studied.

Bolus injection

Fetal exposure is determined by the rate of placental transfer and the time the drug is in the maternal circulation. After an intravenous injection the UV concentration rises because of the M:F gradient. As the drug is cleared from maternal plasma, the maternal concentration decreases and the diffusion gradient is reversed. Hence, the UV concentration depends on the timing of the sample.

A lipophilic drug may approach equilibrium across the placenta in a single circuit, but full equilibration within the fetal compartment takes longer. For relatively lipid soluble compounds the rate of drug elimination from the fetus is dictated mainly by maternal elimination characteristics, i.e. placental clearance is the most important route of elimination from the fetus. With a less lipophilic drug the maternal concentration declines more gradually because of slower distribution. Placental transfer is also slowed and the F:M ratio rises slowly, but fetal exposure may be greater because of more sustained maternal concentrations.

Repeated exposure

When a drug is given continuously or repeatedly a constant maternal concentration is reached and factors other than placental permeability and maternal drug elimination become more important in determining fetal exposure, in particular protein binding and fetal drug elimination. Under steady-state conditions, lower drug concentrations in the fetus do not necessarily imply restricted placental transfer, as the concentration of unbound drug may be the same in mother and fetus.

Fetal elimination

Fetal steady-state plasma concentrations tend to be lower than maternal, possibly due to fetal drug elimination. Fetal hepatic drug metabolising activity is lower than that of the adult and a substantial proportion of umbilical venous blood bypasses the liver through the ductus venosus. Drugs may be metabolised to sulphate and glucuronide complexes in the liver; these conjugates (which have very low placental permeability) are then cleared by renal excretion into the amniotic fluid. Drugs and metabolites may also diffuse into amniotic fluid across chorioallantoic membranes. Peak concentrations in the amniotic fluid may be higher than concurrent values in the maternal and fetal plasma.

Lipid soluble drugs may diffuse back across the chorioallantoic membrane, while less lipid soluble drugs (especially polar metabolites) are swallowed by the fetus, and accumulate in meconium. Metabolites from fetal liver may be excreted in bile and deposited in meconium, which is not normally excreted in utero.

The fetal lung may also play a role in elimination from the circulation into tracheal and then amniotic fluid.

TERATOGENESIS

For a substance to be teratogenic it must be given at appropriate dosage during a particular developmental stage to a susceptible species. Exposure to potential toxins during pregnancy may result in spontaneous abortion, developmental defects (particularly during the critical period of organogenesis, 15–56 days), premature labour, fetal growth retardation, behavioural abnormalities or mutagenesis.

Despite early reports, there is no strong evidence for a greater risk of congenital abnormality in the children of women with occupational exposure to anaesthetic gases. There is possibly a slightly increased risk of miscarriage. An estimated 2% of pregnant women require anaesthesia for surgery. On existing evidence, none of the currently used general or local anaesthetics (except possibly mepivacaine) are human teratogens, though controversy has surrounded the use of nitrous oxide. Nitrous oxide inhibits methionine synthase activity. This enzyme is important in folate metabolism and deoxyribonucleic acid (DNA) synthesis. Long term exposure to nitrous oxide in rats leads to increased abnormalities and fetal loss. However, no changes occur in methionine synthase activity in the human placenta with nitrous oxide exposure times of up to 22 minutes and no significant changes in methionine concentrations occur in humans with exposure to 60–70% nitrous oxide for up to 4 hours. Furthermore, the addition of halothane prevents teratogenicity in rats without altering the change in methionine synthase activity. This suggests that other mechanisms, possibly including decreased uterine blood flow, are involved. Learning difficulties have been noted in rodents exposed to anaesthetic agents in utero, and it has been suggested that psychoactive compounds taken in pregnancy may result in behavioural deficits in human infants. There have, to date, been no well controlled studies to support this allegation.

Surveys of outcome following anaesthesia and surgery during pregnancy show an increase in spontaneous abortion, low birth weight infants (resulting from premature births and intrauterine growth retardation) and increased deaths in the first week of life, but no increase in congenital anomalies, even for surgery in the first trimester. No association between adverse events and type of anaesthesia (including nitrous oxide) has been found. Preterm labour is more likely to follow operations requiring manipulation of the uterus.

Apart from avoiding known toxins, a careful anaesthetic technique avoiding maternal hypoxia, hypotension, hyper- and hypocarbia, prolonged fasting and electrolyte disturbances is important. Lower doses of volatile and local anaesthetic agents are required. Perioperative monitoring of fetal heart rate and uterine contractions, where feasible, is recommended. General anaesthesia and opioids result in loss of beat-to-beat variability but sudden changes in heart rate indicate fetal compromise. Tocolytic therapy may prevent premature labour.

INDIVIDUAL DRUGS

Benzodiazepines

Benzodiazepines have been used for anxiolysis during pregnancy, as premedication, induction agents and anticonvulsants.

Diazepam

This is a lipid soluble basic drug which is virtually unionised at physiological pH. Normally highly bound to albumin, the binding is reduced as gestation proceeds, and the free fraction of the drug is significantly increased in late pregnancy. Diazepam has a number of active metabolites, including the long acting N-desmethyldiazepam. The elimination half-life of diazepam may be double that in non-pregnant women, but clearance is similar. Placental transfer is rapid and, while F:M ratios are less than unity in early pregnancy, increased binding to fetal albumin combined with reduced maternal binding results in fetal accumulation at term and F:M ratios may reach 2. Neonatal elimination is slow and the free fraction increases dramatically after delivery as bound drug is displaced by increasing concentrations of free fatty acids, contributing to neonatal hypotonia, hypothermia and respiratory and neurological depression. Diazepam in early pregnancy has been associated with cleft lip and palate.

Lorazepam

A more polar drug than diazepam, lorazepam is less protein bound in fetal blood than in maternal blood. While it may enhance maternal satisfaction with pethidine analgesia, it readily crosses the placenta and may be associated with neonatal depression. The elimination half-life in the neonate is similar to that in the mother.

Midazolam

This drug is water soluble and, while placental transfer is rapid, it is less than for diazepam and thiopentone. Elimination by the neonate, although slower than maternal elimination, is still relatively rapid and the metabolites are inactive. However, when used to induce anaesthesia for caesarean section, more neonatal depression occurs than with thiopentone.

Onset of anaesthesia is relatively slow when diazepam and midazolam are used for induction of anaesthesia. This, with their unfavourable neonatal effects, precludes their use in pregnancy unless a strong indication, e.g. anticonvulsant action, exists.

Opioids

Some factors influencing the placental transfer of opioids are shown in Table 48.1.

Pethidine

Pethidine is the most commonly used systemic opioid for labour pain and provides satisfactory analgesia in about half the patients. It may cause drowsiness, nausea and vomiting, and greatly slows gastric emptying. Following intramuscular maternal administration, placental transfer is

Table 48.1 Some factors influencing the placental transfer of opioids

Drug	Protein binding		Lipid solubility	F:M ratio
	Main protein	%		
Morphine		Low	Low	0.9
Pethidine	AAG	30–65	Moderate	>1
Fentanyl	Albumin	84	High	0.7
Alfentanil	AAG	92	Moderate	0.3
Sufentanil	AAG	92	Very high	0.3–0 8

AAG, α_1-acid glycoprotein.

rapid, with F:M ratios rising to exceed unity in 2–3 hours. Being basic, it is more ionised in fetal blood, especially with fetal acidosis, and therefore subject to 'ion trapping'.

Maximal neonatal respiratory depression occurs when delivery is approximately 3 hours after maternal dosing, and neurological depression can be demonstrated for up to 3 days. The metabolite norpethidine, which crosses the placenta more slowly but is also produced within the fetoplacental unit, may contribute to this. The elimination half-life of pethidine in the neonate is about 18 hours, while that of norpethidine is 60 hours. Equivalent values for the mother are 3–4 hours and 20 hours, respectively.

Extradural pethidine in combination with a local anaesthetic may improve analgesia, while reducing motor blockade. Placental transfer is of the same order as the intramuscular route.

Morphine

Systemic morphine is rarely used in obstetric practice as it produces greater respiratory depression in the neonate than equipotent doses of pethidine. Although of low lipid solubility, it is only weakly bound to AAG and thus placental transfer is still relatively rapid. Since clearance of morphine back across the placenta from fetus to mother is slow, fetal biotransformation of the drug is important in elimination from the fetal compartment.

Intrathecal morphine has been used in labour. As only a small dose is used, fetal effects are minimal. However, being of low lipid solubility, morphine is less likely to bind with spinal cord receptors and rostral spread with possible respiratory depression is more likely. As larger doses are required by the extradural route, and much of this is absorbed into the systemic circulation, significant transfer to the fetus may occur. The incidence of maternal side-effects with both these routes is high.

Fentanyl

Fentanyl has been used intravenously both at caesarean section, to obtund the hypertensive response to tracheal intubation, and intermittently for labour pain. It has been combined with local anaesthetic to provide analgesia by the extradural route. Placental transfer is rapid and, although equilibration F:M ratios may exceed unity because of relatively increased fetal binding, reported values are generally lower. A single dose ($1 \mu g\,kg^{-1}$) at induction of anaesthesia produces minimal neonatal depression, while repeated small doses during labour provide moderate analgesia with few problems. A linear relationship is found between total dose and cord concentration. Fetal acidosis may lead to greater fentanyl entrapment in the fetal circulation.

When given by the extradural route, fentanyl, being lipophilic, has a faster onset of analgesic action than morphine and there is less likelihood of late respiratory depression because of its more rapid clearance from the cerebrospinal fluid. Respiratory depression has, however, been reported. Extradural fentanyl reduces the total dose of bupivacaine required and results in better analgesia with reduced motor blockade and few side-effects in both mother and neonate. F:M ratios at delivery are similar to those found with intravenous fentanyl.

Alfentanil

Alfentanil is less lipophilic and more highly protein bound (mainly to AAG) than fentanyl. Given intravenously ($10 \mu g\,kg^{-1}$) at caesarean section, it successfully obtunds the hypertensive response to tracheal intubation. Addition of alfentanil to extradural bupivacaine infusion improves analgesia, reduces motor block and causes few side-effects. Volume of distribution, clearance and terminal half-life are similar in pregnant and non-pregnant patients — mainly because of lack of alteration in protein binding and liver blood flow in pregnancy. Free alfentanil rapidly equilibrates across the placenta while F:M ratios for total drug are approximately 0.3, whether given by intravenous bolus injection or extradural infusion — the latter being more representative of a steady-state situation. This low ratio is partly explained by relative fetal and maternal protein binding capacities, and by rapid fetal tissue uptake. Newborn monkeys demonstrate higher plasma alfentanil concentrations 2 hours after birth, suggesting a compartmental shift from tissues to the systemic circulation. Concentrations decline more slowly compared with their mothers. Neonatal respiratory depression and hypotonia occur at higher maternal dose rates.

Sufentanil

Sufentanil has a selective action at the μ receptor. At doses of 10–30 μg, it enhances bupivacaine extradural analgesia and may reduce the number of instrumental deliveries, with no demonstrable depressant effects on neonates. Sensitive assays can detect sufentanil in cord blood, but neonatal exposure is low because of significant maternal uptake. Higher doses, 80 μg, result in neonatal neurobehavioural depression.

Diamorphine

Diamorphine is a moderately lipid soluble drug. It is readily distributed across the placenta, with F:M ratios of morphine equivalents exceeding unity after intramuscular injection. It has been used successfully with extradural bupivacaine and, while Apgar scores and acid–base balance have been satisfactory, transient reductions in neurobehavioural scores can be measured.

Intravenous induction agents

Adequate doses of induction agents at caesarean section are necessary to prevent maternal awareness and increased catecholamine concentrations secondary to light planes of anaesthesia, which may reduce placental perfusion; however, excessive doses may cause cardiovascular depression, with reduced uteroplacental flow, and increased neonatal drug concentrations, with prolonged depression.

Thiopentone

Thiopentone is the most commonly used intravenous anaesthetic induction agent and has not been completely superseded by newer drugs. It is

a lipid soluble weak acid, 75% bound to plasma albumin. It is less than 50% ionised at physiological pH. Placental transfer is rapid and thiopentone is detectable in UV blood within 30 seconds, equilibration between maternal (MV) and umbilical (UV) venous blood occurring at about 3 minutes. UV concentrations decrease rapidly in association with declining maternal concentration, but fetal plasma concentrations may continue to increase for 40 minutes. UA:UV ratio rises from 0.46 with a short induction–delivery (I–D) interval, to 0.87 with longer intervals. Thiopentone decreases cardiac output and transient decreases in uterine blood flow have been demonstrated. Dose related neonatal respiratory and non-specific neurobehavioural depression may occur. Neurobehavioural scores are reduced even with lower doses of 4 mg kg^{-1} at caesarean section when compared with regional block. The neonate eliminates thiopentone more slowly (elimination half-life 14.7 hours) than the mother.

Methohexitone

This also crosses the placenta rapidly, with umbilical venous concentrations peaking at 2–3 minutes after maternal intravenous dosing. Higher induction doses (1.4 mg kg^{-1}) cause more neonatal depression than doses of 1 mg kg^{-1}.

Propofol

Propofol is a low molecular weight, lipid soluble, largely unionised weak acid. Increased clearance in pregnancy contributes to faster recovery. Placental transfer is rapid with UV:MV ratios around 0.6–0.7. Rapid fetal uptake occurs and UA:UV ratios tend to be higher with longer induction–delivery intervals. While neonatal Apgar scores and acid–base status are usually satisfactory, there is a negative correlation between neurobehavioural scores and UV concentrations, and early transient depression has been reported, mainly at higher doses. A propofol total infusion technique is inadvisable because of an increased risk of awareness and neonatal depression compared with a volatile technique. The hypertensive and catecholamine response to tracheal intubation is attenuated. Severe transient bradycardia has been reported after induction with propofol and suxamethonium in the pregnant ewe, but maternal and fetal cardiovascular parameters, acid–base balance and uterine blood flow were well maintained.

Neonatal concentrations at 2 hours old indicate continuing clearance, albeit slower than maternal. Infants exposed to propofol have better nutritive sucking behaviour than those receiving thiopentone.

Etomidate

Etomidate is a lipid soluble weak base which causes minimal cardiovascular depression and is rapidly hydrolysed to an inactive metabolite. It has been suggested as an alternative to thiopentone when the latter is relatively contraindicated. Babies whose mothers have been given the drug compare favourably with those born after thiopentone induction. Cortisol production in the neonate may be suppressed. Relatively low umbilical concentrations are present at delivery, while a mean UA:UV ratio of 0.86 suggests continuing uptake, redistribution and metabolism in the time interval studied.

Ketamine

Ketamine is a lipid soluble weak base, less than 50% protein bound. Placental transfer is rapid and UV levels are greater than MV within minutes. Uterine tone is considerably increased in early pregnancy. Doses of 1–1.5 mg kg^{-1} at caesarean section compare favourably with thiopentone 3–4 mg kg^{-1} but higher doses (2 mg kg^{-1} or greater) may cause a marked, if short-lived, elevation of arterial blood pressure, an unacceptable incidence of dysphoric reactions and neonatal problems. It may have a place in the presence of hypovolaemia.

Inhalational agents

Inhalational agents may be used to provide anal-

gesia in labour or anaesthesia for caesarean section. Low concentrations of volatile agents reduce maternal awareness and obtund the catecholamine response to noxious stimuli, which may lead to uteroplacental vasoconstriction. They also permit the use of higher inspired oxygen concentration, with improved fetal oxygenation. Higher doses may cause cardiovascular depression and thus reduce uterine blood flow, and may also contribute directly to neonatal depression. The neonate can, however, excrete inhalational agents rapidly from the lungs. Blood–gas partition coefficients are significantly less in the newborn than the adult. Pregnancy causes an increase in minute volume and reduction in functional residual capacity so that uptake of inhalational agents is more rapid. Minimum alveolar concentration (MAC) of these agents is reduced in pregnancy (possibly related to progesterone or endorphin levels), returning to normal by 72 hours post partum. Placental transfer of these non-ionised lipid soluble low molecular weight substances readily occurs.

Nitrous oxide

Nitrous oxide is available in a 50% mixture with oxygen (Entonox) to provide analgesia during labour. Because it is relatively insoluble, uptake and excretion are rapid and it is therefore suitable for intermittent use, providing satisfactory pain relief in about 50% of mothers. When used without volatile supplements for caesarean section anaesthesia, a high incidence of maternal awareness is found. Umbilical vein concentrations of nitrous oxide approach 80% of maternal values within 3 minutes of maternal administration, while fetal uptake, as measured by umbilical artery concentration, is also rapid, with UA:UV ratios of 0.6 occurring within 10 minutes, rising to 0.9 with longer induction-delivery (I–D) intervals. Increased nitrous oxide transfer may occur when placental blood flow is high. The neonate rapidly excretes nitrous oxide by the lungs, provided ventilation is quickly established, and the possibility of diffusion hypoxia exists. The short exposure time at caesarean section is unlikely to affect methionine synthase activity (see above).

Halothane

Halothane in low concentrations (0.25–0.5%) reduces the risk of maternal awareness, does not increase uterine bleeding and has no deleterious effect on the neonate when compared with anaesthesia with nitrous oxide and oxygen alone. Predicted MAC values with 50% nitrous oxide are 0.6 after 3 minutes, rising to 0.8 after 10 minutes. Uterine blood flow may be increased. Higher concentrations, above 1.5 MAC, result in maternal hypotension, reduced uterine blood flow and fetal acidosis. Halothane produces a dose related reduction in uterine tone, but does not prevent the response to oxytocin stimulation. The UV concentration increases with duration of anaesthesia, while UV:MA ratio is approximately 0.5 at delivery. Mean UA:UV ratios of 0.5 are found, suggesting continued fetal tissue uptake. Halothane is taken up by the fetal liver, which plays a significant role in decreasing the amount reaching the fetal brain. Halothane and isoflurane produce comparable neonatal outcome at emergency caesarean section.

Enflurane

Enflurane provides anaesthetic conditions and outcome very similar to halothane when used in equipotent doses. Neonatal condition is also satisfactory after vaginal delivery conducted with enflurane anaesthesia. Mean UV:MA ratio at delivery during caesarean section is 0.6, while UA:UV ratio is 0.5. Plasma enflurane concentrations in the neonate decline rapidly after birth and only 9% of the delivery concentration is present at 15 minutes. Renal function is normal, although serum fluoride concentrations are slightly increased.

Isoflurane

Because of its lower blood:gas partition coefficient, maternal uptake of isoflurane is faster than halothane or enflurane. Higher arterial concentrations are rapidly achieved by using an initial inspired concentration of 2% (overpressure technique). Potential advantages of isoflurane include a lower degree of metabolism, better maintenance of cardiac output, increase in uterine blood flow and more rapid elimination. F:M ratios at caesarean delivery are around 0.9. Prolonged anaesthesia with high concentrations of isoflurane (>2 MAC) reduces cardiac output and organ blood flow in the fetal lamb. There has been some recent interest in the supplementation of Entonox with low concentrations of isoflurane for labour analgesia. In clinical practice no observable difference in maternal or neonatal outcome at caesarean section is apparent between halothane, enflurane or isoflurane.

Sevoflurane and desflurane

The place of these newer inhalational agents has not been fully evaluated in obstetric practice. The low blood and tissue:gas solubilities resulting in rapid uptake and recovery would be advantageous in obstetric anaesthesia.

At elective caesarean section, sevoflurane 1% gives comparable results to isoflurane 0.5% in terms of maternal cardiovascular stability, uterine tone, blood loss, neonatal outcome and recovery time. Maternal and umbilical serum concentrations of fluoride are modestly elevated postoperatively.

Muscle relaxants

Neuromuscular blocking drugs are highly ionised molecules of low lipid solubility. Thus, placental transfer is limited and the neonate is clinically unaffected. Umbilical vein concentrations are lower than those producing measurable reduction of twitch height in adults or infants (Table 48.2) and this blood will be further diluted on reaching the fetus. Infants are, however, more sensitive to competitive neuromuscular blockers than adults.

Suxamethonium

Suxamethonium remains the muscle relaxant of choice for rapid tracheal intubation in obstetrics. Despite reduced serum cholinesterase levels in pregnancy, suxamethonium action is rarely pro-

Table 48.2 Placental transfer of non-depolarising muscle relaxants

Drug	Maternal dose (mg kg⁻¹)	Mean plasma concentration at delivery (ng ml⁻¹)		Mean F:M ratio	Plasma concentration (ng ml⁻¹) causing 50% ↓ twitch height
		Maternal	Umbilical vein		
Pancuronium	0.04	115	22	0.2	88 (adults)
	0.1	510	120	0.3	
Vecuronium	0.04	162	18	0.1	94 (adults)
	0.06–0.08	390	40	0.1	
Atracurium	0.3	1829	103	0.1	383 (infants)
Rocuronium	0.6	2412	390	0.16	654* (infants)

*Causes 75% depression in twitch height.

longed. This is probably due to the increased volume of distribution, as prolongation of action can be demonstrated 1–2 days post partum when extracellular fluid volume has returned towards normal but serum cholinesterase activity is still reduced. Because of its rapid hydrolysis, no assay for plasma suxamethonium is available but ¹⁴C-labelled suxamethonium in monkeys shows a peak fetal concentration of approximately 4% the maximum maternal concentration at 5–10 minutes after maternal intravenous administration. Biotransformation is slower in the fetus. The neonate appears unaffected by usual therapeutic doses but neuromuscular block may occur after repeated high doses or in the presence of atypical cholinesterase.

Non-depolarising muscle relaxants

The non-depolarising muscle relaxants cause no demonstrable neonatal problems when used in the normal dose range, although muscle weakness has occurred in a neonate whose mother received tubocurarine 425 mg to control convulsions. In contrast, an infant with normal Apgar scores was born after maternal dosing of atracurium 520 mg over 16 hours.

Limited placental transfer of alcuronium, tubocurarine and pancuronium has been measured. UV:MV ratios tend to rise with prolonged dose to delivery (D–D) intervals. The use of suxamethonium permits the use of a lower dose of pancuronium, a shorter D–D time, lower fetal

blood concentrations and better neonatal condition. No depression of passive or active neonatal tone is apparent. The relatively long action of pancuronium, however, makes it less suitable for caesarean section.

The shorter duration of action and lack of cardiovascular effects of vecuronium enhance its suitability. Placental transfer is minimal with mean UV:MV ratios of 0.1 (Table 48.2) and there is no apparent effect on the neonate. The onset of neuromuscular block is shorter and recovery slower than in non-pregnant patients. The elimination half-life is half that for pancuronium (36 compared to 72 minutes).

Atracurium has a duration of approximately 30 minutes at caesarean section, cardiovascular stability is well maintained and the drug undergoes spontaneous degradation by Hofmann elimination. Neonatal condition at delivery is good. UV:MV ratios at delivery are low (Table 48.2), increasing slightly with D–D time.

Initial studies with rocuronium for caesarean section demonstrate a shorter onset but similar duration of action compared to vecuronium. It is, however, inferior to suxamethonium for rapid sequence induction–intubation in obstetrics. Mean UV:MV ratio at delivery is low (Table 48.2). No correlation between fetal plasma concentrations and neurobehavioural scores is found.

Neostigmine is not given until after delivery of the baby but, being highly ionised in maternal plasma, would be unlikely to undergo significant placental transfer.

Local anaesthetic agents

Regional anaesthesia is widely employed in obstetrics. Well conducted extradural analgesia provides excellent pain relief with a low incidence of maternal and fetal complications. Infusions of dilute local anaesthetic solutions combined with small doses of opioids are commonly used, permitting reduced doses of both drugs with enhanced analgesia, less motor block and less hypotension. The rapid onset of effective block and the improved maternal and neonatal safety when compared with general anaesthesia have greatly increased the popularity of subarachnoid block for caesarean section. With both these techniques it is important to avoid hypotension, which decreases uteroplacental flow and may lead to fetal hypoxia.

Local anaesthetic drugs are lipid soluble weak bases variably bound to AAG, an important factor in the degree of placental transfer (Table 48.3). However, low F:M total concentration ratios do not necessarily imply fetal safety, as pharmacological effects are related to free drug concentrations. Fetal acidosis increases the maternal:fetal pH gradient so, as local anaesthetics are weak bases, free drug can accumulate in the fetus. Local anaesthetic agents are rapidly absorbed after extradural or pudendal injection. Unexpectedly high plasma concentrations of amide-type local anaesthetics associated with fetal bradycardia may occur with paracervical block and have been attributed to diffusion across the uterine arterial wall.

Bupivacaine

Bupivacaine continues to be the most popular agent for extradural analgesia because of its long action, limited motor blocking properties, and lack of tachyphylaxis. No clinically significant neonatal cardiovascular or neurobehavioural depression is found with usual doses, although loss of beat-to-beat variability and late deceleration heart patterns have been reported. Uterine blood flow and tone are not affected. Maternal and fetal plasma concentrations peak at 10–20 minutes. The addition of adrenaline reduces peak maternal concentrations but has less effect on fetal values and F:M ratios may actually be higher. UV:MV ratios remain low even after prolonged extradural analgesia. The low F:M ratios for total drug are due to differential protein binding in maternal (90–95%) and fetal (50–84%) plasma, while F:M ratios for free drug are closer to unity. UA:UV ratios increase towards unity 30–40 minutes after maternal dosing, suggesting equilibration at this time. Fetal concentrations are well below the toxic range. The elimination half-life is longer (6–9 hours) in the mother at term compared with the non-pregnant subject (1–2 hours). Similar values are found in the healthy neonate, increasing to over 9 hours in the acidotic baby.

A number of cases of cardiac arrest have been reported in obstetric patients after inadvertent intravascular injection of bupivacaine. The safety margin, i.e. the ratio of plasma concentration producing convulsions to that causing cardiovascular collapse, is narrower for bupivacaine than for other local anaesthetic agents, and pregnancy may render the myocardium more sensitive to bupivacaine, although studies are conflicting. Bupivacaine 0.75% has been withdrawn from obstetrics use. Extradural dosage should be limited to 2 mg kg^{-1} body weight in any 4 hour period.

Lignocaine

Extradural lignocaine has a relatively short duration of action, may induce tachyphylaxis and causes more motor blockade than bupivacaine. Placental transfer is greater than bupivacaine (Table 48.3). Prolonged use may result in accumulation in mother and fetus, and higher blood

Table 48.3 Relationship between degree of protein binding and placental transfer of local anaesthetic agents

Drug	Protein bound %	F:M ratio
Bupivacaine	90–95	0.2–0.3
Ropivacaine	94	0.2
Etidocaine	90	0.3
Mepivacaine	75	0.6–0.7
Lignocaine	60	0.5–0.6
Prilocaine	55	1

concentrations are found in acidotic babies. The addition of adrenaline reduces maternal plasma concentrations of lignocaine but has little effect on umbilical cord values. Neonatal elimination half-life is 1.5–3 hours. Neonatal hypotonia was associated with lignocaine in earlier, but not more recent, studies.

Other amides

F:M ratios greater than unity have been recorded for *prilocaine*. This factor, plus the development of methaemoglobinaemia in mother and fetus with repeated doses, limits its use in obstetrics. Maternal toxic reactions and neonatal hypotonia have been associated with *mepivacaine*. Elimination half-life is prolonged (9 hours) in the baby. *Etidocaine* has placental transfer characteristics similar to bupivacaine. It produces a high degree of motor block, so is less suitable for use during labour. When used for caesarean section, onset of analgesia is faster but considerably inferior to bupivacaine. *Ropivacaine* is chemically similar to bupivacaine but has a greater therapeutic index. Pregnancy does not enhance its toxicity. Onset and duration of sensory block is similar with epidural ropivacaine but motor block is of slower onset and shorter duration in pregnant patients. F:M concentration ratio is 0.2 in sheep.

Chloroprocaine

The rapid hydrolysis of this ester-linked drug results in minimal placental transfer, with extremely low umbilical cord blood concentrations. No loss of beat-to-beat variability is noted when chloroprocaine is used in labour and neonates perform well in neurobehavioural tests, although subtle changes can be detected. Onset of action is rapid but short lived. Chloroprocaine appears to antagonise epidural opioids. Inadvertent intrathecal injection has resulted in chronic neurological damage. The antioxidant, sodium metabisulphite, may be implicated and has been removed from commercial preparations. It is not available in the UK.

Sympathomimetics

Endogenous catecholamines, produced in response to the stress and pain of labour, may reduce uterine blood flow — an effect attenuated by epidural analgesia. High exogenous adrenaline plasma concentrations, e.g. after accidental intravenous injection of adrenaline-containing local anaesthetic, significantly reduce uterine blood flow. Low plasma concentrations caused by systemic absorption from the extradural space do not decrease intervillous flow in healthy parturients but may increase uteroplacental vascular resistance in patients with pregnancy induced hypertension.

Extradural or spinal anaesthesia may cause maternal hypotension despite careful positioning and fluid preloading. The resultant uteroplacental hypoperfusion, if untreated, causes fetal hypoxia and acidosis.

Ephedrine has both α- and β-adrenergic effects. It augments venoconstriction more than arterial constriction and thus improves venous return and cardiac output, restoring maternal arterial blood pressure and uterine perfusion. It is, however, subject to tachyphylaxis and may cause maternal tachycardia. It undergoes rapid placental transfer and may increase fetal heart rate.

More recently, the α agonists *phenylephrine* and *methoxamine* have been used to successfully treat maternal hypotension associated with regional anaesthesia without adverse fetal effects. However, the healthy placenta has a substantial reserve capacity so that the fetus may tolerate brief periods of reduced perfusion. Doppler velocimetry indicates significant increases in uterine vascular resistance with phenylephrine and methoxamine, but not with ephedrine. In the pregnant ewe, dopamine causes a dose related decrease in uterine blood flow secondary to increased uterine vascular resistance. Higher doses result in fetal acidosis. Low dose ephedrine would therefore seem to be the drug of choice when a vasopressor is required, particularly with pre-existing uteroplacental insufficiency.

Pre-eclampsia: seizure prophylaxis

Traditionally, diazepam and chlormethiazole have

been used to prevent convulsions in patients with severe pre-eclampsia; however, their popularity has been declining because of maternal sedation and fetal effects such as hypotonia, hypothermia and apnoea. Two drugs are now prominent — magnesium sulphate and phenytoin. The recent Collaborative Eclampsia Trial found magnesium sulphate to be the drug of choice in eclampsia because more recurrent convulsions occurred with diazepam and phenytoin and phenytoin also caused more maternal and neonatal morbidity.

Magnesium sulphate

The mechanism of anticonvulsant action is not well understood but may involve a primary central nervous system effect, a peripheral effect at the neuromuscular junction, competition for binding sites with calcium and stimulation of prostacyclin synthesis. It depresses smooth muscle contraction and catecholamine release, leading to mild vasodilatation and some reduction in arterial blood pressure, with improved uterine and renal blood flow. Myometrial contractility is reduced, which is useful if uterine hyperactivity is present, but may prolong labour and predispose to postpartum haemorrhage.

Magnesium sulphate rapidly crosses the placenta by active diffusion and fetal plasma concentrations may be comparable with maternal. Therapeutic plasma concentrations (2–3.5 mmol l^{-1}) in the mother are not associated with adverse neonatal outcome. High (> 4 mmol l^{-1}) maternal concentrations (more common in the presence of impaired renal function) result in muscle weakness and respiratory insufficiency in both mother and baby. Cardiac arrest occurs at very high concentrations. Slow intravenous calcium counteracts toxic effects.

Of importance to anaesthetists is the potentiation of non-depolarising muscle relaxants by magnesium sulphate.

Phenytoin

Phenytoin is an anticonvulsant used for the treatment of epilepsy. It is highly bound to albumin and has a narrow therapeutic index. Serum albumin concentrations may be even lower in severe pre-eclampsia, resulting in a higher free fraction requiring adjustment of dosage. It does not cause uterine relaxation. Phenytoin is given by slow intravenous injection with electrocardiographic control — too rapid injection may cause arrhythmias, hypotension and cardiovascular collapse. Binding is lower in maternal than fetal plasma and total F:M ratio for phenytoin is around unity. Phenytoin undergoes biphasic elimination in the neonate.

Pre-eclampsia: antihypertensive therapy

Severe pre-eclampsia can constitute an obstetric emergency, and safe, efficient lowering of arterial blood pressure is required. Treatment of less severe hypertension during pregnancy, although beneficial to the mother, does not necessarily improve fetal status or neonatal outcome.

Hydralazine

Hydralazine has been the most extensively used drug in pre-eclampsia. It decreases precapillary arteriolar resistance. Maximal effect occurs at 20–30 minutes after an intravenous dose and effect lasts 2–3 hours. Undesirable effects include tachycardia, ventricular arrhythmias and more minor effects, such as headache and nausea. Renal blood flow is increased. Umbilical vein blood flow may be increased without change in intervillous blood flow. Occasionally, arterial pressure reduction is too rapid, leading to diminished uteroplacental flow and exacerbation of fetal hypoxia.

Labetalol

Labetalol has both α- and β-blocking properties. Onset of action is rapid with intravenous infusion and blood pressure control is smoother than with hydralazine. It does not reduce placental perfusion and neonatal outcome is generally not adversely affected. It has relatively low lipid solubility and placental transfer is limited, but fetal exposure is considerable as the drug is only slowly eliminated from the maternal circulation. F:M ratio at delivery is about 0.5. Labetalol can also be used to attenuate the hypertensive response to tracheal intubation. It is comparable to methyldopa for control of moderate hypertension.

Calcium channel blockers

These drugs relax vascular smooth muscle. Uterine muscle is also relaxed and the possibility of postpartum haemorrhage exists. Compared to hydralazine in severe pre-eclampsia, nifedipine gives better blood pressure control, prolongs pregnancy and is associated with considerably less fetal distress episodes. Renal blood flow and urinary output are improved. When used with magnesium sulphate, the hypotensive response is potentiated. Peak blood concentrations occur about 40 minutes after oral ingestion and elimination half-life is 54 minutes.

Other drugs

Methyldopa has commonly been used for the treatment of hypertension during pregnancy and has a proven safety record.

Prolonged treatment with β blockers has been associated with intrauterine growth retardation, fetal bradycardia and neonatal hypoglycaemia and hypoxia. The more cardioselective β_1 blockers, atenolol and metoprolol, have been used successfully to reduce arterial blood pressure without adverse fetal effects. Esmolol, a short acting β blocker, attenuates the hypertensive response to tracheal intubation but may cause fetal β blockade. Oral clonidine appears safe for the mother and fetus during pregnancy but intravenous use has been associated with fetal problems.

The short acting powerful antihypertensive agents trimetaphan (a ganglion blocker), nitroprusside (a directly acting arterial vasodilator) and nitroglycerin (a venodilator) have been used to control sudden rises of blood pressure during general anaesthesia. These require careful monitoring. Nitroprusside cyanide toxicity in the fetus is avoided by short term infusion rates of less than 3 μg kg^{-1} h^{-1}.

Gastrointestinal drugs

Antiemetics

The dreadful teratogenic effects of thalidomide have led to extreme caution in the use of antiemetics (and other drugs) in early pregnancy. The antihistamine, cyclizine, appears safe in human pregnancy, as shown by retrospective and prospective studies, although association with cleft palate has been noted. Phenothiazines have traditionally been used in labour for anxiolysis, possible augmentation of pethidine analgesia and reduction of associated nausea and vomiting. These drugs readily transfer across the placenta and may cause observable depression of neonatal muscle tone and respiration. Metoclopramide markedly reduces the incidence of vomiting during labour, increases the gastric emptying rate, reduces gastric volume and increases the tone of the lower oesophageal sphincter. As a lipid soluble, low molecular weight drug, placental transfer is rapid and fetal plasma concentrations approach maternal within 1 hour. Neonatal parameters (including neurobehavioural tests) are not adversely affected.

Antacid therapy

Attempts are made to reduce gastric acidity routinely in labouring women in some units, and in selected high risk patients in other units, to lessen the risk of the development of Mendelson's syndrome if stomach contents are inhaled during anaesthesia (see also Ch. 40).

Cimetidine and ranitidine are histamine H_2-receptor blockers that have been extensively used in labour. The latter is longer acting: a 150 mg oral dose maintains gastric pH >2.5 for approximately 6 hours. Pethidine administration results in greatly reduced absorption of oral ranitidine. F:M ratios approach unity after 3 hours with intravenous ranitidine. Apgar and neurobehavioural scores, neonatal gastric acidity and blood glucose are similar to babies of untreated mothers.

Omeprazole, a gastric proton pump inhibitor, reduces gastric acidity and volume and is effective given by oral or intravenous routes. Human placental transfer has not been reported in detail but omeprazole concentration in cord blood is approximately half that of maternal after a single 80 mg oral dose on the evening before surgery.

Since the above drugs require time to act and have no effect on existing acid, oral alkalis are usually given preoperatively to raise gastric pH. Particulate antacids may themselves cause a chemical pneumonitis if inhaled, and their use has declined in favour of saline antacids such as sodium citrate or bicarbonate.

Anticholinergic drugs

Atropine and hyoscine freely diffuse across the placenta. After an intravenous dose, the F:M ratio of atropine rapidly approaches unity and fetal tachycardia and mydriasis in the neonate frequently occur. Glycopyrrolate, a quaternary ammonium compound, is highly ionised at maternal pH, so placental transfer is limited, and, although F:M ratios increase with time, fetal serum concentrations (measured in the dog) never rise above 5% of the corresponding maternal value. It is therefore to be preferred where an anticholinergic effect on the fetus is undesirable.

Drugs affecting coagulation

Warfarin is a weak acid bound to albumin with free placental transfer. Use in pregnancy is associated with fetal loss of approximately 40%. There is a low but definite risk of teratogenesis associated with its use in the first trimester, while serious retroplacental and intracerebral fetal bleeding may occur in late pregnancy. Fetal production of clotting factors is deficient, while vitamin K dependent clotting factors do not cross the placenta.

Unfractionated heparin is a polar drug with a variable molecular weight of 3000–30 000. There is no detectable placental transfer. It is recommended that heparin is substituted for warfarin in the first trimester and from 36 weeks onwards.

Low molecular weight heparins (heparin fractions of 4000–6000) selectively inhibit the effect of factor Xa, with less effect on factor IIa. Because of their long half-life, a single daily injection is adequate and clinical trials demonstrate efficacy in preventing thromboembolic morbidity. Placental transfer of these drugs cannot be demonstrated.

In pregnancy complicated by pre-eclampsia, there is a relative decrease in prostacyclin and an increase in thromboxane A_2 synthesis. Low dose aspirin therapy results in irreversible inhibition of thromboxane A_2, while prostacyclin synthesis is less affected. Although high maternal doses of aspirin close to delivery cause abnormalities in neonatal haemostasis, this does not seem to be a problem with the low dose (60 mg) currently being used in trials to assess effect on pre-eclampsia and intrauterine growth retardation. Initial results of these trials are encouraging. Because of concerns regarding possible teratogenic effects, treatment should not start before 15 weeks. Aspirin is discontinued at 37 weeks so that possible prolonged bleeding does not interfere with epidural analgesia.

Drugs used for specific action on the uterus

Uterine stimulants

Ergometrine

Ergometrine is an ergot alkaloid which causes frequent uterine contractions superimposed on a tonic contraction, while higher doses cause sustained contraction, and its use is confined to the postpartum period. Its vasoconstrictor effect increases arterial blood pressure and reduces peripheral blood flow. This pressor effect is more marked in hypertensive states and may precipitate cardiac failure, eclampsia and cerebral haemorrhage in susceptible patients. Nausea and vomiting are common. Ergometrine is active after oral administration, but absorption is variable. The ergot alkaloids are mainly metabolised in the liver and excreted in the bile.

Oxytocin

Oxytocin is a posterior hypothalamic nonapeptide that stimulates rhythmic uterine contractions.

The synthetic preparation is frequently used to induce or augment labour and to treat postpartum haemorrhage. Large doses may cause hypotension secondary to vascular smooth muscle relaxation, more marked in patients with hypovolaemia or cardiac disease. Structurally related to vasopressin, oxytocin has water retaining properties, resulting in overhydration and hyponatraemia when given with electrolyte-free solutions. Acute water intoxication and cerebral oedema have been reported with severe hyponatraemia and convulsions in the newborn. Infants have an increased incidence of hyperbilirubinaemia.

Prostaglandins

These are compounds formed from arachidonic acid. The E and F types are used to ripen the cervix and stimulate uterine contraction. Side-effects include nausea, vomiting, diarrhoea and pyrexia. Use in epilepsy is contraindicated as convulsions have been reported. Bronchoconstriction may occur in asthmatic patients. While mild hypotension and bradycardia commonly occur, severe hypertension has occasionally been seen.

Uterine activity and fetal condition should be carefully monitored when the above agents are used.

Relaxants

β-adrenergic agents with selective β_2 activity are used in the treatment of preterm labour. Ritodrine, terbutaline and salbutamol have all been used for tocolysis.

The clinical side-effects of β-mimetic drugs are dose related maternal tachycardia, hypertension and pulmonary oedema. The last is more likely with steroid therapy, twin pregnancy, anaemia, pre-existing hypertension and crystalloid therapy. Elevations in glucose, free fatty acids, lactic acid and insulin may occur. These agents readily cross the placenta and may increase fetal heart rate and cardiac output. Cerebral haemorrhage has been

reported. Neonatal complications include hypoglycaemia, hypokalaemia and hypertension.

Magnesium sulphate (see above) has also been found useful in suppressing preterm labour. Long term therapy may result in inadequate metaphyseal calcification in the baby.

DRUG THERAPY AND BREAST FEEDING

Drugs pass from plasma into breast milk mainly by passive diffusion down a concentration gradient via multiple lipoprotein cell membranes. Molecular weight, lipid solubility, protein binding and pK_a of the drug all influence the degree of transfer. The average pH of breast milk is 7.08, so basic drugs are subject to 'ion trapping'. Apart from such drugs as chemotherapeutic agents and radioactive isotopes, nursing rarely needs to be stopped because of maternal medication. For analgesia, morphine may be preferred to pethidine, as patient controlled analgesia with the latter causes significant neurobehavioural depression in the baby. Aspirin should probably be avoided because the neonate has immature biotransformation and excretory pathways and platelet dysfunction and metabolic acidosis may occur. Anaesthetic drugs (intravenous induction agents, inhalational agents, muscle relaxants, extradural local anaesthetic agents) are unlikely to cause significant problems in the suckling infant. Diazepam and its long acting metabolite, N-desmethyldiazepam, have been detected in breast milk and the possibility of accumulation in the baby exists.

CONCLUSION

This chapter reviews the effect of drugs most commonly encountered by the anaesthetist treating the pregnant patient. It is not, however, possible to fully cover all aspects of this important topic in the space allocated. The reader is therefore strongly advised to consult some of the excellent books/reviews on the topic, a number of which are listed.

FURTHER READING

Cheek T G, Gutsche B B 1993 Maternal physiologic alterations during pregnancy. In: Shnider S M, Levinson G (eds) Anesthesia for obstetrics, pp 3–17. Williams & Wilkins, Baltimore

Lee J J, Rubin A P 1993 Breast feeding and anaesthesia. Anaesthesia 48: 616–625

Levinson G, Shnider S M (eds) 1993 Anesthesia for surgery during pregnancy. In: Anesthesia for obstetrics, pp 259–280. Williams & Wilkins, Baltimore

Reynolds F 1993 Effects on the baby of maternal analgesia and anaesthesia. Saunders, London

Reynolds F, Knott C 1989 Pharmacokinetics in pregnancy and placental drug transfer. Oxford Reviews of Reproductive Biology 11: 389–449, Oxford University Press

49

Childhood and anaesthetic drugs

T. M. Gallagher

Paediatric physiology represents a continuous process of adaptation from intrauterine life, where the placenta is the principal organ of oxygenation, excretion and detoxification, to extrauterine existence, where the lung, kidneys and liver assume these roles. It could be said that adaptation and development is complete in the young adult, when the process of degeneration begins.

The most important differences between the physiology and pharmacology of the child and the adult are particularly evident in early neonatal life and gradually become less apparent with increasing maturity. For the sake of clarification the following definitions will be used: a *term infant* is one born with a postconceptual age greater than 37 weeks; a *neonate* is a baby less than 1 month old; an *infant* is one aged between 1 month and 1 year; a *child* is between 1 and 12 years of age.

This chapter describes some of the most important physiological differences between children and adults, with particular reference to the neonate, and reviews how these may affect pharmacology in childhood.

RESPIRATORY SYSTEM

Lung development is compatible with successful adaptation to extrauterine life by 24 weeks gestation. However, alveolar capillary units continue to grow and develop for at least 8 years postnatally and the conducting airways only reach full maturity in the early teenage years. Anatomically, the neonatal and infant airway and respiratory apparatus differ in several aspects from the adult's and increase the risk of respiratory problems in the younger age group. The tongue is relatively large; the glottic opening is higher, at the level of C4, and lies anteriorly; the epiglottis is floppy and inclines posteriorly; the subglottic area is the narrowest part of the airway and is especially susceptible to oedema, being completely surrounded by cricoid cartilage. The thoracic cage is softer and less supportive in infancy and the horizontal placement of ribs and poor development of intercostal and diaphragmatic muscles further increase susceptibility to respiratory stresses. With increasing growth, these structures assume adult configuration by early adolescence.

Neonatal respiration differs from the adult's particularly in regard to compliance, airway resistance and central control. The chest wall in infants is very compliant but lung tissue compliance is low. There is a relative deficiency of elastin in neonatal alveoli and airways, which increases the tendency to collapse. Maturity in this respect is not reached until the late teenage years. Pulmonary compliance is further compromised if there is deficiency of the surface tension lowering agent, surfactant, either because of immaturity or disease. Airway resistance is greater in infants because of the smaller calibre of both the airways. Although the functional residual capacity in the neonate and adult are similar ($30 \, ml \, kg^{-1}$), the higher oxygen consumption in the former means that there is little oxygen reserve in the event of stress. Minute ventilation is higher in the neonate at $230 \, ml \, kg^{-1} \, min^{-1}$ compared to the adult $70 \, ml \, kg^{-1} \, min^{-1}$ and is achieved mainly by maintaining a rapid respiratory rate in the range 30–40 breaths per minute.

Unlike adults, neonates can have episodes of periodic breathing or even apnoeic episodes lasting for as long as 15 seconds. Premature infants may have more prolonged episodes, which usually resolve with manual stimulation. The mechanism is unclear but may reflect immaturity of central control of respiration. Furthermore, infants appear to be more sensitive to the inhibitory

effects of laryngeal reflexes and readily develop reflex apnoea in response to stimuli such as severe gastro-oesophageal reflux.

CARDIOVASCULAR SYSTEM

During intrauterine development the essential components of the cardiovascular system are established by the 12th week of gestation, but the distribution of blood flow is quite different to that of the adult circulation. The right and left ventricles function in parallel, linked by two shunts at atrial and aortopulmonary level. The placenta is the oxygenating organ in the fetus. The umbilical vein, carrying oxygenated blood from the placenta, divides at the liver so that 50% of its flow bypasses that organ to enter the inferior vena cava through the ductus venosus.

In the right atrium approximately one-third of inferior vena caval blood is shunted through the foramen ovale to the left atrium, and thence to the left ventricle and the ascending aortic arch for distribution to the upper body. Most of the remaining blood and superior vena caval blood enters the right ventricle and pulmonary artery. Since the pulmonary vascular resistance is high in utero, most of the pulmonary artery blood is shunted through the ductus arteriosus to the descending aorta, effectively bypassing the lungs.

At birth, smooth adaptation to extrauterine life depends on the lungs taking over from the placenta as the organs of oxygenation and on the establishment of serial continuity between the outputs of both ventricles. Pulmonary vascular resistance decreases through various complex mechanisms but in particular by the effect of lung inflation and the establishment of a separate pulmonary circulation driven by the right ventricle. The left atrial pressure increases slightly because of an increase in pulmonary venous return and the foramen ovale closes functionally within 1 hour of birth. The ductus venosus also closes within 1–3 hours of birth as a result of reduced umbilical venous flow. Closure of the ductus arteriosus occurs initially in response to an increase in oxygen tension, usually within 12 hours, but complete anatomical closure does not occur for several days after birth. Although the pulmonary vascular resistance normally reduces after birth, adult values are not established for several months. The first few days of life are critical because during this transitional phase any factor that might cause pulmonary vascular resistance to remain elevated — hypoxia, hypercarbia or congenital anomalies — may result in re-establishment of fetal type circulation.

Cardiac output in the neonate is heart rate dependent, with a very limited ability to increase stroke volume. Sympathetic innervation of the myocardium is not complete until 4–6 months of age and parasympathetic activity is dominant in early infancy. Undue stimulation of the parasympathetic system, which occurs readily with simple manoeuvres such as airway intubation, may induce profound bradycardia with a significant reduction in cardiac output.

TEMPERATURE CONTROL

The ability to maintain a constant body temperature despite fluctuations in environmental temperature is an essential homeostatic mechanism in humans. When the environmental temperature is kept within the thermoneutral range, body heat production is balanced by heat loss to the environment and body temperature remains constant. Although newborns and young infants have some capacity for homeothermy, their control mechanisms are less efficient than adults if exposed to temperatures outside a narrow thermoneutral zone. Although newborns can vasoconstrict skin blood vessels they are not good at conserving heat because (1) their large surface area results in greater heat loss from skin, (2) there is less subcutaneous insulating fat, and (3) their small body size is a poor heat sink. These problems are exacerbated in premature infants, especially in the first 2 weeks of life, because inadequate keratinisation of skin further increases heat loss from evaporation. Moreover, apart from adopting a flexed posture, infants have no other behavioural techniques that conserve heat and their ability to shiver is undeveloped.

Maintenance of a normal core temperature in newborns and young infants depends on increasing body heat production by non-shivering thermogenesis. This occurs especially in brown fat, which is distributed in the axilla, neck and mediastinum. Metabolism of brown fat, which is under sympathetic control, results in increased heat production at the cost of energy utilisation. Although non-shivering thermogenesis is useful in maintaining homeostasis, it is associated with increased oxygen consumption and increased glucose and fatty acid metabolism. Care should be taken to minimise heat loss in neonates and to avoid stimuli for non-shivering thermogenesis. Similarly, an excessively warm environment should be avoided because young babies' ability to sweat is not well developed. In these circumstances body temperature may increase and, in turn, increase oxygen consumption. Non-shivering thermogenesis may become inadequate for maintaining core temperature when brown fat stores are depleted after prolonged exposure to a cold environment or hypoxia.

BODY FLUIDS AND RENAL FUNCTION

In the healthy fetus renal development starts at the third week of gestation and continues until the 34th week. Further development is related to hyperplasia. Although the fetal kidney can produce urine after 11–12 weeks, the placenta is the principal organ of excretion. From the 34th week, when nephrogenesis is complete, the fetal kidney prepares for its role in extrauterine life by increasing glomerular filtration rate and urine production. Renal function in the neonate is a measure of gestational age and the term infant adapts readily to normal postnatal demands. The neonatal kidney can excrete a dilute urine, but tubular function is immature and there is only a limited ability to concentrate urine and to conserve sodium. Adult capabilities are achieved at 1 year.

The main function of the kidney is to maintain the internal environment of the body, especially in maintaining water balance. Infants differ from adults not only in total body water volumes but also in the distribution of fluids in the extracellular and intracellular spaces. In a healthy 70 kg adult man, the total body water is 60%

body weight, with approximately 14 litres in the extracellular and 28 litres in the intracellular compartments.

In utero, the fetus is 80% water: 60% extracellular and 20% intracellular. With increasing maturity and deposition of fat, total body water falls and in the term infant accounts for 75% of body weight. Normal development is associated with redistribution of body fluid compartments, with a relative decrease in extracellular fluid. This process continues until adult values are achieved at adolescence.

These differences have important implications clinically: (1) infants are more readily compromised because they depend on others to ensure adequate fluid intake; (2) are less capable of dealing with either over- or underestimation of fluid requirements; and (3) the large extracellular fluid volume results in a large volume of distribution for drugs, which as a consequence may not achieve therapeutic concentrations.

CENTRAL NERVOUS SYSTEM

Although the central nervous system is already well developed at birth, the first year of life is characterised by further rapid growth and differentiation. The brain, which represents 10% of body weight at birth, doubles its weight in the first 6 months and trebles it by 1 year. Adult proportions are only achieved by 12 years of age, when the brain accounts for 2% body weight. The full complement of adult neurones is in place by the end of the second trimester and postnatal growth comprises mainly glial cell proliferation, further branching of dendritic processes and myelination.

Blood–brain barrier

The endothelial cells of cerebral capillaries are adapted to form tight junctions that prevent diffusion of certain substances from blood into the brain, effectively providing a barrier between brain extracellular fluid and blood. Only water, oxygen and carbon dioxide enter the brain by simple diffusion, but brain tissue needs substrates, such as glucose, lactate and amino acids,

and their entry into the brain has to be facilitated by active transport systems. These processes of specialisation begin in the first trimester and by birth the normal neonate has a functioning blood–brain barrier. The metabolic function and structure of the blood–brain barrier in the neonate is not fully understood and, rather than being simply immature, it is now considered suitable for the metabolic requirements of the developing brain. For instance, transport mechanisms for lactate and ketone bodies are more prominent in neonates and may increase their tolerance to hypoxia and hyperglycaemia. However, the developing blood–brain barrier may be more susceptible to the effects of metabolic toxins, such as lead, than that of an adult.

PHARMACOKINETICS

Absorption

Age related changes in pharmacokinetics are most apparent in the neonate, but by the fifth year of life are less important (Table 49.1). Drug absorption after oral administration may be erratic in the first few days of life but thereafter gastrointestinal absorption is similar to that of adults. Although the clinical effect of anaesthetic drugs and analgesics given by the rectal route in children is unpredictable, this route is useful for administering anticonvulsants for status epilepticus when intravenous access is difficult. The percutaneous route is widely used in adults for drug delivery but its value in infants is limited by the greater risk of toxicity. There are several reports of systemic toxicity after prolonged accidental contact of infant skin with various dyes, antiseptics and alcohol. Although the neonatal epidermis is comparable with that of the adult, the large surface area:weight ratio in the neonate allows increased absorption of drugs applied to the skin, with resultant overdosage. EMLA (eutectic mixture of local anaesthetics) cream contains prilocaine and may cause methaemoglobinaemia in susceptible infants; it is not recommended in infants aged under 3 months.

The transmucosal route — sublingual or nasal — has been used to deliver sedative drugs, such as fentanyl, sufentanil, ketamine or midazolam,

Table 49.1 Pharmacokinetics of drugs in children compared with 'normal' adults

	Age of child					
	Newborn preterm	Term (0–4 weeks)	Infancy	1–4 years	5–12 years	Comments
Absorption	↓	↔	↔	↔	↔	
Distribution Body water	↑↑↑	↑↑	↑	↑	↑	Weight related doses produce lower blood concentrations of water soluble drugs in the newborn
Body fat	↓↓	↓	↓ Slight	?↔	?↔	Minimal clinical effect
Plasma albumin	↓	↓	↓ Slight	↔	↔	Minimal clinical effect
Biotransformation Oxidation hydrolysis	↓↓↓	↓↓	↑↑ (After some weeks)	↑	↑ Slight	Reduce dosage for newborn and early infancy; increase dosage subsequently
N-demethylation	↓↓↓	↓	↑↑	↑	↔	Applies to theophylline, caffeine
Acetylation	↓	↓	↑	↑	↔	Reduce dose in newborn — for example, sulphonamides
Conjugation–glucuronidation	↓↓	↓	↑	↑	↔	Reduce dose in newborn — for example, chloramphenicol
Renal excretion Glomerular filtration	↓↓	↓	↓ Slight to 6 months	↔	↔	Reduce dose in first few months
Tubular secretion	↓↓	↓	↓ Slight to 6 months	↔	↔	Reduce dose in first few months

From Rylance (1988). (BMJ 1988)
↑, Increased; ↓, decreased, ↔, unaltered.

to young children, either for premedication or for sedation for minor surgical procedures. However, these techniques are not widely used because of unpredictable clinical effects and a high incidence of side-effects, especially with opioid drugs.

The intraosseous route is currently recommended for administering fluids and drugs during resuscitation. The technique is most readily performed in children under 5 years. The young marrow is highly vascularised and plasma drug concentrations are achieved that are comparable to those following intravenous administration. The intramuscular route is used very infrequently in infants because of poor muscle bulk, although age alone has little effect on absorption.

Distribution

Since total body water and extracellular fluid volume are relatively large in the neonate, the volume of distribution of water soluble drugs is increased. In order to achieve a particular clinical effect in an infant, and provided receptor capacity is the same, it may be necessary to give a higher loading dose of some drugs.

Protein binding of drugs is reduced in infants because the plasma concentrations of α_1-acid glycoprotein and albumin are also reduced; adult concentrations are achieved by the first year. The availability of binding sites is decreased and there is an increase in the free fraction of some drugs. The most important effect of reduced protein binding capacity is that competition between drugs and endogenous substances such as bilirubin may result in toxic concentrations of bilirubin.

Metabolism and excretion

All the enzymes necessary for hepatic metabolism of drugs are in place in the term neonate, although they are less active than in the adult. The enzyme systems responsible for various phase I reactions mature at different rates, but most are efficient by 2–3 years of age. However, demethylation, necessary for theophylline and caffeine metabolism, is poorly developed and these drugs need to be monitored carefully. Modern techniques for measuring the plasma concentrations of drugs are improving our knowledge of drug metabolism and showing important differences between neonates and older infants. For instance, the half-life of the active metabolite of chloral hydrate is prolonged by a factor of 4 compared with that in older children. The implications of these differences in metabolism are not fully established at present but it is clear that further studies of other commonly used drugs are warranted.

Most drugs or their metabolites are excreted by the kidney. The capacity of the kidney to excrete drugs increases with age. In the neonate glomerular filtration is decreased, leading to delayed excretion of some drugs, including antibiotics and digoxin. By 6 months of age, adults patterns of excretion are achieved.

INHALATIONAL ANAESTHETICS

Inhalational anaesthetics remain popular both for induction and maintenance of anaesthesia in children. In addition to the general features of the ideal anaesthetic, in children the inhaled anaesthetic should not be pungent or irritant to the upper airway and should provide smooth induction of anaesthesia. The more relevant pharmacokinetic and pharmacodynamic differences between adults and children will be discussed and the advantages and disadvantages of individual agents in children will be reviewed. Some of the features of anaesthetic agents in both age groups are shown in Table 49.2.

Uptake and distribution

The uptake of inhaled anaesthetics is greater in infants and children than in adults. This difference is due to several factors: (1) the blood:gas solubility coefficient of the commonly used agents is less in infants than in adults; (2) cardiac output distribution is mainly to vessel-rich tissues, such as brain, heart and lung; and (3) the relatively greater alveolar ventilation in infants. It is important to remember during the administration of volatile anaesthesia to children that uptake is more rapid, tissue saturation more readily achieved and the potential for overdosage greater than in adults.

Minimum alveolar concentration

The minimum alveolar concentration (MAC) of halothane, isoflurane and desflurane is age

Table 49.2 Some features of inhalational anaesthetics in adults and children

	Halothane	Isoflurane	Desflurane	Sevoflurane
Chemical structure	CF_3—CHClBr	CHF_2—O—CHCl—CF_3	CHF_2—O—CHF—CF_3	CH_2F—O—CH(CF_3)CF_3
Boiling point (°C)	50.2	48.5	23.5	58.6
Metabolised (%)	15–20	0.2	0.02	3.3
Blood/gas solubility			0.42	0.66
Adults	2.4	1.4		0.66
Neonates	2.1	1.2	—	
MAC			7.0	2.05
Adults	0.75	1.2	9.2	3.3
Neonates	0.87	1.6		
MAC depression by N_2O (%)			53	—
Adults	53	60	26	24
Children	60	40		
Systolic blood pressure reduction (%)			22	0
Children	13	16	34	34
Neonates	23	—		
Preterm	25	30	—	—
Heart rate	↓	↑	– or ↓	– or ↑
Anaesthetic induction	Smooth	Irritant	Irritant	Smooth (± excitation)

dependent. In general, MAC increases during infancy and decreases after 6 months of age. The variation of MAC with age may be related to differences in cerebral blood flow, the uptake of the anaesthetic agent or the higher metabolic rate in infants. Sevoflurane does not demonstrate a similar increase in MAC in infancy but the mechanism for this difference is not understood.

Halothane

Halothane is probably the most popular inhalational agent used in children. Although it is a potent myocardial depressant and is arrhythmogenic, it has a pleasant odour and is easy to administer. MAC in infants is 1.08%. Children are more tolerant than adults to the myocardial sensitising effects of halothane when vasoconstrictors such as adrenaline are used. Halothane is more likely than isoflurane or sevoflurane to cause bradycardia. Controversies regarding the repeated used of halothane have not been fully resolved. Although there have been sporadic case reports of halothane hepatitis in children after repeated exposure, the general consensus amongst paediatric anaesthetists is that repeat halothane anaesthesia is acceptable practice in children, the advantages of halothane outweighing the theoretical risk of hepatitis.

Enflurane

Enflurane is not a satisfactory agent for induction in children because of its unpleasant odour and the difficulty in delivering sufficiently high inspired concentrations. It is often used instead of halothane when repeat anaesthesia is necessary, but there is no clear evidence that it is a safe alternative. It has a more potent respiratory depressant effect than halothane or isoflurane in children.

Isoflurane

Isoflurane displays many of the features of the ideal anaesthetic but its pungent odour makes induction of anesthesia unpleasant in children. Although increased experience with isoflurane, and premedication with atropine or sedation, may reduce the incidence of troublesome side-effects such as laryngospasm and coughing, the drug lacks the smoothness and safety of halothane.

Sevoflurane

Sevoflurane is a pleasant-smelling ether and studies indicate that it may be a useful alternative to halothane for induction of anaesthesia in children. Despite its lower blood:gas solubility coefficient, the induction time in children is similar to that of halothane. It interacts with soda lime to produce a series of degradation products, the most notable of which is compound A. The implications of this interaction in neonates and children require further investigation.

Desflurane

Desflurane is not suitable for induction of anaesthesia in children because of its pronounced tendency to provoke laryngospasm and breath holding. Although recovery from desflurane anaesthesia is rapid, it may be associated with excitement and restlessness in children; however, desflurane is the least metabolised of all the volatile anaesthetic drugs and this feature may be an advantage for prolonged administration.

INTRAVENOUS ANAESTHETICS

Thiopentone

Intravenous induction of anaesthesia is becoming more popular in infants and children with the advent of EMLA cream. Thiopentone is probably the most useful drug, providing smooth induction of anaesthesia. In neonates, anaesthesia is usually induced at a dose of 3 mg kg^{-1}, whereas older infants and children may require up to 7 mg kg^{-1}. Thiopentone may cause cardiovascular collapse, especially in the presence of hypovolaemia, and it should be used with caution in infants with congenital heart disease.

Propofol

Propofol may be used for induction and maintenance of anaesthesia in children more than 3 years old. Dose requirements are higher in the younger age group, probably because of differences in the volume of distribution. It is associated with pain on injection, which is not always blocked by the addition of lignocaine and which is independent of the use of EMLA cream. The incidence of excitatory effects appears to be greater in children. Propofol is probaby a better choice of induction agent than thiopentone for day care surgery because recovery from anaesthesia is more rapid and more complete.

Propofol is not recommended for sedation by continuous infusion in children, following reports of deaths in children in intensive care when this technique was used. The mechanism by which metabolic acidosis and fatal heart failure developed in these children is unclear.

Ketamine

This phencyclidine derivative is widely used in paediatric anaesthesia, both for induction of anaesthesia in high risk infants and for postoperative analgesia. It is a most versatile drug and may be administered orally, rectally, nasally, intramuscularly or intravenously. Dose requirements are higher in children under 2 years of age. Older children may experience similar dreams and hallucinations as adults and these must be prevented by simultaneous administration of an intravenous benzodiazepine or opioid agonist such as morphine. Ketamine stimulates copious oral and bronchial secretions, which may be prevented by atropine. Although protective reflexes may appear active during ketamine anaesthesia, this is illusory and the drug demands the same standard of care and monitoring in use as any other induction agent.

ANALGESICS

The management of pain in children is hampered by difficulty of assessment of pain in the younger age group and the greater risk of toxicity with potent analgesics. Paracetamol can be given orally or rectally and is widely used for managing minor discomfort or as an adjunct to other analgesics. Aspirin is not recommended in children but non-aspirin-containing non-steroidal anti-inflammatory drugs are being used more frequently for pain relief. Although these drugs can have serious side-effects on the gastro-intestinal tract, renal function and platelets, they are proving useful in combination with other therapies. Their role and safety profile in children requires further evaluation.

Opioids

Opioids form the basis of most analgesic regimens in children. Intravenous morphine, given either by bolus, infusion or patient controlled analgesia systems, is the gold standard and is generally satisfactory in older children. However, in infants under 3 months old the efficacy and toxicity of morphine is unpredictable for the following reasons: (1) the clearance of morphine is slower in this age group, (2) morphine is partly metabolised to morphine-6-glucuronide, a long acting, potent analgesic and respiratory depressant; (3) transfer across the neonatal blood–brain barrier may be greater; and (4) neonates display great variation in their ability to metabolise morphine. For these reasons the drug must be used with caution in spontaneously breathing infants, and the respiratory effects assessed clinically and with the aid of monitors, including pulse oximetry. Opioids can also be administered to children by the epidural route but the optimum drug and dosage is not clearly established.

Bupivacaine

Local anaesthetic techniques are also useful in managing postoperative pain. Bupivacaine, the most popular drug, must be used with caution in neonates because their immature hepatic metabolism, slower clearance and decreased protein binding capacity increase the risk of toxicity. Even in older children continuous infusion techniques with bupivacaine have been associated with systemic toxicity, including seizures and cardiovascular collapse.

MUSCLE RELAXANTS

Suxamethonium

Suxamethonium is a muscle relaxant that acts by causing profound depolarisation at the motor end-plate. It is widely used in paediatric anaesthesia on account of its rapid but short duration of action and the excellent conditions it provides for tracheal intubation. The ED_{90} (90% effective dose) is greater in infants and children than in adults, probably because of the difference in extracellular fluid volumes. Thus, larger doses of the drug are required in infants (2–4 mg kg^{-1}) and children (2 mg kg^{-1}). In view of the risk of bradycardia and cardiac arrest with even a single dose of suxamethonium in the younger age group, atropine (10–20 µg kg^{-1} intravenously) is recommended before giving the relaxant. Infants do not develop fasciculations with suxamethonium, probably as a result of their small muscle bulk. The incidence of muscle pain in children after suxamethonium administration is unknown. Older children approaching adolescence should be pretreated with a small dose of non-depolarising muscle relaxant in the same way as adults, taking other risk factors into consideration. However, it should be remembered that diplopia is an uncomfortable side-effect of this type of pretreatment.

In view of recent reports of fatal hyperkalaemic cardiac arrest with suxamethonium in boys with undiagnosed myopathy, it has been suggested that its use should be restricted to emergencies only. However, because of its many advantages and the lack of a suitable alternative, this suggestion has not met with widespread approval. Anaesthetists should be aware of the possibility of this rare complication and be familiar with the management of cardiac arrest and hyperkalaemia. The relationship between suxamethonium and masseter spasm and the subsequent risk of malignant hyperthermia is still uncertain; however, there is considerable evidence that masseter muscle tone increases briefly after administration of suxamethonium. Apparent spasm or resistance to mouth opening may be the result of premature attempts to intubate the airway while masseter tone is at a maximum. Alternatively, it may represent inadequate neuromuscular blockade due to underdosage with suxamethonium. It seems reasonable to conclude that masseter spasm alone is rarely a sign of malignant hyperthermia. Nevertheless, the management of a child with masseter spasm and the decision to abandon surgery must be judged on an individual basis, taking into account other signs of malignant hyperthermia. Although the evidence is not conclusive, it would seem prudent to avoid suxamethonium after halothane, as this drug combination may be associated with a higher risk of malignant hyperthermia.

Non-depolarising muscle relaxants

The neuromuscular junction of the neonate is more sensitive to the effects of non-depolarising relaxants than that of the adult. Thus the onset of neuromuscular blockade is more rapid in this age group and duration of action is longer. However, there is considerable variation in their response to different relaxants and the influence of age is complex — for instance, although neonates need a smaller dose of atracurium than older children or adults for a similar degree of neuromuscular blockade, the duration of block is shorter, possibly because of an increased rate of metabolism. Conversely, vecuronium block is prolonged in neonates, due perhaps to slower metabolism and a greater volume of distribution. Mivacurium, a short acting relaxant, has a more rapid onset of action in children than in adults and a shorter duration of action. In general, these intermediate acting relaxants are suitable for children because of their wide safety margin. For prolonged surgical procedures continuous infusions of these drugs are satisfactory.

Rocuronium is currently being evaluated in children. Its rapid onset of action makes it an attractive alternative to suxamethonium. There is some evidence that its duration of action is shorter in children than in adults but further studies are necessary before its role in paediatric practice is clear.

FURTHER READING

Gregory G A 1994 Pediatric anesthesia, 3rd edn. Churchill Livingstone, New York

Mayers D J, Hindmarsch K E, Sankaran K, Gorecki D K J, Kasian G F 1991 Chloral hydrate disposition following single-dose administration to critically ill neonates and children. Developmental Pharmacology and Therapeutics 16: 71–77

Morselli P L 1989 Clinical pharmacology of the perinatal period and early infancy. Clinical Pharmacokinetics 17 (suppl 1): 13–28

Rylance G W 1988 Prescribing for infants and children. British Medical Journal 296: 984–986

Steward D J 1995 Manual of pediatric anesthesia. Churchill Livingstone, Edinburgh

Stewart C F, Hampton E M 1987 Effect of maturation on drug disposition in pediatric patients. Clinical Pharmacy 6: 548–564

Tyler, D C 1994 Pharmacology of pain management. Pediatric Clinics of North America 41: 59–72

50

Physiology and pharmacology of ageing

W. F. M. Wallace
R. Dwyer

The elderly account for a large proportion of patients undergoing anaesthesia and surgery, and an even larger proportion of the resulting morbidity and mortality. This chapter deals with the physiological changes brought about by advancing years and the manner in which these affect the body's response to drugs. These changes have implications for the care of patients before, during and after anaesthesia, including intensive care.

PHYSIOLOGY

This section is concerned with the recognised pattern of change with age in the physiological functioning of the body and its various systems. Currently there is no evidence that this process can be interrupted, although its effects may be accelerated or mimicked, e.g. solar radiation has an ageing effect on skin. Theories of ultimate causation will not be considered. The emphasis will be on the consequences of the ageing process and how these may affect the elderly patient's response to anaesthetic and other drugs. The changes described occur throughout life and are remarkably consistent in their 'downhill' nature. Initially, they are balanced by the effects of growth and maturation. It is usual to examine the process from the age of about 20 years onwards. After this, the magnitude and severity of change increase proportionally with the patient's age, although age related disease may accelerate the process.

Patterns of change underlying the ageing process

Four fairly clear cut changes occur with ageing of the tissues and these account for much of the well documented effect of ageing on organ function. These underlying changes are a loss of flexibility, alteration in body composition, loss of cells (and extracellular materials) which are not replaced, and genetic deterioration — mutations which erode the normal control of cellular function.

Loss of flexibility

Several illustrations will be considered, and other examples given when specific systems are discussed. Commonly-known features of ageing are joint stiffness and wrinkled skin, the latter giving a major clue to a person's age. Both indicate loss of the ability of tissues to alter their shape readily and then return to their original state. A more precise example is the compliance of the aorta. This has been measured in postmortem specimens from individuals of varying ages. Compliance is a measure of the response obtained from a given input. In the case of the aorta, the change in volume in response to a change in distending pressure indicates the compliance, which is measured in units of volume/pressure, e.g. ml mmHg^{-1}. (The same units are used for pulmonary compliance.) This loss of aortic compliance reduces the smoothing effect of the aorta on arterial blood pressure, so that in elderly patients the pulse pressure is often much higher than in young people.

Another example is the lens of the eye. In young people the lens has a natural convex shape which is made less convex by the pull of the suspensory ligaments when the ciliary muscle is relaxed, as when the subject focuses at infinity. During focusing at the near point (the minimum distance from the eye where an object can be seen in sharp focus), the circular ciliary muscle contracts maximally, relaxing the suspensory ligaments attached to the lens, and the lens springs into its convex state. With ageing the lens becomes less able to change its shape (accommodate) and the power of the lens (a measure of the range of focal length) decreases. In fact recession of the near point begins in early childhood, an example of the lifelong nature of the ageing process. This lengthening of the distance from the eye to the near point is recognised as an effect of ageing in the term presbyopia (literally, vision in the elderly).

Body composition

One of the reasons for the loss of flexibility with age is almost certainly the progressive loss of body fluids (as a percentage of body weight) from infancy, and indeed from the fetal state. Whereas the percentage of water in the body of a young adult is generally taken as 60–70%, it is actually much higher in the fetus or infant, falling to around 50% in old age. By 60 years, body weight is often some 25% higher in men and 20% higher in women than in mature young adults. After this, however, body weight tends to decrease. In contrast, body composition changes progressively and irreversibly throughout middle age and into old age. Ageing increases the ratio of lipid to aqueous body tissues and thereby increases the fraction of total body mass which serves as a reservoir for anaesthetic and other lipid soluble drugs. Women in particular experience a very marked increase in total body lipid. Simultaneously, osteoporosis reduces bone mass and there is a significant reduction of intracellular water, reflecting the loss of metabolically active tissues. Elderly men undergo a more generalised, multicompartmental loss of tissue mass, with moderate reductions in both adipose tissue and bone. Unlike ageing women, there is a marked diminution of both intracellular and interstitial water in aged men, probably because of a dramatic decrease in skeletal muscle mass.

The functional consequences of this loss of muscle tissue are a 30–50% decrease in maximal oxygen consumption in physically active men, and highly significant reductions in resting oxygen consumption in both men and women.

Overall metabolic activity also decreases in a similar manner. The reduction in resting cardiac output that occurs with age reflects loss of active tissue. Heat production also becomes less effective, contributing to a reduced ability to maintain core temperature in cold environments.

There is some evidence that muscle strength can be usefully improved in the elderly by appropriate physical activity.

Loss of cells

In a number of tissues, including brain, kidney, liver and cardiac muscle, cellular multiplication ceases at or soon after birth, so that cells lost due to injury, wear and tear and disease are not replaced. Similarly, extracellular tissue such as the cartilage of joints is not renewed, contributing to the joint stiffness already mentioned.

Genetic deterioration

There is good evidence that ionising radiation, to which all are exposed, largely from natural sources such as cosmic rays, leads to damage of the immensely complicated deoxyribonucleic acids which constitute the genetic material of cells. Two well known findings support this suggestion. The first is the great increase in the frequency of cancer with increasing age. The second is the increased incidence of the Down syndrome with maternal age. In the mother, the primordial follicles are all present at birth; with increasing age there has therefore been an increased opportunity for genetic deterioration not countered by cell multiplication and chromosomal renewal. The Down syndrome is associated with particulary gross genetic change — trisomy, or tripling, of chromosome 21.

Changes in specific systems

The effects of the above general changes will now be considered in relation to specific body systems.

Nervous system

Here the effect of loss of cells is particularly responsible for changes with ageing. Several examples concerned with patients and with the anaesthetised patient will be considered. Well known but of great importance are the deteriorations in the special senses: vision, hearing, smell and taste. Two major patterns are seen with vision. Firstly, there is loss of visual acuity, i.e. loss of the ability to distinguish two images when they are close together. Secondly, there is the loss of accommodation referred to earlier. The first requires thought to be given to producing larger print for the elderly. The second contributes to the need for large print, in that recession of the near point, which may not be corrected fully with spectacles, means that the angle subtended by a given size of letter is reduced. As well as providing large print for all written medical communications, such as drug labelling, the provision of excellent lighting is important in that this induces pupillary constriction, and the smaller pupil leads to a sharper image, with less spherical aberration.

Deterioration of hearing may increase reliance on the written word. Loss of hearing with age (presbycusis, or the hearing pattern of the elderly) appears to depend largely on deterioration of the most sensitive initial part of the organ of hearing, in that high pitched sounds mediated here are more affected than low pitched sounds detected by a greater length of the more robust regions remote from the oval window. The frequencies lost are particularly those associated with consonants, critical for the interpretation of speech. A lower frequency of voice tends to be more clearly heard.

The autonomic neurones, with relatively small, unmyelinated, slowly conducting C-type axons, are particularly susceptible to ageing, particularly in diabetics. This leads to impairment of the many functions depending on such nerves, such as peripheral vascular control, swallowing and pain from the viscera. Such conditions will affect the patient's responses during and after anaesthesia. The presence of autonomic deterioration (neuropathy) can be detected by physiological tests of reflexes involving these nerves, e.g. changes in peripheral blood flow with cooling, which relies on sympathetic nerves, and respiratory sinus arrhythmia, which relies on the cardiac vagus. Respiratory sinus arrhythmia (the amplitude of heart rate variation during a maximal respiratory cycle at a breathing frequency of 6 breaths per minute) has been reported to diminish from 20–25 in young adults to 10–15 at age 70–80 years.

Temperature regulation depends on widespread autonomic reflexes and deteriorates with ageing. The elderly are less sensitive to small changes in skin temperature than the young, and, as discussed above, the efferent side of the reflexes is also impaired. Thus the elderly are more susceptible to excessive cooling (hypothermia) in cold environments, and to an excessive rise in core temperature (hyperthermia) in an environmental temperature above the thermoneutral.

A major problem with the elderly is disturbance of the sleep–wake patterns. These are established in infancy when the infant moves from a pattern of sleeping and waking every few hours to the adult pattern of a single sleeping period associated with the hours of darkness. Circadian rhythms also become established in synchrony with the sleep–wake rhythm. In old age these patterns begin to fragment. The elderly subject is less alert during the day and may indulge in frequent naps; at night sleep becomes discontinuous and the proportions of deep sleep and of rapid eye movement sleep decrease. Changes in circadian rhythms and frequency of micturition may contribute to poor sleep quality. The effect is distressing and the combination of wakefulness at night and lack of concentration during the day may make the sufferer seek hypnotics, but these cannot restore the normal sleep–wake rhythm and in the long term are likely to impair daytime function without improving night-time sleep.

Cardiovascular system

Impaired function of the cardiovascular system is a major factor limiting activity in the elderly. About 60% of elderly patients have clinical evidence of cardiovascular disease and another 20% may have subclinical disease. It is thought that less than 15% of geriatric patients have cardiovascular systems that are physiologically sound. Cardiovascular disease accounts for approximately 10% of perioperative deaths. In the absence of disease, cardiac function sufficient for a basal level of activity is preserved into advanced old age.

The main age related changes in the heart are ventricular wall thickening, myocardial fibrosis and valvular calcification. The resulting decrease in ventricular compliance, together with the deterioration in baroreceptor responsiveness, makes elderly patients intolerant of changes in blood volume. Thus decreased volume leads more readily to hypotension, and increased volume may precipitate congestive cardiac failure. Reduced compliance of large arteries necessitates a higher left ventricular pressure to achieve a given stroke volume and this, in turn, induces further hypertrophy.

Maximal activity depends on a maximal cardiac output; in the young this is mainly achieved by an increase in heart rate. As an approximation, a person's maximal heart rate declines by one beat per minute for each year of life (maximal heart rate = 220 – age in years) and this decline has been found to be a very constant feature of ageing. Age related cardiac slowing is at least partially compensated for by an increase in stroke volume, according to the Frank–Starling hypothesis, end-diastolic volume increasing due to greater preload. Despite this, maximal cardiac output is said to decrease by 1% per year from the mid-50s.

Loss of autonomic nerves reduces the variability of blood flow. Vasoconstriction is less efficient so heat loss is greater in cool conditions. Similarly, vascular responsiveness to the various controlling chemicals tends to decline, so that vasodilatation is also less effective, leading to inadequate heat loss in hot conditions. These factors also impair baroreflex responses, thus accounting for the much higher incidence of postural hypotension with advancing age. Clearly, loss of autonomic integrity will have widespread consequences for vascular control.

Blood

Ageing alone has a minimal effect on the haematocrit, white cell count, the number or function of platelets, or coagulation. Total bone marrow mass and spleen size reduce progressively with increasing age, and erythrocyte fragility increases. Anaemia and bleeding diatheses are almost always due to disease or dietary factors, although the elderly are slower to restore the circulating red cell mass after haemorrhage. The erythrocyte sedimentation rate increases steadily with age, presumably because of a change in blood constituents which facilitates rouleaux formation. The well known susceptibility of elderly patients to life threatening infection suggests a functional decline in the immune response. Thymic activity declines sharply after adolescence.

Respiratory system

The effects of ageing have probably been more thoroughly documented in the respiratory system than in any other. Patterns of change particularly reflect loss of flexibility, with a loss of elastic tissue in the lungs as ageing progresses. This causes a progressive loss of elastic recoil and increases lung compliance. Loss of elastic tissue leaves small airways poorly supported and there is a tendency for these to collapse. There is also a loss of alveoli due to breakdown of the alveolar septum and this results in increased anatomical and physiological dead space. Since elastic tissue is necessary for holding open the small airways during forced expiration, it is not surprising that the forced expiratory volume in 1 second (FEV_1) declines steadily with age and becomes a decreasing percentage of the vital capacity. Vital capacity also declines with increasing years, airway closure trapping more air distal to closed airways. This trapping steadily increases residual volume, so that there is little age related change in total lung capacity. The lung volume at which this airway closure begins is called the closing volume and, as this increases with age, it may eventually exceed the functional residual capacity. Thus in the elderly small airways may close during normal breathing, and particularly during anaesthesia.

Calcification of costal cartilages decreases chest wall compliance, so, despite increased lung compliance, total pulmonary compliance may change very little. Functional residual capacity (FRC) increases slightly but progressively.

These well documented changes diminish the efficiency of gas exchange in the elderly. The alveolar–arterial oxygen pressure gradient increases and the arterial oxygen tension is about 10% lower than in the young. The amount of ventilation necessary for the uptake of 1 litre of oxygen increases. In a similar manner to the cardiovascular system the reserves of function above the resting state decline and the maximal ventilation rate decreases.

Renal system

The mass of the kidney is reduced by approximately 30% in the very old and there is said to be only half the number of functioning renal glomeruli in octogenarians compared with young adults. Ageing also affects renal function through its effects on the renal vasculature, total renal blood flow decreasing by approximately 10% per decade in the adult years. The glomerular filtration rate (GFR) in the average adult decreases at the rate of some 8 ml min^{-1} per decade. Both GFR and renal plasma flow (RPF) decline more sharply than would be expected from the change in kidney mass because the renal vasculature is compromised preferentially. The GFR decreases more slowly than RPF owing to a compensatory increase in the filtration fraction.

As with other organs, the kidneys have considerable reserves of function, so that in normal conditions blood urea and electrolytes can be maintained. Despite the reduction in GFR, serum creatinine concentrations in the elderly remain within the normal range, probably in part due to the reduction in skeletal muscle mass; however, the ability to deal with severe disturbances of fluids and electrolytes is impaired. One function that tests the kidneys to the limit is production of a maximally concentrated urine. This relies on maximal reabsorption from the collecting ducts in the presence of antidiuretic hormone (vasopressin). Maximal reabsorption relies in turn on the extent of the medullary hypertonicity generated by the thick ascending limb of the loop of Henle. It has been found that maximal urinary osmolality declines steadily with age from a value in young adults of around four times the normal osmolality of the plasma and body fluids. Because dilution of the urine also relies on the loop of Henle, the range of dilution/concentration is constricted at both ends. Thus, as well as having more severe effects on the circulation in the elderly, disturbances of the body fluids are more slowly corrected. Loss of lean body mass reduces total body stores of exchangeable potassium and predisposes to iatrogenic hypokalaemia.

Reduced renal vascularity, changes in regional blood flow and concurrent medication (non-steroidal anti-inflammatory drugs, some antibiotics) increase the likelihood of renal ischaemia, and the risk is heightened by pre-existing renal impairment. Acute renal failure is thought to account for one fifth of perioperative deaths in older patients.

Metabolism

With declining activity in the major organs as cells are lost, it is not surprising that basal metabolic rate and maximal metabolic rate decline with age. The few studies of adrenocortical and endocrine function that have been performed in the elderly indicate that, for the most part, these functions remain intact or only modestly compromised. However, it is recognised that elderly patients exhibit an almost universal and progressive decrease in their ability to handle a glucose load. The mechanism of glucose intolerance is probably insulin antagonism or impairment of insulin function. Age related decrease in lean body mass may also be a factor as these tissues act as glycogen stores. The impairment in glucose utilisation suggests that intravenous carbohydrates should be given cautiously to elderly patients.

Alimentary system

Here again the effect of ageing has been studied by quantitative measures in subjects of differing ages. It has been found that both basal and stimulated gastric acid secretion decline with age. This could have consequences for both digestion and protection against ingested organisms. Impairment of intrinsic nerve function would cause the motility of the gastrointestinal tract to diminish with increasing years and delay gastric emptying, particularly in the presence of autonomic neuropathy, as in diabetes mellitus.

Liver

Microsomal and non-microsomal enzyme activities in liver biopsy specimens from young and elderly adults suggest there is little qualitative change in enzyme function with advancing years. However, elderly men, but not women, frequently have significant reductions in plasma cholinesterase activity. Also, for several of the benzodiazepines, elderly women appear to maintain normal rates of hepatic clearance more frequently than do men. There may therefore be some subtle but important gender-specific changes in enzyme systems, particularly those involved in oxidative phase I forms of drug metabolism.

By 80 years, the mass of the liver has reduced by as much as 40% and there is a corresponding decrease in hepatic blood flow. Liver function studies indicate that loss of liver tissue impairs hepatic function. Healthy patients over 70 years who have no evidence of hepatic dysfunction have bromsulphthalein excretion values in the abnormal range. It would seem likely that it is the quantitative loss of hepatocytes and reduced liver blood flow that contribute most to the age related decrease in the clearance of most drugs that are metabolised by the liver.

Overall effects

The overall effects produced by combined loss of function in the above and other systems can be seen in situations where the body is stressed to the maximum. Two examples will be considered, one related to normal activity and one to disease.

Time to complete long distance races, such as marathons, has been documented for adults of various ages. Completion time is shortest around 20–30 years, where maturity and improved efficiency from practice are optimal. However, above this age completion time increases, and the increase is steep above 40–50 years. For the shorter distance of 1 mile, the world record for subjects around 20–30 years is under 4 minutes, while for subjects of 90 years of age the record is between 13 and 14 minutes. As discussed above, important contributing factors to this general decline of function include decreases in maximal cardiac output and maximal minute volume, which, together with impaired efficiency of the neuromuscular system, bring about an inexorable decline in maximal activity.

Secondly, the response to widespread full thickness burns is an example of the challenge to the combined resources of the body systems — the ability to mount an appropriate neuro-endocrine response to stress, including maintenance of the circulation, and the ability to deal with toxins and infection. As an approximate rule, it has been found that those of age 20 years can survive around 80% destruction of the body surface in this way, whereas, reciprocally, the limit for survival at age 80 years is around 20%.

Another way of looking at the overall response of the body to various stresses is through the homeostatic curve (Fig. 50.1). This can be recognised as applying to many functions, from main-

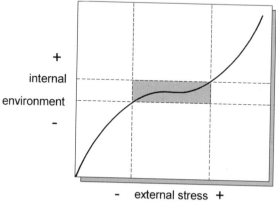

Figure 50.1 The homeostatic curve, whereby external stress on the internal environment of the body fails to produce a significant effect over the normal range of homeostasis but, outside this range, changes in the external environment produce disorders due to dramatic changes in the internal environment of the body cells. The external stress represents a factor that threatens the normal internal environment, e.g. an increase (+) or decrease (–) in temperature, gain (+) or loss (–) of extracellular fluid. Within the shaded zone any change in the internal environment does not interfere with normal function. The effect of age is to narrow the plateau of effective response.

tenance of a normal core temperature to the curve of cerebrovascular autoregulation. In all cases, a stress that challenges normal homeostasis can be resisted over a range of severities to give a plateau of normal function (core temperature, cerebral blood flow), but when the stress becomes too great in any direction (hot environment, cold environment, fall in arterial blood pressure, rise in arterial blood pressure) the expected deviation from normal occurs, with severe deviation leading to fatal changes. The ability of the elderly to adapt psychologically to a change in environment (e.g. hospitalisation) or to a change in lifestyle as a result of surgery (e.g. amputation, colostomy) is similarly reduced.

PHARMACOLOGY

Ageing alters the pharmacokinetics and pharmacodynamics of drugs. Knowledge of these alterations allows a more rational approach when considering anaesthesia for this high risk group of patients.

Ageing may affect drug pharmacokinetics in the following ways:

- uptake (e.g. changes in respiratory function, gastrointestinal absorption)
- rate of redistribution (decreased cardiac output, vascular disease)
- distribution (e.g. increased volume of distribution of lipid soluble drugs, changes in plasma proteins)
- decreased clearance by liver and kidney.

Alterations in drug pharmacokinetics occur as a normal part of ageing and this chapter deals with their effects in the healthy elderly population. The effects of disease must be superimposed on the changes outlined below.

There may be some argument about the definition of an 'elderly patient' and there is no abrupt change in physiology at any given age. The physiological changes described above occur in a gradual fashion after 30 years, with the rate of change increasing somewhat over 70 years. Change occurs at different rates in different individuals: patients who are 'young' or 'old' for their age are commonly observed. Heterogeneity and marked interindividual variability in response to drugs are characteristics of the elderly population.

There is an element of natural selection in the population who survive to reach old age and the physical condition of individual patients is commonly better than that predicted by studying the rate of change in the population as a whole.

Pharmacokinetics: drug absorption, distribution and elimination

Intravenous absorption is immediate in all age groups. Bioavailability of orally administered drugs is not altered by ageing, despite the decrease in function of the gastrointestinal tract. It has been hypothesised that any decrease in absorption of drugs from the gut is counter-balanced by a decrease in first pass metabolism in the liver. The rate of absorption of drugs by inhalation is determined by (1) alveolar ventilation, (2) respiratory function, (3) cardiac output, (4) blood:gas and (5) tissue:blood partition coefficients of drugs. Ageing affects these variables but the changes have opposing effects on the rate of increase in arterial partial pressures, e.g. blood:gas partition coefficients decrease but respiratory function is impaired. The overall effect on the rate of increase in arterial partial pressures compared with the effect on younger people is unchanged when administering isoflurane but slightly slowed with halothane (Fig. 50.2).

The pharmacokinetics of potent, highly lipid soluble anaesthetic agents are greatly influenced by cardiac output. The action of these agents in the central compartment (which includes the brain and heart) is terminated by redistribution to peripheral compartments. Decreases in cardiac output slow redistribution from the central compartment. This increases the magnitude, and prolongs the effect, of anaesthetic agents on the brain and cardiovascular systems. Elderly patients may have a lower cardiac output than the young (unless highly conditioned) and are more sensitive to the cardiovascular depressant effects of anaesthetic agents. A decreased rate of redistribution of drugs from the central compartment is important in decreasing dose require-

ments and increasing the duration of action of anaesthetic agents in the elderly.

Decreased serum albumin concentration leads to reduced plasma protein binding and a smaller initial volume of distribution for injected drugs. This results in increased free drug and an exaggerated pharmacological effect immediately after administration. Decreased serum albumin concentration decreases the blood:gas partition coefficient for volatile agents, which tends to increase the rate of uptake of volatile agents. However, the protein that binds basic drugs, α_1-acid glycoprotein, is present in the same concentrations in the elderly as in younger individuals.

Replacement of protein by lipid and fibrous tissue throughout the body causes an increase in lipid and a decrease in water as proportions of body mass. The volume of distribution of lipid soluble drugs increases, resulting in slower elimination and prolonged effects. This is important for the potent anaesthetic agents which are highly lipid soluble. Conversely, there is a decrease in the volume of distribution of water soluble drugs, such as alcohol, muscle relaxants and digoxin. This tends to increase their initial clinical effect and to decrease dose requirements. However, many factors influence the magnitude and duration of drug effects and the pharmacokinetics of each drug must be considered individually.

In the liver and kidney hepatocytes and nephrons are lost. Hepatic blood flow diminishes and drug elimination is slowed. This is particularly true for drugs with a high hepatic clearance, such as lignocaine and propranolol. It has been suggested that, in the elderly, liver blood flow decreases more in response to abdominal surgery than in the young, thereby reducing hepatic clearance. Increasing age inhibits different hepatic enzyme systems to different degrees, with oxidative enzyme systems being more affected than conjugative systems. The inhibition in oxidative enzyme systems may be more pronounced in males.

Glomerular filtration rate decreases by 50% between the ages of 20 and 90 years, with implications for (1) drugs whose elimination depends on renal function, e.g. digoxin, pancuronium; and (2) drugs whose renally excreted metabolites are pharmacologically active, e.g. morphine. Tubular function also decreases, as shown by diminished capacity of the kidney to concentrate urine and to excrete H^+.

Renal and hepatic function is adequate for normal demands because of the large functional reserve and a generalised decrease in metabolic activity. However, the decrease in function leads to slower elimination and prolonged effect of many drugs used during anaesthesia. Acidosis and hypothermia influence drug disposition and are more likely in the elderly than in healthy young patients because of impaired homeostatic ability. For example, it has been proposed that acidosis causes secondary peaks in fentanyl plasma concentrations.

Hypothermia decreases metabolic rate and the rate of metabolism of drugs.

Pharmacodynamics

Decreased homeostatic ability in the elderly makes them more sensitive to the effects of anaesthetics, including cardiovascular, respiratory and central nervous system depression. There is a loss of functioning neurones in the brain, with decreased numbers of receptors, decreased affinity of receptors for neurotransmitters and a decrease in neurotransmitter concentration. It is well established that brain sensitivity to a given concentration of anaesthetic is greater in the elderly for volatile agents, benzodiazepines and opioids, but surprisingly this has not been shown with intravenous agents. Alterations in brain sensitivity in the elderly have been documented for both receptor mediated and non-receptor mediated agents.

Cardiovascular changes with ageing increase sensitivity to the effects of cardiovascular depressants such as anaesthetic agents. In equipotent concentrations isoflurane decreases cardiac output and tissue perfusion in the elderly more than in the young. Propofol used to maintain anaesthesia decreases blood pressure from baseline values more in the elderly than in the young. This may be related to the greater reliance on preload

to achieve a given stroke volume, a relative resistance to catecholamines and decreased heart rate response to baroreflex stimulation.

Respiratory depression by drugs is more common in the elderly, as evidenced by the increased incidence of apnoea after opioids or intravenous induction agents and increased incidence of aspiration owing to greater depression of airway reflexes after anaesthesia.

Drug toxicity, as evidenced by adverse reactions like bone marrow suppression or renal or hepatic toxicity, is more common in the elderly.

Many elderly patients are already taking medications before presenting for anaesthesia. This increases the possibility of drug interactions by interfering with either the pharmacokinetics or pharmacodynamics of other agents.

Sedatives: benzodiazepines, phenothiazines, droperidol

The benzodiazepines are among the large number of drugs whose effects are increased and more prolonged in the elderly. Nitrazepam 10 mg as night sedation causes prolonged impairment of psychomotor performance in the elderly but not in the young. Drowsiness is 2–3 times more common in elderly patients receiving diazepam compared with patients under 40. A single dose of triazolam caused significantly more psychomotor impairment in elderly subjects. Intramuscular midazolam 1, 2 or 3 mg has anxiolytic, sedative and amnesic effects in the elderly similar to those seen with much larger doses in the young; patients over 70 years may became unresponsive after doses that have little effect in the young. Both pharmacokinetic and pharmacodynamic changes contribute to these increased effects. The elimination half-life of diazepam increases markedly with age and in hours is approximately the same as the patient's age in years. Plasma concentrations of triazolam are higher in the elderly after a single dose. This has been reported to be due to increased volume of distribution or to decreased clearance. Changes in pharmacokinetics are less marked for agents transformed by glucuronide conjugation (temazepam, lorazepam) than by microsomal oxidation (diazepam, midazolam). Oversedation during chronic benzodiazepine use is reduced by using shorter acting agents.

The plasma concentration of midazolam required to prevent response to verbal command in an 80-year-old individual is only 25% of that required in one 40 years old, showing that brain sensitivity to benzodiazepines is markedly increased. Increased pharmacodynamic sensitivity is an important factor, in addition to alterations in pharmacokinetics.

In addition to causing depression of the central nervous system the benzodiazepines cause hypotension and hypoxaemia at lower doses in the elderly.

Data are few on the use of other sedatives in the elderly but clearance of chlordiazepoxide and tricyclic depressants is reduced. It is said that the incidence of hypotension and extrapyramidal side-effects with phenothiazines and butyrophenones is increased in the elderly, and 'high potency' agents like haloperidol may have a decreased incidence of side-effects compared to 'low potency' agents like chlorpromazine.

Intravenous induction agents

Induction dose requirements for thiopentone are 35–60% less in the elderly. It was initially proposed that this was due to decreased initial volume of distribution but is now considered to be due to a decreased rate of redistribution from the central compartment (i.e. blood, heart, brain). This leads to accumulation of thiopentone in the central compartment and higher thiopentone concentrations acting on the brain. Thiopentone causes greater cardiovascular depression in the elderly and this may explain slower redistribution from the central compartment. The onset of action of thiopentone is also slower in the elderly. Whereas time to eye opening is the same in young and elderly, full return of psychmotor skills takes 50–60% longer in the elderly. This may be explained by prolonged elimination half-life.

In contrast to benzodiazepines and volatile agents, brain sensitivity to thiopentone (and other intravenous agents) is unchanged in the elderly.

Blood concentrations of thiopentone were the same in young and elderly patients, in whom the same degree of depression of the electroencephalogram (EEG) was achieved by thiopentone.

Propofol also has decreased dose requirements (15–30%) in the elderly for induction and for maintenance of anaesthesia. The elderly wake more slowly than the young after propofol infusion, even if the total dose is less. Propofol causes an increased incidence of hypotension and apnoea in the elderly but pain on injection is less common. The cardiovascular and respiratory depression associated with propofol may be overcome by slow administration. Initially it was felt that propofol was contraindicated in the elderly but it has been shown that in equipotent doses, thiopentone (2.5 mg kg^{-1}) and propofol (1.5 mg kg^{-1}) have similar depressant effects on arterial blood pressure. Propofol controls heart rate and obtunds the hypertensive response to tracheal intubation better than thiopentone. Propofol used for maintenance of anaesthesia causes a greater decrease in blood pressure from baseline values in the elderly than it does the young.

As with thiopentone, the greater sensitivity to propofol observed in elderly patients is thought to be due to pharmacokinetic rather than pharmacodynamic factors. Blood concentrations of propofol at awakening are similar in young and elderly. Decreased initial volume of distribution and decreased plasma clearance explain the decreased dose requirements and prolonged effect of propofol in the elderly. Dose requirements of etomidate, methohexitone and ketamine are decreased in a similar fashion.

Etomidate is associated with minimal or no cardiovascular depression in the elderly. As a result, it fails to obtund the hypertensive response to tracheal intubation, especially in the elderly, in whom these responses are greater. It may be indicated in patients in whom one wishes to maintain cardiac output. The cardiovascular stimulatory effects of ketamine are retained in the elderly and this agent may be useful in the high risk patient where cardiovascular depression is undesirable, with caution advised in patients with ischaemic heart disease.

Inhalation agents

The pharmacokinetics and pharmacodynamics of volatile agents have been extensively studied in the elderly. Blood:gas partition coefficients of volatile agents decrease, tending to increase alveolar and arterial partial pressures more quickly after introduction of the agent. In addition, greater cardiovascular depression by volatile agents in the elderly should allow arterial partial pressures to increase more quickly. Conversely, decreased respiratory function and increased tissue:blood partition coefficients should slow arterial uptake.

Overall these physiological changes do not change the rate of uptake of isoflurane. Arterial partial pressures of isoflurane increase at the same rate in young and elderly subjects. Arterial partial pressures of the more soluble agent, halothane, increase slightly more slowly in the elderly but the effect is small and of little clinical significance.

Similarly, elimination of volatile agents occurs at the same rate in young and elderly. Arterial partial pressures of halothane and isoflurane decrease at the same rate in young and elderly after discontinuation of the agents (Fig. 50.2). A study over a longer period of time demonstrated greater end-tidal concentrations of volatile agents in the elderly at 2 days after discontinuation of

these agents, consistent with a greater volume of distribution of the agents. Concentrations 2 days after anaesthesia are not clinically relevant and for clinical purposes the rate of elimination of the volatile agents is the same in young and elderly.

Greater sensitivity of the elderly to the volatile agents has been clearly established and minimum alveolar concentration (MAC) for all the volatile agents decreases with increasing age. MAC for isoflurane is 1.05 at age 64 years, 1.15 at 44 years and 1.28 at 26 years. Similarly, MAC for halothane is 0.64 at age 81 years, 0.76 at 42 years and 0.84 at 25 years. Decreased anaesthetic requirement in the elderly is confirmed by studies showing awakening at lower end-tidal concentrations of isoflurane or sevoflurane in the elderly and greater depression of EEG activity at a given end-tidal isoflurane concentration.

Interestingly, nitrous oxide combined with isoflurane produces a constant rather than increasing reduction in isoflurane requirements with increasing age, suggesting that MAC of nitrous oxide is unchanged by ageing.

Because of decreased requirements for anaesthetic agents in the elderly, awareness during anaesthesia is rare in patients over 60 years. In two series which examined a total of 53 patients aware during anaesthesia the oldest was 57 years.

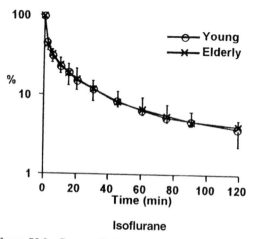

Isoflurane

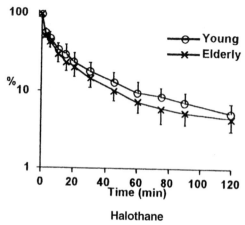

Halothane

Figure 50.2 Decay with time of arterial partial pressures of isoflurane and halothane, taking pressure at discontinuation as 100%.

Cardiovascular depression by isoflurane is greater in the elderly. Cardiac index decreases below baseline values in elderly but not young patients during 1.0 MAC isoflurane anaesthesia (Fig. 50.3). This is due to the absence of compensatory tachycardia (to maintain cardiac output) in the older age group.

Interestingly, halothane has similar cardiovascular depressant effects in both young and elderly. Although halothane depresses cardiovascular function more than isoflurane in the young, the agents have very similar cardiovascular effects in the elderly.

Analgesics

Pain threshold is unchanged in the elderly but the effects of opioids are greater and more prolonged than in younger patients. This often permits a reduction in dosage. Some studies of patient controlled analgesia report the same usage in young and old, with the old achieving better analgesia, others show reduced usage in the older patients but the same degree of pain relief. There is an increase in the incidence of undesirable side-effects in the elderly, with a higher likelihood of apnoeic episodes and hypotension. Because of the elderly's increased proportion of body fat and reduced clearance capacity particular care must be taken to avoid drug cumulation when prescribing repeat doses of powerful respiratory depressants such as opioids.

Morphine 10 mg has a better analgesic effect in the elderly than in the young, and fentanyl 30 μg kg^{-1} induces anaesthesia more reliably. The doses of fentanyl and alfentanil necessary to achieve a given level of depression of the EEG are thought to decrease by a factor of about 50% between the ages of 20 and 90 years. Dose requirements of alfentanil as a supplement to nitrous oxide anaesthesia are about 25% less in the elderly.

There is conflicting evidence as to whether these differences are due to pharmacokinetic or pharmacodynamic factors. Pharmacokinetic alterations explain decreased requirements due to reduced plasma clearance or smaller volume of distribution resulting in increased plasma or tissue concentrations. In addition, elimination of the active metabolite of morphine, morphine-6-glucuronide, may be delayed as a consequence of decreased renal function.

There is evidence suggesting increased brain sensitivity to the effects of opioids in the elderly. In addition, brain concentrations may decrease more slowly than plasma concentrations and these are a poor reflection of clinical effects.

Pethidine is commonly used in the elderly because of a belief that it is safer than other agents in this age group but there are no reliable

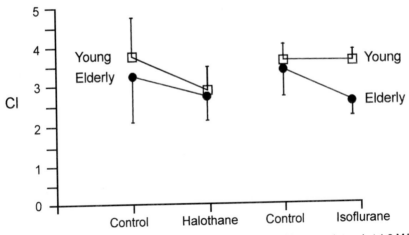

Figure 50.3 Cardiac index (1 min^{-1} m^{-2}) in young and elderly subjects awake and at 1.0 MAC isoflurane or halothane. (Data from McKinney M S, Fee J P H, Clarke R S J 1993 British Journal of Anaesthesia 71: 696–701.)

data to support this. No particular agent is safer in the elderly and all have been associated with toxic effects.

Non-steroidal anti-inflammatory drugs are frequently used for postoperative pain in the elderly and they are effective and useful drugs. Although there is a risk of side-effects such as peptic ulceration and renal impairment with long term treatment, it is not clear to what extent this is likely when these drugs are given over short periods; however, they should be avoided in patients with bleeding or clotting abnormalities, dyspepsia, asthma or renal impairment. Pharmacokinetic or pharmacodynamic interactions may occur with other drugs. Clearance may be prolonged and maximum recommended doses should not be exceeded.

Local anaesthetics

Dose requirements for regional anaesthesia are significantly less in the elderly. Bupivacaine 0.5% 3 ml in the subarachnoid space provides a level of anaesthesia on average two segments higher at age 70 years than 20 years. Onset of block is faster than in the young but duration does not seem to be related to age. The spread of local anaesthetic solution is less predictable in the elderly because of higher specific gravity of cerebrospinal fluid, lower pressure and greater variability of volume.

Hypotension is more common but the incidence of spinal headache is significantly less (10% compared to 25% in the young; 20 gauge needle). The size of needle used makes little difference to the incidence (25 gauge needle; 10%).

Ageing has similar effects on the characteristics of epidural anaesthesia. Onset of block is faster and the block spreads to a higher level. Investigators have noted both a shorter and a longer duration of action in older patients given epidural bupivacaine. Increased effect of epidural local anaesthetics may be explained by changes in the spinal canal, such as degeneration of myelin and connective tissues, decreased volume of the paravertebral space and closure of intervertebral foramina, preventing leakage of solution. Age does not alter the rate of systemic absorption of bupivacaine, and protein binding is

unaltered, presumably because plasma concentrations of α_1-acid glycoprotein do not change with ageing. Plasma clearance of bupivacaine and lignocaine decreases in the elderly and elimination half-life is extended. Studies in primates suggest that the threshold for central nervous system toxicity due to bupivacaine is similar in young and old.

Muscle relaxants

The sensitivity of the neuromuscular receptor to muscle relaxants is the same in young and elderly patients and a given plasma concentration of relaxant causes the same degree of block. Being water soluble the volume of distribution of the commonly used muscle relaxants is relatively unchanged by advancing years. Not surprisingly therefore, the initial dose requirements of muscle relaxants are similar and the ED_{50} and ED_{95} values for atracurium, vecuronium and pancuronium are unchanged.

However, the duration of effect of the commonly used non-depolarising agents is increased and dose requirements to maintain neuromuscular blockade are decreased. Taking vecuronium as an example, the time for recovery from 25 to 75% of twitch height is about 15 minutes in patients aged less than 36 years, compared with 45 minutes in patients over 63 years. Similarly, dosage requirements to maintain blockade at 10% of baseline twitch height were about 2.8 mg m^{-2} h^{-1} in the young group, compared with 1.8 mg m^{-2} h^{-1} in the old. Most other non-depolarising relaxants behave like vecuronium, although atracurium-induced block appears to be unaffected by increasing age.

The prolonged effect in older patients may be explained by reduced clearance and increased elimination half-life. Hepatic and renal clearance of atracurium is also decreased but clearance by Hofmann elimination is increased so that total plasma clearance is unchanged. Mivacurium is metabolised by plasma cholinesterase, the activity of which is diminished in the elderly.

There are few data on the comparative effects of suxamethonium in young and old age groups. It could be postulated that its action might be augmented in the older patient because of diminished plasma cholinesterase activity; alternatively, the slower circulation time might allow a longer time for hydrolysis, thereby increasing dose requirements. Clinical experience suggests that the action of suxamethonium does not differ markedly between young and old. Muscle pains are less likely in the elderly.

Neostigmine and pyridostigmine (but not edrophonium) have a prolonged effect and this is a useful property which tends to balance the prolonged effect of the non-depolarising relaxants.

The chronotroplc effect of atropine is less marked in the elderly. Atropine and hyoscine cross the blood–brain barrier and elimination is delayed. Consequently, these drugs may cause confusion and sedation in the elderly. Conversely, glycopyrrolate does not cross the blood–brain barrier and is devoid of central nervous system effects.

Other drugs

Changes in drug pharmacokinetics and pharmacodynamics occur in the non-anaesthetic drugs to which the elderly are exposed. The same precautions in respect of drug doses and dosage intervals apply. Drugs to which the elderly are notoriously sensitive include digoxin and warfarin, but there is decreased sensitivity to β-adrenergic agonists. In addition, many adverse effects of drugs are more common in the elderly, e.g. the Stevens–Johnson syndrome and agranulocytosis after co-trimoxazole.

FURTHER READING

Bloom H G, Shlom E A 1993 Drug prescribing for the elderly. Raven Press, New York
Dodds C (ed.) 1993 Anaesthesia and the geriatric patient. Baillière's Clinical Anaesthesiology
Muravchick S 1994 Anaesthesia for the elderly. In: Miller R D (ed) Anesthesia, 4th edn Churchill Livingstone, Edinburgh
Smith R B, Gurkowski M A, Bracken C A (eds) 1995 Anesthesia and pain control in the geriatric patient. McGraw-Hill, New York

Drug toxicity

SECTION CONTENTS

51

Adverse reactions and drug interaction

W. McCaughey

The general principles and the mechanisms of drug action have been discussed in the early chapters of this book. In a few cases, a drug may produce the desired effect and no other — the 'magic bullet' that Ehrlich described — but in most cases action is not so selective, and other effects occur. These side-effects may be beneficial, neutral, or potentially or actually harmful.

Adverse reactions are common, and the incidence increases dramatically as a larger number of drugs is given to the patient. Although it undoubtedly overstated the case, an early editorial suggested that as much as one-seventh of all hospital days could be devoted to managing complications of drug interaction. This is a problem particularly in the older age group — the number of patients on concurrent medication increases steadily with age so that by 70 years over 70% are taking one or more drugs. Mainly in younger people, self-medication with alcohol and other 'recreational' drugs is an increasing problem, and poses additional difficulties.

Cardiovascular drugs account for almost one-third of all prescriptions and this is reflected in the high proportion of elderly people presenting for anaesthesia on this type of medication. Diuretics, non-steroidal anti-inflammatory drugs, salbutamol, β-adrenoceptor blocking drugs, calcium channel antagonists, digoxin, tricyclic antidepressants and benzodiazepines may each be taken by at least 10% of all patients. There will obviously be risks associated with these drugs, and potential problems of an interaction with anaesthetic or other drugs given in hospital must be balanced against the risks of omitting the treatment. Problems can also arise due to nurses withholding medication because the patient is fasting, or failure of medical staff to prescribe.

Adverse reactions may take a number of forms, and some definitions are given here.

Overdosage or underdosage. These may occur because of error, or because of a change in the formulation of a drug. This is a potential problem with generic prescribing, where in a small number of cases there are significant differences between preparations from different manufacturers. Relative over- or underdose may also occur because of a change in the pharmacodynamic or pharmacokinetic profile of the patient (see below for some examples).

Intolerance. Here a patient shows a qualitatively normal response to the drug, but at an abnormally low dose. This may simply be a response at the extreme of the normal range of variation. The gaussian distribution of response to a drug includes individuals who are unusually sensitive as well as those who are resistant. On the other hand, the response to some drugs shows two or more genetically determined populations — for example, the response to suxamethonium in normal persons and in those with abnormal variants of cholinesterase.

Idiosyncrasy. This is a response which is qualitatively different from the action of the drug in normal individuals, again often genetically determined. Of importance to anaesthetists are abnormal responses to several drugs in patients with acute intermittent porphyria, and in those susceptible to the malignant hyperpyrexia syndrome.

Allergy and hypersensitivity. These responses are not dose-related, and are not related to the usual mechanisms of action, effects and side-effects of the drug.

Direct organ toxicity. Some substances may directly damage cells of a particular organ or system, either because they are specifically toxic to these cells, or because they are concentrated in one area. Alternatively, a metabolite may be responsible; for example, liver damage occurs in paracetamol overdose because of a toxic intermediate product binding to hepatocytes.

Secondary effects. Some effects are only indirectly related to the action of the drug; for example, vitamin deficiency in patients whose gut flora has been modified by broad spectrum antibiotics.

Drug interaction. When more than one drug is given, one may modify the action of the other in some manner. Predictable drug interactions form the basis of the drug combinations used in anaesthesia. However, with the increasing number of drugs being used in different facets of the patient's management, there is a considerable risk of unexpected interactions occurring before, during or after anaesthesia and surgery. Improved knowledge of the modes of action and pharmacokinetic disposition of drugs is gradually making more of these interactions understandable and thus predictable.

Overall, drug interactions form only a small proportion of all adverse reactions to drugs (6.9% in one large study), but some are important. The number of reported interactions is enormous, and only those of relevance to anaesthesia and intensive care are discussed in this chapter.

Details of adverse reactions to drugs

The majority of the types of adverse reactions listed above are described in the appropriate chapters earlier in this book. Many of them may be anticipated by a clear understanding of the pharmacodynamic and pharmacokinetic principles underlying a drug's action. In the rest of this chapter, interactions between drugs, and allergic and hypersensitivity reactions are discussed in more detail, together with two examples of an idiosyncratic reaction: porphyria and the malignant hyperpyrexia syndrome.

DRUG INTERACTION

Definitions

When drugs interact, there may be an increased action of one or both, a decreased action, or an effect qualitatively different from either. A number of specific terms are used to describe these.

Where the result of interaction is an increased action, this may be of different types. An *additive* effect (or *summation*) occurs when the combined effect of the two drugs is simply the sum of each (2 + 2 = 4) — allowing for the fact that it is generally the log dose which is proportional to effect. In this case there is in fact no real interaction between the drugs. Where the combined effect is greater than this (2 + 2 = 5) the effect is *synergism*. The term *potentiation* is used where one agent shows no appreciable effect on the biological system, but causes an increased response from the second substance (2 + 0 = 3). The more subtle aspects of this are discussed by Halsey (1987) in a review paper. Where one drug opposes all, or part, of the action of another, the term *antagonism* is used. Antagonism at receptor sites may be *competitive* or *non-competitive*; these concepts have been discussed in Chapter 3. Non-competitive antagonism (or potentiation) can also occur for pharmacokinetic reasons if a drug modifies the absorption, transport, biotransformation or excretion of another. Another non-competitive mechanism is *physiological* or *functional* antagonism, where two drugs have directly opposing effects, though at different sites. If the two drugs form an inactive complex, this is chemical antagonism.

Classification

Drug interactions are most easily grouped according to the site at which the interaction takes place. A parallel method of classification is as *pharmacokinetic* or *pharmacodynamic*. Pharmacokinetic interactions occur when one drug interferes with the absorption, distribution, metabolism or excretion of another drug. Such interference may be two way and may involve more than one mechanism. These may augment or counteract each other. This type of drug interaction may increase or decrease the concentration of 'free' drug in the plasma (and at its site of action). Pharmacodynamic interactions, on the other hand, lead to a change in the activity of the drug at the site of action itself. This may be by competition for receptor sites, or by other mechanisms related to the mode of action of the drug at cellular level. Many drug interactions can be predicted from knowledge of the principles of pharmacokinetics and of the mode of action of

the drugs concerned, and so this chapter should be read in conjunction with the chapters which describe these principles.

PHARMACOKINETIC INTERACTIONS

Direct chemical or physical interaction

It is common for drugs to be incompatible when mixed, so that one or either is inactivated. This is particularly obvious when a precipitate results. Additives to intravenous fluids are a particularly fruitful source of such incompatibilities, especially with parenteral nutrition solutions, and in general only additives that have been tested by the manufacturer should be used. Insulin may adsorb to the wall of a container or delivery system so that delivery to the patient is reduced; when insulin is being infused from a syringe driver this problem can be minimised by adding colloid to the solution — the insulin adsorbs to the colloid molecules and is delivered to the patient. Direct inactivation can also occur within the body — for example, if tetanus toxoid and antitoxin are given simultaneously at the same site.

Modified absorption

This will be relatively unimportant in anaesthetic practice, where few drugs are given by the oral route. The factors involved there have been described earlier, in Chapter 4. The absorption of parenterally administered drugs can also be modified — use of a vasoconstrictor with local anaesthetics is a common example.

Transport and distribution

Most drugs are carried by the circulation from their site of administration to their sites of action and elimination. Competition for protein binding sites and other factors have been described in Chapter 4, and some relevant examples are given in Table 51.1.

Modified metabolism

The effects of drugs in inducing and inhibiting

Table 51.1 Drug reactions and interactions and some special risk situations with anaesthetic drugs

Drug	Secondary drug or clinical situation	Site and pharmacology	Potential interaction or risk
Inhalational anaesthetics			
Halothane and other halogenated volatile anaesthetics	Adrenaline and other sympathomimetics	(S) Anaesthetic sensitises myocardium to adrenaline; risk of severe ventricular arrhythmias	Adrenaline solutions should be dilute and not given i.v. Avoid hypercarbia
Cyclopropane Methoxyflurane Enflurane Sevoflurane ?	Renal disease	(M) Renal toxicity from inorganic fluoride	Avoid prolonged exposure in patients with pre-existing renal disease
Diethyl ether Enflurane	Tetracycline β-Adrenergic blockers	(S) Increased risk of renal toxicity Blockade of normal compensation for cardiodepressant effects	Risk of myocardial depression and hypotension
Diethyl ether Enflurane	Epilepsy	(S)	Risk of convulsions
Halothane Enflurane etc.	Nondepolarising relaxants	(S) Potentiation of neuromuscular blockade	Reduction in dosage requirement
All volatile anaesthetics	MHS patients	(S) May trigger malignant hyperthermia	
Intravenous anaesthetics			
Thiopentone	Renal failure Cirrhosis	(B) Decreased protein binding of thiopentone may enhance its activity	Reduced rate of administration
Thiopentone Methohexitone	Metabolic acidosis Acute intermittent porphyria	(B) Enhanced activity (M) Induction of ALA synthase by barbiturates	Precipitation of attacks
Methohexitone Thiopentone Methohexitone	Epilepsy Allergy Asthma	(S) (S) Hypersensitivity	Risk of convulsions Increased risk of anaphylactic response and bronchospasm
Etomidate	Prolonged use	Blockade of corticosteroid synthesis	Impaired stress response. Especially in ITU patients
Local anaesthetics			
All local anaesthetics Amethocaine	Metabolic acidosis Low serum cholinesterase activity	(B) (M)	Increased risk of toxicity Prolonged activity
Procaine Prilocaine	Large or repeated doses Neonates and infants	(M) Methaemoglobinaemia	Care with dosage
Muscle relaxants			
Suxamethonium	Severe liver disease Anticholinesterases	(M) Reduced serum cholinesterase levels	Prolonged block
	Procaine	(M) Competition for plasma cholinesterase	Prolonged block
Non-depolarising relaxants	Diuretics Hypokalaemia	(S) Potentiation of neuromuscular block	Danger of prolonged paralysis
	Antibiotics: Aminoglycosides Polymyxins Tetracyclines Lincomycin Clindamycin	(?S) Depending on group, either or both pre- and postganglionic block and potentiation of nondepolarizing muscle relaxants	Prolonged neuromuscular block. Rarely, muscle weakness caused by antibiotic alone
	Calcium entry blockers	(S) Preganglionic block	Potentiation of block
Analgesic drugs			
1. Opioids			
Morphine, etc.	Diazepam and other CNS depressants	(S) Additive effect	Titrate doses carefully
	Antagonist and agonist-antagonists	(S) Competitive antagonism	Precipitation of abstinence syndrome in addicts
Pethidine (meperidine)	MAOI drugs	See text	Dangerous interaction — see text

Table 51.1 (*contd*)

Drug	Secondary drug or clinical situation	Site and pharmacology		Potential interaction or risk
Alfentanil	Phenobarbitone and other enzyme inducers	(M)	Increased production of norpethidine	Increased sedation, danger of convulsions
	Erythromycin	(M)	Reduced clearance of alfentanil	Prolonged action of alfentanil
2. NSAIDs	Surgery	(S)	Inhibition of prostaglandins (i) in platelets (ii) in kidney	Risk of bleeding Risk of acute renal failure
Antidepressants Monoamine oxidase inhibitors	Pethidine (Meperidine)	(?)	Possibly due to increased 5-HT level in brain; a certain critical level may have to be reached	Severe, potentially fatal reaction in some patients
	Indirectly acting sympathomimetics	(S) (M)	Inhibition of metabolism of noradrenaline which accumulates at sympathetic nerve endings Release leads to overstimulation and adrenergic crisis	
Antihypertensive drugs β-Adrenergic blockers	Diethyl ether Enflurane	(S)	Additive cardiovascular depressant effects	β Blockade not normally a problem during anaesthesia but avoid drugs which are myocardial depressants
	Calcium entry antagonists	(S)	Additive negative inotropic effect on the heart	Severe bradycardia possible Use cautiously together
Clonidine	Withdrawal of treatment	(S)		Rebound hypertension
ACE inhibitors	General anaesthesia	(S)	Renin-angiotensin system blockade	Intra- and postoperative hypotension

(S), at or near site of action; (M), metabolism; MHS, malignant hypertension syndrome; MAOI, monoamine oxidase inhibitors; ACE, angiotensin converting enzyme; 5-HT, 5-hydroxytryptamine.

metabolism of others have again been described in Chapter 4. There are several examples of relevance to anaesthetic practice. The toxicity of pethidine may be enhanced by barbiturates, increasing metabolism to the toxic metabolite norpethidine. Monoamine oxidase inhibition is described below, as is the problem of amino-laevulinic acid synthase induction in porphyria.

Modified excretion

Two main effects occur here: firstly, change in the pH of urine — weak bases such as pethidine are more easily excreted in an acid urine, while alka-linisation promotes excretion of weak acids such as salicylates and phenobarbitone. Secondly, drugs that compete for an active excretion mechanism will reduce each others' elimination — probenecid was used in the early days of peni-

cillin to conserve the drug, while less desirable interactions also occur — for example, chlor-propamide and phenylbutazone interact to give increased levels of chlorpropamide and a danger of hypoglycaemia.

PHARMACODYNAMIC INTERACTIONS

These are defined here as interactions that take place at or near the site of action of the drug at cellular level, and thus represent some modification of the drug–receptor association, or change in the events that occur after the drug acts on its receptor. The complexity of the intracellular pathways involving G protein and other coupling of receptor to effector, and the way in which many different pathways are interdependent — relationships which are only gradually being worked out — give opportunities for a wide range of possible interactions between drugs at this level. The simplest concepts to understand are those of competition for attachment to receptor sites (see Ch. 3), and augmentation of adenylate cyclase activity by phosphodiesterase inhibition, but other interactions occur, involving both G-protein coupled and inositol 1,4,5-triphosphate (IP$_3$) pathways.

Many of the pharmacodynamic interactions of most interest to the anaesthetist occur in pathways associated with the various divisions of the nervous system, central and autonomic, and thus influence the control of the cardiovascular system.

In the rest of the chapter the drugs discussed will be grouped by drug class or by body system, as many may have both a pharmacodynamic and a pharmacokinetic element to their spectrum of interactions, and these will be described together.

CLINICALLY IMPORTANT INTERACTIONS

Psychoactive drugs

A growing number of drugs are used that affect the many neurotransmitters in the brain — benzodiazepines and others act on γ-aminobutyric acid (GABA)ergic transmission; antidepressants such as monoamine oxidase inhibitors and tricyclic antidepressants are thought to increase the concentration of transmitter amines in the brain and so elevate mood — these will also act at peripheral nerve terminals, so interactions with them are a combination of peripheral and central actions. Levodopa increases central as well as peripheral dopamine, and the newest class of psychoactive drugs, the selective serotonin reuptake inhibitors (SSRIs), of which the ubiquitous fluoxetine (Prozac) is best known, act in a similar way on serotonergic pathways.

Monoamine oxidase inhibitors

The monoamine oxidase inhibitor (MAOI) antidepressants have recently enjoyed a resurgence of popularity. Newer drugs are selective for the MAO-A subtype of the enzyme, and are less

likely to interact with foods or other drugs, although they are probably not any more effective as antidepressants than older MAOIs. Monoamine oxidase (MAO) inactivates monoamine substances, many of which are, or are related to, neurotransmitters. The central nervous system (CNS) mainly contains MAO-A, whose substrates are adrenaline, noradrenaline, metanephrine and 5-hydroxytryptamine (5-HT), whereas extraneuronal tissues such as the liver, lung and kidney contain mainly MAO-B, which metabolises β-phenylethylamine, phenylethanolamine *o*-tyramine and benzylamine.

MAO inhibition has been thought to act by increasing levels of transmitter substances such as noradrenaline in the brain. However, the results of their administration are complex. CNS levels of monoamine do increase, but this leads to reduced rates of synthesis. By-products, such as the false transmitter octopamine, accumulate, and slowly displace noradrenaline from storage vesicles. Inhibitory presynaptic α-adrenergic and dopamine receptors may be α$_1$, α$_2$, and β receptors, 5-hydroxytryptamine (5-HT$_1$ and 5-HT$_2$) receptors but not dopamine receptors. Apart from behavioural changes, the main effect of MAO inhibition is a generalised reduction in sympathetic tone, with lower resting blood pressure and a reduced ability to respond to stresses such as postural change. The classic (type I) reaction with MAOIs, although complex, can be regarded as extreme overstimulation of the sympathetic nervous system. Tyramine, one of the main culprits in the 'cheese' reaction, has been shown to act by inhibiting the inhibitory α$_2$-adrenergic pathways in the locus ceruleus. Should it occur, treatment is largely symptomatic: chlorpromazine 50–100 mg may control the central excitatory symptoms, and contribute to control of others, while more specific antihypertensive therapy may be required; labetalol, a combined α and β blocker has been used successfully; arrhythmias may require β blockade.

There are no serious interactions with the commonly used anaesthetic agents, but problems have occurred with pethidine. When a patient on an MAOI is inadvertently given pethidine, either at induction or postoperatively, there follows a reaction characterised by hypertension, hyperthermia, decreased level of consciousness or coma, and even convulsions. This is unlikely to occur with other opioids unrelated to pethidine, although data are scarce, and there has been one report implicating fentanyl. Indirectly acting sympathomimetics (i.e. those that work by stimulating catecholamine release, such as ephedrine) may have an augmented action. Local analgesic solutions that contain adrenaline are unlikely to cause problems, but it may be wise to use a solution containing felypressin instead.

It is less well recognised that in addition to this excitatory response, a 'depressive' type of reaction (type II) can occur as a consequence of reduced metabolism, resulting occasionally in an increased and prolonged response to drugs such as morphine.

Withdrawal of MAOIs can result in severe anxiety, agitation, pressured speech, sleeplessness or drowsiness, hallucinations, delirium and paranoid psychosis, and thus should not be undertaken lightly. The older drugs caused irreversible inhibition of MAO, and it was advisable to stop treatment at least 1 week before operation. Newer MAO-A selective inhibitors should be reversible in 24–48 hours, although, with careful selection of anaesthetic management, it should usually be possible to avoid drugs likely to interact. Patients receiving these newer MAOIs should, however, omit the drug on the morning of operation.

Tricyclic antidepressants

These antidepressant drugs act by blocking the reuptake of noradrenaline into nerve terminals. As would be expected, they enhance the action of noradrenaline, adrenaline and other directly acting sympathomimetic compounds. They also exhibit anticholinergic activity which potentiates the activity of atropine-like drugs and can induce sinus tachycardia, atrial ectopic beats or more dangerous arrhythmias. Tricyclic antidepressants have a high affinity for cardiac muscle and have a negative inotropic effect. They exert a quinidine-like, membrane stabilising action on the heart, which causes delayed conduction manifest on the electrocardiograph as prolonged PR, QRS and QT_c times, the last increasing the risk of sudden ventricular fibrillation. At therapeutic doses, orthostatic hypotension may occur, but severe cardiovascular side-effects are usually only a feature in overdose. Management of overdose is described in the next chapter.

Levodopa

In parkinsonism the basal ganglia are depleted of dopamine. As dopamine does not cross the blood–brain barrier, its precursor levodopa (L-dopa), which does, is used in treatment. About 95% of orally administered levodopa is rapidly decarboxylated in the periphery to dopamine, although this is reduced by giving with a dopa carboxylase inhibitor. Cardiovascular effects occur due to increased circulating levels of dopamine. In particular, myocardial irritability may increase, an effect which is maximal about 1 hour after taking levodopa, and may lead to development of arrhythmias, especially in the presence of halogenated volatile anaesthetics. Sudden withdrawal of levodopa carries the danger not only of worsening of the control of parkinsonism but also of a small risk of development of hyperthermia and a syndrome resembling the malignant hyperthermia syndrome, which may be due to imbalance in central dopaminergic pathways.

Anticonvulsants

Anticonvulsants such as the barbiturates and phenytoin are well known inducers of hepatic enzymes and may increase the dosage requirements of many drugs, including fentanyl. They also cause resistance to non-depolarising muscle relaxants (except atracurium) but the mechanism of the interaction is unclear, and may be pharmacodynamic, perhaps due to a change in the sensitivity of acetylcholine receptors. The benzodiazepines, although inducing dependence with chronic use, do not cause significant enzyme induction. There are no clinically significant interactions between the benzodiazepines and drugs used in anaesthesia, although care should be taken when using flumazenil to avoid precipitating withdrawal symptoms in habituated patients.

Alcohol

The effects of chronic alcohol use differ from those of acute intoxication. Chronic long term intake leads initially to induction of hepatic enzymes, and enhances the metabolism of alcohol itself, together with other drugs. Later the picture may change with the development of cirrhotic damage to the liver. In contrast, acute intake of alcohol tends to inhibit microsomal drug metabolism and enhances the effects of drugs. However, if the toxicity of a drug (e.g. paracetamol) depends on the formation of toxic metabolites, the acute intake of alcohol may, paradoxically, reduce the toxicity, whereas chronic alcohol intake may increase it. Pharmacodynamic alterations may also occur with chronic alcohol abuse, perhaps related to adaptive changes in cell membrane lipids or proteins, leading to tolerance. In the context of anaesthesia, it is important to note that the alcoholic shows tolerance to the CNS effects of anaesthetic drugs, but not to their cardiovascular depressant effects.

Cardiovascular drugs

Antihypertensive drugs

Antihypertensive drugs act by many different mechanisms. Since the mid-1970s there has been a consensus that hypertensive patients are, in general, at less risk if treatment is continued throughout the perioperative period; adequate preoperative antihypertensive treatment may be the most important prophylaxis against postoperative hypertension, with its attendant risks of myocardial ischaemia and infarction. The spectrum of drugs used in treatment of hypertension has changed. Currently diuretics, β-adrenergic and calcium channel blocking drugs (see below), angiotensin converting enzyme (ACE) inhibitors and drugs acting on α-adrenergic receptors are first line treatment, with some differences in prescribing patterns between different countries.

The ACE inhibitors, captopril, enalapril, etc. act on the renin–angiotensin system, inhibiting the formation of the powerful vasoconstrictor angiotensin II. In addition to its systemic effects, angiotensin II causes changes in local, end-organ renin–angiotensin systems which control local perfusion to the kidney, adrenal gland, heart, etc. Thus, the effects of ACE inhibitors are complex.

It is usually recommended that ACE inhibitors be continued perioperatively in common with other antihypertensives. It has been suggested that they improve haemodynamic stability during operation, and there is some evidence that in aortic aneurysm repair or coronary artery bypass grafting, postoperative haemodynamic stability is improved and renal function protected, although data are scanty. Pretreatment with ACE inhibitors may reduce tachyphylaxis to sodium nitroprusside and help to prevent rebound hypertension.

On the other hand, there is evidence that ACE inhibitors may predispose to hypotension during anaesthesia and that they reduce cerebral blood flow during any period of systemic hypotension. Furthermore, the response to and recovery from hypotensive episodes due to blood loss or circulatory depletion may be impaired. At present the advice concerning these drugs would be to continue therapy up to and including the day of operation.

Clonidine is an antihypertensive agent which acts by multiple and complex mechanisms, including a prominent central α_2-agonist action combined with some reduction of peripheral adrenergic transmission. It appears to reduce the incidence of hypertensive episodes during anaesthesia, such as the response to laryngoscopy and intubation. It is recognised that this may be at the expense of an increased incidence of hypotension and bradycardia at other times perioperatively, with the latter being somewhat resistant to atropine. In contrast, pressor responses to indirectly acting vasopressors such as ephedrine may be increased. These factors must be considered in deciding in individual cases whether to continue clonidine treatment up to the day of operation. If it is discontinued abruptly, the release of catecholamines from stores in nerve terminals may lead to a potentially fatal syndrome of rebound hypertension, anxiety, tremor and cardiac arrhythmias. Alternative antihypertensive treatment must be substituted to avoid this danger, preferably well in advance of surgery.

Calcium channel antagonists

Calcium channel antagonists are widely used in patients with cardiac disease, principally in the management of hypertension or ischaemic heart disease. Generally when a patient is taking one of these drugs, it should be continued peri-operatively. They have three main effects:

1. Depression of cardiac conduction, with slowing of the rate of sinoatrial node discharge, prolongation of atrioventricular node refractoriness, and slowing of atrioventricular conduction.
2. A direct negative inotropic effect.
3. Vasodilatation of both coronary and systemic arteries and arterioles. The potential for depression of cardiac function is thus usually offset by afterload reduction, especially in the case of nifedipine, which actually has the most marked negative inotropic effect.

Serious side-effects are rare and result from improper use of these agents, as when intravenous verapamil (or diltiazem) is given to patients with sinus or atrioventricular nodal depression from drugs or disease, or nifedipine to patients with aortic stenosis.

The volatile anaesthetics can interact adversely with calcium blockers. Experimentally, halothane and enflurane have direct cardiac inhibitory effects similar to verapamil and diltiazem, whereas the properties of isoflurane seem closer to the dihydro-pyridines (nifedipine and nicardipine), whose dominant action is vasodilatation. Interactions may cause an additive effect on conduction with, for example, isoflurane or halothane.

Nifedipine, nicardipine and nimodipine are vasodilator drugs with a hypotensive action, which is especially obvious in hypertensive patients and when combined with similarly acting agents, such as sodium nitroprusside or nitroglycerin. The vascular hypotensive effect of calcium channel antagonists may also be intensified by cardiac depressants such as halothane or isoflurane.

Calcium channel antagonists, with their vasodilator effect, and halogenated inhalation anaesthetics both reduce hypoxic pulmonary vasoconstriction, and the depressant effect of the combination of halothane or isoflurane with verapamil is significantly greater than when the drugs are administered alone. This might exacerbate ventilation/perfusion mismatching during anaesthesia.

Drug interactions involving calcium antagonists occur with other cardiovascular agents such as α- and β-adrenergic blocking drugs, digoxin, quinidine and disopyramide. Some of these interactions are pharmacokinetic. For example, plasma concentrations of carbamazepine or phenytoin may rise when calcium channel antagonists are given concurrently; this may result in toxicity and the dosage of the anticonvulsants may need to be reduced. Verapamil can cause an increase in the plasma concentrations of other cardiovascular drugs and digoxin levels may be raised by 50–80%, although the change is relatively small with other calcium channel antagonists. With β-adrenergic blockers the interaction can be mutual (see below).

Combined therapy using calcium antagonists with β blockers is increasingly common, and is probably safest with the dihydropyridines. Synergy occurs, which can lead to marked interference with conduction, leading to bradycardia or even sinus arrest. Caution is needed during anaesthesia in patients receiving such a combination, as conduction disturbances can occur, although very careful monitoring of the electrocardiograph will usually forestall any problems.

The interaction between oral verapamil and propranolol may involve negative chronotropic, inotropic or dromotropic effects. The interaction is partly pharmacokinetic — verapamil increases the AUC and peak concentration C_{max} and shortens the time to peak concentration t_{max} of propranolol, whereas propranolol decreases the AUC and C_{max} of verapamil (Carruthers et al 1989). The greater reduction of heart rate with the combination of verapamil and propranolol is only partly explained by higher plasma concentrations of propranolol, and also represents a synergistic effect on conduction. Some of the depressant effects of the combination may be antagonised by amrinone or glucagon.

There is some evidence that the cardiotoxicity

of bupivacaine may be intensified in patients who are receiving either calcium channel or β-adrenergic blocking drugs (de La Coussaye et al 1990).

β-Adrenergic blocking drugs

These drugs are widely used for a number of medical indications, including hypertension, angina and migraine. Adverse effects can include bronchospasm, heart failure, prolonged hypoglycaemia, bradycardia, heart block, intermittent claudication and Raynaud's phenomenon. Neurological reactions include depression, fatigue and nightmares.

Bradycardia, hypotension and bronchospasm are the main hazards in β-blocker treated patients undergoing anaesthesia. However, continuation of β blockade up to and including the day of operation results in improved perioperative haemodynamic stability and avoids the rebound effect which can result from abrupt withdrawal. There may be a risk of bradycardia following reversal with neostigmine in β-blocked patients, and it is advisable to give the anticholinergic drug first rather than mixed with anticholinesterase.

Bronchospasm is not a direct action of these drugs but blockade of β receptors increases the reactivity of the airway and increases the likelihood of bronchospasm during laryngoscopy and tracheal intubation. It is also possible that the severity, and possibly the incidence of acute anaphylaxis, is increased in patients on large doses of β blockers and that resuscitation may be hampered in these circumstances (Toogood 1987).

Side-effects that occur after systemic use of β blockers can also occur with ophthalmic preparations of these drugs, but treatment should continue in the perioperative period.

Neuromuscular junction

Several different classes of drug given preoperatively or during anaesthesia may affect the duration of neuromuscular blockade. Muscle weakness is not a common result of the use of these drugs, except when function is also compromised by another factor, a neuromuscular

disease for example, or the presence of clinical or subclinical doses of other drugs acting in this region. A number of antibiotics possess neuromuscular blocking activity. The aminoglycoside, polymyxin, lincosamide and tetracycline groups are those most commonly involved, while penicillins, cephalosporins and erythromycin have not caused clinical problems. They have their action at different sites: the aminoglycosides mainly prejunctional, the polymyxins, tetracyclines and lincosamides mainly postjunctional. There are also considerable differences between individual drugs of each group. Because of these complexities, antagonism of this type of block is uncertain, and, although in the experimental setting calcium can achieve a 75% reversal of the effect of aminoglycosides, clinically it is usually safer to continue ventilation until adequate muscle power has returned. Less difficulty might be expected with the newer non-depolarising drugs such as atracurium and vecuronium, but clinical concentrations of aminoglycosides (gentamicin, tobramycin) can prolong blockade.

Calcium channel blockade interferes with prejunctional calcium flux at the neuromuscular junction, and can thus potentiate neuromuscular blockade. Both verapamil and nifedipine have been shown to potentiate the effect of the commonly used non-depolarising muscle relaxants, including vecuronium and atracurium. Magnesium sulphate, used in management of pre-eclampsia, has a similar effect, and the two drugs in combination may themselves cause neuromuscular block.

Suxamethonium breakdown may be delayed by drugs that reduce plasma cholinesterase levels or compete as substrates. Many of the drugs which do this, such as procaine or propanidid, are mainly of historical interest, but metoclopramide, which is often given before obstetric anaesthesia, prolongs the duration of action of suxamethonium by as much as 50%.

Malignant hyperpyrexia

Some susceptible patients, who suffer from an inherited abnormality in muscle membrane, develop a fulminating and often fatal hyperpyrexia when given certain anaesthetic drugs and depolarising muscle relaxants. Most patients develop muscle contracture, acidosis and hyperkalaemia. Unexplained tachypnoea, tachycardia, sweating, cyanosis, or rise in expired carbon dioxide may be non-specific early warnings. A working clinical definition of malignant hyperpyrexia is an unexplained fever during anaesthesia, in which the body temperature rises at a rate of at least 2°C an hour, but sometimes the rise in body temperature can be a late sign.

Malignant hyperpyrexia is due to an abnormality in the calcium channel of the muscle sarcolemma or sarcoplasmic reticulum. The channel, which is responsible for calcium efflux from the sarcoplasmic reticulum, is frequently referred to as the ryanodine receptor, as ryanodine is a specific ligand at this receptor site. The abnormality is inherited, probably in an autosomal dominant manner. In pigs, a single chromosomal defect appears to be responsible, but the human picture is more complicated. An abnormality has been traced to a gene on the long arm of chromosome 19 (at the locus 19q13.1), and is found consistently in subjects susceptible to malignant hyperpyrexia in the families in which it has been found. However, the abnormality in other families investigated appears to lie at a different chromosome location, which not only indicates a more complicated pattern of inheritance — to date at least six different loci have been traced but makes the development of a simple genetic test for susceptibility unlikely for most families in the near future. At present, firm diagnosis still requires muscle biopsy. There is a link with some forms of myopathy, in particular central core disease. The pathophysiology of malignant hyperpyrexia is discussed in more detail in Ch. 19.

Incidence of the condition as diagnosed lies between 1:6000 and 1:200 000, this range indicating different criteria for diagnosis in the absence of a readily available diagnostic test. Mortality in the UK was around 24%, but is improving as increased oxygen and carbon dioxide monitoring allows earlier diagnosis. Triggering agents include volatile anaesthetic agents, cyclopropane, suxamethonium and other depolarising relaxants.

In addition, there is doubt about ketamine, phenothiazines, tricyclic and other antidepressants, and MAOIs, although this may be because of confusion between malignant hyperthermia and *neuroleptic malignant syndrome*, which is now known to be a separate entity. Safe drugs include all local anaesthetics, thiopentone, propofol, opioids, nitrous oxide, all non-depolarising muscle relaxants, and atropine and neostigmine.

Management of the condition consists first in discontinuation of the triggering agent and symptomatic management, including cooling and treatment of the hyperkalaemia, which can be the fatal event. *Dantrolene sodium* is the specific treatment.

Neuroleptic malignant syndrome

A severe and potentially fatal hyperpyrexic reaction following psychotropic medication may be due to the neuroleptic malignant syndrome (NMS). This shows many resemblances to malignant hyperpyrexia, but does not share a common aetiology. Drugs implicated in triggering this reaction include phenothiazines, butyrophenones, thioxanthines, selective serotonin reuptake inhibitors and miscellaneous antipsychotic agents such as loxapine; a drug's potential for inducing NMS may parallel its antidopaminergic potency. Dantrolene may also be of use in management of NMS.

Dantrolene sodium

Dantrolene, a hydantoin derivative, has a low water solubility, and for this reason a lyophilised formulation of its sodium salt is used, and reconstituted with mannitol and sodium hydroxide. It has a high lipid solubility, and thus can cross all membranes easily.

Dantrolene is a directly acting muscle relaxant that acts by dissociating excitation–contraction coupling in the muscle by inhibiting calcium ion release from the sarcoplasmic reticulum. The site of action may be on the transverse tubular–sarcoplasmic reticulum coupling, or on the sarcoplasmic reticulum directly, or both.

Dosage and pharmacokinetics. A dose of

2.4 mg kg^{-1} dantrolene intravenously will cause maximal (75%) depression of twitch response of skeletal muscle, and this appears to be an adequate dose for prevention or initial treatment of malignant hyperpyrexia during anaesthesia. The dose may be infused over 10–15 minutes, and if necessary repeated at 15 minute intervals until a therapeutic effect has been achieved or until a total dose of 10 mg kg^{-1} has been reached. Later treatment is less clearly defined, but a further prophylactic dose of 2.4 mg kg^{-1} after 10–12 hours may be considered (Harrison 1989). In a study of healthy volunteers, the blood level of dantrolene was found to remain relatively steady for about 5.5 hours, and thereafter decline exponentially with an elimination half-life of about 12 hours, but elimination may be more rapid after intravenous administration.

Given orally, dantrolene is 70% absorbed, reaching peak blood concentrations at about 4–6 hours. Dantrolene is metabolised in the liver by both reductive and oxidative pathways, and excreted in both bile and urine, 4% unchanged and the remainder as a reduced acetylated derivative.

Oral dantrolene has been used for prophylaxis of malignant hyperpyrexia, in daily doses ranging from 1 to 12 mg kg^{-1}. One recommended regimen is to give 2.2 mg kg^{-1} orally — half at 8 hours before operation, and half 4 hours before. However, the effectiveness of oral dantrolene is controversial, and it may be better to give it intravenously in all cases.

The main side-effect of dantrolene is muscle weakness, which may be experienced for up to 48 hours, but which is not clinically important. Myocardial depression is not a problem at the doses described, but if given with verapamil, then animal studies have shown marked myocardial depression.

Porphyria

A number of drugs used in anaesthetic practice are highly dangerous in patients suffering from one of the three 'acute' porphyrias — acute intermittent porphyria, variegate porphyria or hereditary coproporphyria — as they may precipitate an acute attack. The mechanism involved is induc-

tion of hepatic δ-aminolaevulinic acid synthase. The status of many drugs is uncertain, and was reviewed by Harrison et al (1993). Barbiturates are the classical example of drugs dangerous in porphyrics. Temazepam is safe, other benzodiazepines less certain. Propofol is the best choice at present for intravenous induction, although raised urinary porphyrins have been reported after its use. Halothane is recommended if a volatile agent is required; morphine and fentanyl are safe; there are insufficient data on some other analgesics to be sure of their position. Suxamethonium and curare are safe and vecuronium probably safe; atropine and neostigmine are safe. Drugs that are unsafe or probably unsafe include barbiturates, etomidate, enflurane, alcuronium, mepivacaine, pentazocine, some benzodiazepines, calcium channel blockers, aminophylline and cimetidine.

HYPERSENSITIVITY REACTIONS

Definitions

This term may be used to cover a type of adverse reaction resembling the effects of histamine liberation ('histaminoid') and unrelated to the mode of action of the drug itself. The term 'anaphylactoid' may equally be used to describe these reactions, meaning simply that they resemble anaphylactic reactions. The term 'anaphylactic' is better restricted to immune mediated phenomena involving previous sensitisation of the patient. Since one does not always know the patient's history, the mechanism, or even with certainty the drug involved, the more general terms are safer for descriptive purposes. Reactions can then be classified according to their severity.

Mechanisms

Hypersensitivity reactions have been classified as types I to IV. Type I, involving IgE or IgG antibodies, is the main mechanism involved in most hypersensitivity to anaesthetic drugs, but type IV, cellular responses mediated by sensitised lymphocytes, may account for as much as 80% of *local* anaesthetic allergic reactions. In type I reactions, the first exposure to the antigen results in the formation of specific IgE antibodies which are firmly fixed to mast cells and basophils. Subsequent exposure results in rapid degranulation of these cells and liberation of vasoactive substances, particularly histamine. This mechanism still only accounts for about 20% of all reactions to thiopentone but is important for reactions to plasma substitutes. Complement based reactions of some type were common with the Cremophorcontaining solutions but are rare with other drugs. Probably the most frequent cause of hypersensitivity reactions is histamine release by the drug or drug combinations concerned. This is therefore related to the dose and rate of administration. It is not predictable in terms of previous exposure and is not reliably detected by skin testing.

Histamine. This appears to be the main factor involved in all types of hypersensitivity reactions and its presence explains most of the manifestations. Plasma histamine levels are difficult to estimate, particularly in the emergency situation, but levels correlate closely with the severity of the reaction, figures above 10 ng ml^{-1} indicating a severe reaction and above 100 ng ml^{-1} being usually fatal.

Predisposing factors

A history of atopy (asthma, hay fever or eczema) or of allergy to any injected substance is frequently seen in patients reacting to anaesthetic drugs and this association can be confirmed statistically. In most of these cases there is probably a raised IgE level, but this is not an essential feature in patients having true hypersensitivity reactions. Repeated exposure to particular drugs is not a predisposing factor to reactions, as judged by the drug history of thiopentone reactors and others. In general, reactions are most common with substances of high molecular weight, but smaller molecules can attach themselves to plasma proteins or polypeptides and become antigenic.

Frequency of reactions

In the field of anaesthesia, hypersensitivity reactions occur most frequently with muscle relaxants, induction agents, plasma substitutes and antibiotics, as well as to latex, and it is often difficult to identify the causative drug. The incidence of reactions is between 1:10 000 and 1:20 000 anaesthetics (Fisher & Baldo 1993), and a muscle relaxant is involved in a majority, perhaps as many as 70%, of these. The most frequently incriminated are alcuronium and suxamethonium, and the lowest number of reactions occurs with pancuronium and vecuronium. The incidence for muscle relaxants is probably higher than for intravenous barbiturates, while the safest of the induction agents appears to be etomidate. Reactions to plasma substitutes are also relatively frequent. A recent French study found rates of 1/300 for gelatins, 1/400 for dextrans, 1/1000 for albumin and 1/1700 for starches, of which about 20% were serious. Figures for penicillin are about 1/5000. The mortality in published reactions to thiopentone is approximately 10% and the same figure applies to penicillin reactions, but this is much lower with other agents.

Clinical features

Cutaneous

The majority of clinically definite and immunologically confirmed reactions have erythema as a main feature. Erythema is, however, a common accompaniment to the administration of many drugs (e.g. tubocurarine) and it should not be regarded as part of a life threatening reaction unless there are changes in other systems of the body. In addition, most reactors have oedema, particularly of the eyelids.

Cardiovascular

Hypotension is the other common feature of hypersensitivity reactions. Its basis is hypovolaemia from extravasation of protein-containing fluid through the capillary wall, together with arteriolar and capillary vasodilatation. Both these are classical features of histamine liberation. There is usually a marked tachycardia which is both histamine induced and compensatory for the hypotension. Plasma loss of up to 35% of circulating blood volume may occur within 10 minutes, due to capillary permeability, and rapid replacement, using colloid for preference, is indicated. Adrenaline, infused intravenously with electrocardiographic monitoring, is the drug treatment of choice. When adrenaline and adequate volume do not produce improvement, noradrenaline may be life saving. Antihistamines and corticosteroids have little effect in the acute stages, although they are worth trying as second line drugs (Fisher 1986).

Respiratory

Bronchospasm has been seen in more than half of the published descriptions of reactions, either on its own or as an accompaniment to other changes. It should, however, only be regarded as indicative of a reaction if other forms of airway obstruction and other causes of tracheal irrita-

tion have been excluded. It is a more common physical sign, as one would expect, in asthmatic patients and in patients receiving muscle relaxants (where tracheal intubation may be a factor).

Gastrointestinal disturbance

Abdominal pain, nausea or vomiting occur in about 10% of published case reports.

Confirmation of reaction

Measurement of plasma tryptase levels immediately after an episode may be useful to confirm that a histaminoid reaction has occurred. Some 4 weeks later, skin tests and specific antibody tests (RAST) may help to identify the causative drug, although these tests do produce false positive and false negative results.

REFERENCES AND FURTHER READING

Carruthers S G, Freeman D J, Bailey D G 1989 Synergistic adverse hemodynamic interaction between oral verapamil and propranolol. Clinical Pharmacology and Therapeutics 46: 469–477

de la Coussaye J E, Eldjan J J, Burgada J et al 1990 Do beta adrenergic receptor blockers increase bupivacaine cardiotoxicity. Annales Françaises d'Anesthésie et de Réanimation 9: 132–136

Fisher M McD 1986 Clinical observations on the pathophysiology and treatment of anaphylactic cardiovascular collapse. Anaesthesia and Intensive Care 14: 17–21

Fisher M M, Baldo B A 1993 The incidence and clinical features of anaphylactic reactions during anesthesia in Australia. Annales Françaises d'Anesthésie et de Réanimation 12: 97–104

Halsey M J 1987 Drug interactions in anaesthesia. British Journal of Anaesthesia 59: 112–123

Harrison G C 1989 Malignant hyperthermia. In: Nunn J F,

Utting J E, Brown B R Jr (eds) General anaesthesia, 5th edn. Butterworth, London.

Harrison G G, Meissner P N, Hift R J 1993 Anaesthesia for the porphyric patient. Anaesthesia 48: 417–421

Laxenaire M C, Charpentier C, Feldman L 1994 [Anaphylactoid reactions to colloid plasma substitutes: incidence, risk factors, mechanisms. A French multicenter prospective study.] Annales Françaises d'Anesthésie et de Réanimation 13: 301–310

McKinnon R P, Wildsmith J A 1995 Histaminoid reactions in anaesthesia (review). British Journal of Anaesthesia 74(2): 217–228

Suspected anaphylactic reactions associated with anaesthesia. Revised Edition 1995. The Association of Anaesthetists of Great Britain and Ireland and The British Society of Allergy and Clinical Immunology.

Toogood J H 1987 Beta-blocker therapy and the risk of anaphylaxis. Canadian Medical Association Journal 136: 929–933

52

Management of drug overdose

J. R. Johnston

Drug overdose is one of the most common causes of admission to hospital and encompasses the following categories.

Self-poisoning or parasuicide

This refers to the ingestion of a drug or toxic substance as a response to a personal or social crisis, and accounts for approximately 10% of all medical admissions. The drugs most commonly incriminated are the psychotropic drugs, benzodiazepines being the most common individual group.

Non-accidental poisoning

This is used to describe the administration of a potentially harmful substance, usually by a parent to a child.

Accidental poisoning

This describes unpremeditated poisoning and is most frequent in children aged between 9 months and 5 years. The substances usually involved are drugs (60%), household cleaning products (35%) and plants (4%). Adults also become poisoned accidentally, generally by ingestion or inhalation of substances at home or at work.

GENERAL PRINCIPLES OF MANAGEMENT

The management of poisoned subjects requires an initial assessment of their vital signs followed by interventions to support life, e.g. maintenance of the airway, breathing and circulation (Collee and Hanson 1993). Measures to obtain a working diagnosis of the cause of the poisoning are also carried out at this time. Specific signs to be looked for and managed during the examination and investigation are summarised in Table 52.1. Laboratory investigations likely to provide useful information include arterial blood gases, electrolytes and urea estimations, blood glucose and in certain circumstances a toxicological screen. Further management involves consideration of prevention of absorption, antidotes and promotion of excretion of the poison.

Prevention of absorption

The methods available to prevent absorption include removal from a toxic atmosphere, decontamination of affected skin and, most commonly, prevention of absorption from the gastrointestinal tract. This last method involves consideration of the following techniques.

Gastric lavage

The stomach may be emptied by lavage or by emetics, except when corrosives or petroleum products have been ingested. Lavage must be performed only if a potentially harmful substance has been taken relatively recently and is probably not of value unless performed within 4 hours of ingestion. Exceptions to this rule include substances that delay gastric emptying, such as salicylates and tricyclic antidepressants. When the patient is unconscious the airway must be

Table 52.1   Clinical effects of the common poisons

Clinical effect	Poison
Skin	
Colour — blue	(Cyanosis, methaemoglobinaemia)
— flushed	Carbon monoxide, anticholinergics, cyanide, alcohol
Puncture marks	Narcotics
Bullae	Barbiturates, carbon monoxide, tricyclics
Sweating	Salicylates, organophosphates, amphetamines, cocaine
Pupils	
Constricted	Narcotics, organophosphates
Dilated	Hypoxia, hypothermia, tricyclics, phenothiazines, anticholinergics
Mouth	
Burns	Corrosives, caustics, paraquat
Flaccidity	Benzodiazepines, barbiturates, alcohol, β blockers
Hyperreflexia	Tricyclics, anticholinergics, phenothiazines
Convulsions	Tricyclics, isoniazid, lithium, amphetamines, theophylline, mefenamic acid, carbon monoxide, phenothiazines, ethylene glycol, cocaine
Specific organ damage	
Renal	Paracetamol, paraquat
Hepatic	Paracetamol, carbon tetrachloride
Temperature	
Pyrexia	Anticholinergics, tricyclics, carbon monoxide, salicylates, amphetamines, cocaine
Hypothermia	Barbiturates, alcohol, narcotics
Cardiac rhythm	
Bradycardia	Digoxin, β blockers, carbamates, organophosphates
Tachycardia	Salicylates, theophylline, cyanide, carbon monoxide, anticholinergics
Arrhythmias	Digoxin, phenothiazines, tricyclics, anticholinergics, quinine
Blood pressure	
Hypotension	Sedatives, hypnotics
Hypertension	Anticholinergics, tricyclics, cocaine

protected using an endotracheal tube. The value, safety and efficacy of routine gastric lavage has been questioned (Merigan et al 1990) and it should no longer be performed automatically. If it is performed, there may be benefit in leaving 50 g activated charcoal in the stomach.

Induced emesis

Induced emesis, predominantly used in children, must not be used if there is a risk of aspiration into the lungs or if substances such as petroleum products or corrosives have been taken The standard emetic is syrup of ipecacuanha (Vale et al 1986). This plant extract has as its active constituents the alkaloids emetine and cephaeline. Both induce vomiting by a central action, cephaeline being twice as potent as emetine and also having a direct irritant action on the gastric mucosa. This results in the initial bout of vomiting, the combined central actions causing the later vomiting.

Problems arise if the administered dose of ipecacuanha is too large, producing prolonged vomiting which may mimic the symptoms of poisoning and confuse the clinical picture. It may also cause diarrhoea and lethargy, again mimicking the signs and symptoms of poisoning. Serious side-effects from forceful vomiting, such as gastric rupture and barotrauma, may occur. Emetine can act as a myocardial depressant.

Allied to these problems is the concern that using ipecacuanha may not be the most effective method for reducing drug absorption. Activated charcoal can reduce the absorption of a range of substances, including paracetamol and aminophylline, more effectively than emesis (Neuvonen et al 1983). It needs to be remembered that administration of emetic agents precludes the use of adsorbents such as methionine or activated charcoal. The use of emetics must be questioned, especially when considering the growing number of poisonings for which activated charcoal is effective.

Whole-gut lavage

Whole-gut lavage is reserved for the elimination of sustained release drug formulations.

Adsorbents

Administration of adsorbents, such as activated charcoal, bentonite, Fuller's earth or cholestyramine, bind poison in the gut. Activated charcoal is available as Medicoal or Carbomix. They have a high adsorptive capacity for a wide range of substances and should be given as an aqueous suspension as soon as possible after the ingestion of the poison.

Later administration of charcoal may result in binding of drug remaining within the gut lumen and also drug returned to the lumen by enterohepatic circulation. It should not be used simultaneously with oral emetics as both substances are rendered ineffective. The degree of adsorption to the poison depends on the degree of ionisation and molecular size of the latter. Many drugs require more than double their dose of charcoal for complete adsorption; a ratio of 10:1 of charcoal:poison is recommended. Its adsorptive capacity for the following compounds is too low to be of use: ferrous sulphate, lithium carbonate, strong acids and alkalis, alcohols, cyanides, sulphonylureas and some insecticides.

Antidotes

Specific antidotes to poisons work in a number of ways:

1. An antidote may interact with a poison to form an inert complex, which is then excreted. Heavy metals (arsenic, copper, gold and mercury) are poisonous because of their ability to interact with sulphydryl groups found on organic enzymes. Dimercaprol, a chelating agent which substitutes its own sulphydryl groups, forms a complex with the heavy metal, thus releasing the enzymatic complex. An alcohol group on the dimercaprol promotes excretion by keeping the complex water soluble. Further examples of inert complex formation are given in Table 52.2.

2. Certain antidotes may accelerate the formation of a less toxic form of the poison. The main route of detoxification of cyanide is the formation of thiocyanate. Thiosulphate is required for this

Table 52.2 Antidotes that act by inert complex formation

Poison	Antidote
Arsenic, copper, gold, mercury	Dimercaprol
Cholinesterase inhibitors	Pralidoxime
Cyanide	Sodium nitrite, dicobalt edetate, thiosulphate
Digoxin	Fab antibody fragments
Lead, copper, mercury, zinc	Penicillamine
Thallium	Prussian blue

process and its administration increases the rate of cyanide metabolism.

3. An antidote can reduce the metabolism of the poison to a more toxic compound. Methanol is metabolised in the liver to formaldehyde and formic acid, which are responsible for its toxic effects. This metabolic step is inhibited by ethanol.

4. Antidotes can compete with the poison at receptor sites. Oxygen is used in the treatment of carbon monoxide poisoning because the half-life of elimination of carbon monoxide is reduced from 250 minutes while breathing room air to 50 minutes when breathing 100% oxygen at 1 atmosphere.

5. Antidotes may cause the blockade of receptor sites for action of the poisons. Organophosphorus compounds act at nicotinic and muscarinic receptor sites causing accumulation of acetylcholine. Atropine will block the effects at the muscarinic receptor and pralidoxime blocks the effects at the neuromuscular junctions.

6. An antidote may bypass the effects of the poison, such as using oxygen for a cyanide poisoning.

Enhancement of drug elimination

Several methods are available to promote excretion of a poison; they differ in complexity and in principle. These measures have a limited role and are most effective in situations where there are high plasma concentrations of the poison (small volume of distribution, minimal protein binding). They will be ineffective where the poison is highly tissue bound (large volume of distribution), e.g. tricyclic antidepressants.

Activated charcoal

Activated charcoal is a fine black powder made by the distillation of certain organic materials (wood pulp, coconut shells or coal), which is activated by the action of steam or strong acids at high temperatures. This gives it a large surface area of 950–1200 $m^2 g^{-1}$, which, along with its electrostatic properties, aids binding. Its absorptive capacity is 500–1000 mg of drug per gram of charcoal. It is available as Carbomix (50 g; may cause nausea, vomiting and constipation) and Medicoal (5 g effervescent powder; may cause diarrhoea).

Repeated oral dosing of the bowel will cause transfer of the poison from the circulation in the gut villi to the charcoal in the lumen, especially the small intestine — 'gastrointestinal dialysis'. This is especially effective for lipophilic compounds which are unionised in plasma, have a long elimination half-life, a small volume of distribution and are not highly tissue bound. Those that undergo enterohepatic recirculation or are actively secreted in the bowel can be particularly easy to clear.

50–100 g activated charcoal is given orally as soon as possible after poisoning, followed by the instillation of 12.5 g h^{-1}. Precautions to protect the airway should be taken if there is a risk of aspiration. The following compounds can be eliminated using this technique: salicylates, benzodiazepines, digoxin, digitoxin, dapsone, meprobamate, phenytoin, phenobarbitone, phenylbutazone, carbamazepine, theophylline and quinine. If Carbomix is used, measures to counteract the constipation should be undertaken. Vomiting may be a problem with both formulations.

There are hazards reported with this technique. It may cause pulmonary aspiration of charcoal, gastrointestinal obstruction and sodium overload.

Forced diuresis

The poison is excreted preferentially in the urine by manipulating urine pH so that the poison becomes fully ionised. The degree of ionisation depends on the ionisation constant (K_a) of the drug and the pH of the solution in which it is dissolved. Thus ionisation of weak acids, and therefore their excretion, will be increased in an alkaline urine; basic drugs are maximally ionised in an acid urine. Alkaline diuresis is useful for poisoning by drugs with a pK_a range of 3.0–7.5, where the pH of urine is maintained at 7.5–8.0, e.g. phenobarbitone, salicylates and phenoxyacetate herbicides. An acid diuresis may be used for drugs with a pK_a range of 7.5–10.5, where the pH of urine is maintained at 5.5–6.5.

It is ineffective for highly protein bound drugs (tricyclic antidepressants) and those with a large volume of distribution (lithium, paracetamol). The potential complications of this technique relate to the amount of fluid used, which may lead to pulmonary and cerebral oedema, cardiac failure and electrolyte disturbances. Its use has declined in recent years.

Peritoneal dialysis or haemodialysis

A drug or poison, if present in quantity in the plasma as low molecular weight particles, will diffuse through the peritoneum or dialysis membrane. Thus if it is highly tissue bound, dialysis will not be effective. Peritoneal dialysis, although a simple technique, has practically been abandoned because of the low clearance obtained. Haemodialysis relies upon diffusion of the poison across a semipermeable cellophane membrane down a concentration gradient from blood to dialysate. Small molecules cross the membrane freely; larger molecules (mol. wt. 2000–10 000) pass with difficulty. The technique is used mainly to increase the elimination of lithium, methanol and ethylene glycol, although some barbiturates and salicylates can be removed. It requires sophisticated equipment and, because of the foreign membrane, either heparin or prostacyclin as anticoagulants.

Haemoperfusion

This technique uses broadly similar apparatus to that of haemodialysis except that the 'membrane' used is a column containing an adsorbent material such as polymer-coated activated charcoal, anion resins and uncharged resins. As with the methods outlined above, it is contraindicated if the ingested poisons have a large volume of distribution; the plasma will contain only a small proportion of the total amount of poison in the body. It is also contraindicated if an antidote is available or if binding to a receptor site can readily be reversed. It is of particular value in treatment of poisoning with all the barbiturates, some hypnotics, carbamazepine, disopyramide, theophyllines and salicylates.

MANAGEMENT OF COMMON POISONINGS

Analgesics

Salicylates

Ingestion of acetylsalicylic acid (aspirin) is the most common form of salicylate poisoning. As an acid with pK_a 3.5 it is unionised in the acidic medium of the stomach and is therefore rapidly absorbed.

If taken in overdose it may precipitate out in the stomach and coat the gastric mucosa. This may produce absorption continuing over many hours, and warrants emptying the stomach after the usually recommended time for complete absorption. It is also readily absorbed from the small intestine and is then hydrolysed to salicylic acid. The main route of excretion of salicylate is conjugation to form salicyluric acid. This step is easily saturated even within the therapeutic dose range. Elimination is slow after overdose and toxicity can arise easily.

The two main toxic effects are direct central stimulation of the respiratory centre and uncoupling of oxidative phosphorylation. The former effect leads to respiratory alkalosis with compensatory excretion of bicarbonate, sodium, potassium and water, leading to dehydration and hypokalaemia. The latter effect leads to interference with carbohydrate, lipid, protein and amino acid metabolism and accumulation of organic acids. Oxygen utilisation and carbon dioxide production are increased. Energy released by the uncoupling is dissipated as heat, manifesting as hyperpyrexia and sweating. Central stimulation also causes nausea and vomiting which, together with decreased oral intake, exacerbate fluid loss. All of these lead to a metabolic acidosis. This will tend to reduce the degree of ionisation of the salicylic acid, which will increase its intracellular concentration, central nervous system (CNS) toxicity and lead to a poorer prognosis.

These two effects usually manifest themselves at different rates, depending on the age of the subject. In adults there is often a first stage of 12–24 hours, which, if left untreated, leads to the second stage of metabolic acidosis. In children below the age of 12 years the first stage of respiratory alkalosisis is short or absent and the more dangerous acidotic stage predominates earlier. Glucose metabolism is also affected and there may be an increased peripheral demand, leading to hypoglycaemia. However, with the increased metabolic rate and increased demand, the combined effects of adrenocortical stimulation, increased glucose 6-phosphatase activity and hepatic glycogenolysis may lead to hyperglycaemia.

Elimination of the drug relies upon the renal pathway; a urinary pH of greater than 6 leading to increased excretion. A stage of respiratory alkalosis tends to protect against serious salicylate toxicity and will also help excretion.

The clinical manifestations of salicylate overdose are summarised in Table 52.3. The therapeutic blood level of aspirin is approximately 150 mg l^{-1}; toxicity becomes apparent at 250–350 mg l^{-1}. Levels between 500 and 750 mg l^{-1} give rise to moderate toxicity and levels of greater than 750 mg l^{-1} indicate severe toxicity. Blood levels must be interpreted in association with the plasma pH because with an acidosis intracellular concentration may rise while blood levels fall. The presence of a metabolic acidosis following salicylate poisoning indicates a poor prognosis.

In patients who present within 24 hours of poisoning, gastric aspiration and lavage should be carried out. If presentation is early, oral activated charcoal should be given and, if clinical conditions allow, repeated. Fluid and electrolyte deficits from the vomiting, sweating and hyperventilation must be corrected; plasma pH should be manipulated if the pH is low and temperature should be reduced using tepid sponging. Vitamin K may be given for hypoprothrombinaemia.

Forced alkaline diuresis should be carried out only in the more severely affected patients (greater than 500 mg l^{-1} in adults or 300 mg l^{-1} in children). Complications are most likely in the very young, in the elderly, in those with pre-existing cardiac and renal disease, and in those severely poisoned (greater than 750 mg l^{-1}). In those patients with an acidosis this must be corrected first. A urinary pH of greater than 7.5 is more effective than a very brisk diuresis. If there is any potassium deficit it will be difficult to obtain a suitably alkaline urine.

With very severely poisoned patients (level greater than 1000 mg l^{-1}) it may be necessary to use haemodialysis or haemoperfusion, with the former technique being preferred because it aids correction of the fluid and electrolyte deficits.

Paracetamol

This drug is now the main cause of acute liver necrosis in the UK; it is taken either alone or in compounds such as Distalgesic (dextropropoxyphene and paracetamol).

Approximately 1–4% of the dose of paracetamol is excreted as the free drug. Of the remainder, the majority (60–90%) is excreted as glucuronide and sulphate conjugates. A small proportion, however, forms an oxidative metabolite (N-

Table 52.3 Clinical features of salicylate poisoning

Poisoning	Features
Mild to moderate (500–750 mg l^{-1})	Irritability, tremor Tinnitus, deafness Nausea, vomiting, epigastric discomfort Hyperventilation Sweating, vasodilatation, (Hyperpyrexia in children)
Severe (750–1200 mg l^{-1})	Confusion, delirium, convulsions, coma Hypotension, cardiac arrest Hyperpyrexia Pulmonary oedema, cerebral oedema Hypoglycaemia Renal failure, liver failure Tetany Gastrointestinal haemorrhage

acetyl-*p*-benzoquinoneimine), which is either excreted as catechol derivatives (5–10%) or conjugated with glutathione and excreted as cysteine or mercapturate conjugates (5–10%).

If an overdose of paracetamol occurs, the stores of glutathione are depleted and the levels of the oxidative metabolite increase; this is free to cause hepatic and renal cell damage. In situations where the microsomal oxidative enzymes are induced the hepatic and nephrotoxic effects of paracetamol are enhanced (Fig. 52.1). This can occur in those, for example, taking barbiturates, anticonvulsants and rifampicin. Other types of patient in this high risk group are alcohol abusers and those with eating disorders.

Within the first 24 hours of poisoning there may only be anorexia, nausea and vomiting, abdominal pain and sweating. By 24–36 hours there may be right subcostal pain due to early hepatic damage. This can occur after as little as 150 mg kg^{-1} body weight, i.e. 10–15 g paracetamol (20–30 tablets of 500 mg). Because the circulating levels of hepatic enzymes do not rise until some days after the damage has been done, great reliance is now placed on estimation of the plasma paracetamol level and relating it to the time after ingestion. This will indicate the potential degree of damage and will influence treatment by allowing reference to a zoned chart (Fig. 52.1) of drug levels against time.

Treatment initially involves gastric lavage if presentation is within 2 hours of ingestion, followed by the instillation of activated charcoal. An estimation of plasma paracetamol level must be made no sooner than 4 hours after ingestion, as levels before this time will not take into account continuing absorption. If presentation is within 8 hours, the history is reliable and greater than 150 mg kg^{-1} body weight has been taken, measures to prevent hepatic damage with either methionine or *N*-acetylcysteine are instituted while awaiting the result.

Oral methionine increases the synthesis of hepatic glutathione. Difficulty with the oral administration of this drug may be encountered because of vomiting or because of unconsciousness. *N*-acetylcysteine is rapidly hydrolysed to cysteine, which is a precursor of glutathione. It

may also act by reducing the oxidative metabolite back to paracetamol. It can be given either by intravenous injection (Vale and Proudfoot 1995) or orally and causes less nausea and vomiting, although its use has been associated with anaphylactoid reactions.

If the ingestion time is greater than 8 hours, *N*-acetylcysteine should be given intravenously immediately on admission if more than 150 mg kg^{-1} body weight of paracetamol has been taken. Management of patients with ingestion times of greater than 24 hours is controversial but consideration should be given to administering *N*-acetylcysteine. It may be continued if the patient has, or is at risk of developing, liver failure.

Forced diuresis and haemodialysis are of limited or no value in treatment of this type of poisoning, although haemoperfusion may be some value in very severe toxicity, especially if presentation is delayed.

Opioid analgesics

This group includes drugs such as morphine, heroin, pethidine and methadone. As potent respiratory depressants, these drugs can be dangerous. Other clinical features include constricted pupils, convulsions, hypotension and coma. Severe intoxication can lead to pulmonary oedema by an unknown mechanism, cardiac arrhythmias and renal failure.

Management is initially supportive until the narcotic antagonist naloxone can be administered. As this drug is a competitive antagonist the dose required for full reversal will be greater than that used to reverse therapeutic doses of morphine. Initial doses of 1.2–2.4 mg are often necessary. It also has a short duration of action (approximately 10 minutes) and an initial bolus dose may need to be followed by an infusion. The dose given must be titrated to effect; up to 5 mg h^{-1} may be needed. Overtreatment with naloxone can produce hyperventilation, tachycardia and hypertension with pulmonary oedema, and even cardiac arrest has been reported in some cases. These features are almost certainly due to a noradrenaline 'storm'. An acute withdrawal in narcotic addicts may also be produced.

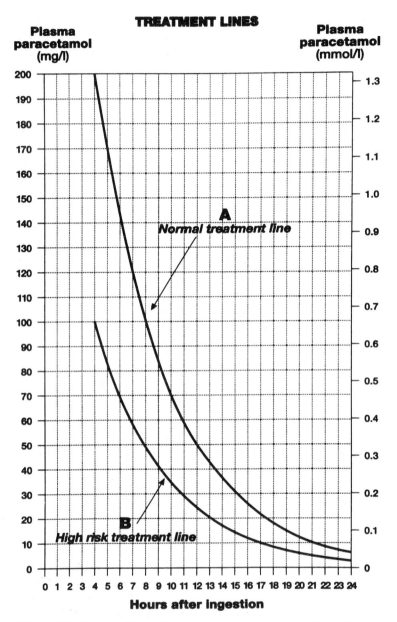

Figure 52.1 Treatment lines after paracetamol overdose in relation to time after ingestion and plasma paracetamol levels. Patients are treated if level lies above and to the right of line A. Use line B in high risk individuals (enzyme induction, malnutrition, AIDS, etc). (Reprinted with permission from the Paracetamol Information Centre, London and the Welsh National Poisons Unit, Cardiff.)

Some combination analgesics contain constituents which can be reversed with naloxone. The combination of dextropropoxyphene and paracetamol (Distalgesic) requires treatment of both drug entities to be successful.

Psychoactive drugs

Approximately 60% of patients admitted with poisoning have taken one of these drugs. Most cause CNS depression, which resolves if supportive measures are undertaken. Barbiturates used to be the 'overdose drug of choice', but have since been replaced by the benzodiazepines.

Benzodiazepines

Benzodiazepines probably act by facilitating the inhibitory effects of the γ-aminobutyric acid (GABA) postsynaptic receptor in the CNS, producing anxiolysis, muscle relaxation and seizure control. Overdose with this group of drugs produces very few serious side-effects. Symptoms include drowsiness, ataxia, dysarthria and nystagmus. The drugs are less likely to cause respiratory depression. Usually supportive measures are all that is needed and active elimination measures are not warranted.

The specific benzodiazepine antagonist, flumazenil, can reverse the effects of benzodiazepines by competitively displacing them at the benzodiazepine–GABA–chloride complex. It has a rapid onset of action of less than 1 minute after an intravenous injection, with an effect maximal at 5 minutes. It has a short duration of action, the elimination half-life being 54 minutes, mainly due to rapid hepatic clearance. It can reverse a comatose state and return respiratory rate and blood pressure towards normal, but because of its short half-life repeat administration is required. It should be used with caution both when used to reverse pure benzodiazepine depression and for mixed drug overdose. Rapid reversal can lead to ventricular fibrillation and status epilepticus.

Phenothiazines

Chlorpromazine is the best known member of this group of drugs which are used to quieten disturbed patients. They are thought to act by blocking dopaminergic D_2 receptors within the CNS but can also affect cholinergic, adrenergic, serotonin and histamine receptors.

They are well absorbed from the alimentary tract and are chiefly metabolised in the liver, with a prominent enterohepatic recirculation occurring. The biological half-life of the phenothiazines is prolonged and metabolites may be excreted

in the urine for months. Blood levels are correspondingly low. Poisoning with this group of drugs gives rise to irritability, lowered level of consciousness, convulsions, hypotension, tachycardia, hypothermia, electrocardiographic (ECG) changes and a range of dystonic reactions. These latter problems can be alleviated by an anticholinergic drug such as benztropine (Cogentin), orphenadrine (Disipal) or procyclidine (Kemadrin). General management measures such as gastric lavage and administration of activated charcoal depend on the individual circumstances. Active elimination measures are ineffective because of the low plasma drug levels. Repeated doses of activated charcoal may bind drug excreted via the enterohepatic route.

Although hypothermia is the norm in overdose, hyperthermia may occur. In rare cases it may be severe — 'neuroleptic malignant syndrome'. This requires active cooling and treatment with dantrolene.

Monoamine oxidase inhibitors

Although the use of this class of antidepressant is limited because of the serious side-effects, renewed interest has occurred because of favourable therapeutic responses in certain psychiatric conditions. Monoamine oxidase inhibitors (MAOIs) act by inhibition of monoamine oxidase and cause an accumulation of amine neurotransmitters. However, they have inhibitory effects throughout the body and can obstruct the first pass metabolism of compounds such as tyramine, resulting in severe sympathetic overactivity. They are readily absorbed from the gastrointestinal tract, metabolised in the liver and rapidly excreted as the acid metabolite, although their effect can be prolonged as a consequence of irreversible inhibition of their target enzyme. A new subgroup of MAOIs, acting by the reversible inhibition of monoamine oxidase type A (termed RIMA) is available. Their interaction profile (see Ch. 51) is similar to the main group but less pronounced.

Overdose with these compounds will result in CNS excitation and sympathetic stimulation. There is a latent phase of 12–24 hours before the onset of toxic symptoms. This is followed by neuromuscular excitation (muscle spasm, rigidity, facial grimacing, opisthotonus) and sympathetic hyperactivity (tremor, irritability and agitation, tachycardia and hypertension and fixed dilated pupils). The core temperature often rises, causing severe hyperglycaemia. Convulsions may occur and precede CNS depression and cardiovascular collapse.

Treatment is predominantly supportive, always remembering that there is a latent period before symptoms appear. The sympathetic overactivity should be controlled with sedatives or β-adrenergic blocking agents. Chlorpromazine can help to control the cerebral excitement and hyperpyrexia. If this is severe, dantrolene (1 mg kg^{-1} bolus repeated as necessary to total of 10 mg kg^{-1}), muscle relaxation, artificial ventilation and active cooling may be necessary for control.

Hypertension should be controlled with a rapid, short acting parenteral agent such as phentolamine or sodium nitroprusside. Hypotension will require volume replacement and agents that act directly on the postsynaptic receptors rather than relying on the release of intracellular amines whose kinetics may be altered by MAOIs (noradrenaline, dopamine). The use of elimination procedures is not warranted.

Tricyclic antidepressants

These are the most commonly prescribed antidepressants and act by blocking the reuptake of noradrenaline and/or 5-hydroxytryptamine, leading to increased amine concentration in certain areas of the brain. As basic compounds they are poorly absorbed from the stomach but much better in the duodenum, and as very lipophilic compounds, they become extensively tissue bound, with a predilection for cardiac tissue. Overdose has wide ranging effects on the central and peripheral nervous system, the parasympathetic system (atropine-like) and on the cardiovascular system (quinine-like). Symptoms appear within 1 hour and are initially anticholinergic in character, such as drowsiness, dry mouth, dilated pupils, tachycardia, blurred vision, urinary retention and an ileus. Convulsions and increased

reflexes with an extensor plantar response associated with hypertension and arrhythmias herald the onset of reduced reuptake of noradrenaline. Once the catecholamine reserves are depleted the stage of cardiorespiratory depression occurs with brainstem areflexia and coma leading to death.

The cardiac effects are varied because of the conflicting influences of the anticholinergic, sympathetic and quinidine-like actions. This last effect probably accounts for the ECG changes and impaired myocardial contractility. In severe intoxication the usually slightly raised heart rate returns to normal, or even slows. There may be widening of the QRS complex and decreases in the size of the P wave. There is an associated fall in blood pressure.

Severity of poisoning can be estimated from the duration of the QRS complex and from plasma levels. Severe poisoning occurs at levels of more than 1 mg l^{-1}. Treatment involves gastric lavage, even up to 12 hours after ingestion, as the anticholinergic effects delay gastric emptying. Supportive measures are necessary and include correction of arterial pH, blood gas tensions and electrolyte levels. Arrhythmia control will be easier when these are normalised. Further treatment of the arrhythmias should be resisted if possible. Treatment with disopyramide, lignocaine, quinidine or procainamide is contraindicated as they potentiate the cardiotoxicity. Bradycardia may be treated by cardiac pacing; ventricular fibrillation should be treated by conventional means.

Tricyclic antidepressants have a large volume of distribution and as such are not readily eliminated by forced diuresis, haemodialysis or haemoperfusion.

Amoxapine

This dibenzoxazepine derivative has a tricyclic structure with a fourth ring as a side structure (Kulig 1986). Unlike other tricyclic agents it blocks dopamine receptors, perhaps resulting in neuroleptic, in addition to is antidepressant, effects. Compared with other tricyclic drugs, features of overdose with amoxapine are its lack of cardiovascular toxicity but a higher incidence of convulsions and acute renal failure. The mortality rate after overdose may be higher. Treatment is supportive, with aggressive convulsion control being predominant.

Maprotiline

This tetracyclic antidepressant, as with the tricyclics, inhibits reuptake of noradrenaline at nerve endings. It may have the advantage of fewer anticholinergic side-effects; conversely, central effects such as delirium and convulsions occur more readily than with tricyclics (Kulig 1986). Thus, maprotiline's toxicity to the CNS may exceed its peripheral anticholinergic effects. Cardiac toxicity is probably similar to that found with tricyclics.

Mianserin

This tetracyclic is thought to act by increasing noradrenaline release and by inhibiting serotonin uptake. It has no anticholinergic properties and appears to be less toxic when taken as an overdose. The clinical features include a lowered level of consciousness, sinus tachycardia, dizziness and ataxia. Treatment is supportive.

Trazodone

This compound has a unique structure among antidepressants and acts by selectively inhibiting serotonin reuptake (Kulig 1986). It has little or no effect on noradrenaline, although it can block adrenergic receptors. It has no anticholinergic properties. It has no active metabolites and also stands out among tricyclics and tetracyclics by having a shorter half-life of 4–6 hours. Its volume of distribution is thought to be smaller than those of tri- or tetracyclics, which have large volumes. Overdose would appear to cause only mild cardiac effects but other symptoms include drowsiness, dizziness and nausea.

Selective serotonin reuptake inhibitors (SSRIs)

This class of antidepressant drugs includes fluoxetine (Prozac), paroxetine (Seroxat), sertraline (Lustral) and venlafaxine (Efexor). They selectively inhibit the reuptake of serotonin with venlafaxine also inhibiting noradrenaline reuptake. Their profile is one of less sedative, membrane stabilising cardiotoxic and antimuscarinic effects than tricyclics. Therefore the toxicity profile for these recently introduced drugs should be safer, although they do cause CNS agitation and convulsions. Because of their effect on serotonin, it might be expected that hyperpyrexia would be a feature of overdose.

Management of overdose is supportive, using activated charcoal to help with adsorption. Convulsions will require benzodiazepines.

Lithium

The salts of this metal are used in the treatment of mania. They have a low therapeutic index and, as the main route of elimination is by the kidneys, reduced renal function can lead to accumulation. Toxicity is worsened by sodium depletion so disruption of water and electrolyte balance (diuretic therapy or water loss by vomiting or diarrhoea) can also promote poisoning. The therapeutic range is $0.6–1.2$ mmol l^{-1}, with poisoning occurring if levels reach 1.5 mmol l^{-1}, becoming severe at 2.0 mmol l^{-1}. Symptoms may be delayed by 12 or more hours and include apathy, followed by thirst, polyuria, diarrhoea and vomiting. In severe cases depressed level of consciousness, hypertonicity and tremor, nystagmus, dysarthria, convulsions and coma occur. Further problems that may arise are oliguria leading to anuria, electrolyte disturbances, hypotension, cardiac conduction defects and arrhythmias.

In mild cases, administration of sodium and fluid may reverse toxicity. Initial management of the more severe cases includes gastric lavage, which can be useful up to 6 hours after ingestion. A plasma estimation should be performed, although its interpretation should be combined with a clinical assessment of the patient. Supportive therapy, including diazepam to control convulsions, is indicated. In the more severe cases with renal impairment, forced diuresis and saline infusions may be dangerous. Haemodialysis removes lithium easily and is the treatment of choice, especially if the plasma level is greater than 5 mmol l^{-1}. It may need to be repeated, as lithium rebounds into the plasma from the extravascular compartment.

Anticonvulsants

Most anticonvulsants are lipid soluble and, although their precise mode of action is not clear, they appear to halt the spread of depolarisation from an epileptic focus. Overdose is more likely to have serious effects if a combination of drugs is taken.

Phenytoin

This is an effective broad spectrum anticonvulsant. The metabolism is mainly hepatic and is saturable. When this occurs it causes a substantial rise in the circulating concentration, leading to toxicity. Nystagmus, ataxia and dysarthria occur at doses (greater than 25 mg l^{-1}) only slightly exceeding those needed therapeutically (10–20 mg l^{-1}), and are the cardinal symptoms of poisoning. Severe overdose may result in coma, with unresponsive pupils and hypotension. Treatment is supportive.

Carbamazepine

This is a first line drug for management of grand mal and focal and temporal lobe seizures, as well as for patients with trigeminal neuralgia. It has a tricyclic structure; it is related to the tricyclic antidepressants and has anticholinergic properties. Absorption from the gastrointestinal tract is slow and probably incomplete. It is metabolised in the liver to an active metabolite, very little unchanged drug appearing in the urine. The therapeutic range is 4–10 mg l^{-1}, although some patients tolerate 16 mg l^{-1} or above. Overdose will cause symptoms ranging from lowered level of consciousness with hyporeflexia to convulsions and coma. Bradycardia or even complete heart block may occur. Treatment involves gastric lavage followed by the regular gastric instillation of activated charcoal, other management being supportive.

Sodium valproate

This drug can be used in a variety of types of seizure. It is rapidly absorbed so gastric emptying procedures may be non-productive. The therapeutic range is 5–100 mg l^{-1}. At plasma levels of 5–6 times the therapeutic maximum the symptoms experienced are nausea, vomiting and dizziness. Levels of 10–20 times the maximum therapeutic levels may be associated with CNS depression. Valproic acid inhibits platelet aggregation and thrombocytopenia may occur, so that bleeding may be a feature of overdose. Treatment is supportive.

Primidone

This is especially indicated for management of grand mal and temporal lobe epilepsy. It is partially metabolised to two active metabolites, phenobarbitone and phenylethylmalonamide. Overdose will lead to ataxia, CNS depression and eventually respiratory depression and coma.

Cardiac drugs

Although uncommon, poisoning with these drugs requires an intimate knowledge of their pharmacodynamic profile for correct management. They often present with hypotension and/or arrhythmias. General management for them all includes gastric lavage, the administration of activated charcoal (5–10 times the suspected overdose) and supportive care of the cardiorespiratory systems. Electrolyte concentrations must be measured and corrected urgently. Invasive measures such as the administration of positive inotropes and temporary cardiac pacing may be necessary.

β-Adrenergic blocking agents

These compounds exert their effect by competing with catecholamines for β-adrenoceptor sites, although most have no stimulatory effect on those sites. Those that do possess intrinsic sympathomimetic activity (pindolol, oxprenolol, acebutolol, alprenolol and oxprenolol) have a low grade stimulatory effect on the β receptor, while inhibiting the much stronger effect of endogenous catecholamines (Weinstein 1984). β-Adrenoceptors exist as two subgroups and certain compounds can selectively inhibit the inotropic and chronotropic effects of catecholamines at the β_1 receptors in the heart. The β_1-selective agents, such as practolol, atenolol and metoprolol, do not usually produce bronchospasm or hypoglycaemia at therapeutic doses, but lose their selectivity at the doses achieved after an overdose; they become the same as the non-selective agents.

The clinical features found after a small overdose are usually bradycardia and hypotension. Larger overdoses can present with convulsions and coma in association with severe bradycardia and hypotension. Other features include hypoglycaemia, hallucinations and a variety of ECG changes such as first degree heart block, prolongation of the QRS complex, absence of the P wave, conduction defects, ventricular tachycardia and fibrillation and asystole.

A patient's clinical picture will depend on the pharmacological properties of the particular agent taken. The widening of the QRS complex seen with propranolol is probably due to its membrane stabilising effect. Overdose with sotalol may cause prolongation of the QT interval, giving rise to life threatening ventricular arrhythmias; the prolongation is related to the drug's ability to prolong the duration of the action potential and lengthen the effective refractory period. Practolol and pindolol both possess a relatively high degree of intrinsic sympathomimetic activity which can help to maintain heart rate and blood pressure during overdose. Both drugs also lack membrane stabilising properties, making overdose induced convulsions unlikely. On the other hand the seizures seen with propranolol overdose are related to its membrane stabilising effect and its strong lipid solubility, allowing easy access to the CNS. The capacity of the other β blockers to cause seizures is probably in direct relation to their membrane-stabilising effect and lipid solubility.

Management involves instituting supportive measures. Gastric lavage should be performed carefully; it may stimulate an overwhelming vagal discharge and should be covered by the administration of atropine (0.6–1.2 mg). A nasogastric tube should be left in situ if glucagon is to be used, as it may produce vomiting.

Many treatments have been tried to reverse the adverse haemodynamic effect of a massive β-blocker overdose. The agents or treatments commonly used are atropine, isoprenaline and dobutamine, and intracardiac pacing. The most successful appears to be glucagon, the polypeptide hormone produced by the α cells of the pancreas with biological half-life of approximately 3–6 minutes. It promotes formation of cyclic adenosine monophosphate (cAMP) from adenosine triphosphate (ATP) and thus exerts a direct stimulating effect on the heart that is independent of the β-adrenergic receptor. As a positive inotrope it is unaffected by β blockade, although as a chronotrope it is partially affected. Glucagon therefore increases cardiac output and decreases total peripheral resistance. It should be given as a dose of 4–10 mg over 30 seconds, followed by an infusion of 1–3 mg h^{-1}. When administered intravenously it elevates the serum glucose and may cause severe nausea and vomiting. During the infusion the serum glucose should be monitored and, after cessation of treatment, a rebound hypoglycaemia should be guarded against.

For those drugs with a high renal excretion (practolol, nadolol, sotalol), promotion of a diuresis may help.

Calcium channel blockers

Calcium antagonists inhibit transmembrane calcium transport, thus reducing peripheral vascular resistance, myocardial contractility, sinus node automaticity and the speed of atrioventricular nodal conduction. As with β blockers there are differences between members of this class of drug. Nifedipine reduces peripheral and coronary vascular resistance more than verapamil, which has its greatest effect on the speed of atrioventricular nodal conduction. In overdose their effects, however, may be similar. This group of drugs are highly protein bound, have a large volume of distribution and are rapidly metabolised to inactive metabolites.

Overdose may produce nausea and vomiting, dizziness, coma, hypotension, bradycardia, atrioventricular block, hyperglycaemia and metabolic acidosis. Treatment is supportive using lavage and activated charcoal, along with measures to combat the cardiovascular effects. Injection of 10–20 ml calcium chloride (10%) intravenously may shorten the intracardiac conduction time. With severe poisoning large amounts of intravenous fluids and inotropic support may be necessary to combat hypotension (Kenny 1994).

Digoxin and digitoxin

Digitalis is widely available and serious overdose is important because it is often fatal. Plasma concentrations become toxic at levels greater than $2.5\,\mu g\,l^{-1}$ but serious problems only arise at levels above $10\,\mu g\,l^{-1}$. However, plasma levels may not correlate closely with severity of poisoning.

Digoxin overdose leads to an inhibition of the Na^+,K^+-ATPase pump, which causes an increase in the plasma potassium level. This rise is correlated strongly with the clinical course. A single ECG recording with only minor changes or only a few symptoms may be misleading, as severe deterioration in cardiac state or rhythm may occur very suddenly.

Nausea and vomiting are constant features of a toxic overdose, with diarrhoea occurring less frequently. Drowsiness, mental confusion and even a psychosis have been observed. Bradycardia and cardiac arrhythmias are common. There may be varying degrees of atrioventricular block. Supraventricular arrhythmias, with or without heart block, and, less commonly, ventricular ectopic beats, ventricular tachycardia and ventricular fibrillation may also occur.

Treatment is supportive. Gastric lavage, if indicated, should be carried out with care because any increase in vagal tone may lead to cardiac arrest. Bradycardia can be treated with atropine which may need to be repeated over a period of several days. In serious poisoning transvenous cardiac pacing may be required. Hyperkalaemia should be treated with intravenous glucose and insulin, although with a large overdose the potassium level may not decrease because of the severe inhibition of the Na^+,K^+ pump. In these cases treatment with Fab digoxin-specific antibody fragments (Digibind-Wellcome Foundation Ltd) is warranted (see below). Hypokalaemia can occur in certain patients receiving chronic diuretic therapy. Ventricular ectopics should be treated only if they are compromising the cardiac output; ventricular tachyarrhythmias may require lignocaine or mexiletine. Should these fail, amiodarone is appropriate.

Measures to increase elimination, such as forced diuresis, haemodialysis or haemoperfusion, are ineffective because the plasma is constantly being replenished from the extensive tissue compartment; the volume of distribution is large, at $7\,l\,kg^{-1}$.

The treatment of choice for the elimination of digoxin is the administration of digoxin-specific Fab antibody fragments (Wenger et al 1985). It is also useful in digitoxin overdose. The specific indications for use are a rising and uncontrollable potassium concentration, life threatening cardiac arrhythmias and a serum digoxin concentration of greater than $20\,\mu g\,l^{-1}$. They work because their affinity for digoxin is greater than that of digoxin for its receptor, but they lack complement fixing activity or immunogenicity. The low molecular weight of the complex (50 000) means it is small enough to cross the glomerular basement membrane. Digoxin is therefore attracted away from the receptor on heart tissues. After administration, improvements in signs and symptoms begin within 30 minutes. At this time the plasma digoxin concentration rises (10–20-fold), the digoxin now being plasma bound and pharmacologically inactive. There is also a decrease in the serum potassium. The plasma elimination half-life after intravenous administration of Fab ranges from 16 to 34 hours in patients with good renal function.

After the administration of Fab fragments, it is not possible to follow serum digoxin concentrations with routine radioimmune assays as most of the digoxin is protein bound and cannot displace radiolabelled digoxin in competitive binding assays.

Amiodarone

This drug is probably the most potent anti-arrhythmic in use for management of tachy-arrhythmias of a paroxysmal nature, including supraventricular, nodal and ventricular tachycardias. It has a slow onset of action and requires a loading dose period to achieve a therapeutic effect, and therefore has a low acute toxicity. The elimination half-life is within the period of 15–30 days so that excessive dosage can lead to toxicity within the maintenance period. Side-effects will disappear slowly as the tissue levels decline after treatment has been withdrawn.

After an acute overdose the signs and symptoms that may be found include nausea and vomiting, headache with flushing, paraesthesia, ataxia, tremor and vertigo, bradycardia and hypotension. Management is supportive, with inotropic agents (dopamine or dobutamine infusions) being necessary to treat hypotension. Glucagon (see β blockers) may be required.

Respiratory drugs

Poisoning with drugs used in respiratory therapy is common. In particular the slow release form of the theophylline derivatives has become a serious and common problem.

Theophyllines

The mechanisms of action of this group of drugs are varied but there are three main ones: increased levels of cAMP due to phosphodiesterase inhibition; catecholamine related increases in cAMP; and effects on calcium kinetics.

Adverse effects occur readily because theophylline has a low therapeutic index, the therapeutic range being 10–20 mg l^{-1}. There is, however, only a general relationship between the features of toxicity and the plasma concentration, with toxic effects becoming evident at 25 mg l^{-1} and convulsions occurring at levels of over 50 mg l^{-1}. Levels of greater than 60 mg l^{-1} are often fatal. If a slow release formulation has been taken, serum levels may continue increasing for a prolonged period, necessitating repeated blood sampling. Drug

metabolism is mainly hepatic and is reduced in cirrhosis, cardiac failure, pulmonary disease, severe renal failure, obesity, in those over 50 years of age and in neonates. Conversely, the half-life is shortened by a high protein diet, in patients who smoke or take phenobarbitone or are aged between 1 and 20 years.

The early clinical features are those of nausea and vomiting, abdominal pain, haematemesis and diarrhoea. With the increased myocardial stimulation and catecholamine release there may be sinus, supraventricular and ventricular tachycardias. Hypotension with a metabolic acidosis may be precipitated by the decline in peripheral resistance or can be a result of a severe gastrointestinal haemorrhage. Stimulation of the CNS may produce headache, restlessness, agitation, hyperventilation with a respiratory alkalosis, tremor, hyperreflexia and convulsions leading to coma. An important feature is the development of hypokalaemia with Na^+,K^+-ATPase causing influx of potassium into the cells. This predisposes to arrhythmias and skeletal muscle damage (rhabdomyolysis).

Gastric lavage should be carried out on all those who present within 12 hours of an overdose, and should be followed by the administration of oral activated charcoal. It is vital that electrolyte and acid–base disturbances are corrected early, as this may be the only aggressive treatment needed. Nausea and vomiting may not respond to antiemetics, although the gastrointestinal haemorrhage may respond to H_2-receptor blockers. Convulsions will require intravenous diazepam. Cardiac arrhythmias should be treated only if severe, and not with β blockers if the patient is an asthmatic. They should initially be managed by correction of pH, Po_2 and electrolytes, and if necessary antiarrhythmics.

Active elimination measures such as haemodialysis and especially haemoperfusion should be reserved for those with uncontrollable severe symptoms, a serum theophylline level of greater than 60 mg l^{-1} 4 hours after ingestion (greater than 30 mg l^{-1} in the elderly; greater than 80 mg l^{-1} in children), in high risk groups, such as those with cardiac/respiratory/hepatic disease, and in the elderly.

β₂ Agonists

Overdose with these agents can occur with the oral, parenteral or even nebulised forms. They all, however, tend to have a wide margin of safety. At high doses β selectivity is lost, producing agitation, excitement, headache with a tachycardia, tremor and peripheral dilatation. More serious complications include ventricular tachyarrhythmias, pulmonary oedema and convulsions. Hyperglycaemia, hypokalaemia and lactic acidosis also occur.

Gastric lavage should be performed if appropriate, and especially if a slow release compound has been taken. Hypokalaemia should be treated with an intravenous potassium infusion. Should any serious cardiac arrhythmias remain after this correction, they may be treated with a cardioselective β blocker such as atenolol (2.5–10 mg).

Alcohols and ethylene glycol

Methanol, ethanol, isopropanol and ethylene glycol are the most commonly ingested aliphatic alcohols. They are rapidly absorbed from the upper gastrointestinal tract and initially oxidised mainly by hepatic alcohol dehydrogenase. With the exception of isopropanol they are further metabolised by aldehyde dehydrogenase to yield acids. Methanol and ethylene will produce a large anion gap metabolic acidosis, whereas isopropanol does not result in an acidosis.

Methanol

Otherwise known as wood alcohol or methyl alcohol, this substance can cause poisoning from an accidental ingestion or when taken in homemade beverages, varnish, paint removers or antifreeze. Antifreeze may also contain ethanol, isopropanol or ethylene glycol. Methylated spirit contains only 5% methanol and 98% ethanol, and is toxic because of its ethanol rather than methanol content.

Methanol is much more toxic than ethanol because it is metabolised to formaldehyde and then to the more toxic compound, formic acid. These two highly reactive compounds readily become tissue bound and interfere with oxidative metabolism. They cause a severe metabolic acidosis by an accumulation of hydrogen ion and by inhibiting gluconeogenesis and lactate conversion.

After a lag period, the patient becomes restless, confused and ataxic, followed by impairment of consciousness. The severe metabolic acidosis that develops after the latent period of 8–12 hours leads to tachypnoea. The distribution of methanol to different tissues is determined by their water content, and thus a high concentration is found in the vitreous body and optic nerve. Impairment of vision is a characteristic feature of the poisoning and may progress to blindness. Methanol can produce gastric irritation, resulting in epigastric pain, nausea and vomiting, and has been associated with acute pancreatitis.

The treatment of methanol poisoning should be centred on gastric lavage followed by correction of the acidosis, inhibition of its metabolism and removal of methanol itself with its metabolites (Kruse 1992). The acidosis will often require large doses of sodium bicarbonate, which may lead to hypernatraemia and fluid overload. The enzymatic oxidation of methanol is inhibited by ethanol because of the saturation of the alcohol dehydrogenase by ethanol. Indeed, methylated spirit drinkers seldom develop toxic effects from methanol because they are protected by the larger amounts of ethanol ingested. Ethanol treatment should be instituted only if there are large amounts of methanol still to be metabolised, and only in adults.

Ethanol should be administered orally or intravenously as a loading dose to achieve a blood level of at least 1000 mg l^{-1}. As the volume of distribution of ethanol is 600 ml kg^{-1}, the dose needed is approximately 600 mg kg^{-1} of ethanol or approximately 1 ml kg^{-1} of a 95% solution. (95% alcohol has a density of 750 mg ml^{-1}.) This could conveniently be given as 125 ml of whisky. This should be followed by an infusion of 10–15 g h^{-1} ethanol or 25 ml h^{-1} whisky. By maintaining an ethanol level of 1000–2000 mg l^{-1}, the metabolism of methanol will be blocked because the alcohol dehydrogenase enzyme will be 90% saturated. The plasma ethanol and methanol concentrations should be frequently measured and the infusion continued until methanol is undetectable and the patient is no longer becoming acidotic, when the infusion is stopped. It is slowly eliminated by renal excretion over a period of days.

Removal of methanol and its metabolites, once its metabolism has been halted by ethanol, may be prompted by haemodialysis. This should be performed if more than 30 g of methanol has been ingested, if the blood concentration is greater than 500 mg l^{-1}, if the patient has a metabolic acidosis, if mental, visual or fundoscopic complications are present or if there is renal failure. Should haemodialysis be undertaken the infusion of ethanol must be increased to 17–22 g h^{-1} to allow for ethanol removed by dialysis. Folinic acid 30 mg intravenously every 6 hours may protect against ocular toxicity by accelerating formate metabolism.

Ethanol

Ethanol or ethyl alcohol is a primary and progressive CNS depressant and, as a frequent companion to other drugs in self-poisoning, ethanol can exacerbate the effects of the other drugs. High concentrations induce pylorospasm, thus retarding gastric emptying. It is rapidly absorbed once in the small intestine and is distributed throughout the body tissues according to their water content; 5% is eliminated intact and the rest is oxidised to acetaldehyde and then to acetate. The fatal dose will vary because of individual tolerance but about 600 ml of pure alcohol consumed in 1 hour will be fatal.

Its effects are related to its blood concentration (Table 52.4). It also produces peripheral vasodilatation, hypothermia and hypotension. In children hypoglycaemia is likely to occur and in adults a lactic acidosis may develop when associated with severe liver disease, pancreatitis, sepsis or hypotension. Dehydration and hypoglycaemia may lead to a ketotic state.

Most patients require only supportive measures. If levels are greater than 7500 mg l^{-1}, haemodialysis should be carried out. Those with an acidosis will require correction of the blood

Table 52.4 Clinical effects of ethanol

Blood ethanol concentration (mg l^{-1})	Clinical effects
0–500	Decreased inhibition, slight incoordination
500–1000	Slowed reaction time, emotional instability, slurred speech
1000–1500	Poor reaction time, poor coordination, personality and behavioural changes
1500–3000	Sensory loss, visual disturbances, ataxia
3000–4000	Hypothermia, hypoglycaemia, severe ataxia, poor recall, blurred vision, stupor
4000–7000	Hyporeflexia, convulsions, respiratory failure, death

glucose concentration and the fluid deficit. If unresponsive to treatment, haemodialysis may be needed.

Isopropanol

This alcohol is found in disinfectants, aftershave lotions and antifreeze. An ingestion of 20 g may produce symptoms; 150–250 g may be fatal, the toxicity being due to the compound rather than its metabolites. Ingestion of this substance does not lead to an acidosis, 20% being excreted unchanged and 15% metabolised to acetone, most of which is excreted in the urine.

The CNS effects resemble those of ethanol. There is often a haemorrhagic gastritis, renal tubular necrosis, an acute myopathy and a haemolytic anaemia. Hypotension occurs with severe intoxication.

Treatment is supportive, with haemodialysis being used to control the serious complications, especially if blood concentrations are greater than 400 mg l^{-1}.

Ethylene glycol

Ethylene glycol is a colourless, odourless liquid with a pleasant taste which is used as an antifreeze compound either alone or with other alcohols. It is metabolised to glycoaldehyde by alcohol dehydrogenase and then to glycolic acid by aldehyde dehydrogenese, in a similar fashion to methanol. Glycolic acid is the major metabolite responsible for the metabolic acidosis; 3% is converted to oxalic acid. This may combine with calcium to cause renal, cardiac and cerebral oxalosis.

Three stages of ethylene glycol poisoning have been identified. An initial period of inebriation is followed several hours later by nausea and vomiting. There may be convulsions leading to coma, and also visual disturbances culminating in optic atrophy. The second stage is manifested by a progressive metabolic acidosis with tachycardia and tachypnoea arising from cardiac failure and pulmonary oedema. A later stage, occurring 1–3 days after poisoning, is distinguished by acute renal failure, often with pain in the renal angle. Calcium oxalate crystals may be found in the urine and there may be hypocalcaemia from chelation by the anionic metabolites of ethylene glycol.

After gastric lavage and instillation of activated charcoal, the treatment of ethylene glycol poisoning is similar to that of methanol poisoning (Walder and Tyler 1994). It is based on inhibiting formation of toxic metabolites with ethanol, thus preventing the acidosis. The acidosis must be controlled with sodium bicarbonate. Haemodialysis will be indicated if more than 30 g of ethylene glycol is ingested, if the plasma concentration is greater than 500 mg l^{-1} and if there are serious clinical effects of the poisoning. Hypocalcaemia will need to be treated by infusions of calcium gluconate, repeated as necessary.

Stimulants

Amphetamines

This class of drug, used as mood elevating and stimulant agents, can also cause paranoia, hallucinations and hypertension, followed by exhaustion, convulsions and coma. Their use is controlled but currently the analogues of methamphetamine have become popular. 3,4-Methylenedioxyamphetamine (MDA), 3,4-methylenedioxymethamphetamine (MDMA, 'Ecstasy', 'E', 'XTC', 'Adam', 'MDM') and 3,4-methylenedioxyethamphetamine (MDEA, 'Eve') are all structurally related to methamphetamine, which has sympathomimetic properties.

MDA, which was a popular recreational drug in the 1960s, can selectively damage serotonin nerve terminals in rat brain. It is a metabolite of the more commonly used MDMA and is also sometimes unwittingly taken as 'Ecstacy' (O'Dwyer et al 1995).

MDMA or 'Ecstasy' was first developed as an appetite depressant in 1914, was used in psychotherapy in the 1970s, and since the 1980s has become a drug of abuse. The usual dose is 200 mg; it has a rapid onset of action in about 30 minutes and probably acts at central serotonin 5-HT$_2$ receptors. It produces stimulation of the serotonergic pathways in association with a rapid fall in CNS serotonin (5-HT) levels. Inhibition of 5-HT reuptake also occurs, leading to increased intracellular calcium, which, by stimulating 5-HT release, further depletes 5-HT stores. As serotonin is an important mediator of temperature-increasing effects, drugs causing increased 5-HT release, e.g. MDMA and fluoxetine, can cause a hyperthermic serotonin syndrome — tremor, rigidity, seizures and hyperthermia.

The initial release of 5-HT produces an early period of disorientation, then a 'rush', when tingling may be experienced and jerking may occur. Finally there is a feeling of 'enhanced sociability'. The effects wear off in 4–6 hours, leaving a state of depression and confusion.

MDEA or 'Eve' was developed as a legal alternative to MDMA when it was banned in the USA in 1985. It has similar effects to MDMA which are reported to be milder, although reactions can still be life-threatening (Tehan et al 1993).

The pattern of toxicity is not usually one of overdose but is of adverse reactions to recreational doses of amphetamine, and particularly its analogues. It is not uncommon for a mixture of drugs including amphetamines, either MDMA or MDEA, and alcohol to be taken, with the risk that tablets may also contain MDA, lysergic acid diethylamide, ketamine or even dried mushrooms. The side-effects include hyperpyrexia, muscle rigidity, sweating, life threatening ventricular arrhythmias and death, some of them occurring after the ingestion of only one tablet. Disseminated intravascular coagulation, acute renal and hepatic failure and rhabdomyolysis may also occur. The particular format of toxicity that occurs may depend on the circumstances of abuse; in the UK they are often taken at 'dance parties' and may be associated with anaesthesia. At these events there is sustained muscular exercise (which is probably an effect of the drug), a high ambient temperature and conditions that favour dehydration. The resultant effect is that these patients commonly present with all the features of malignant hyperpyrexia, although the underlying mechanism is obviously different from the genetically determined malignant hyperthermia associated with anaesthesia (see Chs 19 and 51).

Management requires aggressive fluid replacement and active cooling. Gastric lavage may be useful and activated charcoal should be given together with a purgative. Intravenous dantrolene 1 mg kg^{-1} every 10 minutes should be given early, up to a maximum of 10 mg kg^{-1}, although 3 mg kg^{-1} is the average requirement. It inhibits calcium release from the sarcolemma and reduces the heat production from the increased muscle activity. Even though this action is a peripheral one, and the action of these drugs appears to be central, its use can be life saving (Singarajah and Lavies 1992). Measures to promote and maintain a high alkaline urine output must be made to prevent the onset of acute renal failure secondary to the myoglobinuria from the rhabdomyolysis. Alkalinisation of the urine may decrease the urinary excretion of amphetamine but acidification may increase the chances of myoglobinuric renal failure. Convulsions need to be controlled aggressively, especially because of the extra muscle activity they produce. Other management is supportive.

Cocaine

Benzoylmethylecgonine ('Cocaine') is an ester with a structure similar to local anaesthetics. It is sniffed, smoked or injected. In a highly purified form, when removed from its hydrochloride base, it is known as 'crack'. In this form it is smoked and as a 'free base' its effect is equivalent to the intravenous route.

Cocaine stimulates the CNS initially, produc-ing a state of alertness, euphoria, tremor and dysphoria, which is followed by a depressive and paranoid phase. At higher doses it produces increased motor activity which is associated with sweating and hyperpyrexia. There is also an inhibition of catecholamine reuptake, producing excessive sympathetic activity, hypertension, tachycardia and cardiac dysrhythmias. Seizures are also a feature of central stimulation.

Management of cocaine intoxication involves providing basic life support if consciousness is impaired, controlling the agitation and seizures with benzodiazepines, adopting active cooling measures if there is hyperpyrexia and controlling the cardiovascular manifestations. β Blockade may increase hypertension by unmasking excess α-adrenergic activity, labetalol can be especially useful as it has both β- and α-adrenergic antagonist properties.

Agricultural and horticultural chemicals

Paraquat

This weedkiller is available either as Gramoxone (20% paraquat), Weedol (2.5% paraquat and diquat) or Pathclear (2.5% paraquat and simazine). Its herbicidal action is due to an interference with electron transfer during photosynthesis, causing superoxide and peroxide radical production. In humans, these radicals are also produced in the gastrointestinal tract, kidney, liver and lungs. In the lungs an active transport mechanism results in concentrations at least 6 times that in other tissues. It is corrosive, causing burns and ulceration to the mouth and oesophagus, vomiting and diarrhoea. Absorption is rapid and it is rapidly distributed to tissues. Doses of less than 6 g may lead to death over a period ranging from several days to months. Hepatic, renal or pulmonary damage may appear within 24 hours but is more usual after 3 days. The hepatocellular and renal tubular damage can be mild but pulmonary damage is often severe, with a chemical pneumonitis, leading to progressive fibrosis and death. Ingestion of 6 g or more will lead to rapid death within hours from circulatory failure, convulsions and metabolic acidosis.

Confirmation of paraquat poisoning is made by adding urine to an alkaline solution of sodium diathionite. A green or blue colour is confirmatory; the prognosis can then be estimated by relating the plasma paraquat level to time from ingestion.

Treatment involves gastric lavage followed by instillation of 250 ml solution of Fuller's earth (30%), bentonite (7%) or activated charcoal (50 g), followed by a purgative (magnesium sulphate or mannitol). Further measures, such as whole-gut lavage, forced diuresis, haemodialysis or haemoperfusion, are not warranted unless performed very soon after ingestion, as the poison becomes tissue bound very quickly. Other therapy is supportive, but added oxygen may *increase* the toxicity of paraquat.

Organophosphates and carbamates

These substances are found in a wide range of insecticides and are all cholinesterase inhibitors. They can be absorbed through skin, respiratory tract and gastrointestinal tract and give rise to effects due to accumulation of acetylcholine at nicotinic and muscarinic receptors in autonomic ganglia, neuromuscular junctions, smooth muscle and CNS.

There are considerable differences in toxicity between different members of this group, organophosphates having a longer effect than carbamates. The organophosphate compounds phosphorylate the active site of acetylcholinesterase, forming a stable complex, but the carbamates carbamylate the site, forming a compound which can hydrolyse spontaneously. The earliest features seen are muscarinic effects in the body system where entry was obtained. There is miosis and blurred vision, salivation, nausea and vomiting, abdominal colic and diarrhoea, bradycardia, coughing with frothy secretions and pulmonary oedema. The nicotinic effects are manifested as progressive fasciculation, flaccidity and weakness of all muscle groups, which may proceed to paralysis. In severe poisoning there are CNS effects of anxiety, irritability and dizziness, leading to lowering of the level of consciousness and convulsions.

Treatment initially involves removal of the poison, establishment of an airway, artificial ventilation if needed and removal of bronchial secretions. Atropine inhibits the effects of these agents at the muscarinic receptor. Full atropinisation will require 2 mg repeated at 5–10 minutes intervals until there is evidence of dilated pupils, a dry mouth and a restored or rapid pulse. It may need to be continued for several days but has little effect at the autonomic ganglia or neuromuscular junction.

With carbamate poisoning cholinesterase inhibition reverses spontaneously, but with organophosphate poisoning treatment is needed. Pralidoxime mesylate will regenerate the cholinesterase enzyme and reverse the action of the poison at the neuromuscular junction but not at autonomic or CNS sites. It acts by forming an inert complex with the organophosphate. The antidote (15–30 mg kg^{-1}) is given by slow intravenous injection, which may be repeated. If it is given too quickly it may precipitate further weakness, diplopia, dizziness, headache, nausea and tachycardia. It should be given with the atropine or as soon after as possible, and certainly within 24 hours of poisoning, as the organophosphate–acetylcholinesterase complex becomes resistant to regeneration. Regeneration will allow a reduction in the dose of atropine.

Phenoxyacetates

These compounds are widely used as 'hormone' weedkillers. After ingestion they cause a feeling of burning in the mouth, nausea and vomiting, pyrexia, sweating and hyperventilation, leading to convulsions and coma. An acute myopathy, with pain, fasciculation, weakness and myoglobinuria, may occur. Appropriate steps to empty the stomach should be made. 2,4-D and mecoprop, as acidic compounds, will be eliminated more rapidly with the help of a forced alkaline diuresis.

Asphyxiants

Asphyxiants interfere with tissue oxygenation either by preventing delivery of oxygen to the cell (carbon monoxide) or by interfering with cellular oxygen utilisation (cyanide).

Carbon monoxide

Carbon monoxide (CO) poisoning is the most common type of chemical asphyxiation. It is a colourless, odourless, tasteless, non-irritating gas produced by the incomplete combustion of carbonaceous materials. There is endogenous production of CO, resulting in a normal carboxyhaemoglobin concentration of 1–3% in non-smokers, rising to 5–6% in smokers.

The causes of toxicity from CO are multifactorial. CO combines avidly with haemoglobin to form carboxyhaemoglobin (COHb). The affinity of CO for haemoglobin is 223 times as great as that of oxygen, and thus oxygen is replaced by CO, reducing the total oxygen carrying capacity of blood, producing an 'anaemia'. Moreover the addition of CO to a molecule of haemoglobin shifts the HbO_2 dissociation curve to the left as the affinity of the remaining oxygen molecules for their haem groups is increased. This interferes with the unloading of oxygen at tissue level and results in a greater degree of tissue anoxia than would be expected from a simple loss of oxygen carrying capacity. There is also evidence that CO inhibits cellular respiration by combining with other haem-containing proteins such as myoglobin and the cytochrome system (Meredith and Vale 1988).

The clinical course is directly related to the degree and duration of exposure (Table 52.5).

Table 52.5 Clinical effects of carbon monoxide poisoning

Concentration COHb (%)	Signs and symptoms
0.3–3 0	Normal range
<10	No symptoms
10–20	Slight headache, variable vasodilatation
20–30	Throbbing headache, dyspnoea and angina on exertion
30–40	Severe headache, nausea, vomiting, visual disturbance, weakness, dizziness
40–50	Syncope, tachycardia, tachypnoea
50–60	Coma, convulsions, Cheyne–Stokes respiration
60–70	Cardiorespiratory failure, death

The acute effects of CO poisoning are due to tissue hypoxia, and as the brain and heart are the organs with the highest metabolic rate, they are the organs that demonstrate the major toxic manifestations. Individuals with pre-existing coronary and cerebral artery disease, myocardial insufficiency, pulmonary disease or anaemia are more vulnerable. The CNS, being especially vulnerable to hypoxia, tends to be the most affected, and the effect ranges from lethargy to acute agitation and mental confusion to coma.

Patients in whom consciousness is maintained usually recover rapidly and completely. Those who become unconscious may continue to deteriorate clinically despite a COHb that is returning to normal. This indicates the presence of cerebral oedema and is associated with papilloedema, hypertension and increased reflexes. Some patients may recover completely only to develop a 'delayed posthypoxic encephalopathy' days or weeks later. Myocardial ischaemia is frequent and may precipitate angina, and even progress to infarction. In severe poisoning the marked degree of hypoxia initially causes stimulation of the respiratory centre with hyperventilation. Acute pulmonary oedema may occur and respiratory centre failure may follow. Visual defects, including loss of vision and retinal haemorrhage, may occur. Acute neuropsychiatric findings range from headache and fatigue to epilepsy and chronic cognitive and psychomotor changes, which may be permanent. Many of these abnormalities may be induced at low levels of COHb.

Various types of skin lesion can occur, varying from bullous eruptions to areas of erythema and alopecia. The pink skin colour due to COHb is uncommon unless poisoning is severe. Cyanosis and skin pallor are more common. It should be noted that in cyanide, atropine and phenothiazine poisoning a pink colour is also seen. The distinction between cyanide and CO poisoning is critical because appropriate treatment for one would be inappropriate for the other. Hyperpyrexia following skin sweat gland necrosis may be a feature. Myonecrosis may occur as a compartmental symptom and may even lead to rhabdomyolytic renal failure.

The most reliable method for diagnosis of CO poisoning is direct measurement by spectrophotometry (oximetry). The correlation between COHb concentrations and clinical effects is given in Table 52.5. It must be borne in mind that CO is very rapidly eliminated and the blood level on arrival at hospital does not necessarily reflect the true insult if a delay occurs between exposure and COHb analysis. It should be noted that the arterial P_{O_2} is usually normal in CO poisoning because it reflects dissolved oxygen content of the blood and not haemoglobin saturation.

Treatment is initiated by terminating exposure, securing the airway and administering 100% oxygen as soon as possible, using either a tightly fitting facemask or an endotracheal tube. The half-life of COHb in a patient breathing room air is 5–6 hours; with 100% oxygen the half-life decreases to 45–90 minutes; with a hyperbaric pressure of 3 atmospheres the half-life approximates to 23 minutes. The mechanism of action of a high inspired oxygen fraction is that the CO will be diluted and displaced by oxygen from cytochromes, myoglobin and haemoglobin by a mass action effect. Hyperbaric oxygen will also increase the amount of oxygen dissolved in the blood to a level sufficient to contribute substantially to tissue needs even without functioning haemoglobin. Treatment with hyperbaric oxygen will reduce the duration of coma, the incidence of the delayed encephalopathy and the long term morbidity to less than 5% (Meredith and Vale 1988). Unfortunately it is not widely used because of the lack of suitable facilities close enough to hand. Broome and colleagues (1988) recommend, if consciousness has not been lost and there are no symptoms other than headache or nausea or the COHb level is less than 40%, that normobaric oxygen is sufficient. If there are other symptoms or consciousness has been lost or the COHb is greater than 40%, then hyperbaric oxygen is the treatment of choice. It should be applied at 2.5–3.0 atmospheres for at least 90 minutes and should be repeated until consciousness is normal.

Further supportive treatment should be given as required, especially if there is evidence of myocardial ischaemia or cerebral oedema.

Cyanide

Inhalation, cutaneous absorption or ingestion of cyanide can produce death from asphyxia within a few minutes, although it can be delayed for several hours. Hydrogen cyanide (hydrocyanic acid; prussic acid) or its salts are used in numerous industrial processes including precious metal extraction and electroplating. It is also used as a fumigant and in the extermination of rabbits by farmers. It arises from the combustion of polyurethane foams from furniture upholstery, which is probably a more common cause of cyanide poisoning than is generally appreciated. Cigarette smokers have been found to have mean whole blood cyanide levels of about $0.41\ \mu g\ ml^{-1}$.

Cyanide causes a histotoxic (intracellular) hypoxic poisoning by the binding of the cyanide ion to the ferric (Fe^{3+}) ion of mitochondrial cytochrome oxidase. This causes inhibition of cytochrome oxidase activity, paralysing the tricarboxylic acid cycle and leading to anaerobic metabolism with reduced formation of ATP and lactic acidosis. Cellular utilization of oxygen is severely depressed and the venous P_{O_2} is increased. Indeed the arterial and venous blood samples will demonstrate a similar P_{O_2}. The body has major routes of cyanide detoxication (thiosulphate or rhodanese pathways) and minor routes (cysteine binding, hydroxycobalamin binding, oxidation and excretion via the lungs). These mechanisms may be rapidly overwhelmed in the face of significant quantities of cyanide.

The speed of onset and severity of symptoms and signs depends on the quantity of cyanide absorbed. After exposure to a small amount, the initial features often mimic those of anxiety, with hyperventilation and CNS stimulation. There is cyanide stimulation of the carotid chemoreceptors and the respiratory centres during this early phase. There may also be hypertension with a reflex bradycardia and various degrees of atrioventricular block. Headache, dyspnoea, palpitations, vomiting, ataxia and loss of consciousness may occur gradually. If a large amount is absorbed the features appear very rapidly and the patient becomes deeply unconscious, the limb reflexes are absent and the pupils become dilated. There is hypotension and ECG changes consistent with hypoxia. A metabolic acidosis can present, as can slowing of the respiratory rate, leading to profound respiratory depression. Pulmonary and cerebral oedema may arise. Since the oxygen carrying capacity of haemoglobin is unimpaired, the blood remains well oxygenated and cyanosis does not occur until the stage of circulatory collapse and respiratory depression. The odour of bitter almonds, although pathognomonic, may not necessarily be present.

Blood cyanide levels of below 1 mg l^{-1} are usually associated with the early stage of poisoning, while levels of $1–3 \text{ mg l}^{-1}$ correlate with severe toxicity leading to death. Some cyanide binds to the ferrous (Fe^{2+}) ion of normal haemoglobin. This cyanhaemoglobin cannot transport oxygen and will lead to a discrepancy between the measured (by CO oximeter) arterial oxygen saturation and the calculated (by nomogram) oxygen saturation. If the difference between the two values is 5 or greater it is suggestive of a poison producing an abnormal (non-oxygen transporting) haemoglobin. Poisons that will produce this gap include carbon monoxide, hydrogen sulphide and methaemoglobin producing agents.

Once the diagnosis is suspected, therapy must be instituted rapidly. Firstly, the patient should be removed from the source of exposure or contamination. If poisoning is due to ingestion, the administration of the antidotes should be carried out as soon as possible. Gastric lavage should then be carried out and 300 ml of 25% sodium thiosulphate left in the stomach. Administration of activated charcoal has not yet been shown to be beneficial. Provision of supportive care in the form of 100% oxygen, carefully applied artificial ventilation (avoiding intoxication by the resuscitator), control of seizures, correction of acidosis and cardiovascular support may be sufficient to allow survival in less severe cases.

For severe cases there are three specific types of antidote: thiosulphate and nitrites; dicobalt edetate and hydroxycobalamin. Some of these compounds are extremely toxic in the absence of cyanide ions and it is therefore essential to be certain that the diagnosis of cyanide toxicity is correct, and that free cyanide is still circulating, before administration of the antidote.

Cyanide may be converted to the less toxic thiocyanate by rhodanese. Thiosulphate is required for this reaction and its administration increases the rate of cyanide metabolism; 25 ml of a 50% solution is administered intravenously over 10 minutes. It is not very effective on its own and is usually preceded by sodium nitrite (10 ml of a 3% solution intravenously over 5 minutes), which causes the formation of methaemoglobin. This has iron in the ferric state rather than the ferrous state. It will attach to the cytochrome oxidase–cyanide complex to form the cyanmethaemoglobin, freeing the cytochrome oxidase to take up its normal activity. Methaemoglobinaemia should be reduced to levels of less that 40%. As the cyanide dissociates from the methaemoglobin it is metabolised by rhodanese to thiocyanate.

The methaemoglobin-producing agents have now been superseded by the chelating agent, dicobalt edetate (Kelocyanor). It forms inert complexes with the cyanide. An initial 600 mg is given intravenously over 1 minute, followed by a further 300 mg if there is no improvement within 1 minute. This compound, if administered in the absence of cyanide or when cyanmethaemoglobin has already been produced by nitrite administration, may produce its own toxic effects: hypotension, tachycardia, vomiting, facial and palpebral oedema. It should not be used as a precautionary measure.

Hydroxocobalamin inactivates cyanide by forming cyanocobalamin but this treatment method is not practical because of the relatively large volumes of hydroxycobalamin needed, its brevity of action (half-life 5 minutes) and its high cost.

REFERENCES

Broome J R, Pearson R R, Skrine H 1988 Carbon monoxide poisoning: 'forgotten not gone!'. British Journal of Hospital Medicine 39: 298–305

Collee G G, Hanson G C 1993 The management of acute poisoning. British Journal of Anaesthesia 70: 562–573

Kenny J 1994 Treating overdose with calcium channel blockers. British Medical Journal 308: 992–993

Kruse J A 1992 Methanol poisoning. Intensive Care Medicine 18: 391–397

Kulig K 1986 Management of poisoning associated with 'newer' antidepressant agents. Annals of Emergency Medicine 15: 1039–1045

Meredith T J, Vale J A 1988 Carbon monoxide poisoning. British Medical Journal 296: 77–79

Merigan K S, Woodard M, Hedges J R, Roberts J R, Stuebing R, Rashkin M C 1990 Prospective evaluation of gastric emptying in the self poisoned patient. American Journal of Emergency Medicine 8: 479–483

Neuvonen P J, Vartiainen M, Tokola O 1983 Comparison of activated charcoal and ipecac syrup in prevention of drug absorption. European Journal of Clinical Pharmacology 24: 557–562

O'Dwyer G, Buckley M, O'Morain C, Fitzpatrick G 1995 Multiple organ dysfunction following ingestion of methylenedioxyamphetamine (MDA). Clinical Intensive Care 6: 181–183

Singarajah C, Lavies N G 1992 An overdose of ecstasy. A role for dantrolene. Anaesthesia 47: 686–687

Tehan B, Hardern R, Bodenham A 1993 Hyperthermia associated with 3,4-methylenedioxyethamphetamine ('Eve'). Anaesthesia 48: 507–510

Vale J A, Proudfoot A T 1995 Paracetamol (acetaminophen) poisoning. Lancet 346: 547–552

Vale J A, Meredith T J, Proudfoot A T 1986 Syrup of ipecacuanha: is it really useful? British Medical Journal 293: 1321–1322

Walder A D, Tyler C K G 1994 Ethylene glycol antifreeze poisoning. Anaesthesia 49: 964–967

Weinstein R S 1984 Recognition and management of poisoning with beta-adrenergic blocking agents. Annals of Emergency Medicine 13: 1123–1131

Wenger T L, Butler V P, Haber E, Smith T W 1985 Treatment of 63 severely digitalis-toxic patients with digoxin-specific antibody fragments. Journal of the American College of Cardiology 5: 118a–123a

Index

E

O